CHAPTER 1: **Pectoral Region, Axilla, Shoulder, and Upper Limb**   Plates 1–138

CHAPTER 2: **The Thorax**   Plates 139–218

CHAPTER 3: **The Abdomen**   Plates 219–322

CHAPTER 4: **The Pelvis and Perineum**   Plates 323–370

CHAPTER 5: **The Back, Vertebral Column, and Spinal Cord**   Plates 371–408

CHAPTER 6: **The Lower Limb**   Plates 409–516

CHAPTER 7: **The Neck and Head**   Plates 517–668

CHAPTER 8: **Cranial Nerves**   Plates 669–694

Index   I-1–I-24

Anatomy
A REGIONAL ATLAS OF THE HUMAN BODY

Sixth Edition

Carmine D. C

Distinguished Profe
Professor of Neurol
University of Califor

Professor of Surger
Charles R. Drew Un
Los Angeles, Califo

With More Tha

 Wolters Kluwer | Lippincott Williams & Wilkins
Health

Philadelphia • Baltimore • New York • London
Buenos Aires • Hong Kong • Sydney • Tokyo

Acquisitions Editor: Crystal Taylor
Marketing Manager: Brian Moody
Product Manager: Julie Montalbano
Designer: Terry Mallon
Compositor: Aptara, Inc.

351 West Camden Street   530 Walnut Street
Baltimore, MD 21201   Philadelphia, PA 19106

Printed in China.

9 8 7 6 5 4 3 2 1

This 6th edition of *Anatomy: A Regional Atlas of the Human Body* is published by arrangement with Elsevier Germany GmbH, publisher and copyright holder of *Sobotta Atlas der Anatomie des Menschen, 22. Auflage, Band 1, Band 2; München: Elsevier/ Urban & Fischer* ©2006. The English translation was undertaken by Lippincott Williams & Wilkins.

Most of the illustrations in this atlas have been previously published in the following:
Clemente, Carmine D. *Anatomy: A Regional Atlas of the Human Body,* 4th Edition. Baltimore: Williams & Wilkins, 1997.
Sobotta, J. *Atlas of Human Anatomy,* 21st German Edition/13th English Edition, Volumes 1 and 2. Edited by R. Putz and R. Pabst. Munich: Urban & Fischer, 2000; Baltimore: Lippincott Williams & Wilkins, 2001.
Sobotta, J. *Atlas of Human Anatomy,* 11th English Edition, Volume 1. Edited by J. Staubesand. Baltimore, Munich: Urban & Schwarzenberg, 1990.
Sobotta, J. *Atlas der Anatomie des Menschen, 18. Auflage,* Band 2. Edited by H. Ferner. Munich: Urban & Schwarzenberg, 1982.
Wicke, L. *Atlas of Radiologic Anatomy,* 6th English Edition. Edited and translated by A.N. Taylor. Baltimore: Williams & Wilkins, 1998.

Library of Congress Cataloging-in-Publication Data

Clemente, Carmine D.
  Anatomy : a regional atlas of the human body / Carmine D. Clemente. – 6th ed.
    p. ; cm.
  Includes bibliographical references and index.
  ISBN 978-1-58255-889-9 (alk. paper)
  1. Anatomy, Surgical and topographical–Atlases. I. Title.
  [DNLM: 1. Anatomy, Regional–Atlases. QS 17 C626a 2011]
  QM531.C57 2011
  611–dc22

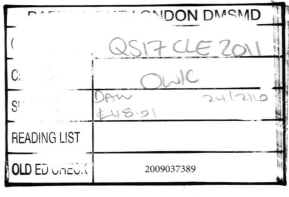

DISCLAIMER

To purchase additional copies of this book, call our customer service department at **(800) 638-3030** or fax orders to **(301) 223-2320**. International customers should call **(301) 223-2300**.

Visit Lippincott Williams & Wilkins on the Internet: http://www.lww.com. Lippincott Williams & Wilkins customer service representatives are available from 8:30 am to 6:00 pm, EST.

Preface to the Sixth Edition

It is always reinforcing and rewarding for an author when the publisher of a book requests another edition. I have now had this pleasure five times after the first edition of this atlas was published 34 years ago in 1975. Previous editions, as well as this edition, have benefited greatly by the many suggestions from colleagues and especially students. Students often approach this in a thoughtful subtle manner. First, the student may say how much he or she has learned from the book and give praise to the nature and color of the figures and then point out a mistaken label in one of the figures that may not have caught my eye. Of course, I am always grateful for these suggestions.

In this edition, I have added many new figures—for example, 14 new figures on 5 plates dealing with the brachial plexus. At the same time, a few figures that did not prove to be excellent teaching items have been removed. Perhaps the most important change in the book is the addition of a significant number of X-rays, CT scans, and ultrasound scans. I am most grateful to Edward J. H. Nathanial, M.D., Ph.D., Emeritus Professor at the University of Winnipeg School of Medicine in Canada, for providing at least 15 figures of clinical significance. Several figures also were contributed by Dr. G.L. Colborn, Emeritus Professor from the Medical College of Georgia in Augusta, Georgia. I have also had the pleasure of discussions with Dr. James D. Collins, Professor of Radiologic Sciences here at UCLA. I thank Dr. Constantine Karakousis, Professor of Surgery and Chief of Surgical Oncology at the University of Buffalo in Buffalo, New York, for the use of several of his figures and for comments on the clinical importance of several plates. Certain X-rays from Dr. Lothar Wicke's 6th English edition of *Atlas of Radiologic Anatomy,* edited by Dr. Anna Taylor here at UCLA, were also used.

There are more than 200 plates of clinical importance in this atlas, and I have benefited greatly from my discussions and collaboration with Professor Gerald Buckberg, M.D., Professor of Cardiac Surgery here at UCLA, and the late Dr. F. Torrent Guasp from Madrid, Spain, on the progressive unfolding of cardiac muscle as shown in Plate 186. These studies have given insightful information on the manner by which the heart muscle develops and matures.

Most of the figures in this atlas come from the Sobotta atlases, recent editions of which have been published by Professor R. Putz in Munich, Germany, and Professor R. Pabst in Hanover, Germany. My deepest appreciation to these two brilliant anatomists knows no bounds. Their German editions of Sobotta have been recently reproduced as the 14th English Edition in 2006. A number of drawings, some of which were also used in the 5th edition, were made by a former resident artist here at UCLA, Ms. Jill Penkhus. I am most grateful for her artistic creativity.

I am most indebted to the editors at Lippincott Williams & Wilkins in Baltimore, and especially to Ms. Crystal Taylor, with whom I have interacted for more than 20 years on several earlier editions of this atlas, and Ms. Julie Montalbano, the Product Manager of this edition. Here at UCLA, I am privileged to have worked with outstanding associates who form the gross anatomy faculty for both the medical and dental school at this university. These include **Dr. Shelley Metten,** the Chairperson of the Anatomy Division, and **Drs. Robert Trelease, Richard Braun, Joseph Miller, Elena Stark, Yau Shi Lin, Jonathan Wisco, Quynh Pham, Guido Zampighi, David Hovda, Anna Taylor, Robin Fisher, Charles Olmstead, Francesco Chiappelli, and Jayc Sedlmayr.** Dr. Sedlmayr is now on the faculty of the Louisiana State University School of Medicine in New Orleans. In my 57 years of active teaching here at UCLA, collectively, these anatomists are the finest anatomy colleagues I have ever worked with.

Finally, but by no means least, I must say that my wife, Julie, has been a steadfast inspiration to me and my academic life, and I am eternally grateful to her.

Carmine D. Clemente
Los Angeles, California—October 2009

From the Preface to the Fifth Edition

I continue to observe the use of this atlas in the anatomy class-room and laboratory here at the UCLA Center for the Health Sciences, and many suggestions I have received over the past six years from students and from friends around the world have been incorporated in this edition. Further, students have convinced me that a **special section on the cranial nerves** would be helpful to them. This has now been included and a series of diagrammatic drawings (patterned after Grant and other authors) along with a number of figures relevant to the cranial nerves have been collected in a group of **29 plates** at the end of the Neck and Head section. Most of the new cranial nerve drawings were done by Ms. Jill Penkhus several years ago when she was the resident artist in the Department of Anatomy here. In addition to these, several new pieces of art have been included in this atlas.

Among the new illustrations in this edition are modified replacements of the nine remaining illustrations in the 4th edition that originated from the controversial atlas *Topographical Human Anatomy* by Pernkopf. These new color illustrations were expertly rendered by the medical illustrators at Anatomical Chart Company (ACC) and David Rini. By far, however, my deepest appreciation is extended to **Professors R. Putz** in Munich and **R. Pabst** in Hanover, Germany, for their exceedingly creative contributions for the 21st German and 13th English editions of the *Sobotta Atlas of Human Anatomy*. More than 325 figures in their most recent two-volume set are the principal new drawings on which this edition is based. The other figures are ones that were used in my 4th edition. I am responsible for all the notes that accompany all of the figures, and any mistakes that may be found in these are mine and those of no one else. I would be most grateful to any student or professor who may have suggestions or who may identify errors, if these were transmitted to me here in Los Angeles.

Many new clinically related plates have been added to those in the 4th edition. This atlas now contains more than 150 plates that are of direct clinical importance. These are listed in the front pages of the book and they include surface anatomy, radiographs (many of which come from the outstanding collection of Professor L. Wicke of Vienna), MRIs, CT scans, arteriograms, lymphangiograms, bronchograms, and even a series of arthroscopic images of the knee joint. These have been added because of the increased emphasis on the clinical relevance to the teaching of Anatomy that has become common in medical schools, not only in the United States but in many other countries as well. One plate (#146) is based on the work of Drs. R. Torrent-Guasp of Madrid and Gerald Buckberg of UCLA here in Los Angeles.

There are many who have helped to make this atlas possible. Among them are Ms. Betty Sun, Ms. Crystal Taylor, Ms. Kathleen Scogna, and Ms. Cheryl Stringfellow at Lippincott Williams & Wilkins in Baltimore and, of course, many at the Elsevier Corporation, the publishers that acquired the Sobotta collection from Urban & Fischer. I am especially grateful to Dr. Constantine Karakousis, Professor of Surgery and Chief of Surgical Oncology at the University of Buffalo in Buffalo, New York, for his recommendations and comments on the clinical importance of several of the plates. Perhaps most of all, my continuing gratitude goes to Julie, my wife, who has helped me both at the computer and in being considerate for all the time it has taken me to do this manuscript, time that could have been given to some of her interests.

Carmine D. Clemente
Los Angeles, California—February 2006

From the Preface to the First Edition

Twenty-five years ago, while a student at the University of Pennsylvania, I marvelled at the clarity, completeness, and boldness of the anatomical illustrations of the original German editions of Professor Johannes Sobotta's atlas and their excellent three-volume English counterparts, the recent editions of which were authored by the late Professor Frank H. J. Figge. It is a matter of record that before World War II these atlases were the most popular ones consulted by American medical students. In the United States, with the advent of other anatomical atlases, the shortening of courses of anatomy in the medical schools, and the increase in publishing cost, the excellent but larger editions of the Sobotta atlases have become virtually unknown to a full generation of students. During the past 20 years of teaching Gross Anatomy at the University of California at Los Angeles, I have found only a handful of students who are familiar with the beautiful and still unexcelled Sobotta illustration.

This volume introduces several departures from the former Sobotta atlases. It is the first English edition that represents the Sobotta plates in a regional sequence—the pectoral region and upper extremity, the thorax, the abdomen, the pelvis and perineum, the lower extremity, the back, vertebral column and spinal cord, and finally, the neck and head. This sequence is consistent with that followed in many courses presented in the United States and Canada and one which should be useful to students in other countries.

Many have contributed to bringing this Atlas to fruition. I thank Dr. David S. Maxwell, Professor and Vice Chairman for Gross Anatomy and my colleague at UCLA, for his encouragement and suggestions. I also wish to express my appreciation to Caroline Belz and Louise Campbell, who spent many hours proofreading and typing the original text. I especially wish to thank Mary Mansor for constructing the index—a most laborious task. I am grateful to Barbara Robins for her assistance in typing some of the early parts of the manuscript, and above all, to her sister Julie, who is my wife and who makes all of my efforts worthwhile through her encouragement and devotion.

Carmine D. Clemente
Los Angeles, California—January 1975

Contents

CHAPTER 1: Pectoral Region, Axilla, Shoulder, and Upper Limb — Plates

Body Regions	1
Anterior Thorax, Superficial Pectoral Region Including Female Breast	2–18
Axilla, Deep Pectoral Region	19–27
Arteries and Superficial Veins of Upper Limb	29–29
Anterior and Posterior Shoulder: Muscles; Neurovascular Structures; Abduction	30–33
Upper Limb: Surface Anatomy and Dermatoses	34–35
Upper Limb: General; Muscles, Vessels and Nerves	36–45
Brachial Plexus	46–53
Shoulder, Anterior and Posterior Arm (Brachium): Muscles, Vessels and Nerves (Detailed)	54–67
Forearm: General (Superficial)	68–69
Forearm: Anterior Aspect, Muscles, Vessels and Nerves	70–79
Forearm: Posterior Aspect, Muscles, Vessels and Nerves	80–89
Hand: Dorsal Aspect	90–93
Hand: Palmar Aspect	94–111
Bones and Joints of the Upper Limb	112–131
Cross Sections of the Upper Limb	132–137
Anatomy of Fingers	90–93; 95–98; 100–105; 107–110; 130

CHAPTER 2: The Thorax — Plates

Surface Anatomy: Thoracic and Abdominal Wall	139
Anterior Thoracic Wall	140–149
Thymus, Pleura, Lungs, Trachea, and Bronchi	150–165
Pericardium and Heart	166–187
Conduction System of the Heart; Heart Valves	188–191
Circulation of Blood	192–195
Posterior and Superior Mediastina	196–205
Sympathetic Trunks and Vagus Nerves	206–209
Thoracic Duct and Lymphatic System	210–211
Frontal Sections and MRIs and Cross Sections of the Chest	212–218

CHAPTER 3: The Abdomen — Plates

Regions of the Body, Diagram of the GI System	219
Anterior Abdominal Wall	220–231

Female Inguinal Region; Autonomic Innervation of Female Genital Organs	232–233
Male Inguinal Region and Genital Organs	234–240
Direct and Indirect Inguinal Hernias	241
Abdominal Structures in the Newborn	242–243
Topographic Views of Thoracic, Abdominal, and Pelvic Organs	244–247
Development of the Mesenteries	248–249
Topographic Views of the Abdominal Organs In Situ	250–253
Stomach: Blood Supply; Surface Projections; X Rays; Lymphatics	254–267
Duodenum	268–269
Liver	270–277
Gallbladder; Bile Duct System; Pancreas; Spleen	278–287
Small Intestine	288–293
Large Intestine	294–305
Posterior Abdominal Wall; Lumbar Nerves	306–317
Cross Sections of Abdomen	318–322

CHAPTER 4: The Pelvis and Perineum

	Plates
Bones of the Pelvis and Sex Differences; Ligaments of the Pelvis	323–329
Female Pelvic Organs	330–335
Placenta; Pregnant Uterus	336–338
Female Pelvic Vessels; Median Sagittal Section of Female Pelvis	339–342
Female Perineum: Muscles, Urogenital Diaphragm; Vessels and Nerves; External Genitalia	343–350
Male Pelvic Organs	351–355
Male Perineum	355–358
Rectum	359–362
Cross Sections and CT Scans: Female and Male Pelvis	363–364
Male Urogenital Region: Surface Anatomy, Vessels and Nerves	365–366
Male External Genitalia: Penis (Corpora), Spermatic Cord, Vessels, Nerves, and Cross Sections	367–370

CHAPTER 5: The Back, Vertebral Column, and Spinal Cord

	Plates
Back: Surface Anatomy; Skeleton; Dermatomes; Cutaneous Nerves; Superficial Muscles	371–373
Back: Superficial and Intermediate Muscle Layers	373–374
Back: Intermediate and Deep Muscle Layers; Semispinalis Capitis Muscle; Muscle Charts	375–381
Upper Back and Suboccipital Triangle	381–385
Cross Sections Showing Typical Spinal Nerve and Deep Back Muscles	386
Vertebral Column and Vertebrae: Ligaments and Intervertebral Disks	387–401
Spinal Cord	402–408

CHAPTER 6: The Lower Limb

	Plates
Anterior and Medial Thigh: Muscles, Vessels, and Nerves	409–427
Gluteal Region and Posterior Thigh	428–439
Anterior, Medial and Posterior Nerves of the Lower Limb	440–441
Popliteal Fossa: Muscles, Vessels and Nerves	442–445
Anterior and Lateral Compartments of the Leg	446–453
Dorsum of the Foot	454–459

Posterior Compartment of the Leg 460–469

Plantar Aspect of the Foot 470–477

Bones and Joints of the Lower Limb 478–509

Cross Sections and MRIs of the Lower Limb 510–516

CHAPTER 7: The Neck and Head   Plates

Surface Anatomy of the Head and Neck 517–518

Triangles of the Neck; Platysma Muscle; Fascias; Nerves and Lymphatics 519–528

Cervical Plexus of Nerves; Trunks of the Brachial Plexus; Accessory Nerve 529–534

Arteries and Veins of the Neck; Thyroid Gland; Lymphatics 535–540

Prevertebral Region; Subclavian and Vertebral Arteries 541–544

Submental and Submandibular Regions 545–546

Superficial Muscles of the Face; Facial Nerve Diagram; Muscle Charts 547–550

Parotid Gland; Muscles of Mastication; Facial Nerve Branches 551–556

Temporomandibular Joint 557–558

Internal Carotid Artery; Superficial and Deep Veins of the Head 559–562

Vessels and Nerves of the Deep Face 563–566

Bones of the Skull: Adult and Newborn 567–572

Scalp; Diploic Veins; Radiographs of the Internal Carotid Artery 573–574

Dura Mater; Dural Sinuses 575–578

Internal Carotid and Vertebral Arteries to the Brain 579–584

Base of the Skulls; Bones, Vessels, Nerves; Inferior Surface of the Brain 585–590

Inferior Surface of the Bony Skull 591–592

Eye: Anterior View; Bony Socket; Nasolacrimal System 593–599

Eye: External Structure and Bones of the Nasal Cavity 600–612

Nose: External Structure and Bones of the Nasal Cavity 613–616

Paranasal Sinuses 617–618

Oral Cavity: Anterior View; Lips; Palatine Tonsil and Oropharynx 619–620

Oral Cavity: Sublingual Region; Palate; Submandibular Gland 621–623

Floor of the Oral Cavity 624–626

Tongue 627–632

Mandibular and Maxillary Teeth 633–640

Pharynx: Muscles, Arteries and Nerves 641–649

Larynx 650–656

External, Middle and Internal Ear 657–668

CHAPTER 8: Cranial Nerves   Plates

Cranial Nerves: Attachments to the Brain, Foramina; Base of Skull 669–670

Cranial Nerves I to XII 671–694

Index   I-1–I-24

Plates of Direct Clinical Importance

Plates 1–3	Male and Female Surface Anatomy	Plate 181	Right Coronary Arteriogram
Plates 4, 6, 7–9	Anatomy of the Female Breast and Lymphatic Channels	Plate 191	Heart Valves: Projection on Chest Wall and Their Structure
Plates 10, 12–14	Surface Vessels and Nerves of the Anterior Trunk	Plate 196	Frontal Section of the Thorax and Upper Abdomen
Plates 22–24	Arteries, Veins, and Nerves of the Axilla	Plate 200	Radiograph of Esophagus and View through Esophagoscope
Plates 28, 29	Arteries and Superficial Veins in the Upper Limb	Plate 205	Angiogram of the Aortic Arch and Its Branches
Plates 30–32, 54, 55	Muscles That Form the Rotator Cuff in the Shoulder	Plates 212, 213, 218	MRIs and CT of the Chest
Plate 35	Dermatomes of the Upper Limb	Plate 219	Surface Anatomy: Regions of the Body; GI System Organs
Plates 36, 37	Vessels and Nerves: Anterior and Posterior Brachium	Plate 229	CT Scans of the Body Wall and Abdomen
Plates 38, 39	Arteries and Nerves of the Upper Limb; Brachial Arteriogram	Plates 240, 241	Descent of Testis and Congenital and Direct Inguinal Hernias
Plate 41	Variations in the Superficial Veins of the Upper Limb	Plate 244	Surface Projections: Thorax, Abdomen, Male Pelvic Organs
Plate 46–53	Brachial Plexus	Plate 245	Surface Projections: Thorax, Abdomen, Female Pelvic Organs
Plate 67	Course of the Radial Nerve Along the Radial Groove	Plates 246, 247	Median and Paramedian Sections of Male Abdomen and Pelvis
Plates 68, 69	Superficial Vessels and Nerves of the Forearm; Cubital Fossa	Plate 256	Celiac Trunk Arteriogram
Plates 77–79	Median, Ulnar, and Radial Nerves in the Forearm; Brachial Artery	Plate 257	Variations in Blood Supply to the Liver and Stomach
Plate 86	Dermatomes on Posterior Aspect of Upper Limb	Plate 261	Surface Projections and Radiographs of the Stomach
Plates 90, 91	Local Anesthesia of Fingers	Plate 263	X-Ray of the Stomach
Plate 99	Synovial Sheaths of the Fingers	Plate 265	X-Ray of the Stomach Showing a Small Ulcer
Plate 115	X-Ray of Should Joint Bones	Plate 267	X-Rays Showing Gastric and Duodenal Ulcers
Plates 120, 121	Radiographic Anatomy of the Right Should Joint Bones	Plate 270	Surface Projections of the Liver
Plate 123	X-Rays of Elbow Joint: Adult and Child	Plate 273	Ultrasound Scans of the Hepatic and Portal Veins
Plate 127	Radiograph of the Wrist and Hand	Plate 275	CT Scan of Upper Abdomen at Level T10-T11
Plate 129	Radiograph of the Right Wrist	Plate 276	CT Scan of Abdomen at Level L1
Plate 131	Radiograph of the Right Hand (Lateral Projection)	Plate 277	Ultrasound Scans: Upper Abdomen and Tumor Mass in Liver
Plates 132, 133, 135, 136	CT Scans of the Arm, Forearm, and Wrist	Plate 279	Cholangiogram and X-Ray of Biliary Duct System
Plate 139	Surface Anatomy of Anterior Body Wall (Male and Female)	Plate 280	Ultrasound Scan: Abdomen Showing Parts of the Gallbladder
Plate 151	Radiograph of the Chest Showing the Heart and Lungs	Plate 281	Ultrasound Scans of Gallbladder and Gallstones
Plates 154–156	Surface Projections of the Pleura and Lungs	Plate 282	Surface Projection: Duodenum and Pancreas
Plate 163	Surface Projection of the Trachea	Plate 284	CT Scan: Abdomen at Level L2 Showing Pancreas, etc.
Plate 165	Bronchogram of Bronchial Tree; Bronchoscope of Trachea	Plate 285	CT Scan Showing a Tumor in the Head of the Pancreas
Plate 168	Radiograph of the Thorax	Plate 286	CT Scan: Diffuse Inflammation of the Pancreas (Pancreatitis)
Plate 171	Anterior Wall Projection of Underlying Heart Valves		
Plate 180	Left Coronary Arteriogram		

Plate 287	CT Scan Showing a Hemorrhage within the Spleen
Plate 289	Radiograph of the Jejunum, Ileum, Cecum, and Ascending Colon
Plate 291	Radiograph of the Small Intestine
Plate 293	Superior Mesenteric Arteriogram
Plate 295	Inferior Mesenteric Arteriogram
Plate 302	Variations in the Location of the Vermiform Appendix
Plate 305	Radiograph of the Large Intestine
Plate 310	Arteriogram of the Renal Artery
Plate 311	Surface Anatomy of the Back Showing Location of the Kidneys
Plate 313	Retrograde Pyelogram
Plates 318–322	CT Scans of the Abdomen
Plate 325	Radiograph of the Pelvis
Plate 330	Uterosalpingogram
Plate 332	Variations in the Position of the Uterus in the Pelvis
Plate 334	CT Scan of the Female Pelvis
Plate 337	X-Ray of the Pregnant Uterus
Plate 338	Pregnant Uterus: Fetal Sonograms
Plate 339	Variations in the Divisions of the Internal Iliac Artery
Plate 340	Arteriogram of the Iliac Arteries in the Female
Plate 344	Female External Genitalia
Plate 353	Peritoneum over Empty and Full Bladders
Plate 356	Radiographs of Male Pelvic Organs
Plates 363, 364	CT Scans of the Female and Male Pelvis
Plate 371	Surface Anatomy of the Back
Plate 372	Cutaneous Nerves and Dermatomes of the Back
Plate 391	Radiograph of Odontoid Process and Atlantoaxial Joints
Plate 398	Intervertebral Disks
Plates 400, 401	Radiograph of the Vertebral Column
Plates 402–407	Spinal Cord
Plate 408	Lumbar and Sacral Punctures into the Spinal Column
Plates 409–412	Lower Limb: Surface Anatomy, Cutaneous Nerves, Bones
Plates 413–415	Lower Limb: Arteries, Muscles: Anterior and Posterior Aspects
Plate 422	Variations in the Deep Femoral Artery and Circumflex Arteries
Plate 428	Surface Vessels and Nerves: Gluteal Region, Posterior Thigh
Plates 434, 435	Safe Zones for Intramuscular Injections in Gluteal Region
Plates 440, 441	Nerves of the Lower Limb
Plate 444	Variations in Branching of Anterior Tibial Fibular Arteries
Plate 446	Superficial Veins and Nerves of Anterior and Medial Leg, Foot
Plate 453	Ankle and Foot Movements
Plate 454	Vessels and Nerves of the Dorsal Foot
Plate 460	Vessels and Nerves on the Posterior Aspect of the Leg (Calf)
Plates 474, 476	Vessels and Nerves on the Plantar Aspect of the Foot
Plates 483	Blood Supply and Radiograph of the Hip Joint
Plate 484	Radiograph of the Knee Joint
Plate 489	Four MRIs of the Knee Joint
Plate 490	Arthrogram of the Knee Joint
Plate 491	Arthroscopic Images of the Knee Joint
Plate 493	Radiographs of the Knee Joint
Plate 494	Movements at the Knee Joint
Plate 498	X-Ray of the Ankle Joint
Plate 508	Radiograph, MRI of Ankle, Subtalar, and Talonavicular Joints
Plates 511–513	CT Scans of the Mid and Distal Thigh and Mid Leg
Plate 515	MRI through the Metatarsal Bones of the Foot
Plates 517, 518	Surface Anatomy of the Face and Neck
Plate 599	Surgical Entry into the Respiratory System
Plate 525	Drainage of Lymph of Superficial Lateral Scalp and Face
Plate 535	Jugular Veins in the Neck
Plates 536–538	Thyroid Gland
Plates 548, 553, 554	Facial Nerve on the Face
Plates 557, 558	Temporomandibular Joint
Plate 560	Variations in the Maxillary Artery
Plate 571, 572	Newborn Skull
Plates 573, 574	Scalp, Diploic Veins, Internal Carotid Artery
Plate 582	Variations in the Formation of the Circle of Willis
Plates 583, 584	Arteriogram of the Internal Carotid and Vertebral Arteries
Plates 588–590	Base of the Skull and Brain: Cranial Nerves and Vessels
Plate 593	Eye from Anterior
Plates 601–604	Nerve in the Orbit
Plate 609	Horizontal Section of the Eyeball
Plates 611, 612	MRI, Vessels and Nerves within the Orbit and Retina
Plate 616	Vessels and Nerves in the Nasal Cavity
Plates 617, 618	Paranasal Sinuses
Plates 619–622	Oral Cavity
Plates 625, 626	Salivary Glands
Plates 633–640	Anatomy of the Dental Arches and Teeth; Their Innervation
Plates 641–648	Pharynx
Plates 649–656	Larynx
Plates 657–668	External, Middle, and Internal Ear
Plate 669–694	Cranial Nerves I–XII

Plates Containing Muscle Charts

Pectoral Muscle	Plates 15, 20
Shoulder Muscles	Plates 30, 33
Anterior Brachial Muscles (Flexors)	Plates 56, 57
Posterior Brachial Muscles (Extensors)	Plate 65
Anterior Forearm Muscles (Flexors)	Plates 73, 74
Posterior Forearm Muscles (Extensors)	Plates 80, 81, 85, 87
Thenar Muscles of the Hand	Plates 96, 97
Hypothenar Muscles of the Hand	Plate 98
Dorsal Interosseous Muscles of the Hand	Plate 102
Palmar Interosseous Muscles of the Hand	Plate 103
Intercostal Muscles	Plate 143
Subclavius Muscles	Plate 148
Anterior Abdominal Wall Muscles	Plates 225–227, 230
Posterior Abdominal Wall Muscles and the Diaphragm	Plate 314
Muscles of the Pelvic Diaphragm and the Urogenital Diaphragm	Plate 346
Intermediate and Deep Back Muscles	Plate 379
Deep Muscles of the Back (Continued)	Plate 380
Muscles of the Suboccipital Region	Plate 385
Anterior Muscles of the Hip and Anterior Thigh Muscles	Plate 426
Medial, Lateral, and Posterior Thigh Muscles	Plate 427
Muscles of the Gluteal Region	Plate 434
Muscles of the Posterior Thigh	Plate 436
Muscles of the Anterior and Lateral Compartments of the Leg	Plate 448
Muscles of the Dorsum of the Foot	Plate 457
Muscles of the Posterior Compartment of the Leg	Plates 468, 469
Muscles of the Sole of the Foot	Plate 477
Infrahyoid Muscles of the Neck	Plate 519
Sternocleidomastoid Muscle	Plate 520
Muscles of the Posterior Triangle of the Neck	Plate 528
Anterior Vertebral Muscles	Plate 542
Muscles of Face and Head: Suprahyoid, Scalp Muscles; Ear, Eyelids	Plate 549
Muscles of Face and Head: Muscles of Nose and Mouth	Plate 550
Muscles of Mastication	Plates 555, 556
Schema of Extraocular Muscles	Plate 607
Extrinsic Muscles of the Tongue	Plate 632
Muscles of the Palate and Pharynx	Plate 648
Muscles of the Larynx (see notes under Figs. 653.1–653.4 and Figs. 654.1–654.3)	Plates 653, 654
Muscles of the Middle Ear	Plates 657, 663–665

Plates

1 Regions of the Body

2 Surface Anatomy of the Male Body

3 Surface Anatomy of the Female Body

4 Superficial Dissection of the Breast; Milk Line

5 Surface Anatomy of Female Thoracic Wall; Female Breast

6 Breast: Nipple and Areola (Sagittal Section)

7 Lymph Nodes that Drain the Breast; Lymphangiogram of the Axilla

8 Lymphatic Drainage from Breast; Medial and Lateral Mammary Arteries

9 Lateral View of the Female Breast and a Dissected Nipple

10 Dermatomes; Anterior Thoracic Segmental Nerves

11 Superficial Thoracic and Abdominal Wall Muscles (Lateral View)

12 Superficial Veins of the Anterior Trunk (Male)

13 Superficial Vessels and Nerves of the Anterior Trunk (Female)

14 A Typical Segmental Spinal Nerve and Intercostal Artery

15 Superficial Thoracic and Abdominal Wall Muscles

16 Pectoral Region: Superficial Vessels and Cutaneous Nerves

17 Pectoral Region: Pectoralis Major and Deltoid Muscles

18 The Pectoralis Major and Minor Muscles

19 The Anterior Surface of the Rib Cage

20 Lateral Thoracic Wall and Superficial Axilla

21 The Pectoral Muscles: Intact and Reflected; Serratus Anterior Muscle

22 Deltopectoral Triangle and the Deep Lateral Thoracic Muscles

23 The Axillary Vein and Its Tributaries

24 The Axillary Artery and Its Branches

25 The Internal Thoracic–Epigastric Anastomosis

26 Dissection of Axilla: Superficial Vessels and Nerves

27 Dissection of Axilla: Deep Vessels and Nerves

28 Arterial Supply to the Upper Extremity

29 Superficial Veins of the Upper Extremity

30 Shoulder Region, Anterior Aspect: Muscles

31 Anterior Shoulder Region: Vessels and Nerves; Shoulder Joint Movements

32 Shoulder Region, Posterior Aspect: Muscles

33 Posterior Shoulder: Vessels and Nerves; Abduction of the Upper Limb

34 Surface Anatomy of the Upper Limb

35 Dermatomes of the Upper Limb

36 Superficial Dissection of the Arm (Anterior View)

37 Superficial Dissection of the Arm (Posterior View)

38 Blood Vessels of the Upper Limb

39 Nerves of the Upper Limb

40 Cutaneous (Superficial) Nerves of the Upper Limb

41 Superficial Venous Patterns in the Upper Limb

42 Surface and Skeletal Anatomy of the Upper Limb

43 Muscular Contours of the Upper Limb: Anterior and Posterior Views

44 Muscles of the Upper Limb: Lateral View

45 Muscles of the Upper Limb: Anterior and Posterior Views

46 The Brachial Plexus and Its Three Cords

47 Brachial Plexus: Roots of Origin and General Schema

48 Complete Brachial Plexus Diagram

49 Musculocutaneous Nerve: Distribution and Spinal Segments

50 Median Nerve: Distribution, Spinal Segments, and Median Nerve Palsy

51 Ulnar Nerve: Distribution, Spinal Segments, and Ulnar Nerve Palsy

52 Axillary Nerve: Distribution, Spinal Segments, and Axillary Nerve Palsy

53 Radial Nerve: Distribution, Spinal Segments, and Radial Nerve Palsy

54 Anterior Dissection of the Shoulder and Arm: Muscles

55 The Shoulder Muscles: Anterior and Posterior Views

56 Muscles of the Anterior Arm (Superficial Dissection)

57 Muscles of the Anterior Arm (Deep Dissection)

58 Brachial Artery and the Median and Ulnar Nerves in the Arm

59 Deep Dissection of the Anterior Arm; Musculocutaneous Nerve

60 Posterior Dissection of Shoulder and Arm: Muscles

61 Shoulder Region: Supraspinatus Muscle and the Rotator Cuff Capsule

62 Muscles on the Lateral and Posterior Aspects of the Arm

63 Posterior Arm; The Three Heads of the Triceps Muscle

64 Attachments of Muscles in Upper Limb: Anterior View

65 Attachments of Muscles in Upper Limb: Posterior View

66 Posterior Arm: Vessels and Nerves (Superficial Dissection)

67 Arteries and Nerves of the Scapular and Posterior Brachial Regions

68 Superficial Dissection of the Anterior Forearm

69 Superficial Dissection of the Posterior Forearm

70 Anterior Forearm: Superficial Muscles

71 Anterior Forearm: Pronator Teres and Flexor Digitorum Superficialis

72 Anterior Forearm: Deep Muscles

73 Anterior Muscles of the Forearm; Flexor Muscle Chart

74 Anterior View of Radius and Ulna: Muscle Attachments; Muscle Chart

75 Fracture of the Radius and the Pronator Teres Muscle

76 Anterior Forearm Vessels and Nerves (Superficial Dissection)

77 Anterior Forearm Vessels and Nerves (Intermediate Dissection)

78 Anterior Forearm Vessels and Nerves (Deep Dissection)

79 Elbow Region: Vessels and Nerves

80 Superficial Extensor Muscles of Forearm (Posterior View)

81 Superficial Extensor Muscles of the Forearm (Lateral View)

82 Deep Extensor Muscles of the Forearm

83 Deep Extensor Muscles of the Forearm

84 Supination and Pronation of the Forearm and Hand

85 Extensor Muscles of the Forearm; Muscle Chart

86 Posterior Upper Limb Muscles and Dermatomes (Review)

87 Posterior Attachments of Muscles on the Ulna and Radius; Muscle Chart

88 Nerves and Arteries of the Posterior Forearm (Superficial Dissection)

89 Nerves and Arteries of the Posterior Forearm (Deep Dissection)

90 Dorsum of the Hand: Veins and Nerves; Finger Injection Site

91 Dorsum of the Hand: Tendons and Interosseous Muscles; Dermatomes

92 Dorsal Synovial Tendon Sheaths at the Wrist; Anatomy of a Finger

93 Dorsum of the Hand: Tendons and Arteries (Superficial and Deep Dissections)

94 Palm of the Hand: Superficial Vessels and Nerves

95 Superficial Dissection of the Palm of the Right Hand and Two Fingers

96 Palm of the Hand: Muscles and Tendon Sheaths

97 Thenar and Hypothenar Muscles; Cutaneous Innervation of the Palm

98 Palm of the Hand: Muscles and Flexor Tendon Insertions

99 Palm of the Hand: Deep Dissection of Muscles and Fingers

100 Muscles of the Deep Palmar Hand Region: Dissection #1

101 Muscles of the Deep Palmar Hand Region: Dissection #2

102 Dorsal Interosseous Muscles in the Deep Hand

103 Palmar Interosseous Muscles in the Deep Hand

104 Lumbrical Muscles; Tendons and Cross Section of the Middle Finger

105 The Carpal Tunnel; More Distal Cross Section of the Middle Finger

106 Carpal Tunnel; Superficial Palmar Arterial Arch

107 Palm of the Hand: Nerves and Arteries (Superficial Dissection)

108 Palmar Arterial Arches

109 Palmar Arteries and Nerves; Variations in the Deep Palmar Arch

110 Sagittal Section through the Middle Finger (Ulnar View)

111 Radial Side of the Hand: Arteries and Superficial Nerves

112 Skeleton of the Thorax; Scapula

113 The Humerus

114 Shoulder Joint: Ligaments and Bony Structures

115 X-Ray of the Right Shoulder Joint

116 Acromioclavicular and Shoulder Joints

117 The Right Shoulder Joint (Anterior and Posterior Views)

118 Glenoid Labrum and Cavity; Clavicular and Scapular Ligaments

119 Lateral View of Shoulder Joint and Frontal Section of the Joint

120 Radiographic Anatomy of the Right Shoulder Joint I

121 Radiographic Anatomy of the Right Shoulder Joint II

122 Bones of the Upper Limb: Radius and Ulna

123 Elbow Joint: Radiographs, Adult and Child

124 Left Elbow Joint (Anterior, Posterior, and Sagittal Views)

125 Elbow Joint: Bones; Ligaments (Medial View)

126 Radioulnar Joints

127 Radiograph of the Wrist and Hand

128 Bones of the Wrist and Hand (Palmar Aspect)

129 Bones of the Wrist and Hand (Dorsal Aspect)

130 Wrist and Hand: Ligaments and Joints

131 Wrist, Hand, and Fingers: Joints and Ligaments

132 Cross Sections of the Upper Limb: Arm

133 Cross Sections of the Lower Third of the Arm

134 Cross Sections of the Upper Limb: Elbow and Upper Forearm

135 Middle Forearm (Cross Section and MRI)

136 Computerized Tomographs of the Wrist

137 Cross Sections of the Upper Limb: Wrist and Hand

138 The Thumb, Index Finger, and Fingernails

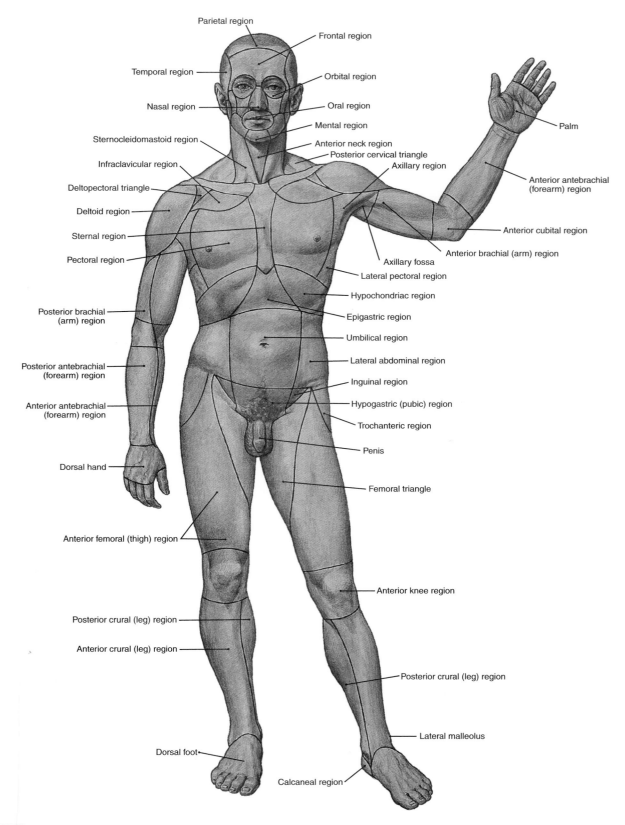

Parietal region
Frontal region
Temporal region
Orbital region
Nasal region
Oral region
Mental region
Sternocleidomastoid region
Anterior neck region
Posterior cervical triangle
Infraclavicular region
Axillary region
Deltopectoral triangle
Palm
Deltoid region
Anterior antebrachial
(forearm) region
Sternal region
Anterior cubital region
Pectoral region
Anterior brachial (arm) region
Axillary fossa
Lateral pectoral region
Hypochondriac region
Posterior brachial
(arm) region
Epigastric region
Umbilical region
Lateral abdominal region
Posterior antebrachial
(forearm) region
Inguinal region
Hypogastric (pubic) region
Anterior antebrachial
(forearm) region
Trochanteric region
Penis
Dorsal hand
Femoral triangle
Anterior femoral (thigh) region
Anterior knee region
Posterior crural (leg) region
Anterior crural (leg) region
Posterior crural (leg) region
Lateral malleolus
Dorsal foot
Calcaneal region

FIGURE 1 **Regions of the Body: Anterior View**

NOTE: (1) Surface areas are identified by specific names to describe the location of structures and symptoms precisely.

(2) Some regions are named after bones (sternal, parietal, infraclavicular, etc.), others for muscles (deltoid, pectoral, sternocleidomastoid), and still others for specialized anatomical structures (umbilical, oral, nasal, etc.).

(3) The principal regions of the body include the pectoral region and upper extremity, thorax, abdomen, pelvis and perineum, lower extremity, back and spinal column, and neck and head.

PLATE 2 **Surface Anatomy of the Male Body**

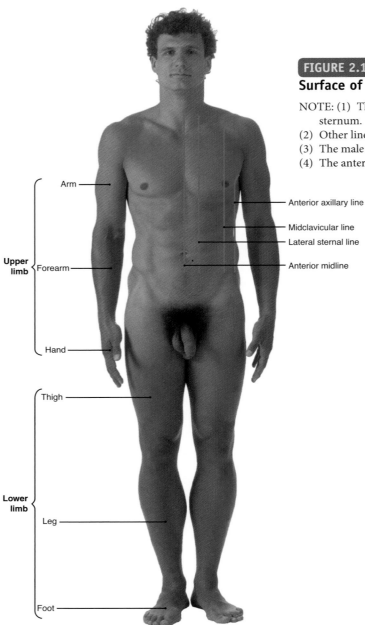

FIGURE 2.1 **Regions and Longitudinal Lines on the Anterior Surface of the Male Body**

NOTE: (1) The lateral sternal line descends along the lateral border of the sternum.
(2) Other lines parallel to this are called parasternal lines.
(3) The male nipple lies near the midclavicular line.
(4) The anterior axillary line descends from the anterior axillary fold.

Arm
Anterior axillary line
Midclavicular line
Lateral sternal line
Upper limb
Forearm
Anterior midline
Hand
Thigh
Lower limb
Leg
Foot

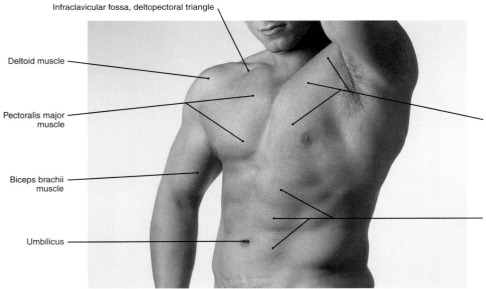

Infraclavicular fossa, deltopectoral triangle

Deltoid muscle

Pectoralis major muscle

Biceps brachii muscle

Umbilicus

Pectoralis major muscle

Rectus abdominis muscle

FIGURE 2.2 **Surface Contours on the Male Thorax**

Certain contours on the chest, upper abdomen, and upper limb reveal the shape of underlying muscles.

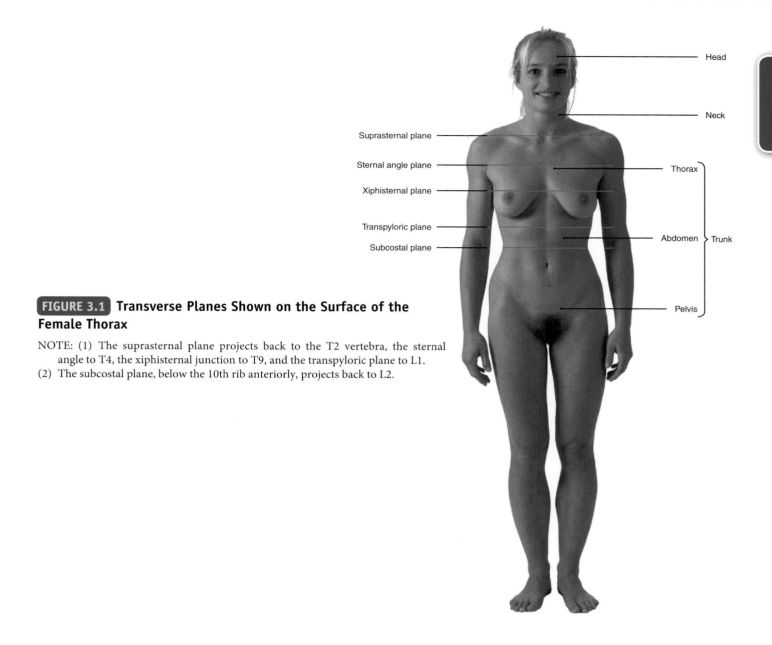

Head

Neck

Suprasternal plane

Sternal angle plane

Thorax

Xiphisternal plane

Transpyloric plane

Abdomen — Trunk

Subcostal plane

Pelvis

FIGURE 3.1 **Transverse Planes Shown on the Surface of the Female Thorax**

NOTE: (1) The suprasternal plane projects back to the T2 vertebra, the sternal angle to T4, the xiphisternal junction to T9, and the transpyloric plane to L1.

(2) The subcostal plane, below the 10th rib anteriorly, projects back to L2.

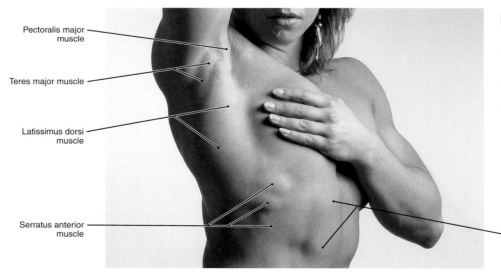

Pectoralis major muscle

Teres major muscle

Latissimus dorsi muscle

Serratus anterior muscle

Rectus abdominis muscle

FIGURE 3.2 **Surface Contours on the Lateral Thorax of a Young Woman**

NOTE the contours of well-developed latissimus dorsi, pectoralis major, teres major, and serratus anterior muscles.

PLATE 4 Superficial Dissection of the Breast; Milk Line

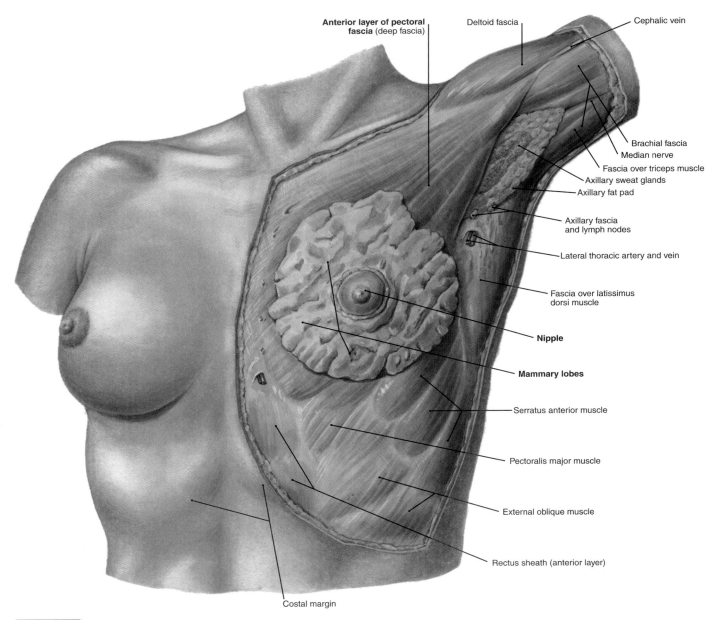

Anterior layer of pectoral fascia (deep fascia)
Deltoid fascia
Cephalic vein
Brachial fascia
Median nerve
Fascia over triceps muscle
Axillary sweat glands
Axillary fat pad
Axillary fascia and lymph nodes
Lateral thoracic artery and vein
Fascia over latissimus dorsi muscle
Nipple
Mammary lobes
Serratus anterior muscle
Pectoralis major muscle
External oblique muscle
Rectus sheath (anterior layer)
Costal margin

FIGURE 4.1 Anterior Pectoral Region and Female Breast ▲

NOTE: (1) The lobular nature of the breast.
(2) It extends from the lateral sternal line to the midaxillary line and from the second to the sixth rib.
(3) The breast is located in the superficial fascia anterior to the pectoral fascia.
(4) Shown are the superficial axillary lymph nodes and the axillary sweat glands.

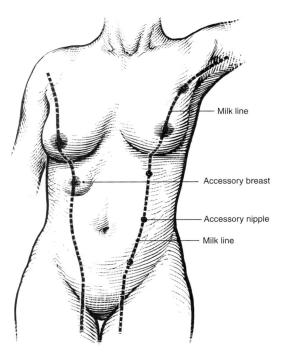

Milk line
Accessory breast
Accessory nipple
Milk line

FIGURE 4.2 Milk Line and Accessory Nipples and Breasts ▶

NOTE: (1) Supernumerary nipples (polythelia) and/or multiple breasts on the same side (polymastia) occur in about 1% of people.
(2) These are found along the curved milk line extending from the axillary fossa to the groin.
(3) This condition occurs slightly more frequently in males than in females and may easily be handled surgically.

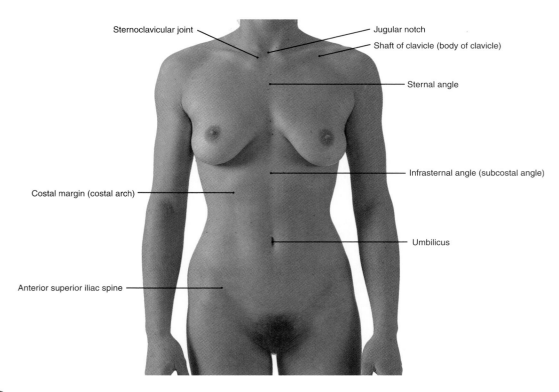

FIGURE 5.1 **Surface Anatomy of the Anterior Thoracic and Abdominal Walls of a Young Female**

NOTE: Bony structures and the umbilicus are labeled.

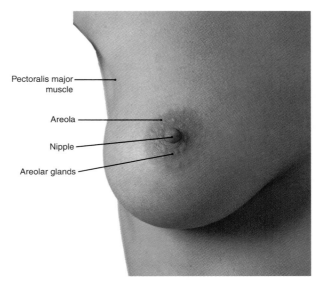

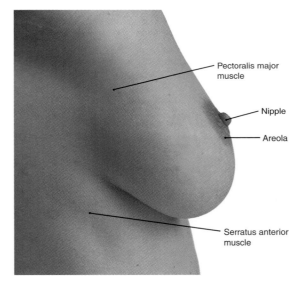

FIGURE 5.2 **Female Breast (Anterior View)**

FIGURE 5.3 **Female Breast (Lateral View)**

NOTE: The nipple and areolar glands project from the surface of the pigmented areola. Also observe the muscular contours of the pectoralis major and serratus anterior muscles.

PLATE 6 **Breast: Nipple and Areola (Sagittal Section)**

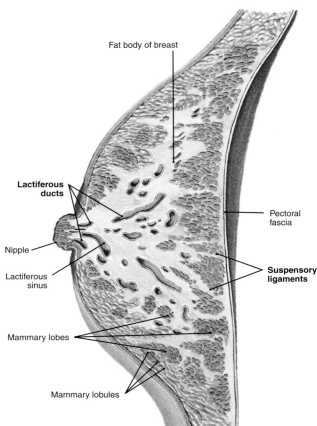

Fat body of breast

Lactiferous ducts

Nipple

Lactiferous sinus

Mammary lobes

Mammary lobules

Pectoral fascia

Suspensory ligaments

FIGURE 6.1 **Sagittal Section through Mammary Gland of Gravid Female**

NOTE: (1) The radial arrangement of the lobes, separated by connective tissue and fat.
(2) In the lactiferous duct system, each of the 15 to 20 lobes has its own duct.
(3) The pectoral fascia separates the breast from the pectoralis major muscle.
(4) The connective-tissue suspensory ligaments (of Cooper) extend to the pectoral fascia.

FIGURE 6.2 **Right Mammary Gland: Dissection of the Nipple ▶**

NOTE: (1) A circular piece of skin has been incised from around the nipple.
(2) The 15 to 20 lactiferous ducts are arranged radially around the nipple and seen just deep to the skin.

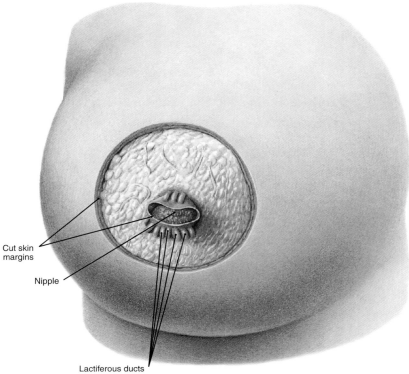

Cut skin margins

Nipple

Lactiferous ducts

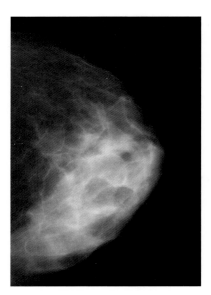

FIGURE 6.3 **Radiograph of Normal Female Breast**

Lateral mammograph of a 47-year-old woman.

Cancer of the Breast

Cancer of the breast usually develops in the epithelial cells that line the ducts of the glandular tissue. Often, the initial clinical sign of breast cancer is a painless lump in the upper lateral quadrant of the organ. This may progress:

(1) to invade the connective tissue between the lobules (suspensory ligaments of Cooper) and cause a **retraction of the nipple;**
(2) to grow more deeply and **fix the breast to the pectoral fascia** overlying the pectoralis major muscle. This causes the breast to be **less movable** and it **tends to elevate** when the underlying pectoralis major contracts;
(3) to cause a **dimpling,** a **thickening,** and a **discoloration of the skin over the tumor.** The skin then assumes an appearance of an orange peel and hence has been called the **peau d'orange sign** of advanced breast carcinoma.

From the local primary tumor site, malignant cells spread by entering lymphatic capillaries and proceed to lymph nodes, where they may multiply to form metastatic secondary tumors. The most frequent routes of early metastatic spread involve the lateral thoracic and axillary lymph nodes as well as nodes that accompany the internal thoracic vessels lateral and parallel to the sternum. Spread of tumor cells also occurs by way of venous capillaries to larger veins and then to more widespread organs.

FIGURE 7.1 **Axillary and Parasternal Nodes and Lymph Channels from the Female Breast**

NOTE the central and anterior axillary nodes. Also observe the deep lateral and deep medial axillary nodes more superiorly along with the parasternal and deep cervical nodes.

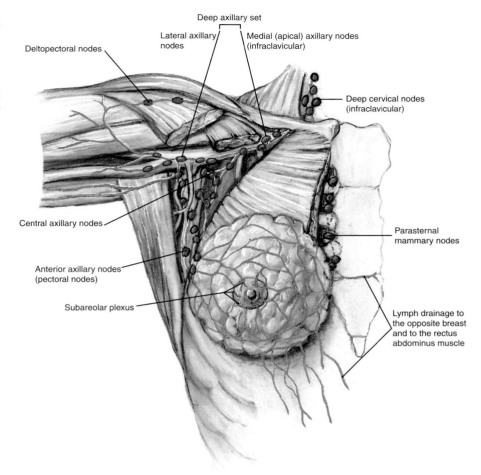

Deep axillary set

Lateral axillary nodes

Medial (apical) axillary nodes (infraclavicular)

Deltopectoral nodes

Deep cervical nodes (infraclavicular)

Central axillary nodes

Parasternal mammary nodes

Anterior axillary nodes (pectoral nodes)

Subareolar plexus

Lymph drainage to the opposite breast and to the rectus abdominus muscle

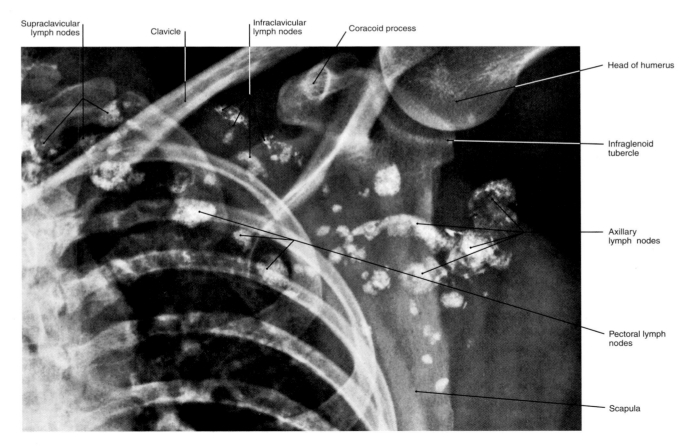

Supraclavicular lymph nodes

Clavicle

Infraclavicular lymph nodes

Coracoid process

Head of humerus

Infraglenoid tubercle

Axillary lymph nodes

Pectoral lymph nodes

Scapula

FIGURE 7.2 **Lymphangiogram of the Pectoral and Axillary Lymph Nodes**

(From Wicke, 6th ed.)

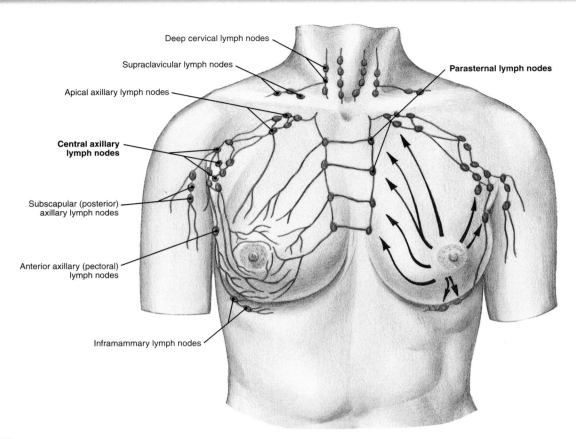

FIGURE 8.1 **Lymphatic Drainage from the Adult Female Breast**

NOTE: (1) Numerous lymph vessels in the breast communicate in a subareolar plexus deep to and around the nipple.
(2) About 85% of the lymph from the breast courses laterally and upward to axillary and infraclavicular nodes.
(3) Most of the remaining lymph passes medially to parasternal nodes along the internal thoracic vessels.
(4) Some lymph vessels drain downward to upper abdominal nodes and some go to the opposite breast.

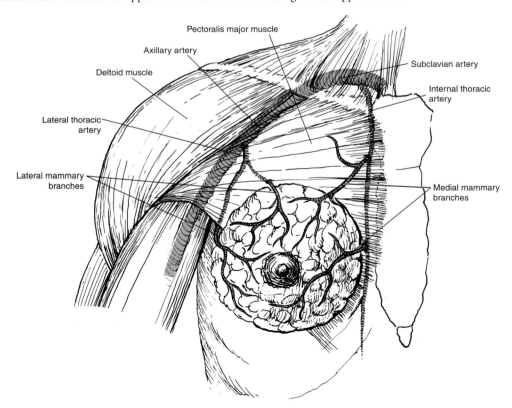

FIGURE 8.2 **Medial and Lateral Mammary Arteries**

NOTE that lateral branches from the lateral thoracic artery and medial perforating branches from the internal thoracic artery supply the breast anteriorly.
(From *Clemente's Anatomy Dissector*, 2nd Edition. Baltimore: Lippincott Williams & Wilkins, 2007.)

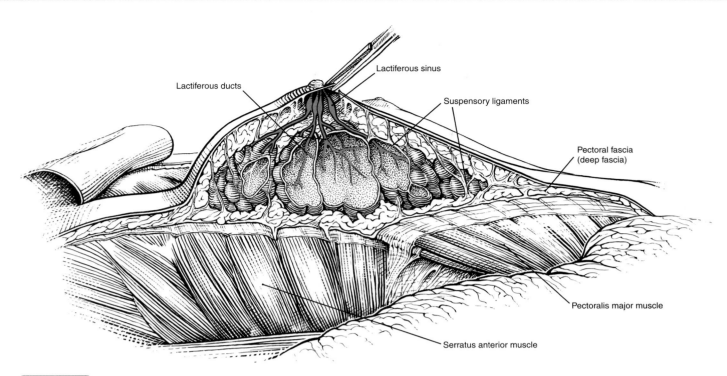

FIGURE 9.1 **Lateral View of the Female Breast in a Reclined Thorax**

NOTE: (1) The duct system originating in the mammary gland lobules. The individual ducts course forward through the superficial fascia of the breast to the nipple.

(2) The **suspensory ligaments** (of Cooper) that separate the mammary lobules. These support the breast by attaching to the deep pectoral fascia. In aging, the ligaments loose strength and result in the characteristic sagging breasts of the elderly.

(From *Clemente's Anatomy Dissector,* 1st Edition. Baltimore: Lippincott Williams & Wilkins, 2002.)

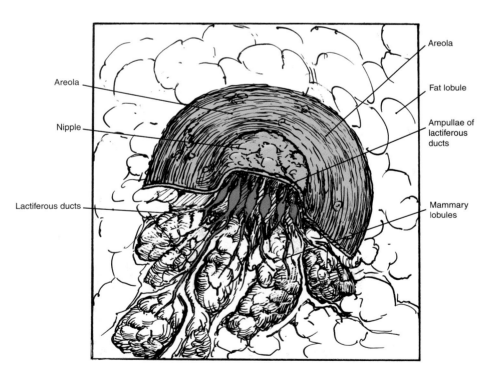

FIGURE 9.2 **The Dissected Nipple and Lactiferous Duct System**

NOTE the lactiferous ducts as they commence in the mammary lobules and course forward to open on the surface of the nipple. Also observe how the ducts enlarge into lactiferous sinuses within which milk collects prior to ejection as the infant suckles.

PLATE 10   **Dermatomes; Anterior Thoracic Segmental Nerves**

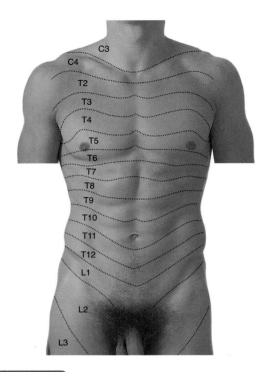

FIGURE 10.1 **Segmental Sensory Innervation of Anterior Body Wall (Dermatomes)**

NOTE: C5 to C8 and most of T1 do not supply the body wall, since they supply the upper limb.

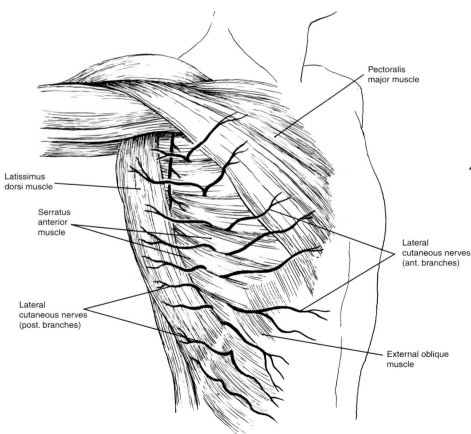

▲ **FIGURE 10.2** **Cutaneous Branches of Spinal Nerves**

NOTE the segmental cutaneous nerves to lateral cutaneous branches in the midaxillary line and anterior cutaneous branches just lateral to the sternum.
(From *Clemente's Anatomy Dissector,* 2nd Edition. Baltimore: Lippincott Williams & Wilkins, 2007.)

FIGURE 10.3 **Lateral Cutaneous Branches of Thoracic Nerves**

NOTE that as the lateral cutaneous nerves penetrate the intercostal space, each divides into anterior and posterior cutaneous branches.

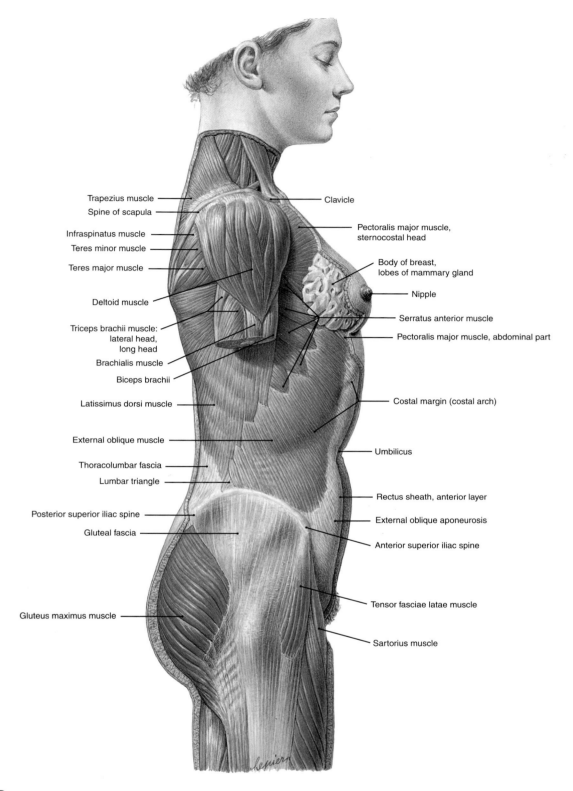

Trapezius muscle
Spine of scapula
Infraspinatus muscle
Teres minor muscle
Teres major muscle
Deltoid muscle
Triceps brachii muscle:
lateral head,
long head
Brachialis muscle
Biceps brachii
Latissimus dorsi muscle
External oblique muscle
Thoracolumbar fascia
Lumbar triangle
Posterior superior iliac spine
Gluteal fascia
Gluteus maximus muscle

Clavicle
Pectoralis major muscle,
sternocostal head
Body of breast,
lobes of mammary gland
Nipple
Serratus anterior muscle
Pectoralis major muscle, abdominal part
Costal margin (costal arch)
Umbilicus
Rectus sheath, anterior layer
External oblique aponeurosis
Anterior superior iliac spine
Tensor fasciae latae muscle
Sartorius muscle

FIGURE 11 **Muscles of the Lateral Thoracic and Abdominal Wall**

NOTE: (1) The interdigitations of the external oblique muscle with the serratus anterior muscle superiorly and the latissimus dorsal muscle inferiorly.
(2) The lumbar triangle. Its boundaries are the external oblique muscle (anteriorly), the latissimus dorsi muscle (posteriorly), and the crest of the ilium (inferiorly).
(3) The external oblique muscle ends in a broad and strong aponeurosis medially.

PLATE 12 Superficial Veins of the Anterior Trunk (Male)

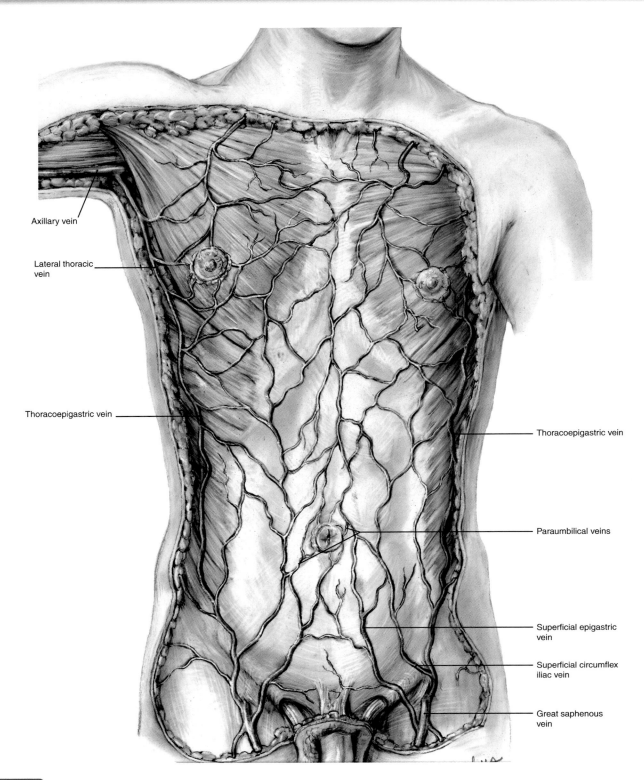

Axillary vein

Lateral thoracic vein

Thoracoepigastric vein

Thoracoepigastric vein

Paraumbilical veins

Superficial epigastric vein

Superficial circumflex iliac vein

Great saphenous vein

FIGURE 12 Anterior Thoracic Wall; Superficial Dissection in the Male

NOTE: (1) The thoracoepigastric veins along both lateral aspects of the thoracic wall; realize that these veins drain superiorly into the lateral thoracic veins, which flow into the axillary veins.

(2) The paraumbilical veins. Surrounding the umbilicus, these form an anastomosis between the systemic anterior abdominal wall veins and the intra-abdominal portal vein.

(3) Usually surface venous blood flow above the umbilicus drains into vessels that feed into the superior vena cava, while surface veins below the umbilicus drain into the femoral veins and thence into the inferior vena cava.

(4) The surface veins can become greatly enlarged if flow through the inferior vena cava is significantly reduced, as in cirrhosis of the liver

(From C.D. Clemente. *Gray's Anatomy,* 30th American Edition. Philadelphia: Lea & Febiger, 1985.)

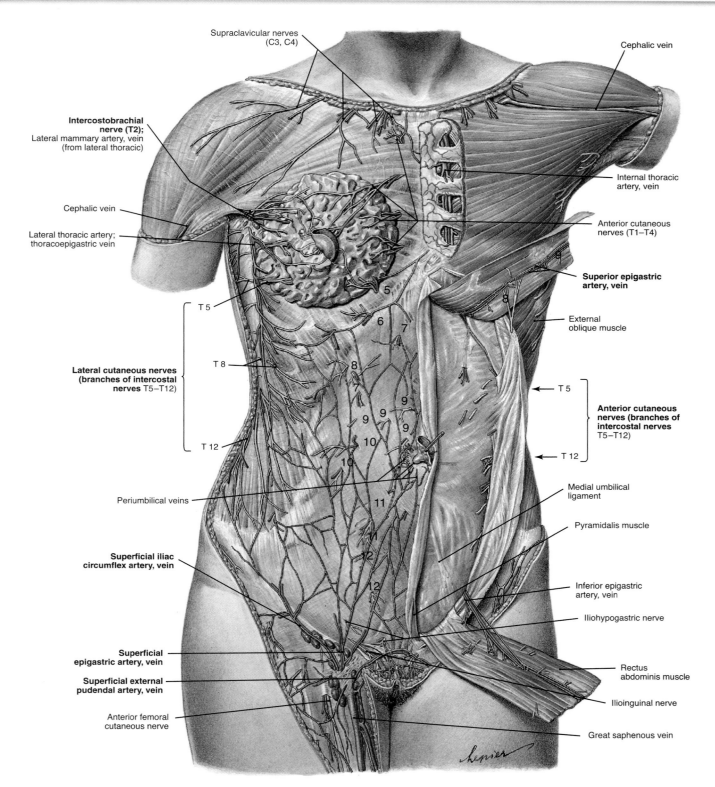

Supraclavicular nerves (C3, C4)

Cephalic vein

Intercostobrachial nerve (T2); Lateral mammary artery, vein (from lateral thoracic)

Cephalic vein

Lateral thoracic artery; thoracoepigastric vein

Internal thoracic artery, vein

Anterior cutaneous nerves (T1–T4)

Superior epigastric artery, vein

External oblique muscle

T 5

Lateral cutaneous nerves (branches of intercostal nerves T5–T12)

T 8

← T 5

Anterior cutaneous nerves (branches of intercostal nerves T5–T12)

← T 12

T 12

Medial umbilical ligament

Periumbilical veins

Pyramidalis muscle

Inferior epigastric artery, vein

Iliohypogastric nerve

Superficial iliac circumflex artery, vein

Superficial epigastric artery, vein

Superficial external pudendal artery, vein

Rectus abdominis muscle

Ilioinguinal nerve

Anterior femoral cutaneous nerve

Great saphenous vein

FIGURE 13 **Superficial Vessels and Nerves of the Anterior Trunk: Pectoral Region and Anterior Abdominal Wall**

NOTE: (1) Cutaneous innervation of the trunk: supraclavicular nerves (C3, C4), intercostal nerves (T1–T12), and the ilioinguinal and iliohypogastric branches of L1.

(2) The intercostal nerves give off lateral and anterior cutaneous branches.

(3) Anastomoses between the thoracoepigastric vein above and the superficial iliac circumflex and inferior epigastric veins below.

(4) The breast, its innervation (T2–T6 intercostal nerves), and its blood supply (internal thoracic artery, lateral thoracic artery, and intercostal arteries).

(5) The nipple at the level of T4 and the umbilicus at the level of T10.

PLATE 14 A Typical Segmental Spinal Nerve and Intercostal Artery

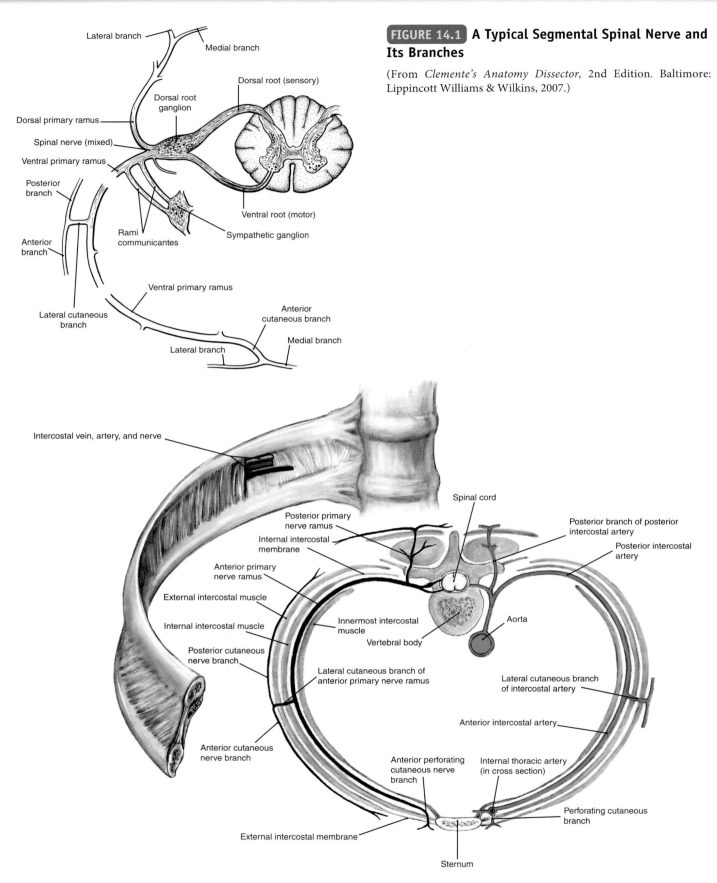

FIGURE 14.1 **A Typical Segmental Spinal Nerve and Its Branches**

(From *Clemente's Anatomy Dissector,* 2nd Edition. Baltimore: Lippincott Williams & Wilkins, 2007.)

FIGURE 14.2 **A Segmental Thoracic Nerve and Intercostal Artery and Their Branches**

NOTE: (1) Segmental intercostal nerves are formed by the junction of dorsal and ventral spinal roots. Distal to this junction, the mixed spinal nerve divides into dorsal and ventral primary rami. The posterior primary ramus courses to the back, while the anterior primary ramus courses between adjacent ribs as an intercostal nerve and gives off lateral and anterior cutaneous branches.

(2) Posterior intercostal arteries are derived from the aorta. Each sends a posterior branch to the back. The anterior branch becomes the anterior **intercostal artery,** and it also gives off lateral and anterior cutaneous branches.

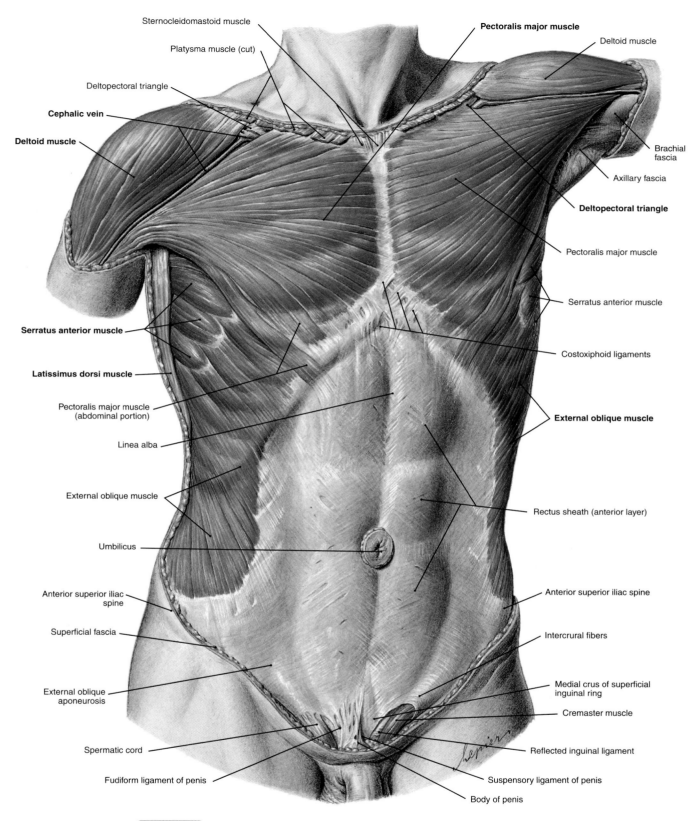

Sternocleidomastoid muscle

Platysma muscle (cut)

Deltopectoral triangle

Cephalic vein

Deltoid muscle

Serratus anterior muscle

Latissimus dorsi muscle

Pectoralis major muscle
(abdominal portion)

Linea alba

External oblique muscle

Umbilicus

Anterior superior iliac
spine

Superficial fascia

External oblique
aponeurosis

Spermatic cord

Fudiform ligament of penis

Pectoralis major muscle

Deltoid muscle

Brachial
fascia

Axillary fascia

Deltopectoral triangle

Pectoralis major muscle

Serratus anterior muscle

Costoxiphoid ligaments

External oblique muscle

Rectus sheath (anterior layer)

Anterior superior iliac spine

Intercrural fibers

Medial crus of superficial
inguinal ring

Cremaster muscle

Reflected inguinal ligament

Suspensory ligament of penis

Body of penis

FIGURE 15 **Muscles of the Superficial Thoracic and Abdominal Walls**

Muscle	Origin	Insertion	Innervation	Action
Pectoralis major	Medial half of clavicle; second to sixth ribs; costal margin of sternum; aponeurosis of external oblique	Humerus, lateral lip of intertubercular sulcus	Lateral (C5, C6, C7) and medial (C8, T1) pectoral nerves	Adducts and rotates arm medially; **sternal part:** helps extend humerus; **clavicular part:** helps flex humerus

PLATE 16 Pectoral Region: Superficial Vessels and Cutaneous Nerves

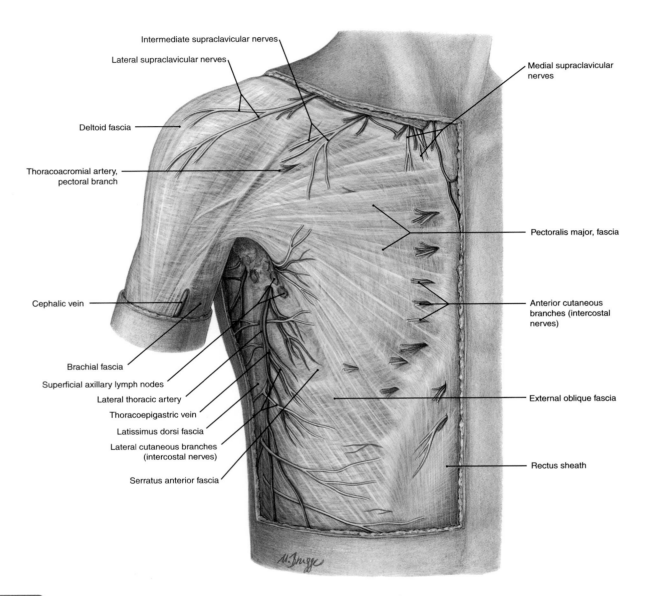

Intermediate supraclavicular nerves

Lateral supraclavicular nerves

Medial supraclavicular nerves

Deltoid fascia

Thoracoacromial artery, pectoral branch

Pectoralis major, fascia

Cephalic vein

Anterior cutaneous branches (intercostal nerves)

Brachial fascia

Superficial axillary lymph nodes

Lateral thoracic artery

Thoracoepigastric vein

Latissimus dorsi fascia

Lateral cutaneous branches (intercostal nerves)

Serratus anterior fascia

External oblique fascia

Rectus sheath

FIGURE 16 **Anterior Thoracic Wall; Superficial Dissection in the Male**

NOTE: (1) The skin and superficial fascia have been removed, but the cutaneous vessels and nerves have been retained.

(2) The cutaneous neurovascular structures penetrate through the deep fascia (pectoral fascia) to get to the superficial fascia and skin.

(3) Most cutaneous vessels and nerves are anterior and lateral cutaneous branches of the intercostal nerves and vessels.

(4) The deep fascia that covers the pectoralis major muscle and the manner in which it blends inferiorly with the sheath of the rectus abdominus muscle (the rectus sheath) and medially across the sternum with the fascia on the opposite side.

(5) The pectoral fascia also has a deep layer that covers the deep surface of the muscle.

(6) The **supraclavicular nerves** are derived from C3 and C4, but overwhelmingly C4.

(7) The **intercostobrachial nerve (T2)** joins the medial brachial cutaneous nerve to supply the skin of the axillary fossa and upper medial arm.

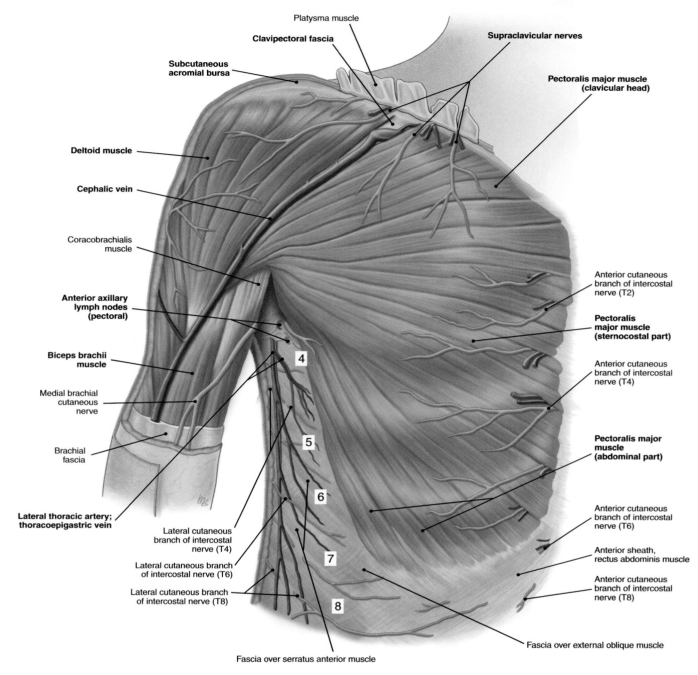

Platysma muscle

Clavipectoral fascia

Subcutaneous
acromial bursa

Supraclavicular nerves

Pectoralis major muscle
(clavicular head)

Deltoid muscle

Cephalic vein

Coracobrachialis
muscle

Anterior axillary
lymph nodes
(pectoral)

Biceps brachii
muscle

Medial brachial
cutaneous
nerve

Brachial
fascia

Lateral thoracic artery;
thoracoepigastric vein

Lateral cutaneous
branch of intercostal
nerve (T4)

Lateral cutaneous branch
of intercostal nerve (T6)

Lateral cutaneous branch
of intercostal nerve (T8)

Fascia over serratus anterior muscle

Anterior cutaneous
branch of intercostal
nerve (T2)

**Pectoralis
major muscle
(sternocostal part)**

Anterior cutaneous
branch of intercostal
nerve (T4)

**Pectoralis major
muscle
(abdominal part)**

Anterior cutaneous
branch of intercostal
nerve (T6)

Anterior sheath,
rectus abdominis muscle

Anterior cutaneous
branch of intercostal
nerve (T8)

Fascia over external oblique muscle

4 5 6 7 8

FIGURE 17 **Pectoralis Major and Deltoid Muscles (Anterior View)**

NOTE: (1) The anterior layer of the pectoral fascia and the deltoid fascia as seen in Figure 16 have been removed.
(2) The lateral cutaneous vessels and nerves penetrating through the intercostal spaces in the midaxillary line.
(3) The anterior cutaneous vessels and nerves piercing the pectoralis major muscle along the lateral border of the sternum.
(4) The clavicular fibers of this muscle course obliquely downward, and laterally, the upper sternocostal fibers are directed nearly horizontally, and the lower sternocostal and abdominal fibers ascend nearly vertically to the humerus.
(5) The natural cleft between the clavicular and sternocostal heads. Detaching the clavicular head uncovers some of the vessels and nerves that supply this muscle (see Fig. 22.1).
(6) The fourth to the eighth ribs are numbered sequentially.

PLATE 18 The Pectoralis Major and Minor Muscles

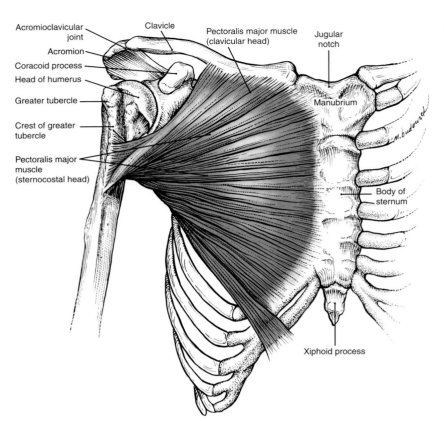

Acromioclavicular joint
Clavicle
Pectoralis major muscle (clavicular head)
Jugular notch
Acromion
Coracoid process
Head of humerus
Manubrium
Greater tubercle
Crest of greater tubercle
Pectoralis major muscle (sternocostal head)
Body of sternum
Xiphoid process

FIGURE 18.1 **The Pectoralis Major Muscle**

NOTE: (1) The pectoralis major muscle has fibers that descend from the clavicle and fibers that ascend from the lower sternum and the aponeurosis of the external oblique muscle. Between these are the transverse fibers that cross the chest.

(2) This broad mass of muscle fibers inserts onto the lateral lip of the intertubercular sulcus of the humerus.

(3) The ascending and lower transverse fibers form a rounded inferior border that becomes the anterior axillary fold. This muscle and the pectoralis minor overlie the nerves of the brachial plexus and the axillary vessels and their branches.

(4) The pectoralis major medially rotates and adducts the humerus. In addition, the clavicular fibers assist in flexing the humerus, while the inferior sternal fibers and those attaching to the aponeurosis of the external oblique assist in extending the humerus.

(Contributed by Dr. Gene L. Colborn, Medical College of Georgia.)

FIGURE 18.2 **The Pectoralis Minor Muscle**

NOTE: (1) The pectoralis minor muscle is often called **"the key to the axilla"**; this is because it crosses the axillary artery, dividing it into three parts, medial, deep, and lateral to the pectoralis minor muscle. There is one branch off of the first part of the axillary artery, two branches off of the second part, and three branches off of the third part.

(2) Deep to the pectoralis minor muscle, the cords of the brachial plexus are found. These are called the **medial, lateral, and posterior cords,** and they are located medial, lateral, and posterior to the axillary artery.

(3) The pectoralis minor muscle can protract the scapula (i.e., draw it forward) when the insertion on the third, fourth, and fifth ribs is fixed. When the attachment to the coracoid process is fixed, the pectoralis minor can help elevate the ribs, and thus, it becomes an accessory muscle of respiration.

(From *Clemente's Anatomy Dissector,* 2nd Edition. Baltimore: Lippincott Williams & Wilkins, 2007.)

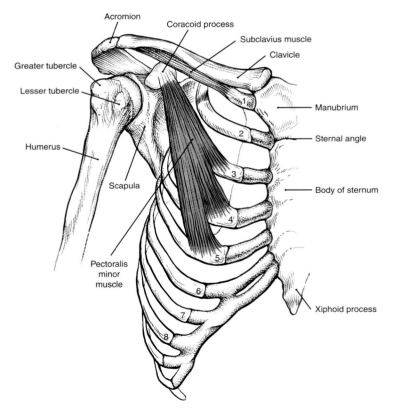

Acromion
Coracoid process
Subclavius muscle
Clavicle
Greater tubercle
Lesser tubercle
Manubrium
Sternal angle
Humerus
Scapula
Body of sternum
Pectoralis minor muscle
Xiphoid process

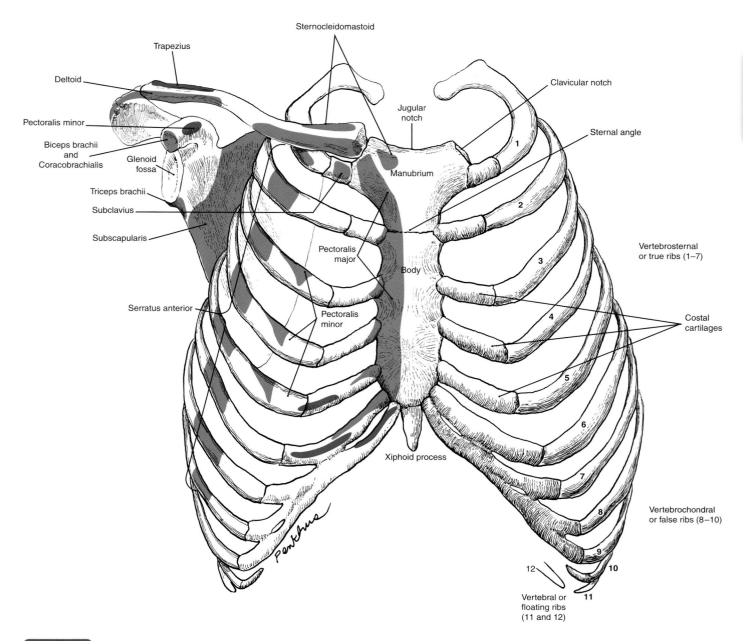

FIGURE 19 **The Anterior Surface of the Sternum and Ribs**

NOTE: (1) The costal cartilages and the manner in which they articulate with the sternum.

(2) The **jugular notch** (also called the suprasternal notch) along the superior border of the manubrium.

(3) Lateral to the manubrium, the clavicle articulates into the clavicular notch, and just below this, the first rib articulates with the lateral surface of the manubrium.

(4) Rib 2 articulates with the sternum lateral to the sternal angle (i.e., between the manubrium and body of the sternum).

(5) Ribs 4, 5, and 6 articulate on the body of the sternum, and rib 7, joined by the costal margins of ribs 8, 9, and 10, attaches to the junction of the **xiphoid process** and sternal body (the **xiphisternal junction**).

(6) The origin of the **pectoralis major muscle** attaches along the medial half of the clavicle and lateral one-third of the manubrium and body of the sternum.

(7) The **pectoralis minor muscle** inserts on the third, fourth, and fifth ribs, and the **biceps brachii** and **coracobrachialis muscles** attach just above the glenoid fossa (supraglenoid tubercle), while the triceps arises from the infraglenoid tubercle below the glenoid fossa.

(From C.D. Clemente. *Gray's Anatomy,* 30th American Edition. Philadelphia: Lea & Febiger, 1985.)

PLATE 20 Lateral Thoracic Wall and Superficial Axilla

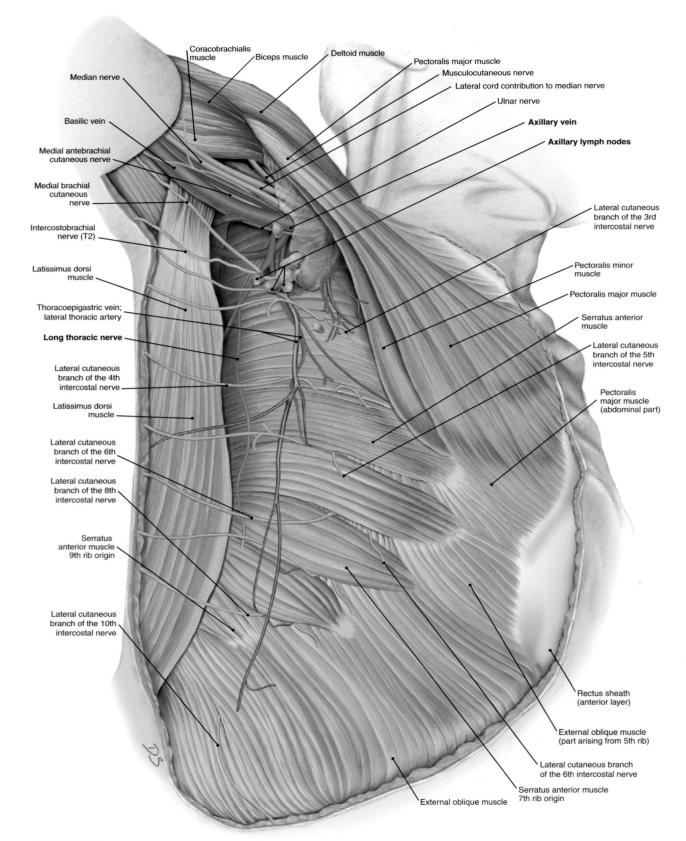

Coracobrachialis muscle
Biceps muscle
Deltoid muscle
Median nerve
Pectoralis major muscle
Musculocutaneous nerve
Lateral cord contribution to median nerve
Basilic vein
Ulnar nerve
Medial antebrachial cutaneous nerve
Axillary vein
Axillary lymph nodes
Medial brachial cutaneous nerve
Intercostobrachial nerve (T2)
Lateral cutaneous branch of the 3rd intercostal nerve
Latissimus dorsi muscle
Pectoralis minor muscle
Thoracoepigastric vein; lateral thoracic artery
Pectoralis major muscle
Long thoracic nerve
Serratus anterior muscle
Lateral cutaneous branch of the 4th intercostal nerve
Lateral cutaneous branch of the 5th intercostal nerve
Latissimus dorsi muscle
Pectoralis major muscle (abdominal part)
Lateral cutaneous branch of the 6th intercostal nerve
Lateral cutaneous branch of the 8th intercostal nerve
Serratus anterior muscle 9th rib origin
Lateral cutaneous branch of the 10th intercostal nerve
Rectus sheath (anterior layer)
External oblique muscle (part arising from 5th rib)
Lateral cutaneous branch of the 6th intercostal nerve
External oblique muscle
Serratus anterior muscle 7th rib origin

FIGURE 20 Lateral Aspect of the Upper Right Thoracic Wall and the Superficial Axillary Structures

Muscle	Origin	Insertion	Innervation	Action
Pectoralis minor	Coracoid process of scapula	Ribs 2 to 5	Medial pectoral nerve (C8, T1)	Protracts scapula; elevates ribs
Serratus anterior	Fleshy slips from upper nine ribs	Medial border of scapula	Long thoracic nerve (C5, C6, C7)	Protracts and rotates scapula; holds scapula close to thoracic wall

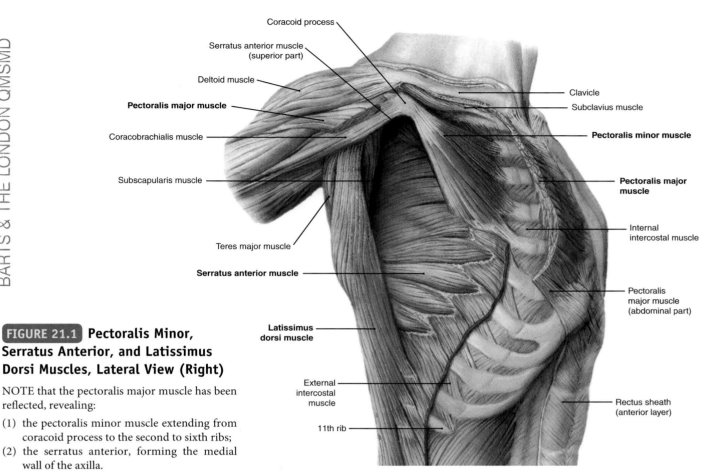

FIGURE 21.1 Pectoralis Minor, Serratus Anterior, and Latissimus Dorsi Muscles, Lateral View (Right)

NOTE that the pectoralis major muscle has been reflected, revealing:

(1) the pectoralis minor muscle extending from coracoid process to the second to sixth ribs;

(2) the serratus anterior, forming the medial wall of the axilla.

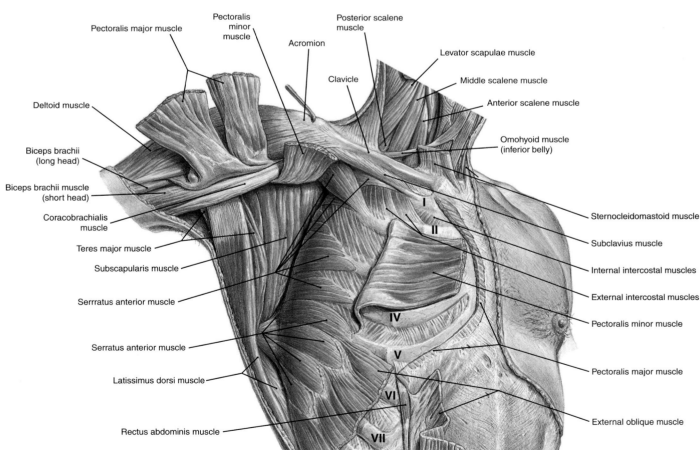

FIGURE 21.2 The Subscapularis and Serratus Anterior Muscles (Right Lateral View)

Chapter 1 Pectoral Region, Axilla, Shoulder, and Upper Limb

PLATE 22 **Deltopectoral Triangle and the Deep Lateral Thoracic Muscles**

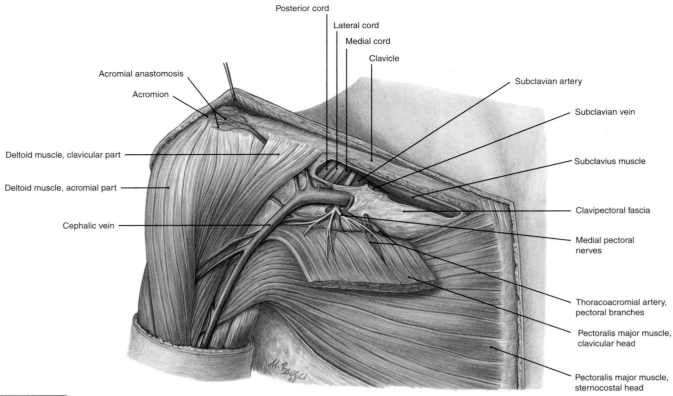

FIGURE 22.1 **Deltopectoral Triangle (Right)**

NOTE: (1) The clavicular head of the pectoralis major muscle has been severed and reflected downward.

(2) The investing layer of deep fascia covering the deep surface of the pectoralis major muscle and the clavipectoral fascia, which extends between the clavicle and the medial border of the pectoralis minor muscle, are exposed.

(3) The cephalic vein pierces the clavipectoral fascia to join the axillary vein.

(4) The thoracoacromial artery (from the axillary artery) and the lateral pectoral nerve (from the lateral cord of the brachial plexus) pierce the fascia from below to supply blood to the region and to innervate the pectoralis major muscle.

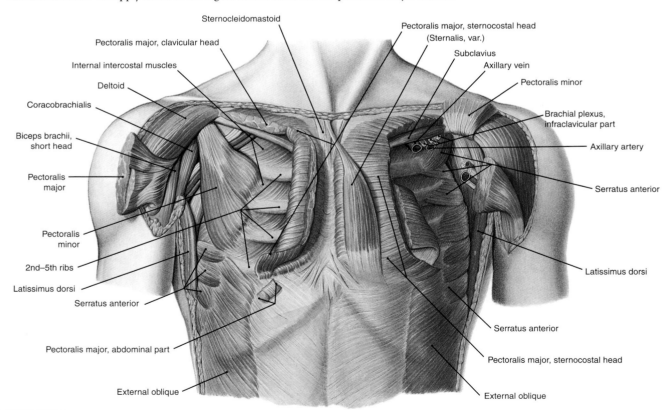

FIGURE 22.2 **Pectoralis Minor, Serratus Anterior, and Latissimus Dorsi Muscles (Right Lateral View)**

NOTE that the pectoralis major muscle has been reflected, revealing the pectoralis minor muscle extending from the second to fifth ribs to the coracoid process. Also note that the serratus anterior muscle forms the medial wall of the axilla.

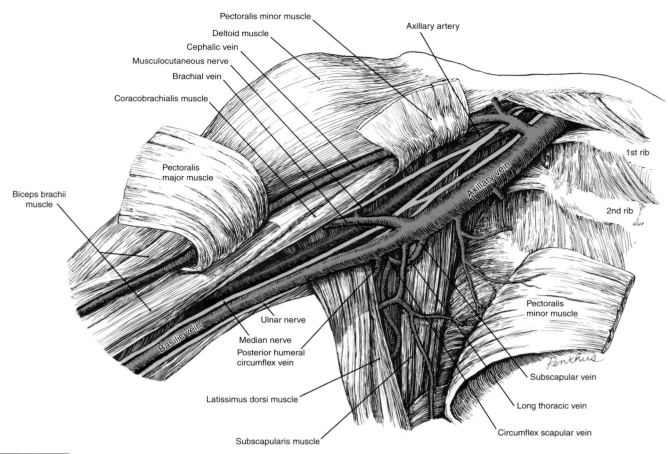

FIGURE 23.1 **The Veins of the Right Axilla**

NOTE the relationship of the axillary vein to the axillary artery and the nerves in the axilla.
(From C.D. Clemente. *Gray's Anatomy,* 30th American Edition. Philadelphia: Lea & Febiger, 1985.)

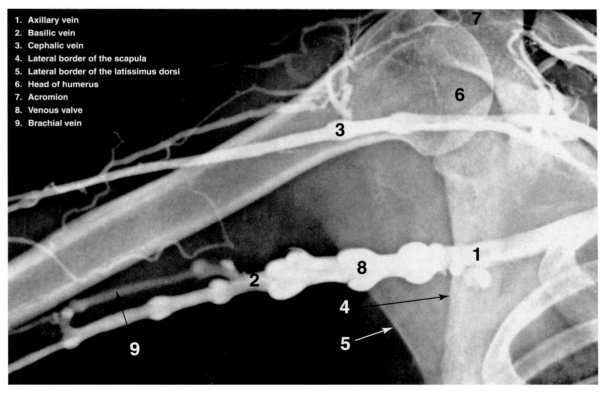

1. **Axillary vein**
2. **Basilic vein**
3. **Cephalic vein**
4. **Lateral border of the scapula**
5. **Lateral border of the latissimus dorsi**
6. **Head of humerus**
7. **Acromion**
8. **Venous valve**
9. **Brachial vein**

FIGURE 23.2 **Radiograph of Veins in the Axillary Region**

NOTE: (1) The basilic vein [2] becomes the axillary vein [1].
(2) One of the brachial veins [9] also flows into the axillary vein, as does the cephalic vein [3], the junction of which is medial to the field shown here.
(3) The venous valves [8] along the course of the axillary vein.

PLATE 24 The Axillary Artery and Its Branches

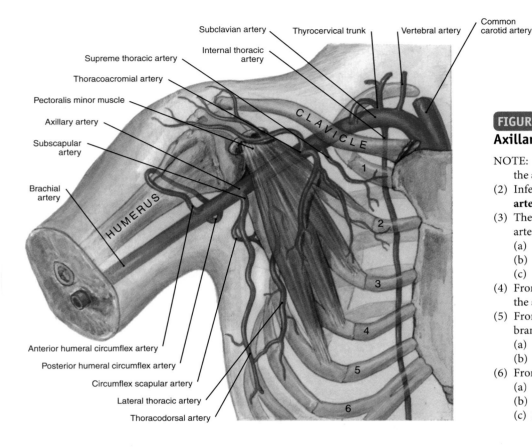

Subclavian artery
Thyrocervical trunk
Vertebral artery
Common carotid artery
Internal thoracic artery
Supreme thoracic artery
Thoracoacromial artery
Pectoralis minor muscle
Axillary artery
Subscapular artery
Brachial artery
HUMERUS
CLAVICLE
Anterior humeral circumflex artery
Posterior humeral circumflex artery
Circumflex scapular artery
Lateral thoracic artery
Thoracodorsal artery

FIGURE 24.1 **Branches of the Axillary Artery**

NOTE: (1) The **subclavian artery** becomes the **axillary artery** distal to the clavicle.
(2) Inferior to the teres major, the **axillary artery** becomes the **brachial artery**.
(3) The pectoralis minor crosses the axillary artery, dividing it into three parts:
  (a) Medial to the muscle
  (b) Beneath the muscle
  (c) Lateral to the muscle
(4) From the first part, there is one branch, the **supreme thoracic artery**.
(5) From the second part are derived two branches:
  (a) **Thoracoacromial artery**
  (b) **Lateral thoracic artery**
(6) From the third part come three branches:
  (a) **Subscapular artery**
  (b) **Anterior humeral circumflex artery**
  (c) **Posterior humeral circumflex artery**

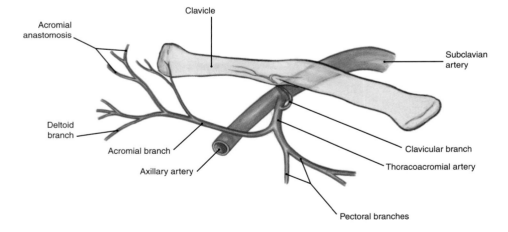

Clavicle
Acromial anastomosis
Subclavian artery
Deltoid branch
Acromial branch
Axillary artery
Clavicular branch
Thoracoacromial artery
Pectoral branches

FIGURE 24.2 **Thoracoacromial Artery and Its Branches**

NOTE that the four branches of the thoracoacromial artery usually are the clavicular, pectoral, acromial, and deltoid.

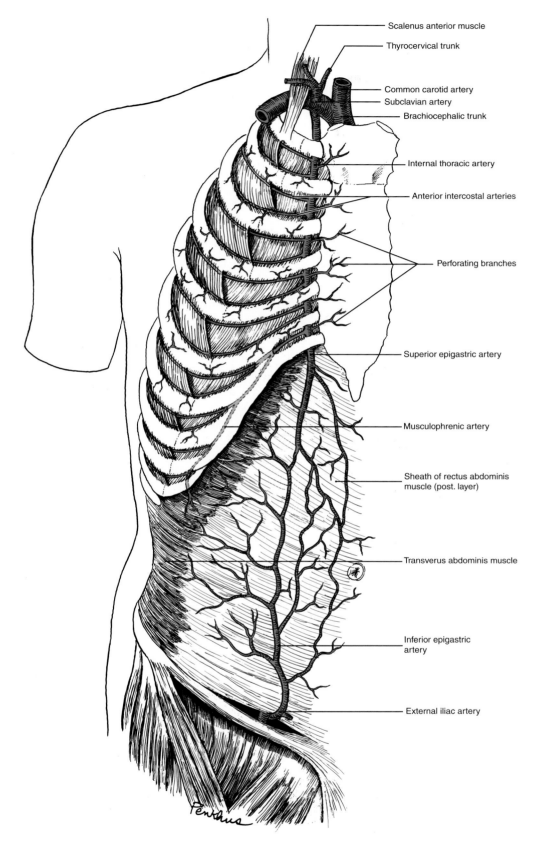

Scalenus anterior muscle

Thyrocervical trunk

Common carotid artery
Subclavian artery
Brachiocephalic trunk

Internal thoracic artery

Anterior intercostal arteries

Perforating branches

Superior epigastric artery

Musculophrenic artery

Sheath of rectus abdominis muscle (post. layer)

Transverus abdominis muscle

Inferior epigastric artery

External iliac artery

FIGURE 25 **The Internal Thoracic and Epigastric Arterial Anastomosis**

NOTE: (1) The **internal thoracic artery** arises from the axillary artery, and in its descent in the chest, it gives off perforating branches segmentally. At the costal margin, the internal thoracic artery terminates by dividing into the **musculophrenic** and **superior epigastric arteries**.

(2) The **inferior epigastric artery** arises from the external iliac artery just superior to the inguinal ligament, and it anastomoses with the superior epigastric branch of the internal thoracic artery.

(3) This arterial anastomosis forms a major interconnection between the subclavian and external iliac systems and, in effect, between the inferior vena cava and the superior vena cava.

(From C.D. Clemente. *Gray's Anatomy,* 30th American Edition. Philadelphia: Lea & Febiger, 1985.)

PLATE 26 **Dissection of Axilla: Superficial Vessels and Nerves**

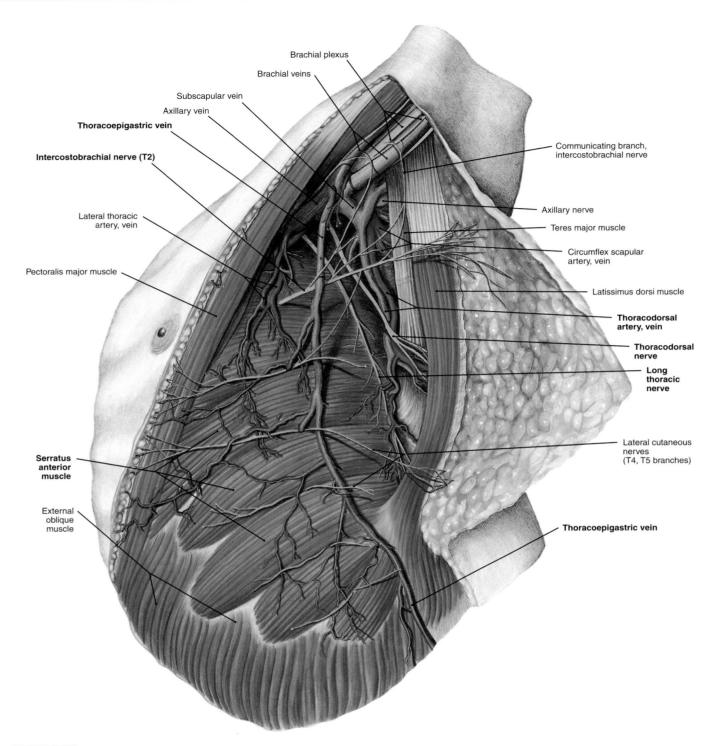

Brachial plexus

Brachial veins

Subscapular vein

Axillary vein

Thoracoepigastric vein

Intercostobrachial nerve (T2)

Lateral thoracic
artery, vein

Pectoralis major muscle

**Serratus
anterior
muscle**

External
oblique
muscle

Communicating branch,
intercostobrachial nerve

Axillary nerve

Teres major muscle

Circumflex scapular
artery, vein

Latissimus dorsi muscle

**Thoracodorsal
artery, vein**

**Thoracodorsal
nerve**

**Long
thoracic
nerve**

Lateral cutaneous
nerves
(T4, T5 branches)

Thoracoepigastric vein

FIGURE 26 **Axilla: Superficial Vessels and Nerves (Left)**

NOTE: (1) The boundaries of the axilla are:
  (a) **Anteriorly**, the pectoralis major muscle
  (b) **Posteriorly**, the subscapularis, teres major, and latissimus dorsi muscles
  (c) **Medially**, the serratus anterior muscle covering the second to the sixth ribs
  (d) **Laterally**, the bicipital groove of the humerus.
(2) The lower part of the serratus anterior muscle arises from the lower ribs as fleshy interdigitations with the external oblique muscle.
(3) The serratus anterior is innervated by the long thoracic nerve, and the latissimus dorsi by the thoracodorsal nerve.
(4) The axillary vein lies medial to the axillary artery and the brachial plexus.
(5) The ascending course of the thoracoepigastric vein and the lateral thoracic vessels.

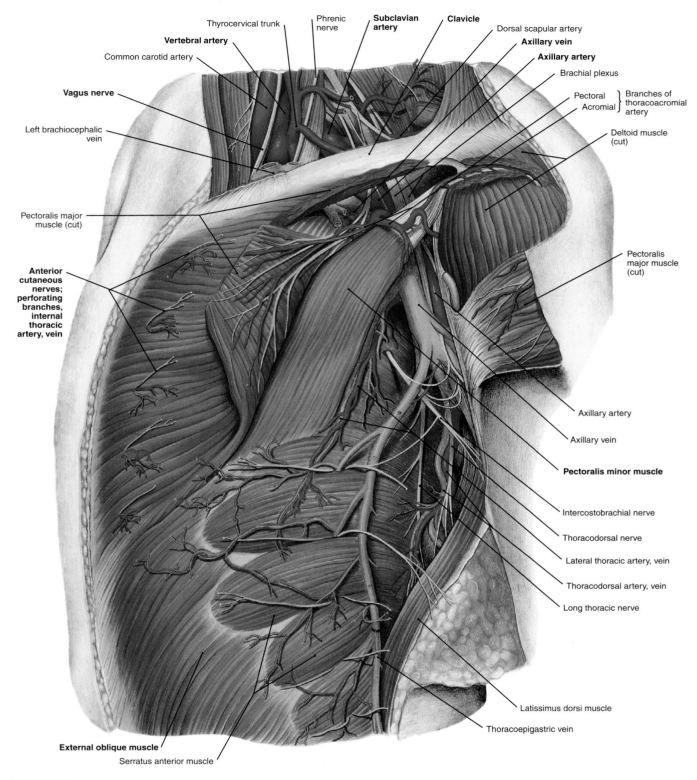

FIGURE 27 Axilla (Left): Deep Vessels and Nerves

NOTE: (1) The subclavian artery becomes the axillary artery distal to the clavicle.
(2) The pectoralis minor muscle is capable of elevating the ribs if the coracoid attachment is fixed or of protracting the scapula if the costal attachment is fixed.
(3) The axillary artery is surrounded by the three cords of the brachial plexus.
(4) The thoracoacromial artery divides into **pectoral, acromial, deltoid,** and small **clavicular** branches.
(5) The intercostobrachial nerve (T2) pierces the second intercostal space in its course toward the axilla and arm, and it communicates with the medial brachial cutaneous nerve.

PLATE 28 Arterial Supply to the Upper Extremity

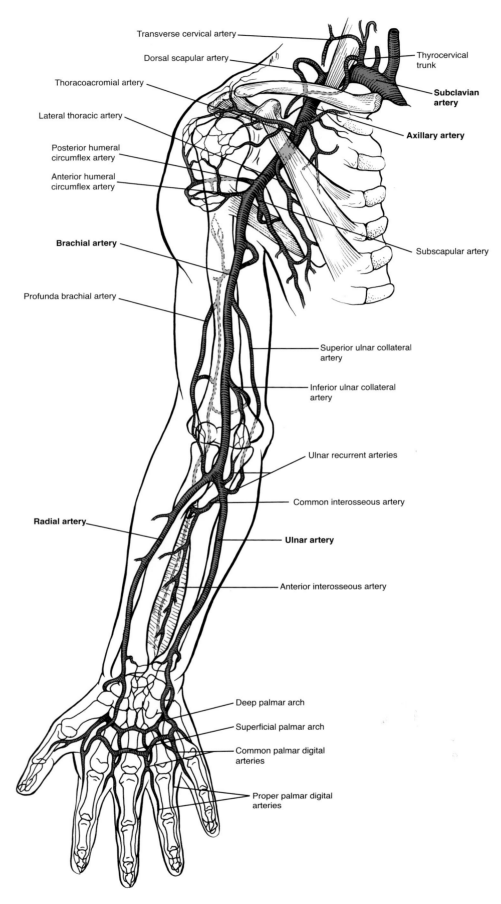

Transverse cervical artery

Dorsal scapular artery

Thoracoacromial artery

Lateral thoracic artery

Posterior humeral circumflex artery

Anterior humeral circumflex artery

Brachial artery

Profunda brachial artery

Thyrocervical trunk

Subclavian artery

Axillary artery

Subscapular artery

Superior ulnar collateral artery

Inferior ulnar collateral artery

Ulnar recurrent arteries

Common interosseous artery

Radial artery

Ulnar artery

Anterior interosseous artery

Deep palmar arch

Superficial palmar arch

Common palmar digital arteries

Proper palmar digital arteries

FIGURE 28 **Arteries of the Upper Limb**

(Contributed by Dr. Gene L. Colborn, Medical College of Georgia.)

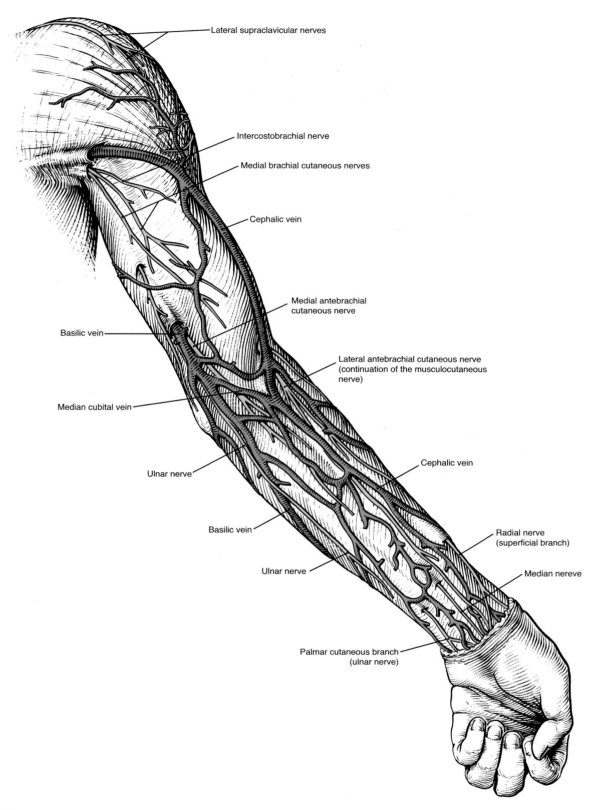

Lateral supraclavicular nerves

Intercostobrachial nerve

Medial brachial cutaneous nerves

Cephalic vein

Medial antebrachial cutaneous nerve

Basilic vein

Lateral antebrachial cutaneous nerve (continuation of the musculocutaneous nerve)

Median cubital vein

Cephalic vein

Ulnar nerve

Basilic vein

Radial nerve (superficial branch)

Ulnar nerve

Median nereve

Palmar cutaneous branch (ulnar nerve)

FIGURE 29 **The Superficial Veins of the Upper Extremity**

NOTE: The **cephalic vein laterally** commencing on the radial (or thumb) side of the hand and the **basilic vein** commencing on the ulnar (or little finger) side of the hand. These channels communicate in the antecubital fossa by the **median cubital vein**. (Contributed by Dr. Gene L. Colborn, Medical College of Georgia.)

PLATE 30 Shoulder Region, Anterior Aspect: Muscles

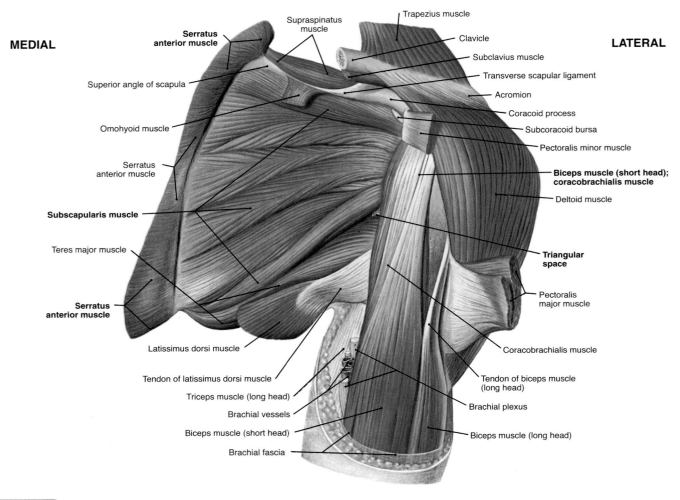

MEDIAL

LATERAL

Trapezius muscle

Supraspinatus muscle

Serratus anterior muscle

Clavicle

Subclavius muscle

Superior angle of scapula

Transverse scapular ligament

Acromion

Omohyoid muscle

Coracoid process

Subcoracoid bursa

Pectoralis minor muscle

Serratus anterior muscle

Biceps muscle (short head); coracobrachialis muscle

Deltoid muscle

Subscapularis muscle

Teres major muscle

Triangular space

Serratus anterior muscle

Pectoralis major muscle

Latissimus dorsi muscle

Coracobrachialis muscle

Tendon of latissimus dorsi muscle

Tendon of biceps muscle (long head)

Triceps muscle (long head)

Brachial vessels

Brachial plexus

Biceps muscle (short head)

Biceps muscle (long head)

Brachial fascia

FIGURE 30 Muscles of Anterior Aspect of the Shoulder (Left)

NOTE: (1) The large triangular mass of the subscapularis muscle occupying the concave subscapular fossa. From this broad origin, its fibers converge toward the humerus, where it inserts on the lesser tubercle.

(2) The subscapularis along with the other muscles that constitute the "rotator cuff" (supraspinatus, infraspinatus, and teres minor) help stabilize the shoulder joint by keeping the head of the humerus in the glenoid fossa.

(3) Both the short head of the biceps and the coracobrachialis have a common origin from the coracoid process.

Muscle	Origin	Insertion	Innervation	Action
Subscapularis	Subscapular fossa of the scapula	Lesser tubercle of humerus	Upper and lower subscapular nerves (C5, C6) from posterior cord of brachial plexus	Medial rotation of humerus
Latissimus dorsi	Thoracolumbar fascia; spinous processes of lower six thoracic and lumbar vertebrae, and the sacrum	Bottom of the intertubercular sulcus of humerus	Thoracodorsal nerve (C6, C7, C8) from posterior cord of brachial plexus	Extends, adducts, and medially rotates the humerus
Deltoid	Lateral third of clavicle; the acromion; spine of the scapula	Deltoid tubercle on lateral surface of humerus	Axillary nerve (C5, C6) from posterior cord of brachial plexus	Abduction of the humerus; anterior fibers assist in flexion and posterior fibers in extension of humerus

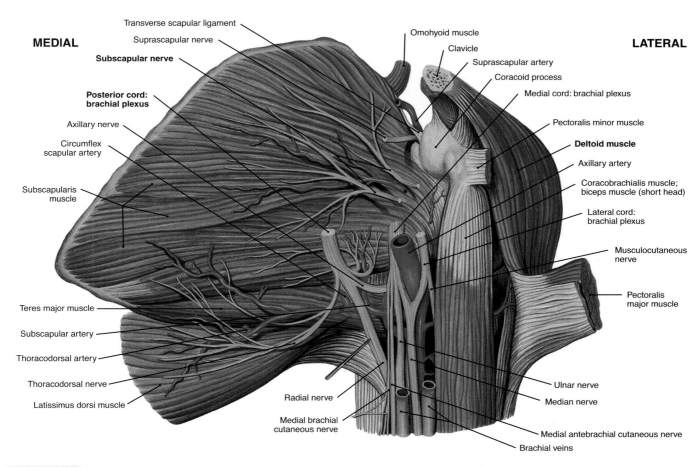

MEDIAL

LATERAL

- Transverse scapular ligament
- Suprascapular nerve
- **Subscapular nerve**
- **Posterior cord: brachial plexus**
- Axillary nerve
- Circumflex scapular artery
- Subscapularis muscle
- Teres major muscle
- Subscapular artery
- Thoracodorsal artery
- Thoracodorsal nerve
- Latissimus dorsi muscle
- Radial nerve
- Medial brachial cutaneous nerve

- Omohyoid muscle
- Clavicle
- Suprascapular artery
- Coracoid process
- Medial cord: brachial plexus
- Pectoralis minor muscle
- **Deltoid muscle**
- Axillary artery
- Coracobrachialis muscle; biceps muscle (short head)
- Lateral cord: brachial plexus
- Musculocutaneous nerve
- Pectoralis major muscle
- Ulnar nerve
- Median nerve
- Medial antebrachial cutaneous nerve
- Brachial veins

FIGURE 31.1 **Nerves and Vessels of Anterior Aspect of the Shoulder (Left)**

NOTE: (1) The relationships of the medial, lateral, and posterior cords of the brachial plexus to the axillary artery.
(2) The posterior cord and its axillary and radial terminal nerves have been pulled medially from behind the axillary artery in this dissection.
(3) The median nerve formed by contributions from the lateral and medial cords. Observe that the median nerve, its two roots of origin and the ulnar and musculocutaneous nerves outline an **M** formation on the anterior aspect of the axillary artery.

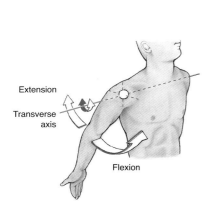

Extension

Transverse axis

Flexion

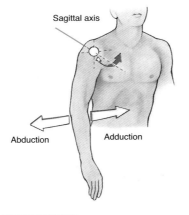

Sagittal axis

Abduction   Adduction

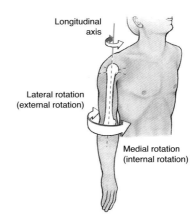

Longitudinal axis

Lateral rotation (external rotation)

Medial rotation (internal rotation)

FIGURE 31.2 **Shoulder Joint: Flexion and Extension**

In **flexion** the upper limb is moved anteriorly (forward), while in **extension** the limb moves posteriorly (backward) in reference to the transverse axis.

FIGURE 31.3 **Shoulder Joint: Abduction and Adduction**

In **abduction**, the upper limb is moved laterally, or away from the midline of the body, with reference to the sagittal axis. In **adduction**, the upper limb is moved medially, or toward the midline of the body.

FIGURE 31.4 **Shoulder Joint: Medial and Lateral Rotation**

Medial rotation at the shoulder joint occurs when the humerus is rotated internally (medially) with reference to the long or longitudinal axis of the bone. In contrast, **lateral rotation** of the upper limb moves the humerus (arm) externally or laterally.

PLATE 32 **Shoulder Region, Posterior Aspect: Muscles**

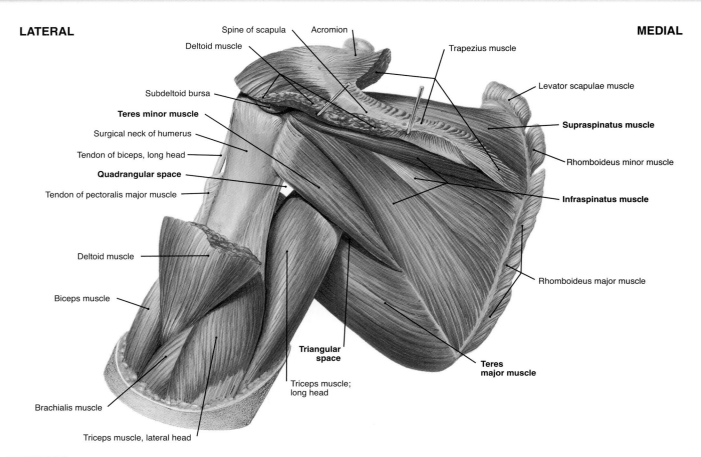

LATERAL

MEDIAL

Spine of scapula
Acromion
Deltoid muscle
Trapezius muscle
Subdeltoid bursa
Levator scapulae muscle
Teres minor muscle
Surgical neck of humerus
Supraspinatus muscle
Tendon of biceps, long head
Rhomboideus minor muscle
Quadrangular space
Tendon of pectoralis major muscle
Infraspinatus muscle
Deltoid muscle
Rhomboideus major muscle
Biceps muscle
Triangular space
Teres major muscle
Triceps muscle; long head
Brachialis muscle
Triceps muscle, lateral head

FIGURE 32 **Posterior Scapular Muscles (Left)**

NOTE: (1) The supraspinatus, infraspinatus, and teres minor muscles all course laterally from the dorsal scapula, and all are considered "rotator cuff" muscles.
(2) These three muscles insert in sequence from above downward on the greater tubercle of the humerus.
(3) The long head of the triceps intersects a space between the teres major and teres minor muscles, forming a **quadrangular space** laterally and a **triangular space** medially.
(4) The posterior humeral circumflex artery and the axillary nerve pass through the quadrangular space.
(5) The circumflex scapular branch of the subscapular artery passes through the triangular space.
(6) Since the lateral border of the quadrangular space is the surgical neck of the humerus, the axillary nerve and posterior humeral circumflex artery are in danger if the bone is fractured at this site.

Muscle	Origin	Insertion	Innervation	Action
Supraspinatus	Supraspinatus fossa of the scapula	Highest facet of the greater tubercle of humerus	Suprascapular nerve (C5)	Initiates abduction of the arm; rotates the humerus laterally
Infraspinatus	Infraspinatus fossa of the scapula	Middle part of greater tubercle of humerus	Suprascapular nerve (C5, C6)	Rotates the humerus laterally
Teres major	Lower lateral border and inferior angle of the scapula	Crest of lesser tubercle and medial lip of intertubercular sulcus of humerus	Lower subscapular nerve (C5, C6)	Adducts and medially rotates the humerus; assists in extension of the arm
Teres minor	Upper part of the lateral border of the scapula	Lower part of the greater tubercle of humerus	Axillary nerve (C5)	Rotates humerus laterally; weakly adducts humerus

LATERAL   **MEDIAL**

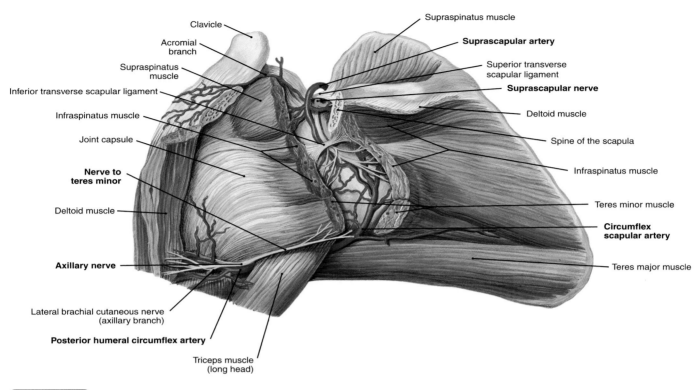

FIGURE 33.1 **Nerves and Vessels of Posterior Scapular Region (Left)**

NOTE: (1) The **superior** transverse scapular ligament bridges the scapular notch, and the suprascapular nerve passes beneath the ligament while the suprascapular artery usually passes above it to reach the supraspinatus fossa.

(2) Both the suprascapular nerve and the artery pass beneath the **inferior** transverse scapular ligament to reach the infraspinatus fossa.

(3) The axillary nerve supplies four structures: (a) the teres minor muscle, (b) the deltoid muscle, (c) the capsule of the shoulder joint, and (d) the skin over the shoulder joint.

(4) The axillary nerve and posterior humeral circumflex artery from the dorsal view. These two structures have passed through the quadrangular space, whereas the circumflex scapular artery reaches the infraspinatus fossa through the triangular space.

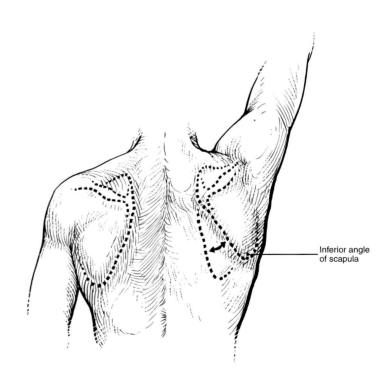

FIGURE 33.2 **Abduction of the Upper Limb**

NOTE: (1) The first 20 degrees of abduction is performed by the supraspinatus muscle.

(2) From 20 to 90 degrees, abduction is almost exclusively the action of the deltoid muscle.

(3) Continuing beyond 90 degrees to 180 degrees (as shown in this figure), the vertebral border and inferior angle of the scapula must rotate laterally as the upper limb is elevated.

PLATE 34 Surface Anatomy of the Upper Limb

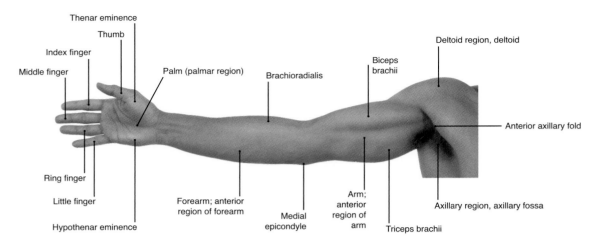

FIGURE 34.1 **Surface Anatomy of the Right Upper Limb (Anterior Aspect)**

NOTE: (1) The vertically oriented **medial bicipital furrow** along the arm. The **basilic vein** and the **medial antebrachial cutaneous nerve** course beneath the skin along this furrow. More deeply are found the brachial artery and vein and the **median** and **ulnar nerves**;
(2) The **cubital fossa** in front of the elbow joint, between the bellies of the flexor and extensor muscles in the upper forearm.

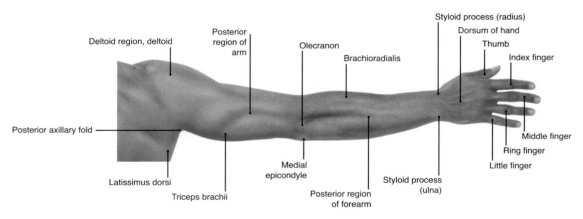

FIGURE 34.2 **Surface Anatomy of the Right Upper Limb (Posterior Aspect)**

NOTE: (1) The surface contours of the **biceps brachii** and **brachioradialis** muscles and the surface projections of the olecranon and the medial epicondyle in the elbow region.
(2) The distal sharp ends of both the radius and the ulna end in a **styloid process**. They are frequently fractured by severe trauma at the wrist.

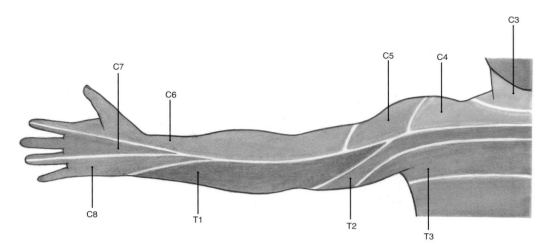

FIGURE 35.1 **Cutaneous Innervation and Dermatomes of the Upper Limb (Anterior Aspect)**

NOTE: (1) An area of skin surface that receives innervation from any single spinal nerve is called a **dermatome**.
(2) The solid lines on this figure and on Figure 35.2 are the boundaries between dermatomes. The boundary between C5 and C6 laterally and T1 and T2 medially is called the **anterior axial line**.
(3) The dermatomes on the anterior aspect of the limb commence over the anterior lateral surface of the brachium with the C5 dermatome.
(4) Continuing down laterally in the forearm is the C6 dermatome, the palmar and radial hand is C7, the ulnar aspect of the hand is C8, and then sequentially up the medial surface of the forearm and arm are the T1 and T2 dermatomes.
(5) Although there is overlap between adjacent dermatomes (such as between C5 and C6), **there is no overlap across the axial** line (such as between C6 and T1). This has important clinical significance, because differences in sensation across the axial line might help localize a problem in the spinal cord.

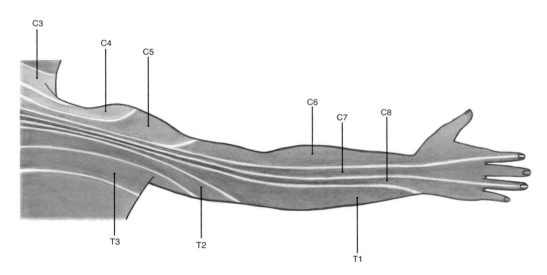

FIGURE 35.2 **Cutaneous Innervation and Dermatomes of the Upper Limb (Posterior Aspect)**

NOTE: (1) Dermatomes on the posterior surface of the upper limb start at the proximal lateral region of the arm with the C5 dermatome.
(2) The C6 dermatome continues down the radial aspect of the forearm and hand; it includes the dorsal thumb and the radial part of the index finger.
(3) The C7 dermatome includes the posterior aspect of the middle finger and the adjacent halves of the index and ring fingers as well as a strip of skin over the intermediate parts of the posterior hand and forearm.
(4) The C8 dermatome includes the little finger and the adjacent part of the ring finger and the ulnar part of the hand, along with a thin region of forearm skin.
(5) Continuing sequentially up the posterior aspect of the medial (ulnar) side of the forearm and arm are the T1 and T2 dermatomes.

PLATE 36 **Superficial Dissection of the Arm (Anterior View)**

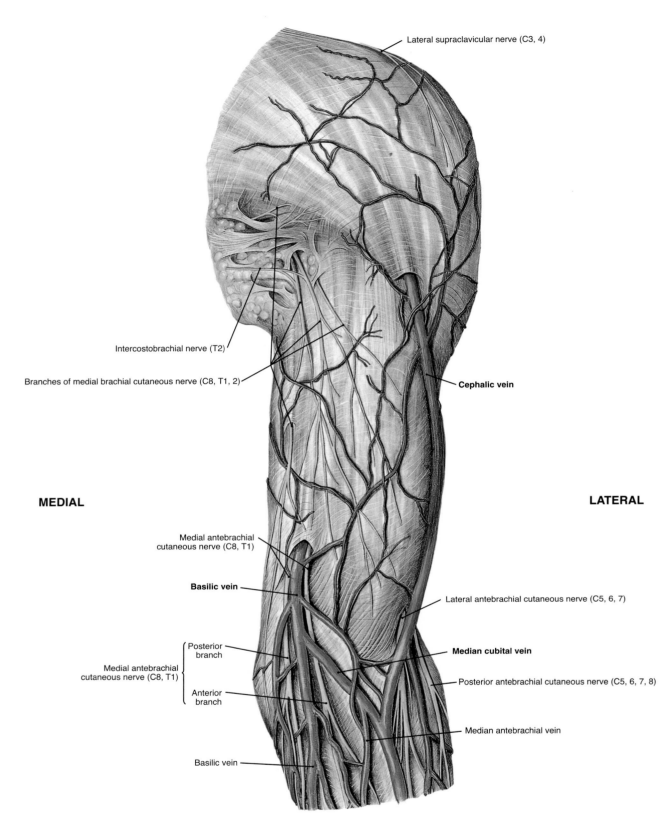

Lateral supraclavicular nerve (C3, 4)

Intercostobrachial nerve (T2)

Branches of medial brachial cutaneous nerve (C8, T1, 2)

Cephalic vein

MEDIAL

LATERAL

Medial antebrachial
cutaneous nerve (C8, T1)

Basilic vein

Lateral antebrachial cutaneous nerve (C5, 6, 7)

Posterior
branch

Median cubital vein

Medial antebrachial
cutaneous nerve (C8, T1)

Posterior antebrachial cutaneous nerve (C5, 6, 7, 8)

Anterior
branch

Median antebrachial vein

Basilic vein

FIGURE 36 **Superficial Veins and Cutaneous Nerves of the Left Upper Arm (Anterior View)**

NOTE: (1) The **basilic vein** ascends on the medial (ulnar) aspect of the arm, pierces the deep fascia, and at the lower border of the teres major, joins the brachial veins to form the axillary vein.

(2) In contrast, the **cephalic vein** ascends along the lateral aspect of the arm toward the axillary vein, which it joins deep to the deltopectoral triangle.

(3) The principal sensory nerves of the anterior arm region are the **medial brachial cutaneous** and **intercostobrachial nerves**.

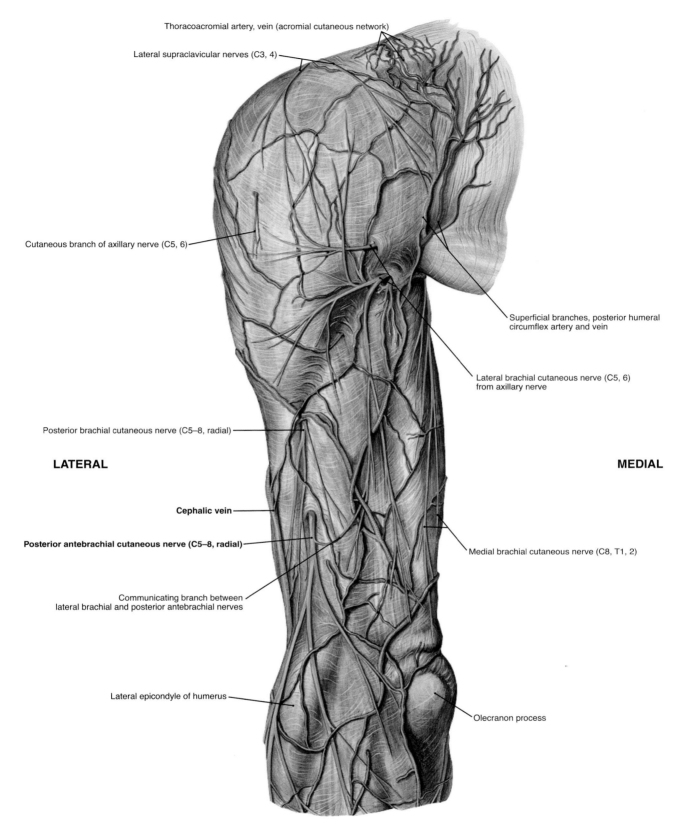

Thoracoacromial artery, vein (acromial cutaneous network)

Lateral supraclavicular nerves (C3, 4)

Cutaneous branch of axillary nerve (C5, 6)

Superficial branches, posterior humeral circumflex artery and vein

Lateral brachial cutaneous nerve (C5, 6) from axillary nerve

Posterior brachial cutaneous nerve (C5–8, radial)

LATERAL

MEDIAL

Cephalic vein

Posterior antebrachial cutaneous nerve (C5–8, radial)

Medial brachial cutaneous nerve (C8, T1, 2)

Communicating branch between lateral brachial and posterior antebrachial nerves

Lateral epicondyle of humerus

Olecranon process

FIGURE 37 Superficial Veins and Cutaneous Nerves of Left Upper Arm (Posterior View)

NOTE: (1) The posterior arm region receives cutaneous innervation from the **radial** (posterior brachial cutaneous nerve) and **axillary** (lateral brachial cutaneous nerve) nerves. Both are derived from the posterior cord of the brachial plexus.

(2) The **posterior antebrachial cutaneous nerve** (from the radial nerve) perforates the lateral head of the triceps about 5 cm above the elbow. Upon piercing the superficial fascia, it sends cutaneous branches to the posterior surface of the forearm as well as a communicating branch to the cutaneous rami of the axillary nerve.

PLATE 38　Blood Vessels of the Upper Limb

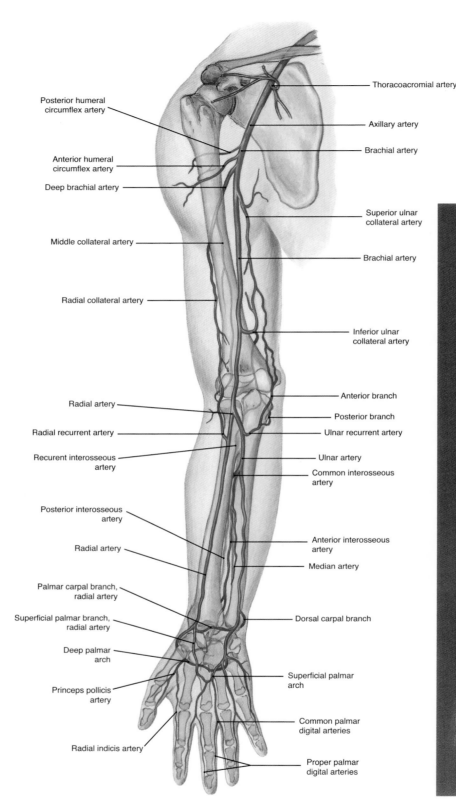

Thoracoacromial artery

Posterior humeral
circumflex artery

Axillary artery

Brachial artery

Anterior humeral
circumflex artery

Deep brachial artery

Superior ulnar
collateral artery

Middle collateral artery

Brachial artery

Radial collateral artery

Inferior ulnar
collateral artery

Anterior branch

Radial artery

Posterior branch

Radial recurrent artery

Ulnar recurrent artery

Recurrent interosseous
artery

Ulnar artery

Common interosseous
artery

Posterior interosseous
artery

Radial artery

Anterior interosseous
artery

Median artery

Palmar carpal branch,
radial artery

Superficial palmar branch,
radial artery

Dorsal carpal branch

Deep palmar
arch

Superficial palmar
arch

Princeps pollicis
artery

Common palmar
digital arteries

Radial indicis artery

Proper palmar
digital arteries

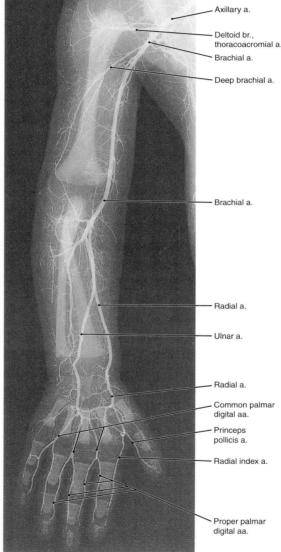

Axillary a.

Deltoid br.,
thoracoacromial a.

Brachial a.

Deep brachial a.

Brachial a.

Radial a.

Ulnar a.

Radial a.

Common palmar
digital aa.

Princeps
pollicis a.

Radial index a.

Proper palmar
digital aa.

FIGURE 38.1 Schematic View of the Arteries of the Upper Limb (Anterior View)

FIGURE 38.2 Arteriogram of the Upper Limb in a Stillborn Infant

NOTE that the arteries of the upper limb derive from the brachial artery and the axillary artery.

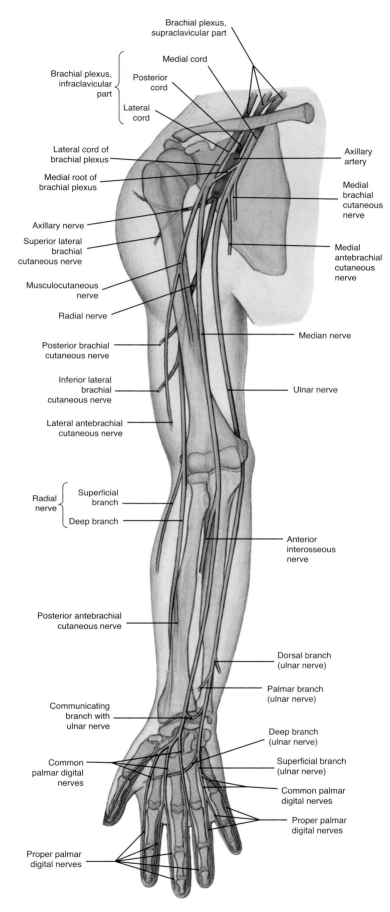

FIGURE 39 **Nerves of the Upper Limb**

NOTE that all of the nerves of the upper limb derive from the brachial plexus in the axilla.

PLATE 40 Cutaneous (Superficial) Nerves of the Upper Limb

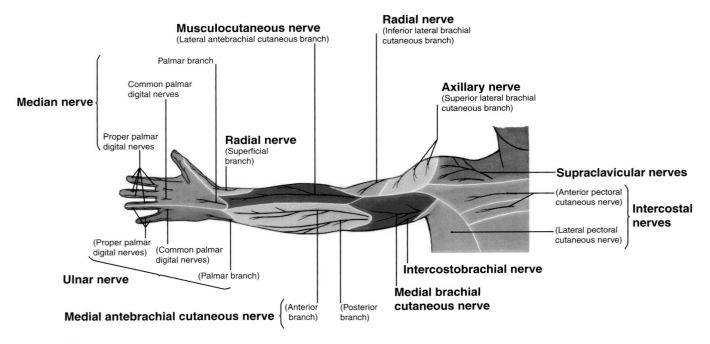

Median nerve
Palmar branch
Common palmar digital nerves
Proper palmar digital nerves

Musculocutaneous nerve
(Lateral antebrachial cutaneous branch)

Radial nerve
(Superficial branch)

Radial nerve
(Inferior lateral brachial cutaneous branch)

Axillary nerve
(Superior lateral brachial cutaneous branch)

Supraclavicular nerves

(Anterior pectoral cutaneous nerve)

(Lateral pectoral cutaneous nerve)

Intercostal nerves

(Proper palmar digital nerves)
(Common palmar digital nerves)

Ulnar nerve

(Palmar branch)

(Anterior branch) (Posterior branch)

Intercostobrachial nerve

Medial brachial cutaneous nerve

Medial antebrachial cutaneous nerve

FIGURE 40.1 Cutaneous Fields and Courses of Cutaneous Nerves in the Upper Limb (Anterior Aspect)

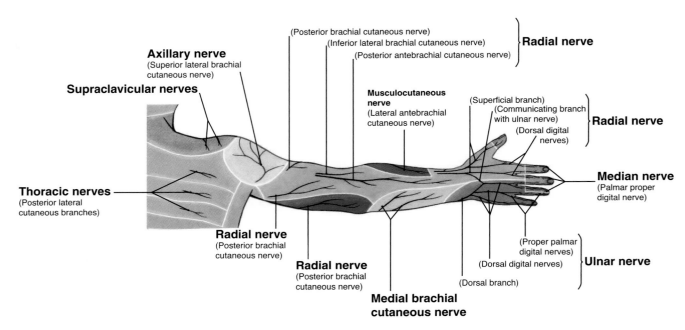

(Posterior brachial cutaneous nerve)
(Inferior lateral brachial cutaneous nerve)
(Posterior antebrachial cutaneous nerve)

Radial nerve

Axillary nerve
(Superior lateral brachial cutaneous nerve)

Supraclavicular nerves

Musculocutaneous nerve
(Lateral antebrachial cutaneous nerve)

(Superficial branch)
(Communicating branch with ulnar nerve)
(Dorsal digital nerves)

Radial nerve

Median nerve
(Palmar proper digital nerve)

Thoracic nerves
(Posterior lateral cutaneous branches)

Radial nerve
(Posterior brachial cutaneous nerve)

Radial nerve
(Posterior brachial cutaneous nerve)

Medial brachial cutaneous nerve

(Proper palmar digital nerves)
(Dorsal digital nerves)
(Dorsal branch)

Ulnar nerve

FIGURE 40.2 Cutaneous Fields and Courses of Cutaneous Nerves in the Upper Limb (Posterior Aspect)

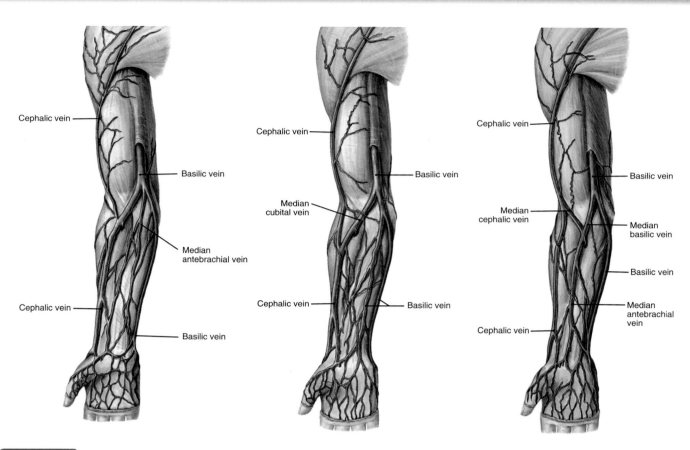

FIGURE 41.1 **Variations in the Venous Pattern of the Upper Extremity**

NOTE: Superficial veins are variable and are of significance clinically. The median cubital vein is often used for the withdrawal of blood and the injection of fluids into the vascular system. Care must be taken not to injure the median nerve or puncture the brachial artery, which lie deep to the median cubital vein and the underlying bicipital aponeurosis.

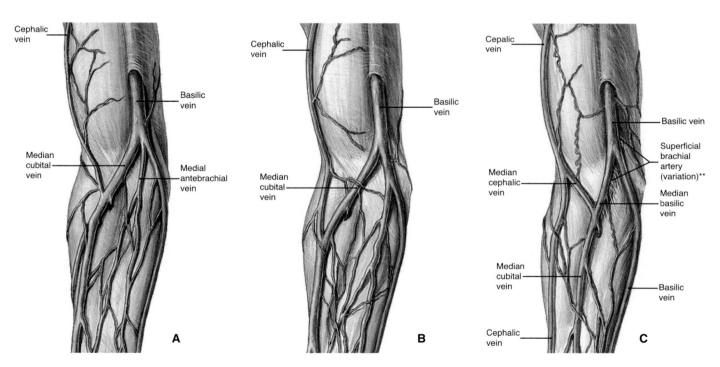

FIGURE 41.2A–C **Variations of the Superficial Veins in the Antecubital Fossa**

NOTE: Each of these three variations is an enlargement of the antecubital region shown in the figure above. **This variation (rare) of a superficial branch of the brachial artery is important to understand. Intended intravenous injections can mistakenly be made into this superficial brachial artery if this variation occurs in a patient.

PLATE 42 **Surface and Skeletal Anatomy of the Upper Limb**

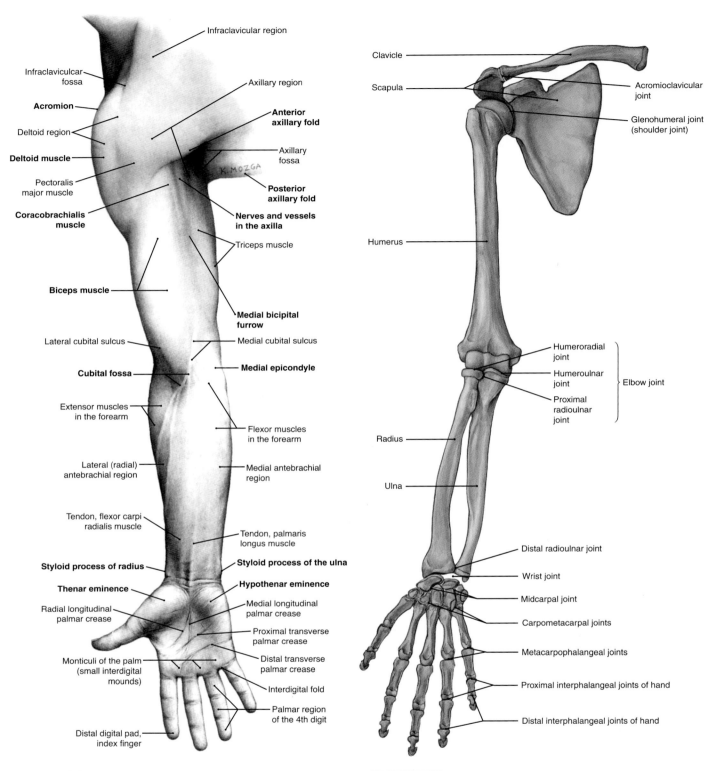

Infraclavicular region

Infraclaviculcar fossa

Acromion

Deltoid region

Deltoid muscle

Pectoralis major muscle

Coracobrachialis muscle

Axillary region

Anterior axillary fold

Axillary fossa

K.MOZGA

Posterior axillary fold

Nerves and vessels in the axilla

Triceps muscle

Biceps muscle

Medial bicipital furrow

Lateral cubital sulcus

Medial cubital sulcus

Cubital fossa

Medial epicondyle

Extensor muscles in the forearm

Flexor muscles in the forearm

Lateral (radial) antebrachial region

Medial antebrachial region

Tendon, flexor carpi radialis muscle

Tendon, palmaris longus muscle

Styloid process of radius

Styloid process of the ulna

Thenar eminence

Hypothenar eminence

Radial longitudinal palmar crease

Medial longitudinal palmar crease

Proximal transverse palmar crease

Monticuli of the palm (small interdigital mounds)

Distal transverse palmar crease

Interdigital fold

Palmar region of the 4th digit

Distal digital pad, index finger

Clavicle

Scapula

Acromioclavicular joint

Glenohumeral joint (shoulder joint)

Humerus

Humeroradial joint

Humeroulnar joint

Elbow joint

Proximal radioulnar joint

Radius

Ulna

Distal radioulnar joint

Wrist joint

Midcarpal joint

Carpometacarpal joints

Metacarpophalangeal joints

Proximal interphalangeal joints of hand

Distal interphalangeal joints of hand

FIGURE 42.1 **Surface Anatomy of the Right Upper Limb, Anterior Aspect**

NOTE: (1) The vertically oriented medial bicipital furrow along the arm. The basilic vein and the medial antebrachial cutaneous nerve course beneath the skin along this furrow. More deeply are found the brachial artery and vein and the median and ulnar nerves;

(2) The cubital fossa in front of the elbow joint, between the bellies of the flexor and extensor muscles in the upper forearm.

FIGURE 42.2 **Bones of the Upper Limb and Pectoral Girdle**

NOTE: The pectoral girdle includes the clavicle and the bones to which it is attached; these are the manubrium of the sternum and the scapula.

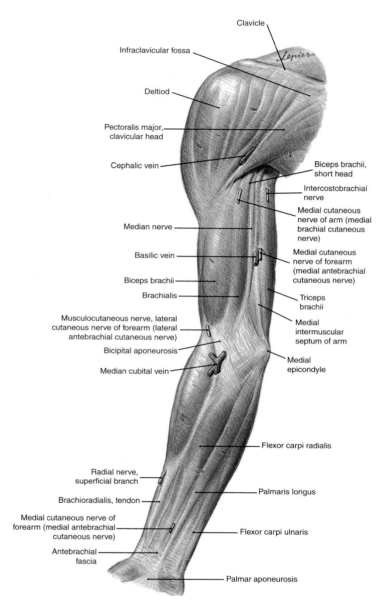

FIGURE 43.1 **Fascia Over the Flexor Compartments of the Right Upper Limb (Anterior View)**

NOTE: (1) The medial neurovascular compartment in the arm showing the median nerve, basilic vein, and medial antebrachial cutaneous nerve.
(2) Observe the flexor muscles of the arm and the flexor muscles of the forearm on the anterior aspect of the upper limb.

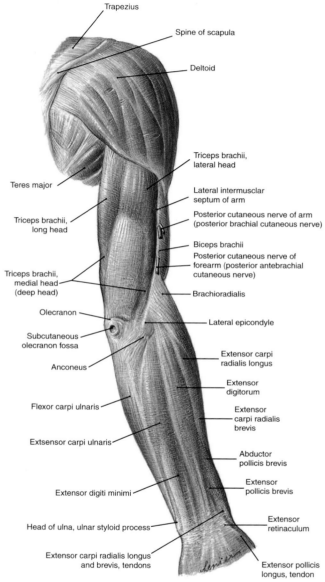

FIGURE 43.2 **Fascia Over the Extensor Muscles of the Right Upper Limb (Posterior View)**

NOTE: (1) The triceps muscle in the posterior compartment of the arm and the extensor muscles of the wrist and fingers on the dorsal aspect of the forearm.
(2) Observe the brachioradialis muscle, which flexes the forearm at the elbow joint when the forearm is pronated. Also note the extensor carpi radialis longus and brevis adjacent to the brachioradialis.

PLATE 44 Muscles of the Upper Limb: Lateral View

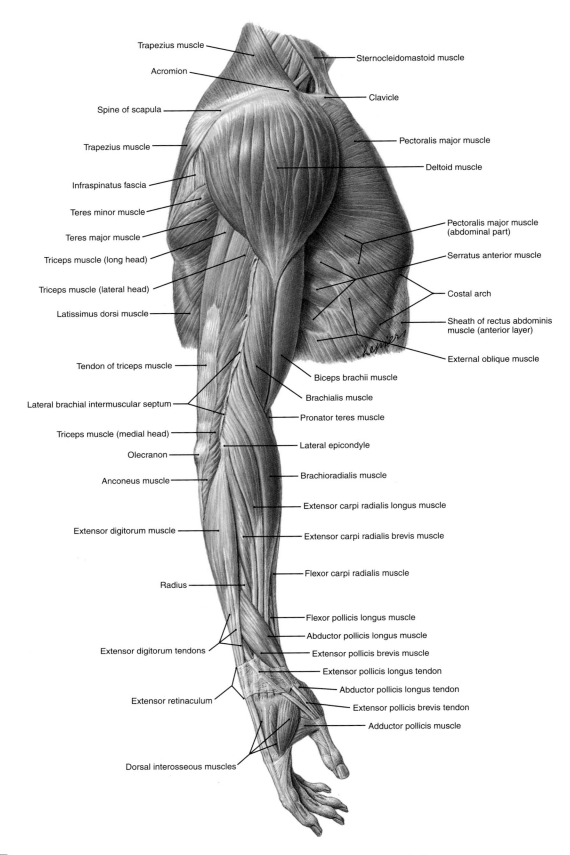

Trapezius muscle

Acromion

Spine of scapula

Trapezius muscle

Infraspinatus fascia

Teres minor muscle

Teres major muscle

Triceps muscle (long head)

Triceps muscle (lateral head)

Latissimus dorsi muscle

Tendon of triceps muscle

Lateral brachial intermuscular septum

Triceps muscle (medial head)

Olecranon

Anconeus muscle

Extensor digitorum muscle

Radius

Extensor digitorum tendons

Extensor retinaculum

Dorsal interosseous muscles

Sternocleidomastoid muscle

Clavicle

Pectoralis major muscle

Deltoid muscle

Pectoralis major muscle (abdominal part)

Serratus anterior muscle

Costal arch

Sheath of rectus abdominis muscle (anterior layer)

External oblique muscle

Biceps brachii muscle

Brachialis muscle

Pronator teres muscle

Lateral epicondyle

Brachioradialis muscle

Extensor carpi radialis longus muscle

Extensor carpi radialis brevis muscle

Flexor carpi radialis muscle

Flexor pollicis longus muscle

Abductor pollicis longus muscle

Extensor pollicis brevis muscle

Extensor pollicis longus tendon

Abductor pollicis longus tendon

Extensor pollicis brevis tendon

Adductor pollicis muscle

FIGURE 44 **Lateral View of the Muscles of the Upper Extremity and Lateral Thorax**

NOTE the lateral view of the **deltoid, triceps brachii, biceps brachii,** and **brachialis** in the arm; the **brachioradialis, extensor carpi radialis longus** and **brevis, extensor digitorum,** and **abductor** and **extensors pollicis longus** and **brevis** in the forearm. Also note the **adductor pollicis** and the **dorsal interosseous muscles** in the hand.

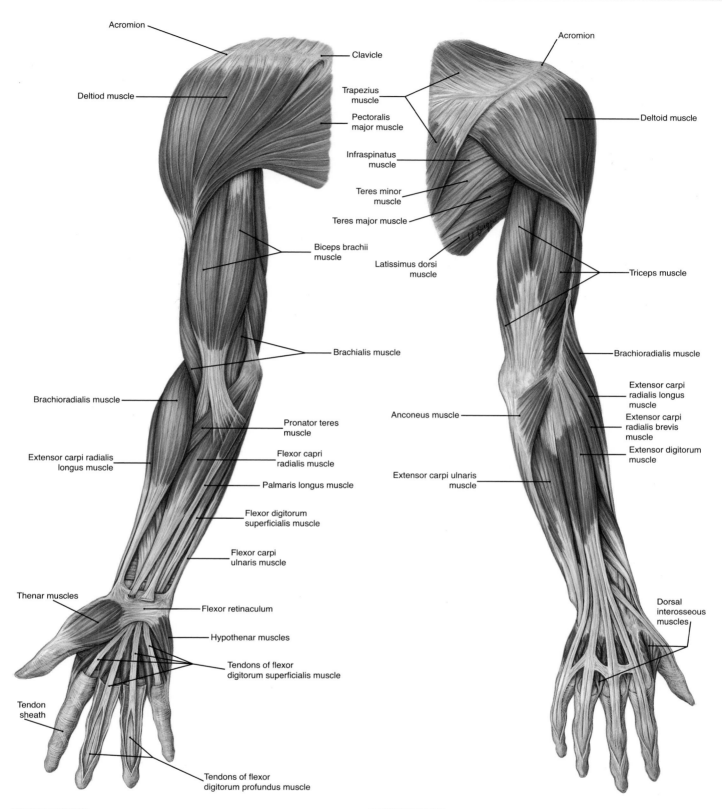

FIGURE 45.1 **Muscles of the Upper Extremity (Anterior View)**

NOTE the **biceps** and **brachialis** muscles in the arm; **pronator teres, flexor carpi radialis, palmaris longus, flexor digitorum,** and **flexor carpi ulnaris** in the forearm; and the **thenar** and **hypothenar** muscles in the hand along with the **flexor tendons.**

FIGURE 45.2 **Muscles of the Upper Extremity (Posterior View)**

NOTE the **triceps** and **brachialis** in the arm; the **brachioradialis, extensor carpi radialis longus** and **brevis, extensor digitorum,** and **extensor carpi ulnaris** muscles in the forearm; and the **dorsal interosseous** muscles in the hand.

PLATE 46 The Brachial Plexus and Its Three Cords

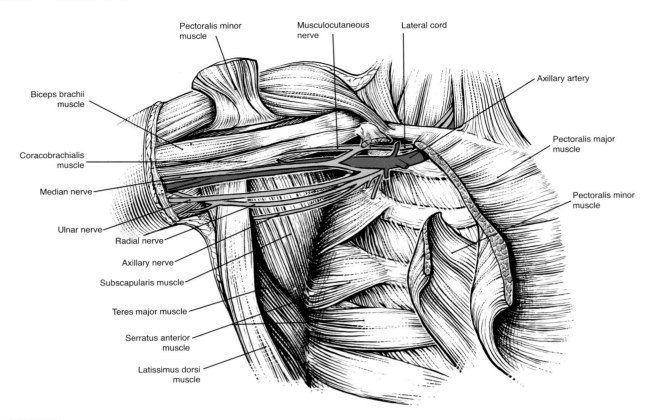

Pectoralis minor muscle

Musculocutaneous nerve

Lateral cord

Axillary artery

Biceps brachii muscle

Pectoralis major muscle

Coracobrachialis muscle

Pectoralis minor muscle

Median nerve

Ulnar nerve

Radial nerve

Axillary nerve

Subscapularis muscle

Teres major muscle

Serratus anterior muscle

Latissimus dorsi muscle

FIGURE 46.1 **The Axillary Artery and the Cords of the Brachial Plexus**

NOTE that the median nerve is formed by contributions from the lateral and medial cords (the **M** of the brachial plexus). (Contributed by Dr. Gene L. Colborn, Medical College of Georgia.)

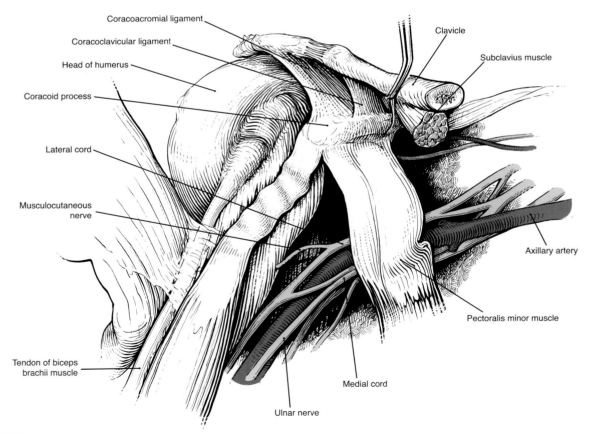

Coracoacromial ligament

Clavicle

Coracoclavicular ligament

Subclavius muscle

Head of humerus

Coracoid process

Lateral cord

Musculocutaneous nerve

Axillary artery

Pectoralis minor muscle

Tendon of biceps brachii muscle

Medial cord

Ulnar nerve

FIGURE 46.2 **The Cords of the Brachial Plexus in the Axilla**

NOTE the musculocutaneous, median, and ulnar nerves. (Contributed by Dr. Gene L. Colborn, Medical College of Georgia.)

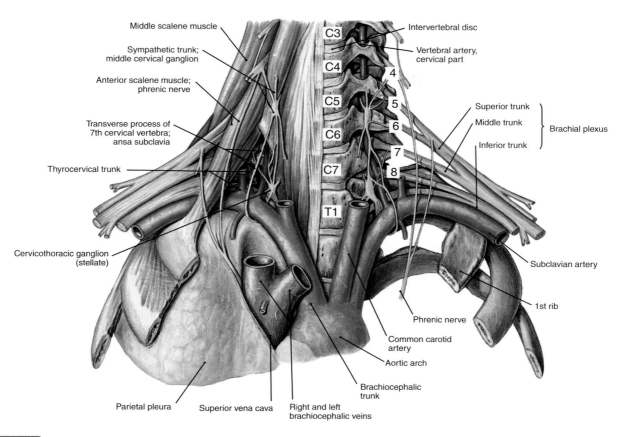

FIGURE 47.1 **Roots of Origin of the Brachial Plexus in the Posterior Lateral Neck Region**

NOTE: (1) The roots of C5, C6, C7, C8, and T1 emerge from the vertebral column and form the upper, middle, and lower trunks of the brachial plexus.
(2) C5 and C6 join to form the upper trunk, C7 forms the middle trunk, and C8 and T1 join to form the lower trunk.
(3) Crossing the first rib under the clavicle with the subclavian artery, each trunk splits into anterior and posterior divisions. The divisions then reassemble to form three cords: **lateral**, **medial**, and **posterior**. Now study Figure 47.2 and read its NOTE.

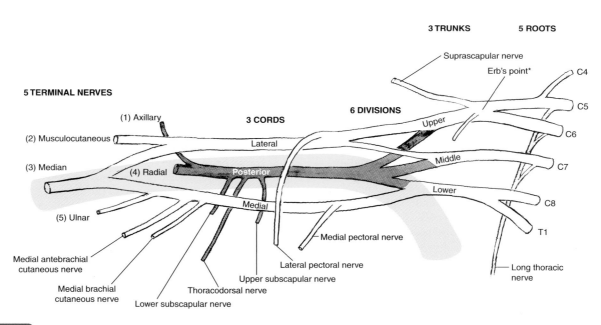

FIGURE 47.2 **Diagrammatic View of the Brachial Plexus with Axillary Artery**

NOTE the **5 roots** (C5, C6, C7, C8, T1), **3 trunks** (upper, middle, and lower), **6 divisions** (3 anterior, 3 posterior), **3 cords** (lateral, medial, and posterior), and **5 terminal nerves** (axillary, musculocutaneous, median, radial, and ulnar). *Erb's point* is a point 2 to 3 cm above the clavicle and lateral to the posterior border of the sternocleidomastoid muscle at which the upper cord of the brachial plexus (C5–C6) can be stimulated electrically to cause certain muscles of the upper limb to contract.
(From *Clemente's Anatomy Dissector*, 2nd Edition. Baltimore: Lippincott Williams & Wilkins, 2007.)

PLATE 48 **Complete Brachial Plexus Diagram**

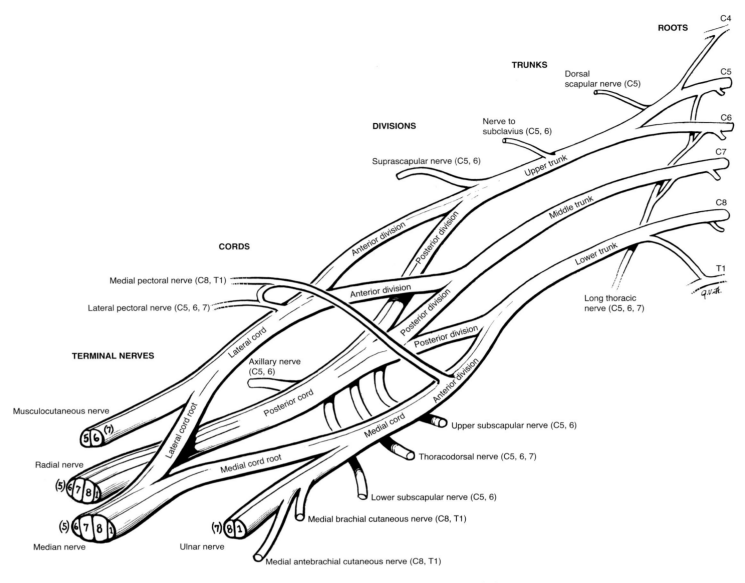

ROOTS

C4

TRUNKS

Dorsal
scapular nerve (C5)

C5

DIVISIONS

Nerve to
subclavius (C5, 6)

C6

Suprascapular nerve (C5, 6)

C7

Upper trunk

Middle trunk

C8

CORDS

Anterior division

Posterior division

Lower trunk

Medial pectoral nerve (C8, T1)

Anterior division

T1

Lateral pectoral nerve (C5, 6, 7)

Posterior division

Long thoracic
nerve (C5, 6, 7)

g.v.t.

Posterior division

TERMINAL NERVES

Lateral cord

Axillary nerve
(C5, 6)

Anterior division

Musculocutaneous nerve

Posterior cord

Lateral cord root

Medial cord

Upper subscapular nerve (C5, 6)

5 6 (7)

Radial nerve

Medial cord root

Thoracodorsal nerve (C5, 6, 7)

(5) 6 7 8 1

Lower subscapular nerve (C5, 6)

(5) 6 7 8 1

(7) 8 1

Medial brachial cutaneous nerve (C8, T1)

Median nerve

Ulnar nerve

Medial antebrachial cutaneous nerve (C8, T1)

FIGURE 48 Formation of the Brachial Plexus

NOTE: (1) The brachial plexus commences with 5 spinal roots (**C5, C6, C7, C8, and T1**).

(2) The 5 roots join to form 3 trunks: **C5** and **C6** form the **upper** trunk, **C7** continues alone as the **middle** trunk, and **C8** and **T1** join to form the **lower** trunk.

(3) Deep to the clavicle, each trunk divides into an **anterior** and a **posterior division**.

(4) These 6 divisions form 3 cords in the axilla: the 3 posterior divisions form the **posterior cord**; the anterior divisions of the upper and middle trunks form the **lateral cord**; and the anterior division of the lower trunk continues as the **medial cord**.

(5) The posterior cord divides into a relatively small branch, the **axillary nerve**, and the large **radial nerve**.

(6) The lateral cord and the medial cord each sends a branch to form the **median nerve**.

(7) The **musculocutaneous nerve** comes off of the lateral cord and the **ulnar nerve** continues from the medial cord down the upper limb.

(8) Eleven other nerves are given off, and they are listed to the right.

Complete brachial plexus:
NOTE: In addition to the 5 terminal nerves discussed to the left, the brachial plexus gives rise to 11 other nerves. These are the:
1. Long thoracic nerve (roots C6, C6, C7)
2. Dorsal scapular nerve (C5 root)
3. Nerve to subclavius muscle (upper trunk)
4. Subscapular nerve (upper trunk)
5. Lateral pectoral nerve (lateral cord)
6. Medial pectoral nerve (medial cord)
7. Medial brachial cutaneous nerve (medial cord)
8. Medial antebrachial cutaneous nerve (medial cord)
9. Upper subscapular nerve (posterior cord)
10. Thoracodorsal nerve (posterior cord)
11. Lower subscapular nerve (posterior cord)

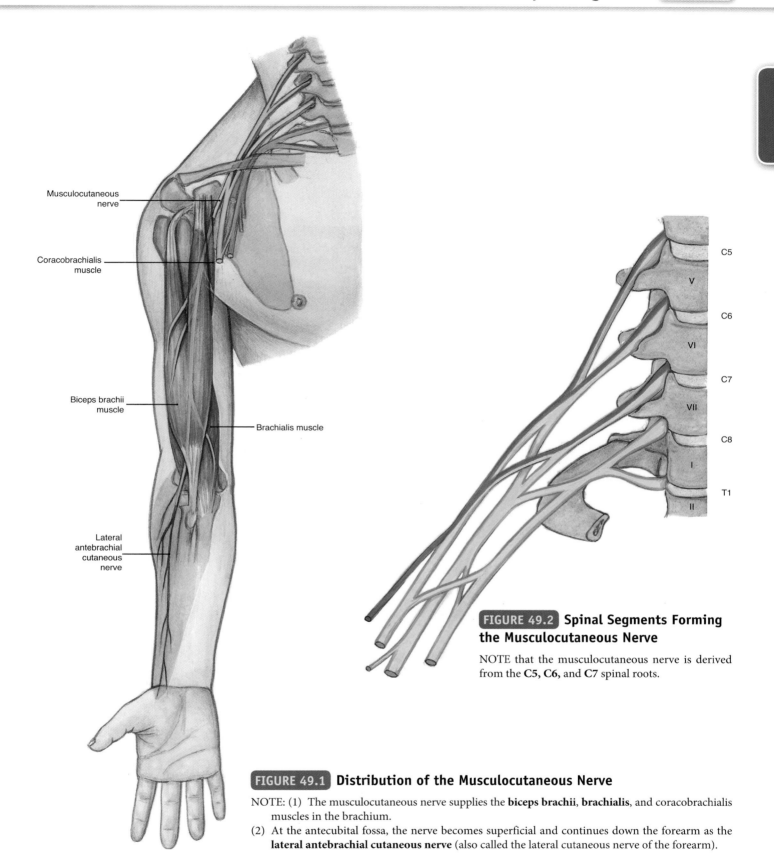

Musculocutaneous nerve

Coracobrachialis muscle

Biceps brachii muscle

Brachialis muscle

Lateral antebrachial cutaneous nerve

C5

V

C6

VI

C7

VII

C8

I

T1

II

FIGURE 49.2 **Spinal Segments Forming the Musculocutaneous Nerve**

NOTE that the musculocutaneous nerve is derived from the **C5, C6,** and **C7** spinal roots.

FIGURE 49.1 **Distribution of the Musculocutaneous Nerve**

NOTE: (1) The musculocutaneous nerve supplies the **biceps brachii**, **brachialis**, and coracobrachialis muscles in the brachium.

(2) At the antecubital fossa, the nerve becomes superficial and continues down the forearm as the **lateral antebrachial cutaneous nerve** (also called the lateral cutaneous nerve of the forearm).

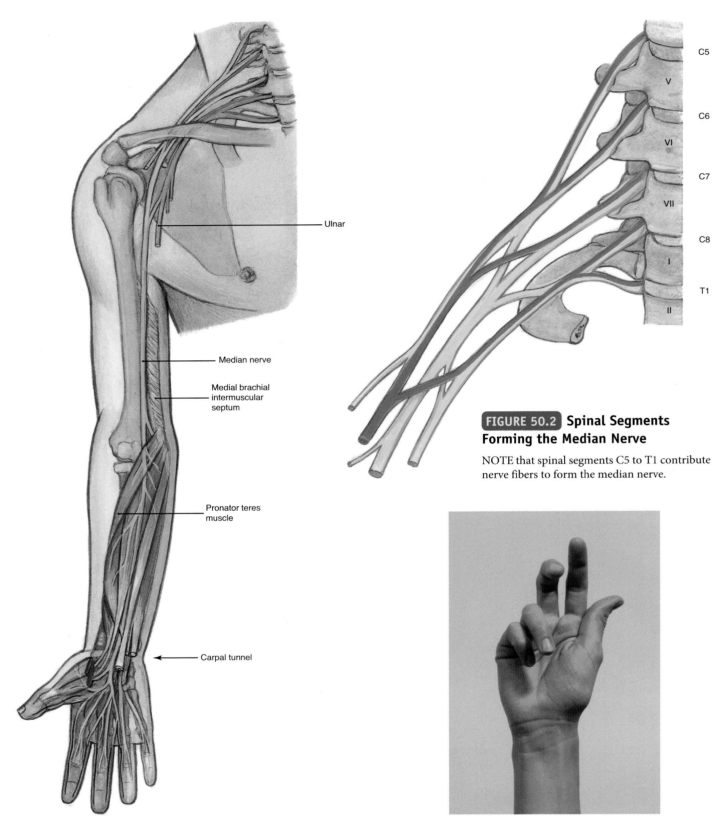

FIGURE 50.2 **Spinal Segments Forming the Median Nerve**

NOTE that spinal segments C5 to T1 contribute nerve fibers to form the median nerve.

FIGURE 50.1 **Median Nerve Distribution in the Forearm and Hand**

NOTE that the median nerve supplies muscles in the anterior forearm, the three thenar muscles to the thumb, and the first two lumbrical muscles in the hand.

FIGURE 50.3 **Median Nerve Palsy**

NOTE that lesions of the median nerve result in an inability to flex the thumb, the index finger, and the middle finger at the metacarpophalangeal joint. The ring and little fingers can still be flexed because the ulnar nerve is intact.

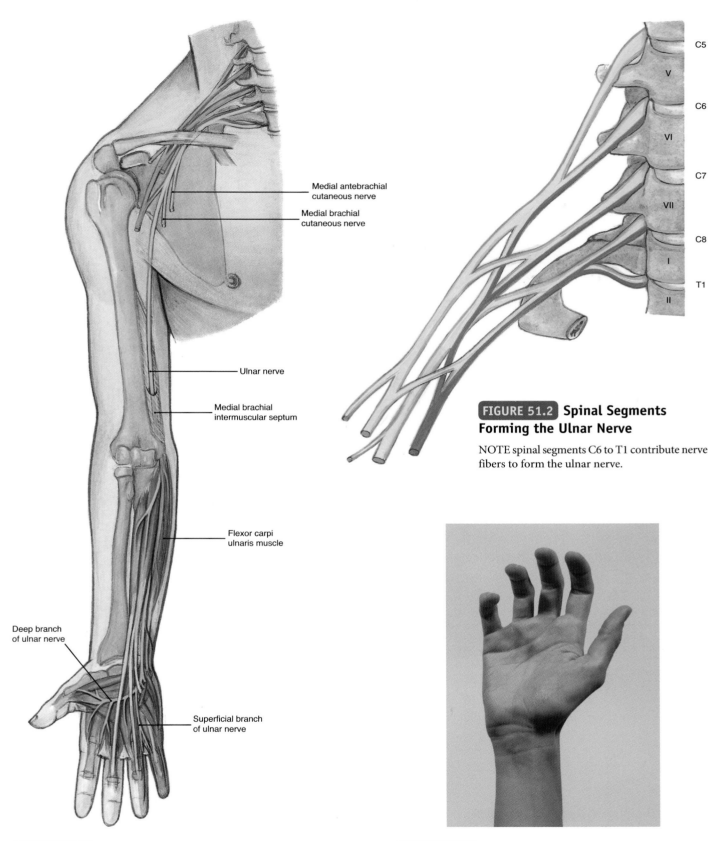

Medial antebrachial
cutaneous nerve

Medial brachial
cutaneous nerve

Ulnar nerve

Medial brachial
intermuscular septum

Flexor carpi
ulnaris muscle

Deep branch
of ulnar nerve

Superficial branch
of ulnar nerve

C5

V

C6

VI

C7

VII

C8

I

T1

II

FIGURE 51.2 **Spinal Segments Forming the Ulnar Nerve**

NOTE spinal segments C6 to T1 contribute nerve fibers to form the ulnar nerve.

FIGURE 51.1 **Ulnar Nerve Distribution in the Forearm and Hand**

NOTE: (1) The ulnar nerve supplies the flexor carpi ulnaris and the medial half of the flexor digitorum profundus in the forearm.

(2) In the hand, the ulnar nerve supplies the three hypothenar muscles, the third and fourth lumbricals, all of the interossei, and sensory innervation to the skin of the ulnar 1½ digits on the palmar and dorsal sides.

FIGURE 51.3 **Ulnar Nerve Palsy**

NOTE: (1) Lesions of the ulnar nerve result in an inability to flex the distal interphalangeal joint of the fourth and fifth digits. Patients cannot make a complete fist. This results in a hand that has a characteristic deformity known as "**claw hand**."

(2) Also, there is loss of sensory innervation to the ulnar aspect of the hand and the medial 1½ digits.

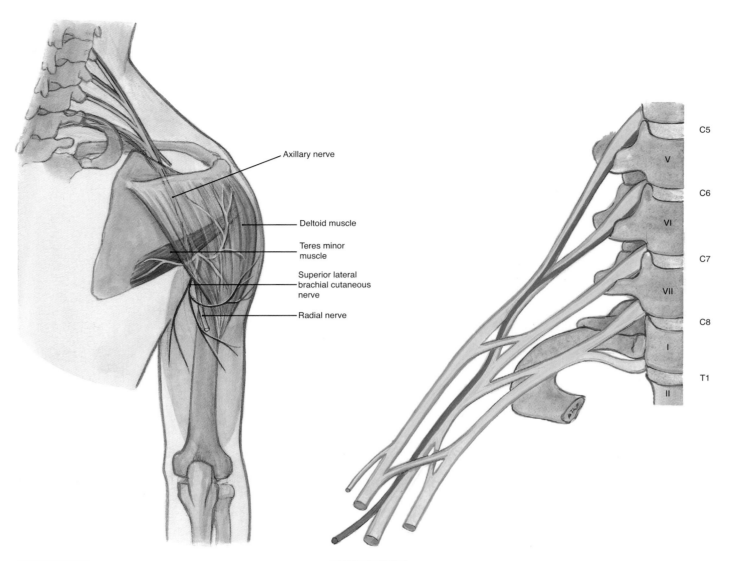

Axillary nerve

Deltoid muscle

Teres minor muscle

Superior lateral brachial cutaneous nerve

Radial nerve

C5

V

C6

VI

C7

VII

C8

I

T1

II

FIGURE 52.1 **Axillary Nerve Distribution in the Arm and Shoulder**

NOTE that the axillary nerve supplies the deltoid and teres minor muscles. It also gives sensory fibers to the shoulder joint and to the skin over the inferior part of the shoulder joint.

FIGURE 52.2 **Spinal Segments Forming the Axillary Nerve**

NOTE that spinal segments C5 and C6 contribute nerve fibers to form the axillary nerve.

FIGURE 52.3 **Ulnar Nerve Palsy**

NOTE that lesions of the axillary nerve result in atrophy of the deltoid muscle that overlies the shoulder region. The teres minor muscle is also denervated. Loss of the deltoid results in a protrusion of the bony structures on the lateral aspect of the shoulder, as seen in this figure.

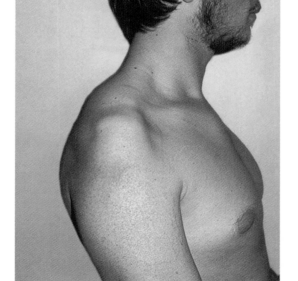

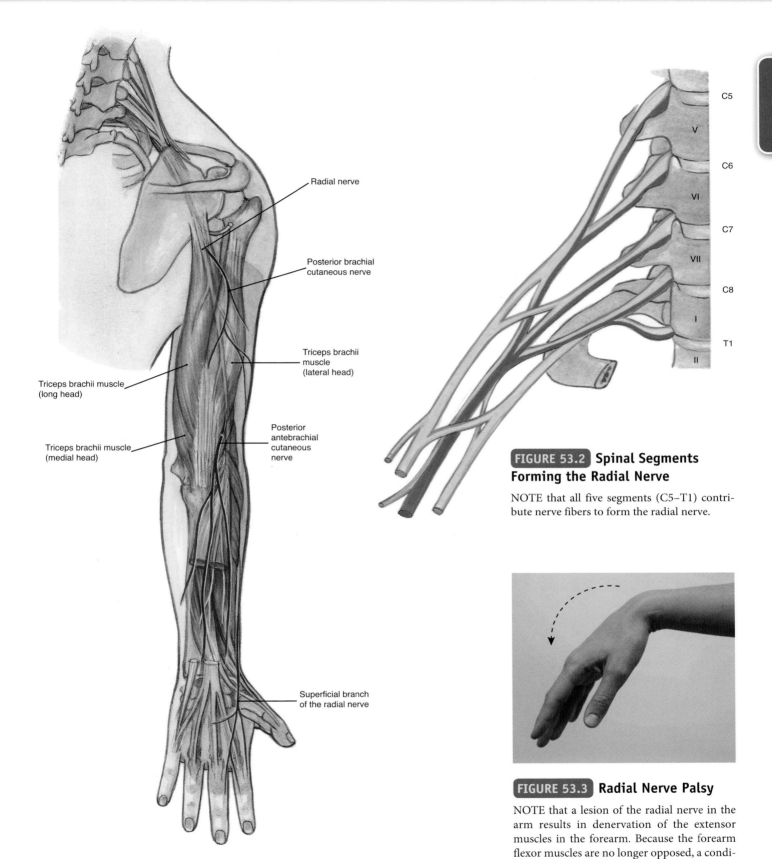

FIGURE 53.2 **Spinal Segments Forming the Radial Nerve**

NOTE that all five segments (C5–T1) contribute nerve fibers to form the radial nerve.

FIGURE 53.3 **Radial Nerve Palsy**

NOTE that a lesion of the radial nerve in the arm results in denervation of the extensor muscles in the forearm. Because the forearm flexor muscles are no longer opposed, a condition called "**wrist drop**" occurs.

FIGURE 53.1 **Radial Nerve Distribution to the Upper Limb**

NOTE: (1) The radial nerve descends from the posterior cord of the brachial plexus to supply the triceps brachii muscle and the extensor muscles in the posterior forearm.

(2) Its sensory branches supply the posterior arm and forearm to the dorsum of the hand. It supplies the thumb, the index and middle fingers, and half of the ring finger down to the distal interphalangeal joint.

PLATE 54 Anterior Dissection of the Shoulder and Arm: Muscles

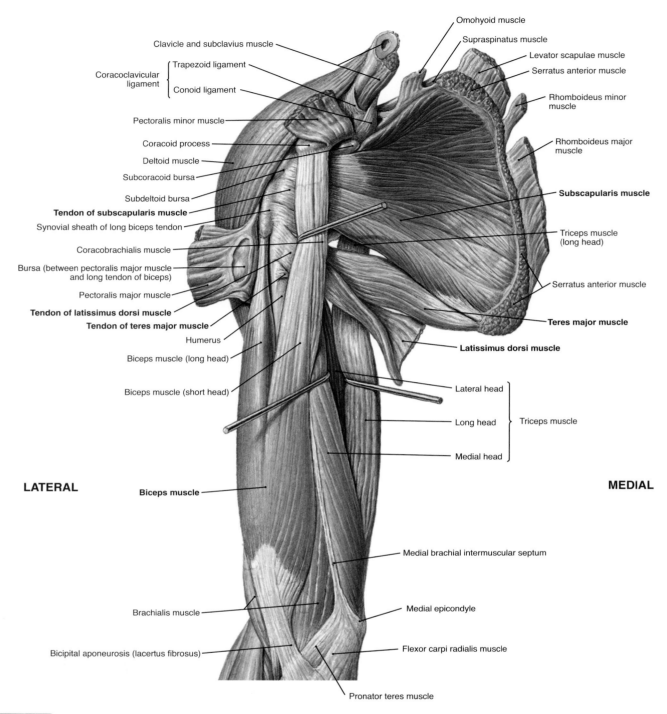

Omohyoid muscle
Supraspinatus muscle
Levator scapulae muscle
Serratus anterior muscle
Rhomboideus minor muscle
Rhomboideus major muscle

Clavicle and subclavius muscle
Coracoclavicular ligament
Trapezoid ligament
Conoid ligament
Pectoralis minor muscle
Coracoid process
Deltoid muscle
Subcoracoid bursa
Subdeltoid bursa
Tendon of subscapularis muscle
Synovial sheath of long biceps tendon
Coracobrachialis muscle
Bursa (between pectoralis major muscle and long tendon of biceps)
Pectoralis major muscle
Tendon of latissimus dorsi muscle
Tendon of teres major muscle
Humerus
Biceps muscle (long head)

Biceps muscle (short head)

Subscapularis muscle
Triceps muscle (long head)
Serratus anterior muscle
Teres major muscle
Latissimus dorsi muscle

Lateral head
Long head } Triceps muscle
Medial head

LATERAL
Biceps muscle

MEDIAL

Medial brachial intermuscular septum

Brachialis muscle

Medial epicondyle

Bicipital aponeurosis (lacertus fibrosus)

Flexor carpi radialis muscle

Pronator teres muscle

FIGURE 54 **Muscles of the Right Shoulder and Arm (Anterior View)**

NOTE: (1) The insertion of the subscapularis muscle on the lesser tubercle of the humerus. Distal to this, from medial to lateral, insert the teres major, latissimus dorsi, and pectoralis major muscles.

(2) The pectoralis minor, coracobrachialis, and short head of the biceps all attach to the coracoid process.

(3) The tendon of insertion of the pectoralis major muscle and the long tendon of the biceps muscle are usually separated by a bursa.

(4) From its origin on the coracoid process, the short head of the biceps courses inferiorly and laterally across the tendons of the subscapularis and latissimus dorsi to join the belly of the long head.

(5) The biceps is a very powerful supinator of the forearm and it is an efficient flexor of the forearm, especially when the forearm is supinated.

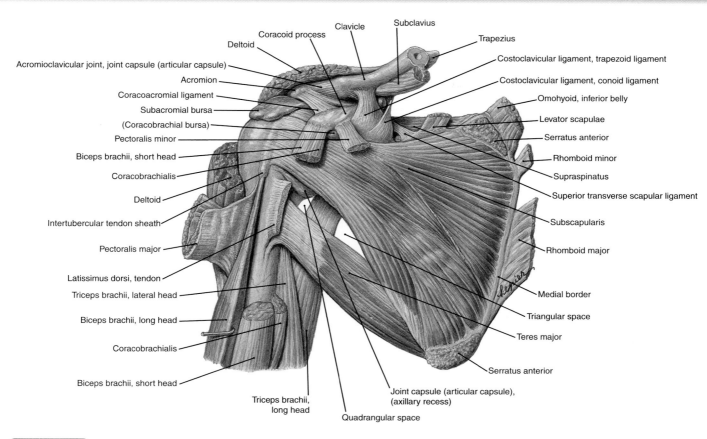

FIGURE 55.1 Anterior View of the Shoulder Muscles

NOTE the subcapularis muscle on the anterior surface of the scapula. It is one of the four muscles that make up the **rotator cuff**. It is a medial rotator of the humerus.

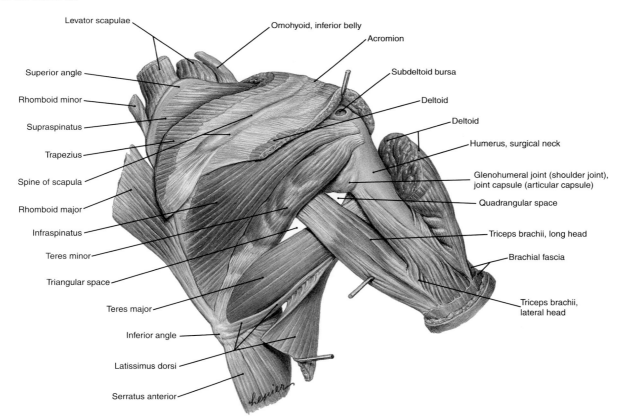

FIGURE 55.2 Posterior View of the Shoulder Muscles

NOTE the **quadrangular space**; through it course the axillary nerve and posterior humeral circumflex artery from the anterior axilla to the posterior surface of the shoulder. Also note the **triangular space** that transmits the circumflex scapular branch of the subscapular artery.

PLATE 56 Muscles of the Anterior Arm (Superficial Dissection)

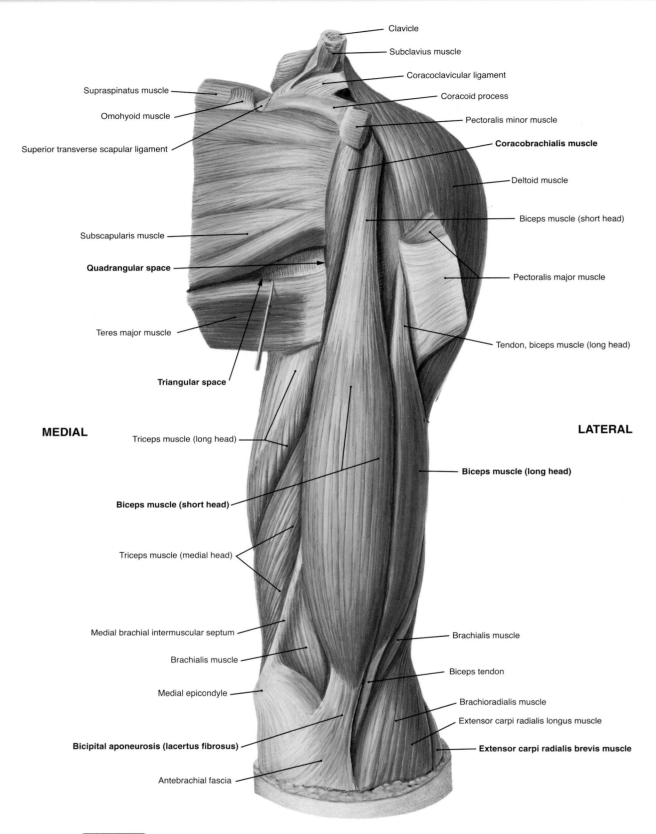

Clavicle

Subclavius muscle

Coracoclavicular ligament

Supraspinatus muscle

Coracoid process

Omohyoid muscle

Pectoralis minor muscle

Superior transverse scapular ligament

Coracobrachialis muscle

Deltoid muscle

Subscapularis muscle

Biceps muscle (short head)

Quadrangular space

Pectoralis major muscle

Teres major muscle

Tendon, biceps muscle (long head)

Triangular space

MEDIAL

LATERAL

Triceps muscle (long head)

Biceps muscle (long head)

Biceps muscle (short head)

Triceps muscle (medial head)

Medial brachial intermuscular septum

Brachialis muscle

Brachialis muscle

Biceps tendon

Medial epicondyle

Brachioradialis muscle

Extensor carpi radialis longus muscle

Bicipital aponeurosis (lacertus fibrosus)

Extensor carpi radialis brevis muscle

Antebrachial fascia

FIGURE 56 Superficial View of Muscles on the Anterior Aspect of the Left Arm

Muscle	Origin	Insertion	Innervation	Action
Biceps brachii	Long head: Supraglenoid tubercle of the scapula. Short head: Coracoid process of the scapula	Tuberosity of the radius and the bicipital aponeurosis	Musculocutaneous nerve (C5, C6)	Flexes and supinates the forearm; long head can also assist in flexing the humerus

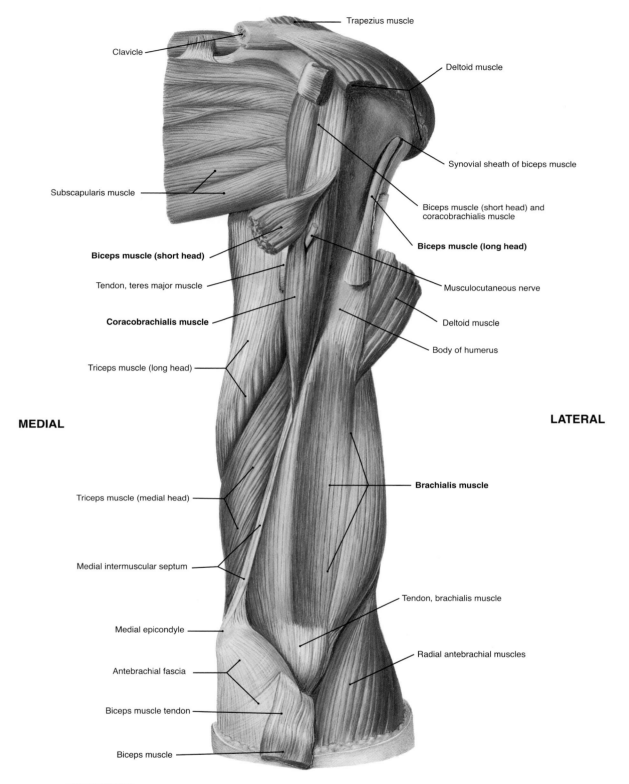

Trapezius muscle

Clavicle

Deltoid muscle

Subscapularis muscle

Synovial sheath of biceps muscle

Biceps muscle (short head) and coracobrachialis muscle

Biceps muscle (short head)

Biceps muscle (long head)

Tendon, teres major muscle

Musculocutaneous nerve

Coracobrachialis muscle

Deltoid muscle

Body of humerus

Triceps muscle (long head)

MEDIAL

LATERAL

Brachialis muscle

Triceps muscle (medial head)

Medial intermuscular septum

Tendon, brachialis muscle

Medial epicondyle

Radial antebrachial muscles

Antebrachial fascia

Biceps muscle tendon

Biceps muscle

FIGURE 57 Deep View of the Muscles on the Anterior Aspect of the Left Arm

Muscle	Origin	Insertion	Innervation	Action
Brachialis	Distal half of anterior surface of the humerus	Tuberosity of the ulna and anterior surface of the coronoid process	Musculocutaneous nerve and often a small branch of the radial nerve (C5, C6)	Powerful flexor of the forearm
Coracobrachialis	Coracoid process of the scapula	Along the medial surface of the humerus near its middle	Musculocutaneous nerve (C6, C7)	Flexes and adducts the arm

PLATE 58 Brachial Artery and the Median and Ulnar Nerves in the Arm

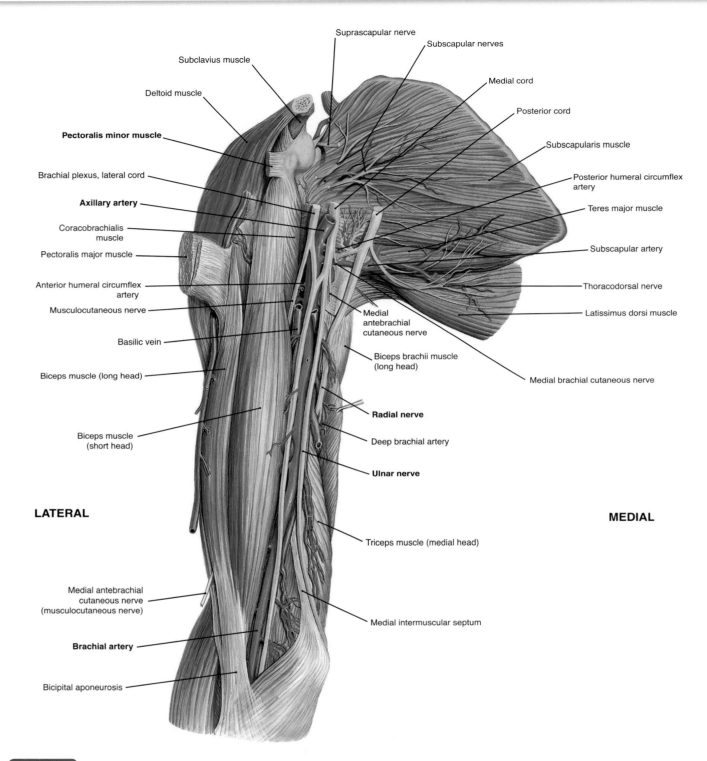

Suprascapular nerve

Subscapular nerves

Subclavius muscle

Medial cord

Deltoid muscle

Posterior cord

Pectoralis minor muscle

Subscapularis muscle

Brachial plexus, lateral cord

Posterior humeral circumflex artery

Axillary artery

Teres major muscle

Coracobrachialis muscle

Subscapular artery

Pectoralis major muscle

Anterior humeral circumflex artery

Thoracodorsal nerve

Musculocutaneous nerve

Latissimus dorsi muscle

Medial antebrachial cutaneous nerve

Basilic vein

Biceps brachii muscle (long head)

Biceps muscle (long head)

Medial brachial cutaneous nerve

Radial nerve

Biceps muscle (short head)

Deep brachial artery

Ulnar nerve

LATERAL

MEDIAL

Triceps muscle (medial head)

Medial antebrachial cutaneous nerve (musculocutaneous nerve)

Medial intermuscular septum

Brachial artery

Bicipital aponeurosis

FIGURE 58 Vessels and Nerves of the Anterior Arm (Right Arm, Superficial Dissection)

NOTE: (1) The **median nerve** crosses the brachial artery anteriorly from lateral to medial just above the cubital fossa.

(2) The median nerve arises by two roots, one each from the medial and lateral cords of the brachial plexus. The lateral cord then continues downward as the **musculocutaneous nerve**, whereas the medial cord becomes the **ulnar nerve** distal to the axilla.

(3) At the origin of the median nerve, its two roots and the musculocutaneous and ulnar nerves combine to form an outline that resembles the letter M.

(4) Neither the ulnar nor the median nerve gives off branches in the arm region.

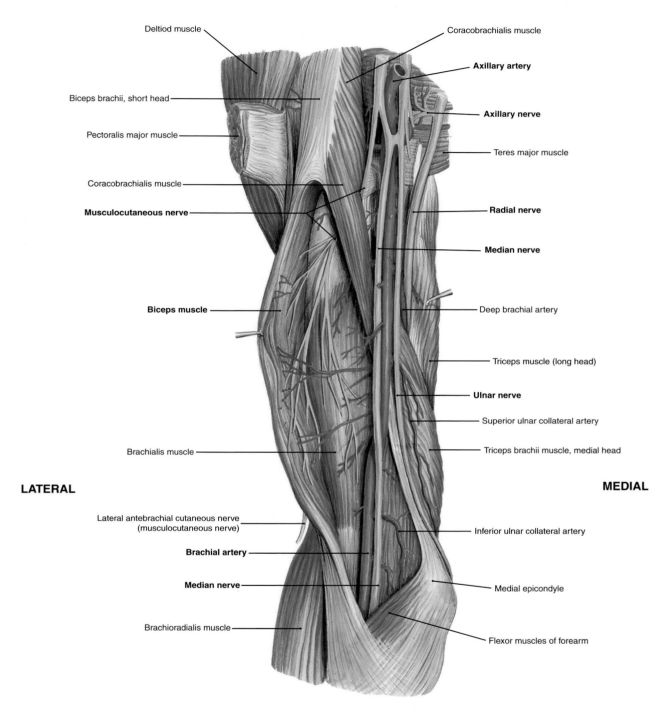

Deltiod muscle

Biceps brachii, short head

Pectoralis major muscle

Coracobrachialis muscle

Musculocutaneous nerve

Biceps muscle

Brachialis muscle

Lateral antebrachial cutaneous nerve
(musculocutaneous nerve)

Brachial artery

Median nerve

Brachioradialis muscle

Coracobrachialis muscle

Axillary artery

Axillary nerve

Teres major muscle

Radial nerve

Median nerve

Deep brachial artery

Triceps muscle (long head)

Ulnar nerve

Superior ulnar collateral artery

Triceps brachii muscle, medial head

Inferior ulnar collateral artery

Medial epicondyle

Flexor muscles of forearm

LATERAL

MEDIAL

FIGURE 59 **Nerves and Arteries of the Anterior Right Arm (Deep Dissection)**

NOTE: (1) The musculocutaneous nerve descends from the lateral cord and perforates the coracobrachialis muscle, which it supplies.

(2) The short head of the biceps muscle has been pulled aside to reveal the musculocutaneous nerve more deeply between the biceps and brachialis muscles, both of which it supplies. This nerve continues into the forearm as the **lateral antebrachial cutaneous nerve**.

(3) The superficial course of the brachial artery in the arm. Its branches include the profunda (deep) brachial artery and the superior and inferior ulnar collateral arteries, in addition to its muscular branches.

PLATE 60 **Posterior Dissection of Shoulder and Arm: Muscles**

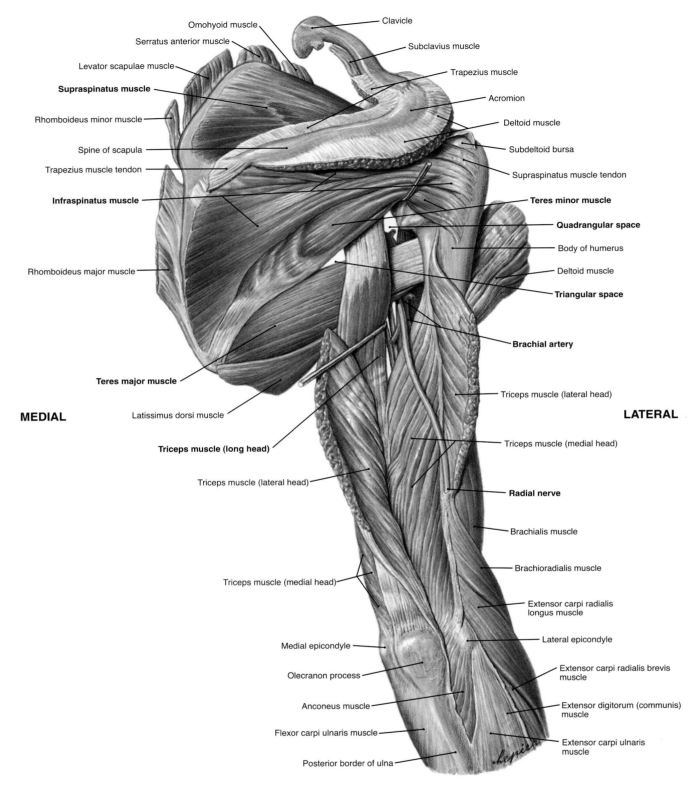

Omohyoid muscle

Clavicle

Serratus anterior muscle

Subclavius muscle

Levator scapulae muscle

Trapezius muscle

Supraspinatus muscle

Acromion

Rhomboideus minor muscle

Deltoid muscle

Spine of scapula

Subdeltoid bursa

Trapezius muscle tendon

Supraspinatus muscle tendon

Infraspinatus muscle

Teres minor muscle

Quadrangular space

Body of humerus

Deltoid muscle

Rhomboideus major muscle

Triangular space

Brachial artery

Triceps muscle (lateral head)

Teres major muscle

MEDIAL

LATERAL

Latissimus dorsi muscle

Triceps muscle (medial head)

Triceps muscle (long head)

Radial nerve

Triceps muscle (lateral head)

Brachialis muscle

Brachioradialis muscle

Triceps muscle (medial head)

Extensor carpi radialis
longus muscle

Medial epicondyle

Lateral epicondyle

Olecranon process

Extensor carpi radialis brevis
muscle

Anconeus muscle

Extensor digitorum (communis)
muscle

Flexor carpi ulnaris muscle

Extensor carpi ulnaris
muscle

Posterior border of ulna

FIGURE 60 **Muscles of the Right Shoulder and Deep Arm (Posterior View)**

NOTE: (1) The deltoid muscle and the lateral head of the triceps have been severed, thereby exposing the course of the radial nerve in the upper arm.

(2) The sequential insertions of the supraspinatus, infraspinatus, and teres minor on the greater tubercle of the humerus.

(3) The boundaries of the quadrangular space: **medial**, long head of triceps; **lateral**, the humerus; **superior**, teres minor; and **inferior**, teres major. The axillary nerve and posterior humeral circumflex vessels course through the space.

(4) The boundaries of the triangular space: **superior**, teres minor; **inferior**, teres major; and **lateral**, long head of triceps. The circumflex scapular vessels course through the space.

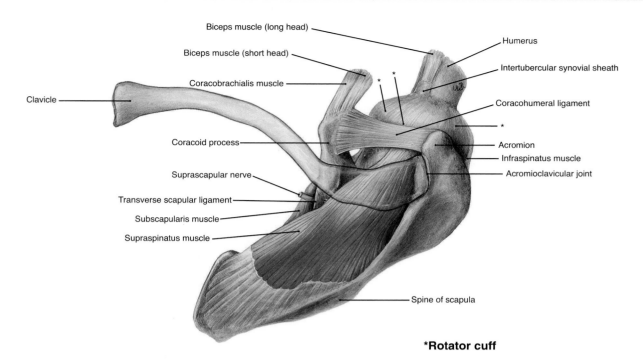

*Rotator cuff

FIGURE 61.1 **The Supraspinatus Muscle Inserting into the Rotator Cuff Tendinous Capsule**

NOTE: (1) The supraspinatus muscle located in the supraspinatus fossa (above the scapular spine) coursing laterally to the head of the humerus.
(2) The tendon of the supraspinatus muscle participates in the formation of the **rotator cuff** (indicated by the asterisks [*]). This is the musculo-tendinous capsule surrounding the head of the humerus.

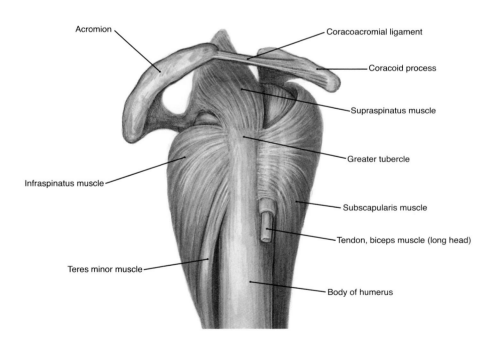

FIGURE 61.2 **Rotator Cuff Muscles (Lateral View of the Humeral Head)**

NOTE: (1) The four muscles—**supraspinatus**, **infraspinatus**, **teres minor**, and **subscapularis**—have tendons of insertion on the head of the humerus. These form a musculotendinous capsule called the **rotator cuff**.
(2) The supraspinatus approaches the humerus superiorly, the infraspinatus and teres minor anteriorly, and the subscapularis posteriorly.

PLATE 62 Muscles on the Lateral and Posterior Aspects of the Arm

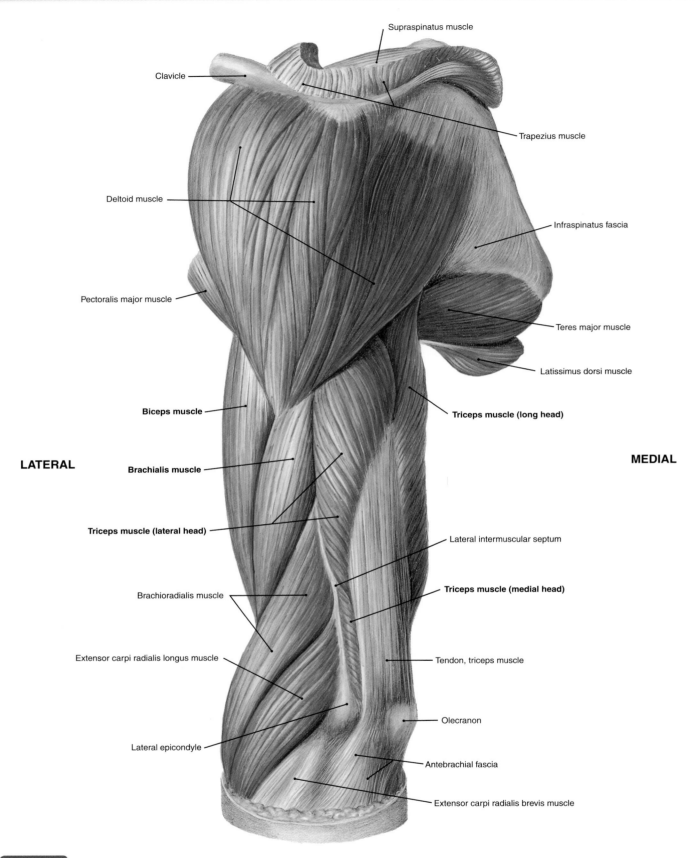

Supraspinatus muscle

Clavicle

Trapezius muscle

Deltoid muscle

Infraspinatus fascia

Pectoralis major muscle

Teres major muscle

Latissimus dorsi muscle

Biceps muscle

Triceps muscle (long head)

LATERAL

MEDIAL

Brachialis muscle

Triceps muscle (lateral head)

Lateral intermuscular septum

Triceps muscle (medial head)

Brachioradialis muscle

Extensor carpi radialis longus muscle

Tendon, triceps muscle

Olecranon

Lateral epicondyle

Antebrachial fascia

Extensor carpi radialis brevis muscle

FIGURE 62 **Muscles of the Arm (Lateral View)**

NOTE: (1) The deltoid muscle acting as a whole abducts the arm. The clavicular portion flexes and medially rotates the arm, whereas the scapular part extends and laterally rotates the arm.

(2) The lateral intermuscular septum separates the anterior muscular compartment from the posterior muscular compartment.

(3) The sequential origin of the brachioradialis and extensor carpi radialis longus from the humerus above the lateral epicondyle; the extensor carpi radialis brevis arises directly from the lateral epicondyle.

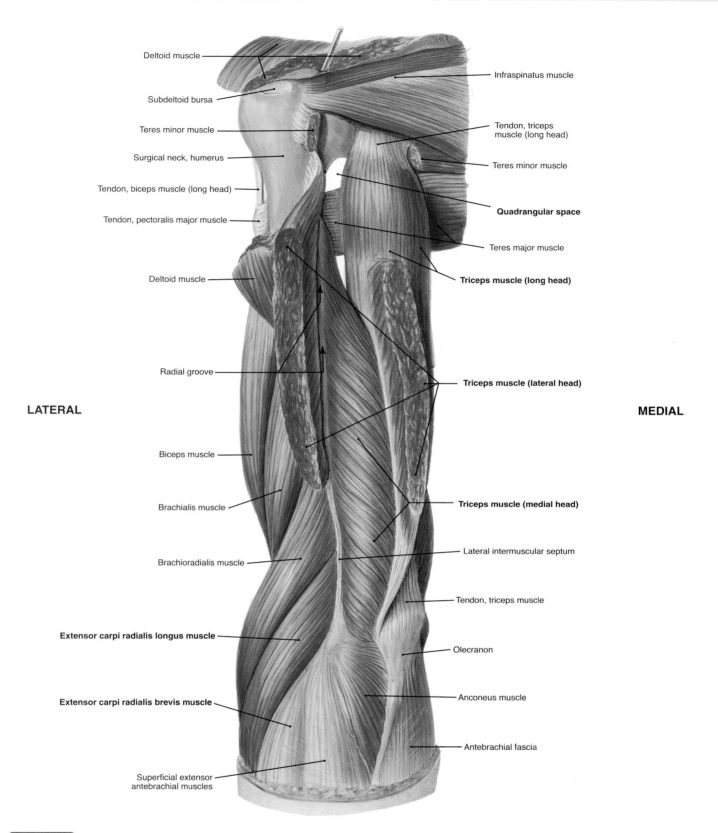

Deltoid muscle

Subdeltoid bursa

Teres minor muscle

Surgical neck, humerus

Tendon, biceps muscle (long head)

Tendon, pectoralis major muscle

Deltoid muscle

Radial groove

LATERAL

Biceps muscle

Brachialis muscle

Brachioradialis muscle

Extensor carpi radialis longus muscle

Extensor carpi radialis brevis muscle

Superficial extensor antebrachial muscles

Infraspinatus muscle

Tendon, triceps muscle (long head)

Teres minor muscle

Quadrangular space

Teres major muscle

Triceps muscle (long head)

Triceps muscle (lateral head)

MEDIAL

Triceps muscle (medial head)

Lateral intermuscular septum

Tendon, triceps muscle

Olecranon

Anconeus muscle

Antebrachial fascia

FIGURE 63 Deep Muscles of the Arm and Shoulder (Posterior View)

NOTE: (1) Much of the deltoid and teres minor muscles has been removed in this dissection, and the lateral head of the triceps muscle was transected and reflected. Observe the radial groove between the medial and lateral heads of the triceps.
(2) The broad origin of the medial and lateral heads of the triceps from the posterior surface of the humerus (see Fig. 65).

PLATE 64 Attachments of Muscles in Upper Limb: Anterior View

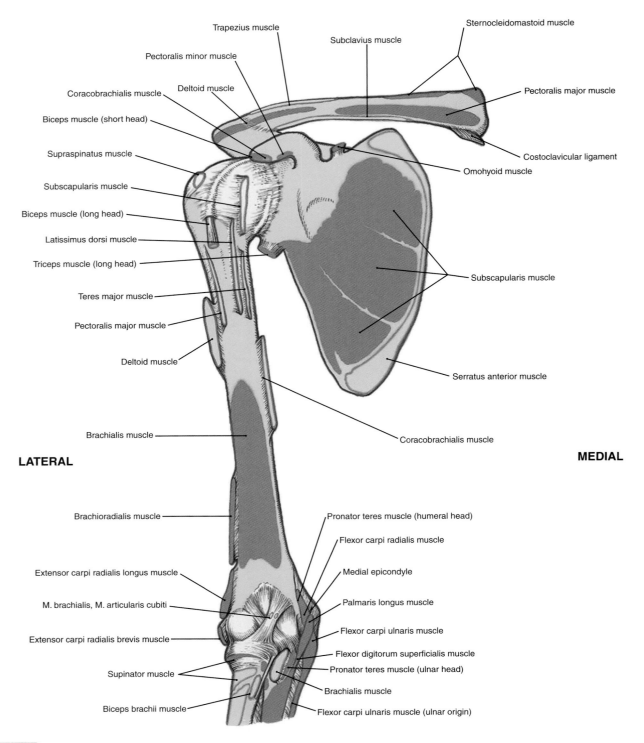

FIGURE 64 Anterior View of Bones of the Upper Limb (Including the Proximal End of the Radius and Ulna) Showing Attachments of Muscles

NOTE: (1) The broad **origin** of the subscapularis muscle in the subscapular fossa of the scapula. Its **insertion** on the lesser tubercle of the humerus is proximal to the insertions of the latissimus dorsi and teres major muscles.

(2) The biceps muscle extends across both the shoulder and elbow joints, but the coracobrachialis muscle crosses only the shoulder joint.

(3) The tendon of the long head of the biceps commences within the capsule of the shoulder joint and immediately becomes enclosed within a sheath formed by the synovial membrane of the joint.

(4) Upon emerging from the joint capsule, the tendon of the long head of the biceps descends in the intertubercular sulcus (bicipital groove). Inflammation of the synovial sheath of this tendon within the sulcus can be exceedingly painful because the tendon is closely bound to bone in this region.

(5) The latissimus dorsi and teres major insert on the humerus medial to the tendon of the long head of the biceps, whereas the pectoralis major inserts lateral to it.

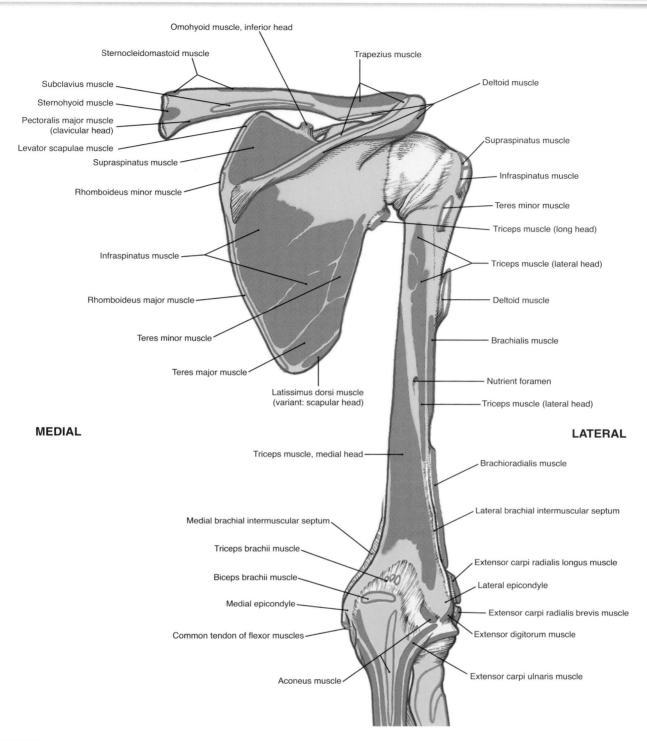

Omohyoid muscle, inferior head

Sternocleidomastoid muscle

Trapezius muscle

Subclavius muscle

Sternohyoid muscle

Pectoralis major muscle
(clavicular head)

Levator scapulae muscle

Supraspinatus muscle

Rhomboideus minor muscle

Deltoid muscle

Supraspinatus muscle

Infraspinatus muscle

Teres minor muscle

Triceps muscle (long head)

Infraspinatus muscle

Triceps muscle (lateral head)

Rhomboideus major muscle

Deltoid muscle

Teres minor muscle

Brachialis muscle

Teres major muscle

Nutrient foramen

Latissimus dorsi muscle
(variant: scapular head)

Triceps muscle (lateral head)

MEDIAL

LATERAL

Triceps muscle, medial head

Brachioradialis muscle

Medial brachial intermuscular septum

Lateral brachial intermuscular septum

Triceps brachii muscle

Biceps brachii muscle

Extensor carpi radialis longus muscle

Medial epicondyle

Lateral epicondyle

Common tendon of flexor muscles

Extensor carpi radialis brevis muscle

Extensor digitorum muscle

Aconeus muscle

Extensor carpi ulnaris muscle

FIGURE 65 **Posterior View of the Bones of the Upper Limb Showing Attachments of Muscles**

NOTE the attachments of the supraspinatus, infraspinatus, teres minor, teres major, and the three heads of the triceps muscle. For the triceps, see below.

Muscle	Origin	Insertion	Innervation	Action
Triceps brachii	**Long head:** Infraglenoid tubercle of the scapula. **Lateral head:** Posterior surface and lateral border of the humerus and the lateral intermuscular septum. **Medial head:** Posterior surface and medial border of the humerus and the medial intermuscular septum.	Posterior part of the olecranon process of the ulna and the deep fascia of the dorsal forearm	Radial nerve (C7, C8)	All three heads extend the forearm at the elbow joint; the long head also extends the humerus at the shoulder joint

PLATE 66 **Posterior Arm: Vessels and Nerves (Superficial Dissection)**

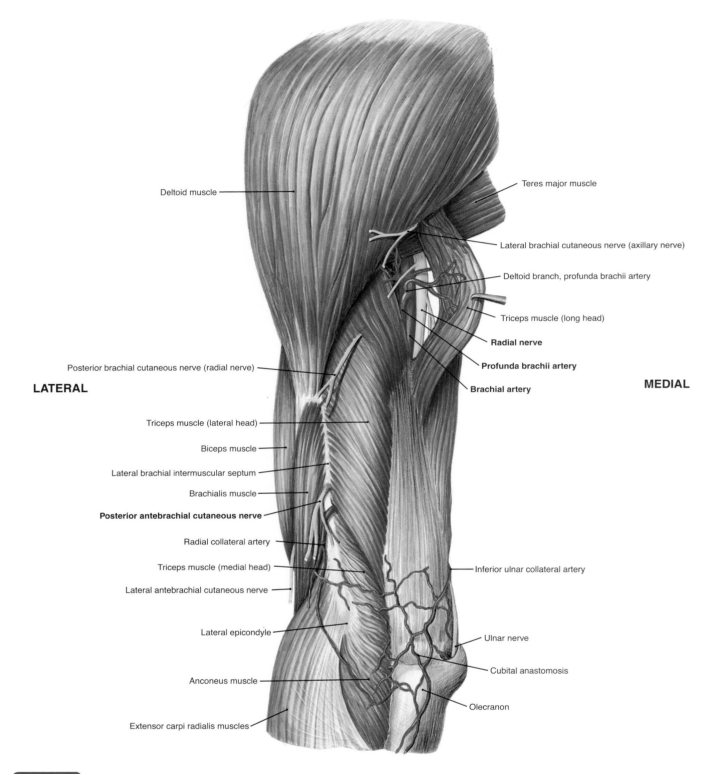

Deltoid muscle

Teres major muscle

Lateral brachial cutaneous nerve (axillary nerve)

Deltoid branch, profunda brachii artery

Triceps muscle (long head)

Radial nerve

Profunda brachii artery

Posterior brachial cutaneous nerve (radial nerve)

LATERAL

Brachial artery

MEDIAL

Triceps muscle (lateral head)

Biceps muscle

Lateral brachial intermuscular septum

Brachialis muscle

Posterior antebrachial cutaneous nerve

Radial collateral artery

Triceps muscle (medial head)

Inferior ulnar collateral artery

Lateral antebrachial cutaneous nerve

Lateral epicondyle

Ulnar nerve

Cubital anastomosis

Anconeus muscle

Olecranon

Extensor carpi radialis muscles

FIGURE 66 **Nerves and Arteries of the Left Posterior Arm (Superficial Branches)**

NOTE: (1) The origin of the profunda brachii artery from the brachial artery and its relationship to the radial nerve. The long head of the triceps has been pulled medially.

(2) The relationship of the ulnar nerve to the olecranon process and the vascular anastomosis around the elbow.

(3) Both the posterior brachial and posterior antebrachial nerves of the radial nerve perforate the lateral head of the triceps muscle to reach the superficial fascia and skin.

(4) The site of attachment of the deltoid muscle on the humerus, and the relationship of this attachment to the uppermost fibers of the brachialis muscle, the lateral intermuscular septum, and the lateral head of the triceps muscle (see Fig. 63).

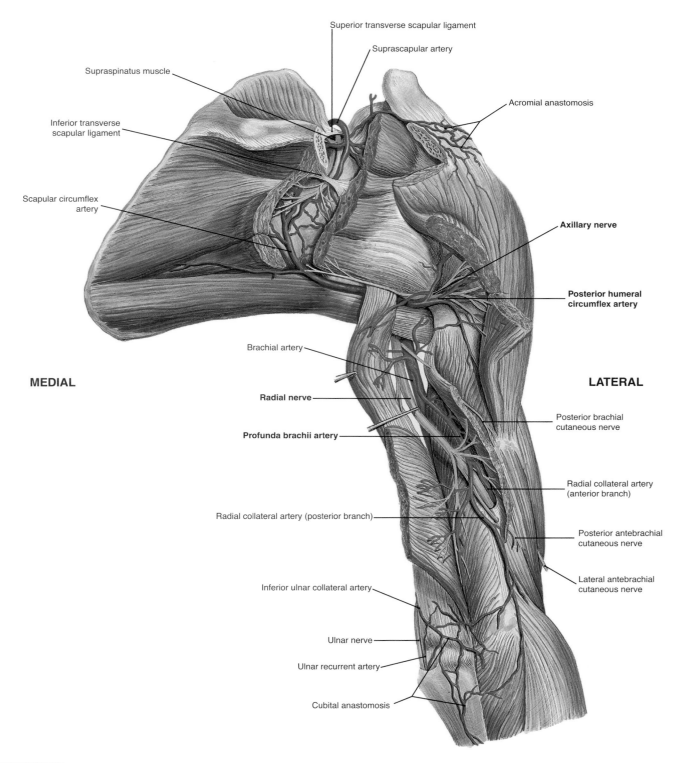

Superior transverse scapular ligament

Suprascapular artery

Supraspinatus muscle

Acromial anastomosis

Inferior transverse scapular ligament

Scapular circumflex artery

Axillary nerve

Posterior humeral circumflex artery

Brachial artery

MEDIAL

LATERAL

Radial nerve

Posterior brachial cutaneous nerve

Profunda brachii artery

Radial collateral artery (anterior branch)

Radial collateral artery (posterior branch)

Posterior antebrachial cutaneous nerve

Lateral antebrachial cutaneous nerve

Inferior ulnar collateral artery

Ulnar nerve

Ulnar recurrent artery

Cubital anastomosis

FIGURE 67 Deep Nerves and Arteries of the Shoulder and Posterior Brachial Regions

NOTE: (1) The course of the axillary nerve and posterior humeral circumflex artery through the quadrangular space to reach the deltoid and dorsal shoulder region.

(2) The course of the radial nerve and profunda brachii artery along the radial (spiral) groove to the posterior brachial region. This groove lies along the body of the humerus between the origins of the lateral and medial heads of the triceps muscle.

(3) The common insertion of the three heads of the triceps muscle onto the olecranon process of the ulna.

(4) In addition to a **deltoid branch**, which anastomoses with the posterior humeral circumflex artery and helps supply the long head of the triceps along with the deltoid muscle, the profunda brachii artery gives off the **middle and radial collateral arteries**.

(5) The latter two vessels and the **superior and inferior ulnar collateral** branches of the brachial artery are the four descending vessels that participate in the anastomosis around the elbow joint (see Fig. 66).

PLATE 68 **Superficial Dissection of the Anterior Forearm**

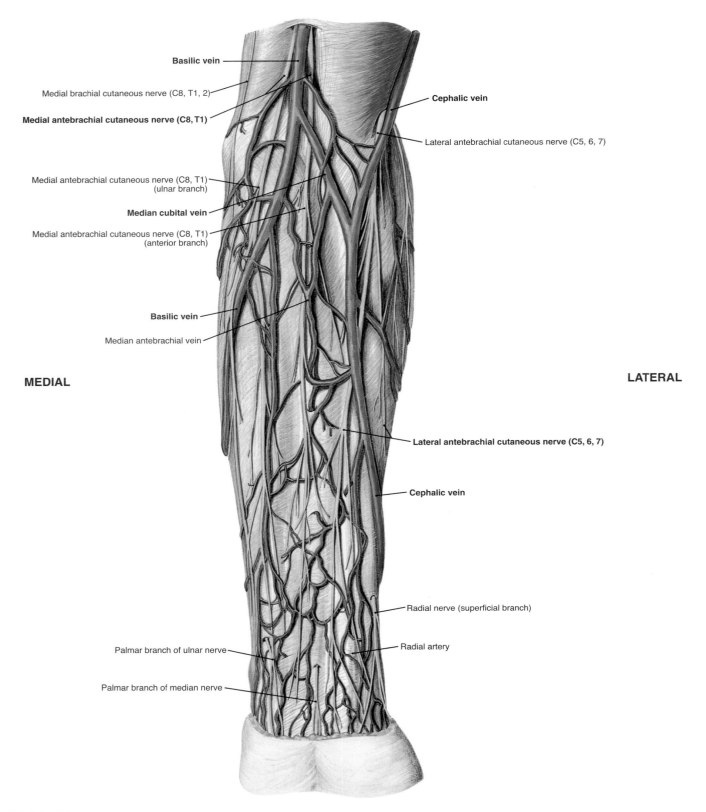

Basilic vein

Medial brachial cutaneous nerve (C8, T1, 2)

Medial antebrachial cutaneous nerve (C8, T1)

Medial antebrachial cutaneous nerve (C8, T1)
(ulnar branch)

Median cubital vein

Medial antebrachial cutaneous nerve (C8, T1)
(anterior branch)

Basilic vein

Median antebrachial vein

MEDIAL

Cephalic vein

Lateral antebrachial cutaneous nerve (C5, 6, 7)

LATERAL

Lateral antebrachial cutaneous nerve (C5, 6, 7)

Cephalic vein

Radial nerve (superficial branch)

Radial artery

Palmar branch of ulnar nerve

Palmar branch of median nerve

FIGURE 68 **Forearm; Superficial Veins and Cutaneous Nerves of Left Upper Limb (Anterior Surface)**

NOTE: (1) The median cubital vein joins the cephalic and basilic veins in the cubital fossa.
(2) The main sensory nerves of the anterior forearm are the medial antebrachial cutaneous nerve (derived from the medial cord of the brachial plexus) and the lateral antebrachial cutaneous nerve, which is a continuation of the musculocutaneous nerve.
(3) The medial antebrachial cutaneous nerve courses with the basilic vein, while the lateral antebrachial cutaneous nerve lies next to the cephalic vein at the elbow.

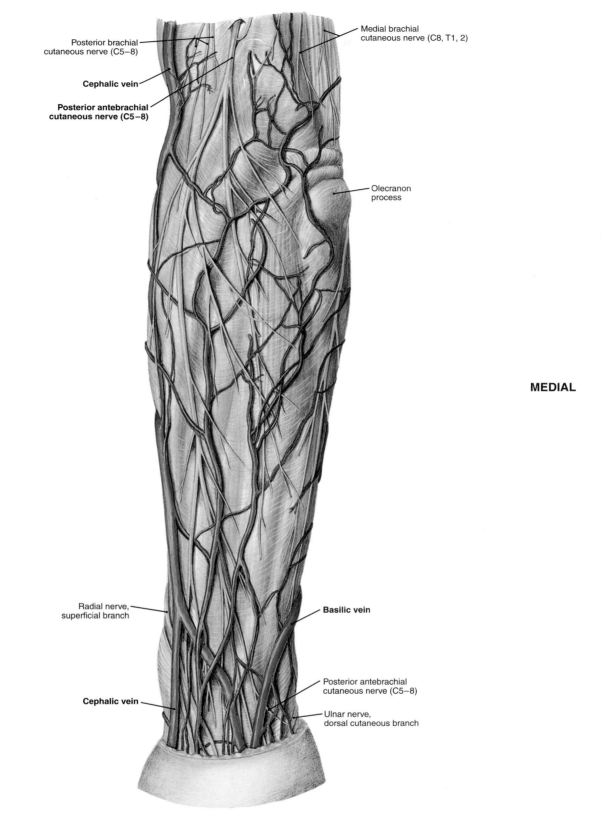

Posterior brachial
cutaneous nerve (C5–8)

Cephalic vein

**Posterior antebrachial
cutaneous nerve (C5–8)**

Medial brachial
cutaneous nerve (C8, T1, 2)

Olecranon
process

LATERAL

MEDIAL

Radial nerve,
superficial branch

Cephalic vein

Basilic vein

Posterior antebrachial
cutaneous nerve (C5–8)

Ulnar nerve,
dorsal cutaneous branch

FIGURE 69 **Forearm; Superficial Veins and Cutaneous Nerves of the Left Upper Limb (Posterior Surface)**

NOTE: (1) Branches of the radial nerve (posterior antebrachial cutaneous and superficial radial) contribute the principal innervation to the skin on the posterior aspect of the forearm.

(2) At the wrist, the dorsal branch of the ulnar nerve passes backward onto the dorsal surfaces of the wrist and hand.

(3) The basilic vein arises on the ulnar (or medial) side of the dorsum of the hand and wrist, while the cephalic vein arises on the radial (lateral) side.

PLATE 70 **Anterior Forearm: Superficial Muscles**

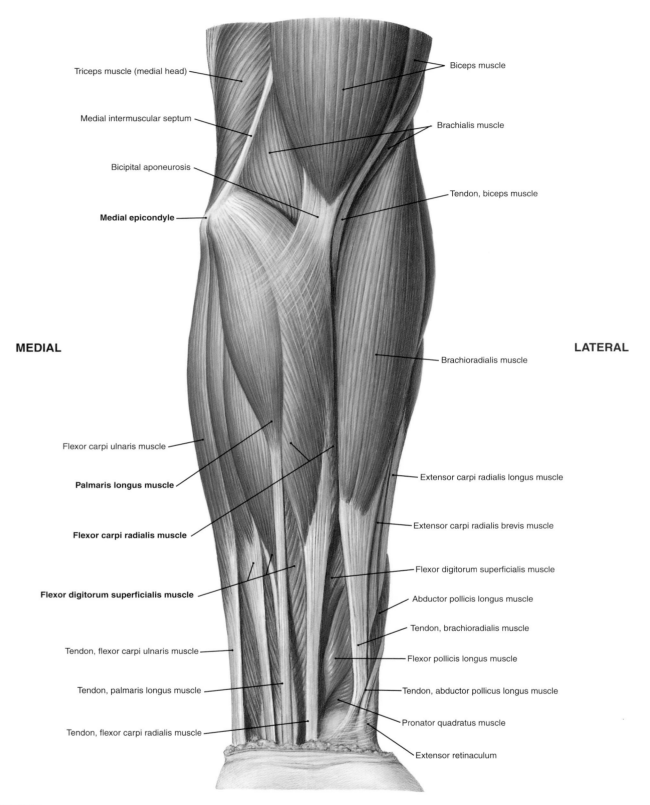

Triceps muscle (medial head)

Biceps muscle

Medial intermuscular septum

Brachialis muscle

Bicipital aponeurosis

Tendon, biceps muscle

Medial epicondyle

MEDIAL

LATERAL

Brachioradialis muscle

Flexor carpi ulnaris muscle

Palmaris longus muscle

Extensor carpi radialis longus muscle

Flexor carpi radialis muscle

Extensor carpi radialis brevis muscle

Flexor digitorum superficialis muscle

Flexor digitorum superficialis muscle

Abductor pollicis longus muscle

Tendon, brachioradialis muscle

Tendon, flexor carpi ulnaris muscle

Flexor pollicis longus muscle

Tendon, palmaris longus muscle

Tendon, abductor pollicus longus muscle

Tendon, flexor carpi radialis muscle

Pronator quadratus muscle

Extensor retinaculum

FIGURE 70 **Left Anterior Forearm Muscles, Superficial Group**

NOTE: (1) The brachioradialis muscle is studied with the posterior forearm muscles and is not included with the flexor muscles of the anterior forearm.

(2) The anterior forearm muscles arise from the medial epicondyle of the humerus and include the pronator teres (not labeled, see Fig. 76), **flexor carpi radialis**, **palmaris longus**, and **flexor carpi ulnaris**. Beneath these is the **flexor digitorum superficialis**.

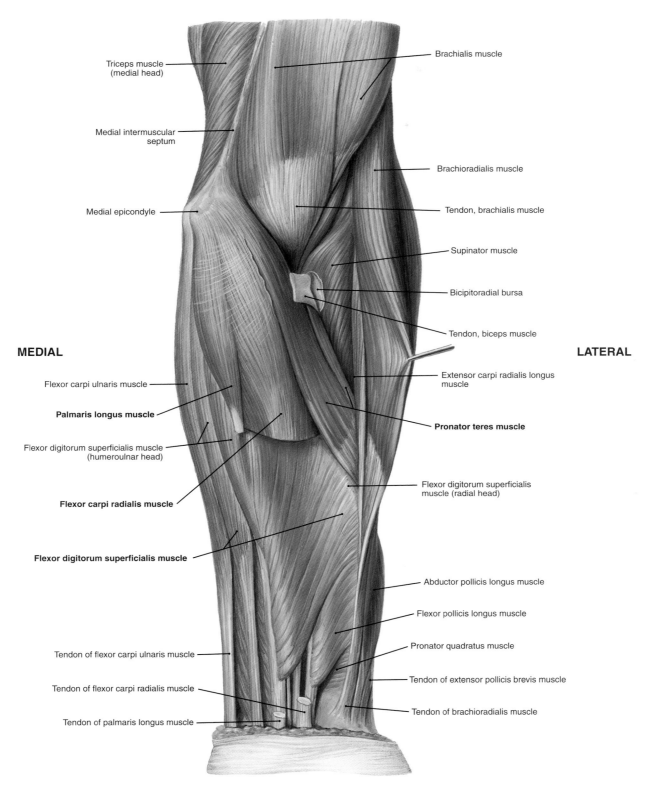

Triceps muscle (medial head)

Medial intermuscular septum

Medial epicondyle

MEDIAL

Flexor carpi ulnaris muscle

Palmaris longus muscle

Flexor digitorum superficialis muscle (humeroulnar head)

Flexor carpi radialis muscle

Flexor digitorum superficialis muscle

Tendon of flexor carpi ulnaris muscle

Tendon of flexor carpi radialis muscle

Tendon of palmaris longus muscle

Brachialis muscle

Brachioradialis muscle

Tendon, brachialis muscle

Supinator muscle

Bicipitoradial bursa

Tendon, biceps muscle

LATERAL

Extensor carpi radialis longus muscle

Pronator teres muscle

Flexor digitorum superficialis muscle (radial head)

Abductor pollicis longus muscle

Flexor pollicis longus muscle

Pronator quadratus muscle

Tendon of extensor pollicis brevis muscle

Tendon of brachioradialis muscle

FIGURE 71 Flexor Digitorum Superficialis Muscle and Related Muscles (Left)

NOTE: (1) The palmaris longus, flexor carpi radialis, and insertion of the biceps have been cut to reveal the flexor digitorum superficialis and pronator teres.

(2) The triangular cubital fossa is bounded medially by the superficial flexors and laterally by the extensors. Its floor is the brachialis muscle.

(3) The pronator teres arises by two heads: a larger **humeral head** from the medial epicondyle and a much smaller **ulnar head** from the coronoid process. It crosses the forearm obliquely to insert on the shaft of the radius.

(4) The flexor digitorum superficialis arises broadly from the humerus and ulna medially (humeral–ulnar head) and from the anterior border of the radius laterally (radial head).

PLATE 72 Anterior Forearm: Deep Muscles

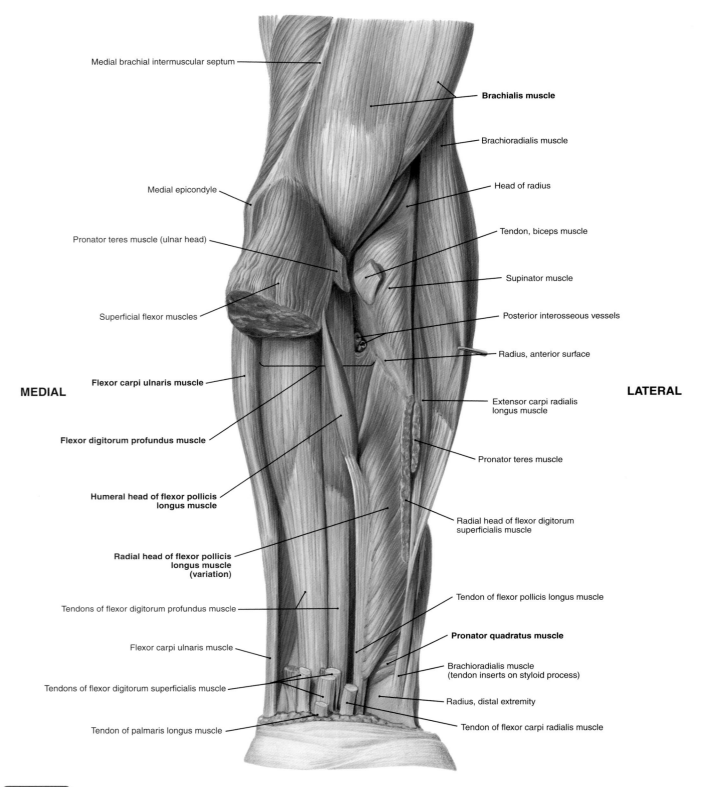

Medial brachial intermuscular septum

Brachialis muscle

Brachioradialis muscle

Medial epicondyle

Head of radius

Pronator teres muscle (ulnar head)

Tendon, biceps muscle

Supinator muscle

Superficial flexor muscles

Posterior interosseous vessels

Radius, anterior surface

Flexor carpi ulnaris muscle

MEDIAL

LATERAL

Extensor carpi radialis longus muscle

Flexor digitorum profundus muscle

Pronator teres muscle

Humeral head of flexor pollicis longus muscle

Radial head of flexor digitorum superficialis muscle

Radial head of flexor pollicis longus muscle (variation)

Tendon of flexor pollicis longus muscle

Tendons of flexor digitorum profundus muscle

Pronator quadratus muscle

Flexor carpi ulnaris muscle

Brachioradialis muscle (tendon inserts on styloid process)

Tendons of flexor digitorum superficialis muscle

Radius, distal extremity

Tendon of palmaris longus muscle

Tendon of flexor carpi radialis muscle

FIGURE 72 **Left Anterior Forearm Muscles, Deep Group**

NOTE: (1) The superficial anterior forearm muscles have been removed to reveal the three muscles of the deep group: the flexor digitorum profundus, the flexor pollicis longus, and the pronator quadratus.

(2) The pronator quadratus is a small quadrangular muscle situated at the distal end of the forearm beneath the tendons of the flexor digitorum profundus and flexor pollicis longus. It is partially shown in this dissection and can be seen better in Figs. 84.1 and 99.1.

(3) In this drawing, the tendons of the flexor digitorum profundus to the ring and little fingers and those to the middle and index fingers appear fused at the wrist, as if they were two structures rather than four.

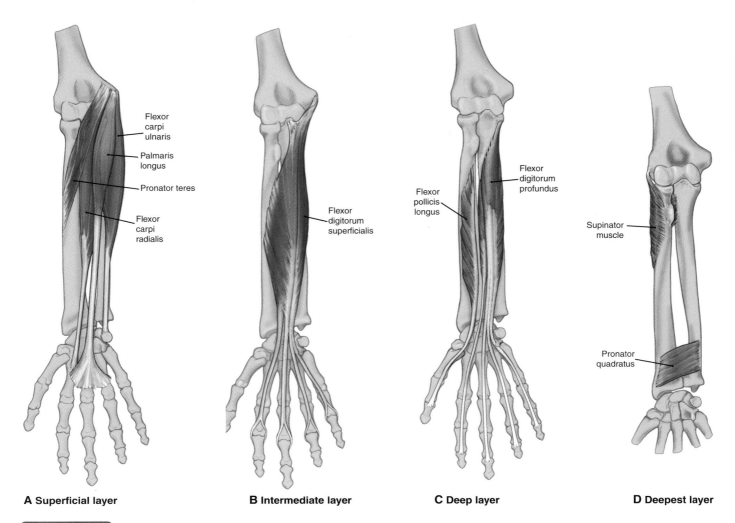

A Superficial layer   **B Intermediate layer**   **C Deep layer**   **D Deepest layer**

FIGURE 73A–D **Anterior Muscles of the Forearm**

NOTE that the supinator muscle shown in **D** is usually classified with the dorsal forearm muscles.

FLEXOR MUSCLES OF FOREARM: SUPERFICIAL GROUP				
Muscle	**Origin**	**Insertion**	**Innervation**	**Action**
Pronator teres	**Humeral head:** Medial epicondyle of humerus. **Ulnar head:** Coronoid process of ulna	Midway along the lateral surface of the radius	Median nerve (C6, C7) (enters the forearm by passing between the two heads)	Pronates and flexes the forearm
Flexor carpi radialis	Medial epicondyle of humerus	Base of the second metacarpal bone	Median nerve (C6, C7)	Flexes the hand at the wrist joint; abducts the hand (radially deviates the hand)
Palmaris longus	Medial epicondyle of humerus	Anterior flexor retinaculum and the palmar aponeurosis	Median nerve (C6, C7)	Flexes the hand at the wrist and tenses the palmar aponeurosis
Flexor digitorum superficialis	**Humeroulnar head:** Medial epicondyle of humerus and the coronoid process of ulna **Radial head:** Anterior surface of the radius below the radial tuberosity	By four long tendons onto the sides of the middle phalanx of the four medial fingers	Median nerve (C7, C8, T1)	Flexes the middle and proximal phalanges of the four medial fingers; also flexes the wrist
Flexor carpi ulnaris	**Humeral head:** Medial epicondyle of humerus **Ulnar head:** Medial margin of olecranon, and upper posterior border of ulna	Pisiform bone and by ligaments to the hamate and fifth metacarpal bone	Ulnar nerve (C7, C8)	Flexes the hand at the wrist joint; adducts the hand (ulnar deviates the hand) **(see also Fig. 72)**

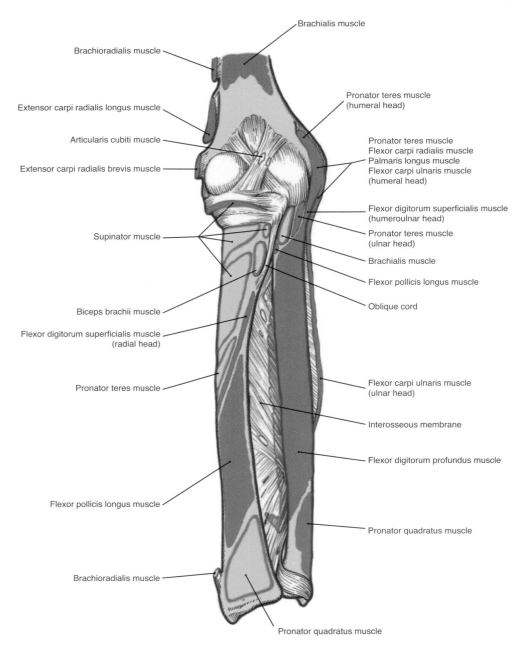

Brachialis muscle

Brachioradialis muscle

Pronator teres muscle
(humeral head)

Extensor carpi radialis longus muscle

Articularis cubiti muscle

Pronator teres muscle
Flexor carpi radialis muscle
Palmaris longus muscle
Flexor carpi ulnaris muscle
(humeral head)

Extensor carpi radialis brevis muscle

Flexor digitorum superficialis muscle
(humeroulnar head)

Pronator teres muscle
(ulnar head)

Supinator muscle

Brachialis muscle

Flexor pollicis longus muscle

Biceps brachii muscle

Oblique cord

Flexor digitorum superficialis muscle
(radial head)

Flexor carpi ulnaris muscle
(ulnar head)

Pronator teres muscle

Interosseous membrane

Flexor digitorum profundus muscle

Flexor pollicis longus muscle

Pronator quadratus muscle

Brachioradialis muscle

Pronator quadratus muscle

FIGURE 74 Muscle Attachments on the Anterior Surface of the Radius and Ulna

NOTE that muscle **origins** are **solid color areas**, while muscle **insertions** are the **open areas** surrounded by red lines.

FLEXOR MUSCLES OF THE FOREARM: DEEP GROUP				
Muscle	**Origin**	**Insertion**	**Innervation**	**Action**
Flexor digitorum profundus	Upper three-fourths of the anterior and medial aspects of the ulna and the ulnar half of the interosseous membrane	Anterior surface of the base of the distal phalanx of the four medial fingers	Median nerve by its interosseous branch; and the ulnar nerve (C8, T1)	Flexes the distal phalanx of the four medial fingers and also flexes the hand at the wrist
Flexor pollicis longus	**Radial head:** Anterior surface of radius and the adjacent part of the interosseous membrane. **Humeral head:** Medial epicondyle of humerus or the coronoid process of the ulna	Base of the distal phalanx of the thumb	Median nerve by its interosseous branch (C8, T1)	Flexes the distal phalanx and helps in flexing the proximal phalanx of the thumb
Pronator quadratus	Distal fourth of anterior surface of the ulna	Distal fourth of anterior surface of the radius	Median nerve by its interosseous branch (C8, T1)	Pronates the hand

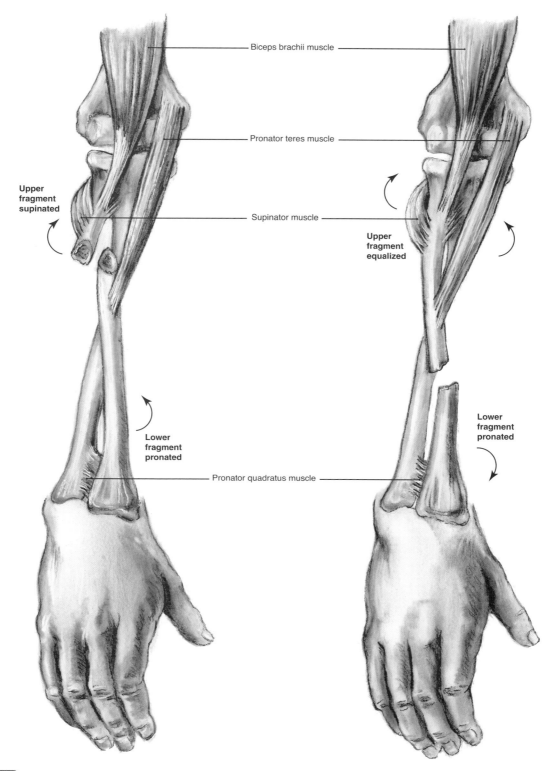

A

B

FIGURE 75A, B **Fracture Site of the Radius Relative to the Pronator Teres Muscle**

NOTE: The pronator teres muscle is important with respect to fractures of the radius.

(1) In **A:** When the fracture is superior to the insertion of the pronator teres, the upper fragment of the radius is pulled into supination by the supinator muscle and the biceps brachii muscle. The inferior fragment is strongly pronated.

(2) In **B:** When the fracture is inferior to the insertion of the pronator teres, the upper fragment's position is equalized between the supinator muscle and the pronator teres muscle, while the lower fragment is fully pronated by the pronator quadratus muscle.

(From P. Thorek. *Anatomy in Surgery*. Philadelphia: J.B. Lippincott, 1958.)

PLATE 76 **Anterior Forearm Vessels and Nerves (Superficial Dissection)**

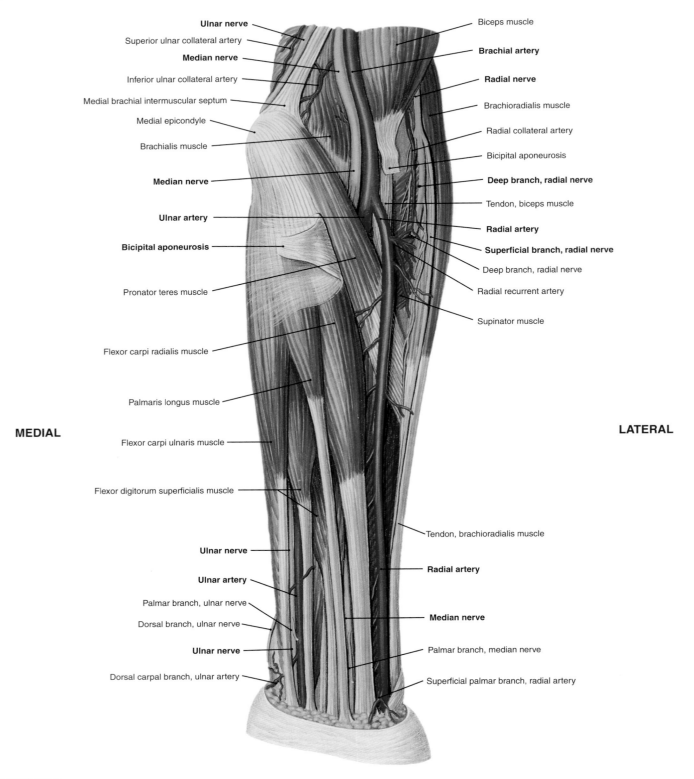

Ulnar nerve
Superior ulnar collateral artery
Median nerve
Inferior ulnar collateral artery
Medial brachial intermuscular septum
Medial epicondyle
Brachialis muscle
Median nerve
Ulnar artery
Bicipital aponeurosis
Pronator teres muscle
Flexor carpi radialis muscle
Palmaris longus muscle
Flexor carpi ulnaris muscle
Flexor digitorum superficialis muscle
Ulnar nerve
Ulnar artery
Palmar branch, ulnar nerve
Dorsal branch, ulnar nerve
Ulnar nerve
Dorsal carpal branch, ulnar artery

Biceps muscle
Brachial artery
Radial nerve
Brachioradialis muscle
Radial collateral artery
Bicipital aponeurosis
Deep branch, radial nerve
Tendon, biceps muscle
Radial artery
Superficial branch, radial nerve
Deep branch, radial nerve
Radial recurrent artery
Supinator muscle
Tendon, brachioradialis muscle
Radial artery
Median nerve
Palmar branch, median nerve
Superficial palmar branch, radial artery

MEDIAL

LATERAL

FIGURE 76 **Anterior Dissection of the Left Forearm Vessels and Nerves, Stage 1**

NOTE: (1) The bicipital aponeurosis has been reflected to reveal the underlying median nerve, brachial artery, and tendon of insertion of the biceps brachii muscle.

(2) The brachioradialis muscle has been pulled laterally (toward the radial side) to expose the course of the radial artery and the division of the radial nerve into its superficial and deep branches.

(3) The radial artery, as it descends in the forearm, courses anterior to the biceps brachii muscle, the supinator muscle, the tendon of insertion of the pronator teres, and the belly of the flexor pollicis longus (the latter is not labeled in this figure, but can be seen in Figs. 72 and 73).

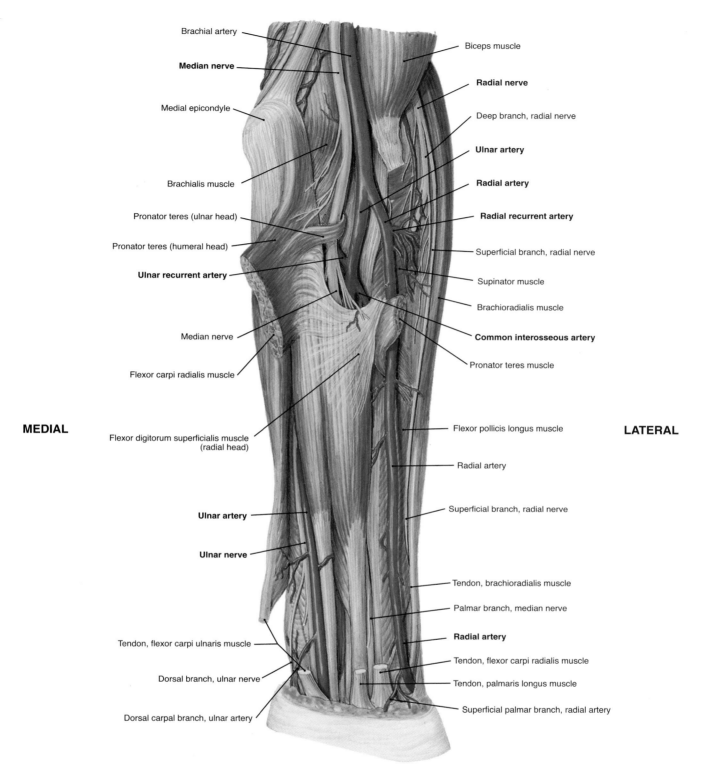

Brachial artery

Median nerve

Medial epicondyle

Brachialis muscle

Pronator teres (ulnar head)

Pronator teres (humeral head)

Ulnar recurrent artery

Median nerve

Flexor carpi radialis muscle

MEDIAL

Flexor digitorum superficialis muscle
(radial head)

Ulnar artery

Ulnar nerve

Tendon, flexor carpi ulnaris muscle

Dorsal branch, ulnar nerve

Dorsal carpal branch, ulnar artery

Biceps muscle

Radial nerve

Deep branch, radial nerve

Ulnar artery

Radial artery

Radial recurrent artery

Superficial branch, radial nerve

Supinator muscle

Brachioradialis muscle

Common interosseous artery

Pronator teres muscle

Flexor pollicis longus muscle

LATERAL

Radial artery

Superficial branch, radial nerve

Tendon, brachioradialis muscle

Palmar branch, median nerve

Radial artery

Tendon, flexor carpi radialis muscle

Tendon, palmaris longus muscle

Superficial palmar branch, radial artery

FIGURE 77 **Anterior Dissection of the Left Forearm Vessels and Nerves, Stage 2**

NOTE: (1) The pronator teres and flexor carpi radialis muscles are reflected just below the cubital fossa to show the bifurcation of the brachial artery into the ulnar and radial arteries.

(2) At the wrist, the tendon of the flexor carpi ulnaris muscle is severed and pulled aside to expose the ulnar nerve and artery.

(3) The median nerve lies deep to the flexor digitorum superficialis muscle along much of its course in the forearm, but just above the wrist it usually becomes visible between the tendons. Observe that the tendons of the flexor pollicis longus and flexor carpi radialis are on its **radial side** and the tendons of the palmaris longus and flexor digitorum superficialis are on its **ulnar side.**

PLATE 78 Anterior Forearm Vessels and Nerves (Deep Dissection)

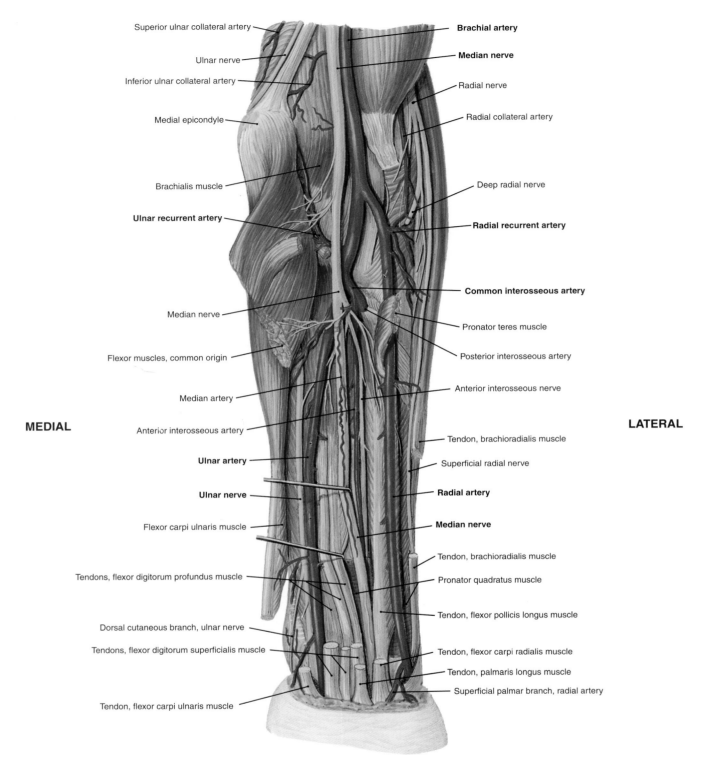

Superior ulnar collateral artery

Ulnar nerve

Inferior ulnar collateral artery

Medial epicondyle

Brachialis muscle

Ulnar recurrent artery

Median nerve

Flexor muscles, common origin

Median artery

MEDIAL

Anterior interosseous artery

Ulnar artery

Ulnar nerve

Flexor carpi ulnaris muscle

Tendons, flexor digitorum profundus muscle

Dorsal cutaneous branch, ulnar nerve

Tendons, flexor digitorum superficialis muscle

Tendon, flexor carpi ulnaris muscle

Brachial artery

Median nerve

Radial nerve

Radial collateral artery

Deep radial nerve

Radial recurrent artery

Common interosseous artery

Pronator teres muscle

Posterior interosseous artery

Anterior interosseous nerve

LATERAL

Tendon, brachioradialis muscle

Superficial radial nerve

Radial artery

Median nerve

Tendon, brachioradialis muscle

Pronator quadratus muscle

Tendon, flexor pollicis longus muscle

Tendon, flexor carpi radialis muscle

Tendon, palmaris longus muscle

Superficial palmar branch, radial artery

FIGURE 78 **Anterior Dissection of the Left Forearm Vessels and Nerves, Stage 3**

NOTE: (1) The division of the **brachial artery** into the **radial** and **ulnar arteries** at the lower end of the cubital fossa.

(2) The **common interosseous artery** branches from the **ulnar artery** and divides almost immediately into the **anterior and posterior interosseous arteries.**

(3) The courses of the ulnar and median nerves. In the lower half of the forearm, the **ulnar nerve** descends with the ulnar artery, whereas the median nerve descends in front of the anterior interosseous nerve and artery.

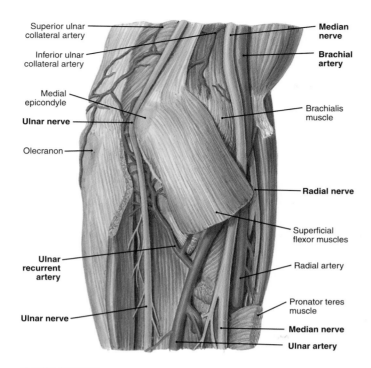

FIGURE 79.1 Nerves and Arteries at the Elbow (Medial View)

NOTE: The **ulnar nerve** enters the forearm directly behind the medial epicondyle, and at this site it is closely related to the **ulnar recurrent artery**.

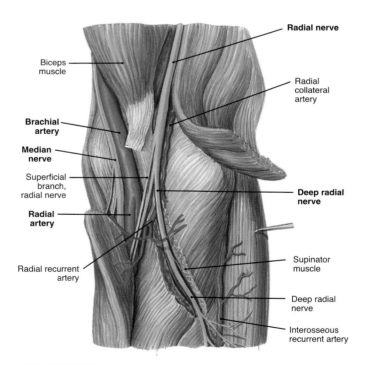

FIGURE 79.2 Nerves and Arteries at the Elbow (Lateral View)

NOTE: The **deep radial nerve** passes into the forearm in front of the lateral part of the elbow joint. It then courses dorsally through the supinator muscle to supply the posterior forearm muscles.

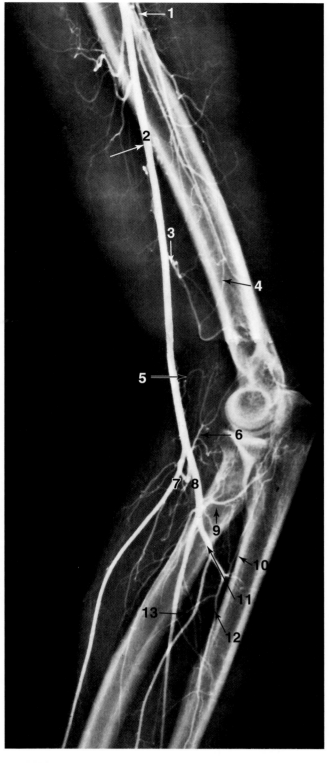

FIGURE 79.3 Brachial Arteriogram Showing the Origins of the Vessels That Supply the Elbow and Forearm

1. Profunda brachii artery
2. Brachial artery
3. Superior ulnar collateral artery
4. Radial collateral artery
5. Inferior ulnar collateral artery
6. Radial recurrent artery
7. Radial artery
8. Ulnar artery
9. Ulnar recurrent artery
10. Interosseous recurrent artery
11. Common interosseous artery
12. Posterior interosseous artery
13. Anterior interosseous artery

PLATE 80 Superficial Extensor Muscles of Forearm (Posterior View)

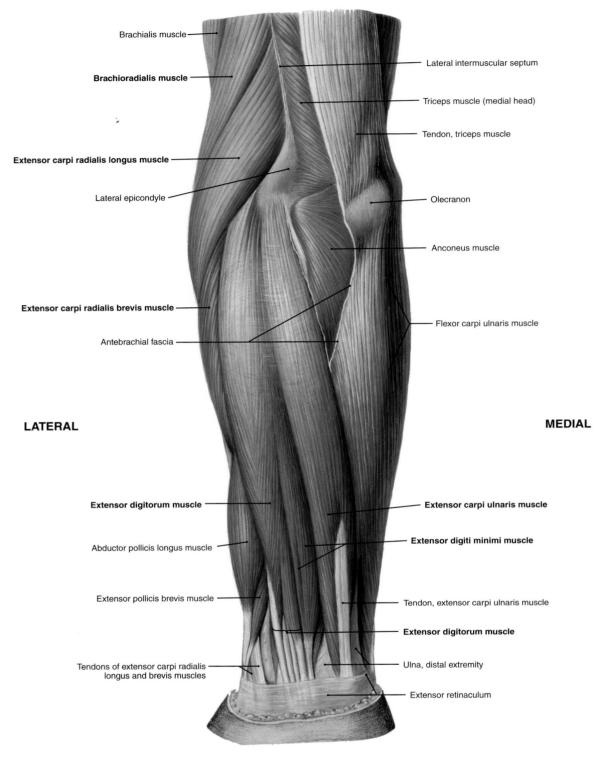

Brachialis muscle

Brachioradialis muscle

Extensor carpi radialis longus muscle

Lateral epicondyle

Extensor carpi radialis brevis muscle

Antebrachial fascia

Lateral intermuscular septum

Triceps muscle (medial head)

Tendon, triceps muscle

Olecranon

Anconeus muscle

Flexor carpi ulnaris muscle

LATERAL

MEDIAL

Extensor digitorum muscle

Abductor pollicis longus muscle

Extensor pollicis brevis muscle

Tendons of extensor carpi radialis
longus and brevis muscles

Extensor carpi ulnaris muscle

Extensor digiti minimi muscle

Tendon, extensor carpi ulnaris muscle

Extensor digitorum muscle

Ulna, distal extremity

Extensor retinaculum

FIGURE 80 Posterior Muscles of the Left Forearm, Superficial Group (Posterior View)

NOTE: The superficial radial group of extensor muscles of the forearm includes the **brachioradialis muscle** and the **extensors carpi radialis longus and brevis**.

Muscle	Origin	Insertion	Innervation	Action
Brachioradialis	Upper two-thirds of lateral supracondylar ridge of humerus	Lateral aspect of the base of the styloid process of the radius	Radial nerve (C5, C6)	Flexes the forearm when the forearm is semipronated

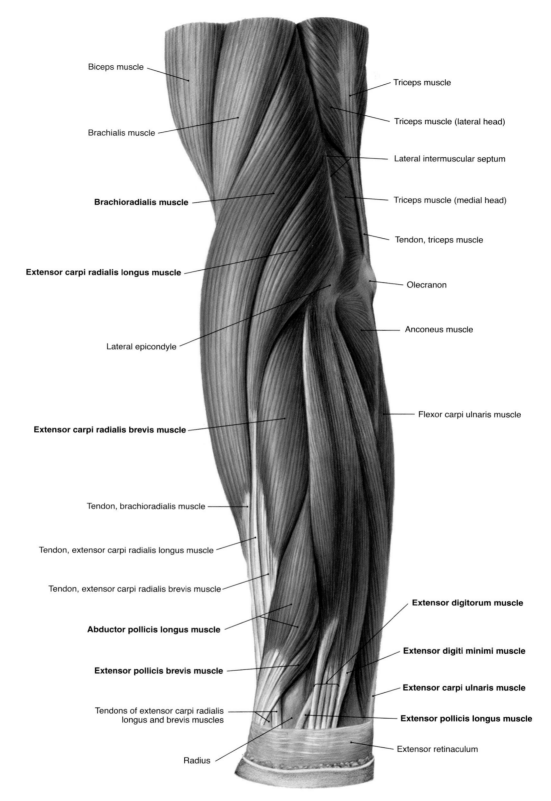

Biceps muscle

Brachialis muscle

Brachioradialis muscle

Extensor carpi radialis longus muscle

Lateral epicondyle

Extensor carpi radialis brevis muscle

Tendon, brachioradialis muscle

Tendon, extensor carpi radialis longus muscle

Tendon, extensor carpi radialis brevis muscle

Abductor pollicis longus muscle

Extensor pollicis brevis muscle

Tendons of extensor carpi radialis longus and brevis muscles

Radius

Triceps muscle

Triceps muscle (lateral head)

Lateral intermuscular septum

Triceps muscle (medial head)

Tendon, triceps muscle

Olecranon

Anconeus muscle

Flexor carpi ulnaris muscle

Extensor digitorum muscle

Extensor digiti minimi muscle

Extensor carpi ulnaris muscle

Extensor pollicis longus muscle

Extensor retinaculum

FIGURE 81 **Posterior Muscles of the Left Forearm, Superficial Group (Lateral View)**

Muscle	Origin	Insertion	Innervation	Action
Extensor carpi radialis longus	Lower third of lateral supracondylar ridge of humerus	Dorsal surface of the base of the second metacarpal bone	Radial nerve (C6, C7)	Extends the hand; abducts the hand at the wrist (radial deviation)
Extensor carpi radialis brevis	Lateral epicondyle of humerus	Dorsal surface of the base of the third metacarpal bone	Radial nerve (C6, C7)	Extends the hand; abducts the hand at the wrist (radial deviation)

PLATE 82 **Deep Extensor Muscles of the Forearm**

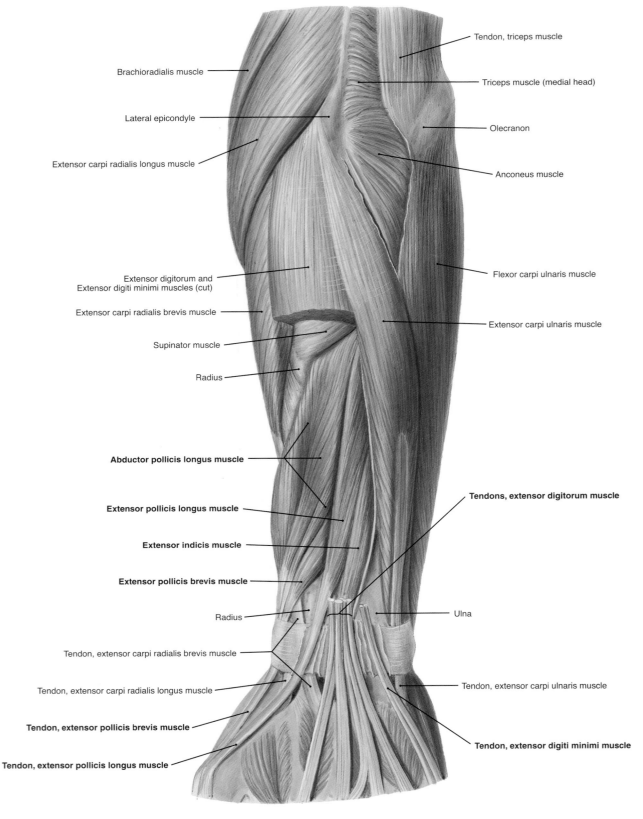

Tendon, triceps muscle

Brachioradialis muscle

Triceps muscle (medial head)

Lateral epicondyle

Olecranon

Extensor carpi radialis longus muscle

Anconeus muscle

Extensor digitorum and
Extensor digiti minimi muscles (cut)

Flexor carpi ulnaris muscle

Extensor carpi radialis brevis muscle

Extensor carpi ulnaris muscle

Supinator muscle

Radius

Abductor pollicis longus muscle

Tendons, extensor digitorum muscle

Extensor pollicis longus muscle

Extensor indicis muscle

Extensor pollicis brevis muscle

Radius

Ulna

Tendon, extensor carpi radialis brevis muscle

Tendon, extensor carpi radialis longus muscle

Tendon, extensor carpi ulnaris muscle

Tendon, extensor pollicis brevis muscle

Tendon, extensor digiti minimi muscle

Tendon, extensor pollicis longus muscle

FIGURE 82 **Deep Extensor Muscles of the Left Posterior Forearm**

NOTE: Four other muscles complete the **superficial** extensor muscles on the posterior aspect of the forearm. These are the **extensor digitorum, extensor digiti minimi, extensor carpi ulnaris,** and the **anconeus.** There are also five **deep** extensor muscles: the **abductor pollicis longus, extensor pollicis longus** and **brevis, extensor indicis,** and the **supinator** muscle.

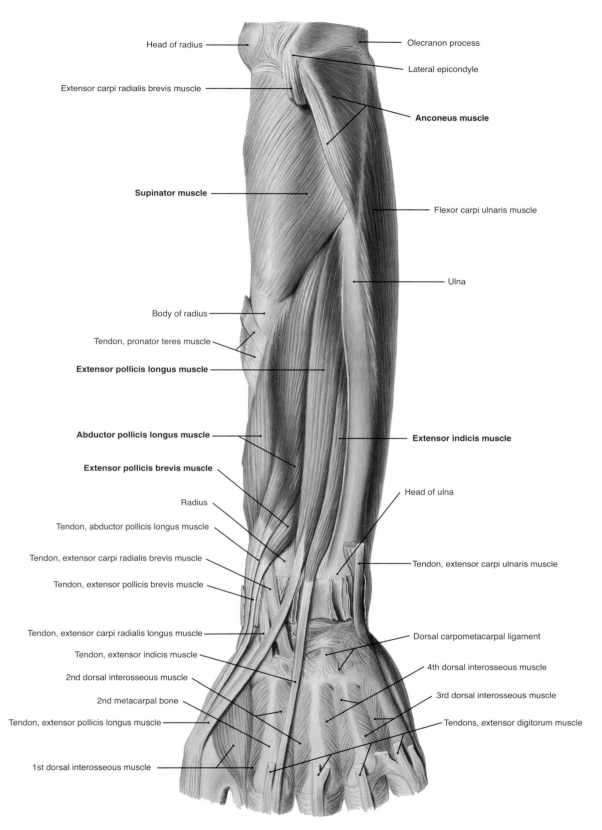

Head of radius

Olecranon process

Lateral epicondyle

Extensor carpi radialis brevis muscle

Anconeus muscle

Supinator muscle

Flexor carpi ulnaris muscle

Ulna

Body of radius

Tendon, pronator teres muscle

Extensor pollicis longus muscle

Abductor pollicis longus muscle

Extensor indicis muscle

Extensor pollicis brevis muscle

Head of ulna

Radius

Tendon, abductor pollicis longus muscle

Tendon, extensor carpi radialis brevis muscle

Tendon, extensor carpi ulnaris muscle

Tendon, extensor pollicis brevis muscle

Tendon, extensor carpi radialis longus muscle

Dorsal carpometacarpal ligament

Tendon, extensor indicis muscle

2nd dorsal interosseous muscle

4th dorsal interosseous muscle

2nd metacarpal bone

3rd dorsal interosseous muscle

Tendon, extensor pollicis longus muscle

Tendons, extensor digitorum muscle

1st dorsal interosseous muscle

FIGURE 83 **Left Posterior Forearm Muscles, Deep Group**

NOTE: (1) The three thumb muscles (abductor pollicis longus and extensors pollicis brevis and longus) are exposed when the extensor digitorum, extensor digiti minimi, and extensor carpi ulnaris are removed.

(2) The extensor indicis courses to the index finger, and the supinator is a broad muscle that stretches across the upper forearm from the humerus and ulna to the upper third of the radius.

PLATE 84 Supination and Pronation of the Forearm and Hand

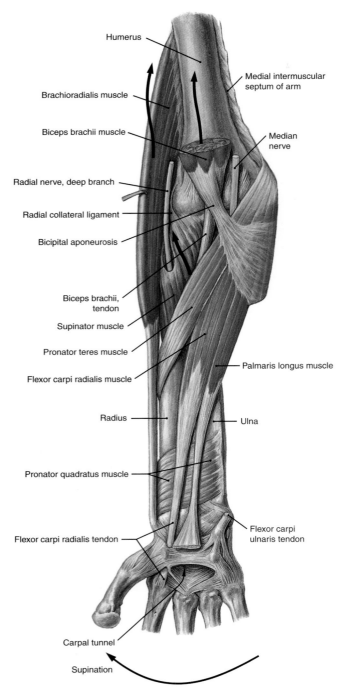

FIGURE 84.1 Supinated Right Forearm (Anterior Aspect)

NOTE: (1) Supination involves turning the pronated forearm and hand over, resulting in the palm being oriented anteriorly and the thumb directed laterally.

(2) In supination, the head of the radius rotates within the annular ligament at the proximal radioulnar joint. The radius then assumes a position lateral to and parallel with the ulna.

(3) The principal muscles that supinate the forearm are the supinator and biceps brachii muscles. In addition, it is thought that the brachioradialis muscle assists in this action, but this has been questioned.

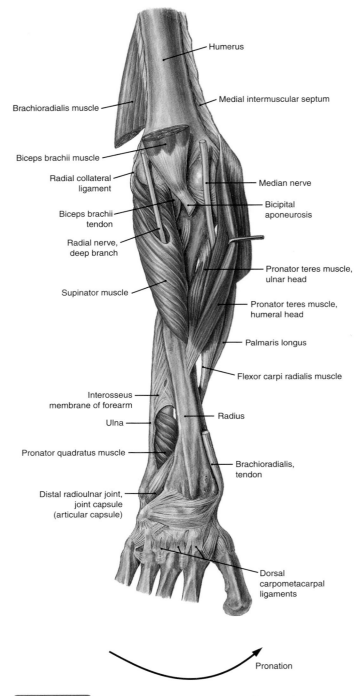

FIGURE 84.2 Pronated Right Forearm (Anterior Aspect)

NOTE: (1) Pronation is the act of turning the supinated forearm and hand over, after which the palm becomes oriented posteriorly and the thumb directed medially.

(2) In pronation of the forearm and hand, the radius turns obliquely across the anterior aspect of the ulna. The proximal end of the radius is still lateral to the ulna, but the distal end is medial to it.

(3) The muscles producing pronation are the **pronator teres** and the **pronator quadratus**. In addition, the **flexor carpi radialis** and the **palmaris longus** may assist.

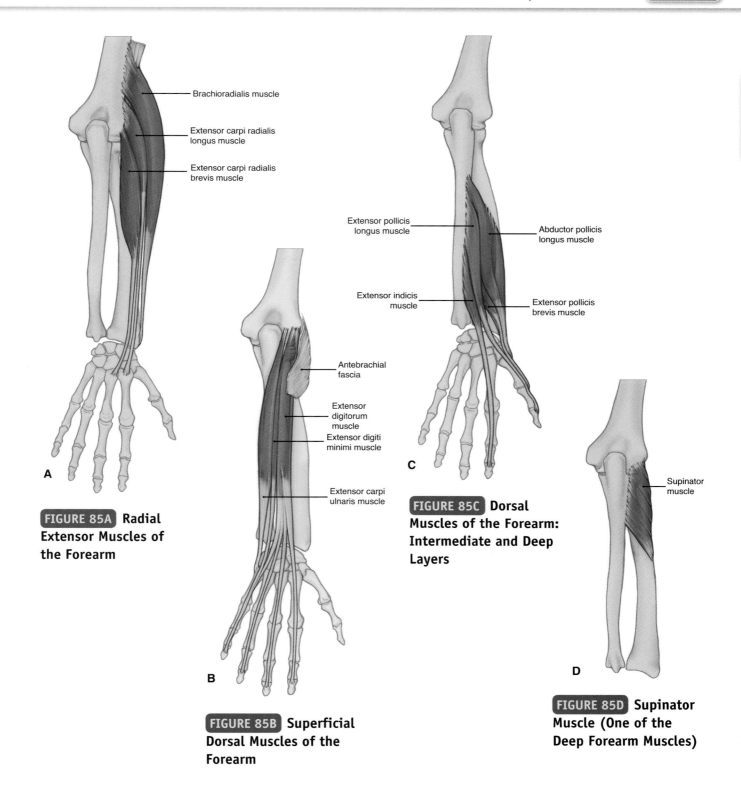

FIGURE 85A Radial Extensor Muscles of the Forearm

- Brachioradialis muscle
- Extensor carpi radialis longus muscle
- Extensor carpi radialis brevis muscle

A

FIGURE 85B Superficial Dorsal Muscles of the Forearm

- Antebrachial fascia
- Extensor digitorum muscle
- Extensor digiti minimi muscle
- Extensor carpi ulnaris muscle

B

FIGURE 85C Dorsal Muscles of the Forearm: Intermediate and Deep Layers

- Extensor pollicis longus muscle
- Abductor pollicis longus muscle
- Extensor indicis muscle
- Extensor pollicis brevis muscle

C

FIGURE 85D Supinator Muscle (One of the Deep Forearm Muscles)

- Supinator muscle

D

SUPERFICIAL EXTENSOR FOREARM MUSCLES				
Muscle	**Origin**	**Insertion**	**Innervation**	**Action**
Extensor digitorum	Lateral epicondyle of humerus	Dorsum of middle and distal phalanges of the four fingers	Posterior interosseous branch of the radial nerve (C7, C8)	Extends the fingers and the hand
Extensor digiti minimi	Lateral epicondyle of humerus	Dorsal digital expansion of little finger	Posterior interosseous branch of the radial nerve (C7, C8)	Extends the little finger and the hand
Extensor carpi ulnaris	Lateral epicondyle of humerus	Medial side of the base of the fifth metacarpal bone	Posterior interosseous branch of the radial nerve (C7, C8)	Extends and adducts the hand (ulnar deviation)
Anconeus	Lateral epicondyle of humerus	Lateral side of olecranon and shaft of ulna	Radial nerve (C7, C8, T1)	Helps extend the forearm at the elbow joint

PLATE 86 Posterior Upper Limb Muscles and Dermatomes (Review)

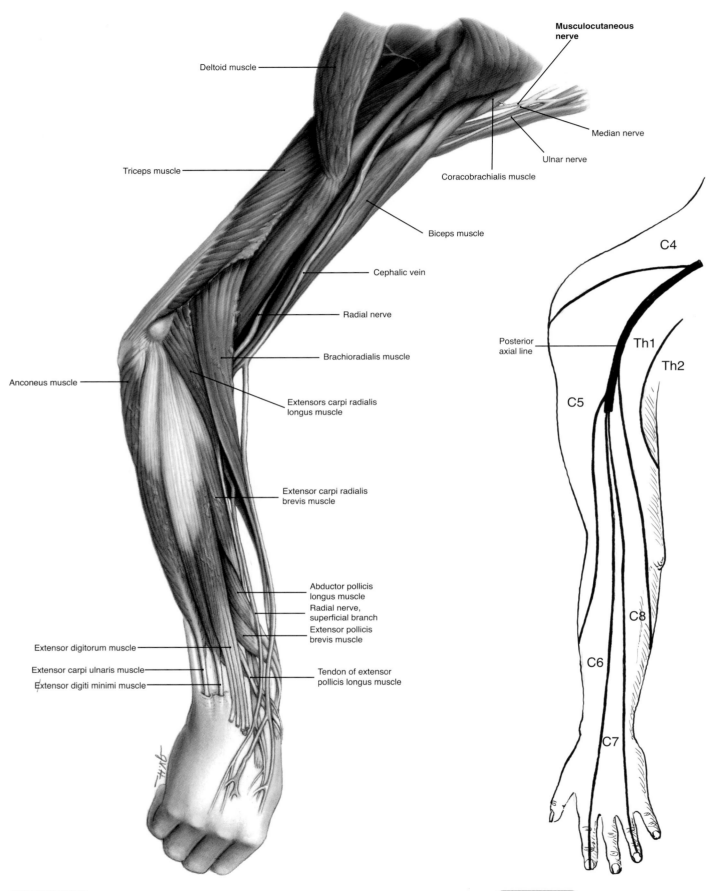

Deltoid muscle

Musculocutaneous nerve

Triceps muscle

Median nerve

Ulnar nerve

Coracobrachialis muscle

Biceps muscle

Cephalic vein

Radial nerve

Brachioradialis muscle

Anconeus muscle

Extensors carpi radialis longus muscle

Extensor carpi radialis brevis muscle

Abductor pollicis longus muscle

Radial nerve, superficial branch

Extensor pollicis brevis muscle

Extensor digitorum muscle

Extensor carpi ulnaris muscle

Extensor digiti minimi muscle

Tendon of extensor pollicis longus muscle

C4

Posterior axial line

Th1

Th2

C5

C8

C6

C7

FIGURE 86.1 **Posterior Muscles on the Dorsal Arm and Forearm**

(Contributed by Dr. Gene L. Colborn, Medical College of Georgia.)

FIGURE 86.2 **Dermatomes as Shown on the Posterior Aspect of the Upper Limb**

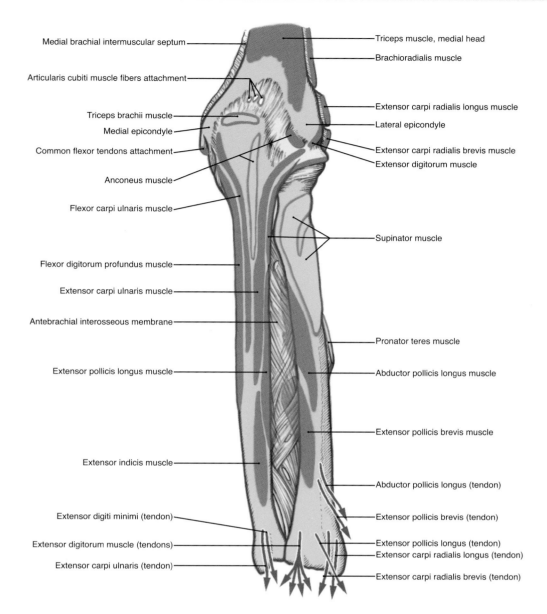

Medial brachial intermuscular septum

Articularis cubiti muscle fibers attachment

Triceps brachii muscle

Medial epicondyle

Common flexor tendons attachment

Anconeus muscle

Flexor carpi ulnaris muscle

Flexor digitorum profundus muscle

Extensor carpi ulnaris muscle

Antebrachial interosseous membrane

Extensor pollicis longus muscle

Extensor indicis muscle

Extensor digiti minimi (tendon)

Extensor digitorum muscle (tendons)

Extensor carpi ulnaris (tendon)

Triceps muscle, medial head

Brachioradialis muscle

Extensor carpi radialis longus muscle

Lateral epicondyle

Extensor carpi radialis brevis muscle

Extensor digitorum muscle

Supinator muscle

Pronator teres muscle

Abductor pollicis longus muscle

Extensor pollicis brevis muscle

Abductor pollicis longus (tendon)

Extensor pollicis brevis (tendon)

Extensor pollicis longus (tendon)

Extensor carpi radialis longus (tendon)

Extensor carpi radialis brevis (tendon)

FIGURE 87 **Attachments of the Extensor Muscles on the Posterior Ulna and Radius**

NOTE that the red arrows (shown inferiorly) indicate the courses of the tendons across the posterior aspect of the wrist joint.

DEEP EXTENSOR FOREARM MUSCLES				
Muscle	**Origin**	**Insertion**	**Innervation**	**Action**
Extensor pollicis longus	Posterior shaft of ulna and interosseous membrane	Base of the distal phalanx of the thumb	Posterior interosseous branch of the radial nerve (C7, C8)	Extends the thumb, and to a minor extent, the hand
Extensor pollicis brevis	Posterior surface of radius and interosseous membrane	Base of the proximal phalanx of the thumb	Posterior interosseous branch of the radial nerve (C7, C8)	Extends the proximal phalanx and metacarpal bone of thumb
Abductor pollicis longus	Posterior surfaces of both radius and ulna and interosseous membrane	Radial side of base of the first metacarpal bone, and on the trapezoid bone	Posterior interosseous branch of the radial nerve (C7, C8)	Abducts and assists in extending the thumb
Extensor indicis	Posterior surface of ulna and interosseous membrane	Into the extensor hood of the index finger	Posterior interosseous branch of the radial nerve (C7, C8)	Extends the index finger and helps extend the hand
Supinator	Lateral epicondyle of humerus; radial collateral ligament; supinator crest of ulna	Lateral surface of the proximal third of the radius	Posterior interosseous branch of the radial nerve (C6)	Rotates the radius to supinate the hand and forearm

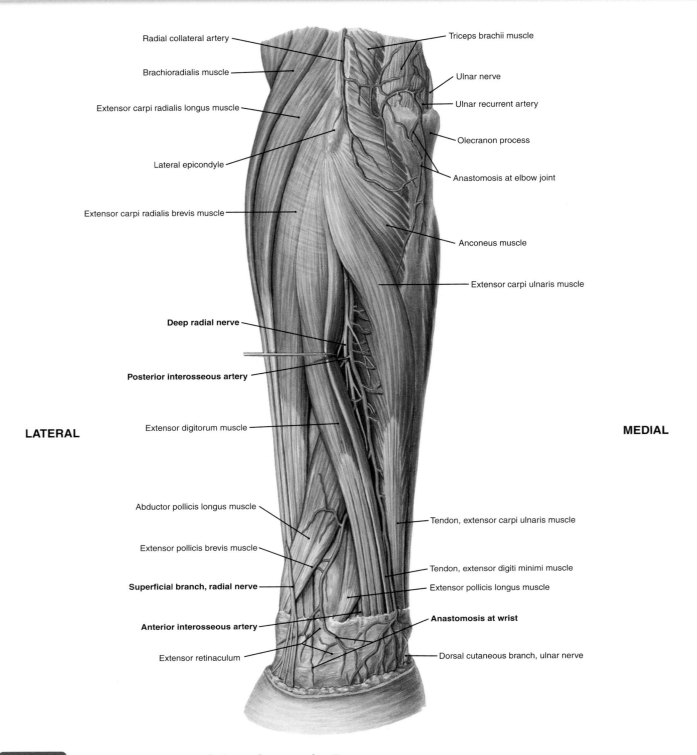

Radial collateral artery

Brachioradialis muscle

Extensor carpi radialis longus muscle

Lateral epicondyle

Extensor carpi radialis brevis muscle

Deep radial nerve

Posterior interosseous artery

LATERAL

Extensor digitorum muscle

Abductor pollicis longus muscle

Extensor pollicis brevis muscle

Superficial branch, radial nerve

Anterior interosseous artery

Extensor retinaculum

Triceps brachii muscle

Ulnar nerve

Ulnar recurrent artery

Olecranon process

Anastomosis at elbow joint

Anconeus muscle

Extensor carpi ulnaris muscle

MEDIAL

Tendon, extensor carpi ulnaris muscle

Tendon, extensor digiti minimi muscle

Extensor pollicis longus muscle

Anastomosis at wrist

Dorsal cutaneous branch, ulnar nerve

FIGURE 88 **Nerves and Arteries of the Left Posterior Forearm**

NOTE: (1) The extensor digiti minimi and extensor digitorum have been separated from the extensor carpi ulnaris to expose the **posterior interosseous artery** and the **deep radial nerve**.

(2) The posterior interosseous artery is derived in the anterior compartment of the forearm from the common interosseous artery, a branch of the ulnar artery, which divides into anterior and posterior interosseous branches (see Fig. 38.1).

(3) The posterior interosseous branch passes over the proximal border of the interosseous membrane to achieve the posterior compartment, and it descends with the deep radial nerve between the superficial and deep extensor forearm muscles.

(4) In the distal forearm, the posterior interosseous artery anastomoses with terminal branches of the anterior interosseous artery to help form the carpal anastomosis at the wrist.

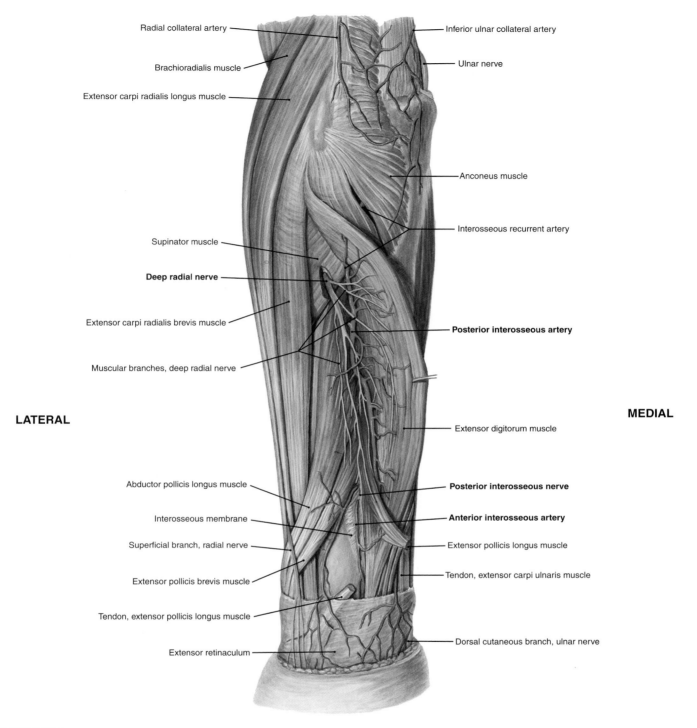

Radial collateral artery

Brachioradialis muscle

Extensor carpi radialis longus muscle

Inferior ulnar collateral artery

Ulnar nerve

Anconeus muscle

Interosseous recurrent artery

Supinator muscle

Deep radial nerve

Extensor carpi radialis brevis muscle

Muscular branches, deep radial nerve

Posterior interosseous artery

LATERAL

MEDIAL

Extensor digitorum muscle

Abductor pollicis longus muscle

Interosseous membrane

Superficial branch, radial nerve

Extensor pollicis brevis muscle

Tendon, extensor pollicis longus muscle

Extensor retinaculum

Posterior interosseous nerve

Anterior interosseous artery

Extensor pollicis longus muscle

Tendon, extensor carpi ulnaris muscle

Dorsal cutaneous branch, ulnar nerve

FIGURE 89 **Nerves and Arteries of the Left Posterior Forearm (Deep Dissection)**

NOTE: (1) The extensor digitorum muscle is separated from the extensor carpi radialis brevis and pulled medially to reveal the **posterior interosseous artery** and **deep radial nerve**.

(2) After the radial nerve leaves the radial groove of the humerus in the lower brachium, it divides into superficial and deep branches.

(3) The **superficial branch** descends along the lateral side of the forearm under cover of the brachioradialis muscle and becomes a sensory nerve to the dorsum of the hand.

(4) The **deep branch** enters the posterior forearm by piercing through the supinator muscle and, coursing along the dorsum of the interosseous membrane, is called the **posterior interosseous nerve**. It supplies all the deep posterior forearm muscles and descends deep to the extensor pollicis longus muscle, which has been cut in this dissection.

PLATE 90 **Dorsum of the Hand: Veins and Nerves; Finger Injection Site**

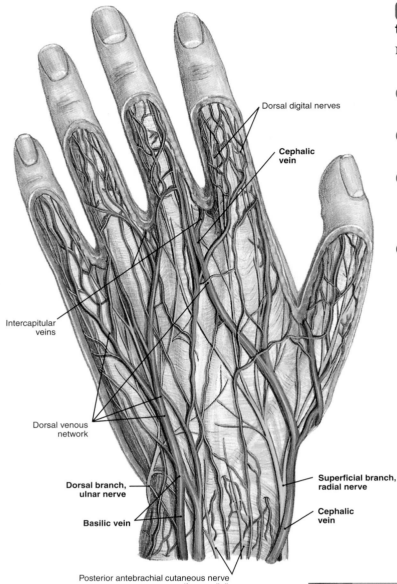

Dorsal digital nerves

Cephalic vein

Intercapitular veins

Dorsal venous network

Dorsal branch, ulnar nerve

Basilic vein

Superficial branch, radial nerve

Cephalic vein

Posterior antebrachial cutaneous nerve (from radial)

FIGURE 90.1 **Superficial Veins and Nerves of the Dorsum of the Left Hand**

NOTE: (1) The **cephalic vein** originates on the radial side of the dorsum of the hand, whereas the **basilic vein** arises on the ulnar side.

(2) The **superficial radial** nerve supplies the dorsum of the radial 3½ digits, whereas the **dorsal branch of the ulnar nerve** supplies the dorsum of the ulnar 1½ digits.

(3) The dorsum of the distal phalanx (not dissected) of the radial 3½ digits is supplied by the **median nerve**, but the same region on the ulnar 1½ digits is supplied by the **ulnar nerve**.

(4) There is a profuse venous plexus on the dorsal surface of the hand but very few small superficial veins on the palmar surface. This is beneficial because the frequent mechanical pressures to which the palmar surface is subjected could injure surface vessels.

(5) Adjacent branches of the radial and ulnar nerve frequently communicate. Observe that the posterior antebrachial cutaneous branches usually terminate at the wrist.

FIGURE 90.2 **Location of Injection Site (X)** ▶ **to Induce Local Sensory Anesthesia of the Middle Finger**

X

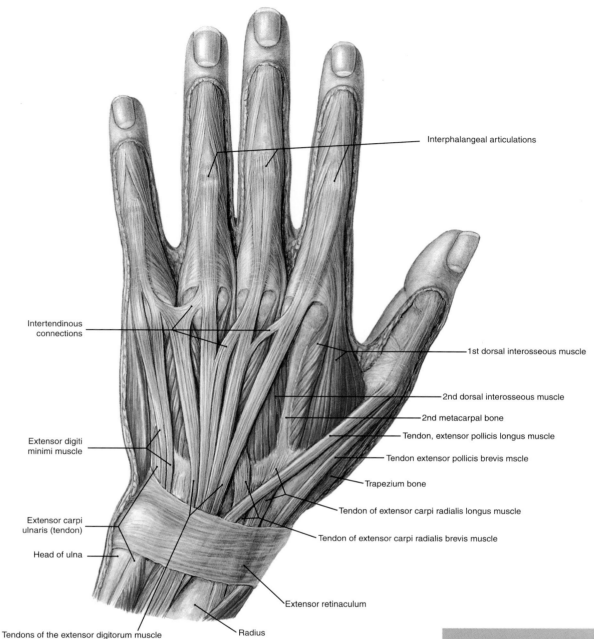

Interphalangeal articulations

Intertendinous connections

1st dorsal interosseous muscle

2nd dorsal interosseous muscle

2nd metacarpal bone

Tendon, extensor pollicis longus muscle

Tendon extensor pollicis brevis mscle

Extensor digiti minimi muscle

Trapezium bone

Tendon of extensor carpi radialis longus muscle

Extensor carpi ulnaris (tendon)

Tendon of extensor carpi radialis brevis muscle

Head of ulna

Extensor retinaculum

Tendons of the extensor digitorum muscle

Radius

FIGURE 91.1 **The Extensor Tendons on the Dorsum of the Left Wrist and Hand**

NOTE: (1) The tendons of the extensor digitorum muscle pass deep to the extensor retinaculum (along with the tendons of the extensors pollicis longus and brevis and extensor digiti minimi).

(2) The extensor digitorum tendons then separate and become inserted onto the middle and distal phalanges of the medial four fingers.

(3) Distal to the metacarpophalangeal joints, the tendons spread into aponeuroses covering the dorsal surfaces of the fingers, thereby helping form the **extensor hood**.

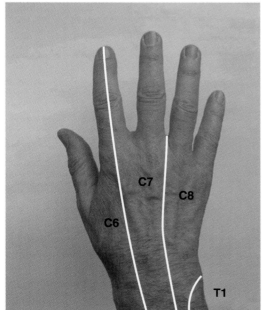

FIGURE 91.2 **Dermatomes on the Dorsal Surface of the Left Hand**

FIGURE 92.1 **Extensor Tendons and Their ▶ Synovial Sheaths of the Left Dorsal Wrist**

NOTE: (1) A synovial sheath is a double mesothelial-lined envelope that surrounds a tendon, allowing it to move more freely beneath the retinaculum.

(2) There are six synovial compartments on the dorsum of the wrist. From radial to ulnar these contain the tendons of:
    (a) Extensor pollicis brevis and abductor pollicis longus
    (b) Extensor carpi radialis longus and brevis
    (c) Extensor pollicis longus
    (d) Extensor digitorum and extensor indicis
    (e) Extensor digiti minimi
    (f) Extensor carpi ulnaris.

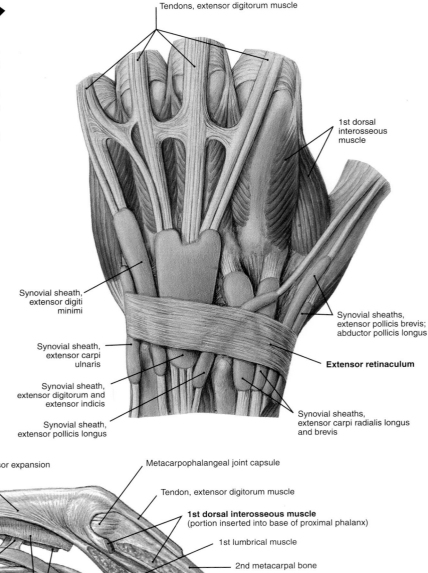

Tendons, extensor digitorum muscle

1st dorsal interosseous muscle

Synovial sheath, extensor digiti minimi

Synovial sheath, extensor carpi ulnaris

Synovial sheath, extensor digitorum and extensor indicis

Synovial sheath, extensor pollicis longus

Synovial sheaths, extensor pollicis brevis; abductor pollicis longus

Extensor retinaculum

Synovial sheaths, extensor carpi radialis longus and brevis

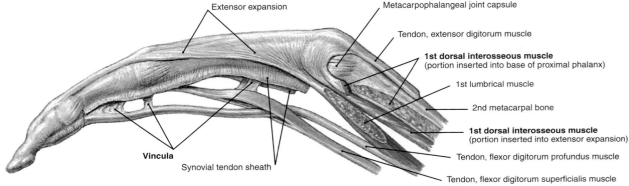

Extensor expansion

Metacarpophalangeal joint capsule

Tendon, extensor digitorum muscle

1st dorsal interosseous muscle (portion inserted into base of proximal phalanx)

1st lumbrical muscle

2nd metacarpal bone

1st dorsal interosseous muscle (portion inserted into extensor expansion)

Tendon, flexor digitorum profundus muscle

Tendon, flexor digitorum superficialis muscle

Vincula

Synovial tendon sheath

FIGURE 92.2 **Tendon Insertions, Index Finger of Right Hand (Radial Side)**

NOTE: (1) The dorsal interosseous and lumbrical muscles join fibers from the extensor tendon in the formation of the dorsal extensor expansion.

(2) The vincula are remnants of mesotendons and attach both superficial and deep tendons to the digital sheath.

(3) The tendon of the flexor digitorum superficialis splits to allow the tendon of the flexor digitorum profundus to reach the distal phalanx of the finger.

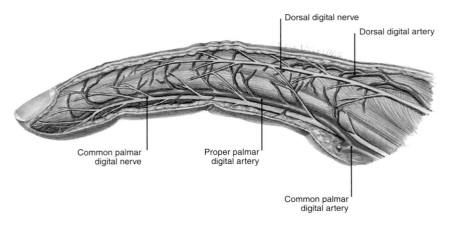

Dorsal digital nerve

Dorsal digital artery

Common palmar digital nerve

Proper palmar digital artery

Common palmar digital artery

FIGURE 92.3 **Nerves and Arteries of the Index Finger**

NOTE: The **dorsal digital nerve** and **artery** extend only two-thirds the length of the finger. The distal third is supplied by the **palmar digital nerve and artery,** which also supplies the entire palmar surface of the finger.

FIGURE 93.1 **Arteries of the Left Dorsal ▶ Wrist and Hand (Deep View)**

NOTE: (1) The transverse course of the dorsal carpal branch of the radial artery.

(2) The princeps pollicis branch of the radial artery coursing deep to the first dorsal interosseous muscle.

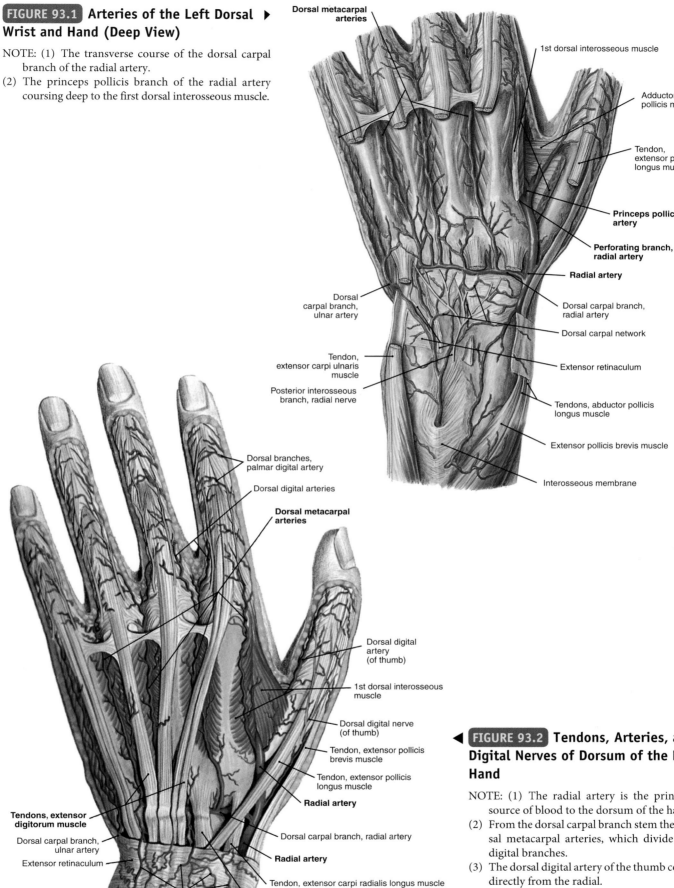

Dorsal metacarpal arteries

1st dorsal interosseous muscle

Adductor pollicis muscle

Tendon, extensor pollicis longus muscle

Princeps pollicis artery

Perforating branch, radial artery

Radial artery

Dorsal carpal branch, radial artery

Dorsal carpal network

Extensor retinaculum

Tendons, abductor pollicis longus muscle

Extensor pollicis brevis muscle

Interosseous membrane

Dorsal carpal branch, ulnar artery

Tendon, extensor carpi ulnaris muscle

Posterior interosseous branch, radial nerve

Dorsal branches, palmar digital artery

Dorsal digital arteries

Dorsal metacarpal arteries

Dorsal digital artery (of thumb)

1st dorsal interosseous muscle

Dorsal digital nerve (of thumb)

Tendon, extensor pollicis brevis muscle

Tendon, extensor pollicis longus muscle

Radial artery

Dorsal carpal branch, radial artery

Radial artery

Tendon, extensor carpi radialis longus muscle

Tendon, extensor carpi radialis brevis muscle

Tendons, extensor digitorum muscle

Dorsal carpal branch, ulnar artery

Extensor retinaculum

Dorsal carpal network

◀ FIGURE 93.2 **Tendons, Arteries, and Digital Nerves of Dorsum of the Left Hand**

NOTE: (1) The radial artery is the principal source of blood to the dorsum of the hand.

(2) From the dorsal carpal branch stem the dorsal metacarpal arteries, which divide into digital branches.

(3) The dorsal digital artery of the thumb comes directly from the radial.

(4) The distal portions of the dorsal aspect of the digits receive both arterial and nerve branches, which curve to the dorsum from the palmar aspect of the fingers.

PLATE 94 Palm of the Hand: Superficial Vessels and Nerves

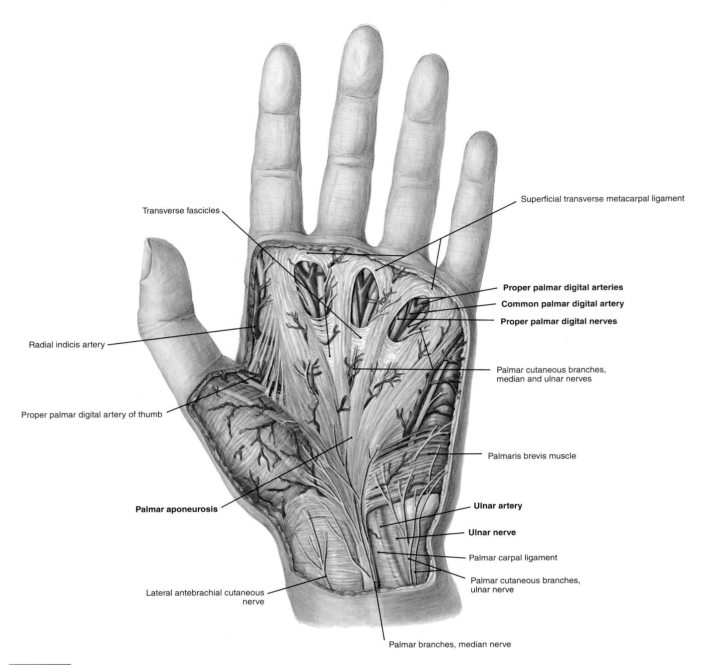

Transverse fascicles

Superficial transverse metacarpal ligament

Proper palmar digital arteries

Common palmar digital artery

Proper palmar digital nerves

Radial indicis artery

Palmar cutaneous branches, median and ulnar nerves

Proper palmar digital artery of thumb

Palmaris brevis muscle

Palmar aponeurosis

Ulnar artery

Ulnar nerve

Palmar carpal ligament

Palmar cutaneous branches, ulnar nerve

Lateral antebrachial cutaneous nerve

Palmar branches, median nerve

FIGURE 94 Superficial Nerves and Arteries of the Palm of the Left Hand

NOTE: (1) The thick and tough fibrous palmar aponeurosis protects the palmar vessels and nerves and strengthens the midportion of the palm. This is of special benefit when the hands are used to push heavy structures or to manually resist an oncoming forceful object (e.g., a fast moving ball in a sport such as baseball).

(2) The radial two-thirds of the surface of the palm is innervated by the median nerve, whereas the ulnar one-third is supplied by the ulnar nerve.

(3) In the distal palm where the palmar aponeurosis is deficient, the vessels and nerves coursing to the fingers are exposed just deep to the skin. This makes them vulnerable to relatively superficial cuts and abrasions.

(4) The three common palmar digital arteries each divides into two proper digital arteries, and their bifurcations occur at the level of the metacarpophalangeal joints.

(5) As each common palmar digital artery divides, the two proper palmar digital arteries course distally on the fingers and supply the adjacent halves of two fingers.

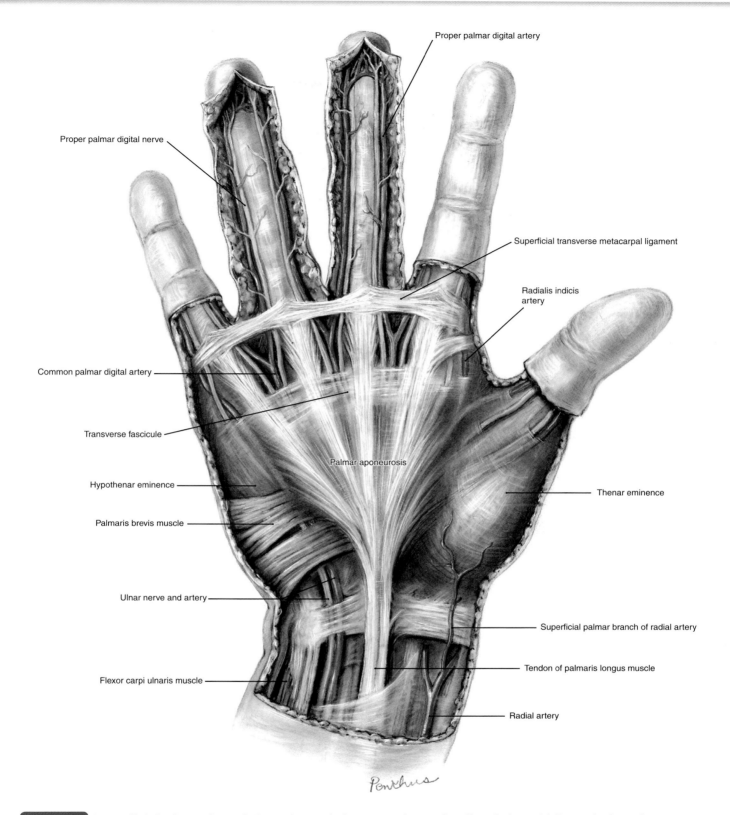

Proper palmar digital artery

Proper palmar digital nerve

Superficial transverse metacarpal ligament

Radialis indicis artery

Common palmar digital artery

Transverse fascicule

Palmar aponeurosis

Hypothenar eminence

Thenar eminence

Palmaris brevis muscle

Ulnar nerve and artery

Superficial palmar branch of radial artery

Tendon of palmaris longus muscle

Flexor carpi ulnaris muscle

Radial artery

FIGURE 95 **Superficial Dissection of the Palm and the Extensions Distally of the Middle and Ring Fingers**

NOTE the distal course of the proper digital nerves and arteries along the fingers. These vessels and nerves are especially vulnerable both proximal and distal to the superficial transverse metacarpal ligaments. There are anastomoses at the distal ends of the fibers beyond the distal phalanx. (From C.D. Clemente. *Gray's Anatomy*, 30th American Edition. Philadelphia: Lea & Febiger, 1985.)

PLATE 96 Palm of the Hand: Muscles and Tendon Sheaths

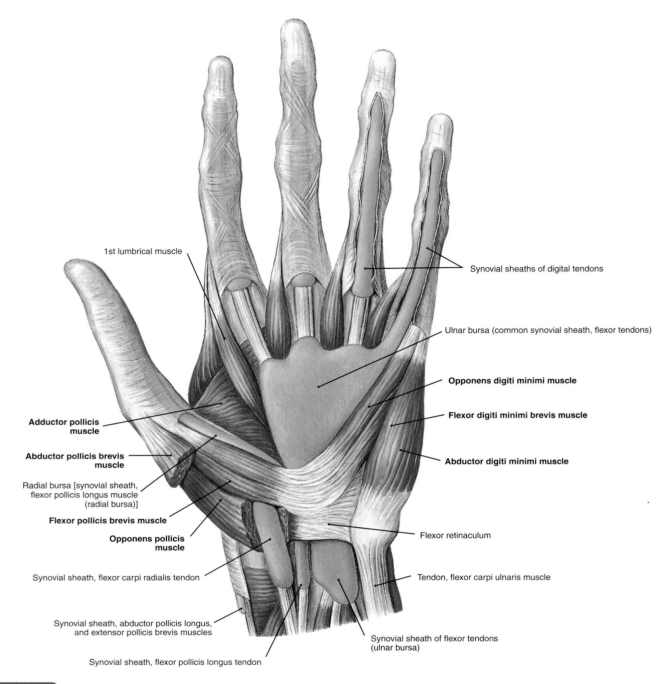

1st lumbrical muscle

Synovial sheaths of digital tendons

Ulnar bursa (common synovial sheath, flexor tendons)

Opponens digiti minimi muscle

Adductor pollicis
muscle

Flexor digiti minimi brevis muscle

Abductor pollicis brevis
muscle

Radial bursa [synovial sheath,
flexor pollicis longus muscle
(radial bursa)]

Abductor digiti minimi muscle

Flexor pollicis brevis muscle

**Opponens pollicis
muscle**

Flexor retinaculum

Synovial sheath, flexor carpi radialis tendon

Tendon, flexor carpi ulnaris muscle

Synovial sheath, abductor pollicis longus,
and extensor pollicis brevis muscles

Synovial sheath of flexor tendons
(ulnar bursa)

Synovial sheath, flexor pollicis longus tendon

FIGURE 96 Muscles, Synovial Sheaths, and Tendons of the Left Wrist and Palm

THENAR MUSCLES Muscle	Origin	Insertion	Innervation	Action
Flexor pollicis brevis	**Superficial head:** Flexor retinaculum and tubercle of the trapezium **Deep head:** Trapezoid and capitate bones	Radial side of base of proximal phalanx of thumb	**Superficial head:** Median nerve (C8, T1). **Deep head:** Deep branch of ulnar nerve (C8, T1).	Flexes proximal phalanx of thumb; flexes metacarpal bone and rotates it medially
Adductor pollicis	**Oblique head:** Capitate bone and bases of second and third metacarpal bones. **Transverse head:** Palmar surface of third metacarpal bone	Ulnar side of base of proximal phalanx of thumb	Deep branch of ulnar nerve (C8, T1)	Adducts the thumb

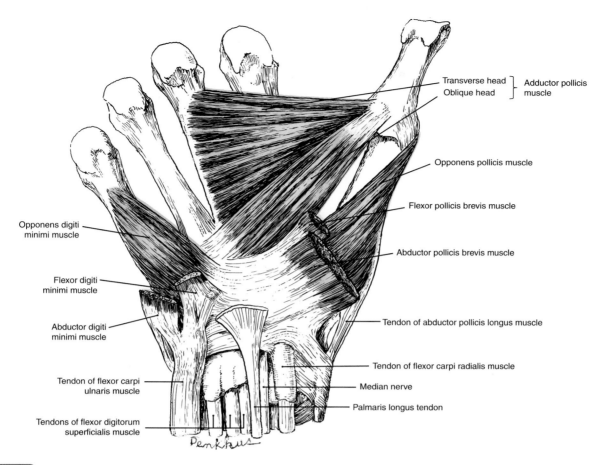

Transverse head ⎤ **Adductor pollicis**
Oblique head ⎦ **muscle**

Opponens pollicis muscle

Flexor pollicis brevis muscle

Abductor pollicis brevis muscle

Opponens digiti minimi muscle

Flexor digiti minimi muscle

Abductor digiti minimi muscle

Tendon of abductor pollicis longus muscle

Tendon of flexor carpi radialis muscle

Median nerve

Tendon of flexor carpi ulnaris muscle

Palmaris longus tendon

Tendons of flexor digitorum superficialis muscle

FIGURE 97.1 **Thenar and Hypothenar Muscles of the Right Hand**

NOTE: (1) The abductor pollicis brevis muscle has been cut and pulled laterally to separate it from the flexor pollicis brevis and to uncover the opponens pollicis.
(2) The flexor digiti minimi brevis has been cut and retracted to show where it separates from the abductor digiti minimi muscle.

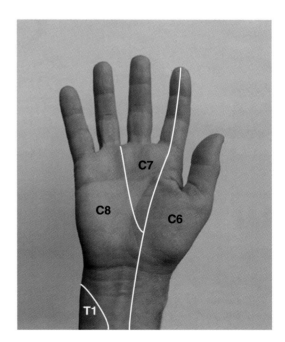

FIGURE 97.2 **Dermatomes on the Palmar Aspect of the Hand**

NOTE that C6, C7, and C8 segmental nerves supply cutaneous innervation to the palmar surface of the hand.

THENAR (THUMB) MUSCLES OF HAND (CONT.)				
Muscle	**Origin**	**Insertion**	**Innervation**	**Action**
Abductor pollicis brevis	Flexor retinaculum and the tubercle of the trapezium	Base of proximal phalanx of thumb; dorsal digital expansion of thumb	Median nerve (C8, T1)	Abducts thumb
Opponens pollicis	Flexor retinaculum and the tubercles of the scaphoid and trapezium bones	Whole length of lateral border of metacarpal bone of the thumb	Median nerve (C8, T1) and often a small branch of deep ulnar nerve	Opposes the thumb to the other fingers

PLATE 98 Palm of the Hand: Muscles and Flexor Tendon Insertions

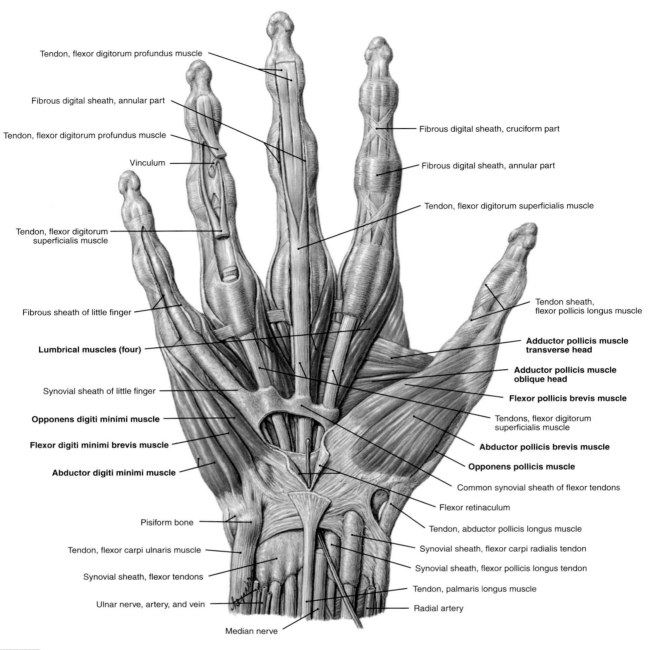

FIGURE 98 Muscles of the Right Hand

HYPOTHENAR (LITTLE FINGER) MUSCLES OF HAND				
Muscle	Origin	Insertion	Innervation	Action
Palmaris brevis (see Fig. 94)	Palmar aponeurosis and flexor retinaculum	Into the dermis on the ulnar side of the hand	Ulnar nerve, superficial branch (C8, T1)	Helps tense the skin over the hypothenar muscles
Abductor digiti minimi	Pisiform bone and tendon of flexor carpi ulnaris	Base of proximal phalanx and dorsal aponeurosis of little finger	Ulnar nerve, deep branch (C8, T1)	Abducts the little finger
Flexor digiti minimi	Hamulus of the hamate bone and flexor retinaculum	Base of proximal phalanx of the little finger	Ulnar nerve, deep branch (C8, T1)	Flexes the little finger at metacarpophalangeal joint
Opponens digiti minimi	Hamulus of the hamate bone and flexor retinaculum	Ulnar side of fifth metacarpal bone	Ulnar nerve, deep branch (C8, T1)	Brings the little finger into opposition with the thumb

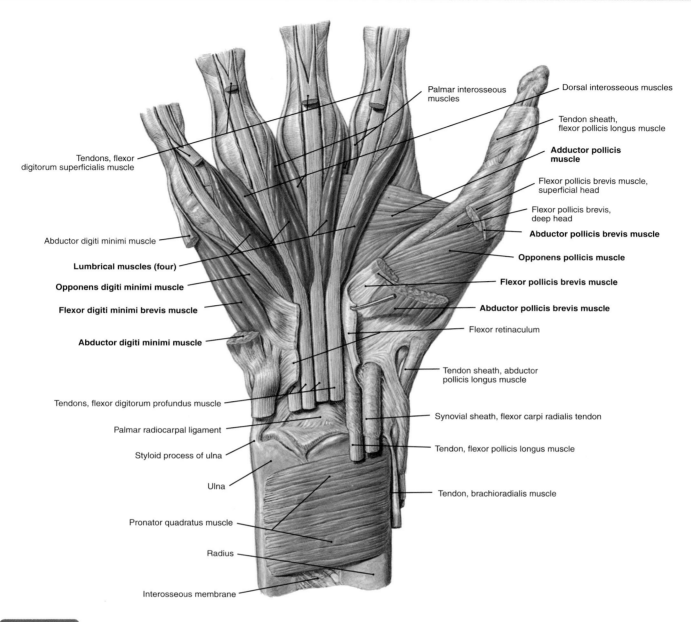

Palmar interosseous
muscles

Dorsal interosseous muscles

Tendon sheath,
flexor pollicis longus muscle

**Adductor pollicis
muscle**

Tendons, flexor
digitorum superficialis muscle

Flexor pollicis brevis muscle,
superficial head

Flexor pollicis brevis,
deep head

Abductor pollicis brevis muscle

Abductor digiti minimi muscle

Opponens pollicis muscle

Lumbrical muscles (four)

Flexor pollicis brevis muscle

Opponens digiti minimi muscle

Abductor pollicis brevis muscle

Flexor digiti minimi brevis muscle

Flexor retinaculum

Abductor digiti minimi muscle

Tendon sheath, abductor
pollicis longus muscle

Tendons, flexor digitorum profundus muscle

Synovial sheath, flexor carpi radialis tendon

Palmar radiocarpal ligament

Styloid process of ulna

Tendon, flexor pollicis longus muscle

Ulna

Tendon, brachioradialis muscle

Pronator quadratus muscle

Radius

Interosseous membrane

FIGURE 99.1 **Deep Muscles of the Right Hand (Palmar View)**

NOTE: (1) The tendon of the flexor digitorum superficialis divides into two slips and allows the flexor digitorum profundus to pass and insert onto the distal phalanx.
(2) In the fingers the tendons are encased in a synovial sheath and then bound by both crossed and transverse (cruciform and annular) fibrous sheaths (see Fig. 98).

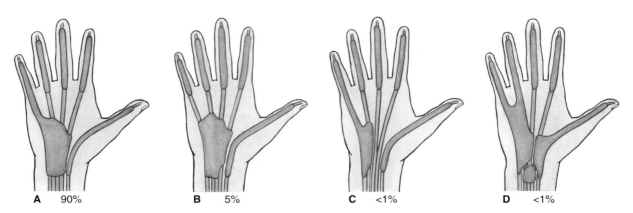

A   90%   B   5%   C   <1%   D   <1%

FIGURE 99.2A–D **Variations in the Synovial Tendon Sheaths within the Carpal Tunnel and Hand**

NOTE that because of these variations the hand surgeon must be careful when repairing carpal tunnel syndrome, since infections spread rapidly within the synovial sheathes of the hand.

PLATE 100 Muscles of the Deep Palmar Hand Region: Dissection #1

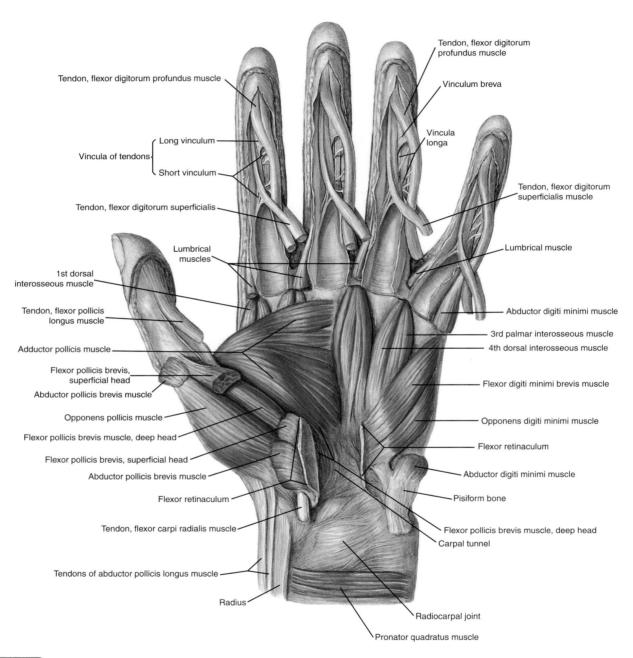

Tendon, flexor digitorum profundus muscle

Tendon, flexor digitorum profundus muscle

Vinculum breva

Vincula longa

Long vinculum

Vincula of tendons

Short vinculum

Tendon, flexor digitorum superficialis muscle

Tendon, flexor digitorum superficialis

Lumbrical muscles

Lumbrical muscle

1st dorsal interosseous muscle

Tendon, flexor pollicis longus muscle

Abductor digiti minimi muscle

Adductor pollicis muscle

3rd palmar interosseous muscle

4th dorsal interosseous muscle

Flexor pollicis brevis, superficial head

Abductor pollicis brevis muscle

Flexor digiti minimi brevis muscle

Opponens pollicis muscle

Opponens digiti minimi muscle

Flexor pollicis brevis muscle, deep head

Flexor pollicis brevis, superficial head

Flexor retinaculum

Abductor pollicis brevis muscle

Abductor digiti minimi muscle

Flexor retinaculum

Pisiform bone

Tendon, flexor carpi radialis muscle

Flexor pollicis brevis muscle, deep head

Carpal tunnel

Tendons of abductor pollicis longus muscle

Radius

Radiocarpal joint

Pronator quadratus muscle

FIGURE 100 **Muscles of the Left Hand: Deep Layer and Superficial and Deep Flexor Tendons**

NOTE: (1) The adductor pollicis muscle. This muscle has oblique and transverse heads that course across and cover the palmar side of the first dorsal and first palmar interosseous muscles.

(2) Observe how the tendons of the flexor digitorum superficialis split in order to allow the tendons of the flexor digitorum profundus to reach the distal phalanx of each finger.

(3) The tendons of the flexor digitorum superficialis insert onto the middle phalanx of the fingers, whereas the tendons of the flexor digitorum profundus insert onto the distal phalanx.

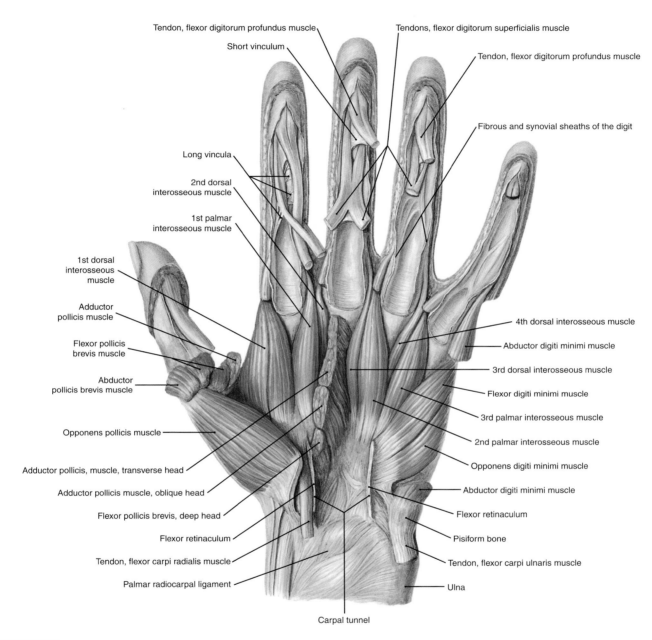

Tendon, flexor digitorum profundus muscle

Short vinculum

Tendons, flexor digitorum superficialis muscle

Tendon, flexor digitorum profundus muscle

Fibrous and synovial sheaths of the digit

Long vincula

2nd dorsal interosseous muscle

1st palmar interosseous muscle

1st dorsal interosseous muscle

Adductor pollicis muscle

Flexor pollicis brevis muscle

Abductor pollicis brevis muscle

Opponens pollicis muscle

Adductor pollicis, muscle, transverse head

Adductor pollicis muscle, oblique head

Flexor pollicis brevis, deep head

Flexor retinaculum

Tendon, flexor carpi radialis muscle

Palmar radiocarpal ligament

4th dorsal interosseous muscle

Abductor digiti minimi muscle

3rd dorsal interosseous muscle

Flexor digiti minimi muscle

3rd palmar interosseous muscle

2nd palmar interosseous muscle

Opponens digiti minimi muscle

Abductor digiti minimi muscle

Flexor retinaculum

Pisiform bone

Tendon, flexor carpi ulnaris muscle

Ulna

Carpal tunnel

FIGURE 101 **Deepest Muscle Dissection of the Left Hand with Adductor Pollicis Muscle Severed**

NOTE: (1) The tendons of the three palmar and four dorsal interosseous muscles are intact and can be seen to course around to the dorsal surface of the fingers to participate in the formation of the dorsal expansion hoods.

(2) Both oblique and transverse heads of the adductor pollicis muscle have been severed to uncover the interosseous muscles more completely.

(3) Each finger requires muscles that allow adduction and abduction. The three palmar interossei adduct the second, fourth, and fifth digits. The four dorsal interossei abduct the second, third laterally, third medially, and fourth digits. To these seven interossei are added the abductor pollicis brevis, adductor pollicis, and abductor digiti minimi, resulting in the required 10 muscles for abduction and adduction of the five digits.

PLATE 102   **Dorsal Interosseous Muscles in the Deep Hand**

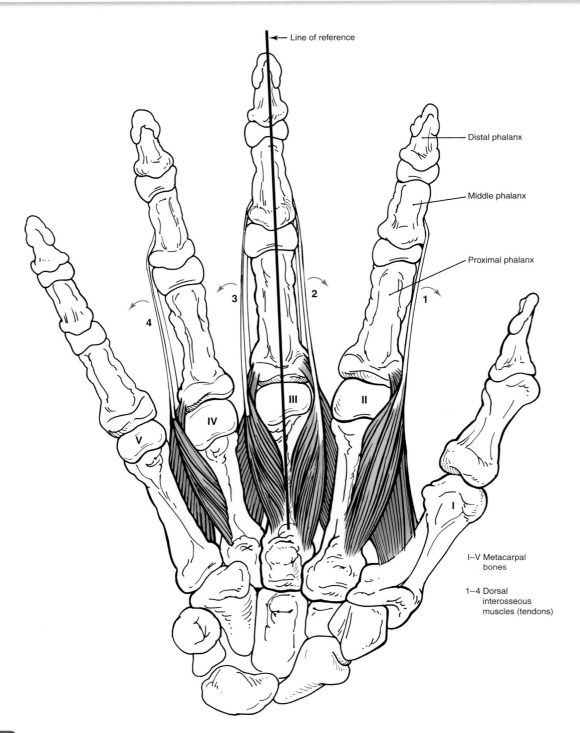

Line of reference

Distal phalanx

Middle phalanx

Proximal phalanx

I–V Metacarpal bones

1–4 Dorsal interosseous muscles (tendons)

FIGURE 102 **The Four Dorsal Interosseous Muscles**

NOTE that the dorsal interosseous muscles abduct the fingers, flex the metacarpophalangeal joints, and extend the interphalangeal joints. Observe that the middle finger (III) has two muscles, one abducting the finger toward the radial side and the other abducting it toward the ulnar side. The line of reference for abduction is midway down the middle finger.

Muscle	Origin	Insertion	Innervation	Action
Dorsal interossei (four)	Each arises by two heads from the adjacent sides of metacarpal bones	Bases of the proximal phalanges and the dorsal expansions of the second, third, and fourth fingers	Ulnar nerve, deep palmar branch (C8, T1)	Abduct fingers; flex at metacarpophalangeal joints and extend at interphalangeal joints

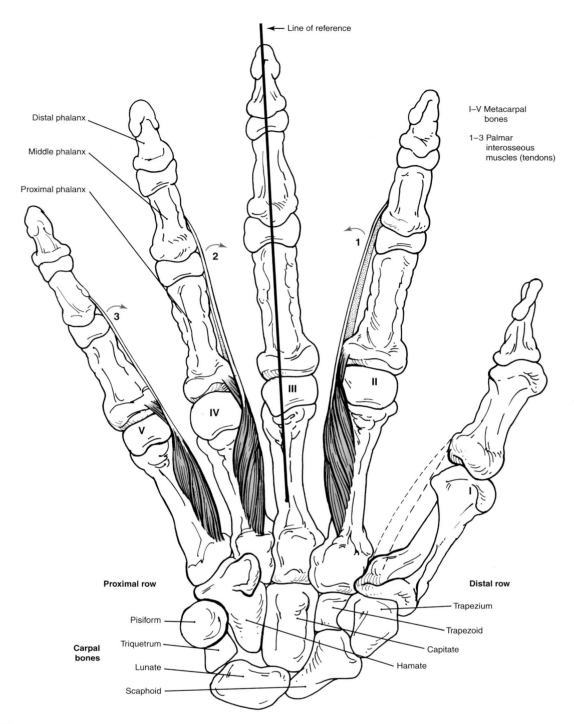

← Line of reference

Distal phalanx

Middle phalanx

Proximal phalanx

I–V Metacarpal bones

1–3 Palmar interosseous muscles (tendons)

2

3

1

III

IV

II

V

I

Proximal row

Distal row

Carpal bones

Pisiform

Triquetrum

Lunate

Scaphoid

Trapezium

Trapezoid

Capitate

Hamate

FIGURE 103 **The Three Palmar Interosseous Muscles**

NOTE: (1) The palmar interosseous muscles adduct the fingers; the middle finger has no palmar interosseous muscle attaching to it. The palmar interosseous muscles also flex the metacarpophalangeal joint and extend the interphalangeal joints. Observe that the line of reference for adduction is midway down the middle finger.

(2) The carpal bones are described as consisting of a **proximal row** of four bones and a **distal row** of four bones, and they articulate proximally with the bones of the forearm and distally with the metacarpal bones of the hand.

Muscle	Origin	Insertion	Innervation	Action
Palmar interossei (three)	Each arises by one head from the second, fourth, and fifth metacarpal bones	Dorsal digital expansions of the second, fourth, and fifth fingers	Ulnar nerve, deep palmar branch (C8, T1)	Adduct fingers; flex at metacarpophalangeal joints and extend at interphalangeal joints

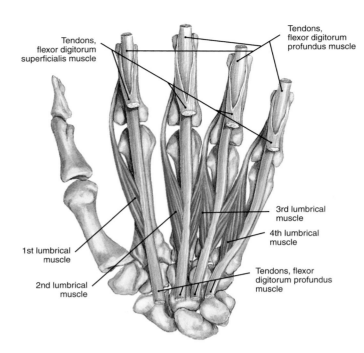

Tendons, flexor digitorum superficialis muscle

Tendons, flexor digitorum profundus muscle

3rd lumbrical muscle

4th lumbrical muscle

Tendons, flexor digitorum profundus muscle

1st lumbrical muscle

2nd lumbrical muscle

FIGURE 104.1 The Lumbrical Muscles

NOTE: (1) The four lumbrical muscles arise from the tendons of the flexor digitorum profundus. Each courses around the radial side of the fingers (i.e., fingers 2, 3, 4, and 5) and inserts on the dorsal digital expansion hood of the same finger.

(2) The lumbricals flex the metacarpophalangeal joints and extend the interphalangeal joints.

(3) The first and second lumbricals are supplied by the median nerve, while the third and fourth lumbricals are supplied by the ulnar nerve.

FIGURE 104.2 Tendon Insertions on the Palmar Surface of the (Index) Finger

NOTE that the dorsal and palmar interosseous muscles course around the palmar side of the finger to insert onto the dorsal expansion hood. The expansion hood cannot be seen from this palmar view.

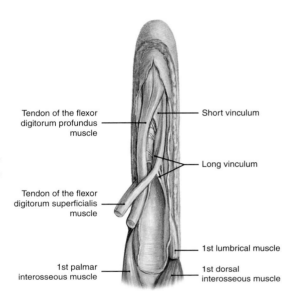

Tendon of the flexor digitorum profundus muscle

Short vinculum

Long vinculum

Tendon of the flexor digitorum superficialis muscle

1st lumbrical muscle

1st palmar interosseous muscle

1st dorsal interosseous muscle

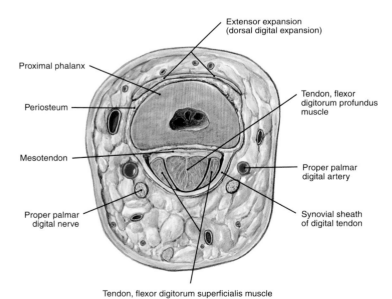

Extensor expansion (dorsal digital expansion)

Proximal phalanx

Periosteum

Tendon, flexor digitorum profundus muscle

Mesotendon

Proper palmar digital artery

Proper palmar digital nerve

Synovial sheath of digital tendon

Tendon, flexor digitorum superficialis muscle

FIGURE 104.3 Cross Section of the Middle Finger through the Proximal Phalanx

NOTE: (1) The extensor expansion (or extensor hood) extends over the dorsal aspect of the proximal phalanx and part of the middle phalanx.

(2) Into the extensor expansion blend the tendon of the extensor digitorum and the tendons of insertion of the adjacent interosseous and lumbrical muscles.

(3) The synovial sheath on the palmar side of the phalanx surrounds the superficial and deep flexor tendons of the digit.

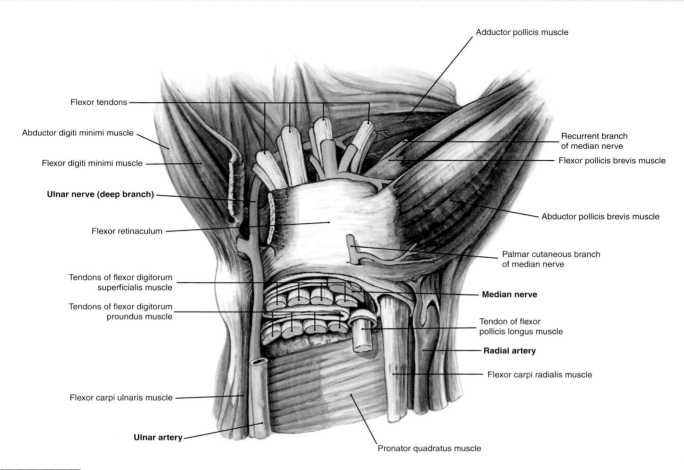

Adductor pollicis muscle

Flexor tendons

Abductor digiti minimi muscle

Flexor digiti minimi muscle

Ulnar nerve (deep branch)

Flexor retinaculum

Tendons of flexor digitorum
superficialis muscle

Tendons of flexor digitorum
proundus muscle

Flexor carpi ulnaris muscle

Ulnar artery

Recurrent branch
of median nerve

Flexor pollicis brevis muscle

Abductor pollicis brevis muscle

Palmar cutaneous branch
of median nerve

Median nerve

Tendon of flexor
pollicis longus muscle

Radial artery

Flexor carpi radialis muscle

Pronator quadratus muscle

FIGURE 105.1 **Flexor Retinaculum and the Carpal Tunnel**

NOTE: (1) The flexor retinaculum anteriorly and the carpal bones posteriorly form a restricted space called the **carpal tunnel** at the anterior
wrist region. Through the space pass the superficial and deep flexor digitorum tendons, the median nerve, and the tendon of the flexor pollicis
longus muscle.

(2) If a pathological process occurs within the space, such as fibrosis due to trauma or an inflammatory process that results in scar formation, the
space could diminish in size and undue pressure could be put on the median nerve. This could result in a wasting of the thenar muscles, and
this condition is called a **carpal tunnel syndrome**.

(3) In addition to the median nerve, the carpal tunnel has coursing through it the tendons of the superficial and deep flexor digitorum muscles,
along with the tendon of the flexor pollicis longus muscle. The ulnar nerve and ulnar artery and the radial artery are NOT structures within the
space.

(Contributed by Dr. Gene L. Colborn, Medical College of Georgia.)

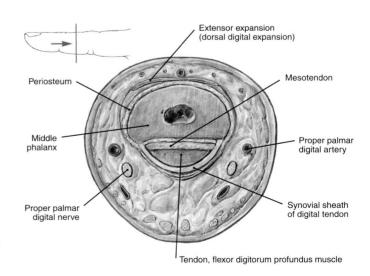

Extensor expansion
(dorsal digital expansion)

Mesotendon

Periosteum

Middle
phalanx

Proper palmar
digital artery

FIGURE 105.2 **Cross Section of the Middle Finger
through the Middle Phalanx**

NOTE: (1) The location of the proper digital nerves and arteries within
the subcutaneous tissue on the sides of the deep flexor tendon.

(2) Knowing the location of these neurovascular structures in the fingers is important both for the application of local anesthesia to the
digit and for the cessation of severe bleeding.

Proper palmar
digital nerve

Synovial sheath
of digital tendon

Tendon, flexor digitorum profundus muscle

PLATE 106 Carpal Tunnel; Superficial Palmar Arterial Arch

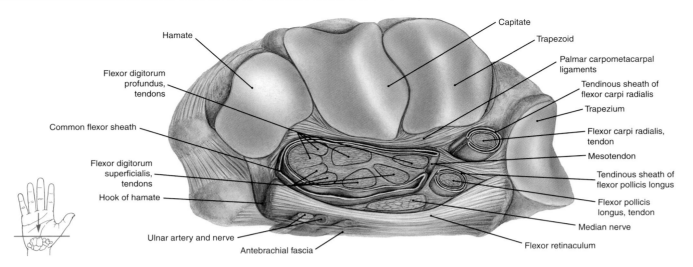

FIGURE 106.1 **Transverse Section through the Right Wrist Showing the Carpal Tunnel and Its Contents**

NOTE that the median nerve can be compressed and, thereby, be functionally compromised if there is edema or fibrosis due to trauma within the carpal tunnel (**carpal tunnel syndrome**). In this condition, weakness is experienced in muscles innervated by the median nerve. Especially reduced are the functions of the abductor pollicis brevis, the flexor pollicis brevis, and the opponens pollicis muscles.

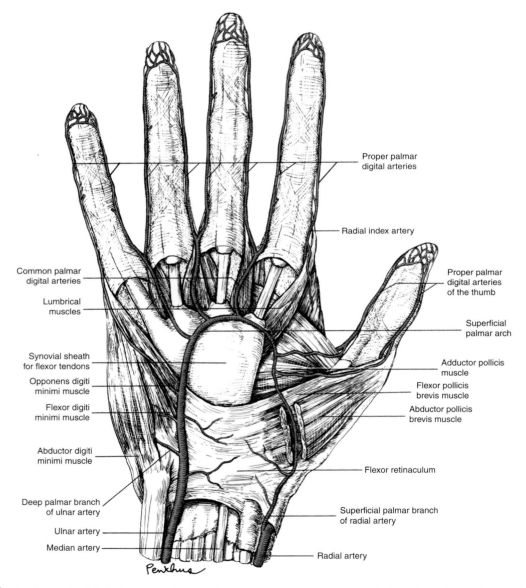

FIGURE 106.2 **The Superficial Palmar Arch and the Common and Proper Digital Arteries of the Right Hand**

NOTE that the ulnar artery is the principal contributor to the superficial palmar arch.
(From C.D. Clemente. *Gray's Anatomy*, 30th American Edition. Philadelphia: Lea & Febiger, 1985.)

Chapter 1 Pectoral Region, Axilla, Shoulder, and Upper Limb

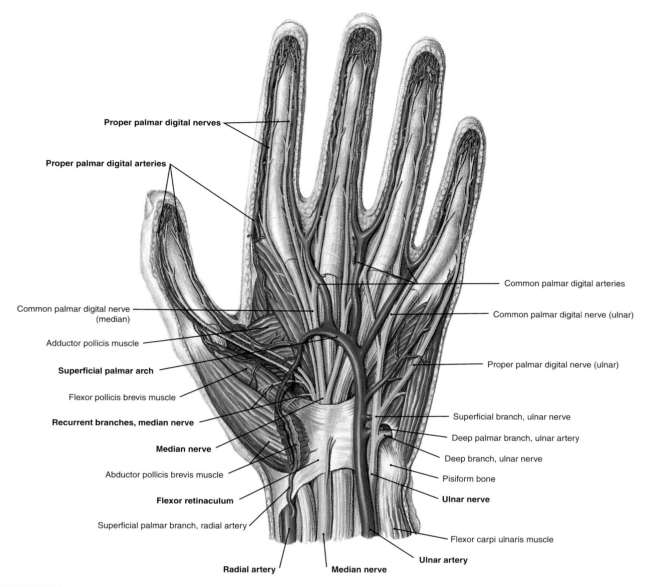

Proper palmar digital nerves

Proper palmar digital arteries

Common palmar digital nerve (median)

Adductor pollicis muscle

Superficial palmar arch

Flexor pollicis brevis muscle

Recurrent branches, median nerve

Median nerve

Abductor pollicis brevis muscle

Flexor retinaculum

Superficial palmar branch, radial artery

Radial artery

Median nerve

Common palmar digital arteries

Common palmar digital nerve (ulnar)

Proper palmar digital nerve (ulnar)

Superficial branch, ulnar nerve

Deep palmar branch, ulnar artery

Deep branch, ulnar nerve

Pisiform bone

Ulnar nerve

Flexor carpi ulnaris muscle

Ulnar artery

FIGURE 107.1 Nerves and Arteries of the Left Palm, Superficial Palmar Arch

NOTE: (1) The **median nerve** enters the palm beneath the flexor retinaculum and supplies the muscles of the thenar eminence: abductor pollicis brevis, opponens pollicis, and the superficial head of the flexor pollicis brevis.

(2) The **median nerve** also supplies the radial (lateral) two lumbrical muscles as well as the palmar surface of the lateral hand and lateral 3½ fingers.

(3) The superficial location of the **recurrent branches of the median nerve,** which supply the thenar muscles. Just deep to the superficial fascia, these branches are easily injured.

(4) The **ulnar nerve** enters the palm superficial to the flexor retinaculum, and it supplies the ulnar 1½ fingers and all the remaining muscles in the hand.

(5) The **superficial palmar arterial arch** is derived principally from the ulnar artery. The arch is completed by the **palmar branch of the radial artery.** From the arch three or four **common palmar digital arteries** course distally and divide into **proper palmar digital arteries.** These accompany the corresponding digital nerves along the fingers.

FIGURE 107.2 Variations of the Superficial Palmar Arch

A: Complete arch
B: Ulnar three fingers supplied by the ulnar artery
C: All fingers supplied by ulnar artery

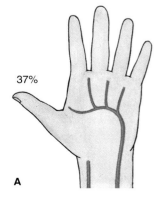

37%

A

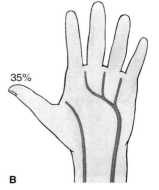

35%

B

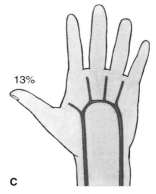

13%

C

PLATE 108 Palmar Arterial Arches

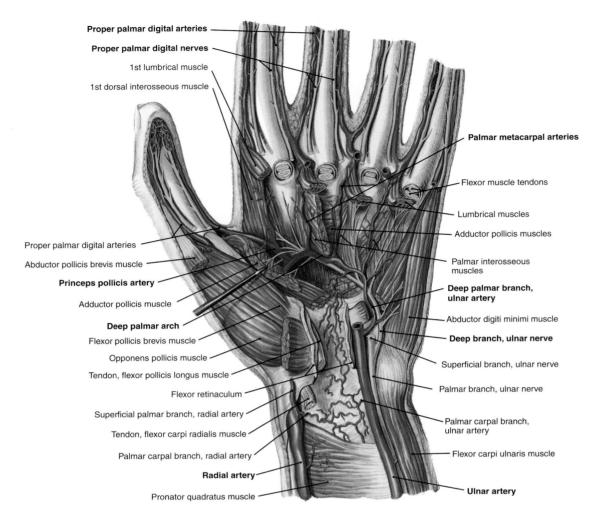

Proper palmar digital arteries
Proper palmar digital nerves
1st lumbrical muscle
1st dorsal interosseous muscle

Palmar metacarpal arteries

Flexor muscle tendons

Lumbrical muscles

Adductor pollicis muscles

Proper palmar digital arteries
Abductor pollicis brevis muscle
Princeps pollicis artery
Adductor pollicis muscle
Deep palmar arch
Flexor pollicis brevis muscle
Opponens pollicis muscle
Tendon, flexor pollicis longus muscle
Flexor retinaculum
Superficial palmar branch, radial artery
Tendon, flexor carpi radialis muscle
Palmar carpal branch, radial artery
Radial artery
Pronator quadratus muscle

Palmar interosseous muscles
Deep palmar branch, ulnar artery
Abductor digiti minimi muscle
Deep branch, ulnar nerve
Superficial branch, ulnar nerve
Palmar branch, ulnar nerve
Palmar carpal branch, ulnar artery
Flexor carpi ulnaris muscle
Ulnar artery

FIGURE 108.1 Nerves and Arteries of the ▲
Left Palm, Deep Palmar Arch

NOTE: (1) The **radial artery** at the wrist enters the
hand dorsally through the "anatomical snuff box"
(see Figs. 93.1 and 93.2) and then passes distally,
perforates the two heads of first dorsal interosseous
muscle, and reaches the palm of the hand.

(2) In the palm, the radial artery forms the **deep palmar arch,** uniting medially with the **deep palmar
branch** of the ulnar artery.

(3) From the deep arch arise the **palmar metacarpal
arteries** as well as the **princeps pollicis artery**.

(4) The **deep branch of the ulnar nerve** courses with
the deep palmar arterial arch. It supplies all the
muscles in the deep palm.

(5) There is a rich anastomosis between the superficial
and deep arches and between the ulnar and radial
arteries.

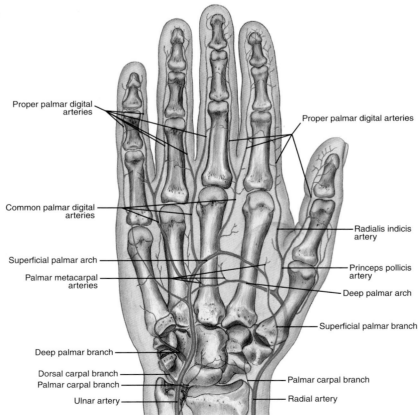

Proper palmar digital arteries

Proper palmar digital arteries

Common palmar digital arteries

Radialis indicis artery

Superficial palmar arch

Palmar metacarpal arteries

Princeps pollicis artery

Deep palmar arch

Superficial palmar branch

Deep palmar branch
Dorsal carpal branch
Palmar carpal branch

Palmar carpal branch

Ulnar artery

Radial artery

FIGURE 108.2 Arteries of the Right ▶
Hand Showing the Palmar Arterial Arches

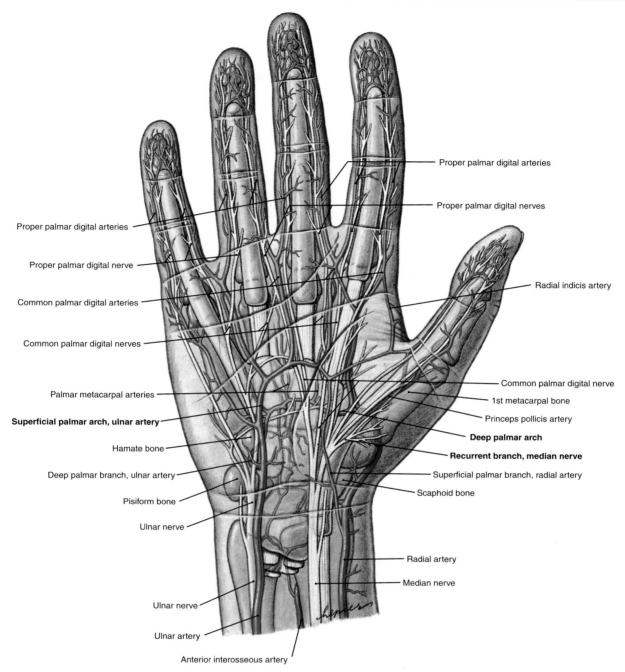

Proper palmar digital arteries

Proper palmar digital nerves

Proper palmar digital arteries

Proper palmar digital nerve

Common palmar digital arteries

Common palmar digital nerves

Palmar metacarpal arteries

Superficial palmar arch, ulnar artery

Hamate bone

Deep palmar branch, ulnar artery

Pisiform bone

Ulnar nerve

Radial indicis artery

Common palmar digital nerve

1st metacarpal bone

Princeps pollicis artery

Deep palmar arch

Recurrent branch, median nerve

Superficial palmar branch, radial artery

Scaphoid bone

Radial artery

Median nerve

Ulnar nerve

Ulnar artery

Anterior interosseous artery

FIGURE 109.1 **Surface Projection of Arteries and Nerves to the Palm of the Hand**

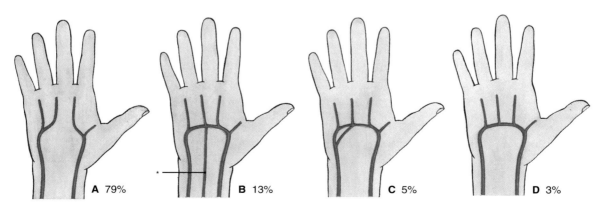

A 79%   **B** 13%   **C** 5%   **D** 3%

FIGURE 109.2 **Variations in the Formation of the Deep Palmar Arch**

A: Complete deep palmar arch. **B:** Double ulnar contribution. **C:** Anastomosis with anterior interosseous artery. **D:** Radial two digits supplied by the radial artery, ulnar three digits supplied by the ulnar artery.

PLATE 110 Sagittal Section through the Middle Finger (Ulnar View)

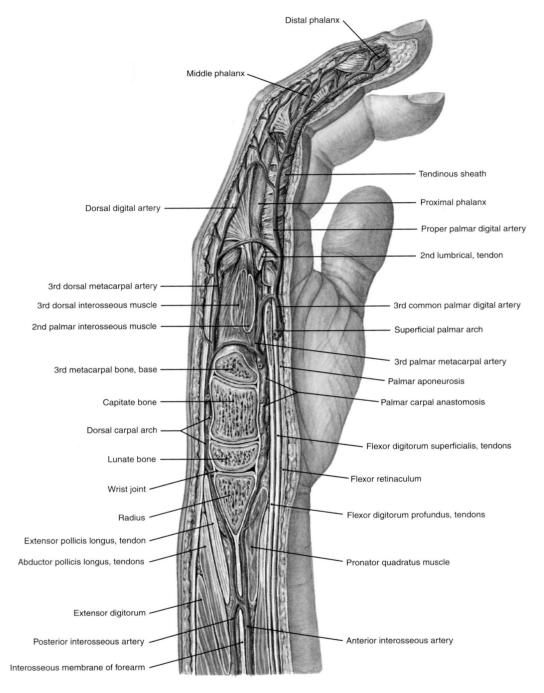

Distal phalanx

Middle phalanx

Tendinous sheath

Dorsal digital artery

Proximal phalanx

Proper palmar digital artery

2nd lumbrical, tendon

3rd dorsal metacarpal artery

3rd dorsal interosseous muscle

2nd palmar interosseous muscle

3rd common palmar digital artery

Superficial palmar arch

3rd metacarpal bone, base

3rd palmar metacarpal artery

Palmar aponeurosis

Capitate bone

Palmar carpal anastomosis

Dorsal carpal arch

Flexor digitorum superficialis, tendons

Lunate bone

Wrist joint

Flexor retinaculum

Radius

Flexor digitorum profundus, tendons

Extensor pollicis longus, tendon

Abductor pollicis longus, tendons

Pronator quadratus muscle

Extensor digitorum

Posterior interosseous artery

Anterior interosseous artery

Interosseous membrane of forearm

FIGURE 110 **Sagittal Section through the Middle Finger: Right Hand (Ulnar View)**

NOTE: (1) There is a rich blood supply and abundant anastomoses along the entire extent of the finger.
(2) The second palmar interosseous muscle of the ring finger and the third dorsal interosseous muscle of the middle finger.
(3) The skeletal continuum from proximal to distal: radius, lunate and capitate bones; the third metacarpal; and the proximal, middle, and distal phalanges.
(4) The anastomosis just proximal to the wrist joint between the anterior and posterior interosseous arteries.

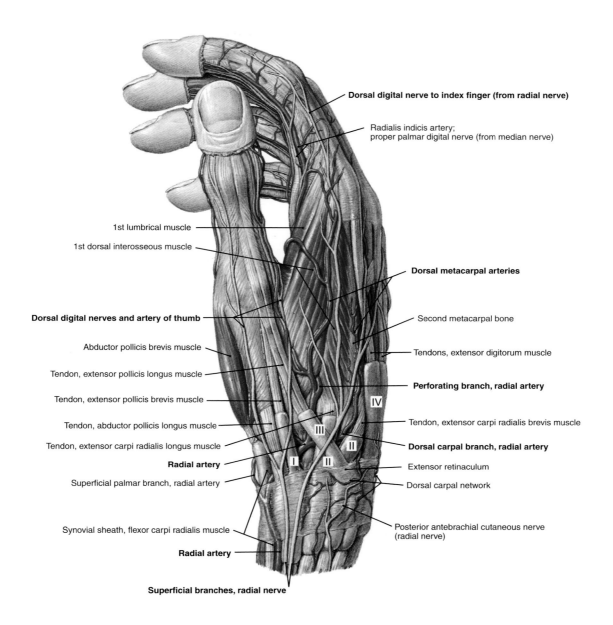

Dorsal digital nerve to index finger (from radial nerve)

Radialis indicis artery;
proper palmar digital nerve (from median nerve)

1st lumbrical muscle

1st dorsal interosseous muscle

Dorsal metacarpal arteries

Dorsal digital nerves and artery of thumb

Second metacarpal bone

Abductor pollicis brevis muscle

Tendons, extensor digitorum muscle

Tendon, extensor pollicis longus muscle

Tendon, extensor pollicis brevis muscle

Perforating branch, radial artery

Tendon, abductor pollicis longus muscle

Tendon, extensor carpi radialis brevis muscle

Tendon, extensor carpi radialis longus muscle

Dorsal carpal branch, radial artery

Radial artery

Extensor retinaculum

Superficial palmar branch, radial artery

Dorsal carpal network

Synovial sheath, flexor carpi radialis muscle

Posterior antebrachial cutaneous nerve
(radial nerve)

Radial artery

Superficial branches, radial nerve

I–IV = Synovial tendon sheaths
I = Abductor pollicis longus and extensor pollicis
brevis tendon sheaths
II = Extensor carpi radialis longus and brevis tendon sheaths
IIII = Extensor pollicis longus tendon sheath
IV = Extensor digitorum and extensor indicis tendon sheath

FIGURE 111 **Superficial Nerves, Arteries, and Tendons on the Radial Aspect of the Right Hand**

NOTE: (1) Only the skin and superficial fascia have been removed in this dissection, and the cutaneous nerves and superficial arteries to the thumb, radial side of the index finger, and dorsum of the hand have been retained.

(2) The **superficial branches of the radial nerve** to the hand (see Figs. 68, 89, and 90.1). These supply the dorsum of the thumb, nearly to the tip, as well as the lateral (radial) half of the dorsum of the hand.

(3) The radial nerve also supplies the proximal part of the dorsum of the index, middle, and lateral half of the ring fingers, as far as the proximal interphalangeal joint because the median nerve sends branches around the digits to supply the more distal parts of the fingers.

(4) The distribution of the radial artery to the thumb and dorsum of the hand (see Figs. 93.1 and 93.2). Observe: (a) the **dorsal digital branch** to the thumb; (b) the **radial indicis branch** to the index finger; (c) the **perforating branch** that penetrates between the two heads of the first dorsal interosseous muscle; and (d) the **dorsal carpal branch,** from which the dorsal metacarpal arteries arise.

PLATE 112 Skeleton of the Thorax; Scapula

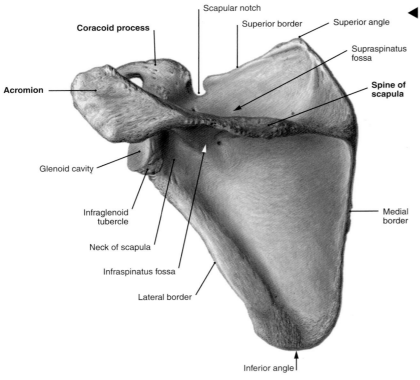

◀ **FIGURE 112.1** **Left Scapula (Dorsal Surface)**

NOTE: (1) The socket for the head of the humerus is formed by the glenoid cavity.

(2) The acromion and coracoid process give additional protection to the socket superiorly, anteriorly, and posteriorly.

(3) The spine of the scapula separates the dorsal surface into supraspinatus and infraspinatus fossae.

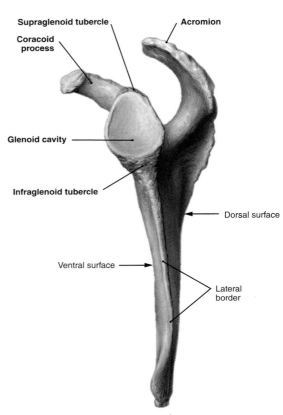

▲ **FIGURE 112.2** **Left Scapula (Lateral View)**

NOTE: (1) The supraglenoid and infraglenoid tubercles from which arise the long heads of the biceps and triceps muscles (see Fig. 118.1).

(2) The anteriorly projecting coracoid process to which are attached the pectoralis minor, short head of biceps, and coracobrachialis muscles.

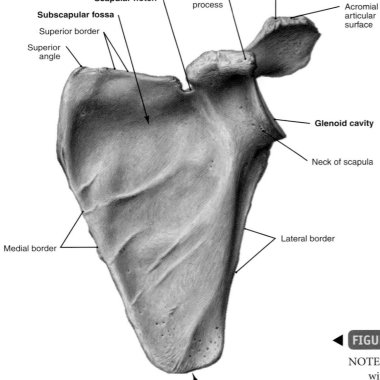

◀ **FIGURE 112.3** **Left Scapula (Ventral Surface)**

NOTE: (1) Much of the ventral surface of the scapula is a concave fossa within which lies the subscapularis muscle.

(2) The scapula has three borders: medial, lateral, and superior; it also has two angles: superior and inferior.

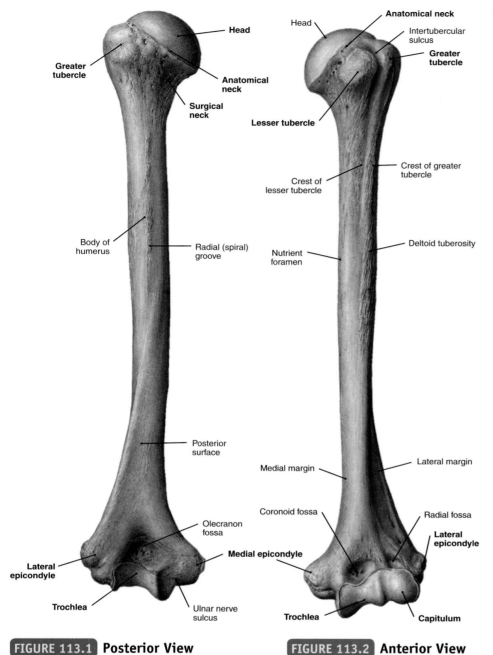

FIGURE 113.1 **Posterior View**

Greater tubercle
Head
Anatomical neck
Surgical neck
Body of humerus
Radial (spiral) groove
Posterior surface
Olecranon fossa
Lateral epicondyle
Trochlea
Medial epicondyle
Ulnar nerve sulcus

FIGURE 113.2 **Anterior View**

Head
Anatomical neck
Intertubercular sulcus
Greater tubercle
Lesser tubercle
Crest of lesser tubercle
Crest of greater tubercle
Nutrient foramen
Deltoid tuberosity
Medial margin
Lateral margin
Coronoid fossa
Radial fossa
Lateral epicondyle
Trochlea
Capitulum

FIGURE 113.1 and 113.2
Left Humerus

NOTE: (1) The hemispheric head of the humerus articulates with the glenoid cavity of the scapula.

(2) The surgical neck of the humerus is frequently a site of fractures.

(3) On the greater tubercle insert the supraspinatus, infraspinatus, and teres minor, in that order. On the lesser tubercle inserts the subscapularis. These four muscles form the **rotator cuff.**

(4) Within the intertubercular sulcus passes the tendon of the long head of the biceps.

(5) Adjacent to the **radial groove** courses the radial **nerve,** which is endangered by fractures of the humerus.

(6) Injury to the radial nerve in the arm results in a condition called **wrist drop,** because innervation to the extensors of the wrist and fingers is lost.

(7) The distal extremity of the humerus articulates with the radius and ulna, the **capitulum** with the head of the radius, and the trochlea with the **trochlear** notch of the ulna.

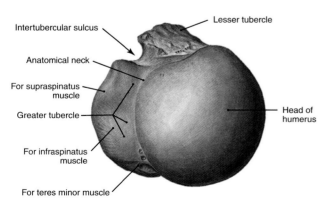

Intertubercular sulcus
Anatomical neck
For supraspinatus muscle
Greater tubercle
For infraspinatus muscle
For teres minor muscle
Lesser tubercle
Head of humerus

FIGURE 113.3 **Head of the Left Humerus (Viewed from Above)**

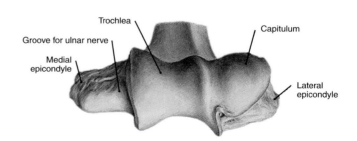

Trochlea
Groove for ulnar nerve
Medial epicondyle
Capitulum
Lateral epicondyle

FIGURE 113.4 **Distal Extremity of the Left Humerus (Viewed from Below)**

PLATE 114 Shoulder Joint: Ligaments and Bony Structures

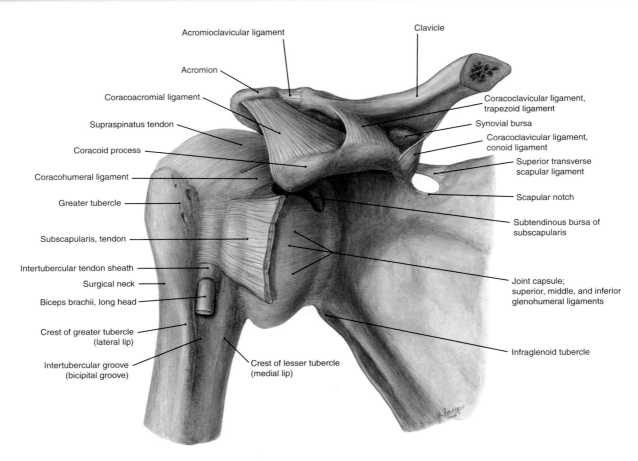

Acromioclavicular ligament

Clavicle

Acromion

Coracoacromial ligament

Coracoclavicular ligament,
trapezoid ligament

Supraspinatus tendon

Synovial bursa

Coracoid process

Coracoclavicular ligament,
conoid ligament

Coracohumeral ligament

Superior transverse
scapular ligament

Greater tubercle

Scapular notch

Subscapularis, tendon

Subtendinous bursa of
subscapularis

Intertubercular tendon sheath

Surgical neck

Biceps brachii, long head

Joint capsule;
superior, middle, and inferior
glenohumeral ligaments

Crest of greater tubercle
(lateral lip)

Infraglenoid tubercle

Intertubercular groove
(bicipital groove)

Crest of lesser tubercle
(medial lip)

FIGURE 114.1 Ligaments of the Right Shoulder (Glenohumeral) Joint (Anterior View)

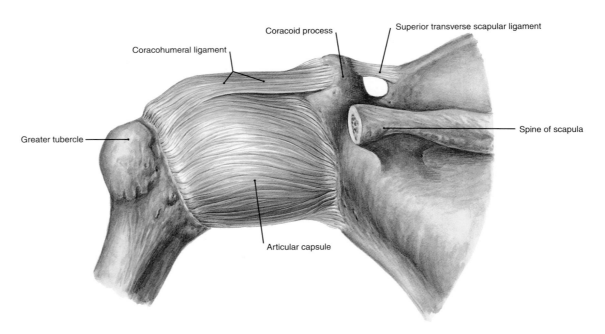

Coracoid process

Superior transverse scapular ligament

Coracohumeral ligament

Greater tubercle

Spine of scapula

Articular capsule

FIGURE 114.2 Capsule of Left Shoulder Joint (Posterior View)

NOTE: (1) The articular capsule completely surrounds the joint. It is attached beyond the glenoid cavity on the scapula above and to the anatomical neck of the humerus below.
(2) The superior part of the capsule is further strengthened by the coracohumeral ligament.

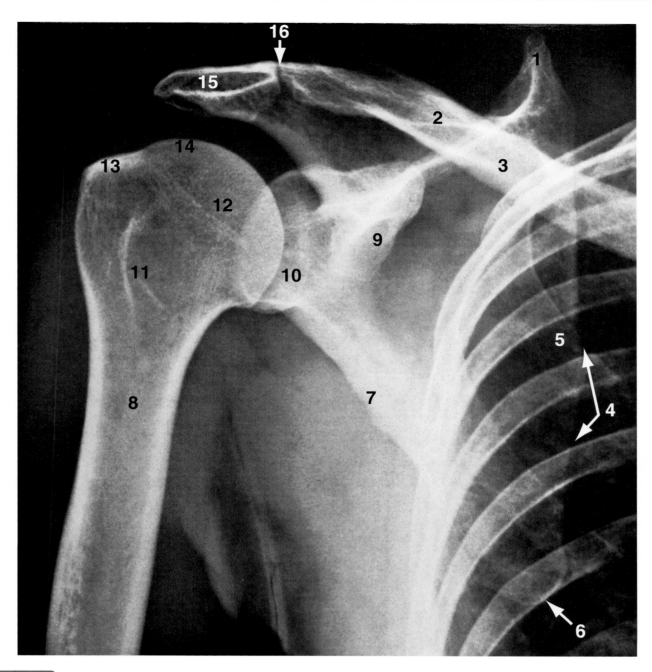

FIGURE 115 **Radiograph of the Right Shoulder Region**

1. Superior angle of scapula
2. Spine of scapula
3. Clavicle
4. Medial margin of scapula
5. Second rib
6. Inferior angle of scapula
7. Lateral margin of scapula
8. Surgical neck of humerus
9. Coracoid process
10. Glenoid cavity
11. Lesser tubercle
12. Anatomical neck of humerus
13. Greater tubercle
14. Head of humerus
15. Acromion
16. Acromioclavicular joint

NOTE: (1) The clavicle, scapula, and humerus are involved in radiography of the shoulder region. The acromioclavicular joint is a **planar** type formed by the lateral end of the clavicle and the medial border of the acromion.

(2) The glenohumeral, or shoulder, joint is remarkably loose and provides a free range of movement. Observe the wide separation between the humeral head and the glenoid cavity.

(3) Inferior **dislocations** of the head of the humerus are common because of minimal protection below. A **shoulder separation** results from a dislocation of the acromion under the lateral edge of the clavicle due to a strong blow to the lateral side of the joint.

(4) The hemispheric smooth surface of the humeral head. Covered with hyalin cartilage, the head of the humerus is slightly constricted at the anatomical neck, where a line separates the articular part superomedially from the greater and lesser tubercles below.

(5) Below these tubercles, the humerus shows another constriction, called the surgical neck, where fractures frequently occur.

(From Wicke, 6th ed.)

PLATE 116 Acromioclavicular and Shoulder Joints

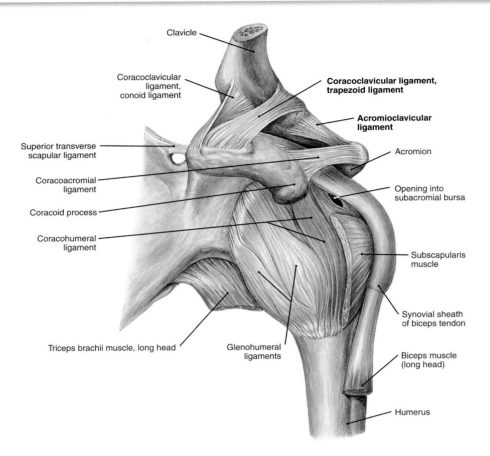

FIGURE 116.1 Left Shoulder Joint and Acromioclavicular Joint (Anterior View)

NOTE: (1) The clavicle is attached to the acromion and coracoid process of the scapula by the **acromioclavicular** and **coracoclavicular ligaments.**

(2) The acromion and coracoid process are interconnected by the **coracoclavicular ligament.**

(3) Neither the acromion nor the clavicle attaches to the humerus, but the glenoid labrum and the coracoid process do.

(4) The acromion, coracoid process, and clavicle protect the shoulder from above. The joint is weakest inferiorly and anteriorly, the directions in which most dislocations occur.

(5) The **glenohumeral ligaments** are thickened bands that tend to strengthen the joint capsule anteriorly.

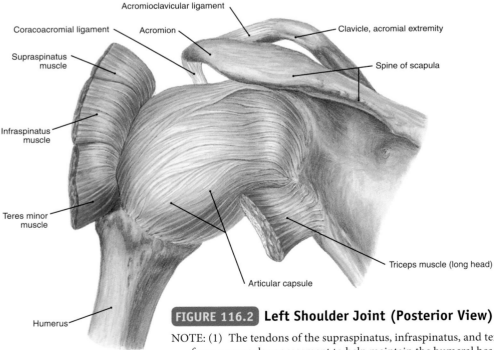

FIGURE 116.2 Left Shoulder Joint (Posterior View)

NOTE: (1) The tendons of the supraspinatus, infraspinatus, and teres minor blend with the joint capsule and form a muscular encasement to help maintain the humeral head in the socket.

(2) The long head of the triceps is attached close to the joint capsule. It is drawn even closer in abduction of the arm and helps prevent dislocation.

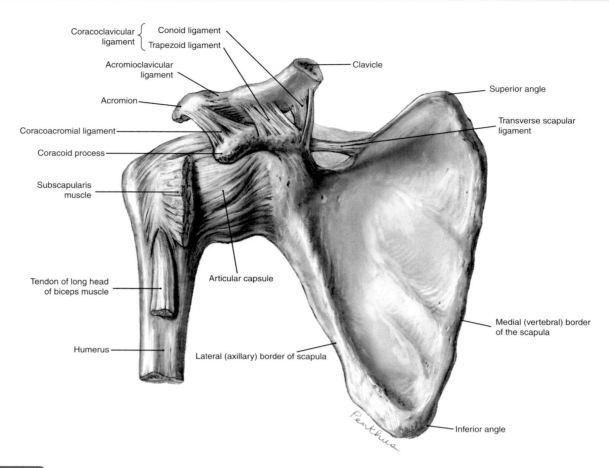

FIGURE 117.1 The Right Shoulder Joint (Anterior View)

Compare this figure with Figure 116.1.

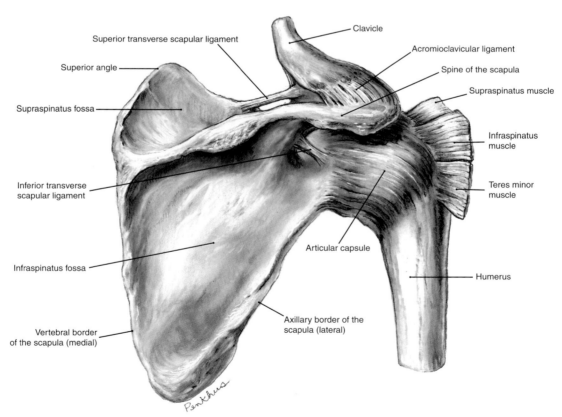

FIGURE 117.2 The Right Shoulder Joint (Posterior View)

Compare this figure with Figure 116.2.

PLATE 118 Glenoid Labrum and Cavity; Clavicular and Scapular Ligaments

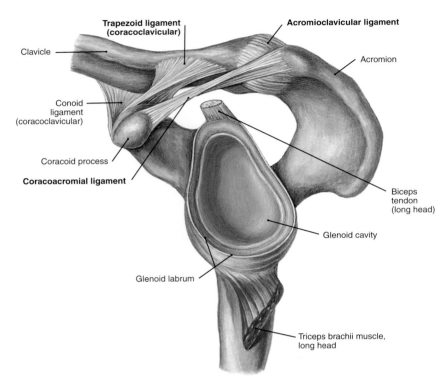

FIGURE 118.1 Left Glenoid Cavity (Lateral View); Scapuloclavicular Joint

NOTE: (1) The glenoid cavity was exposed by removing the articular capsule at the glenoid labrum.

(2) The attachments of the long head of the biceps at the supraglenoid and the long head of the triceps at the infraglenoid tubercles are still intact.

(3) The shallowness of the glenoid cavity is somewhat deepened 3 to 5 mm by the glenoid labrum.

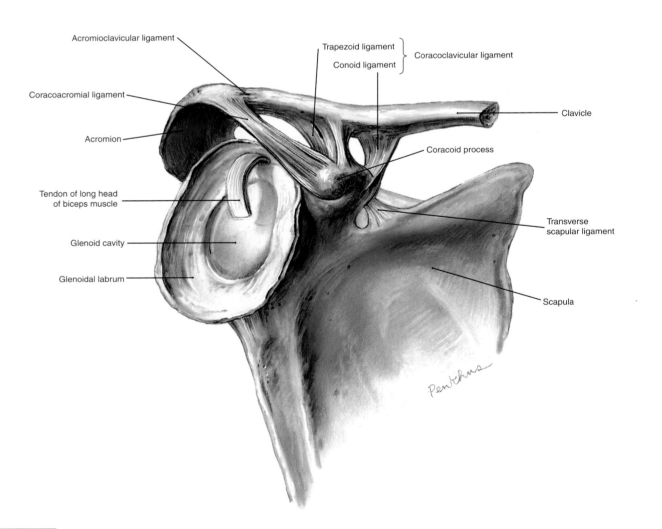

FIGURE 118.2 Right Scapula and Clavicle; Glenoid Fossa (Anterolateral View)

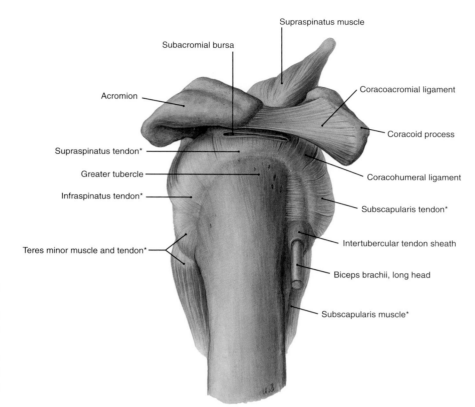

FIGURE 119.1 **Right Shoulder Joint after Removal of the Deltoid Muscle**

NOTE: (1) A fibrous capsule surrounds the shoulder joint.

(2) The tendon of the long head of the biceps enters the capsule on its way to the supraglenoid tubercle of the scapula.

(3) The tendons of the supraspinatus, infraspinatus, teres minor, and subscapularis muscles (noted with asterisks [*]) form the protective "rotator cuff" of the shoulder joint.

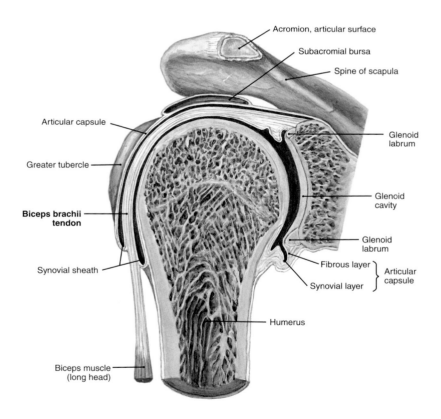

FIGURE 119.2 **Frontal Section through the Right Shoulder Joint**

NOTE: (1) The tendon of the long head of the biceps is enclosed by a synovial sheath. Although the tendon passes through the joint, it is not within the synovial cavity.

(2) The capsule of the joint is composed of a dense outer fibrous layer and a thin synovial inner layer.

(3) A bursa is a sac lined by a synovial-like membrane. It is found at sites subjected to friction and usually does not communicate with the joint cavity.

(4) In the shoulder, bursae are found between the capsule and muscle tendons such as the subscapularis, infraspinatus, and deltoid. The **subacromial bursa** lies deep to the coracoid and acromial processes.

PLATE 120 Radiographic Anatomy of the Right Shoulder Joint I

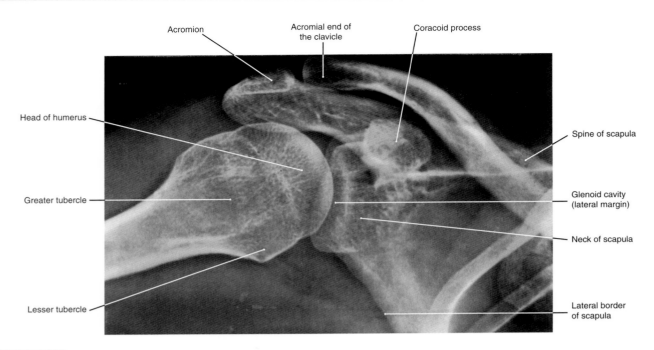

Acromion

Acromial end of
the clavicle

Coracoid process

Head of humerus

Spine of scapula

Greater tubercle

Glenoid cavity
(lateral margin)

Neck of scapula

Lesser tubercle

Lateral border
of scapula

FIGURE 120.1 **Radiograph of the Right Shoulder Joint**

NOTE that this radiograph was taken in an anteroposterior direction. The subject was supine with the upper limb abducted and rotated medially. (From R. Brickner. *Normal Radiologic Patterns and Variations of the Human Skeleton*, Urban and Schwarzenberg, Munich, 1977.)

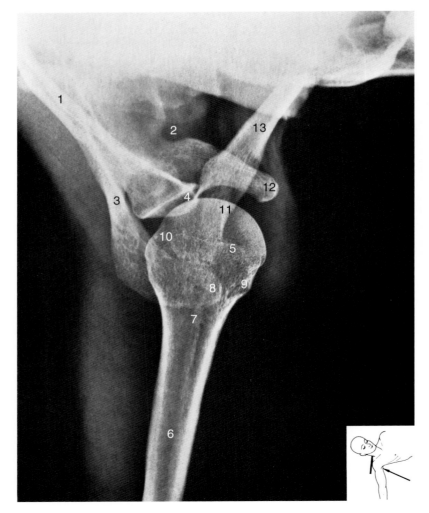

FIGURE 120.2 **Radiograph of the Right Shoulder Joint**

NOTE that this is an axial (longitudinal) view of the shoulder joint with the scapula and clavicle superior and the shaft of the humerus projecting inferiorly.

1. Scapula
2. Scapular notch
3. Spine of the scapula
4. Glenoid fossa
5. Greater tubercle
6. Shaft of the humerus
7. Surgical neck of the humerus
8. Acromion
9. Lesser tubercle
10. Anatomical neck of the humerus
11. Head of the humerus
12. Coracoid process
13. Clavicle

(From Wicke, 6th ed.)

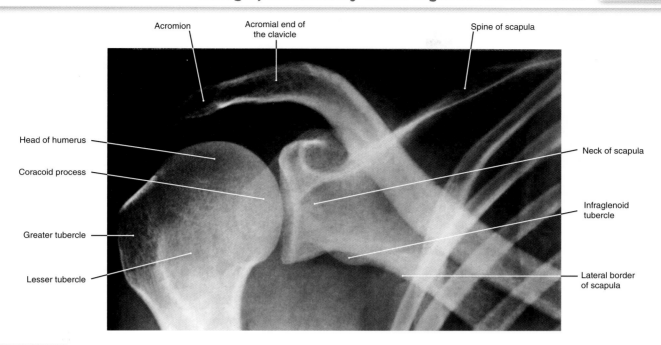

FIGURE 121.1 **Radiograph of the Right Shoulder Joint (Humerus Alongside the Body)**

NOTE that this radiograph was taken in an anteroposterior direction. The subject was supine with the upper arm rotated medially. (From R. Brickner. *Normal Radiologic Patterns and Variations of the Human Skeleton*. Munich: Urban and Schwarzenberg, 1977.)

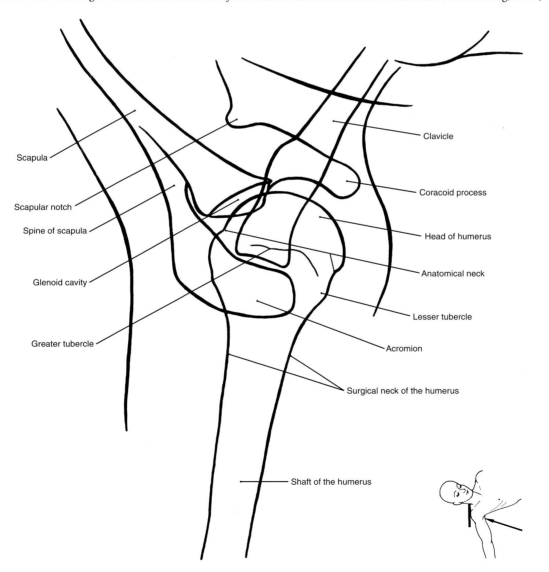

FIGURE 121.2 **Diagrammatic Representation of the Radiograph in Figure 120.2**

PLATE 122 Bones of the Upper Limb: Radius and Ulna

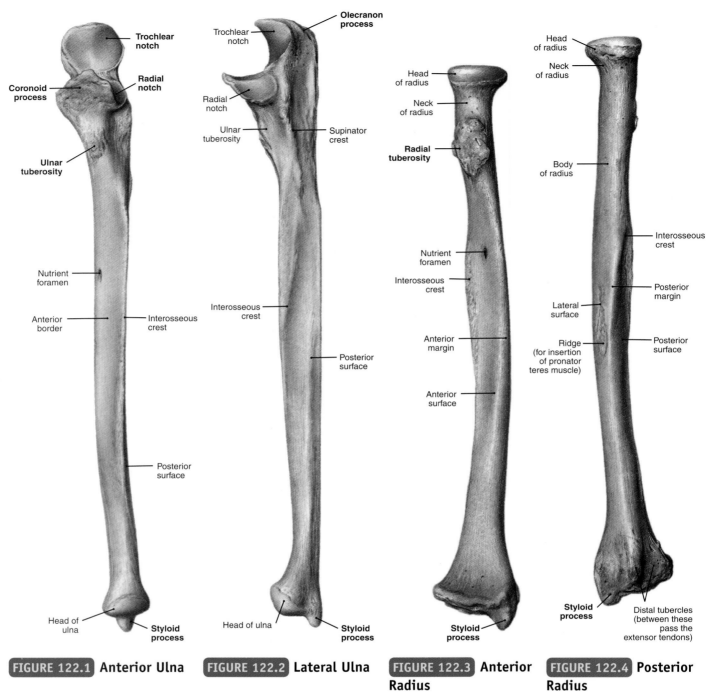

FIGURE 122.1 Anterior Ulna

FIGURE 122.2 Lateral Ulna

FIGURE 122.3 Anterior Radius

FIGURE 122.4 Posterior Radius

Left Ulna (Figs. 122.1 and 122.2)

NOTE: (1) The ulna is the medial bone of forearm. It has a superior extremity, a body or shaft, and an inferior extremity.

(2) The **superior extremity** contains the **olecranon** and **coronoid processes** and two cavities: the **radial notch** for articulation with the radius and the **trochlear notch** for the trochlea of the humerus.

(3) The brachialis muscle inserts on the tuberosity of the ulna.

(4) Along the **body** of the ulna attaches the interosseous membrane.

(5) The **distal extremity** is marked by the **ulnar head** laterally and the **styloid process** posteromedially.

Left Radius (Figs. 122.3 and 122.4)

NOTE: (1) The radius is situated lateral to the ulna, and it has a body and two extremities. Proximally, it attaches to both the humerus and the ulna. Distally, it articulates with the carpal bones (scaphoid, lunate, and triquetrum) and with the ulna.

(2) The **proximal extremity** contains a cylindrical head that articulates with both the **capitulum** of the humerus and the **radial notch** of the ulna.

(3) Onto the **radial tuberosity** inserts the tendon of the biceps brachii.

(4) Onto the **styloid process** attaches the brachioradialis muscle and the radial collateral ligament of the radiocarpal joint.

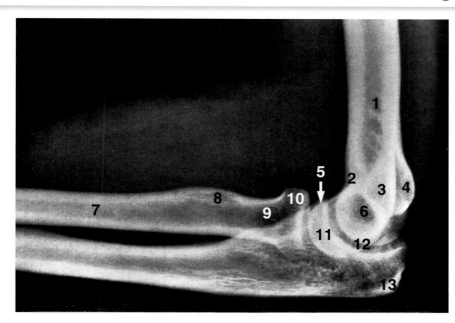

NOTE the following bony structures:

1. Body of humerus
2. Radial fossa
3. Olecranon fossa
4. Medial epicondyle
5. Coronoid process of ulna
6. Trochlea of humerus
7. Body of radius
8. Radial tuberosity
9. Neck of radius
10. Head of radius
11. Capitulum of humerus
12. Trochlear notch
13. Olecranon

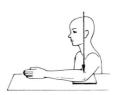

FIGURE 123.1 Radiograph of the Left Elbow Joint in an Adult (Lateral View)

(From Wicke, 6th ed.)

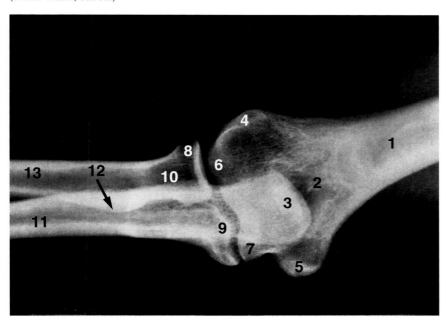

NOTE the following bony structures:

1. Body of humerus
2. Olecranon fossa
3. Olecranon
4. Lateral epicondyle
5. Medial epicondyle
6. Capitulum of humerus
7. Trochlea of humerus
8. Head of radius
9. Coronoid process of ulna
10. Neck of radius
11. Ulna
12. Radial tuberosity
13. Body of radius

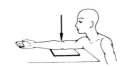

FIGURE 123.2 Radiograph of the Right Elbow Joint in an Adult (Anteroposterior View)

(From Wicke, 6th ed.)

FIGURE 123.3 Radiograph of the Elbow Joint in a 5½-Year-Old Boy

NOTE: (1) The shaft of a long bone is called the **diaphysis,** whereas a center of ossification, distinct from the shaft and usually at the end of a long bone, is called an **epiphysis.**

(2) The epiphysis of the head of the radius is, as yet, not formed in the 5½-year-old child, although ossification has started in the humeral capitulum.

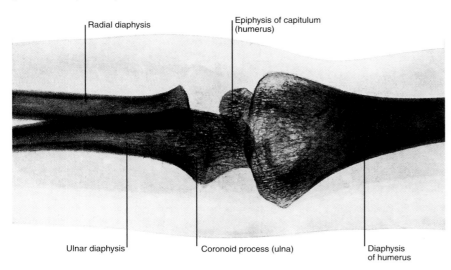

Radial diaphysis

Epiphysis of capitulum (humerus)

Ulnar diaphysis

Coronoid process (ulna)

Diaphysis of humerus

PLATE 124 Left Elbow Joint (Anterior, Posterior, and Sagittal Views)

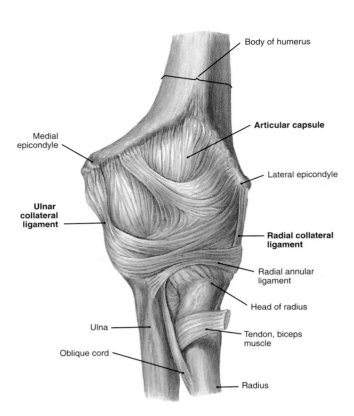

FIGURE 124.1 Left Elbow Joint (Anterior View)

NOTE: (1) The elbow joint is a hinge, or ginglymus, joint.
(2) The **trochlea** of the humerus is received in the trochlear notch of the ulna.
(3) The capitulum of the humerus articulates with the head of the radius.
(4) The articular capsule is loose but is thickened medially and laterally by the ulnar and **radial collateral** ligaments

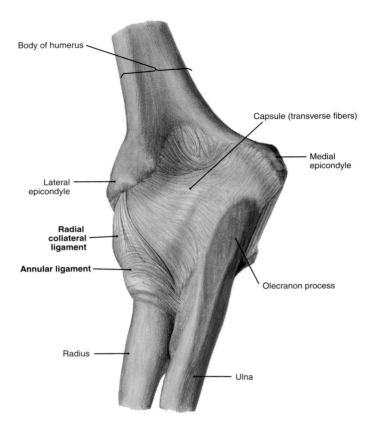

FIGURE 124.2 Left Elbow Joint (Posterolateral View)

NOTE: (1) The fan-shaped **radial collateral ligament** attaches above to the lateral epicondyle and blends with the capsule.
(2) The upper border of the **radial annular ligament** also blends with the joint capsule.

FIGURE 124.3 Left Elbow Joint (Sagittal Section)

NOTE: (1) The adaptation of the trochlea of the humerus with the trochlear notch of the ulna allows only flexion and extension, not lateral displacement.
(2) The posterior surface of the olecranon is separated from the skin by a subcutaneous bursa and the insertion of the triceps.
(3) **Fractures** of the distal end of the humerus occur most often from falls on the outstretched hand, because the force is transmitted through the bones of the forearm to the humerus.
(4) **Fractures** of the olecranon result from direct trauma to the bone by a fall on the point of the elbow.
(5) **Posterior dislocation** of the ulna and attached radius is the most common dislocation at the elbow joint, again from falls on the outstretched and abducted hand.

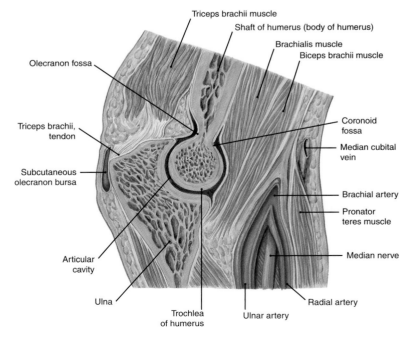

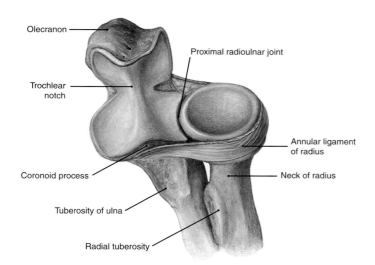

FIGURE 125.1 **Left Proximal Radioulnar Joint**

NOTE: (1) This anterior view of the proximal radioulnar joint (oriented similar to Fig. 124.1) shows the annular ligament surrounding the head of the radius. The ligament attaches to the ulna both anteriorly and posteriorly.

(2) The radial tuberosity onto which inserts the biceps brachii and the olecranon where the triceps brachii inserts

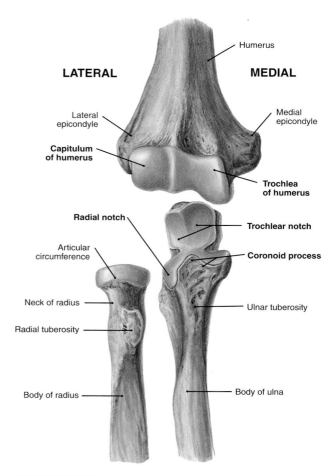

FIGURE 125.2 **Bones of the Right Elbow and Radioulnar Joints (Anterior View)**

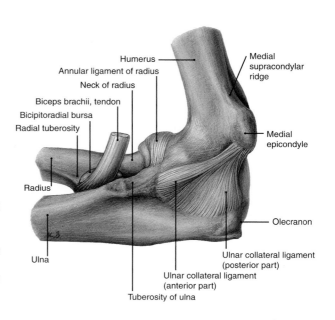

FIGURE 125.3 **Flexed and Supinated Right Elbow Joint (Medial Aspect)**

NOTE: (1) The anterior and posterior parts of the ulnar (medial) collateral ligament.

(2) The annular ligament encasing the head of the radius.

(3) The insertion of the biceps brachii tendon onto the tuberosity of the radius.

(4) The olecranon of the ulna onto which the triceps brachii (not shown) inserts.

PLATE 126 **Radioulnar Joints**

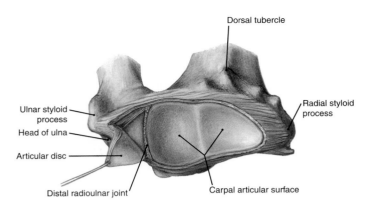

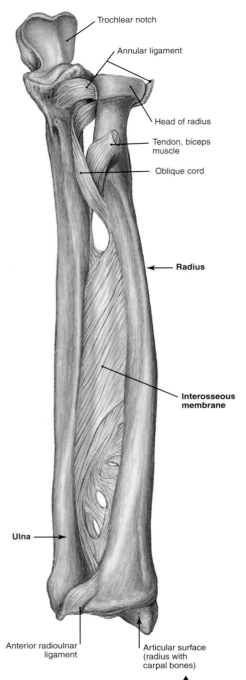

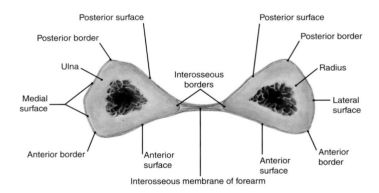

FIGURE 126.2 **Right Radioulnar Joint**

NOTE: (1) The lateral surface of the distal radius and the medial surface of the distal ulna form the distal radioulnar joint.

(2) The synovial cavity at this joint is L-shaped and is interposed between the distal end of the ulna and an articular disk. This cavity extends superiorly between the lateral surface of the distal radius and the medial surface of the distal ulna.

FIGURE 126.3 **Bones of the Forearm (Transverse Section)**

NOTE: (1) The interosseous membrane between the shafts of the radius and ulna. This membrane greatly strengthens the bony structures of the forearm.

(2) If a significant force ascends in the forearm (such as from a fall onto the outstretched hand), the interosseous membrane helps dissipate the impact of the fall. It does this by transmitting a part of the force to the other bone, thereby helping prevent fractures of the forearm bones.

FIGURE 126.1 **Radioulnar Joints (Anterior View, Left)**

NOTE: (1) The radius and ulna articulate proximally, along the shafts of the two bones, and distally.

(2) Proximally, the head of the radius rotates within the radial notch of the ulna (pivot or trochoid joint).

(3) The **annular ligament,** attached at both ends to the ulna, encircles the head of the radius, protecting the joint.

(4) The interosseous membrane extends obliquely between the shafts of the two bones, whereas distally the head of the ulna attaches to the ulnar notch of the radius.

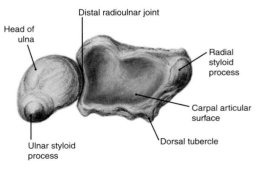

FIGURE 126.4 **Distal Aspect of the Left Radius and Ulna**

NOTE that the distal extremity of both bones is marked by a styloid process. Between the lateral side of the distal end of the ulna and the medial side of the wide lower end of the radius is located the distal radioulnar joint.

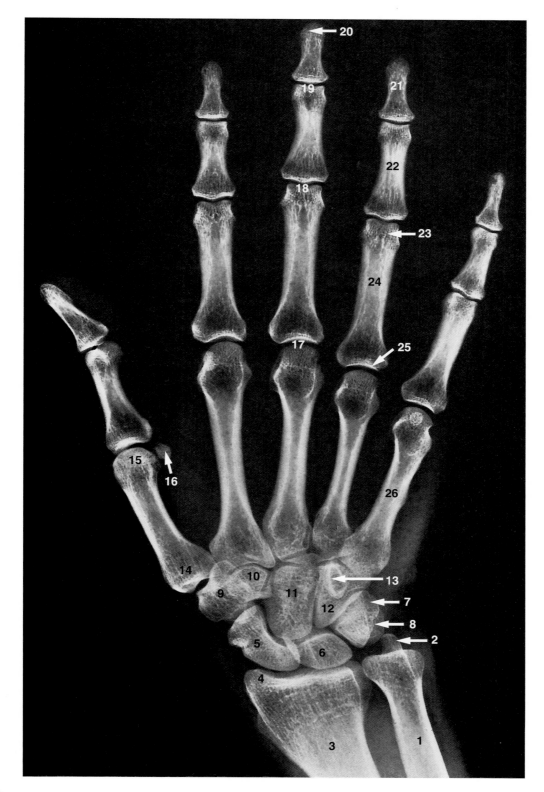

FIGURE 127 **Radiograph of the Right Wrist and Hand (Dorsopalmar View)**

1. Ulna
2. Styloid process of ulna
3. Radius
4. Styloid process of radius
5. Scaphoid
6. Lunate
7. Triquetral

8. Pisiform
9. Trapezium
10. Trapezoid
11. Capitate
12. Hamate
13. Hamulus of hamate
14. Base of first metacarpal bone

15. Head of first metacarpal bone
16. Sesamoid bone
17. Metacarpophalangeal joint
18. Proximal interphalangeal joint
19. Distal interphalangeal joint
20. Tuberosity of distal phalanx
21. Distal phalanx

22. Middle phalanx
23. Head of phalanx
24. Proximal phalanx
25. Base of phalanx
26. Fifth metacarpal bone

(From Wicke, 6th ed.)

PLATE 128 Bones of the Wrist and Hand (Palmar Aspect)

FIGURE 128.1 Skeleton of the Right Wrist and Hand (Palmar View)

NOTE: (1) **Carpal bones:** 8; **metacarpal bones:** 5; **phalanges:** 14 (thumb has 2, each of the other 4 fingers has 3)

(2) **Carpal bones,** lateral to medial:

Proximal Row	**Distal Row**
Scaphoid	Trapezium
Lunate	Trapezoid
Triquetrum	Capitate
Pisiform	Hamate

(3) **Metacarpal bones:**
(a) First is shortest
(b) Second is longest
(c) Each has a **base** (carpal end), a **body,** and a **head** (distal end)

(4) **Phalanges:**
(a) Those of four medial fingers are set in transverse rows—**proximal, middle,** and **distal.**
(b) The thumb has only a proximal and a distal phalanx.

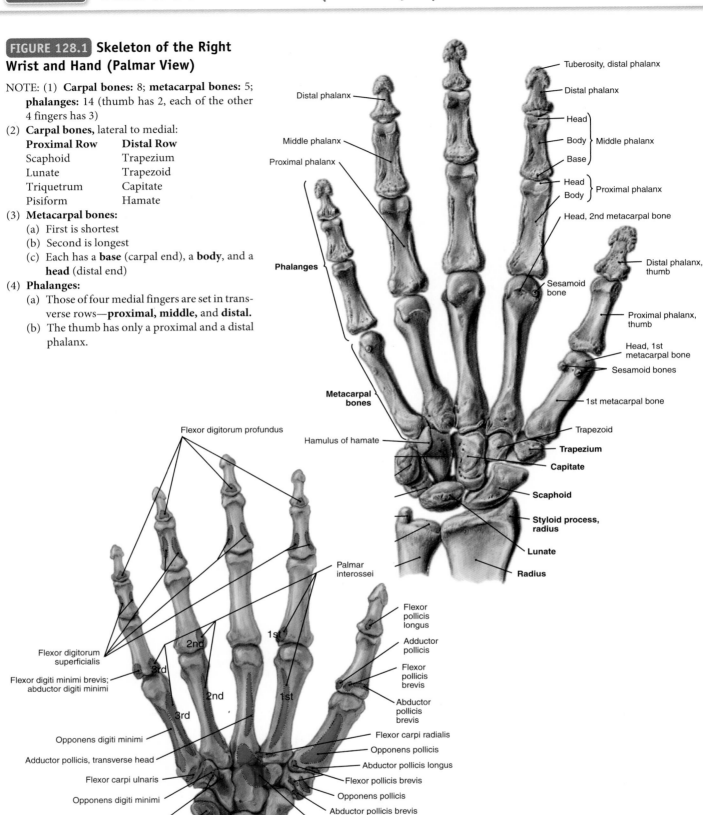

FIGURE 128.2 Bones of the Right Wrist and Hand (Palmar View), Showing the Attachment of Muscles

NOTE: The origins of muscles are in RED, whereas the insertions are in BLUE.

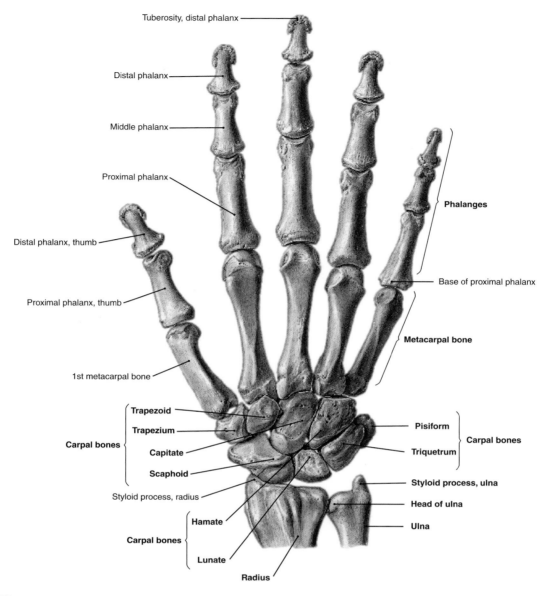

Tuberosity, distal phalanx

Distal phalanx

Middle phalanx

Proximal phalanx

Distal phalanx, thumb

Proximal phalanx, thumb

1st metacarpal bone

Trapezoid

Trapezium

Carpal bones {

Capitate

Scaphoid

Styloid process, radius

Carpal bones {

Hamate

Lunate

Radius

Phalanges

Base of proximal phalanx

Metacarpal bone

Pisiform

Carpal bones

Triquetrum

Styloid process, ulna

Head of ulna

Ulna

FIGURE 129.1 Skeleton of the Right Wrist and Hand (Dorsal View)

FIGURE 129.2 Radiograph of the Right Wrist (Dorsoventral Projection)

NOTE: The following numbered structures:

1. Base of first metacarpal bone (thumb)
2. Trapezium bone
3. Trapezoid bone
4. Capitate bone
5. Hamate bone
6. Hamulus of hamate bone
7. Base of the fifth metacarpal bone (little finger)
8. Scaphoid bone
9. Lunate bone
10. Triquetral bone
11. Pisiform bone
12. Styloid process of radius
13. Ulnar notch (distal radioulnar joint)
14. Styloid process of ulna
15. Radius
16. Ulna

(From Wicke, 6th ed.)

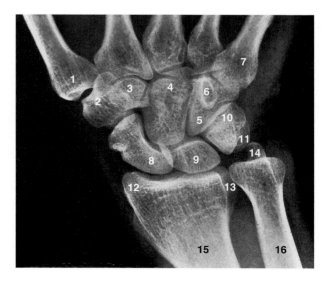

PLATE 130 Wrist and Hand: Ligaments and Joints

FIGURE 130.1 Joints and Ligaments of the ▶
Wrist and Hand (Dorsal View, Left Hand)

NOTE: (1) Most ligaments of joints in the wrist and hand
are named according to the bones they interconnect.

(2) The dorsal radiocarpal ligament strengthens the radiocarpal joint capsule dorsally. It is joined medially and
laterally by the ulnar and radial collateral ligaments (see
Fig. 131.3), which extend distally from the styloid processes of both the radius and the ulna.

(3) The intercarpal and carpometacarpal ligaments are
short, dense connective-tissue strands extending between adjacent bones.

(4) The articular capsule has been cut on the dorsal aspect
of the third metacarpophalangeal joint to reveal the
rounded head of the metacarpal bone and the concave
base of the proximal phalanx.

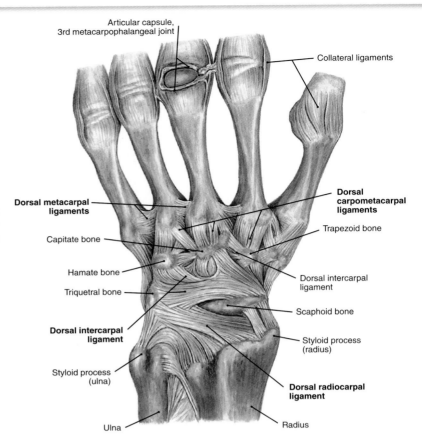

Articular capsule,
3rd metacarpophalangeal joint

Collateral ligaments

**Dorsal
carpometacarpal
ligaments**

Trapezoid bone

**Dorsal metacarpal
ligaments**

Capitate bone

Dorsal intercarpal
ligament

Hamate bone

Triquetral bone

Dorsal intercarpal
ligament

**Dorsal intercarpal
ligament**

Scaphoid bone

Styloid process
(radius)

Styloid process
(ulna)

**Dorsal radiocarpal
ligament**

Ulna

Radius

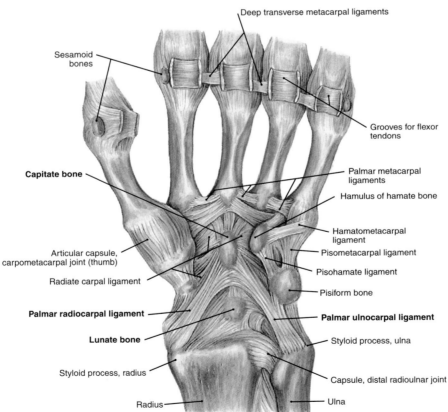

Deep transverse metacarpal ligaments

Sesamoid
bones

Grooves for flexor
tendons

Capitate bone

Palmar metacarpal
ligaments

Hamulus of hamate bone

Hamatometacarpal
ligament

Articular capsule,
carpometacarpal joint (thumb)

Pisometacarpal ligament

Radiate carpal ligament

Pisohamate ligament

Pisiform bone

Palmar radiocarpal ligament

Palmar ulnocarpal ligament

Lunate bone

Styloid process, ulna

Styloid process, radius

Capsule, distal radioulnar joint

Radius

Ulna

FIGURE 130.2 Joints and Ligaments of the Wrist and Hand (Palmar
View, Left Hand)

NOTE: (1) Several strong ligaments in the palmar hand: the radiate ligament surrounding the
capitate bone as well as pisohamate and pisometacarpal ligaments.

(2) The bases of the metacarpal bones are joined by the palmar metacarpal ligaments and the
distal heads by the deep transverse metacarpal ligament.

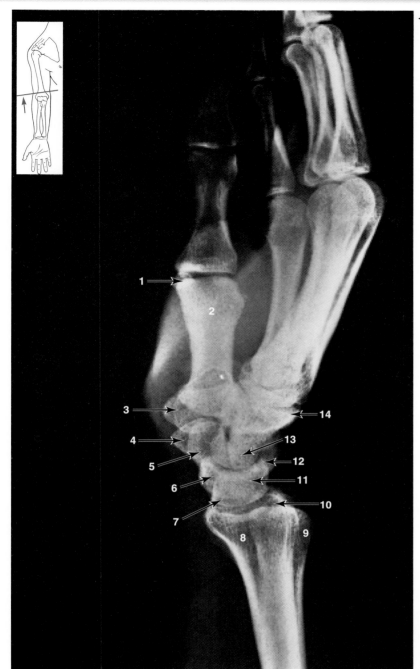

◀ **FIGURE 131.1** Radiograph of the Right Hand (Lateral Projection)

1. Sesamoid bone
2. First metacarpal bone
3. Trapezium bone
4. Tuberosity of scaphoid bone
5. Pisiform bone
6. Styloid process of radius
7. Scaphoid bone
8. Radius
9. Ulna
10. Styloid process of ulna
11. Lunate bone
12. Triquetral bone
13. Head of capitate bone
14. Hamate bone

(From Wicke, 6th ed.)

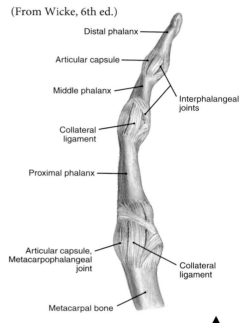

FIGURE 131.2 Joints and Ligaments of the Middle Finger

NOTE: The articular capsules of the joints in the fingers are strengthened by longitudinally oriented collateral ligaments.

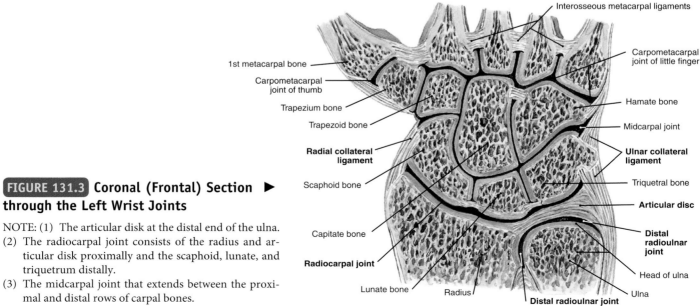

FIGURE 131.3 Coronal (Frontal) Section ▶ through the Left Wrist Joints

NOTE: (1) The articular disk at the distal end of the ulna.
(2) The radiocarpal joint consists of the radius and articular disk proximally and the scaphoid, lunate, and triquetrum distally.
(3) The midcarpal joint that extends between the proximal and distal rows of carpal bones.

Chapter 1 Pectoral Region, Axilla, Shoulder, and Upper Limb

PLATE 132 Cross Sections of the Upper Limb: Arm

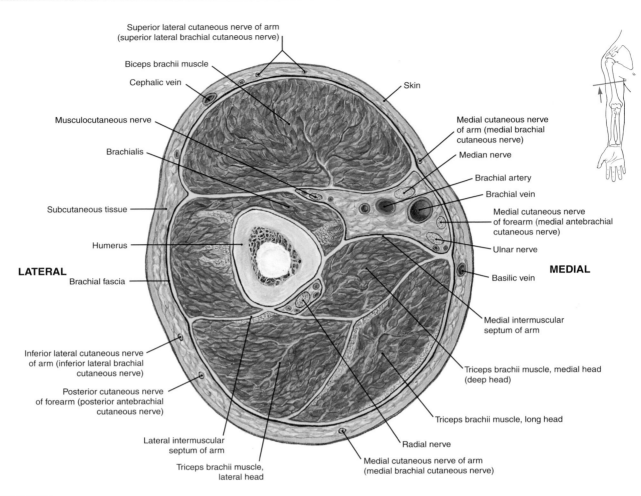

Superior lateral cutaneous nerve of arm
(superior lateral brachial cutaneous nerve)

Biceps brachii muscle

Cephalic vein

Skin

Musculocutaneous nerve

Medial cutaneous nerve
of arm (medial brachial
cutaneous nerve)

Brachialis

Median nerve

Brachial artery

Brachial vein

Subcutaneous tissue

Medial cutaneous nerve
of forearm (medial antebrachial
cutaneous nerve)

Humerus

Ulnar nerve

LATERAL

MEDIAL

Brachial fascia

Basilic vein

Medial intermuscular
septum of arm

Inferior lateral cutaneous nerve
of arm (inferior lateral brachial
cutaneous nerve)

Triceps brachii muscle, medial head
(deep head)

Posterior cutaneous nerve
of forearm (posterior antebrachial
cutaneous nerve)

Triceps brachii muscle, long head

Radial nerve

Lateral intermuscular
septum of arm

Medial cutaneous nerve of arm
(medial brachial cutaneous nerve)

Triceps brachii muscle,
lateral head

FIGURE 132.1 Cross Section of the Right Upper Extremity through the Middle of the Humerus

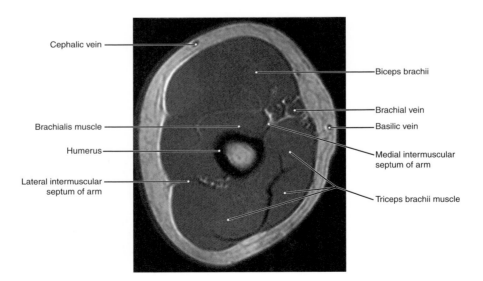

Cephalic vein

Biceps brachii

Brachial vein

Brachialis muscle

Basilic vein

Humerus

Medial intermuscular
septum of arm

Lateral intermuscular
septum of arm

Triceps brachii muscle

FIGURE 132.2 Magnetic Resonance Image (MRI) of the Right Upper Limb through the Middle of the Humerus

NOTE that this MRI may be compared with the cross section in Figure 132.1.

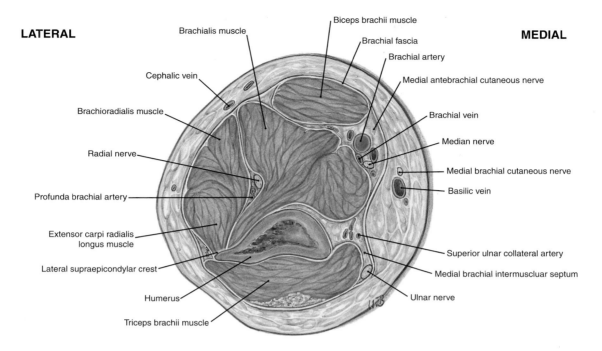

LATERAL

MEDIAL

- Biceps brachii muscle
- Brachialis muscle
- Brachial fascia
- Brachial artery
- Medial antebrachial cutaneous nerve
- Cephalic vein
- Brachioradialis muscle
- Brachial vein
- Median nerve
- Radial nerve
- Medial brachial cutaneous nerve
- Profunda brachial artery
- Basilic vein
- Extensor carpi radialis longus muscle
- Lateral supraepicondylar crest
- Superior ulnar collateral artery
- Medial brachial intermuscluar septum
- Humerus
- Ulnar nerve
- Triceps brachii muscle

FIGURE 133.1 Transverse Section through the Lower Third of the Arm

NOTE the brachial artery, basilic vein, and the median, ulnar, and radial nerves.

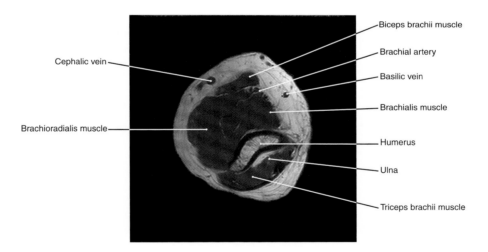

- Cephalic vein
- Brachioradialis muscle
- Biceps brachii muscle
- Brachial artery
- Basilic vein
- Brachialis muscle
- Humerus
- Ulna
- Triceps brachii muscle

FIGURE 133.2 Magnetic Resonance Image (MRI). Cross Section at the Lower Third of the Arm

PLATE 134 Cross Sections of the Upper Limb: Elbow and Upper Forearm

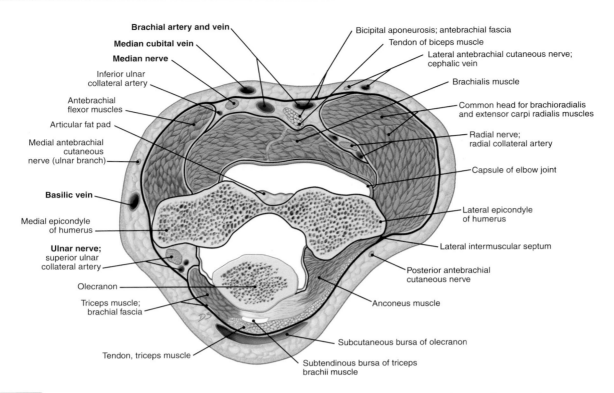

FIGURE 134.1 Cross Section through the Right Upper Extremity at the Level of the Elbow Joint

NOTE: (1) The ulnar nerve and superior ulnar collateral artery lie behind the medial epicondyle of the humerus, medial to the olecranon of the ulna.
(2) The median nerve lies to the ulnar (medial) side of the brachial vein and artery in the cubital fossa, and all three structures lie deep to the cubital fascia and median cubital vein.
(3) At this level, the radial nerve and radial collateral artery lie between the common origins of the extensor muscles and the deeply located brachialis muscle.

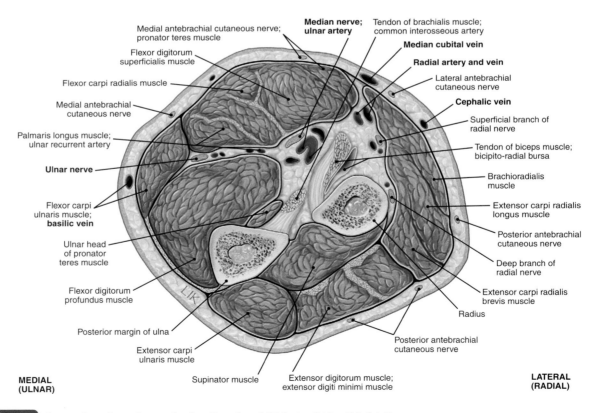

FIGURE 134.2 Cross Section through the Proximal Third of the Right Forearm

NOTE: (1) The common interosseous artery branching from the ulnar artery and the insertions of the biceps brachii and brachialis muscles to the radius and ulna, respectively.
(2) The radial nerve has already divided into its superficial and deep branches.

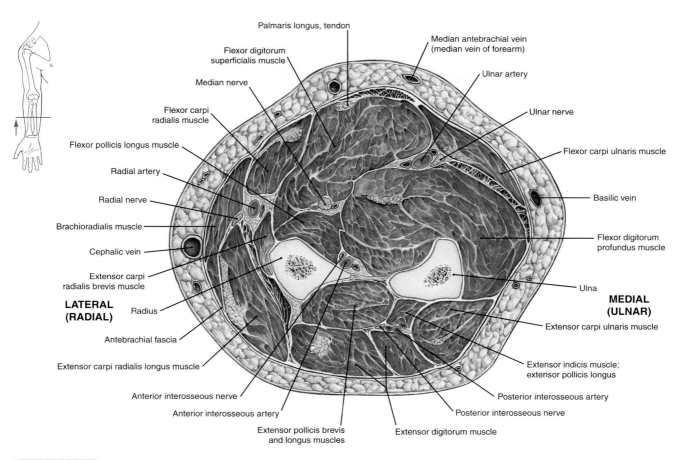

FIGURE 135.1 Cross Section through the Middle Third of the Right Forearm

NOTE: (1) At this level, the ulna, radius, interosseous membrane, and intermuscular septum clearly delineate the **posterior compartment,** extending dorsally and laterally, from the **anterior compartment** located anteriorly and medially.

(2) The **median nerve** coursing down the forearm deep to the flexor digitorum superficialis and anterior to the flexor digitorum profundus and flexor pollicis longus.

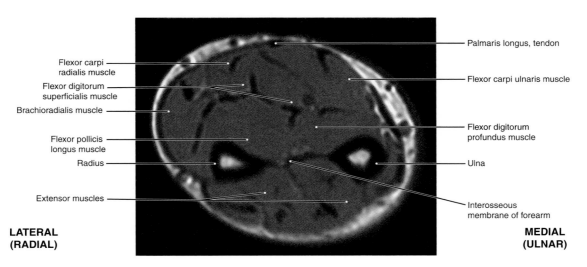

FIGURE 135.2 Transverse MRI Section through the Middle of the Forearm

NOTE that this figure should be compared with Figure 135.1. Observe the locations of the anterior and posterior forearm muscle groups and judge where the important vessels and nerves would be found in the MRI.

Chapter 1 Pectoral Region, Axilla, Shoulder, and Upper Limb

PLATE 136 Computerized Tomographs of the Wrist

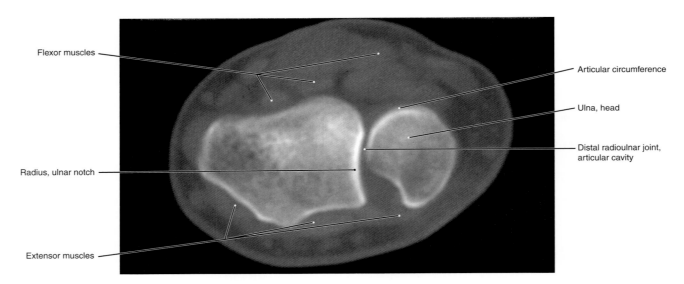

Flexor muscles

Articular circumference

Ulna, head

Distal radioulnar joint, articular cavity

Radius, ulnar notch

Extensor muscles

FIGURE 136.1 **CT of the Right Distal Radioulnar Joint**

NOTE: (1) The **head of the ulna** fits into the **ulnar notch** of the radius and the articular cavity of the distal radioulnar joint between.
(2) The distal end of the radius is large, while its proximal end is relatively small. In contrast, the distal end of the ulna is small in comparison to the proximal end at the elbow joint. Compare with the bones in Figures 137.1 and 137.2.

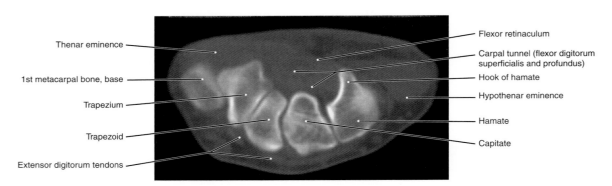

Thenar eminence

Flexor retinaculum

Carpal tunnel (flexor digitorum superficialis and profundus)

1st metacarpal bone, base

Hook of hamate

Hypothenar eminence

Trapezium

Trapezoid

Hamate

Capitate

Extensor digitorum tendons

FIGURE 136.2 **CT of the Right Wrist**

NOTE: (1) This image is taken at the level of the distal row of carpal bones (from lateral to medial: trapezium, trapezoid, capitate, and hamate).
(2) The base of the first metacarpal bone as it articulates proximally with the trapezium to form the carpometacarpal joint of the thumb. Compare this figure with the radiograph in Figure 127.
(3) The hook (hamulus) of the hamate bone projects from the palmar surface of the bone. It can be felt through the skin over the proximal part of the hypothenar eminence.

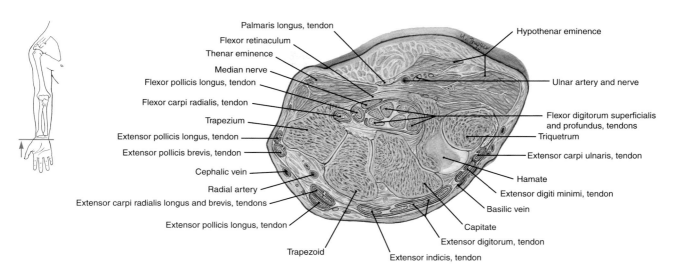

FIGURE 137.1 **Transverse Section through the Wrist Joint**

NOTE: (1) This cross section is at the level of the distal row of carpal bones. Compare the carpal bones in this section with the figures in Plate 91.

(2) The locations of the **median nerve** in the **carpal tunnel** and the ulnar nerve and artery superficial to the carpal tunnel adjacent to the hypothenar muscles.

(3) The strong **flexor retinaculum** bounds the carpal tunnel anteriorly, while the carpal bones bound the tunnel posteriorly. In addition to the median nerve, the flexor tendons enter the hand within the tunnel.

(4) Significant trauma to this region of the hand can result in excessive pressure on the median nerve; this condition is called **carpal tunnel syndrome,** and it severely limits the functions of the thenar muscles supplied by the median nerve.

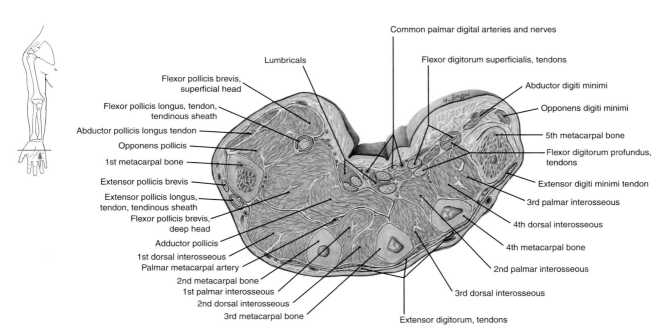

FIGURE 137.2 **Cross Section of the Right Hand through the Metacarpal Bones**

NOTE: (1) The four **dorsal interosseous muscles** that act as abductors of the fingers and fill the intervals between the metacarpal bones.

(2) The three **palmar interosseous muscles** that serve as adductors of the fingers.

(3) The **thenar muscles** on the radial side of the hand and the **hypothenar muscles** on the ulnar side.

(4) There are seven **interosseous muscles**—three palmar and four dorsal. In addition to flexing the metacarpophalangeal joints, these muscles abduct and adduct the fingers. The thumb has its own abductors and adductor and the little finger has its own abductor. This accounts for adduction and abduction actions for the five fingers.

PLATE 138 The Thumb, Index Finger, and Fingernails

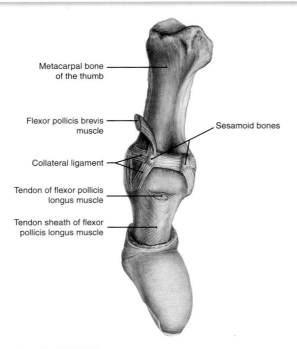

FIGURE 138.1 **Metacarpophalangeal Joint of the Thumb**

NOTE the sesamoid bones, collateral ligaments, and flexor muscle insertions.

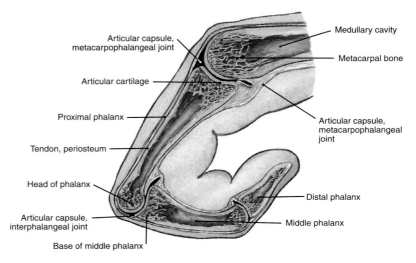

FIGURE 138.2 **Longitudinal Section through a Flexed Finger**

NOTE: The location of the flexion creases in relation to the corresponding joints.

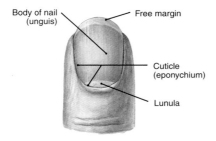

FIGURE 138.3 **Fingernail, Normal Position (Dorsal View) Finger**

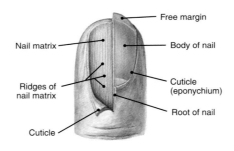

FIGURE 138.4 **Left Half of Finger Nail Bed Exposed**

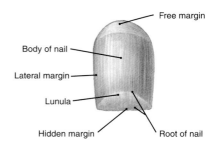

FIGURE 138.5 **Body of Fingernail Removed from the Nail Bed**

CHAPTER 2 The Thorax

Plates

139 Surface Anatomy of the Female and Male Anterior Body Walls

140 Thoracic Cage (Anterior View): Clavicle

141 Thoracic Cage (Posterior View): Sternum

142 Thoracic Cage: Ribs

143 12 Right Ribs and Costal Cartilages

144 Bony Projections onto the Anterior Body Wall

145 Thoracic Cage (Sternocostal Articulations): Clavicle

146 Internal Surface of the Thoracic Cage: Anterior and Posterior Parts

147 Anterior Thoracic and Abdominal Wall: Inner Surface

148 Anterior Thoracic Wall: Muscles

149 Thoracic Cage: Projection of Thoracic and Upper Abdominal Organs

150 Thymus in an Adolescent and from a Young Child

151 Thoracic Cage: Radiograph of the Chest

152 Lungs and Heart In Situ: Anterior Thoracic Wall Removed

153 The Parietal and Visceral Pleurae

154 Reflections of Pleura (Anterior View)

155 Reflections of Pleura (Posterior View)

156 Reflections of Pleura (Lateral Views)

157 Trachea, Bronchi, and Lungs

158 Lungs: Lateral (Sternocostal) View

159 Lungs: Bronchopulmonary Segments (Lateral View)

160 Lungs: Medial (Mediastinal) View

161 Lungs: Bronchopulmonary Segments (Medial View)

162 Trachea and Bronchi

163 Trachea and Bronchi: Surface Projection (Internal Surface)

164 Hilum of Left Lung: Costodiaphragmatic Recess

165 Left Anterior Bronchogram; Bronchoscopy of Tracheal Bifurcation

166 Mediastinum: Right Side, Pleura Removed

167 Mediastinum: Left Side, Pleura Removed

168 Radiograph of the Thorax: Diagram of Cardiac Dimensions and Contours

169 Projection of Heart Valves: Thorax and Heart during Breathing

170 Mediastinum: Great Vessels; Subdivisions of Mediastinum

171 Heart: Surface Projection; Great Vessels

172 Heart and Great Vessels (Anterior View)

173 Heart and Great Vessels (Posterior View)

174 Heart and Great Vessels with the Pericardium Opened

175 Pericardium with the Heart Removed

176 Heart, Blood Supply (Anterior and Superior Surfaces)

177 Heart, Blood Vessels: Posterior (Diaphragmatic) Surface

178 Heart: Coronary Arteries

179 Variations in Coronary Artery Distribution

180 Heart: Arteriogram of the Left Coronary Artery

181 Heart: Arteriogram of the Right Coronary Artery

182 Heart: Right Atrium and Ventricle

183 Heart: Right Ventricle and Pulmonary Trunk

184 Heart: Left Atrium and Ventricle

185 Heart: Left Ventricle and Ascending Aorta

186 Unfolding the Muscular Anatomy of the Heart

187 Heart: Papillary Muscles and Chordae Tendineae

188 Heart: Frontal Section; Conduction System

189 Heart: Conduction System

190 Atrioventricular Bundle System; Cusps of the Aortic Valve

191 Four Heart Valves: Projection and Auscultation Sites

192 Circulation of Blood in the Fetus

193 Simplified Schema of Fetal Circulation

194 Systemic Arteries in the Adult

195 Systemic and Portal Venous Systems in the Adult

196 Mediastinum and Lungs and the Upper Abdomen (Posterior View)

197 Posterior Mediastinum: Esophagus, Aorta, and Trachea

198 Esophageal Blood Supply and Lymph Nodes

199 Posterior Mediastinum (Dorsal View)

200 Radiographs of the Esophagus; Esophagoscopy

201 Esophagus: Sites of Constrictions and Common Sites of Diverticula

202 Superior and Posterior Mediastina: Vessels and Sympathetic Trunk

203 Posterior Thoracic Wall: Azygos System of Veins

204 Veins of the Esophagus

205 Branches from the Aortic Arch and Variations

206 Mediastinum: Sympathetic Trunks and Vagus Nerves (Anterior View)

207 Sympathetic Trunks, Spinal Cord; Vertebral Column: Thoracic Level

208 Autonomic Nervous System: Sympathetic and Parasympathetic Parts

209 Autonomic Nervous System (Diagram)

210 Thoracic Duct and Lymphatic Drainage

211 Regional Lymph Nodes and Principal Lymph Vessels

212 Frontal Section through the Thorax; MRI of Thorax

213 Frontal Section through Lower Left Thorax; MRI of Thorax

214 Cross Section of the Thorax (Third Thoracic Vertebra Level)

215 Transverse Sections through the Thorax

216 Transverse Sections through the Thorax

217 Transverse Sections through the Thorax

218 Tomographic Cross Section of the Thorax; the Diaphragm

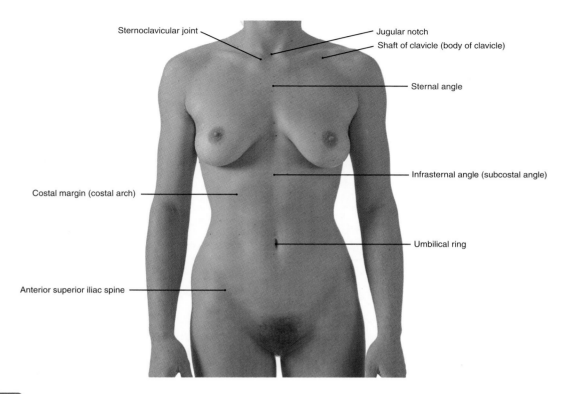

FIGURE 139.1 **Surface Anatomy of the Thoracic and Abdominal Walls in a Young Female**

NOTE that the prominent bony structures are labeled along with the jugular notch and umbilicus.

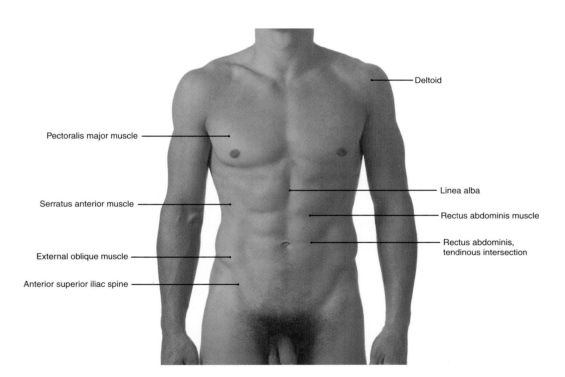

FIGURE 139.2 **Surface Anatomy of the Thoracic and Abdominal Walls in a Young Male**

NOTE that the surface contours of prominent muscles are labeled.

PLATE 140 Thoracic Cage (Anterior View): Clavicle

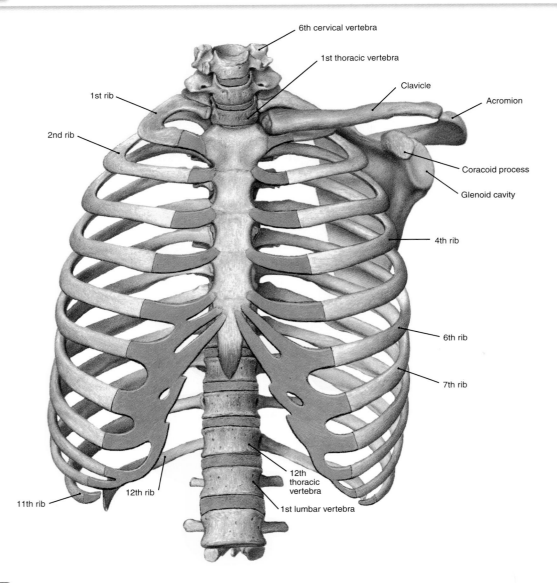

FIGURE 140.1 **Thoracic Skeleton (Anterior View)**

Left clavicle and scapula are shown in yellow; costal cartilages and intervertebral disks are in blue.

NOTE: (1) The skeleton of the thorax protects the thoracic organs. It is formed by 12 pairs of ribs that articulate posteriorly with the 12 thoracic vertebrae. Anteriorly, the bony parts of the ribs are continued as cartilages, the upper seven pairs of which are attached directly to the sternum.

(2) The bony parts of the ribs fall progressively more lateral to the sternum from above downward, resulting in longer costal cartilages in lower ribs than in higher ones.

(3) The thoracic cage is narrow superiorly at its inlet, but is more broad inferiorly, where it is closer to abdominal structures.

FIGURE 140.2 **Sternoclavicular and the First Two Sternocostal Joints**

NOTE: (1) The sternoclavicular joint is formed by the junction of the clavicle with (a) the upper lateral aspect of the manubrium and (b) the cartilage of the 1st rib.

(2) An articular disk is interposed between the clavicle and the sternum, and an articular capsule and fibrous ligamentous bands protect the joint.

(3) The cartilages of the 2nd to the 7th ribs (see Fig. 140.1) articulate with the sternum by movable (diarthrodial) joints. The cartilage of the 1st rib, however, directly joins the sternum and, without a joint cavity, forms an immovable joint (synarthrosis).

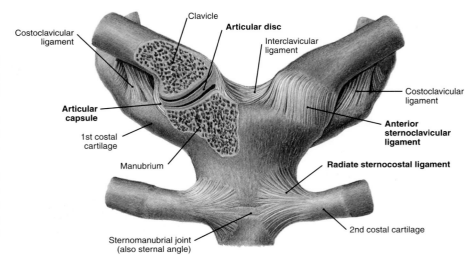

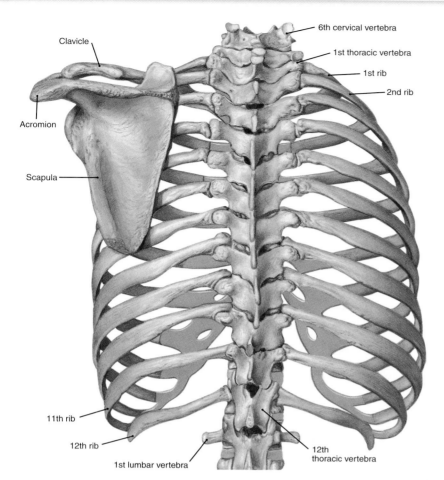

Clavicle

Acromion

Scapula

6th cervical vertebra

1st thoracic vertebra

1st rib

2nd rib

11th rib

12th rib

1st lumbar vertebra

12th thoracic vertebra

FIGURE 141.1 Thoracic Skeleton (Posterior View)

Left clavicle and scapula are shown in yellow.

NOTE: (1) The posterior skeleton of the thoracic cage consists of 12 thoracic vertebrae and the posterior parts of 12 pairs of ribs.

(2) The extremity on the head of typical ribs possesses two articular facets separated by a crest (see Fig. 142: eighth rib).

(3) These two facets articulate with the bodies of two adjacent vertebrae, whereas the crest is attached to the intervertebral disk. The lower facet articulates with the vertebra that corresponds with the rib, whereas the upper facet articulates with the adjacent vertebra above.

(4) The crest between the facets articulates with the intervertebral disk.

(5) The scapula affords some bony protection posteriorly to the upper lateral aspect of the thoracic cage.

FIGURE 141.2 Sternum (Anterior View)

NOTE: (1) The sternum consists of the manubrium, the body, and the xiphoid process and forms the middle portion of the anterior thoracic wall.

(2) The manubrium articulates with the body at the **sternal angle.** The xiphoid process is thin and often cartilaginous.

(3) The concave jugular notch, two clavicular notches, and 1st costal notches on the manubrium.

FIGURE 141.3 Sternum (Lateral View)

NOTE: (1) The clavicle and the 1st rib articulate with the manubrium. The 2nd rib articulates at the sternal angle. The 3rd to the 6th ribs articulate with the body of the sternum, whereas the 7th rib joins the sternum at the junction of the xiphoid process.

(2) A line projected backward through the sternal angle crosses at the 4th thoracic level, whereas the xiphisternal junction lies at T9.

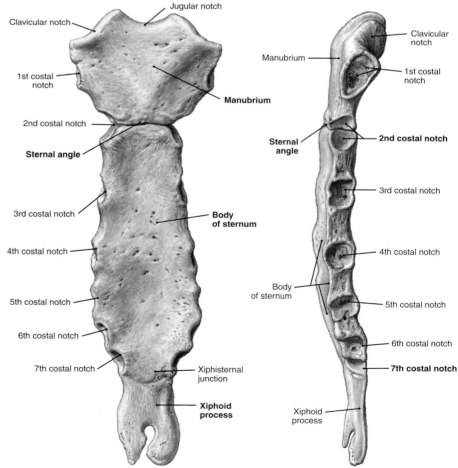

Jugular notch

Clavicular notch

1st costal notch

2nd costal notch

Sternal angle

3rd costal notch

4th costal notch

5th costal notch

6th costal notch

7th costal notch

Manubrium

Sternal angle

Body of sternum

Xiphisternal junction

Xiphoid process

Clavicular notch

Manubrium

1st costal notch

2nd costal notch

Sternal angle

3rd costal notch

4th costal notch

Body of sternum

5th costal notch

6th costal notch

7th costal notch

Xiphoid process

FIGURE 141.2

FIGURE 141.3

PLATE 142 **Thoracic Cage: Ribs**

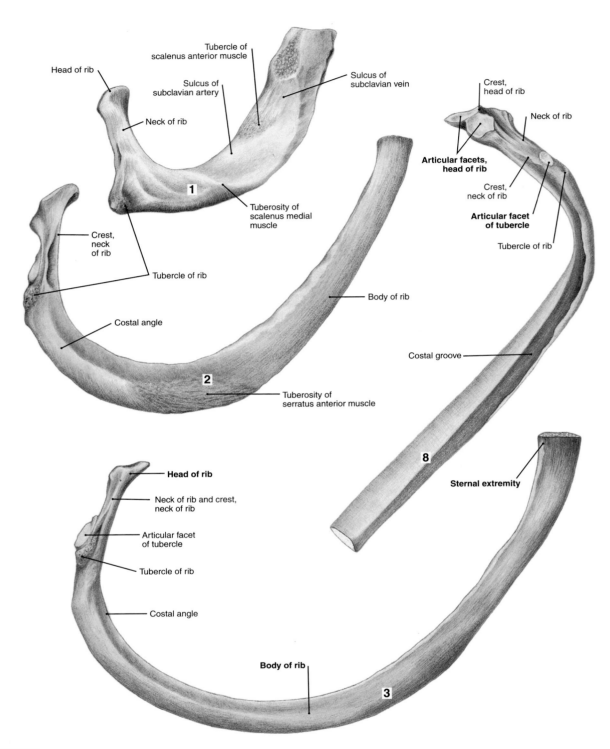

Tubercle of
scalenus anterior muscle

Head of rib

Sulcus of
subclavian artery

Tubercle of
scalenus anterior muscle

Sulcus of
subclavian vein

Neck of rib

Crest,
head of rib

Neck of rib

1

**Articular facets,
head of rib**

Crest,
neck of rib

**Articular facet
of tubercle**

Tuberosity of
scalenus medial
muscle

Tubercle of rib

Crest,
neck
of rib

Tubercle of rib

Body of rib

Costal angle

Costal groove

2

Tuberosity of
serratus anterior muscle

8

Head of rib

Neck of rib and crest,
neck of rib

Sternal extremity

Articular facet
of tubercle

Tubercle of rib

Costal angle

Body of rib

3

FIGURE 142 **1st, 2nd, 3rd, and 8th Right Ribs**

NOTE: (1) The superior surfaces of the 1st, 2nd, and 3rd ribs are illustrated, whereas the inferior surface of the 8th rib is shown.

(2) Each rib has a vertebral extremity directed posteriorly and a sternal extremity directed anteriorly. The body of the rib is the shaft that stretches between the extremities.

(3) The vertebral end is marked by a **head,** a **neck,** and a **tubercle.** The head contains two facets for articulation with the bodies of the thoracic vertebrae, whereas the tubercle has a nonarticular roughened elevation and an articular facet, which attaches to the transverse process of thoracic vertebrae.

(4) The 1st, 2nd, 10th, 11th, and 12th ribs present certain structural differences from the 3rd through the 9th ribs. The 1st rib is the most curved, and the 2nd is shaped similar to the 1st, but it is longer. The 10th, 11th, and 12th ribs also have only a single facet on the rib head.

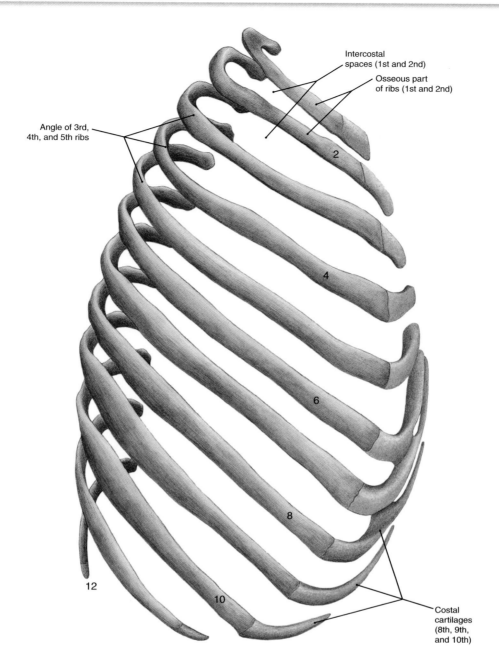

Intercostal
spaces (1st and 2nd)

Osseous part
of ribs (1st and 2nd)

Angle of 3rd,
4th, and 5th ribs

2

4

6

8

12

10

Costal
cartilages
(8th, 9th,
and 10th)

FIGURE 143 **12 Right Ribs Showing the Natural Contour of the Thoracic Cage (Lateral View)**

NOTE: (1) The posterior end of each rib is located more superiorly than the costal end that attaches to the costal cartilage; thus, as each rib leaves its vertebral articulation, it courses around the chest in a rounded, descending manner.

(2) Ribs 5 to 10 are longer than ribs 1 to 4 and 11 and 12. The latter two ribs are considered "floating ribs" because they do not attach to the sternum or the costal margin.

Muscle	Origin	Insertion	Innervation	Action
External intercostal (11 muscles)	Lower border of a rib	Upper border of the rib below	Intercostal nerves	Elevate the ribs; active during normal inspiration
	Within intercostal space, each extends from the tubercle of the rib dorsally to the cartilage of the rib ventrally			
Internal intercostal (11 muscles)	Ridge on the inner surface near lower border of the rib	Upper border of the rib below	Intercostal nerves	Elevate the ribs; active during inspiration and expiration
	Within intercostal space, each extends from the sternum ventrally to the angle of the rib dorsally			

PLATE 144 **Bony Projections onto the Anterior Body Wall**

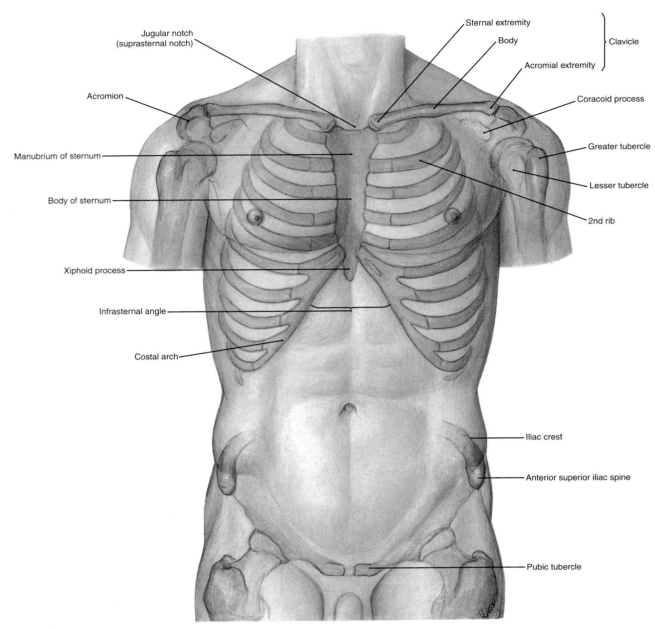

Jugular notch
(suprasternal notch)

Sternal extremity

Body

Acromial extremity

Clavicle

Acromion

Coracoid process

Manubrium of sternum

Greater tubercle

Lesser tubercle

Body of sternum

2nd rib

Xiphoid process

Infrasternal angle

Costal arch

Iliac crest

Anterior superior iliac spine

Pubic tubercle

FIGURE 144 **Projection of the Skeleton onto Both the Thoracic and Abdominal Walls**

NOTE: (1) The clavicular attachments to the sternum medially and the acromion process of the scapula laterally.
(2) The cartilaginous margin that bounds the infrasternal angle.
(3) The costal cartilage of the 2nd rib articulates with the sternum at the junction of the manubrium with the body of the sternum.
(4) Inferiorly, observe the projection of the iliac crest and the anterior superior iliac spine.

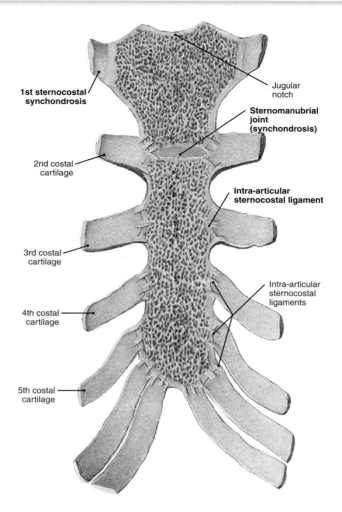

FIGURE 145.1 Sternocostal Articulations, Frontal Section (Posterior View)

NOTE: (1) The articulations of the first pair of ribs do not have joint cavities, but are direct cartilaginous unions (synchondroses), similar to the joint between the manubrium and body of the sternum.

(2) Each of the other sternocostal joints contains a true joint cavity surrounded by a capsule. Intra-articular sternocostal ligaments also attach the rib cartilage to the sternum. These are most frequently found at the junctions of the 2nd and 3rd cartilages with the sternum but may also be seen in lower sternocostal joints.

FIGURE 145.2 Left Clavicle (Inferior View) ▼

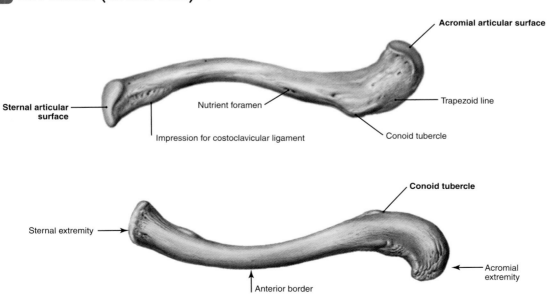

FIGURE 145.3 Left Clavicle (Superior View) ▲

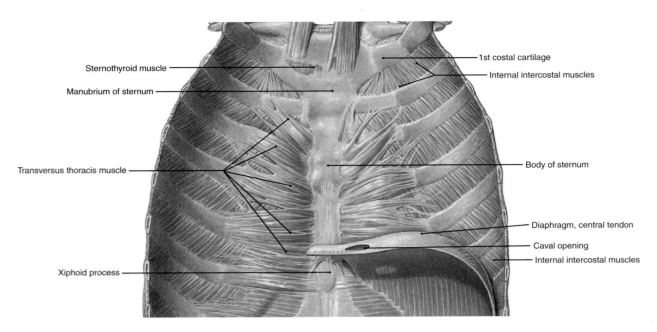

FIGURE 146.1 **Internal Surface of the Thoracic Cage (Anterior Part)**

NOTE: (1) The transversus thoracis muscle. It arises from the inferior half of the body of the sternum and the xiphoid process. Its fibers course laterally and superiorly to insert on the inner surfaces of the 2nd to the 6th ribs and their costal cartilages.

(2) The intercostal nerves supply the transversus thoracis muscle and its fascicles depress the costal cartilages to which the fibers attach.

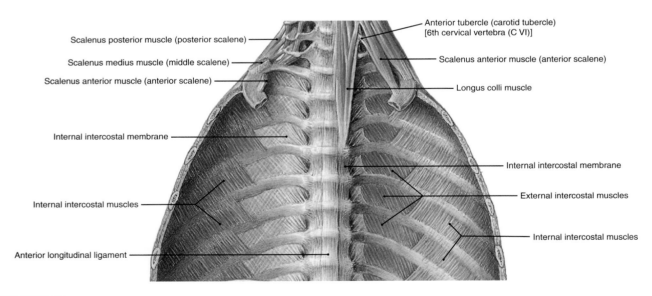

FIGURE 146.2 **Internal Surface of the Thoracic Cage (Posterior Part)**

NOTE: (1) The internal intercostal muscle fibers can be seen to extend between the ribs as far posteriorly as the bodies of the thoracic vertebrae.

(2) In contrast to the external intercostal muscle fibers, the internal intercostal muscle fibers are replaced by the internal intercostal membrane medial to the posterior costal angles of the ribs and as far as the bodies of the thoracic vertebrae.

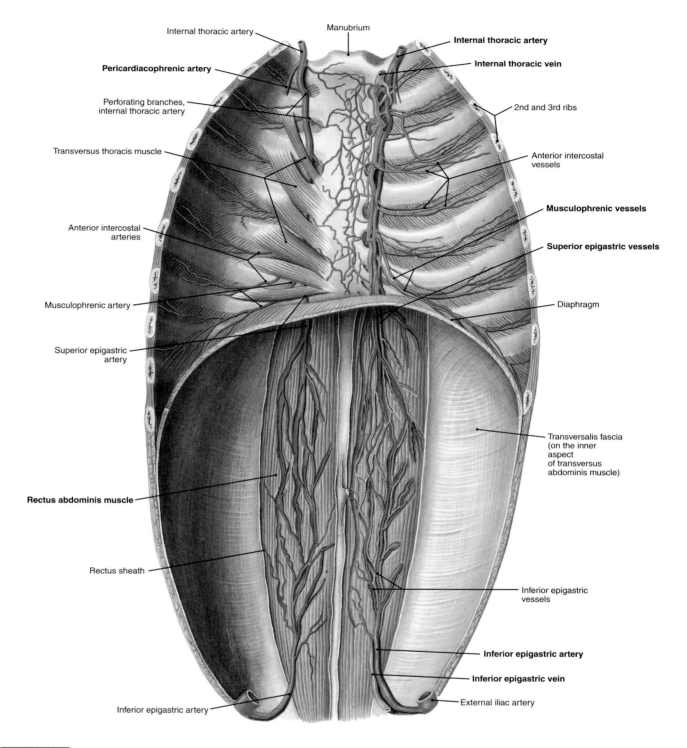

Internal thoracic artery

Manubrium

Internal thoracic artery

Pericardiacophrenic artery

Internal thoracic vein

Perforating branches, internal thoracic artery

2nd and 3rd ribs

Transversus thoracis muscle

Anterior intercostal vessels

Anterior intercostal arteries

Musculophrenic vessels

Superior epigastric vessels

Musculophrenic artery

Diaphragm

Superior epigastric artery

Rectus abdominis muscle

Transversalis fascia (on the inner aspect of transversus abdominis muscle)

Rectus sheath

Inferior epigastric vessels

Inferior epigastric artery

Inferior epigastric vein

External iliac artery

Inferior epigastric artery

FIGURE 147 **Muscles and Blood Vessels of the Thoracic and Abdominal Wall, Viewed from the Inside**

NOTE: (1) The principal vessels dissected include the **internal thoracic** and **inferior epigastric** arteries and veins and their terminal branches.

(2) The internal thoracic artery is a branch of the subclavian artery, and it descends behind the costal cartilages along the inner surface of the anterior thoracic wall in front of the transversus thoracis muscle and parallel to the margin of the sternum.

(3) The internal thoracic artery gives rise to (a) the pericardiacophrenic artery, (b) small vessels to the thymus and to bronchial structures, (c) perforating branches to the chest wall, (d) anterior intercostal branches, and finally it terminates as (e) **the musculophrenic** and **superior epigastric arteries**.

(4) The superior epigastric artery anastomoses with the **inferior epigastric artery**, a branch of the external iliac artery. The anastomosis occurs within the rectus abdominis muscle.

PLATE 148 Anterior Thoracic Wall: Muscles

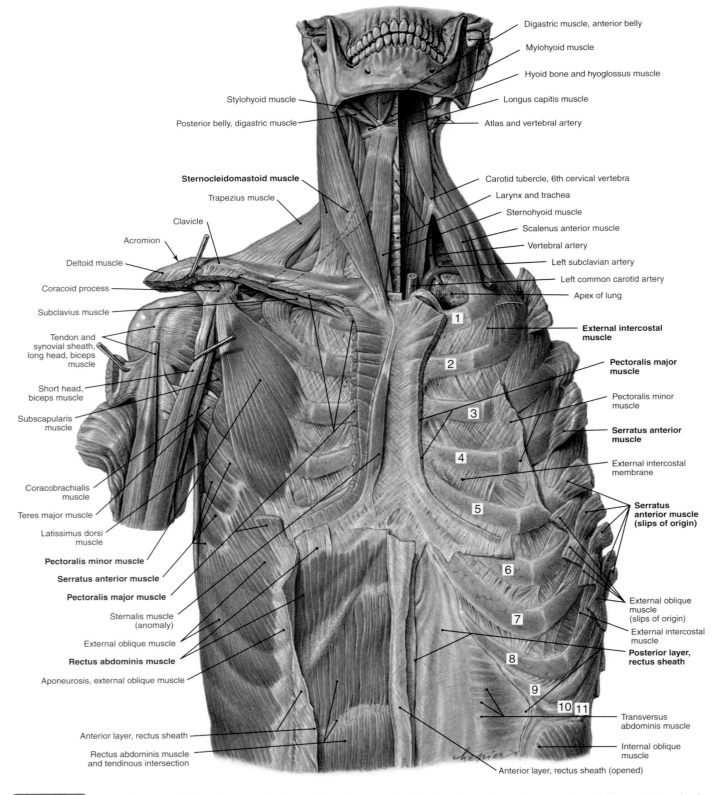

Digastric muscle, anterior belly

Mylohyoid muscle

Hyoid bone and hyoglossus muscle

Longus capitis muscle

Atlas and vertebral artery

Stylohyoid muscle

Posterior belly, digastric muscle

Carotid tubercle, 6th cervical vertebra

Larynx and trachea

Sternohyoid muscle

Scalenus anterior muscle

Vertebral artery

Left subclavian artery

Left common carotid artery

Apex of lung

Sternocleidomastoid muscle

Trapezius muscle

Clavicle

Acromion

Deltoid muscle

Coracoid process

Subclavius muscle

Tendon and synovial sheath, long head, biceps muscle

Short head, biceps muscle

Subscapularis muscle

External intercostal muscle

Pectoralis major muscle

Pectoralis minor muscle

Serratus anterior muscle

External intercostal membrane

Serratus anterior muscle (slips of origin)

Coracobrachialis muscle

Teres major muscle

Latissimus dorsi muscle

Pectoralis minor muscle

Serratus anterior muscle

Pectoralis major muscle

Sternalis muscle (anomaly)

External oblique muscle

Rectus abdominis muscle

Aponeurosis, external oblique muscle

External oblique muscle (slips of origin)

External intercostal muscle

Posterior layer, rectus sheath

Transversus abdominis muscle

Internal oblique muscle

Anterior layer, rectus sheath

Rectus abdominis muscle and tendinous intersection

Anterior layer, rectus sheath (opened)

FIGURE 148 Musculature of the Anterior Thoracic Wall Deep to the Pectoralis Major and the Adjacent Cervical and Abdominal Muscles

NOTE: (1) On the right side (reader's left), the anterior thoracic wall and upper arm are shown after removal of the pectoralis major muscle.
(2) On the left (reader's right), the upper limb and the superficial trunk and cervical muscles have been removed, exposing the ribs and intercostal tissues.

Muscle	Origin	Insertion	Innervation	Action
Subclavius	First rib and its cartilage at their junction	Groove on the lower surface of middle third of the clavicle	Nerve to subclavius from upper trunk of brachial plexus (C5, C6)	Depresses and pulls clavicle forward

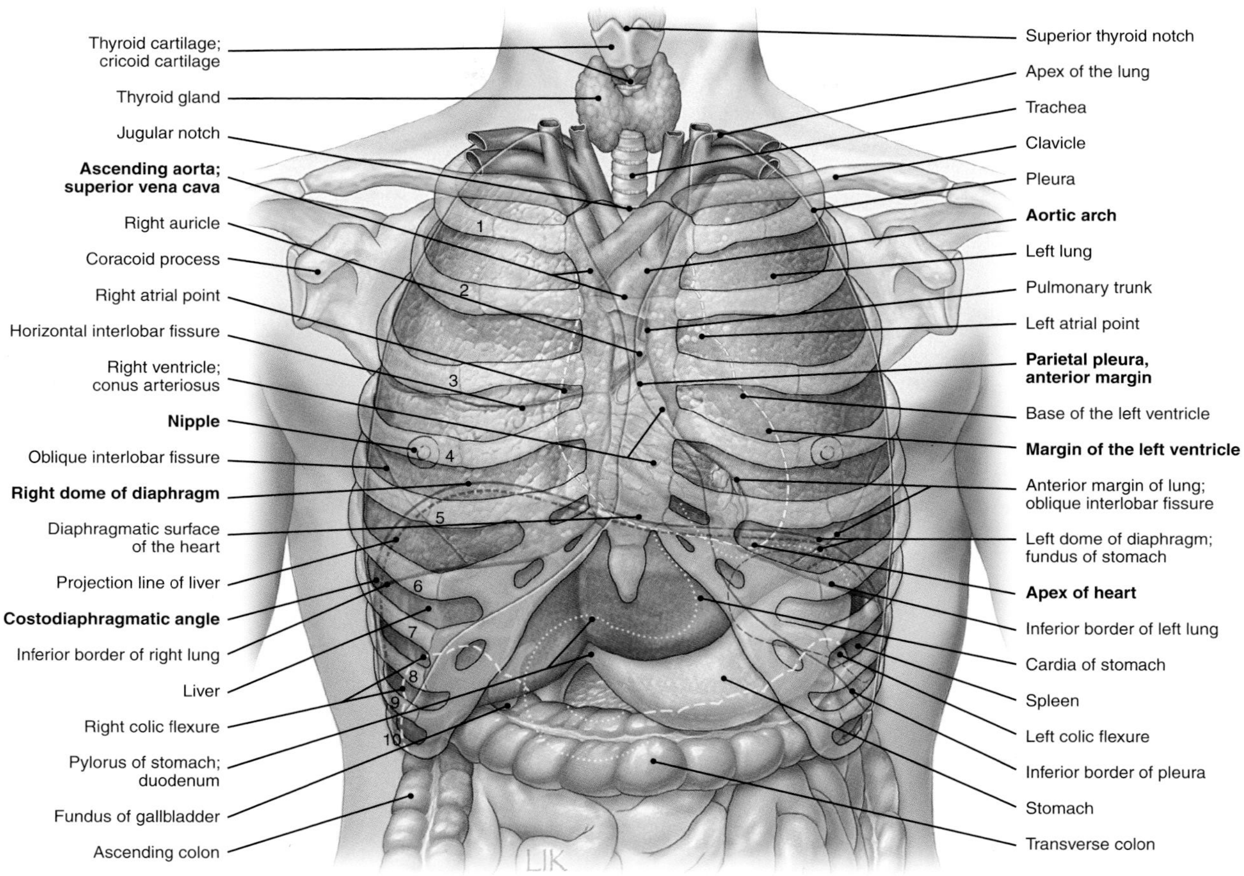

Thyroid cartilage; cricoid cartilage
Thyroid gland
Jugular notch
Ascending aorta; superior vena cava
Right auricle
Coracoid process
Right atrial point
Horizontal interlobar fissure
Right ventricle; conus arteriosus
Nipple
Oblique interlobar fissure
Right dome of diaphragm
Diaphragmatic surface of the heart
Projection line of liver
Costodiaphragmatic angle
Inferior border of right lung
Liver
Right colic flexure
Pylorus of stomach; duodenum
Fundus of gallbladder
Ascending colon
Superior thyroid notch
Apex of the lung
Trachea
Clavicle
Pleura
Aortic arch
Left lung
Pulmonary trunk
Left atrial point
Parietal pleura, anterior margin
Base of the left ventricle
Margin of the left ventricle
Anterior margin of lung; oblique interlobar fissure
Left dome of diaphragm; fundus of stomach
Apex of heart
Inferior border of left lung
Cardia of stomach
Spleen
Left colic flexure
Inferior border of pleura
Stomach
Transverse colon
1
2
3
4
5
6
7
8
9
10

FIGURE 149.1 Thoracic and Upper Abdominal Viscera Projected onto the Anterior Surface of the Body

NOTE: (1) The outline of the heart and great vessels (white broken line) deep to the anterior border of the lungs.

(2) The liver, lying below the diaphragm, extends upward as high as the 4th interspace on the right and to the 5th interspace on the left (red broken line).

(3) The superficial location of the superior vena cava and ascending aorta just deep to the manubrium of the sternum.

(4) A triangular region containing the great vessels above and a lower triangular region over the heart (area of superficial cardiac dullness) are not covered by pleura.

(5) The reflections of the pleura over the lungs. Observe that the anterior margins of the lung and pleura on the left side are indented to form the cardiac notch.

(6) The position of the nipple over the 4th rib (or 4th intercostal space) in the male and in the young female. Also observe the apex of the heart deep to the 5th interspace.

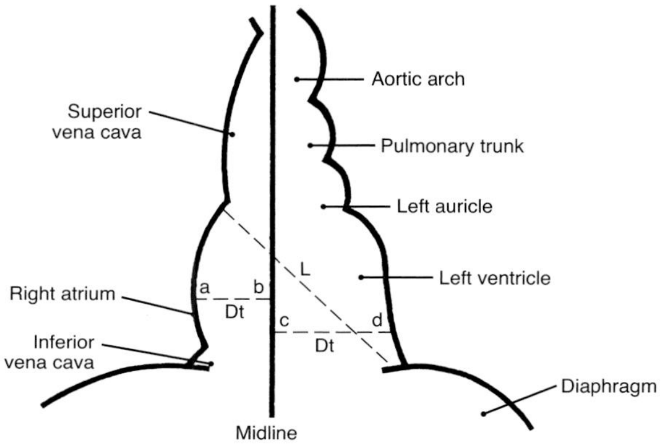

Superior vena cava
Aortic arch
Pulmonary trunk
Left auricle
Left ventricle
Right atrium
Inferior vena cava
a
b
Dt
c
d
Dt
L
Diaphragm
Midline

FIGURE 149.2 Shadow Outline of Heart and Great Vessels in Radiograph of the Thorax

Dt: Transverse diameter (normal)
a to b: about 4 cm
c to d: about 9 cm

L: Longitudinal axis of heart: 15 to 16 cm
(measured from the upper end of the right atrial shadow to the apex of the heart)

PLATE 150 Thymus in an Adolescent and from a Young Child

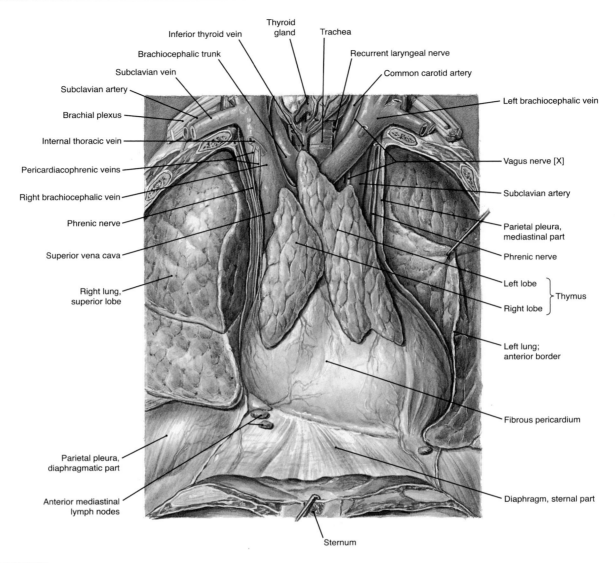

Thyroid gland
Inferior thyroid vein
Trachea
Brachiocephalic trunk
Recurrent laryngeal nerve
Subclavian vein
Common carotid artery
Subclavian artery
Brachial plexus
Left brachiocephalic vein
Internal thoracic vein
Pericardiacophrenic veins
Vagus nerve [X]
Right brachiocephalic vein
Subclavian artery
Phrenic nerve
Parietal pleura, mediastinal part
Superior vena cava
Phrenic nerve
Right lung, superior lobe
Left lobe ⎫
⎬ Thymus
Right lobe ⎭
Left lung; anterior border
Fibrous pericardium
Parietal pleura, diaphragmatic part
Anterior mediastinal lymph nodes
Diaphragm, sternal part
Sternum

FIGURE 150.1 Thymus in an Adolescent

NOTE that the chest wall is removed and the parietal pleura has been opened.

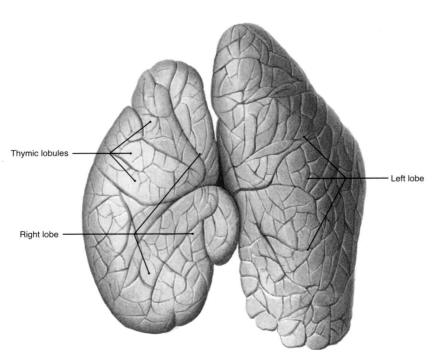

Thymic lobules
Left lobe
Right lobe

FIGURE 150.2 Thymus of a 2-Year-Old Child

NOTE: (1) The thymus is the central organ of the immune-lymphoid system.

(2) At birth it weighs under 15 g and at puberty it has grown to about 35 g. In the adult it diminishes in size, becoming atrophic and being replaced by fat.

(3) The thymus lies in the anterior and superior mediastina, and it receives branches from the internal thoracic and inferior thyroid arteries. Its veins drain into the brachiocephalic, internal thoracic, and inferior thyroid veins.

(4) The thymus differentiates lymphocytes into thymocytes (T cells), which are released into peripheral blood and become capable of cell-mediated immunologic responses to antigenic foreign substances. Also, these cells act with B lymphocytes for humoral responses.

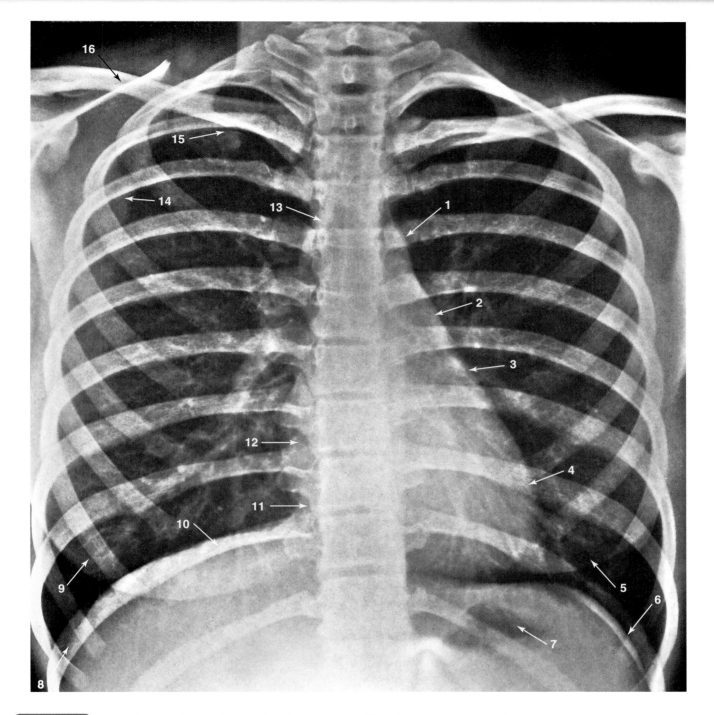

FIGURE 151 **Posterioanterior Radiograph of the Thorax Showing the Heart and Lungs**

NOTE: (1) The contour of the heart and great vessels: arch of aorta [1], pulmonary trunk [2], inferior vena cava [11], and superior vena cava [13], and the relationship of these structures to the vertebral column.

(2) The left margin of the heart is formed by the left auricle [3] and left ventricle [4], and it slopes toward the apex, which usually lies about 9 cm to the left of the midsternal line, deep to the 5th intercostal space.

(3) The right margin of the heart [12] projects as a curved line slightly to the right of the vertebral column (and sternum). Observe that the heart rests on the diaphragm [6], and note the contours of the left [5] and right [9] breasts.

(From Wicke, 6th ed.)

1. Arch of aorta	5. Contour of left breast	9. Contour of right breast	13. Superior vena cava
2. Pulmonary trunk	6. Diaphragm	10. Diaphragm	14. Medial border of scapula
3. Left auricle	7. Air in fundus of stomach	11. Inferior vena cava	15. First rib
4. Left ventricle	8. Costodiaphragmatic recess	12. Right atrium	16. Right clavicle

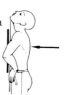
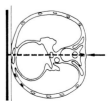

PLATE 152 Lungs and Heart In Situ: Anterior Thoracic Wall Removed

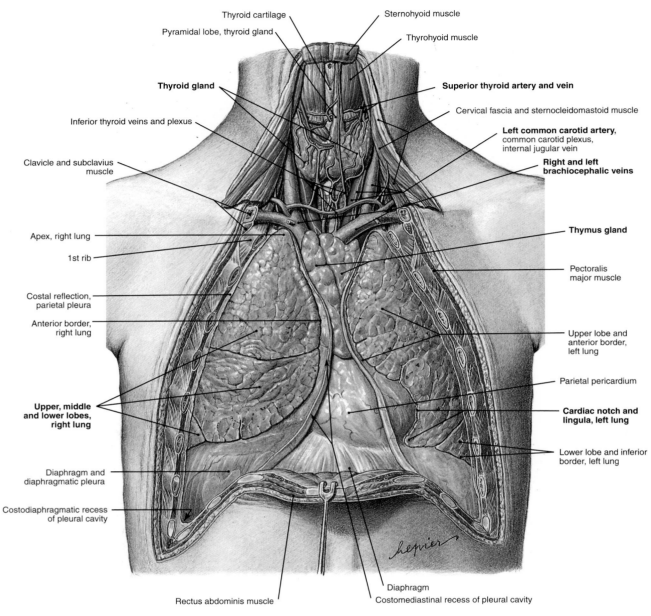

Thyroid cartilage

Sternohyoid muscle

Pyramidal lobe, thyroid gland

Thyrohyoid muscle

Thyroid gland

Superior thyroid artery and vein

Inferior thyroid veins and plexus

Cervical fascia and sternocleidomastoid muscle

Left common carotid artery,
common carotid plexus,
internal jugular vein

Clavicle and subclavius
muscle

**Right and left
brachiocephalic veins**

Apex, right lung

Thymus gland

1st rib

Pectoralis
major muscle

Costal reflection,
parietal pleura

Anterior border,
right lung

Upper lobe and
anterior border,
left lung

Parietal pericardium

**Upper, middle
and lower lobes,
right lung**

**Cardiac notch and
lingula, left lung**

Lower lobe and inferior
border, left lung

Diaphragm and
diaphragmatic pleura

Costodiaphragmatic recess
of pleural cavity

Diaphragm

Rectus abdominis muscle

Costomediastinal recess of pleural cavity

FIGURE 152 **Thoracic Viscera and the Root of the Neck (Anterior Exposure)**

NOTE: (1) The anterior thoracic wall has been removed along with the medial parts of both clavicles to reveal the normal position of the heart, lungs, thymus, and thyroid gland. The great vessels in the superior aperture of the thorax are also exposed.

(2) The parietal pleura has been removed anteriorly. The thymus is situated between the two lungs superiorly, whereas inferiorly is found the bare area of the heart. Observe the **cardiac notch** along the anterior border of the left lung adjacent to the heart.

(3) The basal surface of both lungs and the inferior aspect of the heart rest on the diaphragm, whereas the apex of each lung extends superiorly above the level of the 1st rib.

(4) The rather transverse course in the superior mediastinum of the left brachiocephalic vein in contrast to the nearly vertical course of the right brachiocephalic vein. The two brachiocephalic veins join, deep to the thymus, to form the superior vena cava.

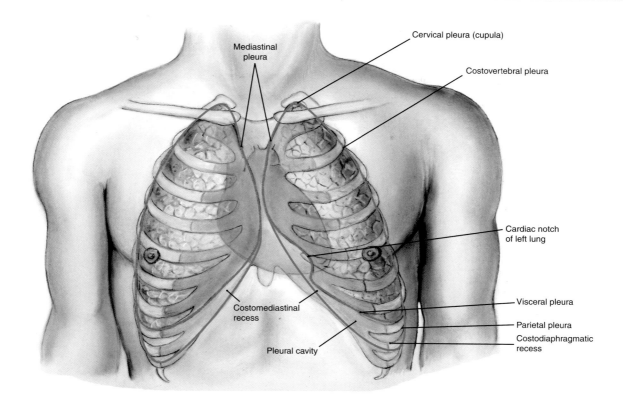

FIGURE 153.1 Projections of the Lungs, Pleura, and Heart onto the Anterior Thoracic Wall

NOTE: (1) The borders of the parietal and visceral layers of pleura. The **parietal layer** on each side completely lines the internal surface of the thorax, and it consists of a **costal** portion lining the ribs, a **mediastinal** portion adjacent to the mediastinum, a **diaphragmatic** part over the diaphragm, and a **cervical** part that ascends into the lower neck.

(2) The **visceral layer** closely adheres to the lungs, and the potential space between the two layers of pleura is called the **pleural cavity**.

(3) The apex of each lung ascends above the medial one-third of the clavicle on that side, and at these sites, the lungs are covered by the **cervical pleura**.

(4) The parietal and visceral layers of the pleura are continuous at the hilum of the lung on each side as shown in the figure below.

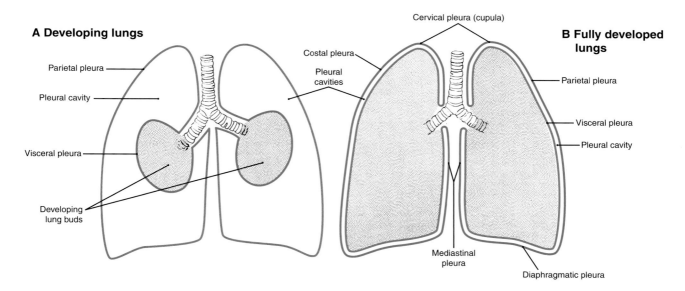

FIGURE 153.2 Diagrammatic Representation of Lung Development into the Pleural Membranes

NOTE: (1) The primordium of each lung (**A**) develops soon after the trachea bifurcates, and it grows on both left and right sides into the pleural membranes. In this manner, the primitive lung buds get surrounded by the visceral pleura.

(2) As the lung growth continues (**B**), the organs fill the pleural coeloms and a potential space develops on both sides between the lung buds (covered by visceral pleura) and parietal pleurae that line the inner surface of the developing thoracic cage. This results in the formation of a pleural cavity between the visceral and parietal layers of pleura.

PLATE 154 Reflections of Pleura (Anterior View)

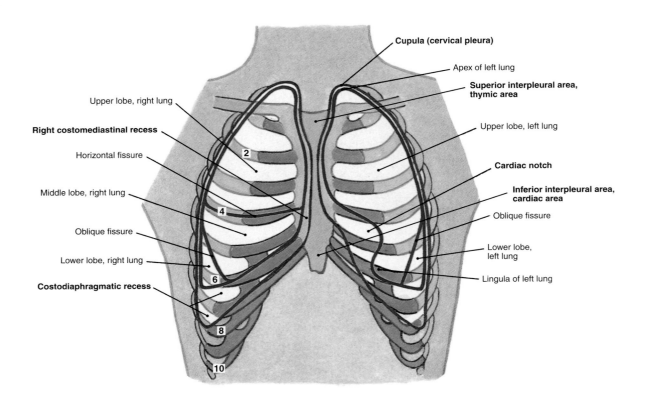

Cupula (cervical pleura)

Apex of left lung

Superior interpleural area, thymic area

Upper lobe, right lung

Upper lobe, left lung

Right costomediastinal recess

Cardiac notch

Horizontal fissure

2

Inferior interpleural area, cardiac area

Middle lobe, right lung

Oblique fissure

4

Oblique fissure

Lower lobe, left lung

Lower lobe, right lung

6

Lingula of left lung

Costodiaphragmatic recess

8

10

FIGURE 154.1 Parietal (Green) and Visceral (Red) Pleural Reflections Projected onto the Anterior Thoracic Wall

NOTE: (1) Each lung is invested by two layers of pleura that are continuous at the hilum of the lung, and thereby form an invaginated sac.

(2) The **parietal layer of pleura** (shown in green) is the outermost of the two layers, and it lines the inner surface of the thoracic wall and the superior surface of the diaphragm. The **visceral layer** of **pleura** closely invests and adheres to the surfaces of the lungs (in red).

(3) The potential space between the two pleural layers is called the **pleural cavity** and contains only a small amount of serous fluid in the healthy person, but it may contain considerable fluid and blood in pathologic conditions.

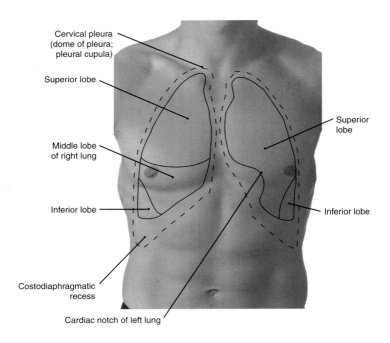

Cervical pleura (dome of pleura; pleural cupula)

Superior lobe

Superior lobe

Middle lobe of right lung

Inferior lobe

Inferior lobe

Costodiaphragmatic recess

Cardiac notch of left lung

FIGURE 154.2 Outline Directly onto the Anterior Thoracic Wall of Pleural Reflections

NOTE: The boundaries of the lungs are shown by solid lines, while those of the parietal pleura are shown by broken lines.

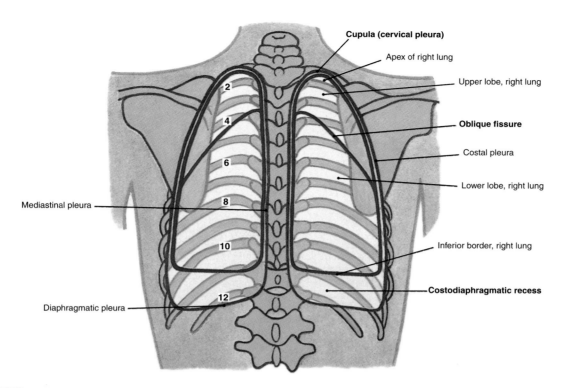

FIGURE 155.1 **Parietal (Green) and Visceral (Red) Pleural Reflections onto the Posterior Thoracic Wall**

NOTE: (1) The parietal pleura is a continuous sheet, but parts of it are named in relation to their adjacent surfaces. Lining the inner surface of the ribs is the **costal pleura**, while the **diaphragmatic** and **mediastinal pleurae** are found on the surfaces of the diaphragm and mediastinum. Overlying the apex of each lung is the **cupula** or **cervical pleura**.

(2) Because of the curvature of the diaphragm, a narrow recess is formed around its periphery into which the lung (visceral pleura) does not extend. An important potential space lies between the costal and diaphragmatic pleurae called the **costodiaphragmatic recess,** which may be punctured and drained of fluid without damage to the lung tissue.

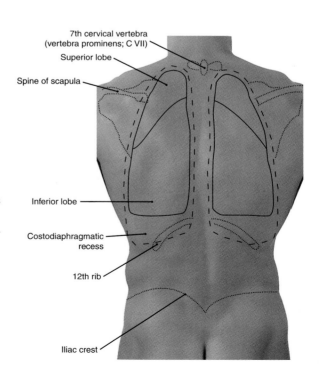

FIGURE 155.2 **Outline of Pleural Reflections Directly ▶ onto the Posterior Thoracic Wall**

NOTE: (1) The boundaries of the lungs are the solid lines, while the boundaries of the pleura are the broken (dash) lines.

(2) The "rib-level" relationships of the lungs (visceral pleura) and the parietal pleura are as follows:

	Visceral pleura	Parietal pleura
(a) Anterior (midclavicular line)	6th rib	8th rib
(b) Lateral (midaxillary line)	8th rib	10th rib
(c) Posterior (medial border of the scapula)	10th rib	12th rib
(Summary of Rib Levels)	**Visceral Pleura**	**Ribs 6, 8, 10**
	Parietal Pleura	**Ribs 8, 10, 12**

PLATE 156 Reflections of Pleura (Lateral Views)

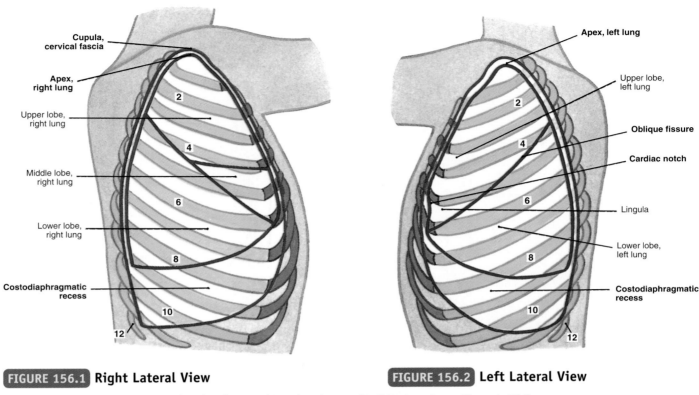

Cupula, cervical fascia

Apex, right lung

Upper lobe, right lung

Middle lobe, right lung

Lower lobe, right lung

Costodiaphragmatic recess

Apex, left lung

Upper lobe, left lung

Oblique fissure

Cardiac notch

Lingula

Lower lobe, left lung

Costodiaphragmatic recess

FIGURE 156.1 Right Lateral View

FIGURE 156.2 Left Lateral View

Pleural Reflections (Green) and Lungs (Red) Projected onto Thoracic Wall

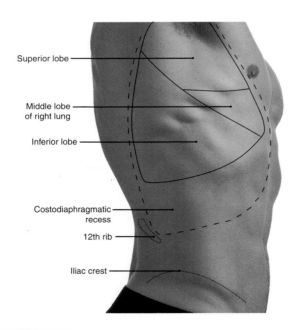

Superior lobe

Middle lobe of right lung

Inferior lobe

Costodiaphragmatic recess

12th rib

Iliac crest

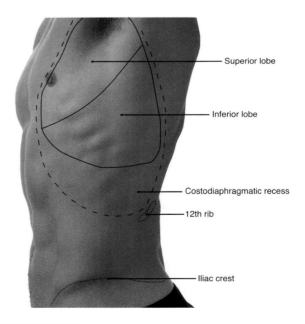

Superior lobe

Inferior lobe

Costodiaphragmatic recess

12th rib

Iliac crest

FIGURE 156.3 Projection of Pleural and Pulmonary Borders (Right Lateral Aspect)

NOTE that the borders of the lung are shown by solid lines, while borders of the pleura are shown by broken (dashed) lines.

FIGURE 156.4 Projection of Pleural and Pulmonary Borders (Left Lateral Aspect)

NOTE that the borders of the lung are shown by solid lines, while borders of the pleura are shown by broken (dashed) lines.

RIGHT LUNG   LEFT LUNG

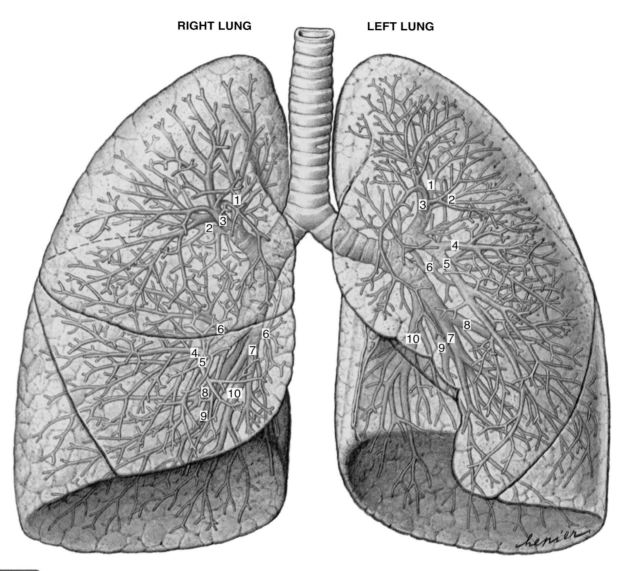

FIGURE 157 **Bronchial Tree and Its Lobar and Bronchopulmonary Divisions (Anterior View)**

NOTE: (1) As the trachea divides, the **left primary bronchus** diverges at a greater angle than the **right primary bronchus** to reach the left lung. The left bronchus, therefore, is directed more transversely and the right bronchus more inferiorly.

(2) **On the right side,** the upper lobar bronchus branches from the primary bronchus almost immediately, even above the pulmonary artery (eparterial), while the bronchus is directed toward the middle and lower lobes branches below the main stem of the pulmonary artery (hyparterial).

(3) **On the left side,** the initial lobar bronchus, branching from the primary bronchus, is directed upward and lateral to the upper lobe segments and its lingular segments. The remaining lobar bronchus is directed inferiorly and soon divides into the segmental bronchi of the lower lobe.

(4) The segmental bronchi numbered in the figure above are as follows:

Right lung		**Left lung**	
1. Apical	6. Superior	1. Apical	6. Superior
2. Posterior	7. Medial basal	2. Posterior	7. Medial basal
3. Anterior	8. Anterior basal	3. Anterior	8. Anterior basal
4. Lateral	9. Lateral basal	4. Superior lingular	9. Lateral basal
5. Medial	10. Posterior basal	5. Inferior lingular	10. Posterior basal

PLATE 158 Lungs: Lateral (Sternocostal) View

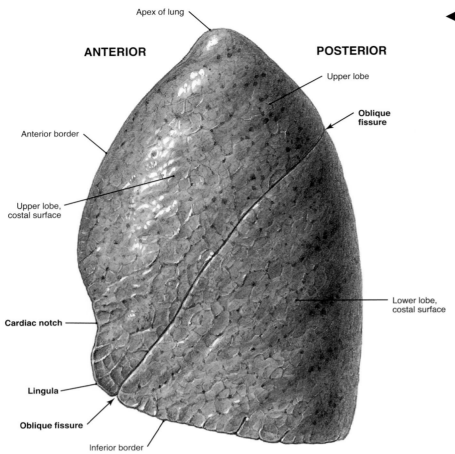

Apex of lung

ANTERIOR

POSTERIOR

Upper lobe

Oblique fissure

Anterior border

Upper lobe, costal surface

Lower lobe, costal surface

Cardiac notch

Lingula

Oblique fissure

Inferior border

◀ **FIGURE 158.1** **Left Lung (Lateral View)**

NOTE: (1) The lateral view of the left lung shows a rounded convex costal surface directed toward the thoracic wall and divided into upper and lower lobes by the **oblique fissure.**

(2) The **upper lobe** has a rounded apex, which is pointed above. The upper lobe forms virtually all of the **anterior border** of the left lung and, inferiorly, it is indented by the **cardiac notch.** A small tongue-like anterior projection below the cardiac notch is called the **lingula.**

(3) The **lower lobe** is somewhat larger than the upper, and its base is the **diaphragmatic surface** of the left lung. This is adapted to the dome shape of the diaphragm.

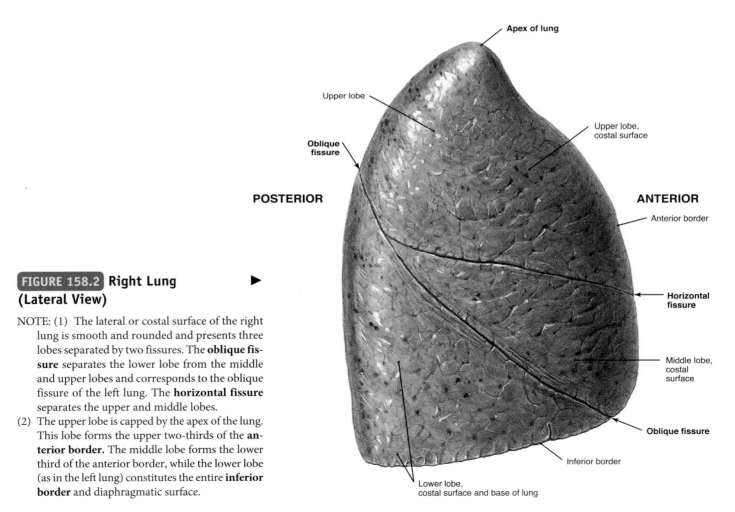

Apex of lung

Upper lobe

Upper lobe, costal surface

Oblique fissure

POSTERIOR

ANTERIOR

Anterior border

Horizontal fissure

Middle lobe, costal surface

Oblique fissure

Inferior border

Lower lobe, costal surface and base of lung

FIGURE 158.2 **Right Lung (Lateral View)** ▶

NOTE: (1) The lateral or costal surface of the right lung is smooth and rounded and presents three lobes separated by two fissures. The **oblique fissure** separates the lower lobe from the middle and upper lobes and corresponds to the oblique fissure of the left lung. The **horizontal fissure** separates the upper and middle lobes.

(2) The upper lobe is capped by the apex of the lung. This lobe forms the upper two-thirds of the **anterior border.** The middle lobe forms the lower third of the anterior border, while the lower lobe (as in the left lung) constitutes the entire **inferior border** and diaphragmatic surface.

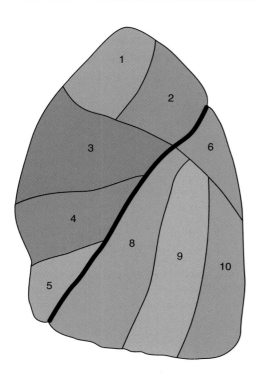

FIGURE 159.1 Left Lung, Bronchopulmonary Segments (Lateral View)

NOTE: (1) Bronchopulmonary segments are anatomical subdivisions of the lung, each supplied by its own segmental (tertiary) bronchus and artery and drained by intersegmental veins.

(2) The trachea divides into two primary bronchi, each of which serves an entire lung. The primary bronchi divide into secondary, or lobar, bronchi. There are two lobar bronchi on the left and three on the right, each supplying a separate lobe.

(3) Secondary bronchi divide into segmental or tertiary bronchi, distributed to the bronchopulmonary segments. Usual descriptions of the bronchopulmonary segments define 8 to 10 segments in the left lung.

(4) In the left lung, the segments are numbered and named as follows:

Upper lobe
1. Apical ⎤
2. Posterior ⎥ Frequently considered as a single segment
3. Anterior ⎦
4. Superior ⎤ Lingular
5. Inferior ⎦

Lower lobe
6. Superior
7. Medial basal ⎤ Usually considered as a single segment;
8. Anterior basal ⎦ medial basal cannot be seen from lateral view.
9. Lateral basal
10. Posterior basal

(5) In the left lower lobe the medial basal bronchus arises separately from the anterior basal bronchus in only about 13% of humans studied.

FIGURE 159.2 Right Lung, Bronchopulmonary Segments (Lateral View) ▶

NOTE: (1) Subdivision of the lungs into functional bronchopulmonary segments allows the surgeon to determine whether segments of lung might be resected in operations in preference to entire lobes.

(2) Although minor variations exist in the division of the bronchial tree, a consistency has become accepted in the naming of bronchopulmonary segmentation. The nomenclature used here was published by Jackson and Huber (Dis Chest 1943;9:319–326) and is now used because it is the simplest and most straightforward of those that have been suggested.

(3) The bronchopulmonary segments of the right lung are numbered and named as follows:

Upper lobe	**Middle lobe**
1. Apical	4. Lateral
2. Posterior	5. Medial
3. Anterior	

Lower lobe
6. Superior
7. Medial basal (cannot be seen from lateral view)
8. Anterior basal
9. Lateral basal
10. Posterior basal

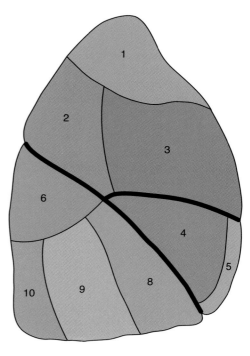

PLATE 160 Lungs: Medial (Mediastinal) View

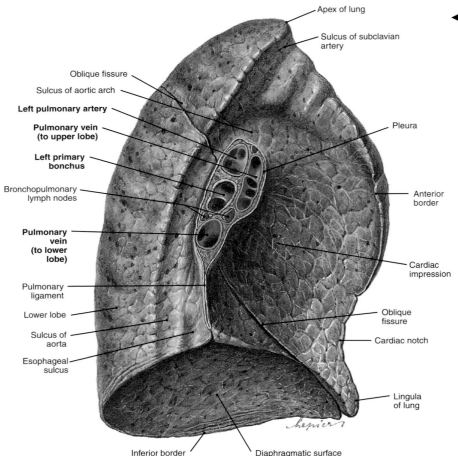

Apex of lung

Sulcus of subclavian artery

Oblique fissure

Sulcus of aortic arch

Left pulmonary artery

Pulmonary vein (to upper lobe)

Left primary bonchus

Bronchopulmonary lymph nodes

Pulmonary vein (to lower lobe)

Pulmonary ligament

Lower lobe

Sulcus of aorta

Esophageal sulcus

Inferior border

Diaphragmatic surface

Pleura

Anterior border

Cardiac impression

Oblique fissure

Cardiac notch

Lingula of lung

FIGURE 160.1 Left Lung, Mediastinal and Diaphragmatic Surfaces

NOTE: (1) The concave diaphragmatic surface on the left lung covers most of the convex dome of the diaphragm, which is completely covered by parietal diaphragmatic pleura.

(2) The mediastinal (or medial) surface of the left lung is also concave and presents the contours of the organs of the mediastinum. The large anterior concavity is the cardiac impression. Observe the grooves for the aortic arch, the aorta, and the subclavian artery as well as the esophagus inferiorly.

(3) The structures at the hilum of the left lung include the **left pulmonary artery**, found superiorly, and below this the **left primary bronchus**. The **left pulmonary veins** lie anterior and inferior to the artery and bronchus. The **oblique fissure** completely divides the lung into two lobes.

FIGURE 160.2 Right Lung, Mediastinal and Diaphragmatic Surfaces

NOTE: (1) The **diaphragmatic surface** of the right lung, similar to the left, is shaped to the contour of the diaphragm, while the **mediastinal surface** shows grooves for the superior vena cava and subclavian artery.

(2) Above the **hilum** of the right lung is the arched sulcus for the azygos vein, which continues inferiorly behind the hilum of the lung. The cardiac impression on the right lung is more shallow than on the left.

(3) The right bronchus frequently branches before the right pulmonary artery. Thus, often the most superior structure at the hilum of the right lung is the bronchus to the upper lobe (eparterial bronchus). The pulmonary artery lies anterior to the bronchus, while the pulmonary veins are located anterior and inferior to these structures.

(4) The root of the lung is ensheathed by parietal pleura, the layers of which come into contact below to form the **pulmonary ligament.** This extends from the inferior border of the hilum to a point just above the diaphragm.

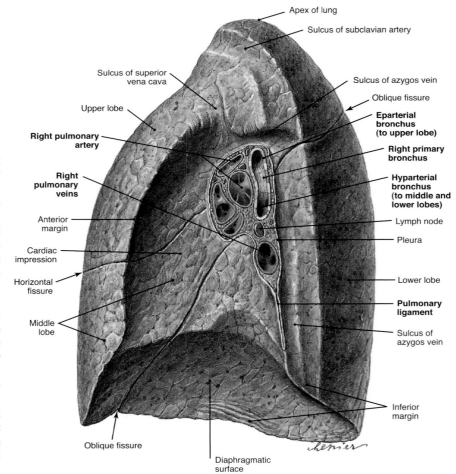

Apex of lung

Sulcus of subclavian artery

Sulcus of superior vena cava

Sulcus of azygos vein

Oblique fissure

Upper lobe

Eparterial bronchus (to upper lobe)

Right pulmonary artery

Right primary bronchus

Right pulmonary veins

Hyparterial bronchus (to middle and lower lobes)

Anterior margin

Lymph node

Pleura

Cardiac impression

Horizontal fissure

Lower lobe

Pulmonary ligament

Sulcus of azygos vein

Middle lobe

Oblique fissure

Inferior margin

Diaphragmatic surface

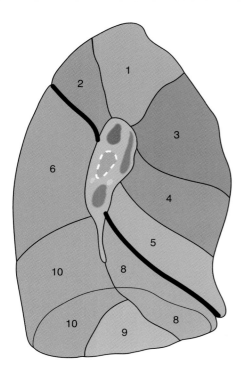

FIGURE 161.1 **Left Lung: Bronchopulmonary Segments (Medial View)**

NOTE: The bronchopulmonary segments of the left lung are identified as follows:

Upper lobe
1. Apical ⎤ Frequently considered
2. Posterior ⎦ as a single segment
3. Anterior
4. Superior ⎤ Lingular
5. Inferior ⎦

Lower lobe
6. Superior
7. Medial basal*
8. Anterior basal*
9. Lateral basal
10. Posterior basal

* The medial basal and anterior basal segments were at one time frequently considered as a single bronchopulmonary segment. Today, however, they have been recognized as separate segments in a majority of left lungs. Therefore, on this figure, the portion of segment 8 just inferior to the oblique fissure should be marked 7 and identified as medial basal.

FIGURES 161.1 and 161.2 **Bronchopulmonary Segments: General Statements**

NOTE: (1) Bronchopulmonary segments are separated by connective-tissue septa that are continuous with the visceral pleura. These septa maintain the air content of each segment and prevent leakage of air into adjacent segments.
(2) Each segment is pyramidal in shape. The apex of each pyramid is oriented toward the hilum of the lung, while the base faces the surface of the pulmonary lobe.
(3) It is important to know the bronchopulmonary segmental patterns in order, accurately, to read and interpret radiographs of the lungs.
(4) Knowledge of segmental anatomy is also important for the localization of pathologic conditions such as tumors, abscesses, or bronchiectasis or small foreign objects that have been aspirated into a lung.

FIGURE 161.2 **Right Lung: Bronchopulmonary Segments (Medial View)** ▶

NOTE: The bronchopulmonary segments of the right lung are identified as follows:

Upper lobe
1. Apical
2. Posterior
3. Anterior

Middle lobe
4. Lateral (not seen from this view)
5. Medial

Lower lobe
6. Superior
7. Medial basal
8. Anterior basal
9. Lateral basal
10. Posterior basal

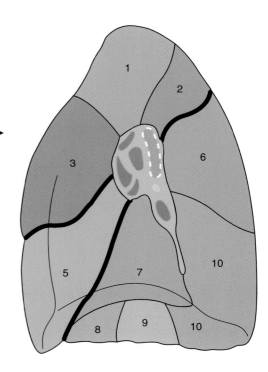

PLATE 162 Trachea and Bronchi

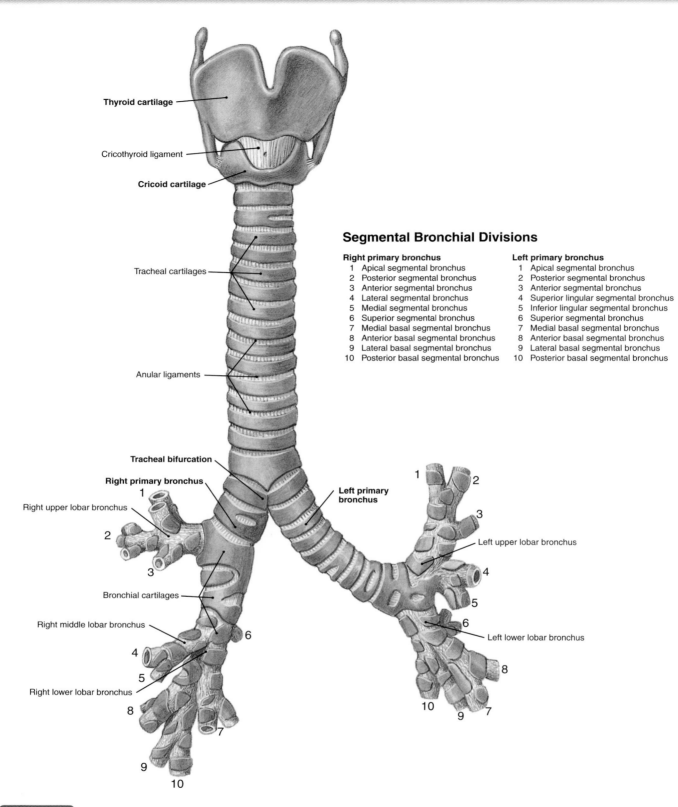

Segmental Bronchial Divisions

Right primary bronchus
1. Apical segmental bronchus
2. Posterior segmental bronchus
3. Anterior segmental bronchus
4. Lateral segmental bronchus
5. Medial segmental bronchus
6. Superior segmental bronchus
7. Medial basal segmental bronchus
8. Anterior basal segmental bronchus
9. Lateral basal segmental bronchus
10. Posterior basal segmental bronchus

Left primary bronchus
1. Apical segmental bronchus
2. Posterior segmental bronchus
3. Anterior segmental bronchus
4. Superior lingular segmental bronchus
5. Inferior lingular segmental bronchus
6. Superior segmental bronchus
7. Medial basal segmental bronchus
8. Anterior basal segmental bronchus
9. Lateral basal segmental bronchus
10. Posterior basal segmental bronchus

FIGURE 162 **Anterior Aspect of Larynx, Trachea, and Bronchi**

NOTE: (1) The **trachea** bifurcates into two **principal** (primary) **bronchi.** These then divide into **lobar** (secondary) **bronchi,** which give rise to **segmental** (tertiary) **bronchi.**

(2) The larynx is located in the anterior aspect of the neck, and its thyroid and cricoid cartilages can be felt through the skin.

(3) The **thyroid cartilage,** projected posteriorly, lies at the level of the fourth and fifth cervical vertebrae, while the **cricoid cartilage** is at the sixth cervical level.

(4) The trachea commences at the lower end of the cricoid cartilage and extends slightly more than 4 in. before bifurcating into the two primary bronchi at the level of T4 to T5 intervertebral disc. Two inches of the trachea lie above the suprasternal notch in the neck, and about 2 in. of trachea are within the thorax above the tracheal bifurcation.

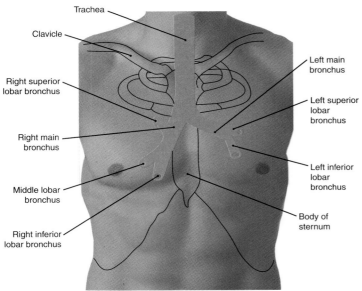

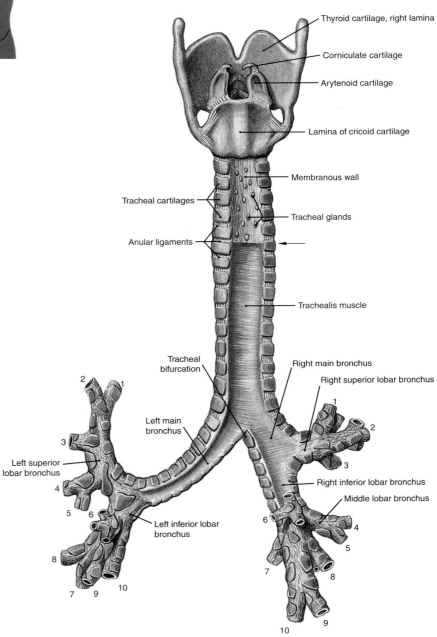

FIGURE 163.1 **Surface Projection of the Trachea and Bronchi in a Living Person**

NOTE that the bifurcation occurs at approximately the level of the sternal angle located anteriorly on the sternum.

FIGURE 163.2 **Opened Trachea and Bronchi (Posterior View)**

NOTE: (1) The numbers refer to the bronchopulmonary segments listed in Plate 162.

(2) Below the arrow, observe the trachealis muscle along the posterior surface of the trachea. It is composed of nonstriated muscle fibers, and it extends along the posterior surface of the bronchi.

PLATE 164 Hilum of Left Lung: Costodiaphragmatic Recess

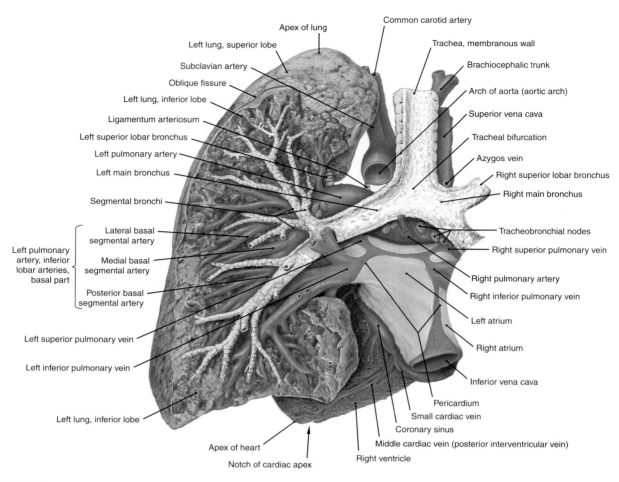

Apex of lung

Common carotid artery

Left lung, superior lobe

Trachea, membranous wall

Subclavian artery

Brachiocephalic trunk

Oblique fissure

Arch of aorta (aortic arch)

Left lung, inferior lobe

Superior vena cava

Ligamentum arteriosum

Left superior lobar bronchus

Tracheal bifurcation

Left pulmonary artery

Azygos vein

Left main bronchus

Right superior lobar bronchus

Right main bronchus

Segmental bronchi

Lateral basal segmental artery

Tracheobronchial nodes

Right superior pulmonary vein

Left pulmonary artery, inferior lobar arteries, basal part

Medial basal segmental artery

Right pulmonary artery

Posterior basal segmental artery

Right inferior pulmonary vein

Left atrium

Left superior pulmonary vein

Right atrium

Left inferior pulmonary vein

Inferior vena cava

Pericardium

Small cardiac vein

Left lung, inferior lobe

Coronary sinus

Apex of heart

Middle cardiac vein (posterior interventricular vein)

Right ventricle

Notch of cardiac apex

FIGURE 164.1 **Dissected Hilum of the Left Lung (Posterior View)**

NOTE that the bronchus is more posterior to the pulmonary vessels.

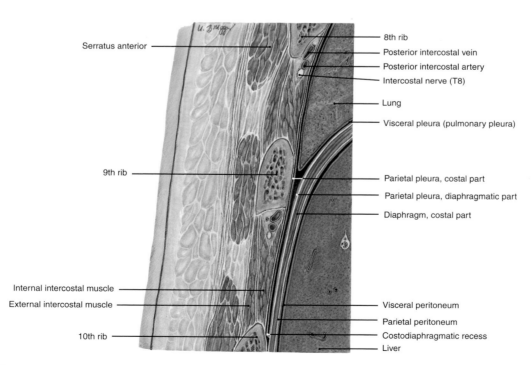

Serratus anterior

8th rib

Posterior intercostal vein

Posterior intercostal artery

Intercostal nerve (T8)

Lung

Visceral pleura (pulmonary pleura)

9th rib

Parietal pleura, costal part

Parietal pleura, diaphragmatic part

Diaphragm, costal part

Internal intercostal muscle

External intercostal muscle

Visceral peritoneum

Parietal peritoneum

10th rib

Costodiaphragmatic recess

Liver

FIGURE 164.2 **Costodiaphragmatic Recess (Frontal Section of Region)**

NOTE: (1) The costodiaphragmatic recesses are located in the lowest lateral regions of the two pleural cavities.
(2) When aspiration of fluid is necessary, care must be taken not to puncture the liver or right lung on the right side, or the spleen or left lung on the left side.

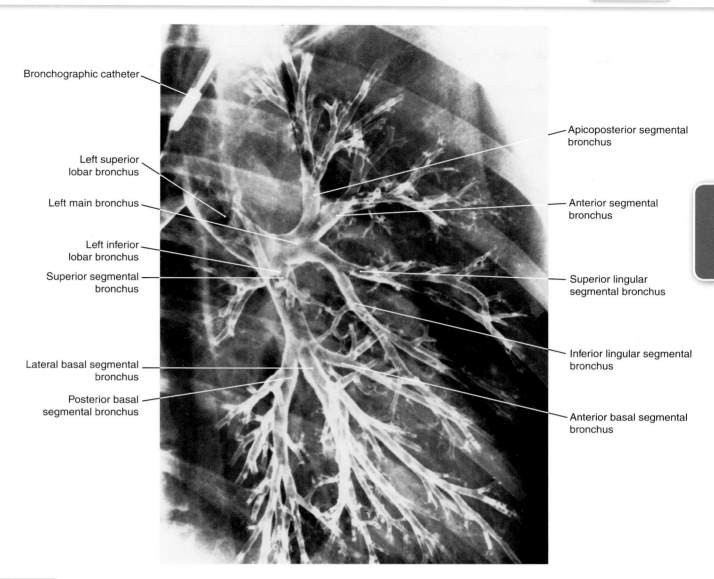

Bronchographic catheter

Left superior lobar bronchus

Left main bronchus

Left inferior lobar bronchus

Superior segmental bronchus

Lateral basal segmental bronchus

Posterior basal segmental bronchus

Apicoposterior segmental bronchus

Anterior segmental bronchus

Superior lingular segmental bronchus

Inferior lingular segmental bronchus

Anterior basal segmental bronchus

FIGURE 165.1 **Left Bronchogram Showing the Bronchial Tree**

NOTE: (1) A powder was administered through the trachea by a catheter to visualize the bronchial tree.

(2) The apical and posterior segmental bronchi (apicoposterior) and the anterior segmental bronchus of the **superior lobe.**

(3) The superior and inferior segmental bronchi of the **lingular part** of the **superior lobe.**

(4) The superior segment and the lateral, posterior, and anterior basal segments of the **inferior lobe.** The medial basal segment of the inferior lobe is mostly missing in this bronchogram. (Compare this bronchogram with Plate 157.)

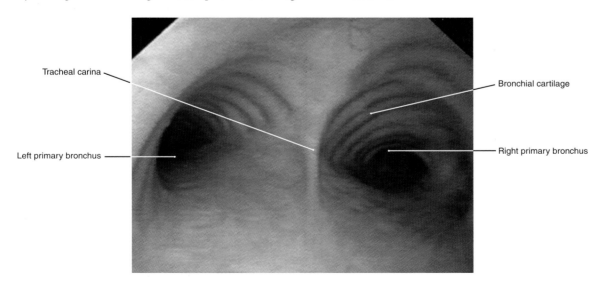

Tracheal carina

Bronchial cartilage

Left primary bronchus

Right primary bronchus

FIGURE 165.2 **Bronchoscopy of a Healthy Individual Showing the Tracheal Bifurcation and the Carina of the Trachea**

PLATE 166 Mediastinum: Right Side, Pleura Removed

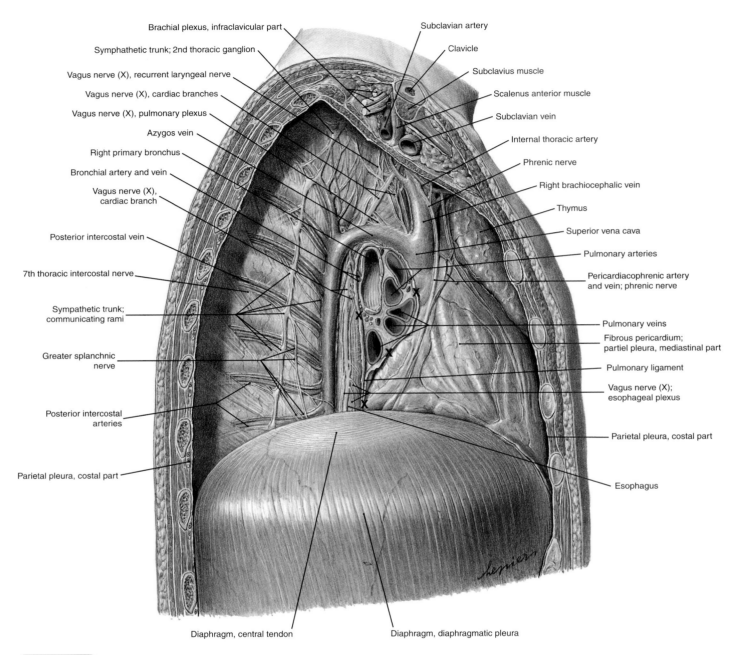

Brachial plexus, infraclavicular part

Symphathetic trunk; 2nd thoracic ganglion

Vagus nerve (X), recurrent laryngeal nerve

Vagus nerve (X), cardiac branches

Vagus nerve (X), pulmonary plexus

Azygos vein

Right primary bronchus

Bronchial artery and vein

Vagus nerve (X), cardiac branch

Posterior intercostal vein

7th thoracic intercostal nerve

Sympathetic trunk; communicating rami

Greater splanchnic nerve

Posterior intercostal arteries

Parietal pleura, costal part

Diaphragm, central tendon

Subclavian artery

Clavicle

Subclavius muscle

Scalenus anterior muscle

Subclavian vein

Internal thoracic artery

Phrenic nerve

Right brachiocephalic vein

Thymus

Superior vena cava

Pulmonary arteries

Pericardiacophrenic artery and vein; phrenic nerve

Pulmonary veins

Fibrous pericardium; partiel pleura, mediastinal part

Pulmonary ligament

Vagus nerve (X); esophageal plexus

Parietal pleura, costal part

Esophagus

Diaphragm, diaphragmatic pleura

FIGURE 166 **Right Side of the Mediastinum with the Mediastinal Pleura and Some Costal Pleura Removed**

NOTE: (1) The lung has been removed, the structures at the hilum transected, and the mediastinal pleura stripped away. This exposes the organs of the mediastinum, and their right lateral surface is presented.

(2) The right side of the heart is covered by pericardium and the course of the **phrenic nerve** and **pericardiacophrenic vessels** is visible.

(3) The ascending course of the **azygos vein,** its arch, and its junction with the superior vena cava.

(4) The **right vagus nerve** descends in the thorax behind the root of the right lung to form the **posterior pulmonary plexus.** It then helps form the **esophageal plexus** and leaves the thorax on the posterior aspect of the esophagus.

(5) The **dome of the diaphragm** on the right side as it takes the rounded form of the underlying liver. The inferior (diaphragmatic) surface of the heart rests on the diaphragm.

(6) The position of the thoracic **sympathetic chain** of ganglia coursing longitudinally along the inner surface of the thoracic wall. Observe the **greater thoracic splanchnic nerve.**

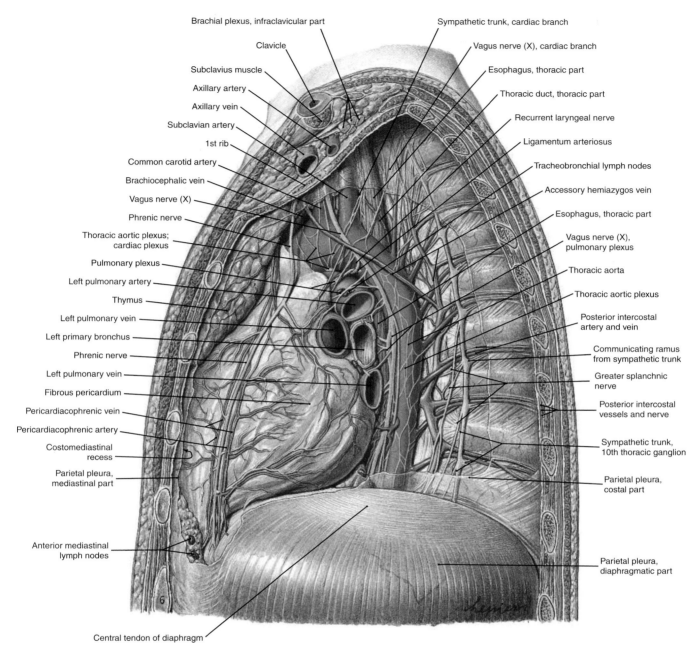

Brachial plexus, infraclavicular part

Clavicle

Subclavius muscle

Axillary artery

Axillary vein

Subclavian artery

1st rib

Common carotid artery

Brachiocephalic vein

Vagus nerve (X)

Phrenic nerve

Thoracic aortic plexus;
cardiac plexus

Pulmonary plexus

Left pulmonary artery

Thymus

Left pulmonary vein

Left primary bronchus

Phrenic nerve

Left pulmonary vein

Fibrous pericardium

Pericardiacophrenic vein

Pericardiacophrenic artery

Costomediastinal
recess

Parietal pleura,
mediastinal part

Anterior mediastinal
lymph nodes

Central tendon of diaphragm

Sympathetic trunk, cardiac branch

Vagus nerve (X), cardiac branch

Esophagus, thoracic part

Thoracic duct, thoracic part

Recurrent laryngeal nerve

Ligamentum arteriosus

Tracheobronchial lymph nodes

Accessory hemiazygos vein

Esophagus, thoracic part

Vagus nerve (X),
pulmonary plexus

Thoracic aorta

Thoracic aortic plexus

Posterior intercostal
artery and vein

Communicating ramus
from sympathetic trunk

Greater splanchnic
nerve

Posterior intercostal
vessels and nerve

Sympathetic trunk,
10th thoracic ganglion

Parietal pleura,
costal part

Parietal pleura,
diaphragmatic part

FIGURE 167   **Left Side of the Mediastinum with the Mediastinal Pleura and Some Costal Pleura Removed**

NOTE: (1) With the left lung removed along with most of the mediastinal pleura, the structures of the mediastinal pleura and the structures of the mediastinum are observed from their left side.

(2) The **left phrenic nerve** and **pericardiacophrenic vessels** course to the diaphragm along the pericardial covering over the left side of the heart.

(3) The **aorta** ascends about 2 in. before it arches posteriorly and to the left of the vertebral column.

(4) The descending **thoracic aorta** commences at about the level of the fourth thoracic vertebra. As it descends, it comes to lie anterior to the vertebral column.

(5) The **intercostal arteries** branch directly from the thoracic aorta. The typical intercostal artery and vein course along the inferior border of their respective rib. Because the superior border of the ribs is free of vessels and nerves, it is a safer site for injection or drainage of the thorax.

(6) The **left vagus nerve** lies lateral to the aortic arch and gives off the **recurrent laryngeal branch,** which passes inferior to the **ligamentum arteriosum.** The main trunk then continues to descend, contributes to the esophageal plexus, and enters the abdomen on the anterior aspect of the esophagus.

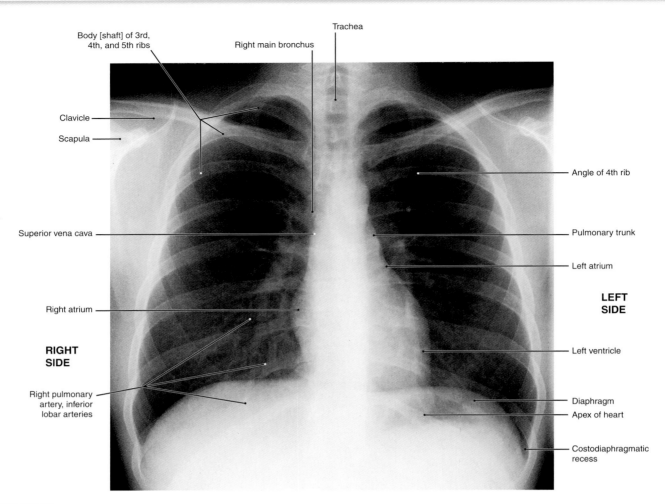

FIGURE 168.1 **Posteroanterior Radiograph of the Thorax in a 27-Year-Old Male**

NOTE: (1) A normal-appearing heart within the chest. Realize that it lies substernally with about two-thirds of the normal heart to the left of the midline and one-third to the right.
(2) Compare the labeled structures on the x-ray with those on the diagram seen in Figure 168.2.
(3) The right dome of the diaphragm is somewhat more superior than the dome on the left. This is because of the liver in the right upper abdomen.

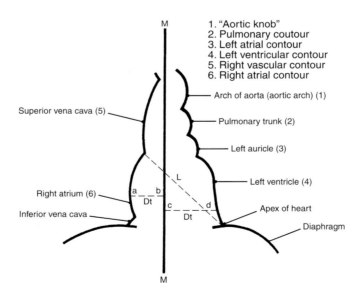

1. "Aortic knob"
2. Pulmonary coutour
3. Left atrial contour
4. Left ventricular contour
5. Right vascular contour
6. Right atrial contour

FIGURE 168.2 **Schematic Diagram of the Heart Seen in the Radiograph of Figure 168.1**

NOTE: (1) The midline of the body (**M**) and the longitudinal (**Ld**) and transverse (**ab** + **cd**) dimensions (**Dt**) of the heart.
(2) Transverse diameter: ab + cd = 13 to 14 cm. Longitudinal axis (Ld): From the superior contour of the right atrium to the apex: 15 to 16 cm.

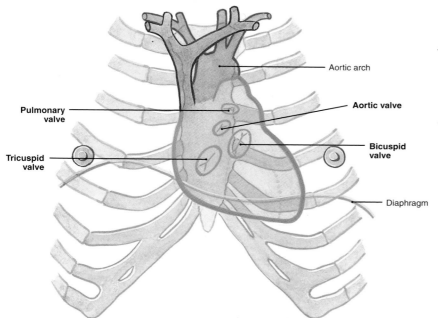

◄ FIGURE 169.1 **Projection of the Heart and Its Valves onto the Anterior Thoracic Wall**

NOTE: (1) The **pulmonary valve** lies behind the sternal end of the third left costal cartilage. The **aortic valve** is behind the sternum at the level of the third intercostal space. The **mitral valve** (bicuspid) lies behind the fourth left sternocostal joint, and the **tricuspid valve** lies posterior to the middle of the sternum at the level of the fourth intercostal space.

(2) The unbroken blue line indicates the **area of deep cardiac dullness,** which produces a dull resonance by percussion. Lung tissue covers this area but does not cover the area limited by the blue dotted line from which a less-resonant **superficial cardiac** dullness is obtained.

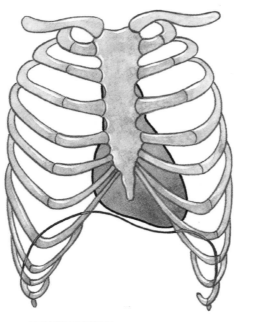

FIGURE 169.2 **Inspiration**

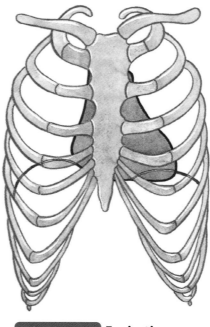

FIGURE 169.3 **Expiration**

FIGURES 169.2 and 169.3 **Positions of the Heart during Full Inspiration (Fig. 169.2) and during Full Expiration (Fig. 169.3)**

NOTE: (1) During **full inspiration (Fig. 169.2).**
 (a) The thorax is enlarged by a lowering of the diaphragm due to contraction of its muscle fibers and by elevation and expansion of the thorax (ribs and sternum).
 (b) The chest expands anteroposteriorly, transversely, and vertically, resulting in the heart becoming more oblong (i.e., its transverse diameter is decreased), and its apex and diaphragmatic surface are lowered.
 (c) Inspiration is accompanied by relaxation of the anterior abdominal wall muscles, protrusion of the abdomen, and a lowering of abdominal viscera.

(2) During **full expiration (Fig. 169.3).**
 (a) The diaphragm is elevated because its muscle fibers relax and because the ribs and sternum contract the size of the thorax.
 (b) With the capacity of the thoracic cage diminished, there is an elevation of the diaphragmatic surface of the heart and the apex of the heart. This results in an increase in the transverse diameter of the heart.
 (c) Expiration is accompanied by contraction of the anterior abdominal wall muscles and an elevation of the abdominal viscera, which also pushes the relaxed diaphragm upward.

PLATE 170 Mediastinum: Great Vessels; Subdivisions of Mediastinum

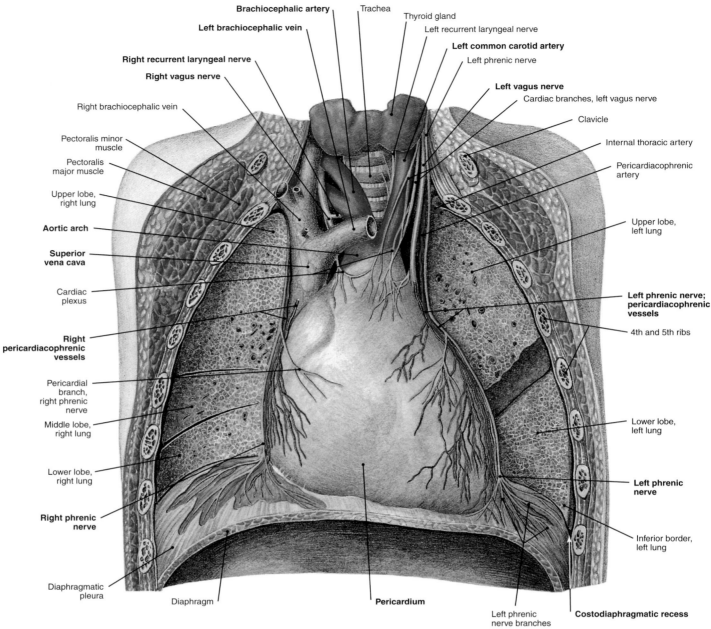

▲

FIGURE 170.1 **Adult Heart, Pericardium, and Superior Mediastinum (Anterior View)**

NOTE: (1) In this frontal section, the anterior thoracic wall and the anterior part of the lungs and diaphragm have been removed, leaving the **pericardium** and its vessels and nerves intact. The **vagus nerves** and some of their branches are also shown.

(2) The **phrenic nerves** form in the neck (C3, C4, and C5) and descend with the pericardiacophrenic vessels to innervate the diaphragm, but they also send some sensory fibers to the pericardium.

(3) The pericardium is formed by an outer **fibrous layer,** which is lined by an inner serous sac. As the heart develops, it invaginates into the serous sac and becomes covered by a **visceral layer of serous pericardium** (epicardium) and a **parietal layer of serous pericardium.**

(4) The visceral layer clings closely to the heart, while the parietal layer lines the inner surface of the fibrous pericardium. The potential space between the visceral and parietal layers contains a little serous fluid and is called the **pericardial cavity.**

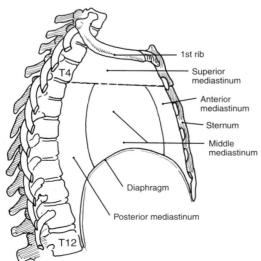

FIGURE 170.2 **Subdivisions of the Mediastinum**

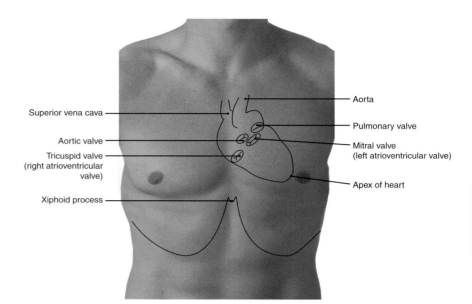

▲

FIGURE 171.1 **Projection of the Heart and Cardiac Valves onto the Thoracic Wall**

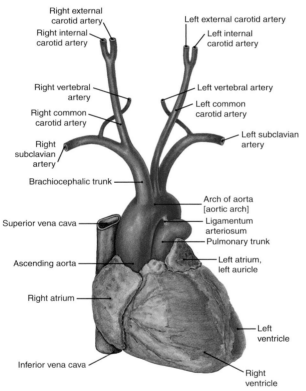

◄ **FIGURE 171.2** **Heart, Aortic Arch, and the Great Arteries from the Arch**

NOTE also the pulmonary trunk and the superior and inferior vena cavae.

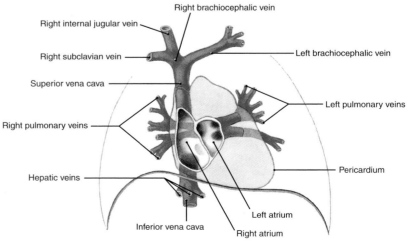

FIGURE 171.3 **Great Veins That Drain into ► the Heart (Anterior View)**

PLATE 172 **Heart and Great Vessels (Anterior View)**

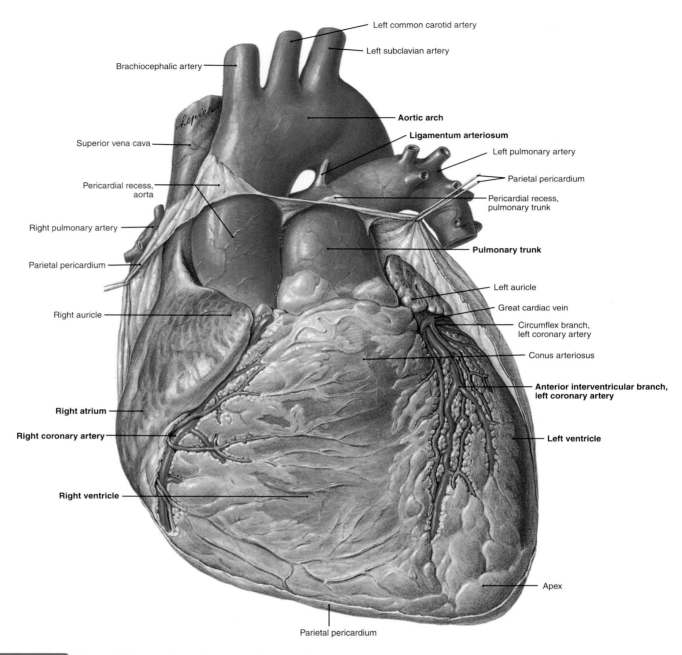

Left common carotid artery

Left subclavian artery

Brachiocephalic artery

Aortic arch

Ligamentum arteriosum

Superior vena cava

Left pulmonary artery

Pericardial recess, aorta

Parietal pericardium

Pericardial recess, pulmonary trunk

Right pulmonary artery

Pulmonary trunk

Parietal pericardium

Left auricle

Great cardiac vein

Right auricle

Circumflex branch, left coronary artery

Conus arteriosus

Anterior interventricular branch, left coronary artery

Right atrium

Right coronary artery

Left ventricle

Right ventricle

Apex

Parietal pericardium

FIGURE 172 **Ventral View of the Heart and Great Vessels**

NOTE: (1) The heart is a muscular organ in the middle mediastinum, and its **apex** points inferiorly, to the left, and slightly anteriorly. The **base** of the heart is opposite to the apex and is directed superiorly and to the right.

(2) The great vessels attach to the heart at its base, and the pericardium is reflected over these vessels at their origin.

(3) The anterior surface of the heart is its **sternocostal surface.** The auricular portion of the **right atrium** and much of the **right ventricle** is seen from this anterior view; also a small part of the **left ventricle** is visible along the left border.

(4) The **pulmonary trunk** originates from the right ventricle. To its right can be seen the **aorta,** which arises from the left ventricle. The **superior vena cava** can be seen opening into the upper aspect of the right atrium.

(5) The **ligamentum arteriosum.** This fibrous structure between the left pulmonary artery and the aorta is the remnant of the fetal **ductus arteriosus,** which, before birth, served to shunt blood directed to the lungs back into the aorta for systemic distribution.

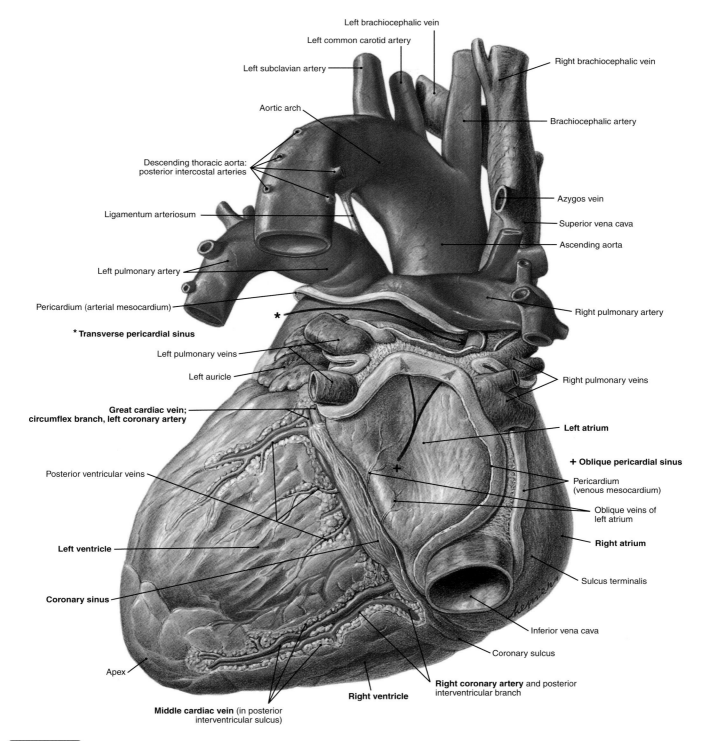

Left brachiocephalic vein

Left common carotid artery

Left subclavian artery

Right brachiocephalic vein

Aortic arch

Brachiocephalic artery

Descending thoracic aorta:
posterior intercostal arteries

Azygos vein

Ligamentum arteriosum

Superior vena cava

Ascending aorta

Left pulmonary artery

Pericardium (arterial mesocardium)

Right pulmonary artery

*Transverse pericardial sinus

Left pulmonary veins

Left auricle

Right pulmonary veins

Great cardiac vein;
circumflex branch, left coronary artery

Left atrium

+ Oblique pericardial sinus

Posterior ventricular veins

Pericardium
(venous mesocardium)

Oblique veins of
left atrium

Right atrium

Left ventricle

Sulcus terminalis

Coronary sinus

Inferior vena cava

Coronary sulcus

Apex

Right coronary artery and posterior
interventricular branch

Right ventricle

Middle cardiac vein (in posterior
interventricular sulcus)

FIGURE 173 **Heart and Great Vessels (Posterior View)**

NOTE: (1) The two pericardial sinuses. The black horizontal arrow indicates the **transverse pericardial sinus,** which lies between the arterial mesocardium and the venous mesocardium. The vertical diverging double arrows lie in the **oblique pericardial sinus,** the boundary of which is limited by the pericardial reflections around the pulmonary veins.

(2) The transverse sinus can be identified by placing your index finger behind the pulmonary artery and aorta with the heart in place. The oblique sinus is open inferiorly and can be felt by cupping your fingers behind the heart and pushing upward; superiorly this sinus forms a closed cul-de-sac.

(3) The **coronary sinus** is a large vein, and it separates the posterior atrial and ventricular surfaces. The posterior atrial surface consists principally of the left atrium, into which flow the pulmonary veins, but also note the right atrium and its superior vena cava below and to the right.

(4) The posterior ventricular surface is formed principally by the left ventricle, and this surface lies over the diaphragm.

PLATE 174 **Heart and Great Vessels with the Pericardium Opened**

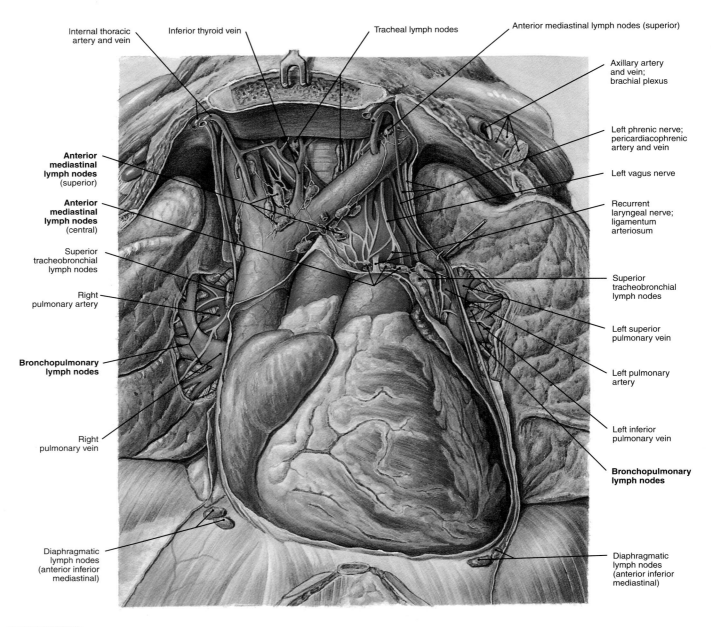

Internal thoracic artery and vein

Inferior thyroid vein

Tracheal lymph nodes

Anterior mediastinal lymph nodes (superior)

Axillary artery and vein; brachial plexus

Anterior mediastinal lymph nodes (superior)

Anterior mediastinal lymph nodes (central)

Superior tracheobronchial lymph nodes

Right pulmonary artery

Bronchopulmonary lymph nodes

Right pulmonary vein

Diaphragmatic lymph nodes (anterior inferior mediastinal)

Left phrenic nerve; pericardiacophrenic artery and vein

Left vagus nerve

Recurrent laryngeal nerve; ligamentum arteriosum

Superior tracheobronchial lymph nodes

Left superior pulmonary vein

Left pulmonary artery

Left inferior pulmonary vein

Bronchopulmonary lymph nodes

Diaphragmatic lymph nodes (anterior inferior mediastinal)

FIGURE 174 **Lymphatics of the Thorax (Anterior Aspect)**

NOTE: (1) The anterior thoracic wall was removed, along with the ventral portion of the fibrous pericardium. The anterior borders of the lungs have been pulled laterally to reveal the lymph nodes at the roots of the lungs.

(2) Removal of the thymus and its related fat and reflection of the manubrium superiorly exposes the organs at the thoracic inlet and their associated lymphatics.

(3) Lymph nodes in the anterior part of the thorax may be divided into those associated with the thoracic cage (parietal) and those associated with the organs (visceral). Probably all the nodes indicated in this figure are visceral nodes.

(4) Situated ventrally are the **anterior mediastinal nodes,** which include a superior group, which lies ventral to the brachiocephalic veins and a more centrally located group that lies ventral to the arch of the aorta. Inferiorly, anterior diaphragmatic nodes are sometimes also classified as part of the anterior mediastinal nodes.

(5) Large numbers of lymph nodes are associated with the trachea, the bronchi, and the other structures at the root of the lung. These nodes have been aptly named **tracheal, tracheobronchial, bronchopulmonary,** and **pulmonary.**

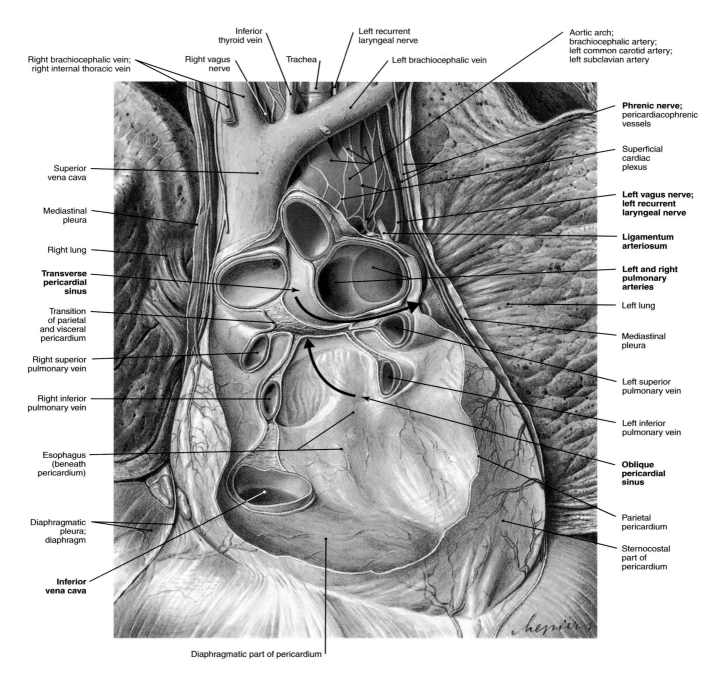

Inferior thyroid vein

Left recurrent laryngeal nerve

Right vagus nerve

Trachea

Left brachiocephalic vein

Aortic arch; brachiocephalic artery; left common carotid artery; left subclavian artery

Right brachiocephalic vein; right internal thoracic vein

Superior vena cava

Mediastinal pleura

Right lung

Transverse pericardial sinus

Transition of parietal and visceral pericardium

Right superior pulmonary vein

Right inferior pulmonary vein

Esophagus (beneath pericardium)

Diaphragmatic pleura; diaphragm

Inferior vena cava

Phrenic nerve; pericardiacophrenic vessels

Superficial cardiac plexus

Left vagus nerve; left recurrent laryngeal nerve

Ligamentum arteriosum

Left and right pulmonary arteries

Left lung

Mediastinal pleura

Left superior pulmonary vein

Left inferior pulmonary vein

Oblique pericardial sinus

Parietal pericardium

Sternocostal part of pericardium

Diaphragmatic part of pericardium

FIGURE 175 **Interior of the Pericardium (Anterior View)**

NOTE: (1) The pericardium has been opened anteriorly, and the heart has been severed from its attachment to the great vessels and removed. Eight vessels have been cut: the superior and inferior venae cavae, the four pulmonary veins, the pulmonary artery, and the aorta.

(2) The **oblique pericardial sinus** is located in the central portion of the posterior wall of the pericardium and is bounded by the pericardial reflections over the pulmonary veins and the venae cavae (venous mesocardium).

(3) With the heart in place and the pericardium opened anteriorly, the oblique pericardial sinus may be palpated by inserting several fingers behind the heart and probing superiorly until the blind pouch (cul-de-sac) of the sinus is felt.

(4) The **transverse pericardial sinus** lies behind the pericardial reflection surrounding the aorta and pulmonary artery (arterial mesocardium). It may be located by probing with the index finger from right to left immediately behind the pulmonary trunk.

(5) The site of bifurcation of the pulmonary trunk beneath the arch of the aorta and the course of the **left recurrent laryngeal nerve** beneath the **ligamentum arteriosum.**

PLATE 176 Heart, Blood Supply (Anterior and Superior Surfaces)

FIGURE 176.1 Coronary Vessels (Anterior View)

NOTE: (1) Both the left and right coronary arteries arise from the ascending aorta. The **left coronary** is directed toward the left and soon divides into an **anterior interventricular branch,** which descends toward the apex, and a **circumflex branch,** which passes posteriorly to the back of the heart.

(2) The **right coronary** is directed toward the right and passes to the posterior heart within the coronary sulcus. In its course, branches from the right coronary supply the anterior surface of the right side (anterior cardiac artery). Its largest branch is the **posterior interventricular artery,** which courses toward the apex on the posterior or diaphragmatic surface of the heart.

(3) The principal veins of the heart drain into the **coronary sinus,** which flows into the right atrium. The distribution and course of the veins is similar to the arteries (see Figs. 177.1 and 177.2).

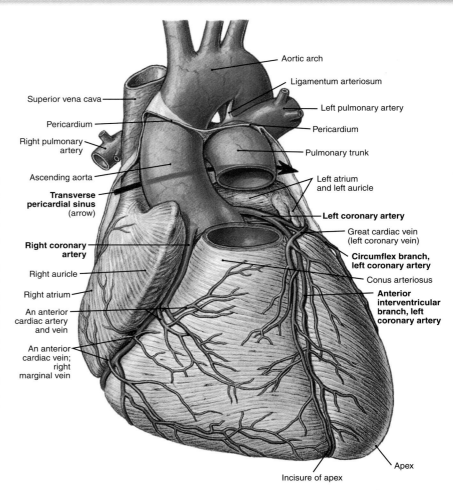

Aortic arch
Ligamentum arteriosum
Left pulmonary artery
Pericardium
Pulmonary trunk
Left atrium and left auricle
Left coronary artery
Great cardiac vein (left coronary vein)
Circumflex branch, left coronary artery
Conus arteriosus
Anterior interventricular branch, left coronary artery

Superior vena cava
Pericardium
Right pulmonary artery
Ascending aorta
Transverse pericardial sinus (arrow)
Right coronary artery
Right auricle
Right atrium
An anterior cardiac artery and vein
An anterior cardiac vein; right marginal vein

Apex
Incisure of apex

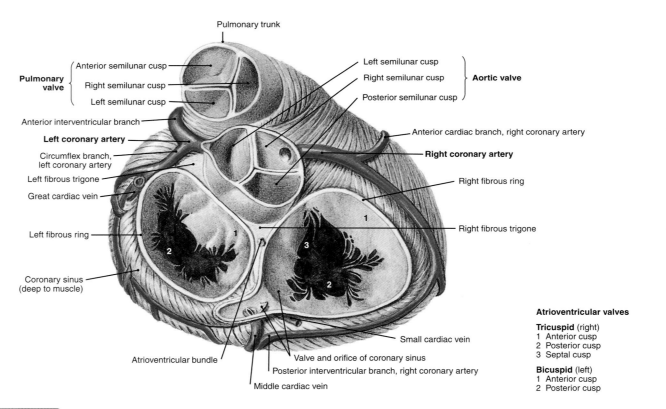

Pulmonary trunk

Pulmonary valve
Anterior semilunar cusp
Right semilunar cusp
Left semilunar cusp

Left semilunar cusp
Right semilunar cusp   **Aortic valve**
Posterior semilunar cusp

Anterior interventricular branch
Left coronary artery
Circumflex branch, left coronary artery
Left fibrous trigone
Great cardiac vein
Left fibrous ring
Coronary sinus (deep to muscle)

Anterior cardiac branch, right coronary artery
Right coronary artery
Right fibrous ring
Right fibrous trigone

Atrioventricular bundle
Valve and orifice of coronary sinus
Posterior interventricular branch, right coronary artery
Middle cardiac vein
Small cardiac vein

Atrioventricular valves

Tricuspid (right)
1 Anterior cusp
2 Posterior cusp
3 Septal cusp

Bicuspid (left)
1 Anterior cusp
2 Posterior cusp

FIGURE 176.2 Valves of the Heart and the Origin of the Coronary Vessels (Superior View)

NOTE that the left coronary artery arises from the aortic wall in the left aortic sinus behind the left semilunar cusp, and the right coronary artery stems from the aorta behind the right aortic sinus and right semilunar cusp.

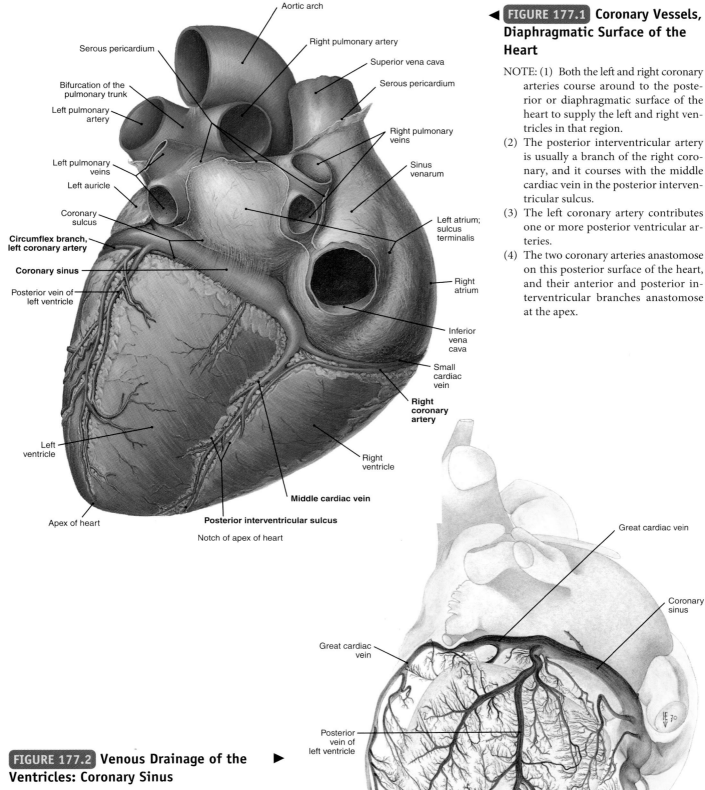

FIGURE 177.1 label references (Figure 177.1):

Aortic arch
Serous pericardium
Right pulmonary artery
Superior vena cava
Serous pericardium
Bifurcation of the pulmonary trunk
Left pulmonary artery
Right pulmonary veins
Left pulmonary veins
Sinus venarum
Left auricle
Coronary sulcus
Left atrium; sulcus terminalis
Circumflex branch, left coronary artery
Coronary sinus
Posterior vein of left ventricle
Right atrium
Inferior vena cava
Small cardiac vein
Right coronary artery
Left ventricle
Right ventricle
Middle cardiac vein
Apex of heart
Posterior interventricular sulcus
Notch of apex of heart

◄ FIGURE 177.1 Coronary Vessels, Diaphragmatic Surface of the Heart

NOTE: (1) Both the left and right coronary arteries course around to the posterior or diaphragmatic surface of the heart to supply the left and right ventricles in that region.

(2) The posterior interventricular artery is usually a branch of the right coronary, and it courses with the middle cardiac vein in the posterior interventricular sulcus.

(3) The left coronary artery contributes one or more posterior ventricular arteries.

(4) The two coronary arteries anastomose on this posterior surface of the heart, and their anterior and posterior interventricular branches anastomose at the apex.

Figure 177.2 labels:
Great cardiac vein
Coronary sinus
Great cardiac vein
Posterior vein of left ventricle
Anterior interventricular vein
Middle cardiac vein

FIGURE 177.2 Venous Drainage of the Ventricles: Coronary Sinus ►

NOTE: (1) The left side and left margin of the heart are oriented forward such that the anterior interventricular vein is seen on the left and the middle cardiac vein is seen on the right.

(2) The anterior **interventricular** vein becomes the **great cardiac vein.** As the great cardiac vein courses in the coronary sulcus, it gradually enlarges to form the **coronary sinus** and receives the **posterior vein of the left ventricle.** The **middle cardiac vein,** which runs in the posterior interventricular sulcus, also drains directly into the coronary sinus.

(3) The coronary sinus opens into the right atrium.

PLATE 178 Heart: Coronary Arteries

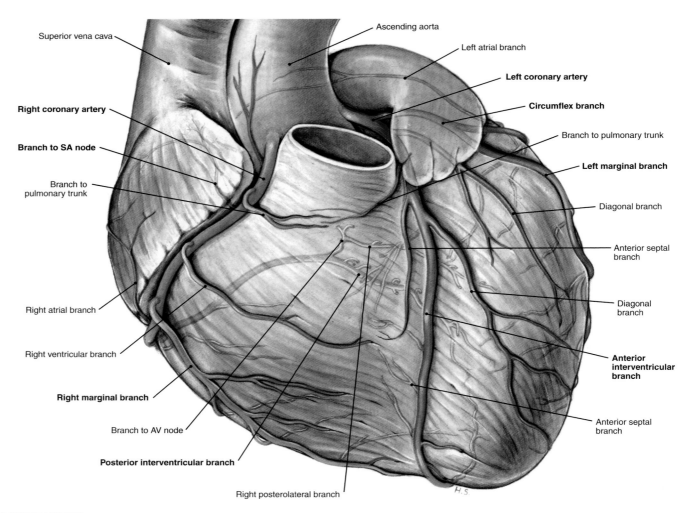

Superior vena cava

Ascending aorta

Left atrial branch

Left coronary artery

Right coronary artery

Circumflex branch

Branch to SA node

Branch to pulmonary trunk

Left marginal branch

Branch to pulmonary trunk

Diagonal branch

Anterior septal branch

Right atrial branch

Diagonal branch

Right ventricular branch

Anterior interventricular branch

Right marginal branch

Anterior septal branch

Branch to AV node

Posterior interventricular branch

Right posterolateral branch

FIGURE 178.1 **Complete Coronary Arterial System** ▲

NOTE: (1) Anastomoses between branches from the left and right coronary arteries (LCA and RCA) are visible in the substance of the posterior wall of the heart. These occur between the posterior interventricular branch of the RCA and the anterior interventricular branch of the LCA, which continues around the apex of the heart to the posterior wall.

(2) Vessels from the circumflex and left marginal branches of the LCA also anastomose with branches from the RCA in the posterior wall.

(3) Branches supplying the sinoatrial (SA) node and the atrioventricular (AV) node arise from the RCA. In about 35% of cases, however, the artery to the SA node comes from the circumflex branch of the LCA. Similarly, in about 20% of specimens, the vessel to the AV node is derived from the circumflex branch of the LCA. (From a drawing by Professor Helmut Ferner at the University of Vienna.)

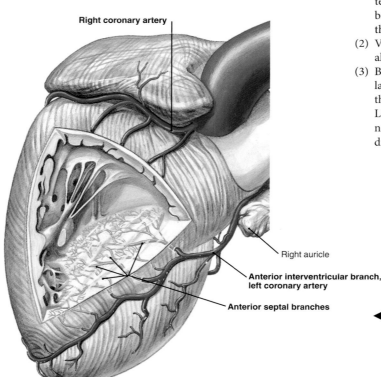

Right coronary artery

Right auricle

Anterior interventricular branch, left coronary artery

Anterior septal branches

◄ **FIGURE 178.2** **Blood Supply to the Interventricular Septum**

Note that the **anterior septal branches** of the anterior interventricular artery course backward and downward to supply the interventricular septum.

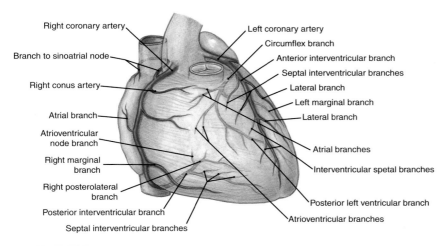

FIGURE 179A Balanced Distribution of the Left and Right Coronary Arteries

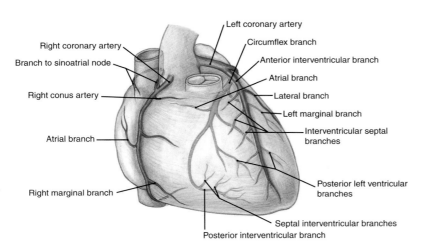

FIGURE 179B Left Dominant Distribution of the Coronary Arteries

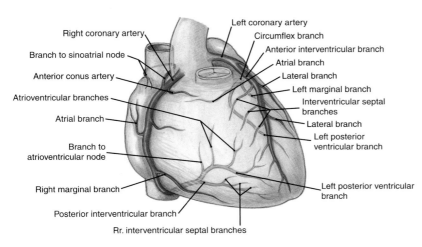

FIGURE 179C Right Dominant Distribution of the Coronary Arteries

≈70%

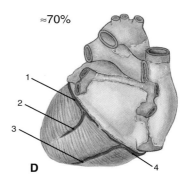

D

≈20%

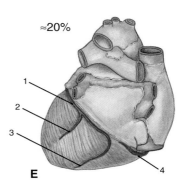

E

≈10%

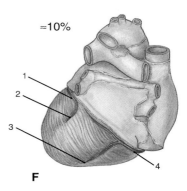

F

FIGURE 179D–F Variations in the Arterial Supply on the Posterior Wall of the Heart (Dorsal View)

1. Circumflex branch (left coronary artery)
2. Left posterior ventricular branch (left coronary artery)
3. Posterior ventricular branch of right coronary artery
4. Right coronary artery

PLATE 180 **Heart: Arteriogram of the Left Coronary Artery**

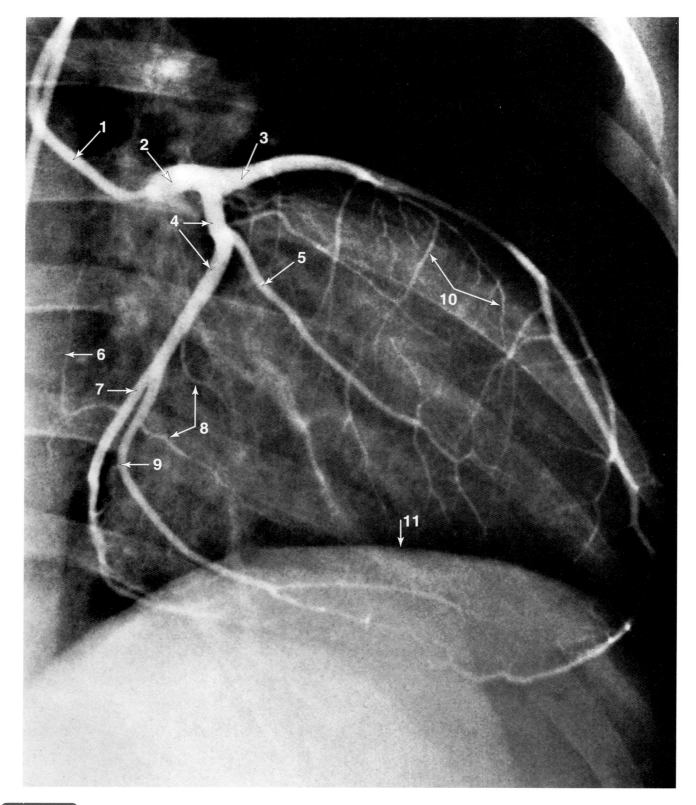

FIGURE 180 **Left Coronary Arteriogram**

NOTE that this arteriogram of the left coronary artery is viewed from a right anterior oblique direction.

1. Catheter
2. Left coronary artery
3. Anterior interventricular branch

4. Circumflex branch
5. Left marginal branch of circumflex
6. Posterior atrial branch

7. Left posterolateral branch of circumflex
8. Posterior ventricular branches
9. Posterior interventricular branch

10. Septal branches
11. Diaphragm

(From Wicke, 6th ed.)

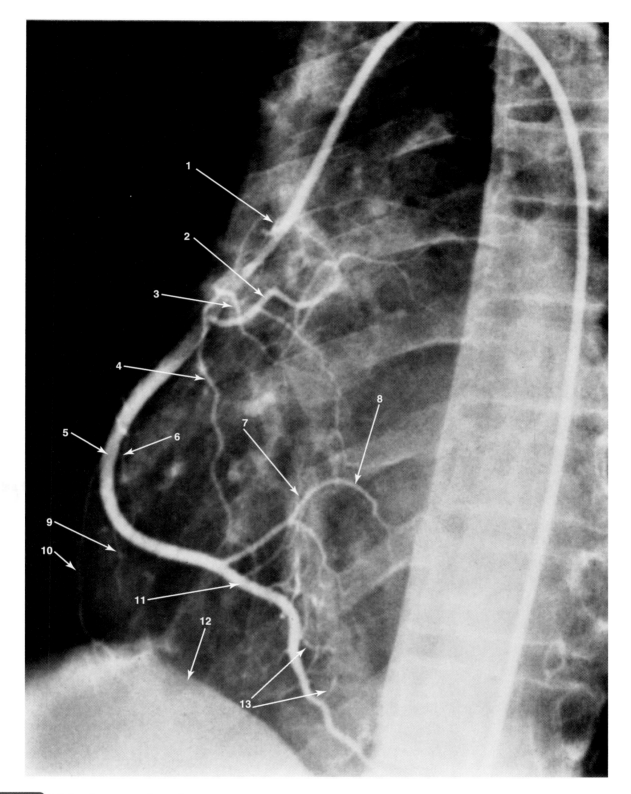

FIGURE 181 **Right Coronary Arteriogram**

NOTE that this arteriogram of the right coronary artery is viewed from the left anterior oblique direction.

1. Catheter
2. Sinoatrial node branch
3. Conus arteriosus branch
4. Anterior ventricular branch

5. Right coronary artery
6. Anterior ventricular branch
7. Atrioventricular node branch
8. Posterior ventricular branch

9. Posterior ventricular branch
10. Right marginal branch
11. Posterior interventricular branch
12. Diaphragm
13. Posterior septal branches

(From Wicke, 6th ed.)

PLATE 182 Heart: Right Atrium and Ventricle

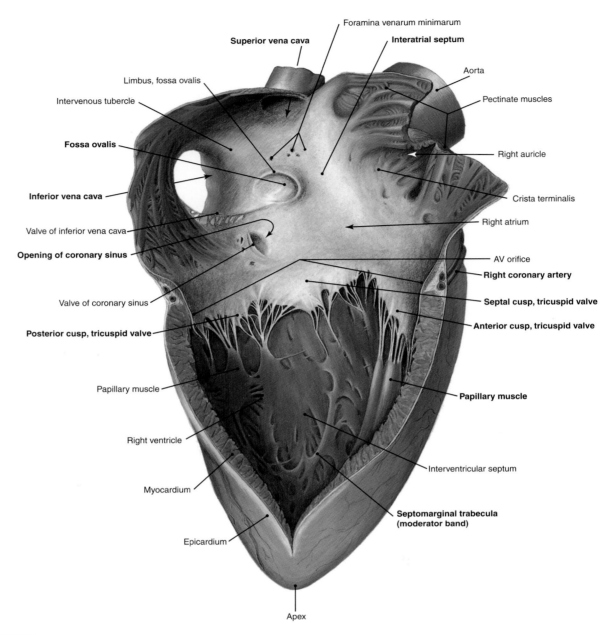

Foramina venarum minimarum
Superior vena cava
Interatrial septum
Aorta
Limbus, fossa ovalis
Pectinate muscles
Intervenous tubercle
Fossa ovalis
Right auricle
Inferior vena cava
Crista terminalis
Valve of inferior vena cava
Right atrium
Opening of coronary sinus
AV orifice
Right coronary artery
Valve of coronary sinus
Septal cusp, tricuspid valve
Posterior cusp, tricuspid valve
Anterior cusp, tricuspid valve
Papillary muscle
Papillary muscle
Right ventricle
Interventricular septum
Myocardium
Septomarginal trabecula (moderator band)
Epicardium
Apex

FIGURE 182 **Right Atrium and Right Ventricle**

NOTE: (1) The right atrium consists of (a) a smooth area (at times called the **sinus venarum**) located between the openings of the superior vena cava and the inferior vena cava and (b) the **right auricle,** which is marked by parallel muscle ridges called the **pectinate muscles.**

(2) Opening into the right atrium are the **superior vena cava,** the **inferior vena cava,** the **coronary sinus,** and the small **venarum minimarum** (Thebesian veins).

(3) Crescent-shaped valves are found at the right atrial openings of both the inferior vena cava and the coronary sinus.

(4) The right atrioventricular (AV) opening is surrounded by the three cusps of the **tricuspid valve.** These are called the **anterior, posterior,** and **septal** cusps, and they are attached to the heart wall by way of the **chordae tendineae** and papillary **muscles.**

(5) The thickness of the right ventricular wall (4–5 mm) is about one-third that of the left ventricle. Normal right ventricular systolic blood pressure ranges between 25 and 30 mm Hg, and it is also much less than normal left ventricular systolic pressure, which ranges between 120 and 140 mm Hg.

(6) The **septomarginal trabecula** (moderator band) within which courses the right crus, or branch, of the **atrioventricular bundle** (of His).

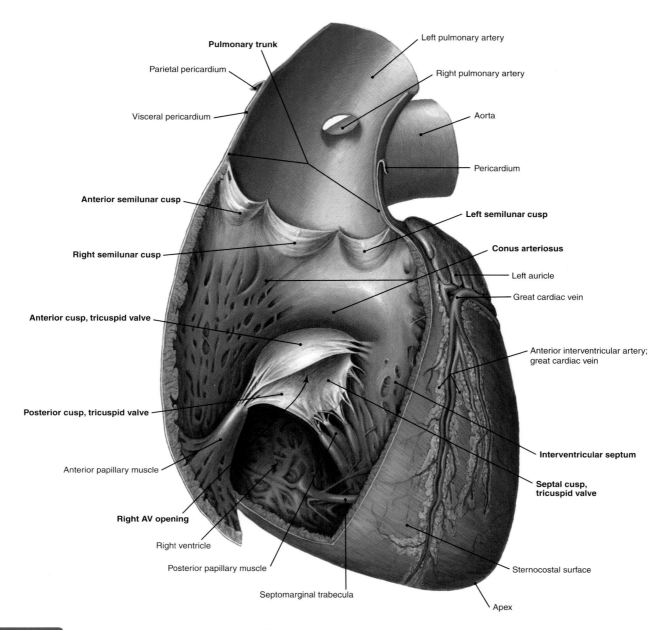

Pulmonary trunk

Parietal pericardium

Visceral pericardium

Anterior semilunar cusp

Right semilunar cusp

Anterior cusp, tricuspid valve

Posterior cusp, tricuspid valve

Anterior papillary muscle

Right AV opening

Right ventricle

Posterior papillary muscle

Septomarginal trabecula

Left pulmonary artery

Right pulmonary artery

Aorta

Pericardium

Left semilunar cusp

Conus arteriosus

Left auricle

Great cardiac vein

Anterior interventricular artery; great cardiac vein

Interventricular septum

Septal cusp, tricuspid valve

Sternocostal surface

Apex

FIGURE 183 **Right Ventricle and Pulmonary Trunk**

NOTE: (1) The musculature of the right ventricle has been cut along a V-shaped incision, thereby forming a flap in the anterior wall of the ventricle. As the flap is reflected to the right, the origin of the **pulmonary trunk** and the cusps of its valve are exposed.

(2) The three semilunar pulmonary cusps—the **right, left,** and **anterior** semilunar pulmonary cusps—are interposed between the right ventricle and the pulmonary artery. Together they comprise the **pulmonary valve.**

(3) The **septal, anterior,** and **posterior cusps** form the **right atrioventricular** (AV) or **tricuspid valve.** Note their attachments to the papillary muscles.

(4) The smooth surface of the right ventricular wall at the site of origin of the pulmonary trunk. This is called the **conus arteriosus** of the right ventricle.

(5) The attachment and shape of the tricuspid valve allow the cusps to open into the right ventricle when blood pressure in the atrium exceeds that in the ventricle. At some point during the cardiac cycle, ventricular pressure exceeds atrial pressure, and the cusps close. Blood is prevented from regurgitating into the atrium because the perimeter of the cusps is secured to the heart wall and the free edges of the cusps are attached to the papillary muscles in the ventricle below.

PLATE 184 Heart: Left Atrium and Ventricle

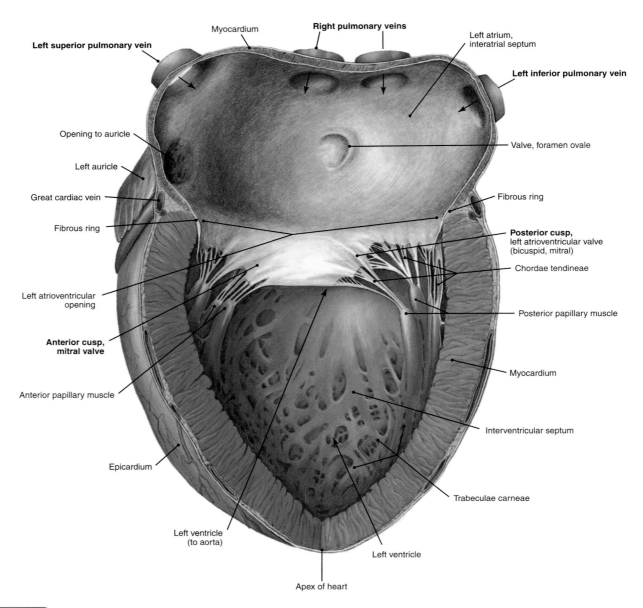

Myocardium

Right pulmonary veins

Left atrium, interatrial septum

Left superior pulmonary vein

Left inferior pulmonary vein

Opening to auricle

Left auricle

Great cardiac vein

Fibrous ring

Left atrioventricular opening

Anterior cusp, mitral valve

Anterior papillary muscle

Epicardium

Left ventricle (to aorta)

Apex of heart

Valve, foramen ovale

Fibrous ring

Posterior cusp, left atrioventricular valve (bicuspid, mitral)

Chordae tendineae

Posterior papillary muscle

Myocardium

Interventricular septum

Trabeculae carneae

Left ventricle

FIGURE 184 Left Atrium and Left Ventricle (Internal Surface)

NOTE: (1) In this specimen, the heart has been opened to expose the inner surface of the left atrium and left ventricle. Likewise, the left atrioventricular opening has been cut behind the **posterior cusp of the mitral valve,** thereby making that cusp visible.

(2) The left atrium receives the four **pulmonary veins** (two from each lung), while the left ventricle leads into the aorta (arrow).

(3) The **interatrial septum** on the left side is marked by the valve of the foramen ovale (falx septi), which represents the remnant of the **septum primum** during the development of the interatrial septum. The crescent-shaped structure around the border of the valve is the limbus of the fossa ovalis and is the remnant of the **septum secundum.**

(4) The mitral valve consists of **anterior** and **posterior cusps**. The cusps are attached to the left ventricular wall by means of chordae tendineae and papillary muscles in a manner similar to that seen in the right ventricle.

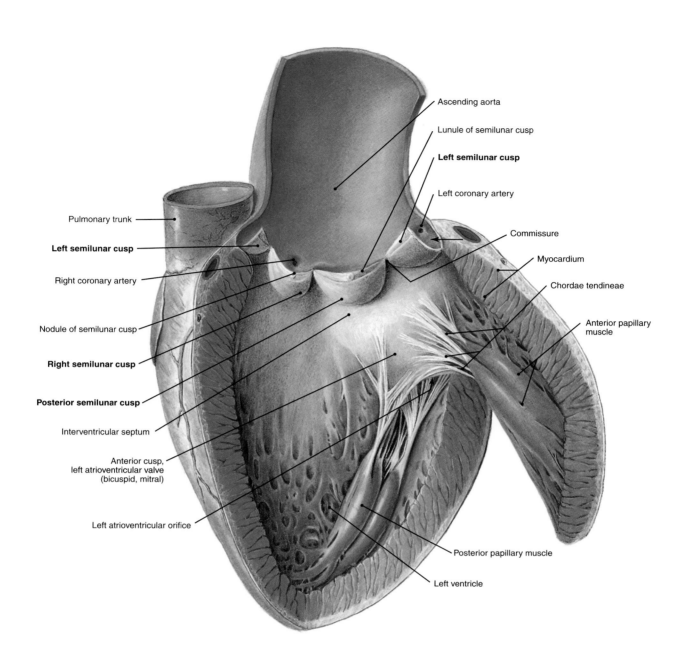

FIGURE 185 **Opened Left Ventricle and Aorta**

NOTE: (1) In this dissection, the left ventricle was opened first to show the anterior and posterior papillary muscles that are related to the cusps of the left AV valve. A second cut was then made in the wall of the left ventricle (near the interventricular septum) that extends through the aortic opening to show the cusps of the **aortic valve.**

(2) The opening of the left coronary artery in the aortic wall behind the (cut) left **semilunar cusp.** Also see the opening of the right coronary artery behind the **right semilunar cusp.** The **posterior cusp** of the aortic valve is the noncoronary cusp.

(3) Between the cusps and the wall of the aorta are pockets called the **aortic sinuses.** These trap blood during the cardiac cycle, thereby closing the valve.

(4) Each cusp is marked by a thickened fibrocartilaginous **nodule** at the center of its free margin. Extending out from the nodule on each side of the cusp are clear crescentic areas of thinning of the free edges called **lunulae,** while the points at which two adjacent cusps come together are called **commissures.**

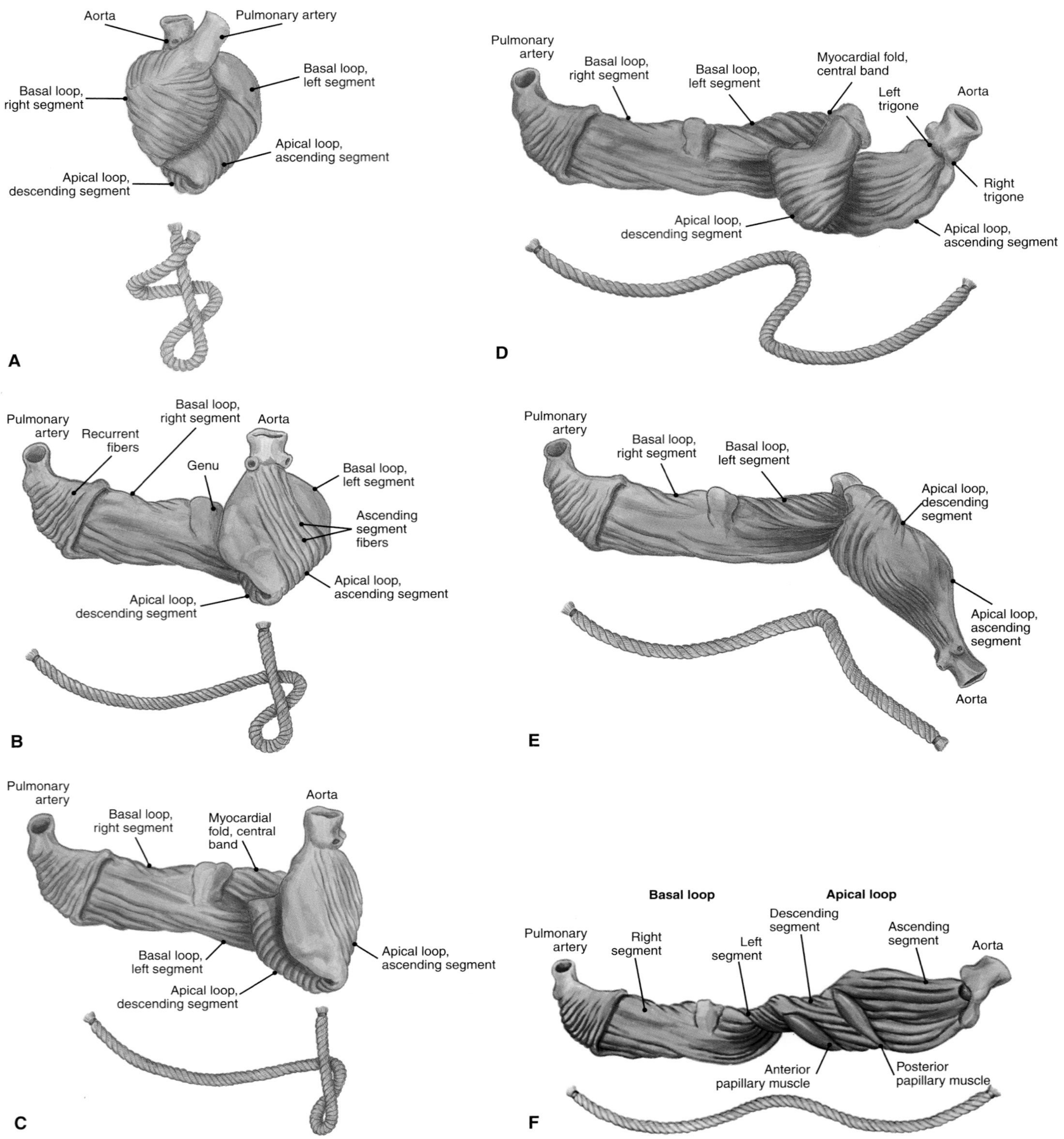

PLATE 186 | Unfolding the Muscular Anatomy of the Heart

A

B

C

D

E

F

FIGURE 186A–F Progressive Unscrolling of the Cardiac Muscle that Forms the Heart (from F. Torrent-Guasp)

NOTE: (1) Upon unscrolling the muscle that forms the heart, the unfolded myocardium has a rope-like configuration (shown by the rope model) comprising a **transverse basal loop,** with fibers running almost horizontally, and a **longitudinal apical loop,** with fibers that course almost vertically from apex to base. **Figure 186A** shows the intact heart. **Figure 186B** shows that detachment of the right ventricular free wall exposes the transverse orientation of the basal loop fibers. The pulmonary outflow tract is limited by **recurrent fibers** coming from the right free wall. These bend all along the anterior interventricular groove to ascend toward the ventricular base. A **genu** at the basal extreme of the posterior interventricular sulcus separates the right and left ventricles or segments of the basal loop.

(2) **Figure 186C:** Further unfolding of the basal loop displays the **left basal segment,** beyond the genu (left), and exposes the central band **myocardial fold** by which fibers of the left segment, subendocardially, become nearly vertical fibers of the descending segment. These course deeper, subendocardially, toward the region of the apex, where they reflect and ascend to become the ascending segment fibers that connect to the aorta. In **Figure 186D,** both **trigones of the aorta** are detached and the ascending segment is unfolded and moved laterally, thereby demonstrating the deeper descending segment of the apical loop. **(Continued on next page.)**

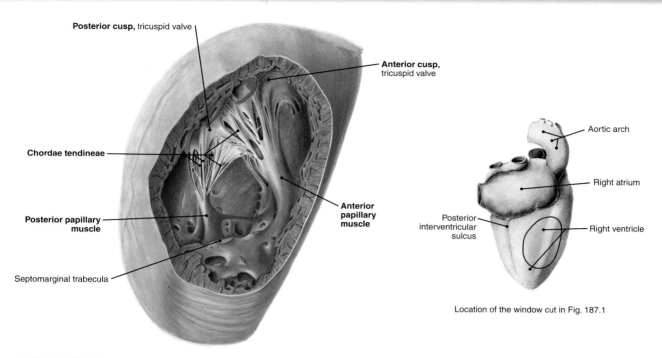

Location of the window cut in Fig. 187.1

FIGURE 187.1 **Right Ventricle: View of the Tricuspid Valve**

NOTE: (1) The anterior and posterior cusps (two of the three) of the tricuspid valve and their attached papillary muscles are exposed.

(2) The **anterior papillary muscle** arises from the anterior and septal walls and attaches to both the anterior and posterior cusps, while the **posterior papillary muscle** arises from the anterior and septal walls and attaches to both the anterior and posterior cusps. Observe the septomarginal trabeculae, or moderator bands, that contain the atrioventricular bundle.

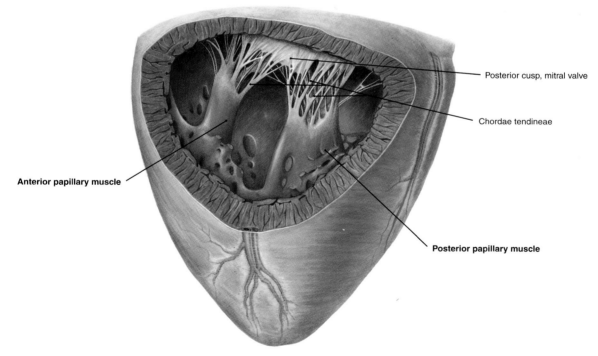

FIGURE 187.2 **Left Ventricle: View of the Mitral Valve**

NOTE that the **posterior and anterior papillary muscles** attach to the cusps of the mitral valve.

(Continued from the previous page.)

(3) **Figure 186E** shows the further unwrapping of the helix to clarify the apical loop that now is seen to be composed of the outer surfaces of descending and ascending segments. **Figure 186F:** The complete transverse myocardial band is seen with the central muscle twist that separates the basal and apical loops. In this figure can be seen the anterior and posterior papillary muscles in the apical loop. The left component is the transverse basal loop, and the right component is the apical loop. Observe that before this folding, both segments have a transverse orientation. The oblique orientation of the unscrolled descending and ascending segments derives from the spiral architectural folding of the myocardial band between the basal and apical loops. (From Buckberg GD, Clemente CD, Cox JL, Coghlan HC, Castella M, Torrent-Guasp F, Gharib M. The structure and function of the helical heart and its buttress wrapping. IV. Concepts of dynamic function from the normal macroscopic helical structure. Semin Thorac Cardiovasc Surg 2001;14:342–357.)

PLATE 188 Heart: Frontal Section; Conduction System

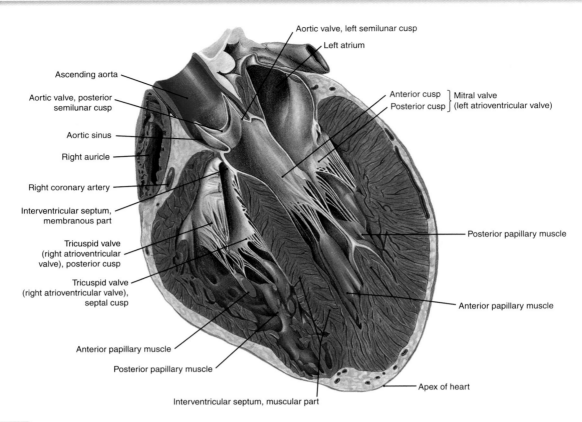

Aortic valve, left semilunar cusp

Left atrium

Ascending aorta

Aortic valve, posterior semilunar cusp

Anterior cusp ⎤ Mitral valve
Posterior cusp ⎦ (left atrioventricular valve)

Aortic sinus

Right auricle

Right coronary artery

Interventricular septum, membranous part

Posterior papillary muscle

Tricuspid valve (right atrioventricular valve), posterior cusp

Tricuspid valve (right atrioventricular valve), septal cusp

Anterior papillary muscle

Anterior papillary muscle

Posterior papillary muscle

Apex of heart

Interventricular septum, muscular part

FIGURE 188.1 Frontal Section through the Heart

NOTE: (1) This frontal section exposes both atria and both ventricles.
(2) The right and left atrioventricular valves (tricuspid and mitral valves) and their cusps. Observe the papillary muscles attached to these cusps by way of the chordae tendineae (the latter are not labeled).
(3) The muscular and membranous parts of the interventricular septum. Observe the difference in thickness of the muscular walls of the two ventricles.
(4) The aorta emerging from the left ventricle and the cusps of the aortic valve.

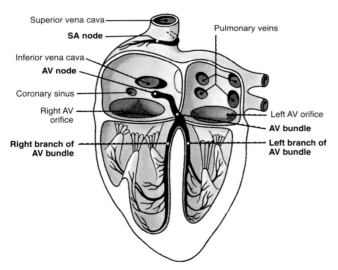

Superior vena cava

SA node

Pulmonary veins

Inferior vena cava

AV node

Coronary sinus

Right AV orifice

Left AV orifice

AV bundle

Right branch of AV bundle

Left branch of AV bundle

FIGURE 188.2 Diagram of the Conduction System of the Heart

NOTE: (1) The cardiac cycle begins at the SA (sinoatrial) node located in the sulcus terminalis between the superior vena cava and the right atrium.
(2) From this pacemaker, a wave of negativity (excitation) spreads over both atria and initiates atrial contraction, thereby increasing atrial blood pressure.
(3) When atrial pressure exceeds ventricular pressure, both atrioventricular (AV) valves open and blood rushes into both ventricles. Soon the impulse reaches the AV node and is passed along the AV bundle to the two ventricles, causing them to contract.
(4) When ventricular pressure exceeds atrial pressure, the AV valves close, and this can be heard with a stethoscope as the first of the two heart sounds of the heartbeat.
(5) Continued ventricular contraction forces the pulmonary and aortic valves to open, and blood rushes simultaneously into the pulmonary artery and the aorta.
(6) When the pressure in these vessels exceeds ventricular pressure, blood tends to rush back into the ventricles, but it gets trapped in the sinuses behind the semilunar cusps. This closes both the pulmonary and aortic valves, resulting in the second of the two heart sounds heard with the stethoscope.

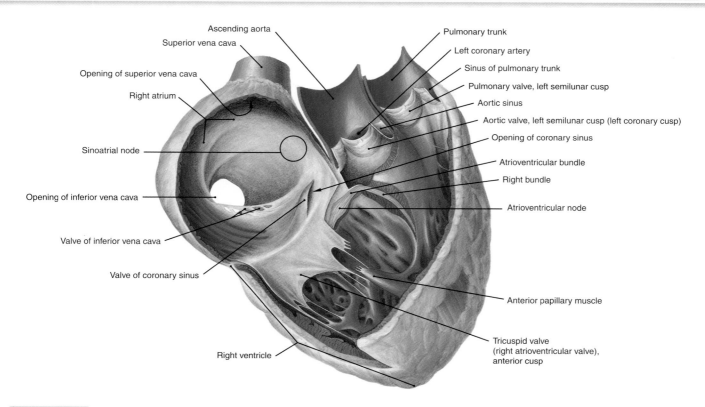

Ascending aorta
Superior vena cava
Opening of superior vena cava
Right atrium
Sinoatrial node
Opening of inferior vena cava
Valve of inferior vena cava
Valve of coronary sinus
Right ventricle

Pulmonary trunk
Left coronary artery
Sinus of pulmonary trunk
Pulmonary valve, left semilunar cusp
Aortic sinus
Aortic valve, left semilunar cusp (left coronary cusp)
Opening of coronary sinus
Atrioventricular bundle
Right bundle
Atrioventricular node
Anterior papillary muscle
Tricuspid valve
(right atrioventricular valve),
anterior cusp

FIGURE 189.1 **Atrioventricular Bundle Dissected in the Right Ventricle**

NOTE: (1) The atrioventricular (AV) bundle forms a part of the conduction system of the heart. It is formed by modified cardiac muscle fibers called Purkinje fibers. It commences at the AV node in the interatrial septum near the opening of the coronary sinus in the right atrium.

(2) The bundle is then directed toward the interventricular septum, where it divides into right and left branches. The **right** branch, dissected in this figure, courses in the wall of the right ventricle and is distributed toward the apex.

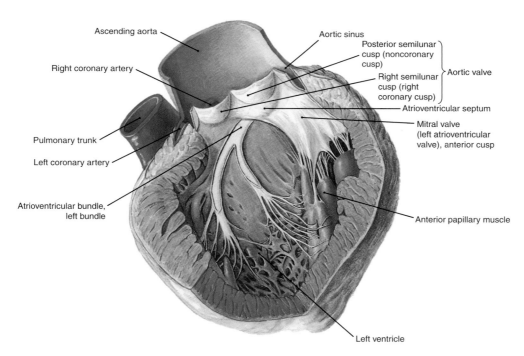

Ascending aorta
Right coronary artery
Pulmonary trunk
Left coronary artery
Atrioventricular bundle,
left bundle

Aortic sinus
Posterior semilunar
cusp (noncoronary
cusp)
Right semilunar
cusp (right
coronary cusp)
Aortic valve
Atrioventricular septum
Mitral valve
(left atrioventricular
valve), anterior cusp
Anterior papillary muscle
Left ventricle

FIGURE 189.2 **Atrioventricular Bundle Dissected in the Left Ventricle**

NOTE: (1) The left branch of the atrioventricular bundle is dissected on the left side of the interventricular wall. It commences as a rather wide band of tissue and soon divides into several strands. These fan out to become distributed among the papillary muscles and trabeculae carneae of the left ventricle.

(2) The conduction system of the heart transmits to the cardiac muscle the rhythmic impulses that characterize the rate of the heartbeat. This rhythm is superimposed on the natural contractile property of cardiac musculature, and the rate responds to regulation by cardiac nerves that innervate the heart.

PLATE 190 Atrioventricular Bundle System; Cusps of the Aortic Valve

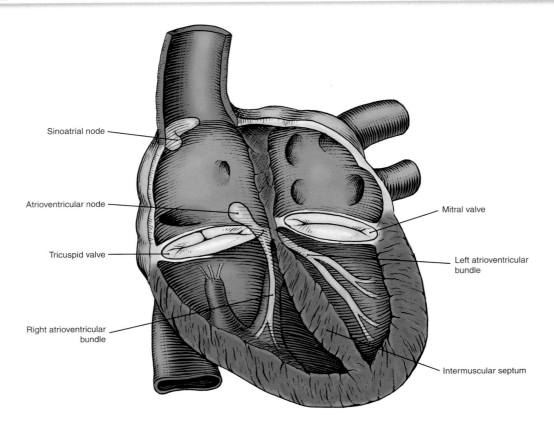

Sinoatrial node

Atrioventricular node

Tricuspid valve

Right atrioventricular bundle

Mitral valve

Left atrioventricular bundle

Intermuscular septum

FIGURE 190.1 Sinoatrial and Atrioventricular Nodes and the Atrioventricular Bundles (Frontal View)

(Contributed by Dr. Gene L. Colborn, Medical College of Georgia.)

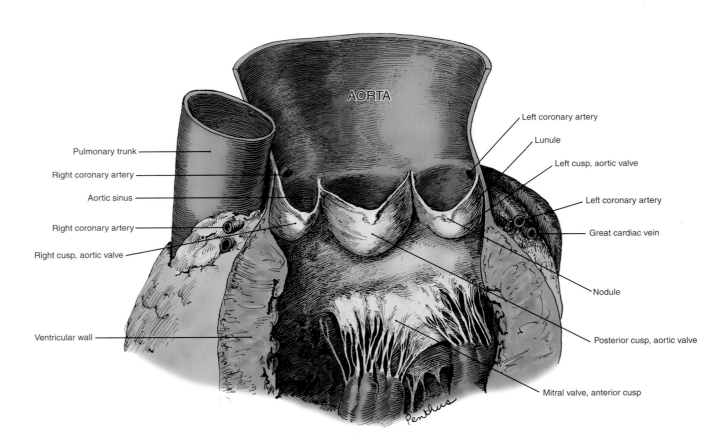

AORTA

Pulmonary trunk

Right coronary artery

Aortic sinus

Right coronary artery

Right cusp, aortic valve

Ventricular wall

Left coronary artery

Lunule

Left cusp, aortic valve

Left coronary artery

Great cardiac vein

Nodule

Posterior cusp, aortic valve

Mitral valve, anterior cusp

FIGURE 190.2 Left Ventricular and Aortic Junction and the Cusps of the Aortic Valve (Frontal Section)

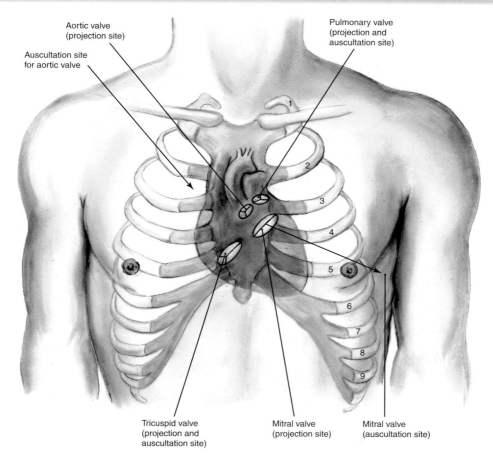

Aortic valve
(projection site)

Auscultation site
for aortic valve

Pulmonary valve
(projection and
auscultation site)

Tricuspid valve
(projection and
auscultation site)

Mitral valve
(projection site)

Mitral valve
(auscultation site)

FIGURE 191.1 Projection and Auscultation Sites of the Four Heart Valves (Anterior View)

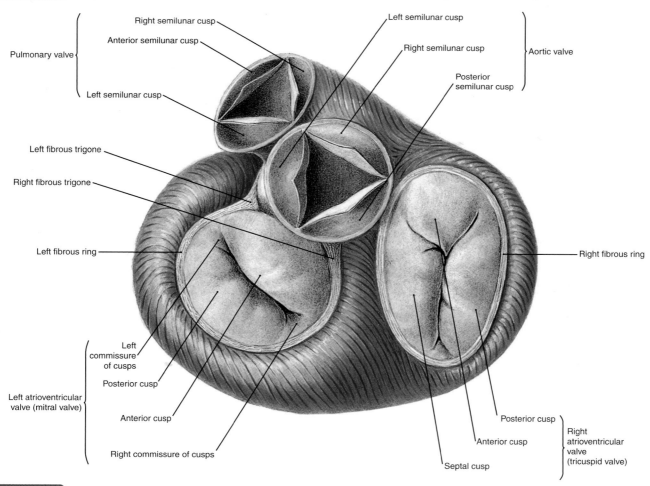

Pulmonary valve

Right semilunar cusp

Anterior semilunar cusp

Left semilunar cusp

Left semilunar cusp

Right semilunar cusp

Posterior
semilunar cusp

Aortic valve

Left fibrous trigone

Right fibrous trigone

Left fibrous ring

Right fibrous ring

Left
commissure
of cusps

Posterior cusp

Left atrioventricular
valve (mitral valve)

Anterior cusp

Right commissure of cusps

Posterior cusp

Anterior cusp

Right
atrioventricular
valve
(tricuspid valve)

Septal cusp

FIGURE 191.2 Four Heart Valves and Their Cusps; Fibrous Rings and Trigones (Superior View)

PLATE 192 Circulation of Blood in the Fetus

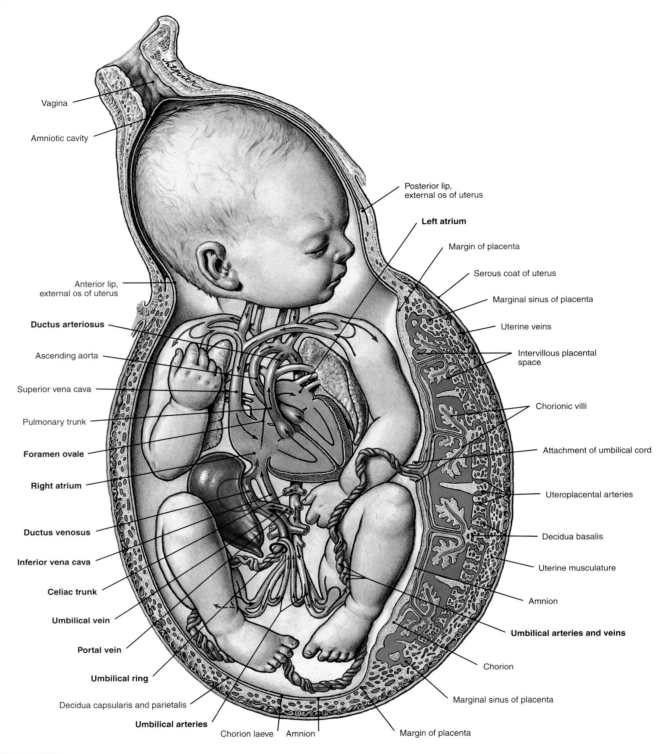

FIGURE 192 Circulation in the Fetus, as Seen in Utero

NOTE: In the fetus:

(1) Deoxygenated blood courses to the placenta by way of the **umbilical arteries.** It is then both nourished and oxygenated and leaves the placenta by way of the **umbilical vein.**

(2) Much of the oxygenated blood bypasses the liver, coursing from the umbilical vein, through the **ductus venosus,** to reach the inferior vena cava.

(3) From the inferior vena cava, blood enters the right atrium, as does blood from the superior vena cava. Right atrial blood bypasses the lungs by two routes:

    (a) across to the left atrium through the **foramen ovale,** then to the left ventricle and out the aorta to the rest of the fetal body, and

    (b) to the right ventricle, out the pulmonary artery and through the **ductus arteriosus** to reach the aorta, and then to the rest of the fetal body (also see Fig. 193).

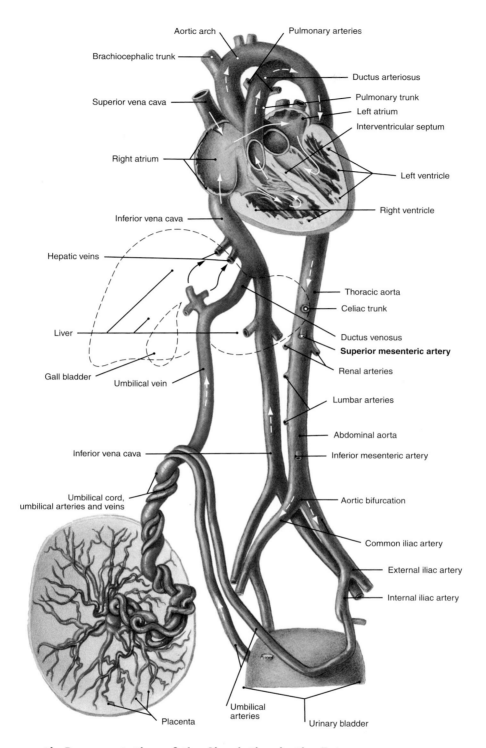

FIGURE 193 **Diagrammatic Representation of the Circulation in the Fetus**

NOTE the changes in the vascular system after birth. The colors indicate the degree of oxygen saturation of the blood, **red** being highest, **blue** the lowest, and **violet,** an intermediate level. Because the newborn infant becomes dependent on the lungs for oxygen:

(1) Breathing commences and the lungs begin to function, thereby oxygenating the blood and removing carbon dioxide.
(2) The **foramen ovale** decreases in size, and blood ceases to cross from the right atrium to the left atrium.
(3) The **ductus arteriosus** that interconnected the pulmonary artery and aorta constricts and gradually closes to become a fibrous cord called the **ligamentum arteriosum.**
(4) The **umbilical arteries** cease to carry blood to the placenta, and they become fibrosed, to form the **medial umbilical ligaments.**
(5) The umbilical vein becomes fibrosed and forms the **ligamentum teres** (of the liver), while the **ductus venosus** is no longer functional and forms the **ligamentum venosum.**

PLATE 194 Systemic Arteries in the Adult

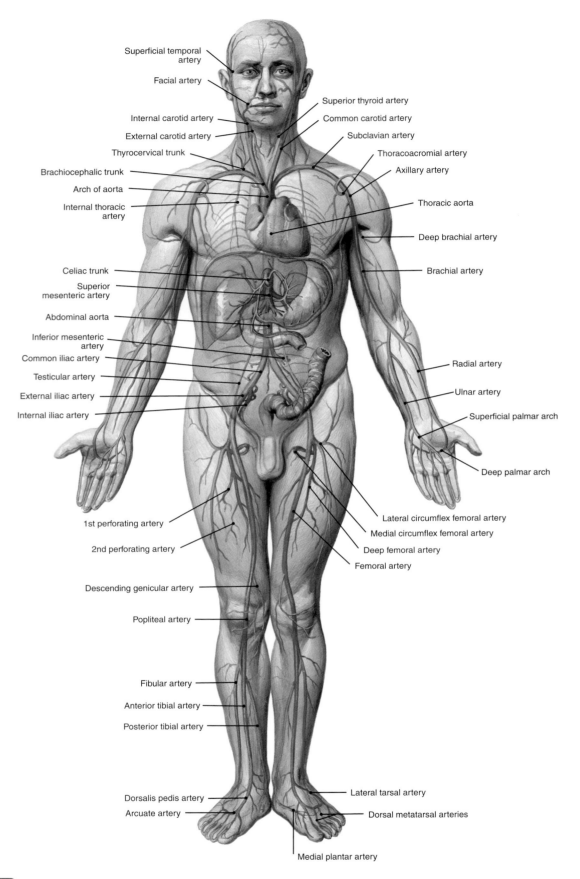

FIGURE 194 Adult Systemic Arterial System (Male)

NOTE: Most, but not all, of the named arteries in the systemic circulation are shown in this figure. In addition, the pulmonary arteries coursing to the lungs from the right ventricle are not included.

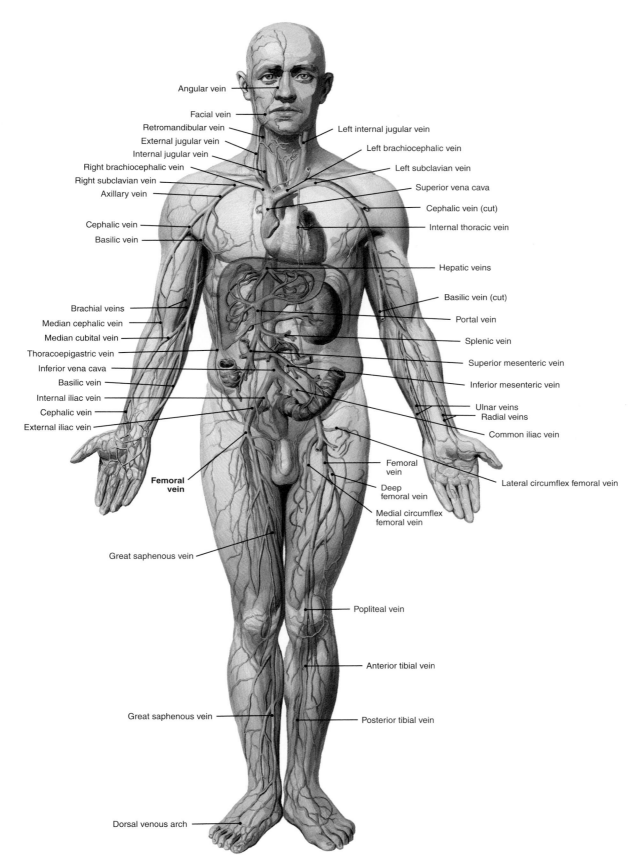

Angular vein

Facial vein

Retromandibular vein

External jugular vein

Internal jugular vein

Right brachiocephalic vein

Right subclavian vein

Axillary vein

Left internal jugular vein

Left brachiocephalic vein

Left subclavian vein

Superior vena cava

Cephalic vein (cut)

Internal thoracic vein

Cephalic vein

Basilic vein

Hepatic veins

Basilic vein (cut)

Brachial veins

Median cephalic vein

Median cubital vein

Thoracoepigastric vein

Inferior vena cava

Basilic vein

Internal iliac vein

Cephalic vein

External iliac vein

Portal vein

Splenic vein

Superior mesenteric vein

Inferior mesenteric vein

Ulnar veins

Radial veins

Common iliac vein

Femoral vein

Deep femoral vein

Medial circumflex femoral vein

Lateral circumflex femoral vein

Femoral vein

Great saphenous vein

Popliteal vein

Anterior tibial vein

Great saphenous vein

Posterior tibial vein

Dorsal venous arch

FIGURE 195 **Adult Systemic and Portal Venous Systems (Male)**

NOTE: Many, but not all, of the named veins are shown in this figure. The pulmonary veins that return blood to the left atrium from the lungs are not included. The portal system is shown in purple, while the other veins are shown in blue.

PLATE 196 Mediastinum and Lungs and the Upper Abdomen (Posterior View)

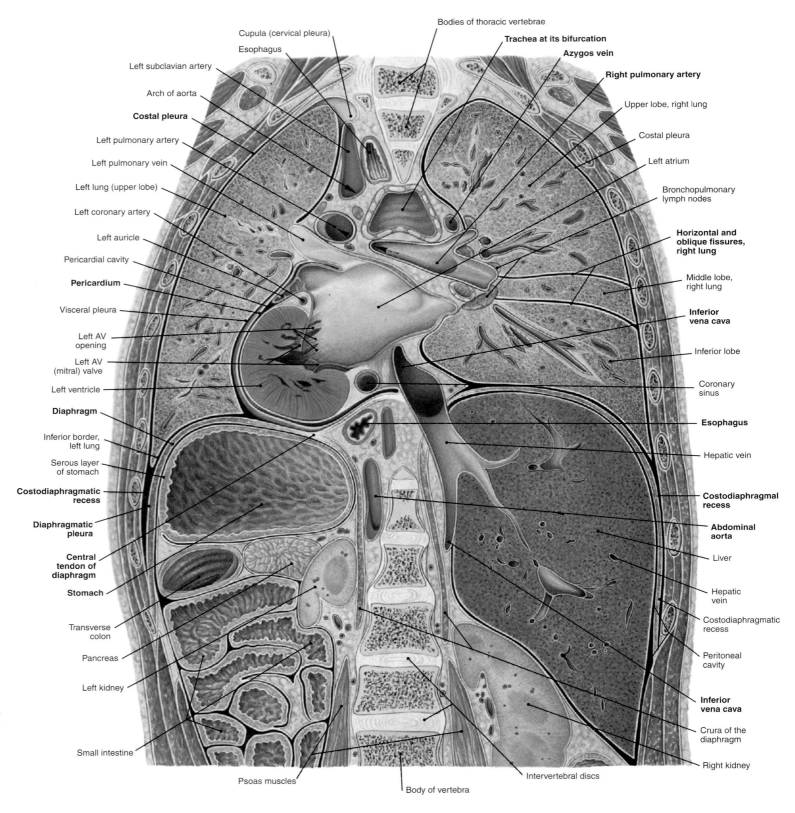

Bodies of thoracic vertebrae

Cupula (cervical pleura)

Esophagus

Trachea at its bifurcation

Azygos vein

Left subclavian artery

Right pulmonary artery

Arch of aorta

Upper lobe, right lung

Costal pleura

Costal pleura

Left pulmonary artery

Left atrium

Left pulmonary vein

Bronchopulmonary lymph nodes

Left lung (upper lobe)

Left coronary artery

Horizontal and oblique fissures, right lung

Left auricle

Middle lobe, right lung

Pericardial cavity

Pericardium

Inferior vena cava

Visceral pleura

Left AV opening

Inferior lobe

Left AV (mitral) valve

Coronary sinus

Left ventricle

Diaphragm

Esophagus

Inferior border, left lung

Hepatic vein

Serous layer of stomach

Costodiaphragmatic recess

Costodiaphragmal recess

Diaphragmatic pleura

Abdominal aorta

Central tendon of diaphragm

Liver

Stomach

Hepatic vein

Transverse colon

Costodiaphragmatic recess

Pancreas

Peritoneal cavity

Left kidney

Inferior vena cava

Small intestine

Crura of the diaphragm

Psoas muscles

Intervertebral discs

Body of vertebra

Right kidney

FIGURE 196 Frontal Section of the Thorax and Abdomen from Behind (Dorsal View)

NOTE: (1) From this dorsal view, the right side of the specimen is on the reader's right. The pulmonary arteries and their branches are shown in blue, as are veins (such as the hepatic veins) that also carry blood with low levels of oxygen saturation.

(2) The anteroposterior plane of this frontal section in the thorax lies through the inferior vena cava and in front of the descending aorta. The esophagus is seen only in the superior mediastinum and at its entrance into the abdomen just below the diaphragm, while the trachea has been cut at its point of bifurcation.

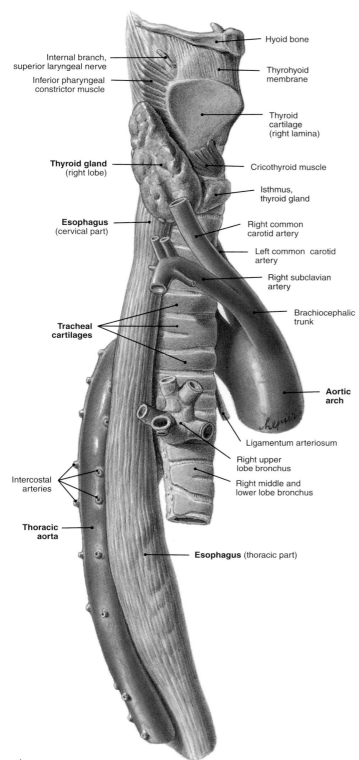

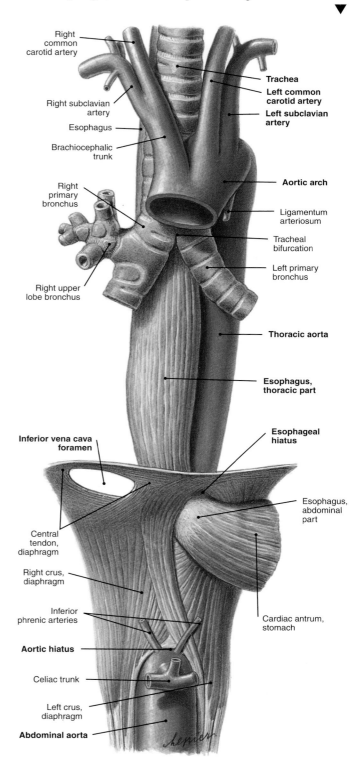

FIGURE 197.2 **Aorta and Lower Esophagus at the Tracheal Bifurcation and Diaphragm**

NOTE: (1) At the level of the bifurcation of the trachea (T5), the esophagus lies between the trachea and the thoracic aorta. It then descends into the thorax with the aorta somewhat to its left. In the lower thorax, the esophagus bends to the left and crosses the aorta anteriorly from right to left.

(2) The esophagus enters the abdomen through the **esophageal hiatus** of the diaphragm, while the aorta passes through the **aortic hiatus.**

▼

FIGURE 197.1 **Relationship of the Esophagus to the Aorta and Trachea, Viewed from Right Side**

NOTE: (1) The **esophagus** commences above as an inferior extension of the pharynx, and it is initially in relationship with the larynx and thyroid gland.

(2) Its **middle third** courses in relation to the trachea, bronchi and the arch of the aorta, while its lower third descends with the thoracic aorta.

PLATE 198 Esophageal Blood Supply and Lymph Nodes

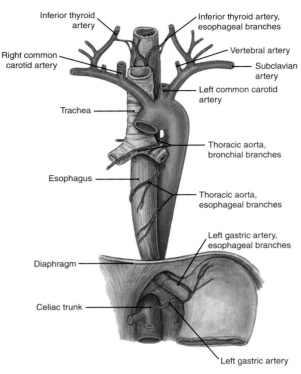

Inferior thyroid artery

Inferior thyroid artery, esophageal branches

Right common carotid artery

Vertebral artery

Subclavian artery

Left common carotid artery

Trachea

Thoracic aorta, bronchial branches

Esophagus

Thoracic aorta, esophageal branches

Left gastric artery, esophageal branches

Diaphragm

Celiac trunk

Left gastric artery

FIGURE 198.1 Arterial Blood Supply of the Esophagus

NOTE: (1) Because the esophagus is an elongated organ extending from the neck to the abdomen, it receives arterial blood from at least three sources:
  (a) **In the neck:** most frequently from the **inferior thyroid** of the **thyrocervical trunk,** but it may come from the subclavian or vertebral arteries or from the costocervical trunk.
  (b) **In the thorax:** multiple **esophageal branches** coming directly from the **aorta.**
  (c) **In the abdomen:** from the **inferior phrenic artery** or the **left gastric artery.**
(2) These vessels anastomose with each other in the substance of the esophagus.

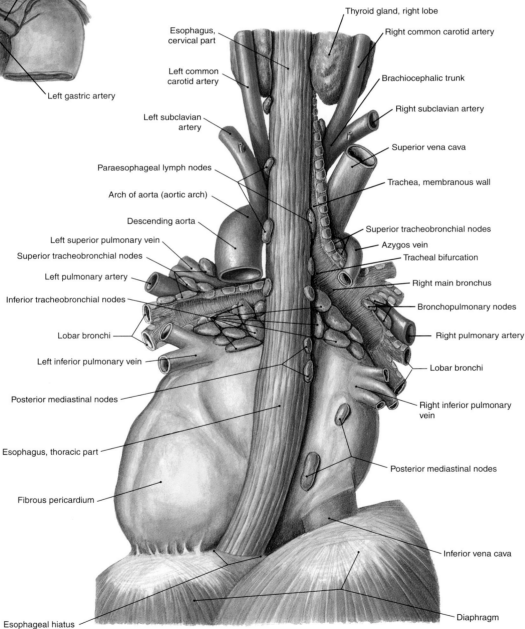

Esophagus, cervical part

Thyroid gland, right lobe

Right common carotid artery

Left common carotid artery

Brachiocephalic trunk

Right subclavian artery

Left subclavian artery

Superior vena cava

Paraesophageal lymph nodes

Trachea, membranous wall

Arch of aorta (aortic arch)

Descending aorta

Superior tracheobronchial nodes

Left superior pulmonary vein

Azygos vein

Superior tracheobronchial nodes

Tracheal bifurcation

Left pulmonary artery

Right main bronchus

Inferior tracheobronchial nodes

Bronchopulmonary nodes

Lobar bronchi

Right pulmonary artery

Left inferior pulmonary vein

Lobar bronchi

Posterior mediastinal nodes

Right inferior pulmonary vein

Esophagus, thoracic part

Posterior mediastinal nodes

Fibrous pericardium

Inferior vena cava

Esophageal hiatus

Diaphragm

FIGURE 198.2 **Posterior View of the Esophagus and the Paraesophageal and Tracheobronchial Lymph Nodes**

NOTE the large number of nodes near the bifurcation of the trachea (into the two primary bronchi). These many nodes may be located at this site for the receipt of macrophages coursing from the lungs, which may have ingested foreign elements from the air we breathe.

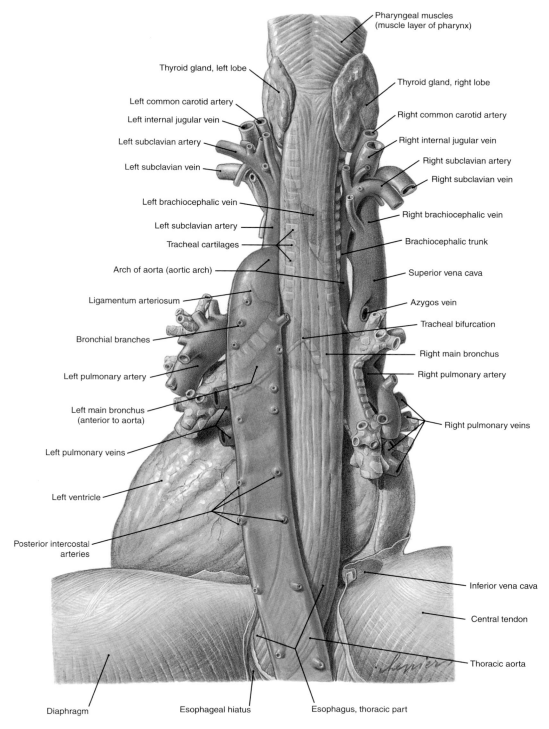

Pharyngeal muscles
(muscle layer of pharynx)

Thyroid gland, left lobe

Thyroid gland, right lobe

Left common carotid artery

Right common carotid artery

Left internal jugular vein

Right internal jugular vein

Left subclavian artery

Right subclavian artery

Left subclavian vein

Right subclavian vein

Left brachiocephalic vein

Right brachiocephalic vein

Left subclavian artery

Brachiocephalic trunk

Tracheal cartilages

Superior vena cava

Arch of aorta (aortic arch)

Ligamentum arteriosum

Azygos vein

Tracheal bifurcation

Bronchial branches

Right main bronchus

Left pulmonary artery

Right pulmonary artery

Left main bronchus
(anterior to aorta)

Right pulmonary veins

Left pulmonary veins

Left ventricle

Posterior intercostal
arteries

Inferior vena cava

Central tendon

Thoracic aorta

Diaphragm   Esophageal hiatus   Esophagus, thoracic part

FIGURE 199 **Posterior View of the Esophagus, Aorta, and Pericardium**

NOTE: (1) The origins of the intercostal arteries from the posterior aspect of the thoracic aorta.

(2) The relationship of the esophagus and the thoracic aorta is well shown in this dorsal view. Observe how the aorta courses posterior to the esophagus from left to right. It then descends in the midline ventral to the vertebral column to the level of L1, where it enters the posterior abdomen.

PLATE 200 Radiographs of the Esophagus; Esophagoscopy

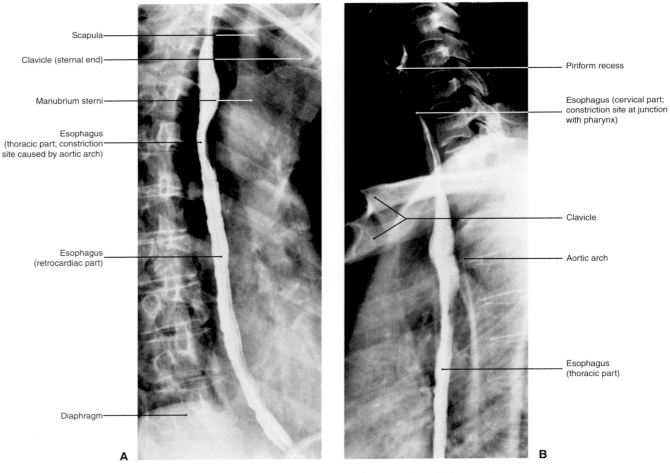

Scapula

Clavicle (sternal end)

Manubrium sterni

Esophagus (thoracic part; constriction site caused by aortic arch)

Esophagus (retrocardiac part)

Diaphragm

Piriform recess

Esophagus (cervical part; constriction site at junction with pharynx)

Clavicle

Aortic arch

Esophagus (thoracic part)

A

B

Right anterior oblique view   **Left anterior oblique view**

FIGURE 200.1AB **Radiographic Views of the Esophagus After Swallowing Contrast Medium**

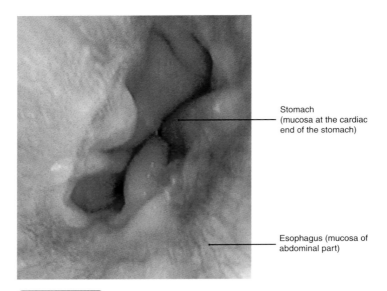

Stomach (mucosa at the cardiac end of the stomach)

Esophagus (mucosa of abdominal part)

FIGURE 200.2 **Esophagus As Seen through an Esophagoscope, Superior View**

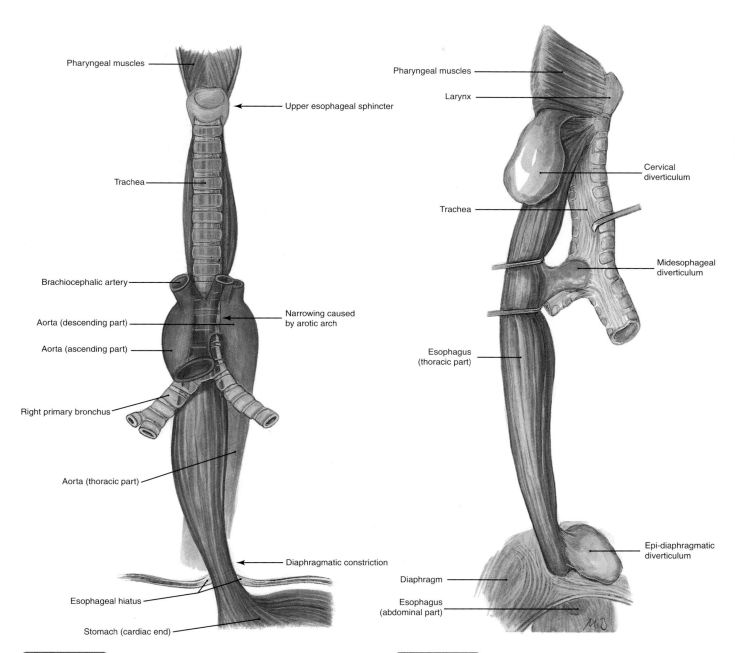

Pharyngeal muscles

Upper esophageal sphincter

Trachea

Brachiocephalic artery

Aorta (descending part)

Narrowing caused by arotic arch

Aorta (ascending part)

Right primary bronchus

Aorta (thoracic part)

Diaphragmatic constriction

Esophageal hiatus

Stomach (cardiac end)

Pharyngeal muscles

Larynx

Cervical diverticulum

Trachea

Midesophageal diverticulum

Esophagus (thoracic part)

Epi-diaphragmatic diverticulum

Diaphragm

Esophagus (abdominal part)

FIGURE 201.1 Esophagus Showing Sites of Constrictions

Three sites:

(1) Constriction caused by upper esophageal sphincter
(2) Narrowing caused by aortic arch
(3) Constriction at the esophageal-diaphragmatic junction

FIGURE 201.2 Esophagus Showing Typical Locations of Diverticula

Cervical diverticula (most frequent; 70%)
Midesophageal diverticula (22%)
Epidiaphragmatic diverticula (8%)

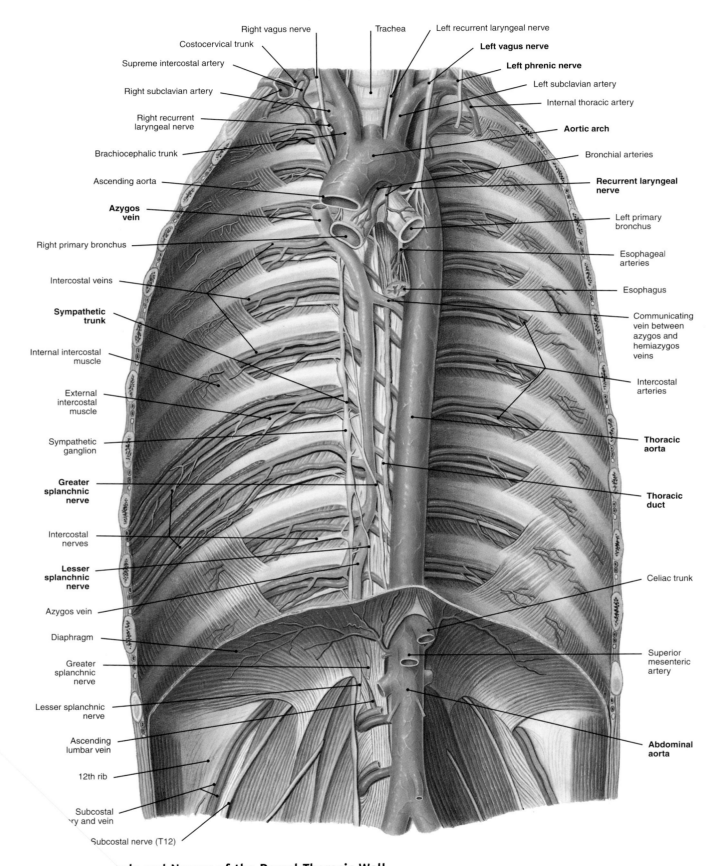

Right vagus nerve

Costocervical trunk

Supreme intercostal artery

Right subclavian artery

Right recurrent
laryngeal nerve

Brachiocephalic trunk

Ascending aorta

**Azygos
vein**

Right primary bronchus

Intercostal veins

**Sympathetic
trunk**

Internal intercostal
muscle

External
intercostal
muscle

Sympathetic
ganglion

**Greater
splanchnic
nerve**

Intercostal
nerves

**Lesser
splanchnic
nerve**

Azygos vein

Diaphragm

Greater
splanchnic
nerve

Lesser splanchnic
nerve

Ascending
lumbar vein

12th rib

Subcostal
ry and vein

Subcostal nerve (T12)

Trachea

Left recurrent laryngeal nerve

Left vagus nerve

Left phrenic nerve

Left subclavian artery

Internal thoracic artery

Aortic arch

Bronchial arteries

**Recurrent laryngeal
nerve**

Left primary
bronchus

Esophageal
arteries

Esophagus

Communicating
vein between
azygos and
hemiazygos
veins

Intercostal
arteries

**Thoracic
aorta**

**Thoracic
duct**

Celiac trunk

Superior
mesenteric
artery

**Abdominal
aorta**

els and Nerves of the Dorsal Thoracic Wall

ds from the left ventricle, arches behind the left pulmonary hilum, and descends through most of the thorax just to the
lumn.

terior mediastinum, the aorta gradually shifts toward the midline, which it has achieved when it traverses the
enter the abdomen.

2 The Thorax

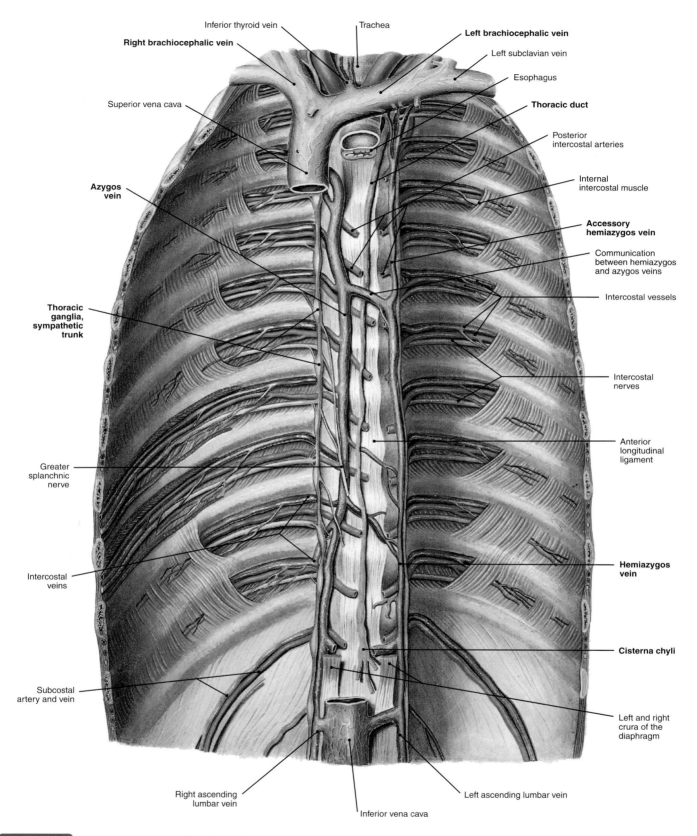

Inferior thyroid vein

Trachea

Left brachiocephalic vein

Right brachiocephalic vein

Left subclavian vein

Esophagus

Superior vena cava

Thoracic duct

Posterior intercostal arteries

Azygos vein

Internal intercostal muscle

Accessory hemiazygos vein

Communication between hemiazygos and azygos veins

Intercostal vessels

Thoracic ganglia, sympathetic trunk

Intercostal nerves

Greater splanchnic nerve

Anterior longitudinal ligament

Hemiazygos vein

Intercostal veins

Cisterna chyli

Subcostal artery and vein

Left and right crura of the diaphragm

Right ascending lumbar vein

Left ascending lumbar vein

Inferior vena cava

FIGURE 203 **Azygos System of Veins, the Thoracic Duct, and Other Posterior Thoracic Wall Structures**

NOTE: (1) With most of the organs of the thorax and mediastinum removed or cut, the **hemiazygos and accessory hemiazygos veins** to the left of the vertebral column are seen communicating across the midline with the larger **azygos vein.**

(2) The azygos vein is seen ascending in the right thorax to open into the superior vena cava.

(3) The **thoracic duct** arises from the cisterna chyli at the first lumbar level and ascends in the thorax anterior to the vertebral column.

PLATE 204 **Veins of the Esophagus**

FIGURE 204.1 **Veins That Drain the Esophagus** ▶

NOTE: (1) Veins that drain the **cervical part** of the esophagus empty into the inferior thyroid vein, while those from the **thoracic part** drain into the azygos, hemiazygos, and accessory hemiazygos veins.

(2) Veins that drain the **abdominal part** of the esophagus drain partially into the left gastric vein and partially into the azygos vein.

(3) In this figure, the inferior part of the esophagus has been severed just above the diaphragm.

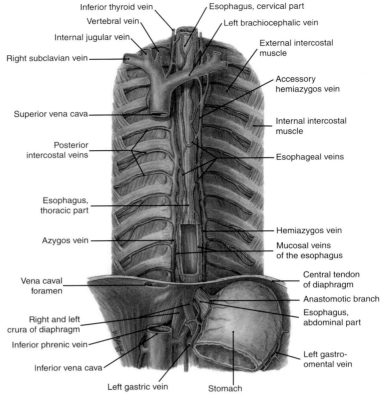

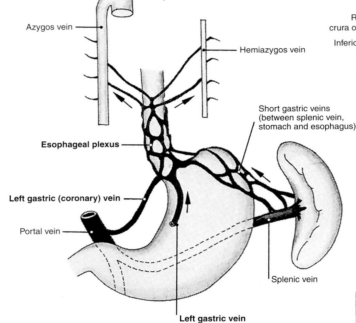

◀ **FIGURE 204.2** **Anastomosis between the Portal Vein and the Superior Vena Cava through the Esophageal Venous Plexus**

This figure shows the anastomosis often used to return blood from the portal vein to the inferior vena cava. Persons who have hypertension in the portal system may have blood diverted from the **portal vein** to the **coronary** and **left gastric veins.** Blood then ascends through the **hemiazygos** and **azygos veins** and finally into the **superior vena cava.**

FIGURE 204.3 **Portal-Caval Shunt** ▶
Dissection

NOTE: (1) This figure shows the hepatic portal vein in the color purple and the inferior vena cava in blue. Observe the anastomosis between the portal vein and the coronary and left gastric veins (also in blue).

(2) Esophageal veins from these two vessels anastomose through the diaphragm with the azygos and hemiazygos veins in the chest.

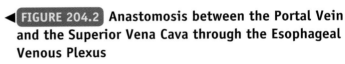

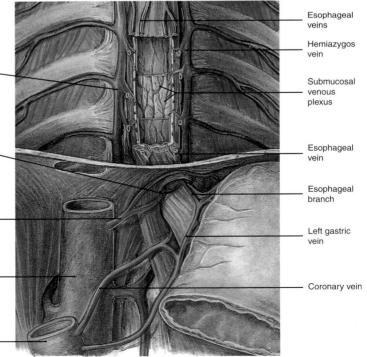

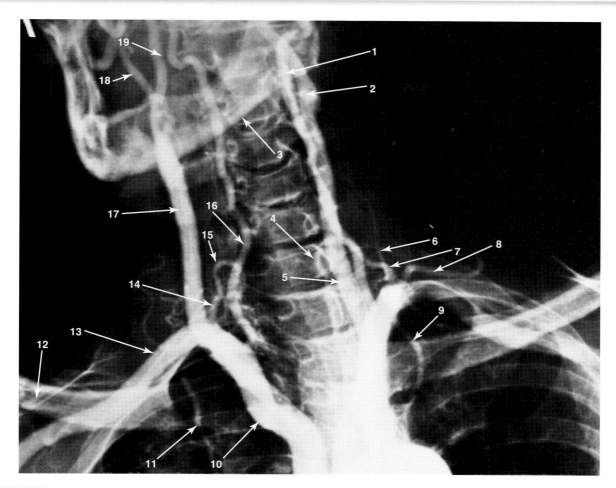

FIGURE 205.1 **Angiogram of the Aortic Arch and Its Branches**

1. Left vertebral artery
2. Left internal carotid artery
3. Body of the mandible
4. Left inferior thyroid artery
5. Left common carotid artery
6. Left ascending cervical artery

7. Left thyrocervical trunk
8. Left transverse cervical artery
9. Left internal thoracic artery
10. Brachiocephalic trunk
11. Right internal thoracic artery
12. Clavicle

13. Right subclavian artery
14. Right thyrocervical trunk
15. Right inferior thyroid artery
16. Right vertebral artery
17. Right common carotid artery
18. Right external carotid artery
19. Right internal carotid artery

(From Wicke, 6th ed.)

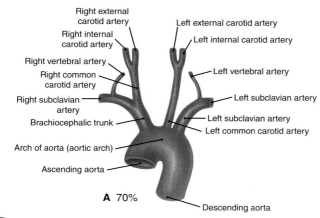

A 70%

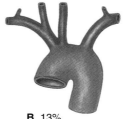
B 13%

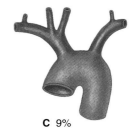
C 9%

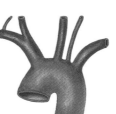
D 3%

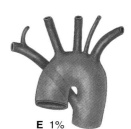
E 1%

FIGURE 205.2 **Variations in Branches from the Arch of the Aorta**

A: Normal
B: Common origin of the brachiocephalic trunk and common carotid artery
C: Common stem for right vessels
D: Left vertebral from the aorta
E: Right subclavian arises below the aortic arch.

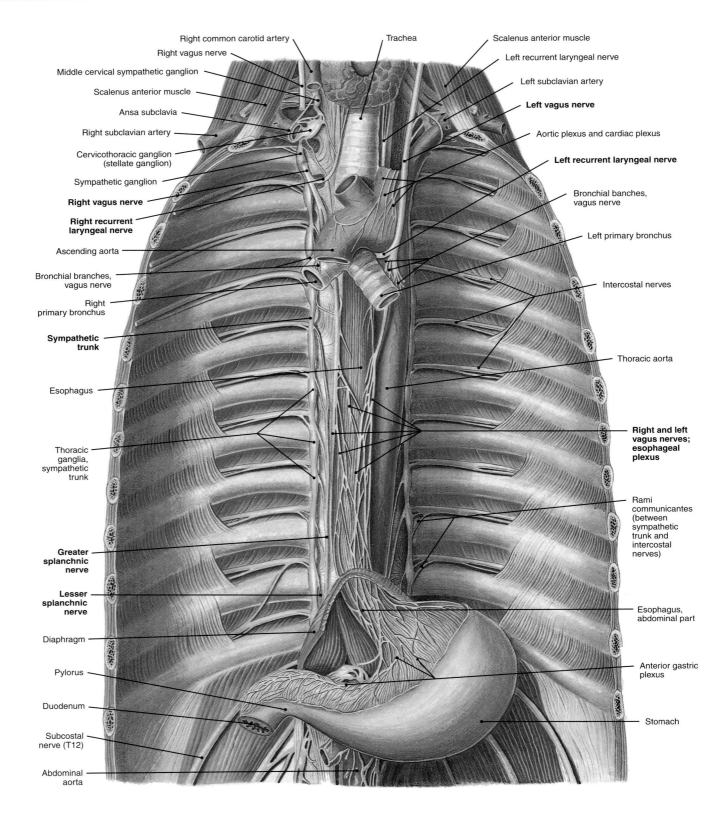

Right common carotid artery

Right vagus nerve

Middle cervical sympathetic ganglion

Scalenus anterior muscle

Ansa subclavia

Right subclavian artery

Cervicothoracic ganglion (stellate ganglion)

Sympathetic ganglion

Right vagus nerve

Right recurrent laryngeal nerve

Ascending aorta

Bronchial branches, vagus nerve

Right primary bronchus

Sympathetic trunk

Esophagus

Thoracic ganglia, sympathetic trunk

Greater splanchnic nerve

Lesser splanchnic nerve

Diaphragm

Pylorus

Duodenum

Subcostal nerve (T12)

Abdominal aorta

Trachea

Scalenus anterior muscle

Left recurrent laryngeal nerve

Left subclavian artery

Left vagus nerve

Aortic plexus and cardiac plexus

Left recurrent laryngeal nerve

Bronchial banches, vagus nerve

Left primary bronchus

Intercostal nerves

Thoracic aorta

Right and left vagus nerves; esophageal plexus

Rami communicantes (between sympathetic trunk and intercostal nerves)

Esophagus, abdominal part

Anterior gastric plexus

Stomach

FIGURE 206 Sympathetic Trunks and Vagus Nerves in the Thorax and Upper Abdomen

NOTE: (1) The ganglionated sympathetic trunks lie lateral to the bodies of the thoracic vertebrae on each side and are continued into the neck superiorly and the abdomen inferiorly.

(2) Each ganglion is connected to an intercostal nerve by means of **rami communicantes. White rami** consist principally of preganglionic sympathetic fibers coursing to the ganglia, while the **gray rami** carry postganglionic fibers back to the spinal nerves.

(3) The course of the vagus nerves in the thorax. Below the aortic arch they send branches to the bronchi and then descend to form much of the esophageal plexus.

(4) Below the diaphragm, most of the fibers of the **left vagus** form the **anterior gastric nerve,** while most of the fibers of the **right vagus** form the **posterior gastric nerve.**

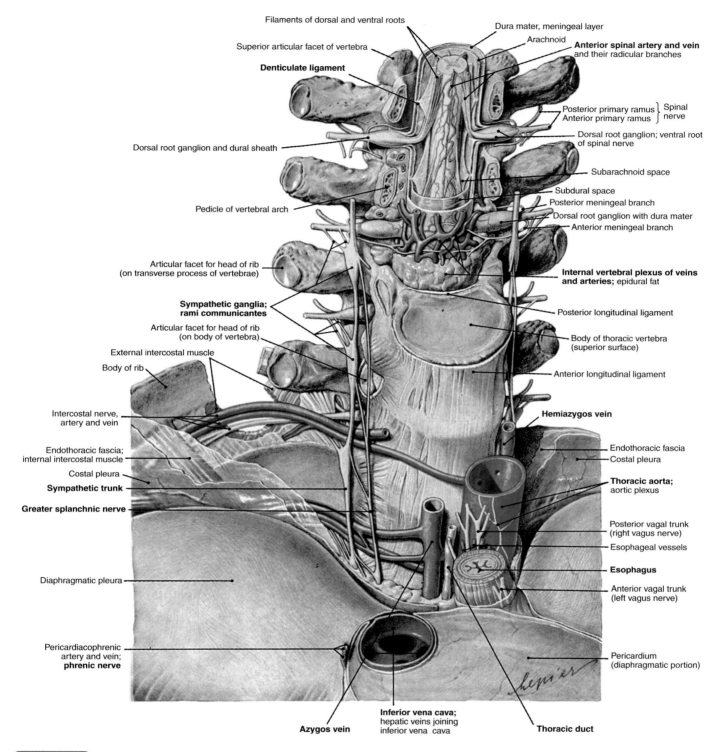

Filaments of dorsal and ventral roots

Superior articular facet of vertebra

Denticulate ligament

Dorsal root ganglion and dural sheath

Pedicle of vertebral arch

Articular facet for head of rib
(on transverse process of vertebrae)

**Sympathetic ganglia;
rami communicantes**

Articular facet for head of rib
(on body of vertebra)

External intercostal muscle

Body of rib

Intercostal nerve,
artery and vein

Endothoracic fascia;
internal intercostal muscle

Costal pleura

Sympathetic trunk

Greater splanchnic nerve

Diaphragmatic pleura

Pericardiacophrenic
artery and vein;
phrenic nerve

Dura mater, meningeal layer

Arachnoid

Anterior spinal artery and vein
and their radicular branches

Posterior primary ramus ⎱ Spinal
Anterior primary ramus ⎰ nerve

Dorsal root ganglion; ventral root
of spinal nerve

Subarachnoid space

Subdural space

Posterior meningeal branch

Dorsal root ganglion with dura mater

Anterior meningeal branch

**Internal vertebral plexus of veins
and arteries;** epidural fat

Posterior longitudinal ligament

Body of thoracic vertebra
(superior surface)

Anterior longitudinal ligament

Hemiazygos vein

Endothoracic fascia

Costal pleura

Thoracic aorta;
aortic plexus

Posterior vagal trunk
(right vagus nerve)

Esophageal vessels

Esophagus

Anterior vagal trunk
(left vagus nerve)

Pericardium
(diaphragmatic portion)

Azygos vein

Inferior vena cava;
hepatic veins joining
inferior vena cava

Thoracic duct

FIGURE 207 **Anterior Dissection of Vertebral Column, Spinal Cord, and Prevertebral Structures at a Lower Thoracic Level**

NOTE: (1) The internal vertebral plexus of veins and arteries that lie in the epidural space, where the epidural fat is also found. These should not be confused with the spinal vessels, which are situated in the pia mater and which are seen to be intimately applied to the spinal cord tissue.

(2) The ganglionated sympathetic chain observable here in the thoracic region receiving and giving communicating rami with the spinal nerves. Also note the formation of the greater splanchnic nerve and its descent prevertebrally into the abdomen.

(3) The aorta, inferior vena cava, azygos and hemiazygos veins, esophagus, and thoracic duct all lying anterior or somewhat to the left of the vertebral column and passing through the diaphragm.

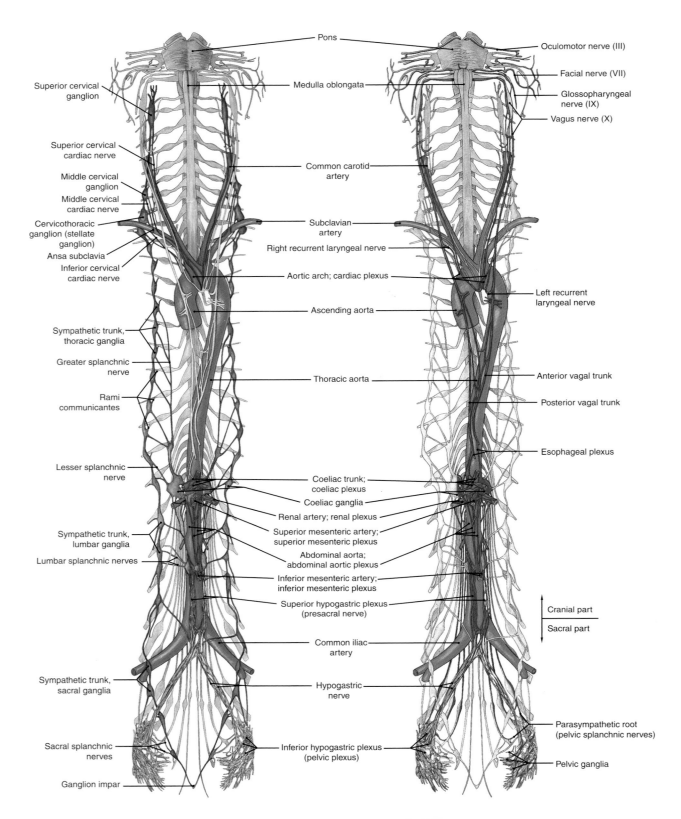

Pons

Superior cervical ganglion

Superior cervical cardiac nerve

Middle cervical ganglion

Middle cervical cardiac nerve

Cervicothoracic ganglion (stellate ganglion)

Ansa subclavia

Inferior cervical cardiac nerve

Sympathetic trunk, thoracic ganglia

Greater splanchnic nerve

Rami communicantes

Lesser splanchnic nerve

Sympathetic trunk, lumbar ganglia

Lumbar splanchnic nerves

Sympathetic trunk, sacral ganglia

Sacral splanchnic nerves

Ganglion impar

Medulla oblongata

Common carotid artery

Subclavian artery

Right recurrent laryngeal nerve

Aortic arch; cardiac plexus

Ascending aorta

Thoracic aorta

Coeliac trunk; coeliac plexus

Coeliac ganglia

Renal artery; renal plexus

Superior mesenteric artery; superior mesenteric plexus

Abdominal aorta; abdominal aortic plexus

Inferior mesenteric artery; inferior mesenteric plexus

Superior hypogastric plexus (presacral nerve)

Common iliac artery

Hypogastric nerve

Inferior hypogastric plexus (pelvic plexus)

Oculomotor nerve (III)

Facial nerve (VII)

Glossopharyngeal nerve (IX)

Vagus nerve (X)

Left recurrent laryngeal nerve

Anterior vagal trunk

Posterior vagal trunk

Esophageal plexus

Cranial part

Sacral part

Parasympathetic root (pelvic splanchnic nerves)

Pelvic ganglia

FIGURE 208.1 Sympathetic Division of the Autonomic Nervous System

NOTE that the sympathetic chain and its ganglia and branches are shown in green. Preganglionic sympathetic fibers emerge from the spinal cord between the T1 and L3 spinal levels. Also called the **thoracolumbar out-flow.**

FIGURE 208.2 Parasympathetic Division of the Autonomic Nervous System

NOTE that the parasympathetic fibers are shown in purple. Preganglionic fibers emerge from the central nervous system in cranial nerves III, VII, IX, and X and the sacral levels S2, S3, and S4. Also called **craniosacral outflow.**

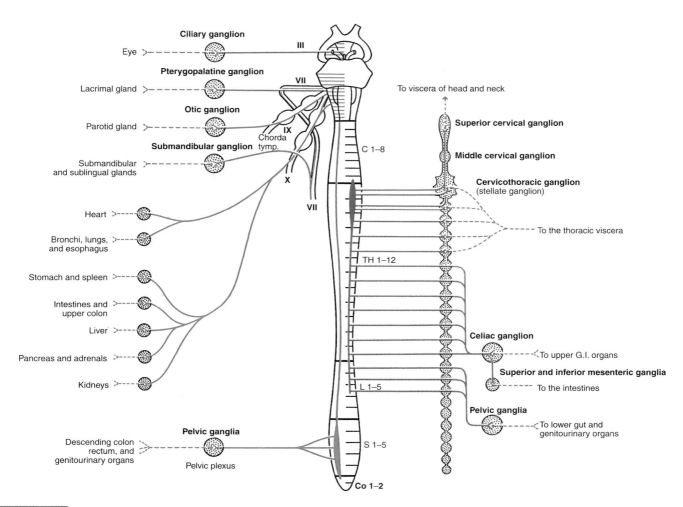

FIGURE 209 **Diagram of the Autonomic Nervous System**

Blue = parasympathetic; red = sympathetic; solid lines = presynaptic neurons; broken lines = postsynaptic neurons.

NOTE: (1) The autonomic nervous system, by definition, is a two-motor neuron system with the neuron cell bodies of the *presynaptic neurons* (solid lines) somewhere within the central nervous system and the cell bodies of the *postsynaptic neurons* (broken lines) located in ganglia distributed peripherally in the body.

(2) The autonomic nervous system comprises the nerve fibers, which supply all the glands and blood vessels of the body, including the heart. In doing so, all the smooth and cardiac muscle tissues (sometimes called involuntary muscles) are thereby innervated.

(3) The autonomic nervous system is composed of two major divisions, called the parasympathetic (in blue) and sympathetic (in red) divisions. The autonomic regulation of visceral function is, therefore, a dualistic control—that is, most organs receive postganglionic fibers of both parasympathetic and sympathetic sources.

(4) The *parasympathetic division* is sometimes called a craniosacral outflow because the preganglionic cell bodies of this division lie in the brainstem and in the sacral segments of the spinal cord. Parasympathetic preganglionic fibers are found in four cranial nerves, III (oculomotor), VII (facial), IX (glossopharyngeal), and X (vagus) and in the second, third, and fourth sacral nerves.

(5) These *pre*ganglionic parasympathetic fibers then synapse with *post*ganglionic parasympathetic cell bodies in peripheral ganglia. From these ganglia the *post*ganglionic nerve fibers innervate the various organs.

(6) The *sympathetic division* is sometimes called the thoracolumbar outflow because the *pre*ganglionic sympathetic neuron cell bodies are located in the lateral horn of the spinal cord between the first thoracic spinal segment and the second or third lumbar spinal segment (i.e., from T1 to L3).

(7) These *pre*ganglionic fibers emerge from the cord with their corresponding spinal roots and communicate with the sympathetic trunk and its ganglia, where some *pre*synaptic sympathetic fibers synapse with *post*ganglionic sympathetic neurons. Other presynaptic fibers (especially those of the upper thoracic segments) ascend in the sympathetic chain and synapse with *post*ganglionic neurons in the cervicothoracic and middle and superior cervical ganglia. *Post*ganglionic fibers from these latter ganglia are then distributed to the viscera of the head and neck. Still other *pre*synaptic sympathetic fibers do not synapse in the sympathetic chain of ganglia at all but collect to form the splanchnic nerves. These nerves course to the collateral sympathetic ganglia (celiac, superior and inferior mesenteric, and aorticorenal ganglia), where they synapse with the *post*ganglionic neurons. The *post*ganglionic neurons of the sympathetic division then course to the viscera to supply sympathetic innervation.

(8) The functions of the parasympathetic and sympathetic divisions of the autonomic nervous system are antagonistic to each other. The parasympathetic division constricts the pupil, decelerates the heart, lowers blood pressure, relaxes the sphincters of the gut, and contracts the longitudinal musculature of the hollow organs. It is the division that is active during periods of calm and tranquility, and it aids in digestion and absorption. In contrast, the *sympathetic division* dilates the pupil, accelerates the heart, increases blood pressure, contracts the sphincters of the gut, and relaxes the longitudinal musculature of hollow organs. It is active when the organism is challenged. It prepares for fight and flight and generally comes to the individual's defense during periods of stress and adversity.

PLATE 210 Thoracic Duct and Lymphatic Drainage

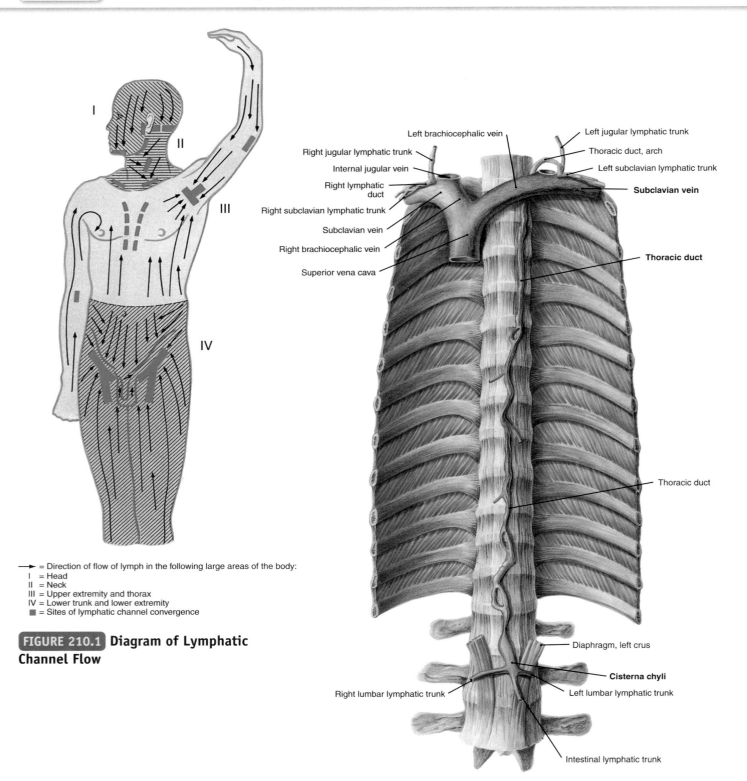

= Direction of flow of lymph in the following large areas of the body:
I = Head
II = Neck
III = Upper extremity and thorax
IV = Lower trunk and lower extremity
■ = Sites of lymphatic channel convergence

FIGURE 210.1 Diagram of Lymphatic Channel Flow

FIGURE 210.2 Thoracic Duct: Its Origin and Course

NOTE: (1) The **thoracic duct** collects lymph from most of the body regions and conveys it back into the bloodstream. The duct originates in the abdomen anterior to the second lumbar vertebra at the **cisterna chyli.**

(2) The thoracic duct enters the thorax through the **aortic hiatus** of the diaphragm, slightly to the right of the midline. Within the posterior mediastinum of the thorax, still coursing just ventral to the vertebral column, it gradually crosses the midline from right to left.

(3) The duct then ascends into the root of the neck on the left side and opens into the **left subclavian vein** near the junction of the **left internal jugular vein.**

(4) The **right lymphatic duct** receives lymph from the right side of the head, neck, and trunk and from the right upper extremity. It empties into the **right subclavian vein.**

FIGURE 211.1 Certain Lymphatics of the Head, Abdomen, Pelvis, and Limbs

NOTE: (1) In addition to its physiologic importance in returning tissue fluids and cells to the blood vascular system, the lymphatic system may serve as pathways for the spread of disease.

(2) Lymph channels may be used as preformed tubes for the spread of infectious diseases as well as metastatic cells from established tumors.

(3) Enlarged or painful lymph nodes are often clinical signs of disease processes elsewhere in the body or of the lymphoid organs themselves.

(4) This figure shows the lymphatic channels that drain the upper limb into axillary nodes and those of the lower limb into the inguinal nodes. Also seen are the iliac and lumbar nodes as well as the mesenteric nodes. Not shown are the deep nodes of the head, neck, and thorax or many of the visceral nodes of the thorax, abdomen, and pelvis.

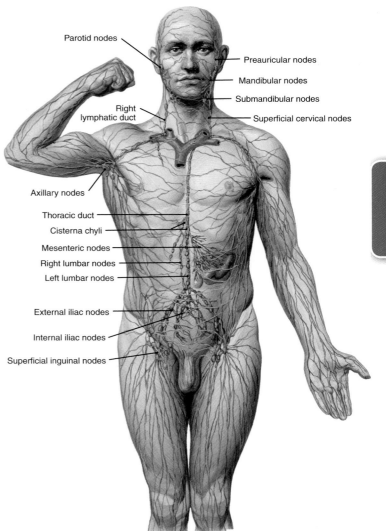

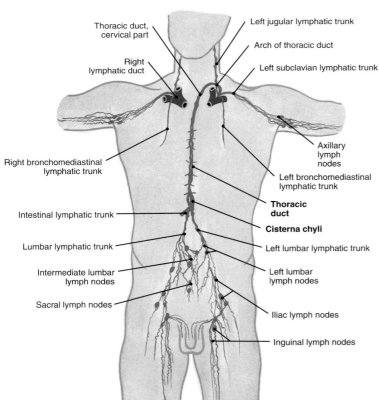

FIGURE 211.2 Large Lymphatic Vessels

NOTE: (1) The **inguinal lymph nodes** drain the lower limb. The inguinal nodes drain into the **iliac nodes,** which also receive lymph from the pelvic organs.

(2) The iliac nodes drain into the **right** and **left lumbar nodes.** The lumbar lymphatic trunks join the **intestinal trunk(s)** to form the **cisterna chyli,** which opens into the **thoracic duct.**

(3) The thoracic duct receives the **left jugular** and **left subclavian trunks** as well as the **left bronchomediastinal trunk** before it opens into the **left subclavian vein.**

(4) The **right lymphatic duct** drains the **right jugular trunk** and the **right subclavian trunk** (shown but not labeled), as well as the **right bronchomediastinal** trunk before opening into the **right subclavian vein.**

PLATE 212 Frontal Section through the Thorax; MRI of Thorax

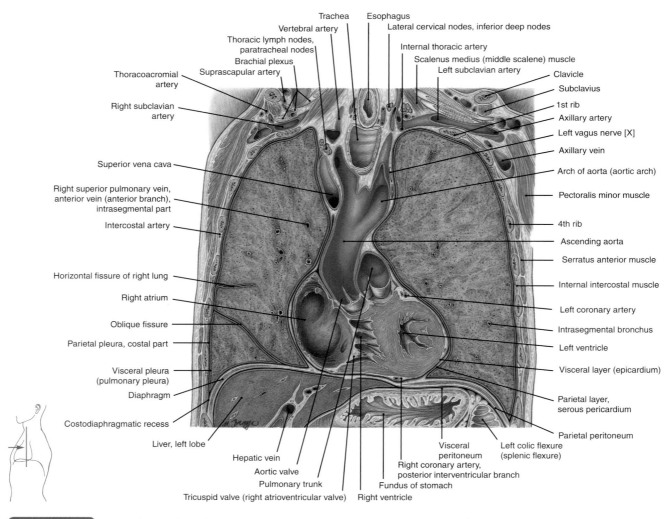

Trachea
Esophagus
Vertebral artery
Lateral cervical nodes, inferior deep nodes
Thoracic lymph nodes, paratracheal nodes
Internal thoracic artery
Brachial plexus
Scalenus medius (middle scalene) muscle
Thoracoacromial artery
Suprascapular artery
Left subclavian artery
Clavicle
Right subclavian artery
Subclavius
1st rib
Axillary artery
Superior vena cava
Left vagus nerve [X]
Axillary vein
Right superior pulmonary vein, anterior vein (anterior branch), intrasegmental part
Arch of aorta (aortic arch)
Pectoralis minor muscle
Intercostal artery
4th rib
Ascending aorta
Serratus anterior muscle
Horizontal fissure of right lung
Internal intercostal muscle
Right atrium
Left coronary artery
Oblique fissure
Intrasegmental bronchus
Parietal pleura, costal part
Left ventricle
Visceral pleura (pulmonary pleura)
Visceral layer (epicardium)
Diaphragm
Parietal layer, serous pericardium
Costodiaphragmatic recess
Parietal peritoneum
Liver, left lobe
Visceral peritoneum
Left colic flexure (splenic flexure)
Hepatic vein
Right coronary artery, posterior interventricular branch
Aortic valve
Pulmonary trunk
Fundus of stomach
Tricuspid valve (right atrioventricular valve)
Right ventricle

FIGURE 212.1 Frontal Section through the Thoracic Cavity (Anterior View)

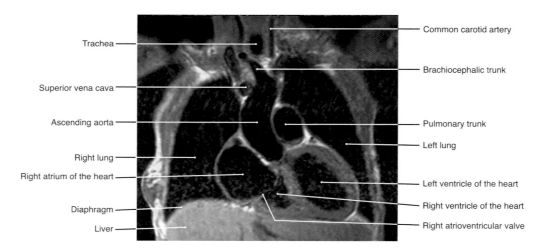

Trachea
Common carotid artery
Brachiocephalic trunk
Superior vena cava
Ascending aorta
Pulmonary trunk
Left lung
Right lung
Right atrium of the heart
Left ventricle of the heart
Diaphragm
Right ventricle of the heart
Liver
Right atrioventricular valve

FIGURE 212.2 MRI of Thorax at the Level of the Superior Vena Cava (Anterior View)

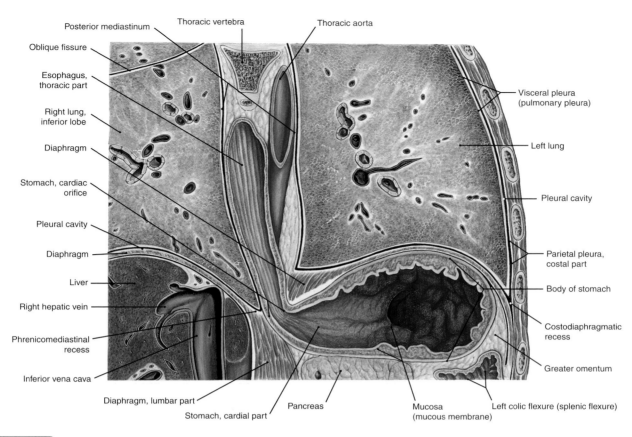

Posterior mediastinum — Thoracic vertebra — Thoracic aorta

Oblique fissure

Esophagus, thoracic part

Right lung, inferior lobe

Diaphragm

Stomach, cardiac orifice

Pleural cavity

Diaphragm

Liver

Right hepatic vein

Phrenicomediastinal recess

Inferior vena cava

Diaphragm, lumbar part

Stomach, cardial part

Pancreas

Mucosa (mucous membrane)

Visceral pleura (pulmonary pleura)

Left lung

Pleural cavity

Parietal pleura, costal part

Body of stomach

Costodiaphragmatic recess

Greater omentum

Left colic flexure (splenic flexure)

FIGURE 213.1 **Frontal Section through the Lower Left Thorax and Upper Left Abdomen (Anterior View)**

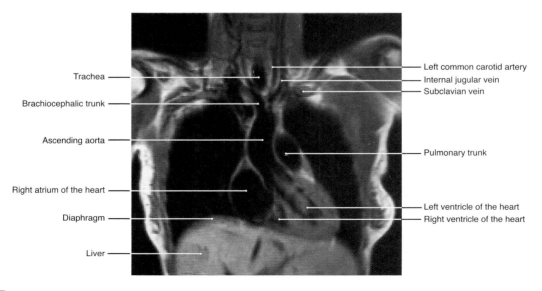

Trachea

Brachiocephalic trunk

Ascending aorta

Right atrium of the heart

Diaphragm

Liver

Left common carotid artery

Internal jugular vein

Subclavian vein

Pulmonary trunk

Left ventricle of the heart

Right ventricle of the heart

FIGURE 213.2 **MRI of Thorax at the Level of the Aortic Valve (Superior View)**

PLATE 214 Cross Section of the Thorax (Third Thoracic Vertebra Level)

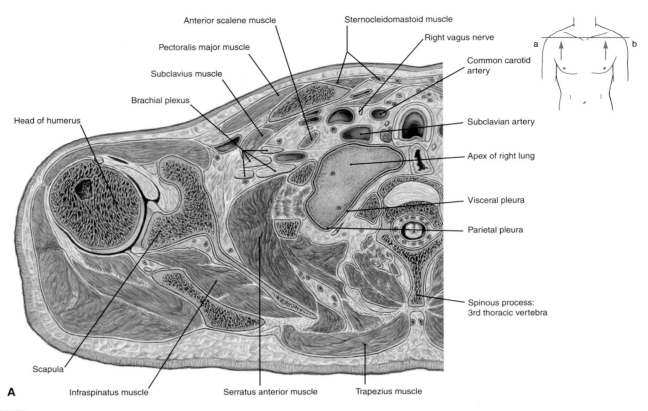

Anterior scalene muscle

Pectoralis major muscle

Subclavius muscle

Brachial plexus

Head of humerus

Sternocleidomastoid muscle

Right vagus nerve

Common carotid artery

Subclavian artery

Apex of right lung

Visceral pleura

Parietal pleura

Spinous process: 3rd thoracic vertebra

Scapula

Infraspinatus muscle

Serratus anterior muscle

Trapezius muscle

A

FIGURE 214A Right Side of Body

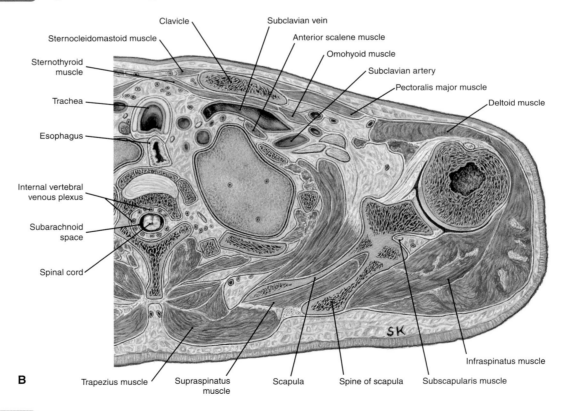

Clavicle

Subclavian vein

Sternocleidomastoid muscle

Anterior scalene muscle

Sternothyroid muscle

Omohyoid muscle

Subclavian artery

Trachea

Pectoralis major muscle

Deltoid muscle

Esophagus

Internal vertebral venous plexus

Subarachnoid space

Spinal cord

Infraspinatus muscle

B

Trapezius muscle

Supraspinatus muscle

Scapula

Spine of scapula

Subscapularis muscle

FIGURE 214B Left Side of Body

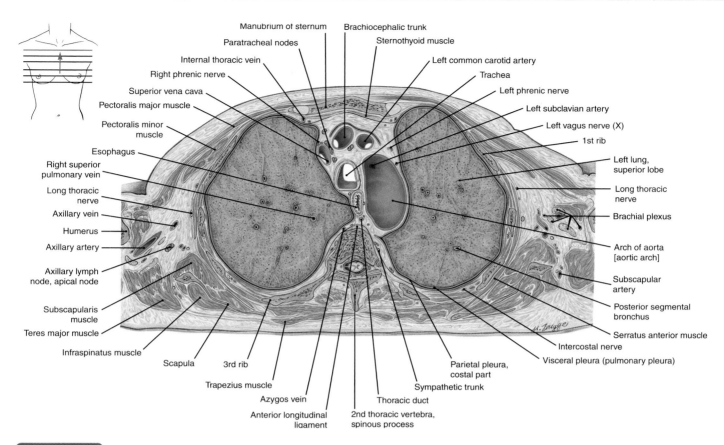

FIGURE 215.1 Horizontal Section through the Thorax at the Level of the Arch of the Aorta (Caudal View)

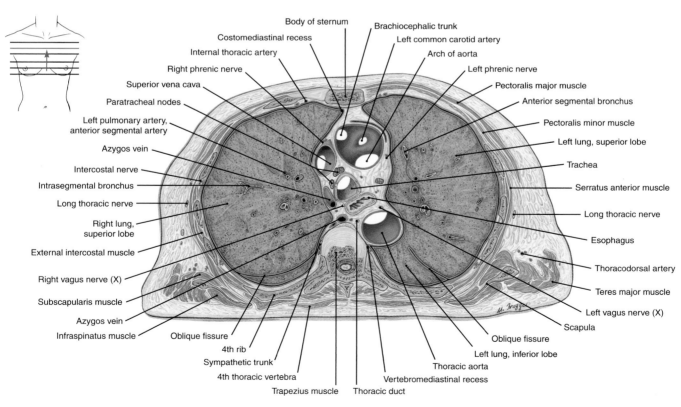

FIGURE 215.2 Horizontal Section through the Thorax at the Level of the Fourth Thoracic Vertebra (Caudal View)

PLATE 216   Transverse Sections through the Thorax

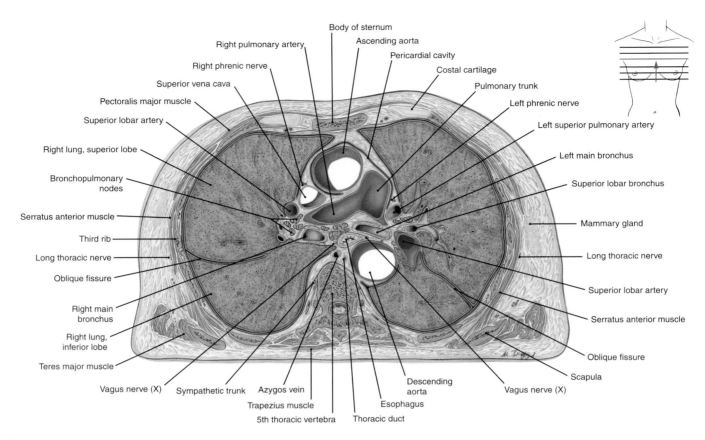

FIGURE 216.1 Horizontal Section through the Thorax at the Bifurcation of the Pulmonary Trunk (Caudal View)

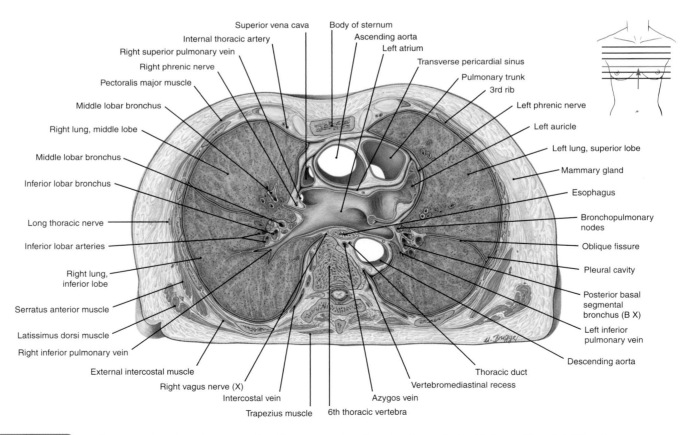

FIGURE 216.2 Horizontal Section through the Thorax at the Level of the Left Atrium (Caudal View)

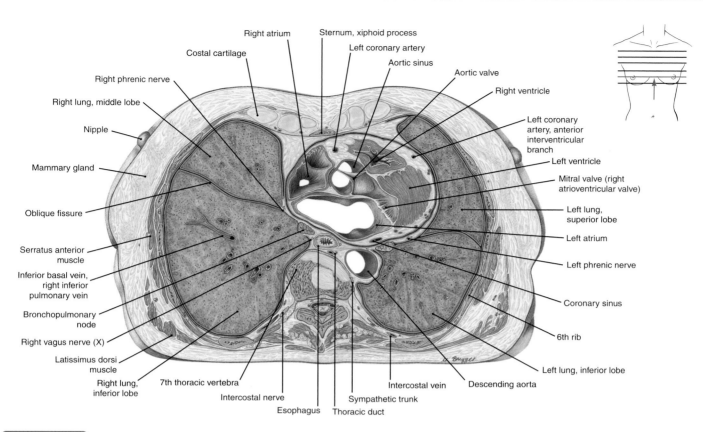

FIGURE 217.1 Horizontal Section through the Thorax at the Level of the Seventh Thoracic Vertebra (Caudal View)

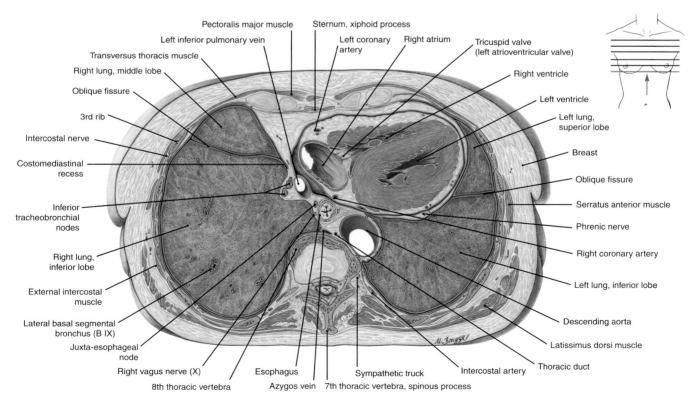

FIGURE 217.2 Horizontal Section through the Thorax at the Level of the Eighth Thoracic Vertebra (Caudal View)

PLATE 218 Tomographic Cross Section of the Thorax; the Diaphragm

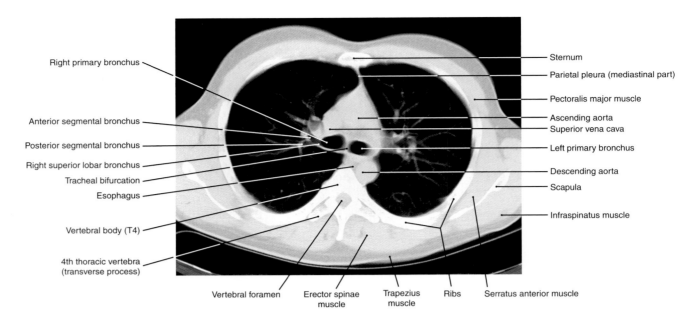

Right primary bronchus

Anterior segmental bronchus

Posterior segmental bronchus

Right superior lobar bronchus

Tracheal bifurcation

Esophagus

Vertebral body (T4)

4th thoracic vertebra
(transverse process)

Vertebral foramen

Erector spinae
muscle

Trapezius
muscle

Ribs

Serratus anterior muscle

Sternum

Parietal pleura (mediastinal part)

Pectoralis major muscle

Ascending aorta

Superior vena cava

Left primary bronchus

Descending aorta

Scapula

Infraspinatus muscle

FIGURE 218.1 Computed Tomographic Cross Section of the Thorax

NOTE that this CT is just inferior to the bifurcation of the trachea.

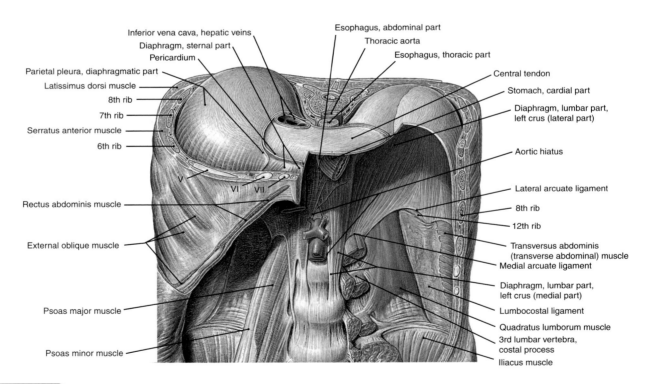

Inferior vena cava, hepatic veins

Diaphragm, sternal part

Pericardium

Parietal pleura, diaphragmatic part

Latissimus dorsi muscle

8th rib

7th rib

Serratus anterior muscle

6th rib

Rectus abdominis muscle

External oblique muscle

Psoas major muscle

Psoas minor muscle

Esophagus, abdominal part

Thoracic aorta

Esophagus, thoracic part

Central tendon

Stomach, cardial part

Diaphragm, lumbar part,
left crus (lateral part)

Aortic hiatus

Lateral arcuate ligament

8th rib

12th rib

Transversus abdominis
(transverse abdominal) muscle

Medial arcuate ligament

Diaphragm, lumbar part,
left crus (medial part)

Lumbocostal ligament

Quadratus lumborum muscle

3rd lumbar vertebra,
costal process

Iliacus muscle

FIGURE 218.2 The Diaphragm

NOTE the inferior vena cava (**vena caval orifice: level of T8**), the esophagus (**esophageal hiatus: level of T10**), and the aorta
(**aortic hiatus: at the level of L1**).

CHAPTER 3 The Abdomen

Plates

219 Regions of the Body: Gastrointestinal Tract

220 Anterior Abdominal Wall: Superficial Vessels and Nerves

221 Anterior Abdominal Wall: External Oblique Muscle

222 Inner Surface of the Anterior Abdominal Wall

223 Superficial Inguinal Ring with Spermatic Cord

224 Anterior Abdominal Wall: Internal Oblique Muscle

225 Anterior Abdominal Wall: Rectus Abdominis and Internal Oblique Muscles

226 Anterior Abdominal Wall: Rectus Sheath; Second Muscle Layer

227 Anterior Abdominal Wall: Transversus and Rectus Abdominis Muscles

228 Muscles of the Abdomen: Transverse Sections

229 Abdominal Muscles: Frontal Section (Computed Tomography)

230 Anterior Abdominal Wall: Rectus Sheath

231 Anterior Abdominal Wall: Epigastric Anastomosis

232 Female Inguinal Region: Superficial Inguinal Ring

233 Innervation of Female Genital Organs

234 Ligaments in the Inguinal Region; Spermatic Cord

235 Innervation of the Male Genital Organs

236 Male Inguinal Region: Superficial Rings and Spermatic Cord

237 Spermatic Cord and Cremaster Muscle

238 Testis: Anterior and Lateral Views and Longitudinal Section

239 Testis and Epididymis

240 Testes in the Scrotum and Their Descent During Development

241 The Inguinal Canal; Indirect and Direct Inguinal Hernias

242 Newborn Child: Anterior Abdominal Wall and Scrotum

243 Newborn Child: Thoracic and Abdominal Viscera

244 Abdominal, Thoracic, and Male Urogenital Organs (Projections)

245 Abdominal, Thoracic, and Female Urogenital Organs (Projections)

246 Median Sagittal Section: Male Abdomen and Pelvis

247 Paramedian Section: Male Abdomen and Pelvis

248 Development of Gastrointestinal System: Mesogastria and Mesenteries

249 Development of the Omental Bursa: Adult Peritoneal Reflections

250 Abdominal Cavity 1: Greater Omentum

251 Abdominal Cavity 2: Omentum Reflected; Large and Small Intestine

252 Abdominal Cavity 3: Celiac Trunk and Its Branches (Anterior View)

253 Abdominal Cavity 4: Splenic and Gastroduodenal Vessels

254 Stomach: Arteries and Veins

255 Stomach and Upper Duodenum: Internal Structure

256 Celiac Trunk and Its Branches

257 Variations in the Blood Supply to the Liver and Stomach

258 Stomach, In Situ; the Omental Foramen

259 Omental Bursa (Opened); Structures in the Porta Hepatis

260 Omental Bursa; Lymphatics of the Stomach and Porta Hepatis

261 Surface Projection and Radiograph of the Stomach

262 The Stomach: Anterior Surface and External Muscle Layers

263 X-Ray of the Stomach

264 Blood Supply to the Stomach; the Stomach and Greater Omentum

265 X-Ray of the Stomach Showing a Small Ulcer

266 Lymphatic Vessels and Nodes of the Stomach, Duodenum, and Pancreas

267 X-Rays Showing Gastric and Duodenal Ulcers

268 The Duodenum: Anterior View and Longitudinal Section

269 Arteries Supplying the Pyloric-Duodenal Region

270 Liver: Surface Projection (Dorsocranial View)

271 Liver: Anterior and Posterior Surfaces

272 Branching Patterns: Portal Vein, Hepatic Artery, and Hepatic Veins

273 Ultrasound Scans of the Hepatic and Portal Veins

274 Segments of the Liver

275 CT of Upper Abdomen; Variations in Shape of the Liver

276 CT of Upper Abdomen

277 Ultrasound of Upper Abdomen and of Metastatic Tumor in the Liver

278 Gallbladder and Biliary Ducts; Variations in Cystic and Hepatic Ducts

279 Radiographs of Biliary Ducts and Gallbladder

280 Blood Supply to the Gallbladder; Ultrasound of Gallbladder

281 Gallbladder Disease: Cholycystitis; Multiple Gallstones

282 Pancreas and Duodenum

283 Pancreatic Duct System: Head of Pancreas (Dorsal View)

284 CT of Second Lumbar Vertebra; Gallbladder, Common Bile Duct, and Pancreatic Duct

285 CT of Tumor in Head of Pancreas; Variations in Common Bile and Pancreatic Ducts

286 CT of Abdomen Showing Pancreatitis; Spleen: Diaphragmatic Surface

287 CT of Abdomen Showing Splenic Hemorrhage; Spleen: Visceral Surface

288 Abdominal Cavity 5: Jejunum, Ileum, and Ascending and Transverse Colons

289 Radiograph of the Jejunum and Ileum

290 Abdominal Cavity 6: Duodenojejunal Junction and Large Intestine

291 Double Contrast Image of the Small Intestine

292 Abdominal Cavity 7: Superior Mesenteric Vessels and Their Branches

293 Radiograph of the Superior Mesenteric Artery and Its Branches

294 Abdominal Cavity 8: Inferior Mesenteric Vessels and Their Branches

295 Radiograph of the Inferior Mesenteric Artery and Its Branches

296 The Abdominal Arteries

297 Variations in the Branching of the Mesenteric Arteries

298 The Hepatic Portal Vein and Its Tributaries

299 The Hepatic Portal Vein and the Inferior Vena Cava

300 Abdominal Cavity 9: Mesocolons and Mesentery of Small Intestine

301 Ileocecal Junction and Cecum

302 Vermiform Appendix

303 Vermiform Appendix: Variations in Its Location; Blood Supply

304 Large Intestine

305 Large Intestine (Radiograph)

306 Abdominal Cavity 10: Roots of the Mesocolons and Mesentery

307 Abdominal Cavity 11: Posterior Abdominal Wall, Retroperitoneal Organs

308 Kidneys: Ventral and Dorsal Relationship; Kidney Segmentation

309 Suprarenal Glands and Kidneys

310 Suprarenal Vessels; Renal Arteriogram

311 Kidneys: Hilar Structures and Surface Projection

312 Kidneys: Internal Structure, Longitudinal Section

313 Retrograde Pyelogram; Kidney Malformations

314 Diaphragm and Other Muscles of the Posterior Abdominal Wall

315 Posterior Abdominal Wall Muscles, Including the Diaphragm

316 Lumbar and Sacral Plexuses within Abdominopelvic Cavity

317 Posterior Abdominal Wall: Vessels and Nerves

318 CT (T10) and Transverse Section (T11) of Abdomen

319 CT (T11) and Transverse Section (T12–L1) of Abdomen

320 Transverse Section of the Abdomen at L1; CT of Abdomen at L1

321 Abdomen: Transverse Section, L3; CT of Abdomen at L3

322 Cross Section and CT of Abdomen at L5 Level

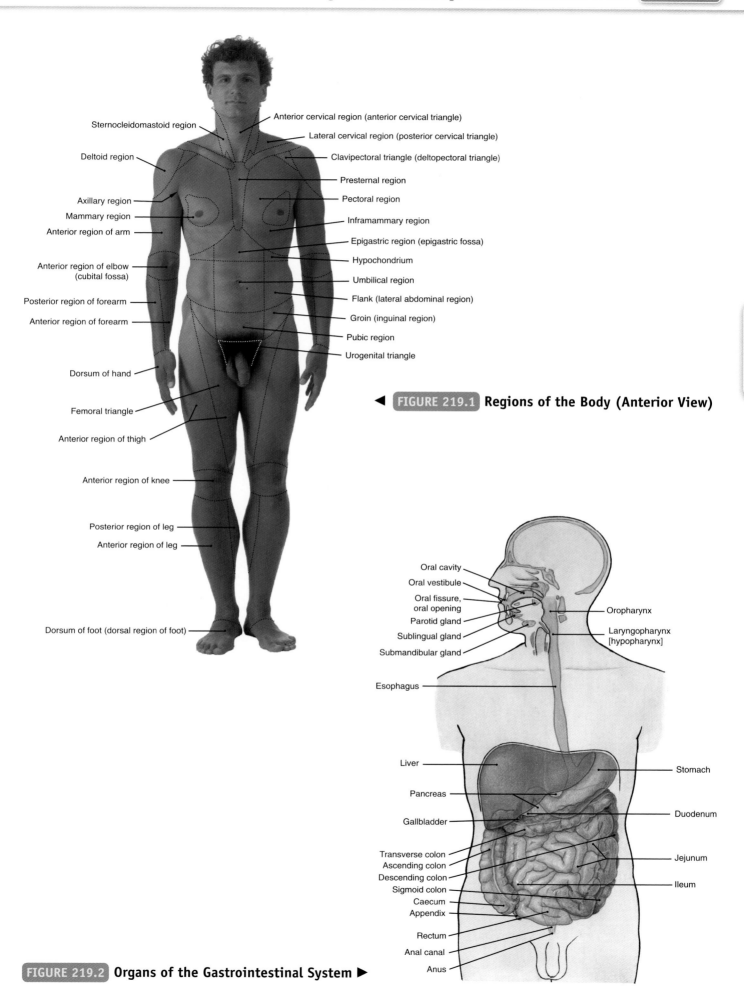

Sternocleidomastoid region

Deltoid region

Axillary region

Mammary region

Anterior region of arm

Anterior region of elbow
(cubital fossa)

Posterior region of forearm

Anterior region of forearm

Dorsum of hand

Femoral triangle

Anterior region of thigh

Anterior region of knee

Posterior region of leg

Anterior region of leg

Dorsum of foot (dorsal region of foot)

Anterior cervical region (anterior cervical triangle)

Lateral cervical region (posterior cervical triangle)

Clavipectoral triangle (deltopectoral triangle)

Presternal region

Pectoral region

Inframammary region

Epigastric region (epigastric fossa)

Hypochondrium

Umbilical region

Flank (lateral abdominal region)

Groin (inguinal region)

Pubic region

Urogenital triangle

◄ **FIGURE 219.1** **Regions of the Body (Anterior View)**

Oral cavity

Oral vestibule

Oral fissure,
oral opening

Parotid gland

Sublingual gland

Submandibular gland

Oropharynx

Laryngopharynx
[hypopharynx]

Esophagus

Liver

Pancreas

Gallbladder

Transverse colon

Ascending colon

Descending colon

Sigmoid colon

Caecum

Appendix

Rectum

Anal canal

Anus

Stomach

Duodenum

Jejunum

Ileum

FIGURE 219.2 **Organs of the Gastrointestinal System** ▶

PLATE 220 Anterior Abdominal Wall: Superficial Vessels and Nerves

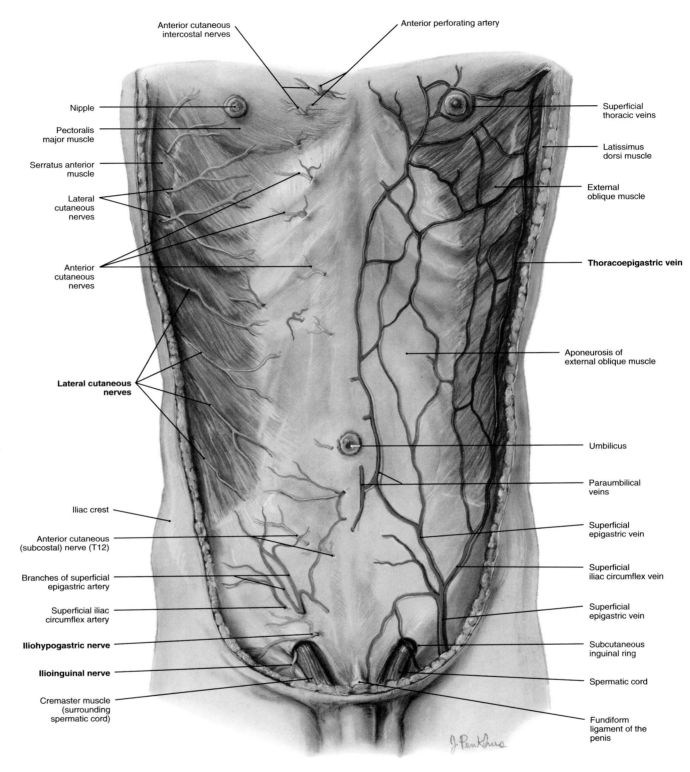

Anterior cutaneous intercostal nerves

Anterior perforating artery

Nipple

Pectoralis major muscle

Serratus anterior muscle

Lateral cutaneous nerves

Anterior cutaneous nerves

Lateral cutaneous nerves

Iliac crest

Anterior cutaneous (subcostal) nerve (T12)

Branches of superficial epigastric artery

Superficial iliac circumflex artery

Iliohypogastric nerve

Ilioinguinal nerve

Cremaster muscle (surrounding spermatic cord)

Superficial thoracic veins

Latissimus dorsi muscle

External oblique muscle

Thoracoepigastric vein

Aponeurosis of external oblique muscle

Umbilicus

Paraumbilical veins

Superficial epigastric vein

Superficial iliac circumflex vein

Superficial epigastric vein

Subcutaneous inguinal ring

Spermatic cord

Fundiform ligament of the penis

FIGURE 220 **Superficial Nerves and Vessels of the Anterior Abdominal Wall**

NOTE: (1) The distribution of the superficial vessels and cutaneous nerves upon the removal of the skin and fascia from the lower thoracic and anterior abdominal wall.

(2) The intercostal nerves supply the abdominal surface with lateral and anterior cutaneous branches.

(3) The ilioinguinal and iliohypogastric branches of the first lumbar nerve become superficial in the region of the **superficial inguinal ring.**

(4) The branches of the **superficial epigastric artery** (which arises from the femoral artery) ascending toward the umbilicus from the inguinal region.

(5) The **thoracoepigastric vein** serves as a means of communication between the femoral vein and the axillary vein. In cases of portal vein obstruction, these superficial veins become greatly enlarged (varicosed), a condition called caput medusae.

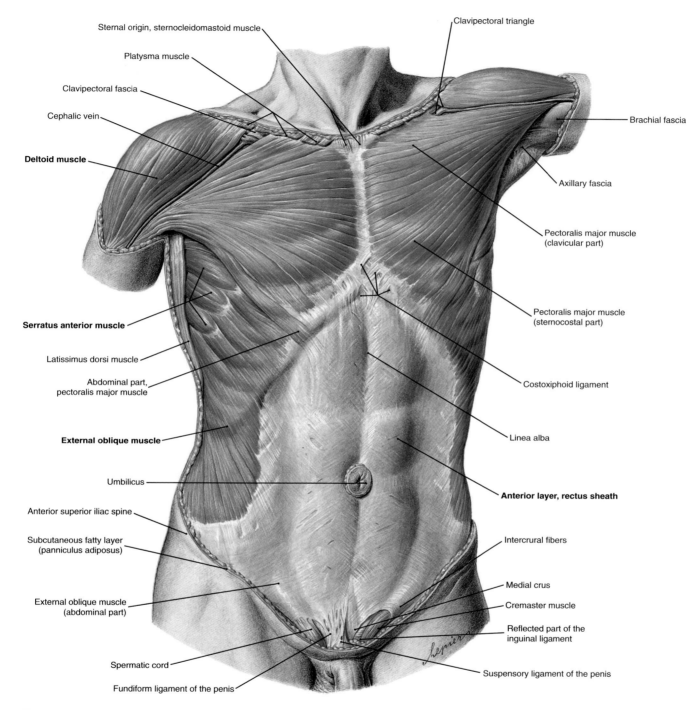

Sternal origin, sternocleidomastoid muscle

Platysma muscle

Clavipectoral fascia

Cephalic vein

Deltoid muscle

Serratus anterior muscle

Latissimus dorsi muscle

Abdominal part, pectoralis major muscle

External oblique muscle

Umbilicus

Anterior superior iliac spine

Subcutaneous fatty layer (panniculus adiposus)

External oblique muscle (abdominal part)

Spermatic cord

Fundiform ligament of the penis

Clavipectoral triangle

Brachial fascia

Axillary fascia

Pectoralis major muscle (clavicular part)

Pectoralis major muscle (sternocostal part)

Costoxiphoid ligament

Linea alba

Anterior layer, rectus sheath

Intercrural fibers

Medial crus

Cremaster muscle

Reflected part of the inguinal ligament

Suspensory ligament of the penis

FIGURE 221 **Superficial Musculature of the Anterior Abdominal and Thoracic Wall**

NOTE: (1) The first layer on the anterior abdominal wall consists of the **external oblique muscle** and its broad flat aponeurosis. Medially, this aponeurosis helps form the sheath of the rectus abdominis muscle, and inferiorly, it becomes the **inguinal ligament.**

(2) The external oblique muscle arises by means of seven or eight fleshy slips from the outer surfaces of the lower seven or eight ribs, thereby interdigitating with the fleshy origin of the **serratus anterior muscle.**

(3) The fibers of the external oblique muscle course inferomedially, or in the same direction as you would insert your hands in the side pockets of your trousers or slacks.

PLATE 222 Inner Surface of the Anterior Abdominal Wall

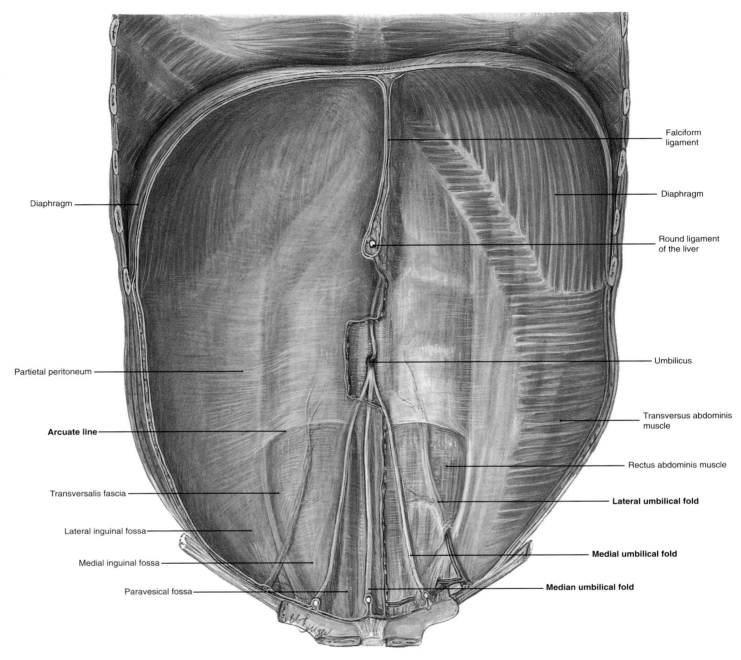

Diaphragm

Partietal peritoneum

Arcuate line

Transversalis fascia

Lateral inguinal fossa

Medial inguinal fossa

Paravesical fossa

Falciform ligament

Diaphragm

Round ligament of the liver

Umbilicus

Transversus abdominis muscle

Rectus abdominis muscle

Lateral umbilical fold

Medial umbilical fold

Median umbilical fold

FIGURE 222 **Inner Aspect of the Anterior Abdominal Wall**

NOTE: (1) This posterior view of the anterior abdominal wall shows to good advantage, inferiorly, the posterior layer of the rectus sheath and the relationship of the **arcuate line** to the umbilicus.

(2) The breadth of the transversus abdominis, which lies adjacent to the next inner layer, the fascia transversalis, deep to which is the parietal peritoneum.

(3) The **median umbilical fold,** which is the remnant of the **urachus** that extended between the apex of the fetal bladder and the umbilicus during development.

(4) The **medial umbilical folds,** which are the obliterated umbilical arteries, covered by a peritoneal layer. These vessels were the continuation of the superior vesical arteries to the umbilicus in the fetus.

(5) The **lateral umbilical folds,** which are folds of parietal peritoneum covering the inferior epigastric arteries and veins.

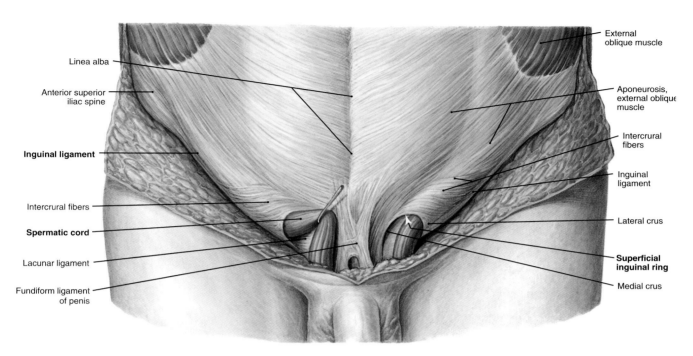

FIGURE 223.1 Superficial Inguinal Ring and Spermatic Cord

NOTE: (1) The superficial inguinal ring transmits the **spermatic cord** in the male and the **round ligament of the uterus** in the female. In this dissection, the right spermatic cord has been lifted to show the border of the ring as well as the **lacunar ligament.**

(2) The tendinous fibers of the aponeurosis are continuous with the fleshy fibers of the external oblique. They are directed inferomedially and decussate across the linea alba.

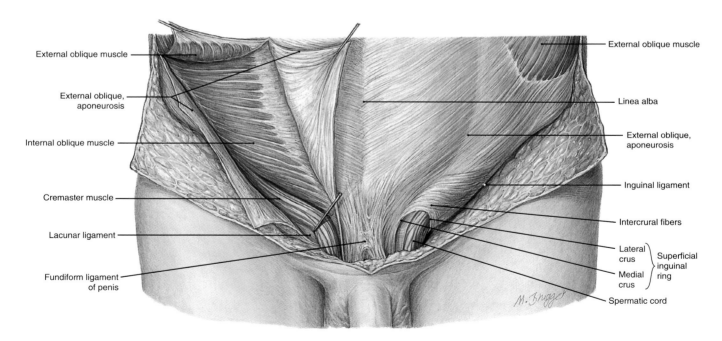

FIGURE 223.2 Right Internal Oblique Muscle (Inferior Part) and the Superficial Inguinal Ring

NOTE: (1) The aponeurosis of the external oblique muscle (reader's left) has been severed and lifted to show the inferior part of the internal oblique muscle.

(2) The right superficial inguinal ring has been opened and the right spermatic cord has been hooked and lifted.

(3) The superficial inguinal ring is a slit-like opening in the external oblique muscle. Observe how **the intercrural fibers** strengthen the lateral aspect of the superficial ring by extending between the **medial and lateral crura.**

(4) The **inguinal ligament** extends between the anterior superior iliac spine and the pubic tubercle. This ligament is formed by the lowermost fibers of the external oblique aponeurosis and **lends** support to the inferior part of the anterior abdominal wall.

(5) The fundiform ligament of the penis extends downward from the aponeurosis of the external oblique muscle.

PLATE 224 Anterior Abdominal Wall: Internal Oblique Muscle

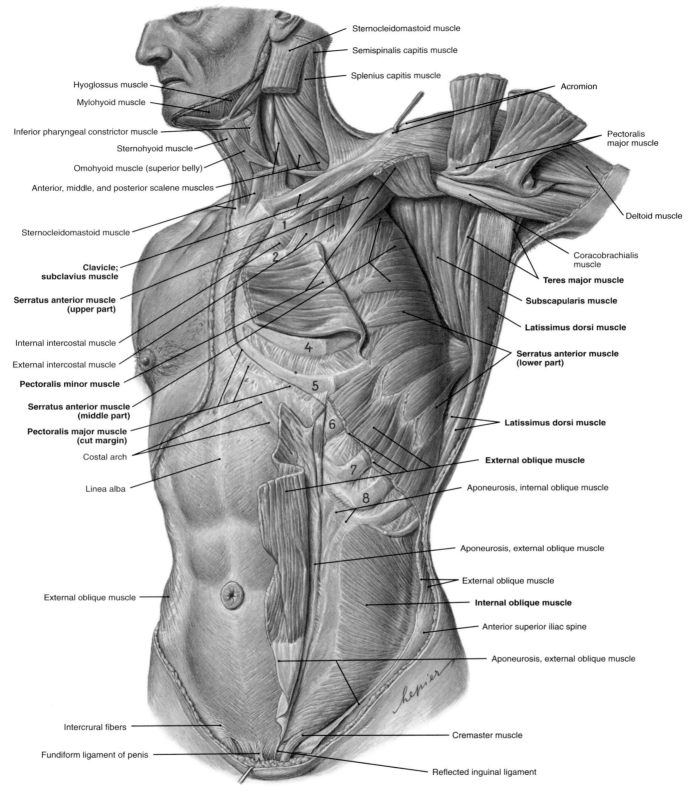

Sternocleidomastoid muscle
Semispinalis capitis muscle
Splenius capitis muscle
Acromion
Hyoglossus muscle
Mylohyoid muscle
Inferior pharyngeal constrictor muscle
Sternohyoid muscle
Omohyoid muscle (superior belly)
Anterior, middle, and posterior scalene muscles
Sternocleidomastoid muscle
Pectoralis major muscle
Deltoid muscle
Coracobrachialis muscle
Clavicle; subclavius muscle
Serratus anterior muscle (upper part)
Teres major muscle
Subscapularis muscle
Latissimus dorsi muscle
Internal intercostal muscle
External intercostal muscle
Serratus anterior muscle (lower part)
Pectoralis minor muscle
Serratus anterior muscle (middle part)
Pectoralis major muscle (cut margin)
Latissimus dorsi muscle
Costal arch
External oblique muscle
Linea alba
Aponeurosis, internal oblique muscle
Aponeurosis, external oblique muscle
External oblique muscle
Internal oblique muscle
External oblique muscle
Anterior superior iliac spine
Aponeurosis, external oblique muscle
Intercrural fibers
Cremaster muscle
Fundiform ligament of penis
Reflected inguinal ligament

FIGURE 224 **Deeper Layers of the Musculature of the Trunk, Axilla, and Neck**

NOTE: (1) The pectoralis major and minor muscles have been reflected to expose the underlying digitations of the serratus anterior muscle, which attaches to the upper nine ribs.
(2) The external oblique muscle and the lower lateral part of its aponeurosis have been severed in a semicircular manner near their origin to reveal the underlying internal oblique muscle, which comprises the second layer of anterior abdominal wall muscles.
(3) The fibers of the external oblique muscle course inferomedially (or in the same direction as you would put your hands in your side pockets), whereas **most** of the fibers of the internal oblique muscle course in the opposite direction, at a 90-degree angle to the external oblique fibers.

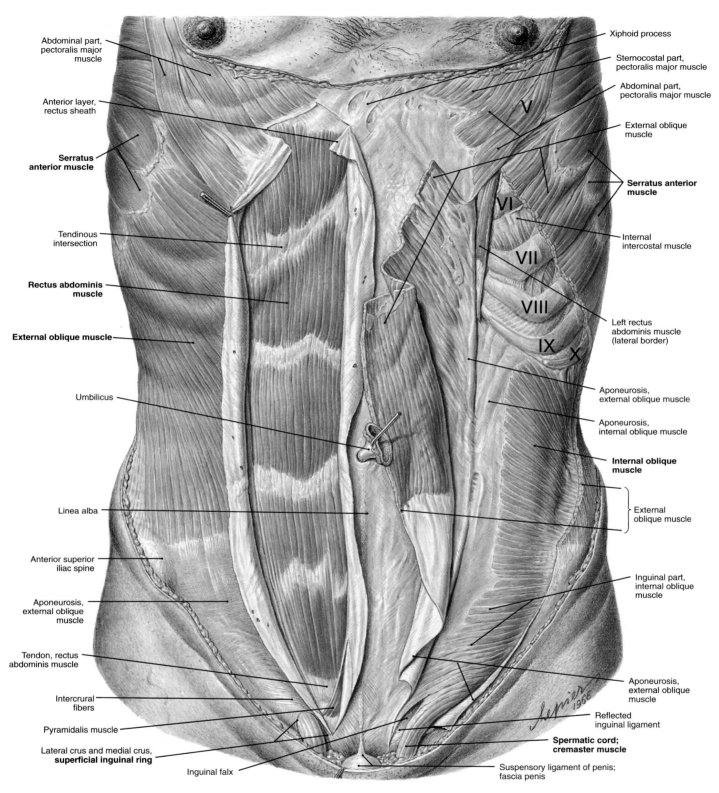

FIGURE 225 **Anterior Abdominal Wall: Rectus Abdominis and Internal Oblique Muscles**

Muscle	Origin	Insertion	Innervation	Action
External oblique	Fleshy slips from the outer surface of the lower eight ribs (ribs 5 to 12)	Outer lip of the iliac crest; aponeurosis of external oblique, which ends in a midline raphe, the **linea alba**	Lower seven thoracic nerves (T6–T12)	Compresses the abdominal viscera; **both muscles:** flex the trunk forward; **each muscle:** bends the trunk to that side and rotates the front of the abdomen to the **opposite** side

PLATE 226 Anterior Abdominal Wall: Rectus Sheath; Second Muscle Layer

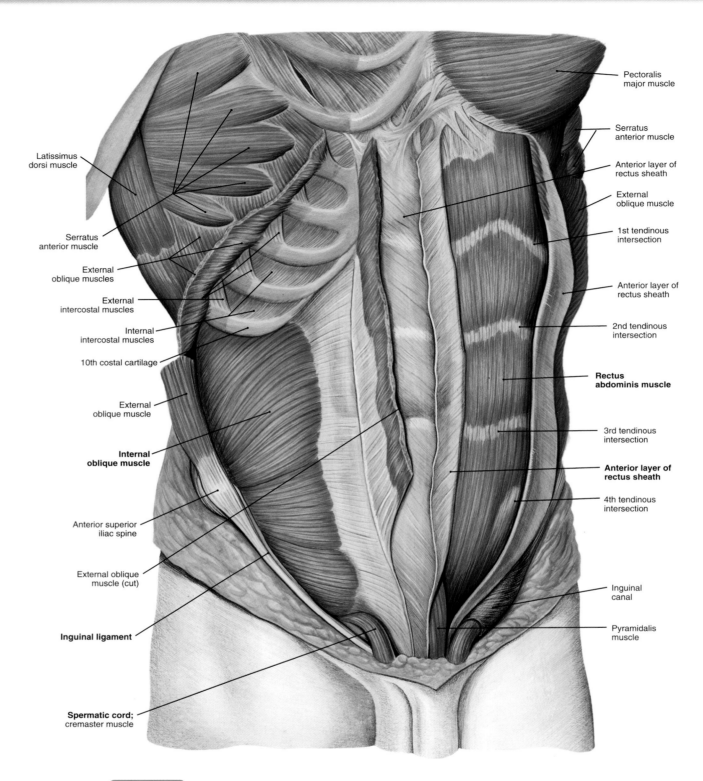

Pectoralis
major muscle

Serratus
anterior muscle

Anterior layer of
rectus sheath

External
oblique muscle

1st tendinous
intersection

Anterior layer of
rectus sheath

2nd tendinous
intersection

**Rectus
abdominis muscle**

3rd tendinous
intersection

**Anterior layer of
rectus sheath**

4th tendinous
intersection

Inguinal
canal

Pyramidalis
muscle

Latissimus
dorsi muscle

Serratus
anterior muscle

External
oblique muscles

External
intercostal muscles

Internal
intercostal muscles

10th costal cartilage

External
oblique muscle

**Internal
oblique muscle**

Anterior superior
iliac spine

External oblique
muscle (cut)

Inguinal ligament

Spermatic cord;
cremaster muscle

FIGURE 226 Middle Layer of Abdominal Musculature: Internal Oblique Muscle

Muscle	Origin	Insertion	Innervation	Action
Internal oblique	Lateral two-thirds of inguinal ligament; the middle lip of the iliac crest; the thoracolumbar fascia	Inferior border of the lower three or four ribs; the **linea alba;** aponeurosis fuses with that of the external oblique to help form the rectus sheath	Lower five thoracic nerves and the first lumbar nerve (T8–L1)	Compresses the abdominal viscera; **both muscles:** flex the trunk forward; **each muscle:** bends the trunk to that side but rotates the front of the abdomen toward the **same** side

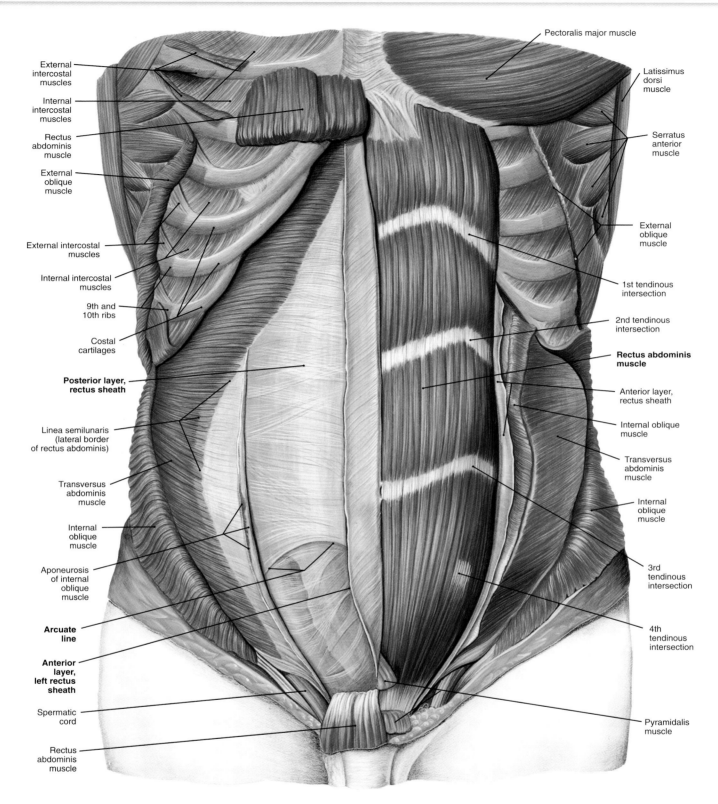

External intercostal muscles

Internal intercostal muscles

Rectus abdominis muscle

External oblique muscle

External intercostal muscles

Internal intercostal muscles

9th and 10th ribs

Costal cartilages

Posterior layer, rectus sheath

Linea semilunaris (lateral border of rectus abdominis)

Transversus abdominis muscle

Internal oblique muscle

Aponeurosis of internal oblique muscle

Arcuate line

Anterior layer, left rectus sheath

Spermatic cord

Rectus abdominis muscle

Pectoralis major muscle

Latissimus dorsi muscle

Serratus anterior muscle

External oblique muscle

1st tendinous intersection

2nd tendinous intersection

Rectus abdominis muscle

Anterior layer, rectus sheath

Internal oblique muscle

Transversus abdominis muscle

Internal oblique muscle

3rd tendinous intersection

4th tendinous intersection

Pyramidalis muscle

FIGURE 227 Deep Layer of Abdominal Musculature: Transversus Abdominis Muscle

Muscle	Origin	Insertion	Innervation	Action
Transversus abdominis	Lateral third of inguinal ligament and inner lip of iliac crest; thoracolumbar fascia; inner surface of lower six ribs	Ends in an aponeurosis; **upper fibers:** to linea alba, help form posterior layer of rectus sheath; **lower fibers:** attach to pubis to form **conjoined tendon**	Lower six thoracic and first lumbar nerves (T7–L1)	Tenses abdominal wall; compresses abdominal contents

PLATE 228 Muscles of the Abdomen: Transverse Sections

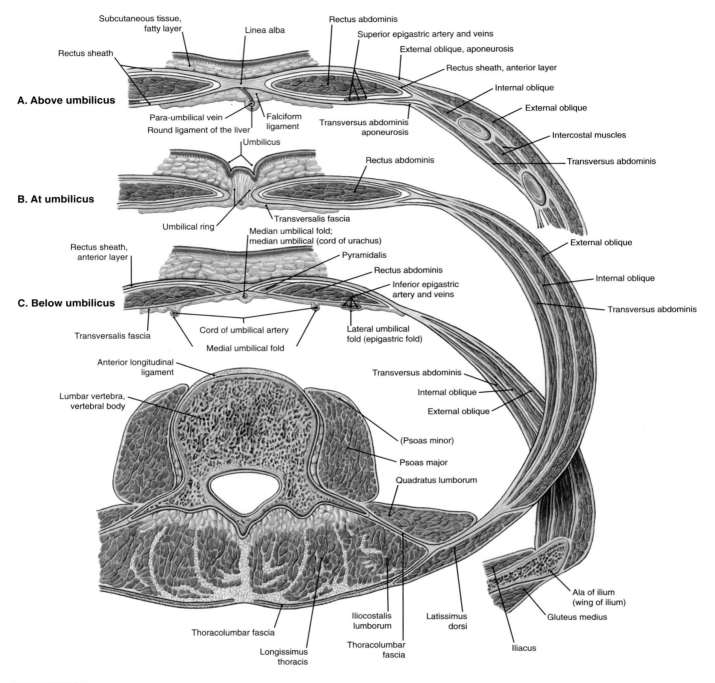

A. Above umbilicus

Subcutaneous tissue, fatty layer
Linea alba
Rectus sheath
Rectus abdominis
Superior epigastric artery and veins
External oblique, aponeurosis
Rectus sheath, anterior layer
Internal oblique
External oblique
Para-umbilical vein
Round ligament of the liver
Falciform ligament
Transversus abdominis aponeurosis
Intercostal muscles
Transversus abdominis
Umbilicus

B. At umbilicus

Rectus abdominis
Transversalis fascia
Umbilical ring
Median umbilical fold; median umbilical (cord of urachus)
External oblique

Rectus sheath, anterior layer
Pyramidalis
Rectus abdominis
Inferior epigastric artery and veins
Internal oblique
Transversus abdominis

C. Below umbilicus

Transversalis fascia
Cord of umbilical artery
Medial umbilical fold
Lateral umbilical fold (epigastric fold)

Anterior longitudinal ligament
Lumbar vertebra, vertebral body
Transversus abdominis
Internal oblique
External oblique
(Psoas minor)
Psoas major
Quadratus lumborum
Thoracolumbar fascia
Longissimus thoracis
Iliocostalis lumborum
Latissimus dorsi
Thoracolumbar fascia
Iliacus
Ala of ilium (wing of ilium)
Gluteus medius

FIGURE 228 **Transverse Sections of the Abdomen at Three Different Levels**

NOTE: (1) In **A,** the section is above the umbilicus; in **B,** the section is at the level of the umbilicus; in **C,** the section is below the umbilicus and below the arcuate line. Observe that in **C** only the **transversalis fascia** is found deep to the rectus abdominis muscle and that the posterior layer of the rectus sheath is absent.

(2) The complete transaction seen at the bottom of the figure is continuous with the lateral and anterior muscles at the level of the umbilicus (**B**).

(3) The differences in the sheath of the rectus abdominis (see Figs. 230.1 and 230.2).

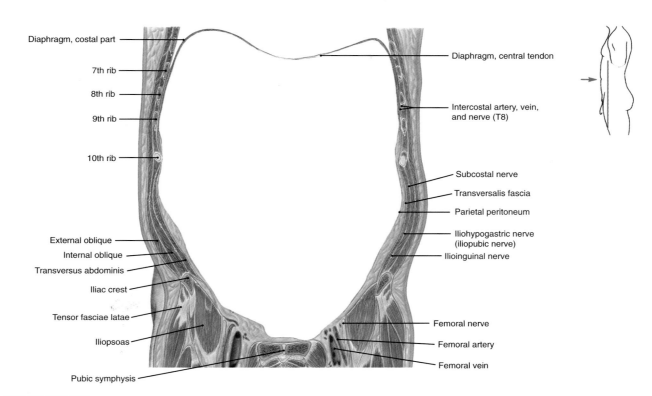

Diaphragm, costal part

7th rib

8th rib

9th rib

10th rib

External oblique

Internal oblique

Transversus abdominis

Iliac crest

Tensor fasciae latae

Iliopsoas

Pubic symphysis

Diaphragm, central tendon

Intercostal artery, vein, and nerve (T8)

Subcostal nerve

Transversalis fascia

Parietal peritoneum

Iliohypogastric nerve (iliopubic nerve)

Ilioinguinal nerve

Femoral nerve

Femoral artery

Femoral vein

FIGURE 229.1 **Frontal Section of the Abdomen through the Iliac Crest and Symphysis Pubis**

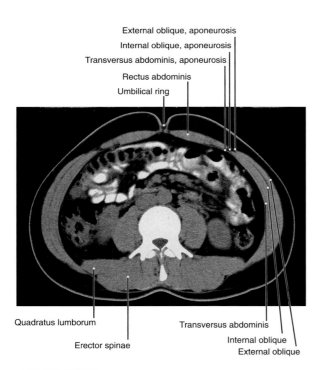

External oblique, aponeurosis

Internal oblique, aponeurosis

Transversus abdominis, aponeurosis

Rectus abdominis

Umbilical ring

Quadratus lumborum

Erector spinae

Transversus abdominis

Internal oblique

External oblique

FIGURE 229.2 **Computed Tomography (CT) of the Muscles of the Abdomen at the Level of the Umbilicus**

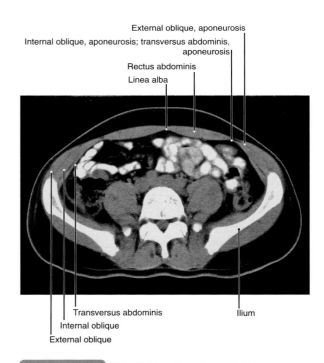

External oblique, aponeurosis

Internal oblique, aponeurosis; transversus abdominis, aponeurosis

Rectus abdominis

Linea alba

Transversus abdominis

Internal oblique

External oblique

Ilium

FIGURE 229.3 **CT of the Muscles of the Abdomen at the Level of the Fifth Lumbar Vertebra**

PLATE 230 Anterior Abdominal Wall: Rectus Sheath

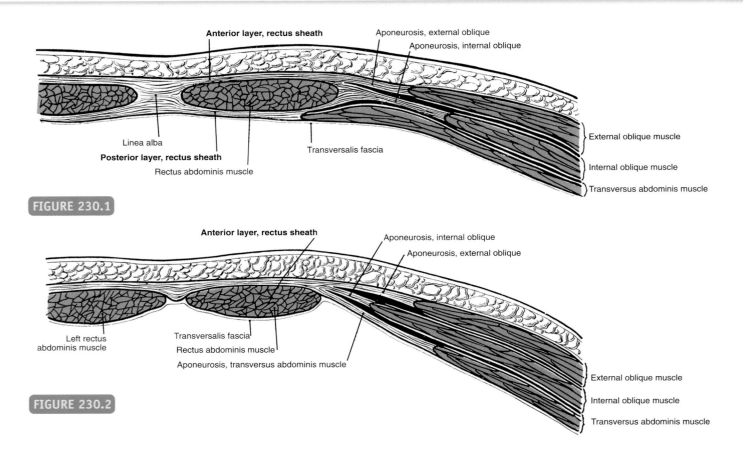

FIGURE 230.1

FIGURE 230.2

FIGURES 230.1 and 230.2 **Transverse Sections of the Anterior Abdominal Wall: Above the Umbilicus (Fig. 230.1) and Below the Arcuate Line (Fig. 230.2)**

NOTE: (1) The sheath of the rectus abdominis is formed by the aponeurosis of the external oblique, internal oblique, and transversus abdominis muscles.

(2) The upper two-thirds of the sheath encloses the rectus muscle both anteriorly and posteriorly. To accomplish this, the internal oblique aponeurosis splits. Part of the internal oblique aponeurosis joins the aponeurosis of the external oblique to form the **anterior layer**, while the other portion joins the aponeurosis of the transversus abdominis to form the **posterior layer** (Fig. 230.1).

(3) The lower third of the sheath, located below the arcuate line, is deficient posteriorly, since the aponeuroses of all three muscles pass anterior to the rectus abdominis muscle (Fig. 230.2).

(4) Deep to the sheath and transversus muscle is located the **transversalis fascia,** interposed between the peritoneum and the anterior wall structures.

Muscle	Origin	Insertion	Innervation	Action
Rectus abdominis	Fifth, sixth, and seventh costal cartilages; costoxiphoid ligaments and xiphoid process	Crest of pubis and pubic tubercle; front of symphysis pubis	Lower seven thoracic nerves (T6–T12)	Flexes vertebral column; tenses anterior abdominal wall; compresses abdominal contents
Cremaster	Midway along the inguinal ligament as a continuation of internal oblique muscle	Onto tubercles and crest of pubis and sheath of rectus abdominis muscle (forms loops over spermatic cord that reach as far as testis)	Genital branch of genitofemoral nerve (L1, L2)	Pulls the testis upward toward the superficial inguinal ring
Pyramidalis	Anterior surface of pubis and anterior pubic ligament	Into **linea alba** between umbilicus and symphysis pubis (muscle variable in size; average, 6 to 7 cm in length)	12th thoracic nerve (T12)	Tenses **linea alba**

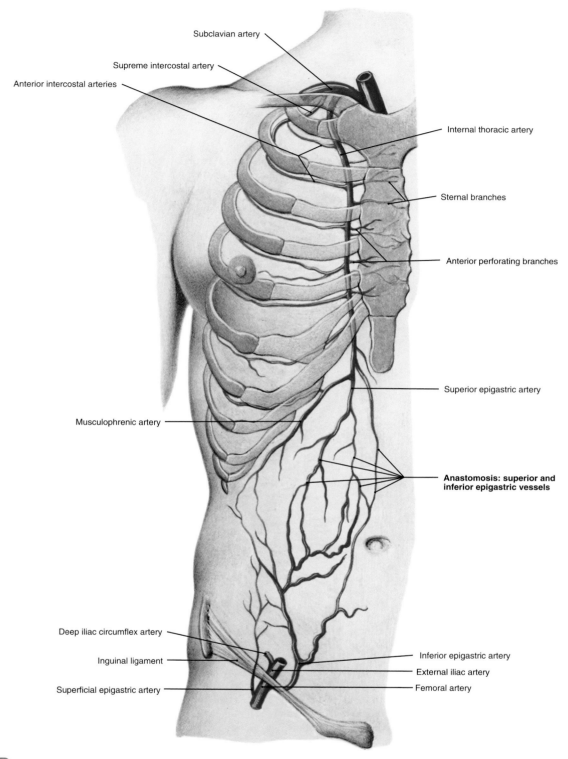

FIGURE 231 **Schematic Diagram of the Epigastric Anastomosis**

NOTE: (1) The **internal thoracic artery** arises from the subclavian artery and descends behind the ribs parallel to the sternum.

(2) Below the sternum, the internal thoracic artery terminates by dividing into the **musculophrenic** and **superior epigastric arteries**.

(3) The musculophrenic artery courses laterally adjacent to the costal margin and helps supply the diaphragm, while the superior epigastric artery descends within the rectus sheath, where it enters the substance of the rectus abdominis muscle.

(4) The inferior epigastric artery is a branch of the external iliac artery. It ascends and enters the rectus sheath at the arcuate line and also ramifies within the rectus abdominis muscle, where it anastomoses with the superior epigastric artery. This anastomosis forms a functional interconnection between arteries that serve the upper and lower limbs.

PLATE 232 Female Inguinal Region: Superficial Inguinal Ring

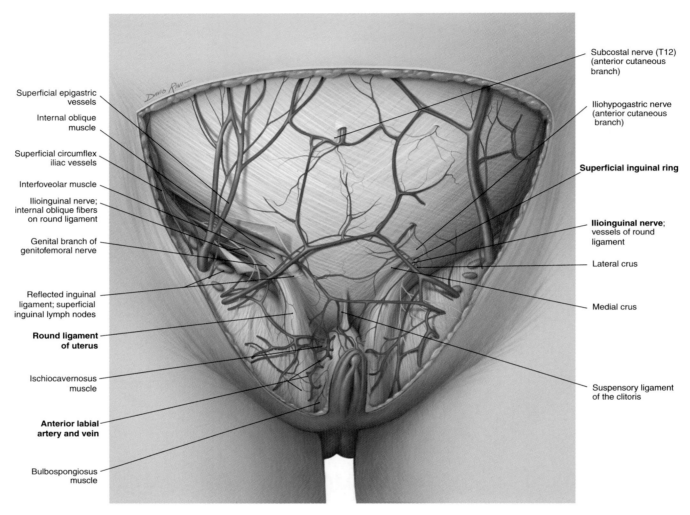

Superficial epigastric vessels

Internal oblique muscle

Superficial circumflex iliac vessels

Interfoveolar muscle

Ilioinguinal nerve; internal oblique fibers on round ligament

Genital branch of genitofemoral nerve

Reflected inguinal ligament; superficial inguinal lymph nodes

Round ligament of uterus

Ischiocavernosus muscle

Anterior labial artery and vein

Bulbospongiosus muscle

Subcostal nerve (T12) (anterior cutaneous branch)

Iliohypogastric nerve (anterior cutaneous branch)

Superficial inguinal ring

Ilioinguinal nerve; vessels of round ligament

Lateral crus

Medial crus

Suspensory ligament of the clitoris

FIGURE 232 **Inguinal Region of the Anterior Abdominal Wall in the Female: Aponeurosis of the External Oblique**

NOTE: (1) The skin and superficial fascia have been reflected from the inguinal region, exposing the aponeurosis of the external oblique muscle, the superficial inguinal ring, the superficial vessels and nerves of the lower abdominal wall, and the muscles and nerves of the clitoris.

(2) The **superficial inguinal ring** is an opening in the aponeurosis of the external oblique muscle. On the specimen's left (reader's right) the ring has been opened to reveal the lower course of the round ligament and the ilioinguinal nerve.

(3) The iliohypogastric nerve (branch of L1) as it penetrates the aponeurosis to become a sensory nerve after supplying motor fibers to the underlying musculature.

(4) Of the superficial vessels, observe the **superficial external pudendal**, the **superficial iliac circumflex**, and the **superficial epigastric.** The latter vessels ascend within the superficial fascia between its superficial fatty (Camper's) and deep (Scarpa's) layers.

(5) The **superficial dorsal vein of the clitoris,** which may drain into either the left or right superficial external pudendal vein.

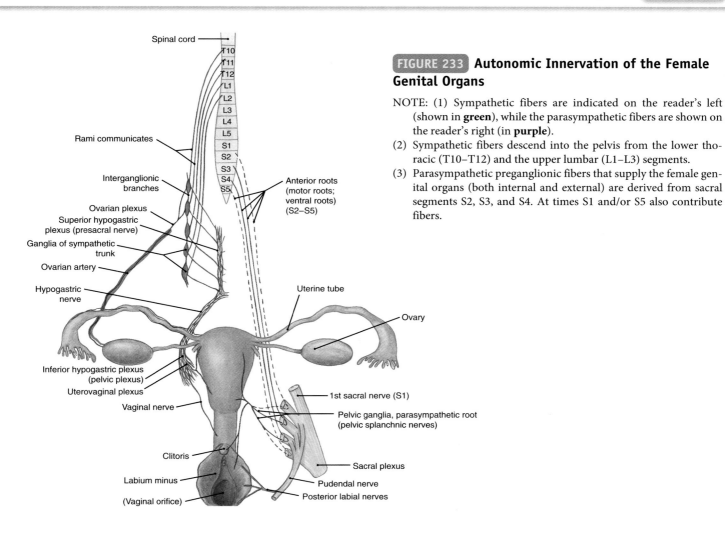

FIGURE 233 **Autonomic Innervation of the Female Genital Organs**

NOTE: (1) Sympathetic fibers are indicated on the reader's left (shown in **green**), while the parasympathetic fibers are shown on the reader's right (in **purple**).

(2) Sympathetic fibers descend into the pelvis from the lower thoracic (T10–T12) and the upper lumbar (L1–L3) segments.

(3) Parasympathetic preganglionic fibers that supply the female genital organs (both internal and external) are derived from sacral segments S2, S3, and S4. At times S1 and/or S5 also contribute fibers.

Labels on figure:

Spinal cord — T10, T11, T12, L1, L2, L3, L4, L5, S1, S2, S3, S4, S5
Rami communicates
Interganglionic branches
Ovarian plexus
Superior hypogastric plexus (presacral nerve)
Ganglia of sympathetic trunk
Ovarian artery
Hypogastric nerve
Inferior hypogastric plexus (pelvic plexus)
Uterovaginal plexus
Vaginal nerve
Clitoris
Labium minus
(Vaginal orifice)
Anterior roots (motor roots; ventral roots) (S2–S5)
Uterine tube
Ovary
1st sacral nerve (S1)
Pelvic ganglia, parasympathetic root (pelvic splanchnic nerves)
Sacral plexus
Pudendal nerve
Posterior labial nerves

INNERVATION OF FEMALE GENITAL ORGANS (BOTH INTERNAL AND EXTERNAL)			
Origin	**Course**	**Organ**	**Function**
Parasympathetic part Spinal cord, sacral part (S1) **S2, S3, S4,** (S5)	Pelvic ganglia, parasympathetic root [pelvic splanchnic nerves] ↓	Uterine tube Uterus	Vasodilatation Vasodilatation
	Cavernous nerves of clitoris	Vagina Clitoris	Production of fluid (transudate) Erection
Sympathetic part Spinal cord, thoracic part **(T10 to T12)** Spinal cord, lumbar part **(L1 to L2 or L3)**	Superior mesenteric plexus ↓ Ovarian plexus ↓ Renal plexus Sympathetic trunk ↓ Superior hypogastric plexus ↓ Hypogastric nerve ↓ Inferior hypogastric plexus ↓ Uterovaginal plexus	Ovary Uterine tube Uterus Vagina	Vasoconstriction Contraction
Somatic efferent **Somatic afferent**	Pudendal nerve Dorsal nerve of clitoris Posterior labial nerves	Clitoris Labia majora Ischiocavernosus Bulbospongiosus	Contraction

PLATE 234 Ligaments in the Inguinal Region; Spermatic Cord

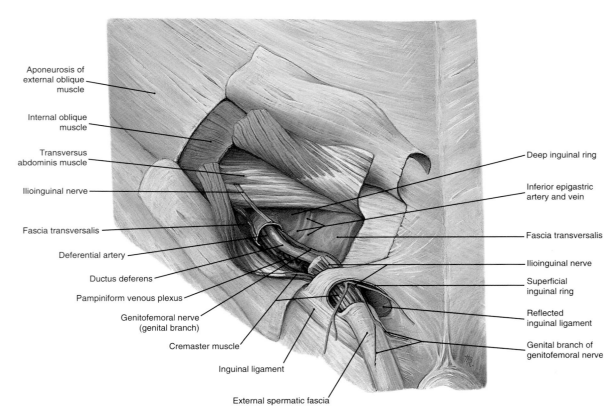

External oblique muscle

Aponeurosis of external oblique muscle

Inguinal ligament

Femoral nerve

Femoral artery and vein

Pectineal ligament (of Cooper)

Lacunar ligament

Intercrural fibers

Superficial inguinal ring

Medial (superior) crus

Reflex inguinal ligament

Lateral (inferior) crus

FIGURE 234.1 Ligaments in the Inguinal Region

NOTE the inguinal, lacunar, and pectineal ligaments and the superficial inguinal ring.

(From *Clemente's Anatomy Dissector,* 2nd Edition. Baltimore: Lippincott Williams & Wilkins, 2007.)

Aponeurosis of external oblique muscle

Internal oblique muscle

Transversus abdominis muscle

Ilioinguinal nerve

Fascia transversalis

Deferential artery

Ductus deferens

Pampiniform venous plexus

Genitofemoral nerve (genital branch)

Cremaster muscle

Inguinal ligament

External spermatic fascia

Deep inguinal ring

Inferior epigastric artery and vein

Fascia transversalis

Ilioinguinal nerve

Superficial inguinal ring

Reflected inguinal ligament

Genital branch of genitofemoral nerve

FIGURE 234.2 The Walls of the Inguinal Canal

NOTE: (1) That the aponeurosis of the external oblique muscle and the internal abdominal oblique muscle have both been opened and the structures of the **spermatic cord** have been exposed.

(2) That the **ilioinguinal** and **genitofemoral nerves** along with the **ductus deferens** and **deferential artery** are all shown and labeled.

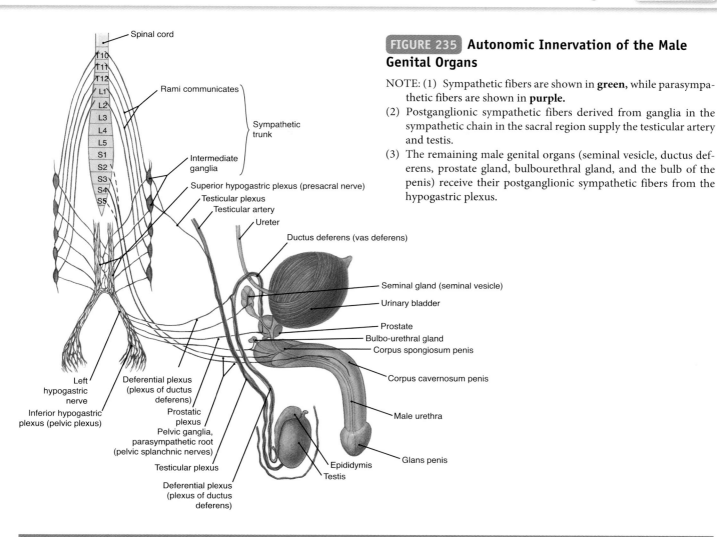

FIGURE 235 **Autonomic Innervation of the Male Genital Organs**

NOTE: (1) Sympathetic fibers are shown in **green**, while parasympathetic fibers are shown in **purple**.

(2) Postganglionic sympathetic fibers derived from ganglia in the sympathetic chain in the sacral region supply the testicular artery and testis.

(3) The remaining male genital organs (seminal vesicle, ductus deferens, prostate gland, bulbourethral gland, and the bulb of the penis) receive their postganglionic sympathetic fibers from the hypogastric plexus.

INNERVATION OF MALE GENITALS				
	Origin	**Course**	**Organ**	**Function**
Parasympathetic part	Spinal cord, sacral part (S1) **S2, S3, S4,** (S5)	Pelvic ganglia, parasympathetic root [pelvic splanchnic nerves]	Penis Corpora cavernosa and spongiosum	Vasodilatation Erection
Sympathetic part	Spinal cord, thoracic part (T10–T12) Spinal cord, lumbar part (L1–L2)	Superior and inferior mesenteric plexus ↓ Sympathetic trunk ↓ Testicular plexus ↓ Superior hypogastric plexus ↓ Hypogastric nerve ↓ Inferior hypogastric plexus	Testis Bulbo-urethral gland Ductus deferens [vas deferens] Seminal gland [seminal vesicle] Prostate	Regulation of blood flow Secretion Contraction, transportation of sperm into urethra Ejaculation into urethra
Somatic efferent Somatic afferent	Spinal cord, sacral part (S2–S4)	Pudendal nerve Posterior scrotal nerves Dorsal nerve of penis	(Sphincter of bladder) Ischiocavernosus Bulbospongiosus Skin of scrotum Skin of penis	Closure of bladder prevents retrograde ejaculation into the bladder Expulsion of ejaculate from urethra

PLATE 236 Male Inguinal Region: Superficial Rings and Spermatic Cord

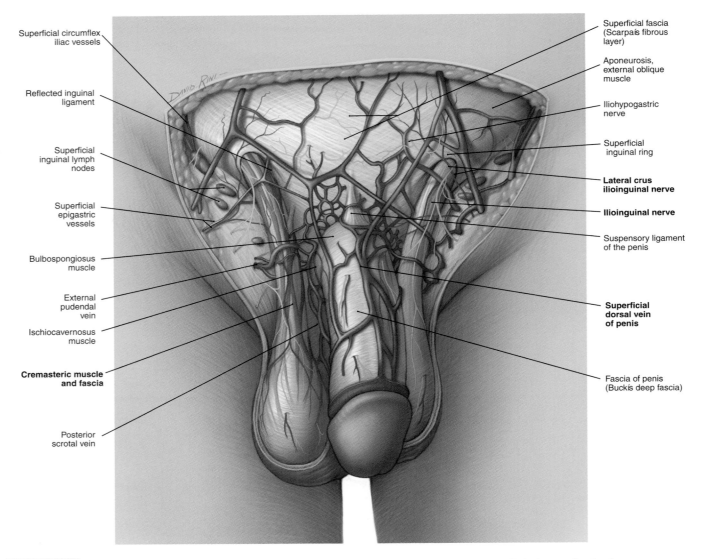

Superficial circumflex iliac vessels

Reflected inguinal ligament

Superficial inguinal lymph nodes

Superficial epigastric vessels

Bulbospongiosus muscle

External pudendal vein

Ischiocavernosus muscle

Cremasteric muscle and fascia

Posterior scrotal vein

Superficial fascia (Scarpa's fibrous layer)

Aponeurosis, external oblique muscle

Iliohypogastric nerve

Superficial inguinal ring

Lateral crus ilioinguinal nerve

Ilioinguinal nerve

Suspensory ligament of the penis

Superficial dorsal vein of penis

Fascia of penis (Buck's deep fascia)

FIGURE 236 **Inguinal Region of the Anterior Abdominal Wall in the Male: Superficial Inguinal Rings and the Cremaster Muscle**

NOTE: (1) On the specimen's right (reader's left), the skin and superficial fatty layer (Camper's) has been removed, while on the left side the skin, fatty layer, and superficial fibrous layer (Scarpa's) have been resected, revealing the aponeurosis of the external oblique muscle.

(2) The superficial inguinal rings have been exposed and the scrotal sacs opened. Observe the course of the **spermatic cord** from the scrotum to the superficial inguinal ring and the cremaster muscle and fascia surrounding the spermatic cord on the left.

(3) The **iliohypogastric nerve** penetrates the aponeurosis of the external oblique just above the superficial inguinal ring, and the **ilioinguinal nerve** emerges from the ring to supply the inguinal region and then continues as the **anterior scrotal nerve.**

(4) The external spermatic fascia (not labeled) covering the spermatic cord is seen on the right, while the cremasteric fascia and cremaster muscle are seen on the left after removal of the external spermatic fascia.

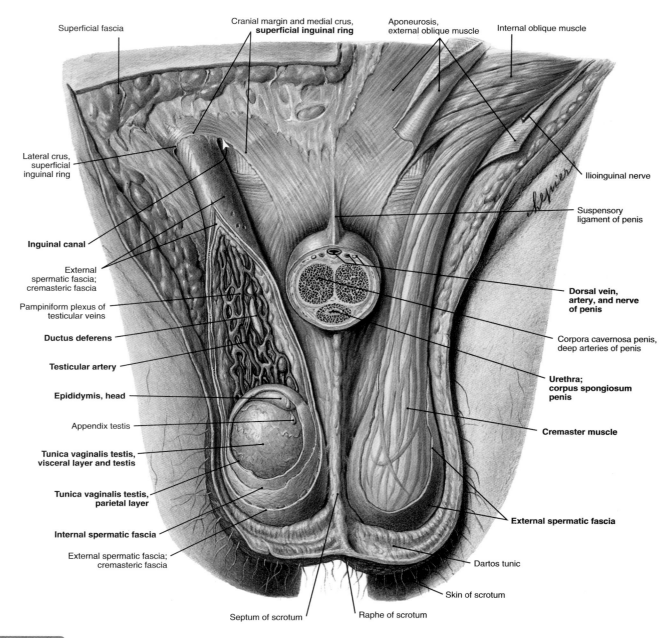

Superficial fascia

Cranial margin and medial crus,
superficial inguinal ring

Aponeurosis,
external oblique muscle

Internal oblique muscle

Lateral crus,
superficial
inguinal ring

Ilioinguinal nerve

Inguinal canal

Suspensory
ligament of penis

External
spermatic fascia;
cremasteric fascia

**Dorsal vein,
artery, and nerve
of penis**

Pampiniform plexus of
testicular veins

Ductus deferens

Corpora cavernosa penis,
deep arteries of penis

Testicular artery

Epididymis, head

**Urethra;
corpus spongiosum
penis**

Appendix testis

Cremaster muscle

**Tunica vaginalis testis,
visceral layer and testis**

**Tunica vaginalis testis,
parietal layer**

External spermatic fascia

Internal spermatic fascia

External spermatic fascia;
cremasteric fascia

Dartos tunic

Skin of scrotum

Septum of scrotum

Raphe of scrotum

FIGURE 237 **Spermatic Cord, Testis, Scrotum, and Cross Section of the Penis (Anterior View)**

NOTE: (1) The **cremaster muscle** descends within the spermatic cord to the testis. It represents a continuation of muscle fibers of the internal oblique muscle of the anterior abdominal wall.

(2) The **testicular vessels** and **ductus deferens** within the spermatic cord. Observe the covering layers of the right testis, the innermost one of which is the **visceral layer of the tunica vaginalis testis.**

(3) Venous blood from the **pampiniform plexus of veins** ascends in the testicular vein. On the right side this vein drains into the inferior vena cava, while on the left side it drains into the left renal vein. If the veins of the left scrotum become varicosed, it may indicate a problem with the left kidney or in the left pelvis along the course of the vein. This could be due to a renal tumor.

(4) The cremaster muscle is responsible for elevating the testis in the scrotal sac when the testicular environment is especially cold (as in a cold shower). It also elevates if the skin of the upper medial thigh is stimulated. This reaction is due to the so-called cremasteric reflex.

PLATE 238 Testis: Anterior and Lateral Views and Longitudinal Section

FIGURE 238.1 Right Testis and Epididymis (Anterior View) ▶

NOTE: The testis is suspended by its efferent duct system, which consists of the head, body, and tail of the epididymis, and this convoluted organ eventually leads to the ductus deferens (see Fig. 239.1).

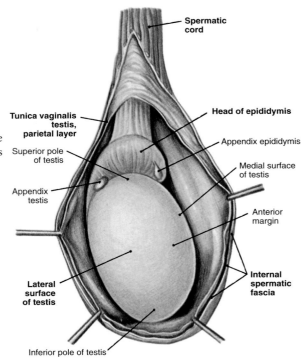

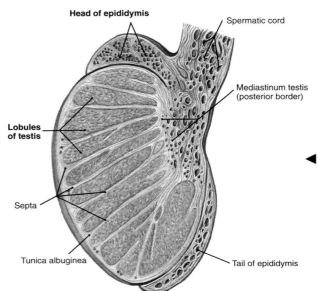

FIGURE 238.2 Longitudinal Section of Testis and Epididymis

NOTE: The lobular separation of the testis by the septa, and the thickened **tunica albuginea,** which encases the lobules. The vessels supplying the testis can be seen at its posterior border (mediastinum).

FIGURE 238.3 Right Testis and Epididymis (Lateral View) ▶

NOTE: The coverings of the testis represent evaginations of the layers forming the anterior abdominal wall. These evaginations precede the testis during its descent in the latter half of gestation. The comparable layers are as follows:

Anterior Abdominal Wall	Coverings of Testis
1. Skin	1. Skin ⎱ Scrotum
2. Superficial fascia	2. Dartos tunic ⎰
3. External oblique	3. External spermatic fascia
4. ⎰ Internal oblique	4. ⎰ Cremaster muscle and
5. ⎱ Transversus abdominis	5. ⎱ Cremasteric fascia
6. Transversalis fascia	6. Internal spermatic fascia
7. Extraperitoneal fat	7. Fatty layer
8. Peritoneum	8. Processus vaginalis

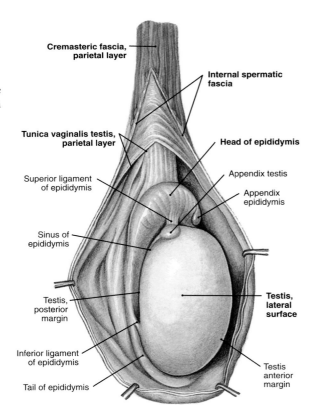

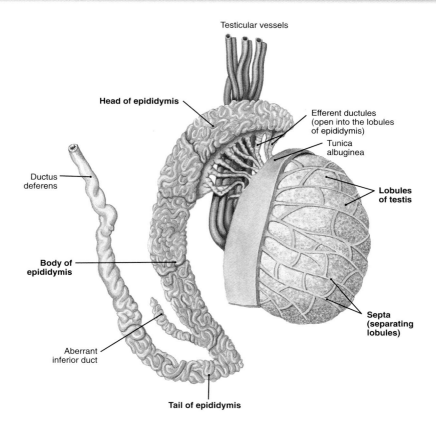

Testicular vessels

Head of epididymis

Efferent ductules
(open into the lobules
of epididymis)

Tunica
albuginea

Ductus
deferens

Lobules
of testis

Body of
epididymis

Septa
(separating
lobules)

Aberrant
inferior duct

Tail of epididymis

FIGURE 239.1 **Testis, Epididymis, and the Beginning of the Ductus Deferens**

NOTE: (1) With the tunica vaginalis and tunica albuginea removed, the testicular lobules, separated by septa and containing the seminiferous
tubules, are exposed.
(2) From the lobules a group of 8 to 10 fine efferent ductules open into the **head of the epididymis.** Observe the highly convoluted nature of the
epididymis. The head of the epididymis leads into the **body** and **tail,** which becomes the **ductus deferens.**
(3) The **testicular artery** (from the aorta) courses with the spermatic cord and the **pampiniform plexus** of veins.

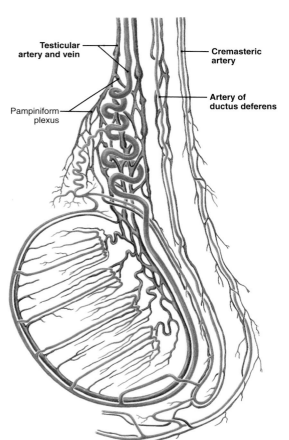

Testicular
artery and vein

Cremasteric
artery

Artery of
ductus deferens

Pampiniform
plexus

FIGURE 239.2 **Schematic Representation of the Blood Supply of
the Testis and Epididymis**

(1) The testis and epididymis are served by the **testicular artery** (from the aorta), the
artery of the ductus deferens (usually from the superior vesical artery), and the
cremasteric artery (from the inferior epigastric artery).
(2) The **pampiniform plexus** of veins drains into the testicular vein, which on the left
side flows into the left renal vein and on the right side opens into the inferior vena
cava.

PLATE 240 Testes in the Scrotum and Their Descent During Development

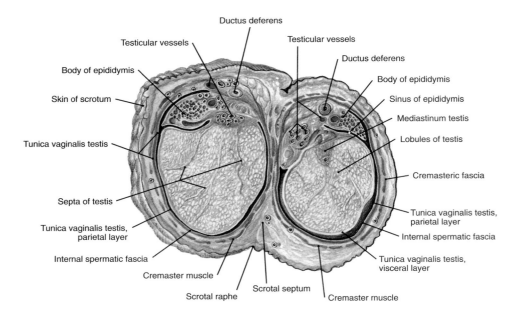

FIGURE 240.1 **Cross Section of Testis and Scrotum**

NOTE: (1) The scrotum is divided by the median raphe and septum into two lateral compartments, each surrounding an ovoid-shaped testis. The two scrotal compartments normally do not communicate.

(2) The **tunica vaginalis testis** consists of a **visceral layer** closely adherent to the testis and a **parietal layer,** which lines the inner surface of the internal spermatic fascia in the scrotum. A serous cavity or potential space between these two layers is a site where fluid might collect to form a **hydrocele.** These may be acquired or congenital.

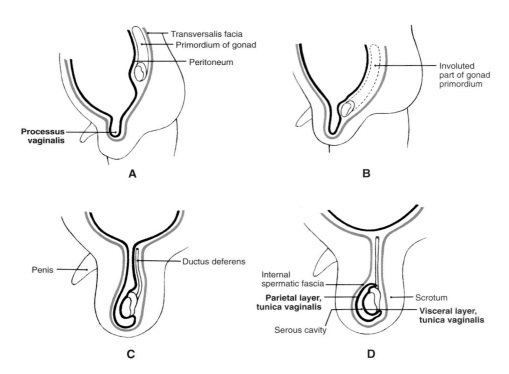

FIGURE 240.2 **Diagrammatic Representation of Four Stages in the Descent of the Testis**

NOTE: (1) (**A**) The testes commence development on the posterior wall of the fetus; (**B**) during the second trimester they attach to the posterior wall of the lower trunk at the boundary between the abdomen and pelvis in what is often called the "false pelvis."

(2) During the latter half of the seventh month of gestation, the testes begin their descent into the scrotum (**B** and **C**); this is normally completed by the ninth month (**D**).

(3) Attached to the peritoneum, each testis carries with it a peritoneal sac that surrounds the organ in the scrotum as the **parietal and visceral layers of the tunica vaginalis.** The peritoneum lining the inguinal canal then fuses, closing off its communication with the abdominal cavity.

(4) When this fusion does not occur, the pathway may be used by a loop of intestine to enter the scrotum, forming **an indirect or congenital hernia.**

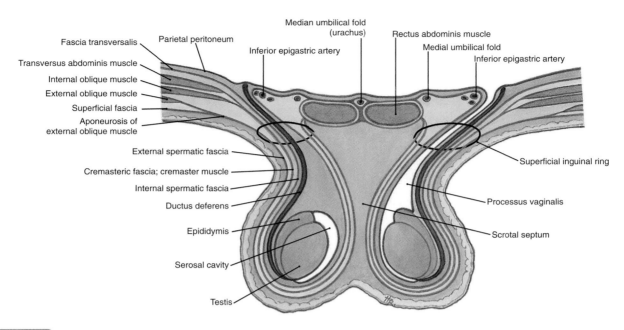

FIGURE 241.1 **Diagram of the Inguinal Canal**

NOTE: (1) On the right side (reader's left), the testis is descended into the scrotum, and the processus vaginalis is sealed, thereby obliterating the pathway of the testis into the scrotum. This situation would not allow a loop of intestine to descend into the scrotum.

(2) On the left side (reader's right), the processus vaginalis is still open. This could allow a loop of intestine the opportunity to descend into the scrotum, thereby creating an indirect (congenital) hernia (also see left side of Fig. 241.2).

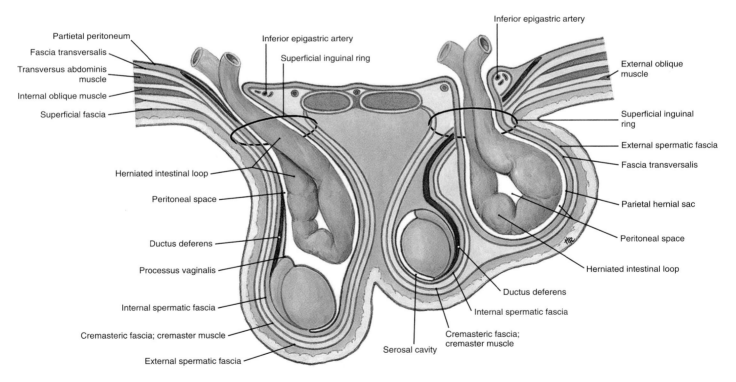

FIGURE 241.2 **Congenital (Indirect) and Acquired (Direct) Inguinal Hernias**

NOTE: (1) On the reader's left, a loop of intestine is shown entering the inguinal canal lateral to the inferior epigastric artery through the abdominal inguinal ring, thereby creating an indirect, congenital hernia.

(2) On the reader's right, a loop of intestine is shown herniated medial to the inferior epigastric artery (within the inguinal triangle), thereby forming a direct (acquired) inguinal hernia.

PLATE 242 Newborn Child: Anterior Abdominal Wall and Scrotum

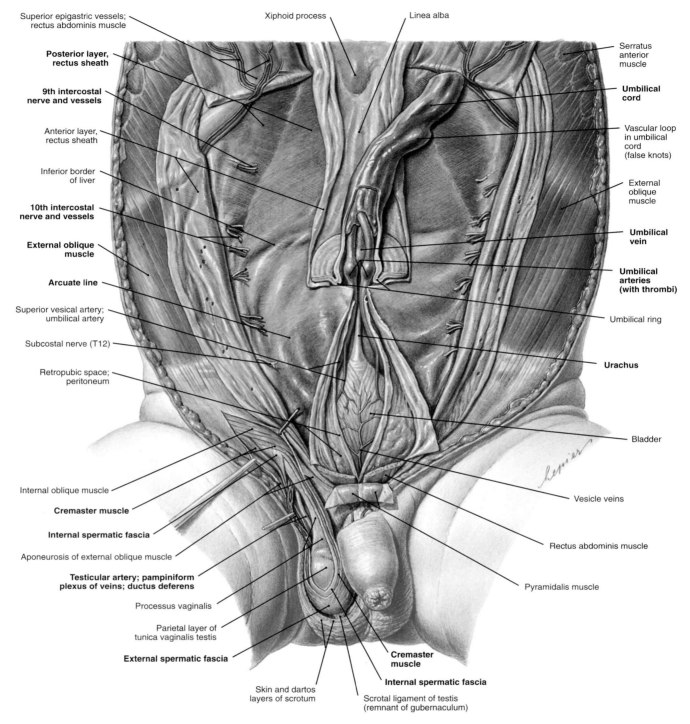

Superior epigastric vessels; rectus abdominis muscle

Posterior layer, rectus sheath

9th intercostal nerve and vessels

Anterior layer, rectus sheath

Inferior border of liver

10th intercostal nerve and vessels

External oblique muscle

Arcuate line

Superior vesical artery; umbilical artery

Subcostal nerve (T12)

Retropubic space; peritoneum

Internal oblique muscle

Cremaster muscle

Internal spermatic fascia

Aponeurosis of external oblique muscle

Testicular artery; pampiniform plexus of veins; ductus deferens

Processus vaginalis

Parietal layer of tunica vaginalis testis

External spermatic fascia

Skin and dartos layers of scrotum

Scrotal ligament of testis (remnant of gubernaculum)

Cremaster muscle

Internal spermatic fascia

Xiphoid process

Linea alba

Serratus anterior muscle

Umbilical cord

Vascular loop in umbilical cord (false knots)

External oblique muscle

Umbilical vein

Umbilical arteries (with thrombi)

Umbilical ring

Urachus

Bladder

Vesicle veins

Rectus abdominis muscle

Pyramidalis muscle

FIGURE 242 **Deep Dissection of the Anterior Abdominal Wall and the Umbilical Region in the Newborn**

NOTE: (1) The anterior layer of the rectus sheath is reflected laterally, and the two rectus abdominis muscles have been cut near the symphysis pubis and turned upward (almost out of view). This exposes the posterior layer of the rectus sheath and the **arcuate line.**

(2) An incision has been made in the midline between the umbilicus and the pubic symphysis exposing the **bladder, urachus,** the **umbilical arteries,** and the **umbilical vein.**

(3) The anterior aspect of the right spermatic cord and scrotal sac have been opened to show the ductus deferens and the **tunica vaginalis testis** surrounding the testis.

(4) The severed umbilical cord, usually 1 to 2 cm in diameter and about 50 cm, or 20 in., long. It contains the two umbilical arteries and the umbilical vein surrounded by a mucoid form of connective tissue called Wharton's jelly.

(5) At times, the umbilical vessels form harmless loops in the umbilical cord called "false knots." More rarely, looping of the cord may be of functional significance and such "true knots" may alter the circulation to and from the fetus.

(6) The bulges in the umbilical arteries. These are in situ blood clots that occlude the arteries but which are probably postmortem phenomena in this dissection.

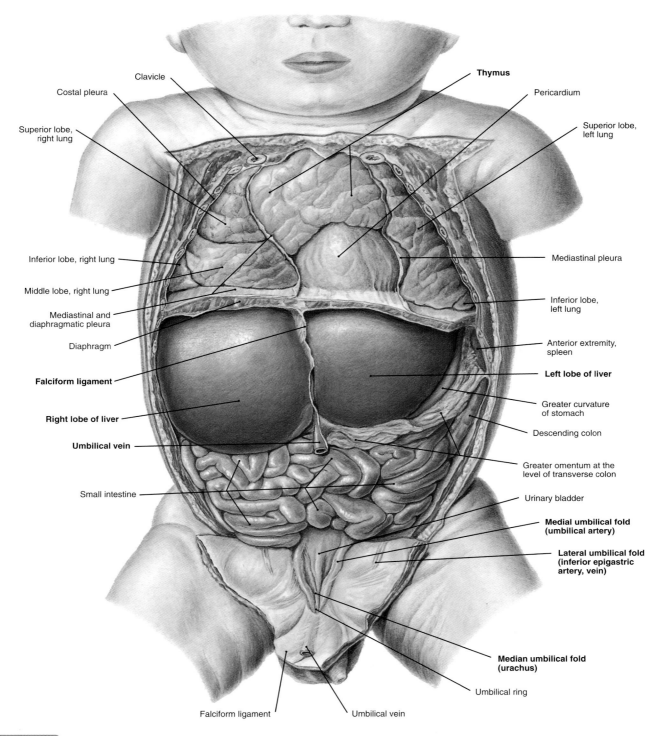

Clavicle

Costal pleura

Superior lobe,
right lung

Inferior lobe, right lung

Middle lobe, right lung

Mediastinal and
diaphragmatic pleura

Diaphragm

Falciform ligament

Right lobe of liver

Umbilical vein

Small intestine

Thymus

Pericardium

Superior lobe,
left lung

Mediastinal pleura

Inferior lobe,
left lung

Anterior extremity,
spleen

Left lobe of liver

Greater curvature
of stomach

Descending colon

Greater omentum at the
level of transverse colon

Urinary bladder

**Medial umbilical fold
(umbilical artery)**

**Lateral umbilical fold
(inferior epigastric
artery, vein)**

**Median umbilical fold
(urachus)**

Umbilical ring

Falciform ligament

Umbilical vein

FIGURE 243 Abdominal and Thoracic Viscera Observed In Situ in the Newborn Child

NOTE: (1) The anterior body wall has been removed in this newborn child, uncovering the viscera. Observe the umbilical ligaments on the inner surface of the lower wall.

(2) The average newborn child weighs about 3300 g (7 lb) and measures about 50 cm (20 in.) from the top of the head to the sole of the foot. The umbilicus is located about 1.5 cm below the midpoint of this crown-to-heel length.

(3) The transverse diameter of the abdomen in the newborn is greatest above the umbilicus due to the inordinate proportion of the abdomen occupied by the liver. The average weight of the liver in the neonate is about 120 g (4% of the body weight). In the adult the liver weighs 12 to 13 times that at birth (but only 2.5%–3.5% of the body weight).

(4) The truncated shape of the thorax and the large thymus, weighing about 10 g at birth (0.42% of body weight at birth compared with 0.03%–0.05% in the adult).

(5) The facts above are taken from: Crelin ES. Functional anatomy of the newborn, New Haven, CT: Yale University Press, 1973, which is an excellent short monograph (87 pages).

PLATE 244 | Abdominal, Thoracic, and Male Urogenital Organs (Projections)

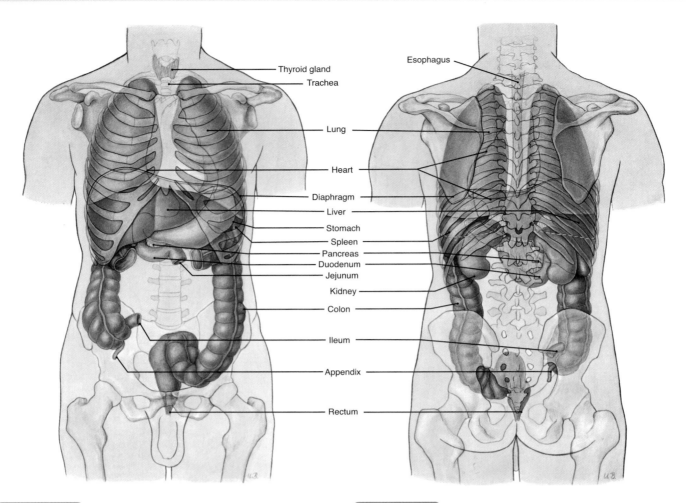

FIGURE 244.1 Surface Projection of Thoracic and Abdominal Organs (Anterior View)

FIGURE 244.2 Surface Projection of Thoracic and Abdominal Organs (Posterior View)

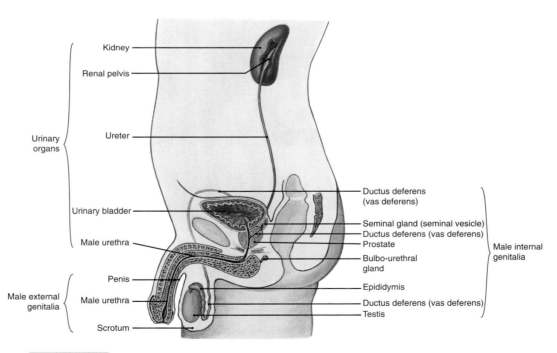

FIGURE 244.3 Surface Projection of Male Urogenital Organs (Left Lateral View)

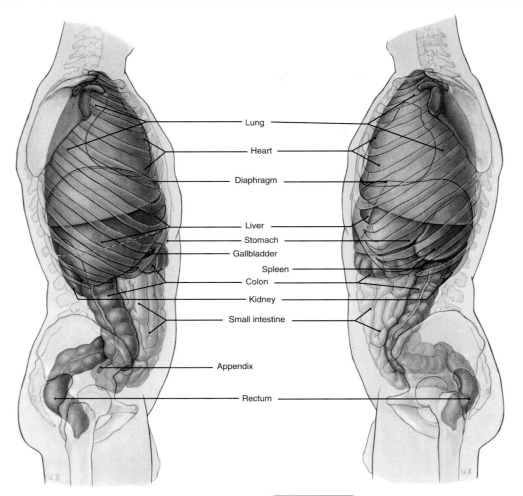

FIGURE 245.1 Surface Projection of Thoracic and Abdominal Organs (Right Lateral View)

FIGURE 245.2 Surface Projection of Thoracic and Abdominal Organs (Left Lateral View)

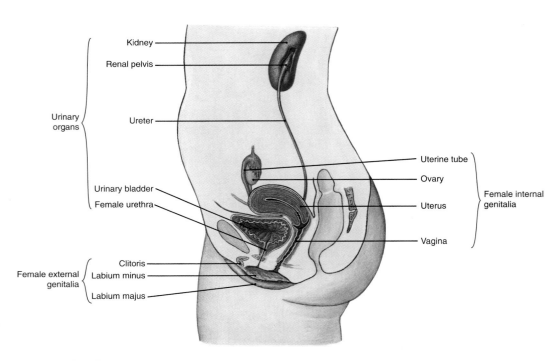

FIGURE 245.3 Surface Projection of Female Urogenital Organs (Left Lateral View)

PLATE 246 Median Sagittal Section: Male Abdomen and Pelvis

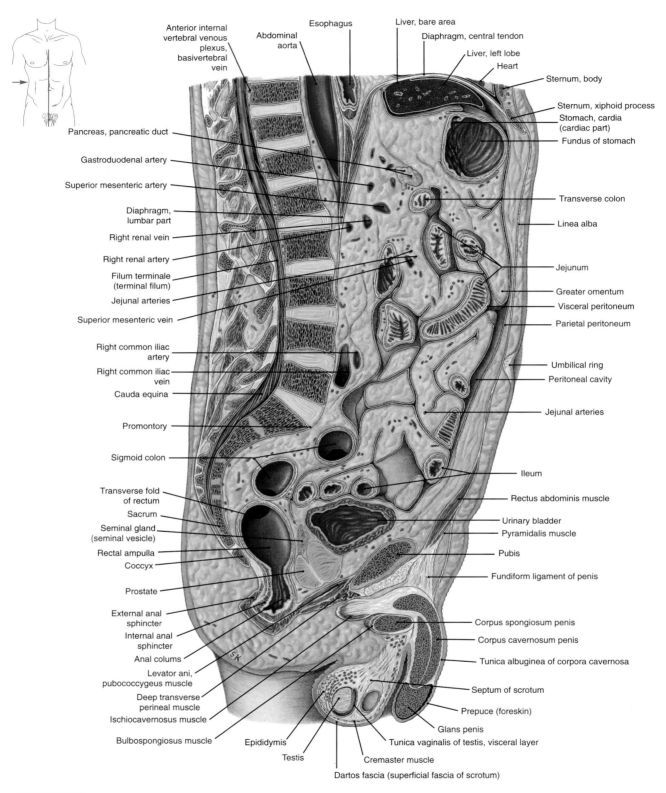

Anterior internal
vertebral venous
plexus,
basivertebral
vein

Esophagus

Abdominal
aorta

Liver, bare area

Diaphragm, central tendon

Liver, left lobe

Heart

Sternum, body

Sternum, xiphoid process

Stomach, cardia
(cardiac part)

Fundus of stomach

Pancreas, pancreatic duct

Gastroduodenal artery

Superior mesenteric artery

Diaphragm,
lumbar part

Right renal vein

Right renal artery

Filum terminale
(terminal filum)

Jejunal arteries

Superior mesenteric vein

Right common iliac
artery

Right common iliac
vein

Cauda equina

Promontory

Sigmoid colon

Transverse fold
of rectum

Sacrum

Seminal gland
(seminal vesicle)

Rectal ampulla

Coccyx

Prostate

External anal
sphincter

Internal anal
sphincter

Anal colums

Levator ani,
pubococcygeus muscle

Deep transverse
perineal muscle

Ischiocavernosus muscle

Bulbospongiosus muscle

Epididymis

Testis

Transverse colon

Linea alba

Jejunum

Greater omentum

Visceral peritoneum

Parietal peritoneum

Umbilical ring

Peritoneal cavity

Jejunal arteries

Ileum

Rectus abdominis muscle

Urinary bladder

Pyramidalis muscle

Pubis

Fundiform ligament of penis

Corpus spongiosum penis

Corpus cavernosum penis

Tunica albuginea of corpora cavernosa

Septum of scrotum

Prepuce (foreskin)

Glans penis

Tunica vaginalis of testis, visceral layer

Cremaster muscle

Dartos fascia (superficial fascia of scrotum)

FIGURE 246 **Median Sagittal Section of the Male Abdomen and Pelvis**

NOTE: (1) This figure is viewed from the right lateral aspect. Observe, however, that the external genitalia and anterior aspect of the pelvis are sectioned to the left of the median plane.

(2) The **filum terminale** and **cauda equina** within the central canal of the vertebral column. Also observe the seminal vesicle and prostate gland on the posterior aspect of the urinary bladder.

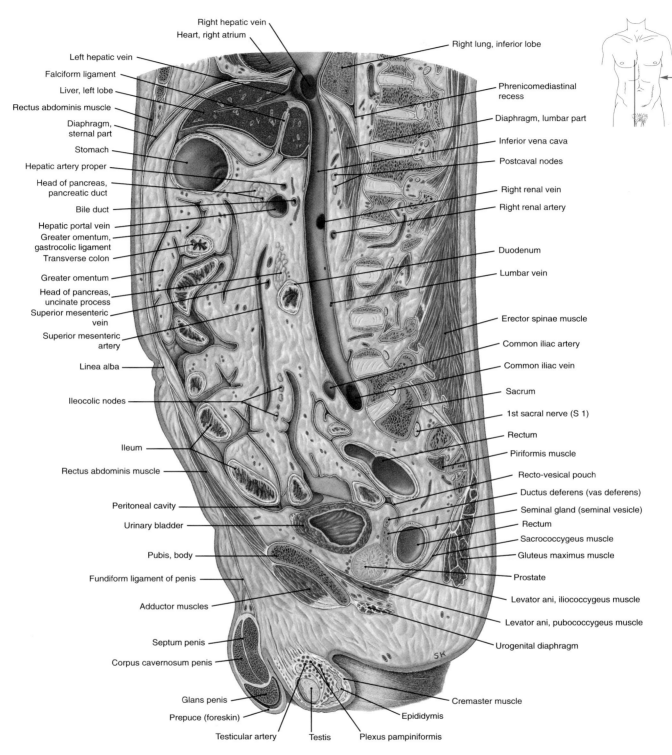

Right hepatic vein
Heart, right atrium
Left hepatic vein
Falciform ligament
Liver, left lobe
Rectus abdominis muscle
Diaphragm, sternal part
Stomach
Hepatic artery proper
Head of pancreas, pancreatic duct
Bile duct
Hepatic portal vein
Greater omentum, gastrocolic ligament
Transverse colon
Greater omentum
Head of pancreas, uncinate process
Superior mesenteric vein
Superior mesenteric artery
Linea alba
Ileocolic nodes
Ileum
Rectus abdominis muscle
Peritoneal cavity
Urinary bladder
Pubis, body
Fundiform ligament of penis
Adductor muscles
Septum penis
Corpus cavernosum penis
Glans penis
Prepuce (foreskin)
Testicular artery
Testis
Plexus pampiniformis

Right lung, inferior lobe
Phrenicomediastinal recess
Diaphragm, lumbar part
Inferior vena cava
Postcaval nodes
Right renal vein
Right renal artery
Duodenum
Lumbar vein
Erector spinae muscle
Common iliac artery
Common iliac vein
Sacrum
1st sacral nerve (S 1)
Rectum
Piriformis muscle
Recto-vesical pouch
Ductus deferens (vas deferens)
Seminal gland (seminal vesicle)
Rectum
Sacrococcygeus muscle
Gluteus maximus muscle
Prostate
Levator ani, iliococcygeus muscle
Levator ani, pubococcygeus muscle
Urogenital diaphragm
Cremaster muscle
Epididymis

FIGURE 247 **Paramedian Section of the Male Abdomen and Pelvis**

NOTE: (1) This section bisects the inferior vena cava longitudinally as that vessel ascends along the posterior abdominal wall. Thus, this section was made to the right of the midline, and it is viewed from the left side.

(2) The head and the uncinate process of the pancreas, the hepatic artery, and the portal vein, all right-sided structures.

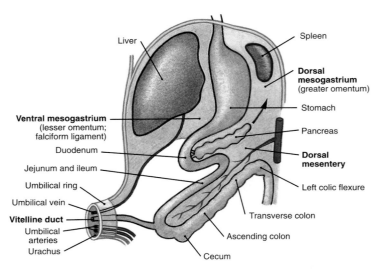

FIGURE 248.1 Developing Gastrointestinal Organs and Their Mesenteries

NOTE: (1) As the primitive gastrointestinal tube develops within the abdominal celom, it is suspended from the body wall by primitive peritoneal reflections, both ventrally and dorsally. The early peritoneal attachments to the expanding stomach are called the ventral mesogastrium and dorsal mesogastrium, whereas the dorsal mesentery develops on the posterior aspect of the primitive small and large intestine.

(2) The embryonic liver develops into the ventral mesogastrium, thereby dividing this ventral peritoneal attachment into:
- (a) A portion between the anterior body wall and the liver, which eventually becomes the falciform ligament and
- (b) A portion between the liver and the stomach, which becomes the lesser omentum.

(3) On the dorsal aspect:
- (a) The pancreas develops in relation to the primitive duodenum, both of which lose their mesenteries during gut rotation to become retroperitoneal.
- (b) The dorsal mesogastrium, attaching along the greater curvature of the stomach and, rotating with the stomach, becomes the greater omentum. This eventually encases the transverse colon.
- (c) The dorsal mesentery remains attached to the small intestine, while the ascending and descending colon become displaced to the right and left side, respectively, becoming adherent to the posterior body wall.
- (d) The sigmoid colon usually retains its mesentery, while that of the rectum becomes obliterated.

(4) Near the cecal end of the small intestine, the developing gastrointestinal canal communicates with the vitelline duct. Before birth, this duct usually becomes resorbed; when it persists (3% of cases), it results in a diverticulum of the ileum called Meckel's diverticulum.

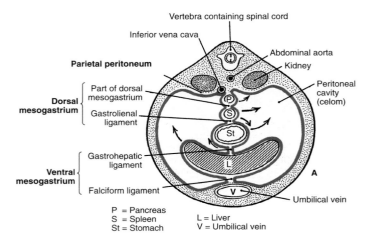

FIGURE 248.2A Cross-Sectional Diagram of Development of Mesogastria: Early Stage (Approximately 6 Weeks)

NOTE: (1) The primitive peritoneal reflections are indicated in red. The arrows show the direction of growth and movement by the various organs shown in Figure 249.1B.

(2) At this early stage, the peritoneum completely surrounds the organs in the upper abdominal region (visceral peritoneum) and attaches peripherally to the body wall (parietal peritoneum). Attaching along the posterior border of the stomach, the dorsal mesogastrium then surrounds the spleen and pancreas. Anterior to the stomach, the liver becomes interposed between the stomach and the anterior body wall. This forms the gastrohepatic ligament (also called the lesser omentum) between the lesser curvature of the stomach and the liver and the falciform ligament between the liver and the anterior body wall.

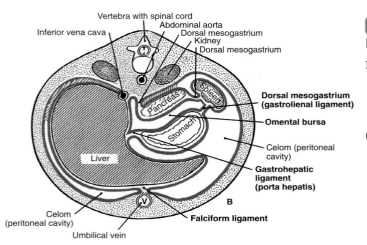

FIGURE 248.2B Cross-Sectional Diagram of Development of Mesogastria: Late Fetal Stage

NOTE: (1) With the rotation of the organs (in the direction of the arrows in Fig. 248.2A), the liver grows into the celomic cavity toward the right and contacts the inferior vena cava, while the stomach rotates such that its dorsal mesogastrium (greater curvature) is shifted to the left.

(2) The reflection of dorsal mesogastrium between the stomach and the spleen becomes established as the gastrolienal ligament, while one layer of mesogastrium surrounding the pancreas and duodenum fuses to the posterior body wall. This fixates these two organs with a layer of peritoneum on their anterior surface, causing them to become retroperitoneal. The omental bursa also develops posterior to the stomach and anterior to the pancreas.

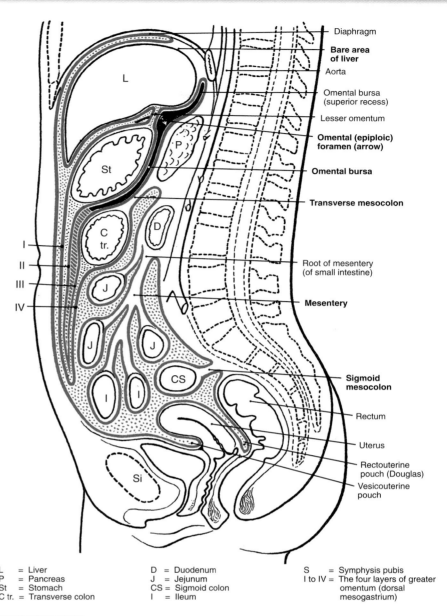

L	= Liver	D	= Duodenum	S	= Symphysis pubis
P	= Pancreas	J	= Jejunum	I to IV =	The four layers of greater
St	= Stomach	CS	= Sigmoid colon		omentum (dorsal
C tr.	= Transverse colon	I	= Ileum		mesogastrium)

FIGURE 249.2 Peritoneal Reflections in Adult Female ▲

NOTE: (1) The greater peritoneal sac (red stippled) lies between the layers of visceral and parietal peritoneum. The greater peritoneal sac communicates with the lesser peritoneal sac (omental bursa; black) through the omental (epiploic) foramen (of Winslow).
(2) Dorsally, the roots of three distinct peritoneal mesenteries can be observed:
    (a) The transverse mesocolon,
    (b) The mesentery surrounding the small intestine, and
    (c) The sigmoid mesocolon.
(3) Behind the stomach and transverse colon, observe the retroperitoneal pancreas and duodenum. A portion of the liver is not surrounded by peritoneum (bare area of the liver) and lies adjacent to the diaphragm.

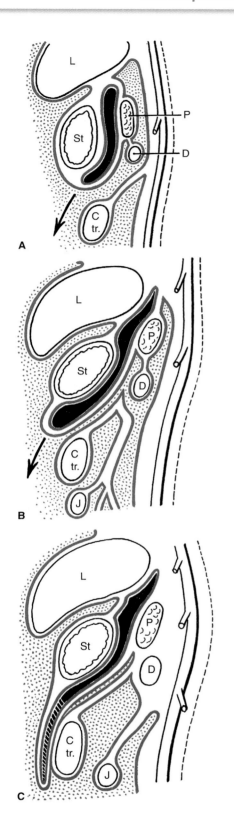

FIGURE 249.1A–C Stages in the Development of the Omental Bursa (Sagittal Diagrams)

NOTE: (1) At 4 weeks, the dorsal border of the stomach grows faster than the ventral border, assisting in the rotation of the stomach on its long axis. The greater curvature and its dorsal mesogastrium become directed to the left, whereas the lesser curvature and the ventral mesogastrium are directed to the right.
(2) By 8 weeks (**A**), the omental bursa (black) forms behind the stomach between the two leaves of dorsal mesogastrium. The pancreas and duodenum are still surrounded by dorsal mesentery. As gut rotation continues, the dorsal mesogastrium extends inferiorly (**B,** arrow) to form the greater omentum, which becomes a double reflection (four leaves) of the dorsal mesogastrium "trapping" the cavity of the omental bursa between the second and third leaves.
(3) Continued development (**C**) results in a further descent of the greater omentum over the abdominal viscera and a fusion (cross-hatched) of the second and third leaves inferiorly.

PLATE 250 Abdominal Cavity 1: Greater Omentum

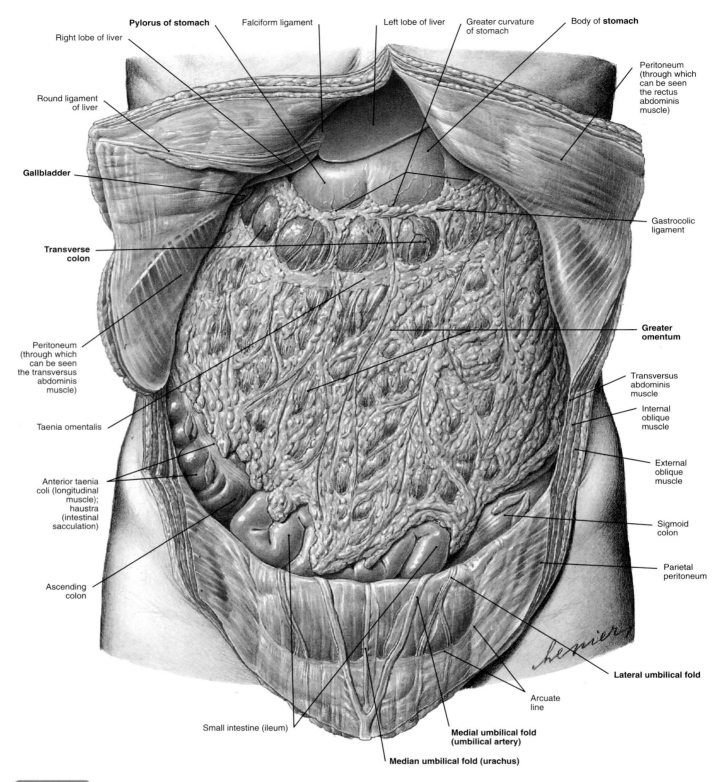

Pylorus of stomach
Right lobe of liver
Round ligament of liver
Gallbladder
Transverse colon
Peritoneum (through which can be seen the transversus abdominis muscle)
Taenia omentalis
Anterior taenia coli (longitudinal muscle); haustra (intestinal sacculation)
Ascending colon
Small intestine (ileum)

Falciform ligament
Left lobe of liver
Greater curvature of stomach
Body of stomach
Peritoneum (through which can be seen the rectus abdominis muscle)
Gastrocolic ligament
Greater omentum
Transversus abdominis muscle
Internal oblique muscle
External oblique muscle
Sigmoid colon
Parietal peritoneum
Lateral umbilical fold
Arcuate line
Medial umbilical fold (umbilical artery)
Median umbilical fold (urachus)

FIGURE 250 Abdominal Cavity, Viscera Left Intact

NOTE: (1) The **greater omentum.** It attaches along the greater curvature of the stomach, covers the intestines like an apron, and extends inferiorly almost to the pelvis.

(2) The **falciform ligament,** a remnant of the ventral mesogastrium, extends between the liver and the anterior body wall and separates the left and right lobes of the liver. The **round ligament** is the remnant of the obliterated umbilical vein.

(3) On the inner surface of the anterior abdominal wall, identify the following folds:
   (a) **Median umbilical fold:** remnant of the urachus, which extended between the bladder and the umbilicus in the fetus.
   (b) **Medial umbilical folds:** the obliterated umbilical arteries, which were the continuation of the superior vesical arteries to the umbilicus in the fetus.
   (c) **Lateral umbilical folds:** a folds of peritoneum over the inferior epigastric vessels.

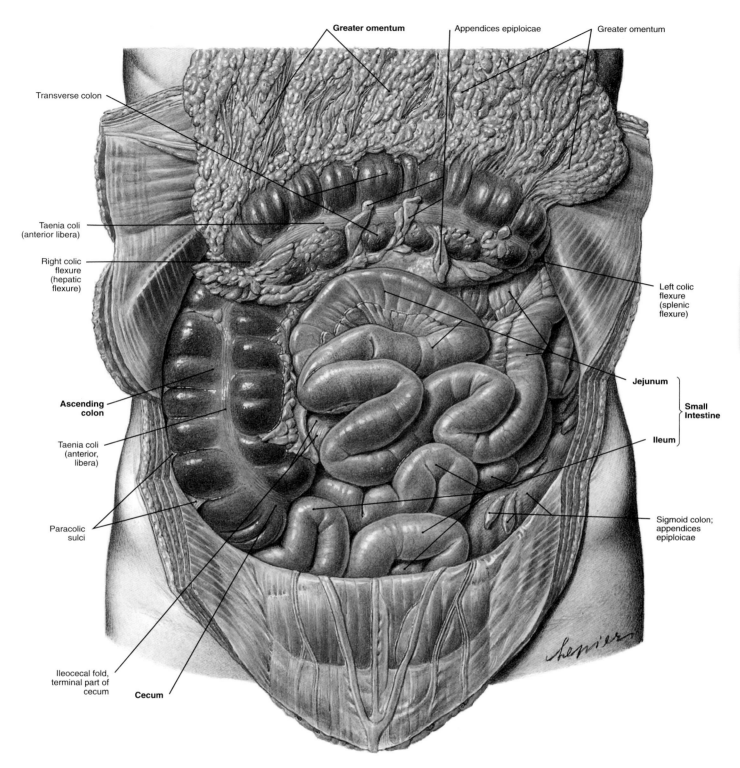

Greater omentum   Appendices epiploicae   Greater omentum

Transverse colon

Taenia coli
(anterior libera)

Right colic
flexure
(hepatic
flexure)

Left colic
flexure
(splenic
flexure)

Jejunum

Ascending
colon

Small
Intestine

Ileum

Taenia coli
(anterior,
libera)

Paracolic
sulci

Sigmoid colon;
appendices
epiploicae

Ileocecal fold,
terminal part of
cecum

Cecum

FIGURE 251 **Abdominal Cavity, Ascending Colon, and Transverse Colon and Its Mesocolon**

NOTE: (1) With the greater omentum reflected upward, the transverse colon is crossing the abdominal cavity from right to left in continuity with
the ascending colon on the right and the descending colon on the left.

(2) Longitudinal muscles called **taeniae,** along the outer surface of the colon. These muscles are shorter than the other coats of the large intestine
causing sacculations, which are called **haustrae.**

(3) Smooth irregular fatty masses called **appendices epiploicae** are suspended from the large intestine. These assist in the identification of the
large gut.

(4) Below the mesocolon (inframesocolic) can be seen the small intestine, which consists of three portions: the **duodenum, jejunum,** and **ileum.**
The outer wall of the small intestine is smooth and glistening and is not sacculated.

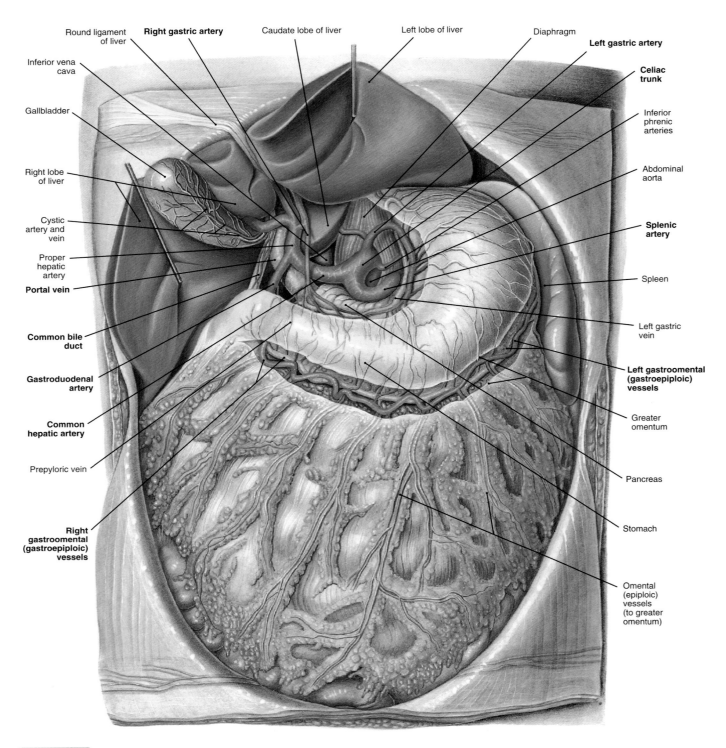

Round ligament of liver
Right gastric artery
Caudate lobe of liver
Left lobe of liver
Diaphragm
Left gastric artery
Inferior vena cava
Celiac trunk
Gallbladder
Inferior phrenic arteries
Right lobe of liver
Abdominal aorta
Cystic artery and vein
Splenic artery
Proper hepatic artery
Portal vein
Spleen
Common bile duct
Left gastric vein
Gastroduodenal artery
Left gastroomental (gastroepiploic) vessels
Common hepatic artery
Greater omentum
Prepyloric vein
Pancreas
Right gastroomental (gastroepiploic) vessels
Stomach
Omental (epiploic) vessels (to greater omentum)

FIGURE 252 Abdominal Cavity: Celiac Trunk and Its Branches

NOTE: (1) The lobes of the liver have been elevated and the lesser omentum has been removed between the lesser curvature of the stomach and the liver to reveal the **celiac trunk** (located anterior to the T12 vertebra) and its branches. These are:

(a) The **left gastric artery,** which courses along the lesser curvature of the stomach and anastomoses with the right gastric artery, a branch of the hepatic artery.

(b) The **splenic artery,** which courses to the left toward the hilum of the spleen.

(c) The **hepatic artery,** which courses to the right and gives off the gastroduodenal artery before dividing to enter the lobes of the liver.

(2) The **gastroduodenal artery** gives rise to the **right gastroomental (gastroepiploic) artery,** which follows along the greater curvature of the stomach to anastomose with the **left gastroomental (gastroepiploic) branch** of the splenic artery.

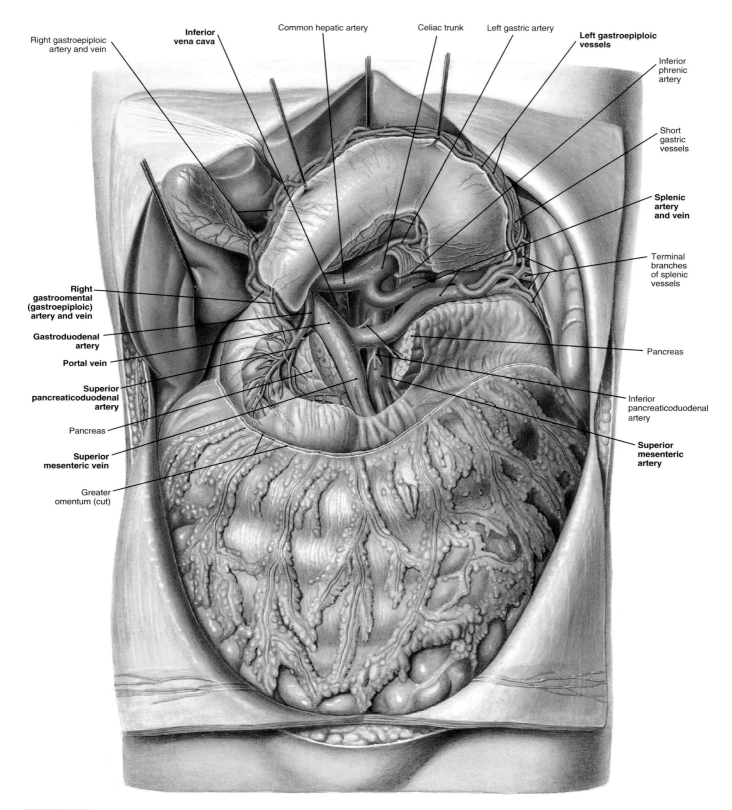

Right gastroepiploic artery and vein

Inferior vena cava

Common hepatic artery

Celiac trunk

Left gastric artery

Left gastroepiploic vessels

Inferior phrenic artery

Short gastric vessels

Splenic artery and vein

Terminal branches of splenic vessels

Right gastroomental (gastroepiploic) artery and vein

Gastroduodenal artery

Portal vein

Superior pancreaticoduodenal artery

Pancreas

Superior mesenteric vein

Greater omentum (cut)

Pancreas

Inferior pancreaticoduodenal artery

Superior mesenteric artery

FIGURE 253 **Abdominal Cavity (4): Splenic Vessels and Formation of the Portal Vein**

NOTE: (1) The greater omentum has been cut along the greater curvature of the stomach. The stomach is lifted to expose its posterior surface and the underlying pancreas, duodenum, and blood vessels. A part of the pancreas has been removed to reveal the **portal vein** formed by the junction of the **splenic and superior mesenteric veins.**

(2) The tortuous **splenic artery** in its course to the splenic hilum, and the **gastroduodenal artery,** behind the pyloric end of the stomach dividing into **right gastroomental** and **superior pancreaticoduodenal arteries.**

PLATE 254 Stomach: Arteries and Veins

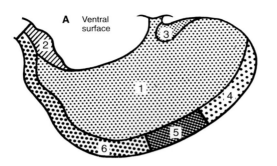
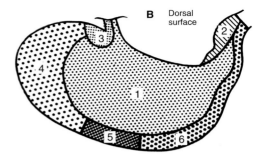

FIGURE 254.1A, B **Regional Arterial Supply to the Stomach**

1. Left gastric artery
2. Right gastric artery
3. Left inferior phrenic artery
4. Short gastric artery
5. Left gastroomental artery
6. Right gastroomental artery

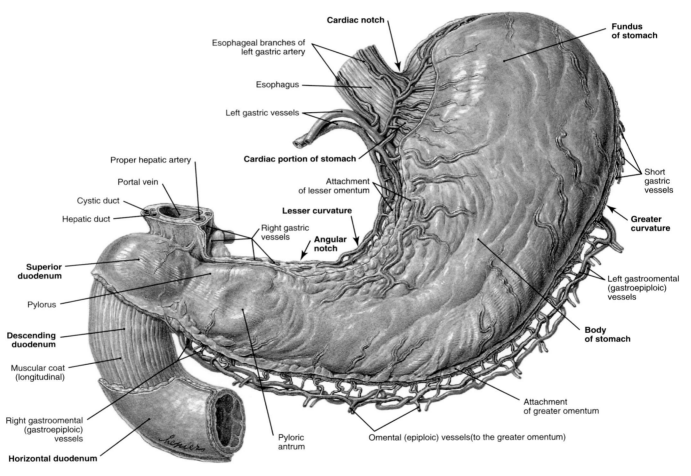

FIGURE 254.2 **Anterior View of Stomach**

NOTE: (1) The stomach is a dilated muscular sac situated in the gastrointestinal tract between the esophagus (cardiac end) and the duodenum (pyloric end). It consists of an upper portion called the **fundus,** a middle portion, the **body,** and a tapering lower part, the **pyloric region.**

(2) Although the shape of the stomach varies, it presents two curvatures as borders. The **greater curvature** is directed toward the left and to it is attached the **greater omentum.** This border forms an acute angle with the esophagus called the **cardiac notch.**

(3) The **lesser curvature** constitutes the right border of the stomach and along this edge the **lesser omentum** is attached.

(4) The blood vessels supplying the stomach include:

    (a) The **left and right gastric arteries** along the lesser curvature,

    (b) The **left and right (gastroepiploic) arteries** along the greater curvature, and

    (c) The **short gastric branches** of the **splenic artery.** Observe that the **esophageal branches** of the left **gastric artery** supply the cardiac end of the stomach.

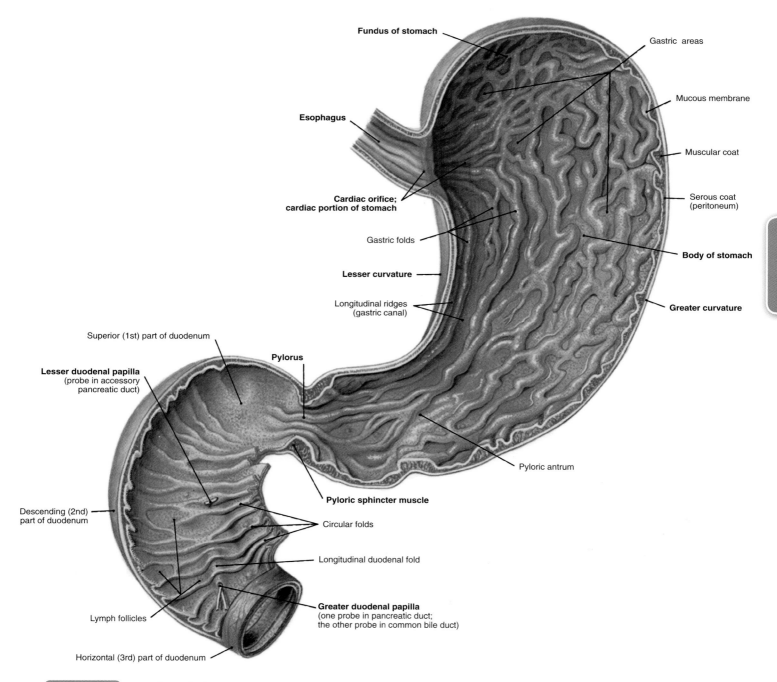

Fundus of stomach

Gastric areas

Mucous membrane

Esophagus

Muscular coat

Cardiac orifice;
cardiac portion of stomach

Serous coat
(peritoneum)

Gastric folds

Body of stomach

Lesser curvature

Greater curvature

Longitudinal ridges
(gastric canal)

Superior (1st) part of duodenum

Pylorus

Lesser duodenal papilla
(probe in accessory
pancreatic duct)

Pyloric antrum

Pyloric sphincter muscle

Descending (2nd)
part of duodenum

Circular folds

Longitudinal duodenal fold

Greater duodenal papilla
(one probe in pancreatic duct;
the other probe in common bile duct)

Lymph follicles

Horizontal (3rd) part of duodenum

FIGURE 255 **Interior of the Stomach and Upper Duodenum**

NOTE: (1) The mucosal lining of the stomach shows a series of longitudinally oriented gastric folds or empty rugae, which tend to disappear when the stomach is full and distended. These folds are more regular along the lesser curvature and form the grooved gastric canal. Food does not travel along this canal (magenstrasse).

(2) The surface of the first part of the duodenum is smooth, but the circular ridges characteristic of the small intestine commence in the second, or descending, portion of the duodenum.

(3) A circular muscle, the **pyloric sphincter,** guards the pyloric junction of the stomach with the duodenum. It diminishes the lumen of the gastrointestinal tract at this point. The pylorus is to the right of midline at the level of the first lumbar vertebra.

(4) The openings in the wall of the duodenum. The **greater duodenal papilla** serves as the site of the openings of both the common bile duct and the main pancreatic duct. The accessory pancreatic duct opens 2 cm more proximally through the lesser duodenal papilla.

PLATE 256 Celiac Trunk and Its Branches

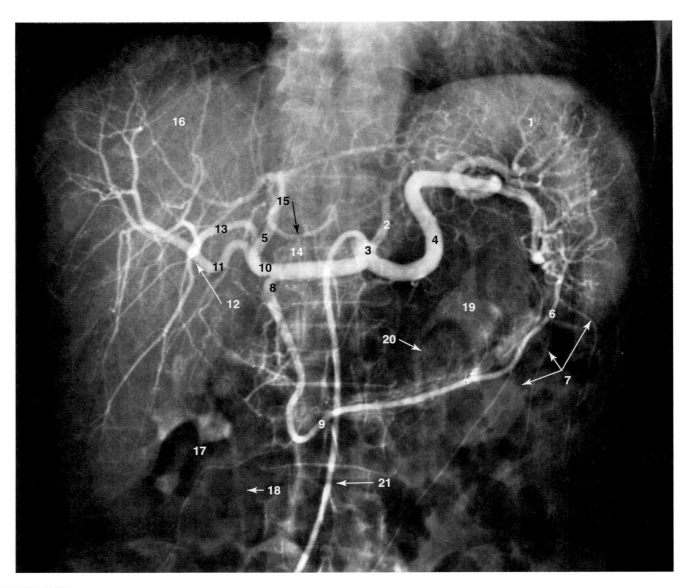

FIGURE 256 Celiac Trunk Arteriogram

NOTE: (1) This figure is a negative print from a radiograph of the upper abdomen after injection of a contrast medium through a catheter (21, arrow) in the abdominal aorta directed upward to the point where the **celiac trunk** [3] branches from the aorta.

(2) The three primary vessels arising from the celiac trunk [3] are the **left gastric artery** [2], the **splenic artery** [4], directed toward the spleen [1], and the **common hepatic artery** [5], which courses directly to the right toward the liver [16].

(3) The **left gastroomental (gastroepiploic) artery** arises from one of the lower hilar branches of the splenic artery. As it courses along the greater curvature to anastomose with the **right gastroomental (gastroepiploic) artery,** the **left gastroomental (gastroepiploic)** artery gives rise to omental **(epiploic) arteries** [7, arrows], which descend to supply the greater omentum. The right gastroomental (gastroepiploic) artery [9] arises from the **gastroduodenal artery** [8], which courses downward from the **common hepatic artery** [5].

(4) Beyond the origin of the gastroduodenal artery [8] the common hepatic artery [5] is called the **proper hepatic artery** [10].

(5) The proper hepatic artery [10] divides into the **right hepatic artery** [11], from which branches the **cystic artery** [12] to the gallbladder, the **middle hepatic artery** [13], and the **left hepatic artery** [14, arrow]. The hepatic vessels supply the liver.

(6) From the right hepatic artery [14] in this individual branches the **right gastric artery** [15, arrow]. Just as frequently, the right gastric artery arises from the common hepatic artery [5]. The right gastric artery courses along the lesser curvature of the stomach to anastomose with the **left gastric artery** [2].

(7) The right renal pelvis [17] and the right ureter [18, arrow] can be seen inferiorly. Because of the liver, these structures on the right side are significantly lower than the left renal pelvis [19] and the origin of the left ureter [20, arrow].

(From Wicke, 4th ed.)

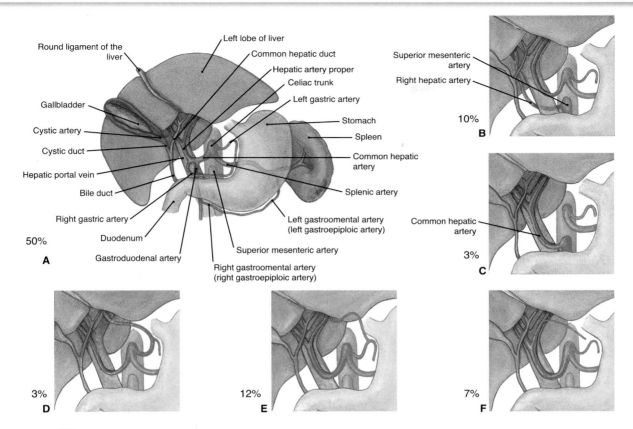

FIGURE 257.1A–F **Variations in the Blood Supply to the Liver**

A: Normal pattern as shown in most diagrams.
B: Superior mesenteric artery helping to supply the liver.
C: Common hepatic artery arising from the superior mesenteric artery.
D: Left gastric artery supplying the left lobe of the liver.
E: Branch of the left gastric artery helping to supply the left lobe of the liver (with the left branch of the hepatic artery).
F: An accessory branch from the proper hepatic artery supplying the lesser curvature of the stomach.

(In 25% of cases, the superior mesenteric artery participates in the arterial supply to the liver.)

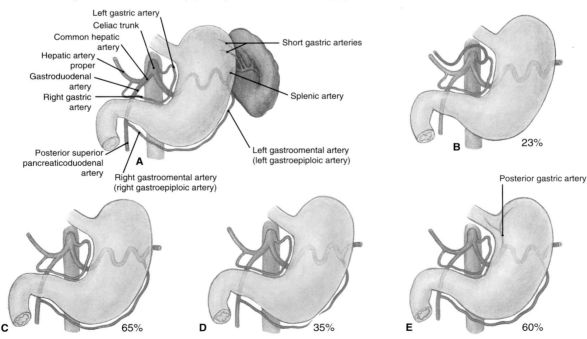

FIGURE 257.2A–E **Variations in the Arterial Blood Supply to the Stomach**

A: Normal pattern as shown in most diagrams.
B: Left gastric artery participating in the supply of the left lobe of the liver.
C: Anastomosis between the right and left gastroomental (gastroepiploic) arteries along the greater curvature.
D: No anastomosis between the right and left gastroomental (gastroepiploic) arteries along the greater curvature.
E: An accessory posterior gastric artery (from the splenic) that helps supply the posterior surface of the stomach.

PLATE 258 Stomach, In Situ; the Omental Foramen

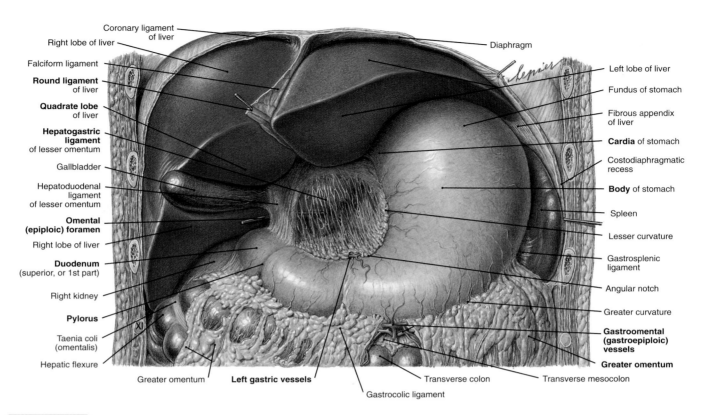

Coronary ligament of liver
Right lobe of liver
Falciform ligament
Round ligament *of liver*
Quadrate lobe *of liver*
Hepatogastric ligament *of lesser omentum*
Gallbladder
Hepatoduodenal ligament of lesser omentum
Omental (epiploic) foramen
Right lobe of liver
Duodenum *(superior, or 1st part)*
Right kidney
Pylorus
Taenia coli (omentalis)
Hepatic flexure
Greater omentum   **Left gastric vessels**
Gastrocolic ligament

Diaphragm
Left lobe of liver
Fundus of stomach
Fibrous appendix of liver
Cardia *of stomach*
Costodiaphragmatic recess
Body *of stomach*
Spleen
Lesser curvature
Gastrosplenic ligament
Angular notch
Greater curvature
Gastroomental (gastroepiploic) vessels
Greater omentum
Transverse mesocolon
Transverse colon

FIGURE 258.1 **Lesser Omentum, Stomach, Liver, and Spleen**

NOTE: (1) The liver is elevated and a probe inserted through the **omental (epiploic) foramen** into the vestibule of the **omental bursa.** By way of this opening, the greater peritoneal sac communicates with the lesser peritoneal sac (omental bursa). The **lesser omentum** consists of the **hepatogastric** and **hepatoduodenal ligaments.**

(2) The omental (epiploic) foramen is situated just below the liver and readily admits two fingers. It is bound **superiorly** by the caudate lobe of the liver, **inferiorly** by the superior part of the duodenum, **posteriorly** by the inferior vena cava, and **anteriorly** by the lesser omentum, which ensheathes the hepatic artery, portal vein, and bile ducts at the **porta hepatis.**

(3) The greater omentum extends along the greater curvature from spleen to duodenum.

(4) The gallbladder is situated between the right and quadrate lobes of the liver and projects just beyond the inferior border of the liver, thereby coming into contact directly with the anterior abdominal wall at this site.

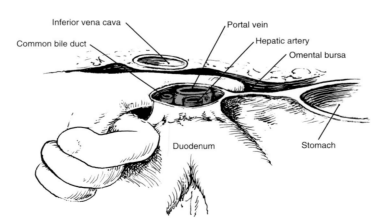

Inferior vena cava
Common bile duct
Portal vein
Hepatic artery
Omental bursa
Duodenum
Stomach

FIGURE 258.2 **Structures at the Porta Hepatis**

NOTE that the finger is entering the **omental foramen (of Winslow)** that allows communication between the **greater peritoneal sac** and the **omental bursa** or **lesser peritoneal sac.**

(From *Clemente's Anatomy Dissector,* 2nd Edition, Lippincott Williams & Wilkins, Baltimore, 2007.)

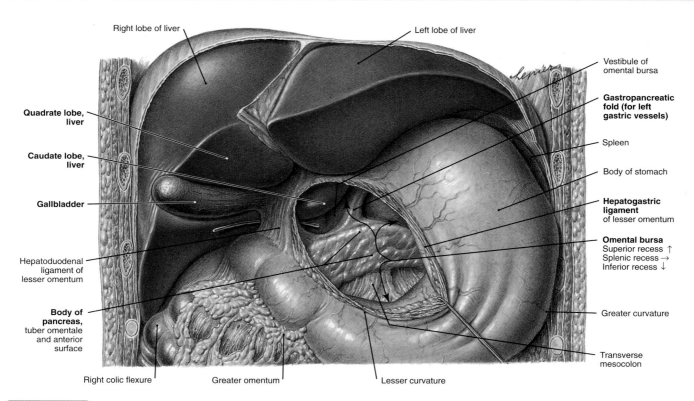

Right lobe of liver

Quadrate lobe, liver

Caudate lobe, liver

Gallbladder

Hepatoduodenal ligament of lesser omentum

Body of pancreas, tuber omentale and anterior surface

Right colic flexure

Greater omentum

Lesser curvature

Left lobe of liver

Vestibule of omental bursa

Gastropancreatic fold (for left gastric vessels)

Spleen

Body of stomach

Hepatogastric ligament of lesser omentum

Omental bursa Superior recess ↑ Splenic recess → Inferior recess ↓

Greater curvature

Transverse mesocolon

FIGURE 259.1 **Omental Bursa, Caudate Lobe of Liver, and Body of Pancreas**

NOTE: (1) With the liver elevated and the lesser curvature of the stomach pulled to the left, the exposure obtained by opening the omental bursa through the hepatogastric part of the lesser omentum has been enlarged. The superior, splenic, and inferior recesses of this bursa are indicated by arrows.

(2) The portion of the omental bursa adjacent to the omental (epiploic) foramen is called the **vestibule.** Observe the **gastropancreatic fold,** which crosses the dorsal wall of the bursa. This fold is a reflection of peritoneum covering the left gastric artery coursing from the celiac trunk to its destination, the lesser curvature of the stomach.

(3) Exposure of the omental bursa reveals the **caudate lobe** of the liver situated on the dorsal surface of the **right lobe.** Also seen is the anterior surface of the body of the pancreas coursing transversely behind the stomach.

(4) The **left lobe** of the liver overlies the lesser curvature, the fundus, and part of the body of the stomach. The **caudate lobe** behind the porta hepatis and the **quadrate lobe,** located between the fossa of the gall bladder and the round ligament, come into contact with the pylorus and the first part of the duodenum.

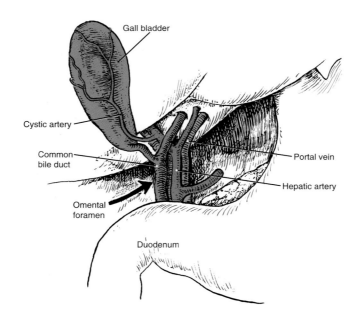

Gall bladder

Cystic artery

Common bile duct

Omental foramen

Duodenum

Portal vein

Hepatic artery

FIGURE 259.2 **The Omental Foramen (of Winslow)**

NOTE the black arrow behind (posterior to) the hepatic artery, portal vein, and common bile duct, thereby demonstrating the omental foramen. Through this foramen, the greater peritoneal sac communicates with the omental bursa, or lesser peritoneal sac.

(From *Clemente's Anatomy Dissector,* 2nd Edition, Lippincott Williams & Wilkins, Baltimore, 2007.)

PLATE 260 Omental Bursa; Lymphatics of the Stomach and Porta Hepatis

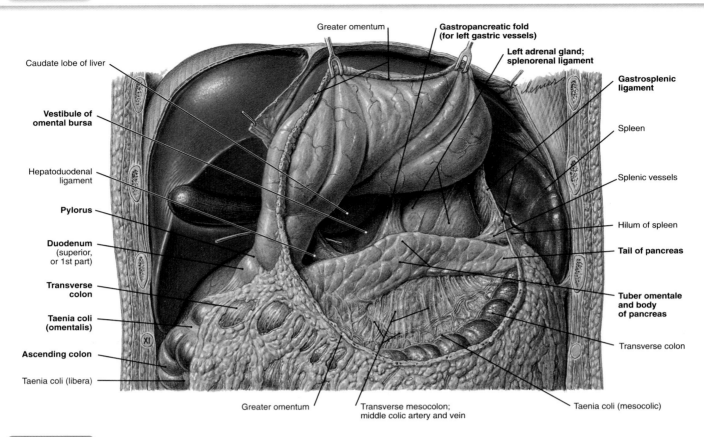

Greater omentum

Gastropancreatic fold (for left gastric vessels)

Left adrenal gland; splenorenal ligament

Caudate lobe of liver

Gastrosplenic ligament

Vestibule of omental bursa

Spleen

Splenic vessels

Hepatoduodenal ligament

Hilum of spleen

Pylorus

Tail of pancreas

Duodenum (superior, or 1st part)

Transverse colon

Tuber omentale and body of pancreas

Taenia coli (omentalis)

Transverse colon

XI

Ascending colon

Taenia coli (libera)

Greater omentum

Transverse mesocolon; middle colic artery and vein

Taenia coli (mesocolic)

FIGURE 260.1 **Omental Bursa and Structures in the Stomach Bed**

NOTE that the greater omentum has been cut along the entire greater curvature of the stomach, and the organ has been lifted to expose the omental bursa. Also note that the **gastrosplenic** and **splenorenal** ligaments have been cut, and that the tail of the pancreas is oriented toward the hilum of the spleen.

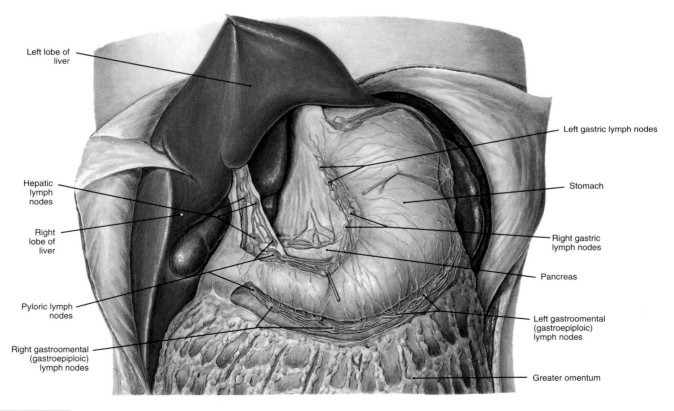

Left lobe of liver

Left gastric lymph nodes

Hepatic lymph nodes

Stomach

Right lobe of liver

Right gastric lymph nodes

Pancreas

Pyloric lymph nodes

Left gastroomental (gastroepiploic) lymph nodes

Right gastroomental (gastroepiploic) lymph nodes

Greater omentum

FIGURE 260.2 **Lymph Vessels and Nodes of the Stomach, Porta Hepatis, and Pancreas**

NOTE that lymph nodes lie along the greater and lesser curvatures of the stomach with the gastroomental (gastroepiploic) and left gastric vessels. Those in the porta hepatis follow the branches of the hepatic artery and posterior to the stomach the pancreatic nodes are located along the splenic vessels. Most of these nodes drain to the **preaortic nodes.**

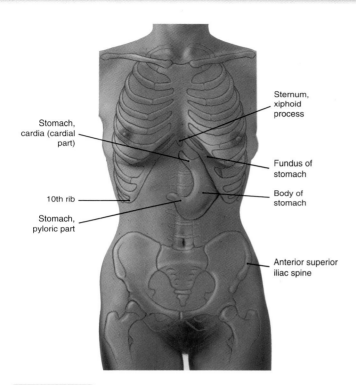

FIGURE 261.1 **Surface Projection of "Normal" Stomach**

NOTE: (1) In this figure the person is standing upright.
(2) The shape and positioning of the stomach are often altered by changes in its content and by organs surrounding the stomach.
(3) The adult stomach has a capacity of about 1500 ml, while at birth it is only about 30 ml.

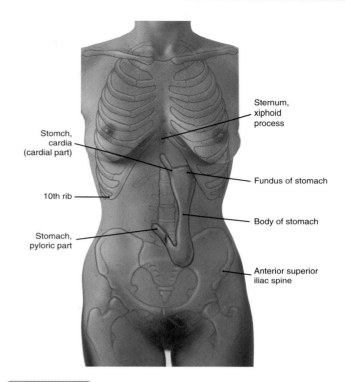

FIGURE 261.2 **Surface Projection of "Normal Fishhook" Stomach**

NOTE: (1) In this figure the person is standing upright.
(2) A "long stomach" of the type shown here can extend as far inferiorly as the upper pelvis (see radiograph in Fig. 261.3)

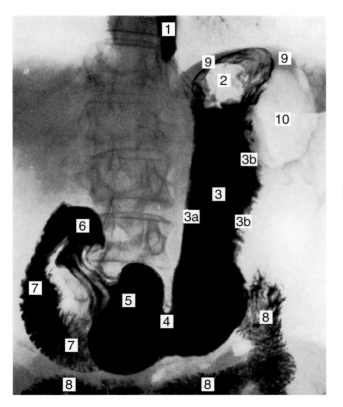

FIGURE 261.3 **Radiograph of the Lower Esophagus, Stomach, Duodenum, and Proximal Jejunum**

NOTE: This is a normal "J-shaped" or "fishhook" stomach. The cardiac and pyloric ends of the stomach are more securely attached to the posterior body wall, whereas the body and pyloric parts are more mobile. Frequently in the upright position, the greater curvature hangs as low as the brim of the pelvis.

1. Esophagus
2. Stomach fundus (air bubble)
3. Body of stomach
3a. Lesser curvature
3b. Greater curvature
4. Peristaltic constriction at angular notch
5. Pyloric antrum (expanded)
6. Bulb of superior duodenum (first part)
7. Descending duodenum (second part)
8. Jejunum
9. Left dome of diaphragm
10. Gas in left colic flexure

PLATE 262 The Stomach: Anterior Surface and External Muscle Layers

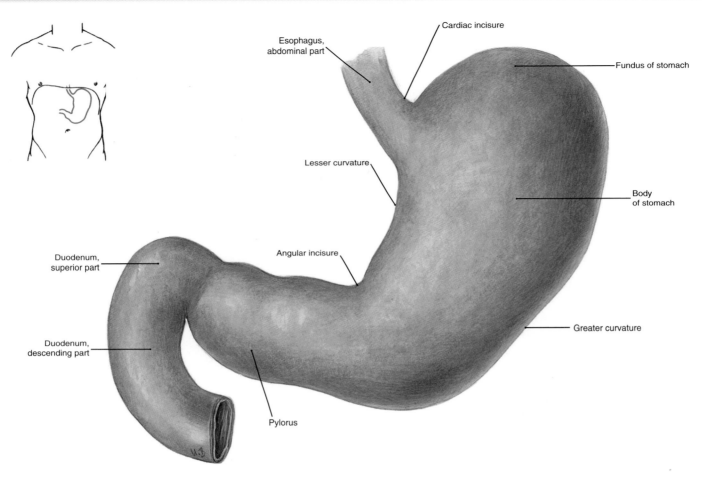

FIGURE 262.1 **Anterior View of the Stomach and Its Junction with the Duodenum**

NOTE the **cardiac incisure, greater and lesser curvatures, angular incisure,** and **pylorus.**

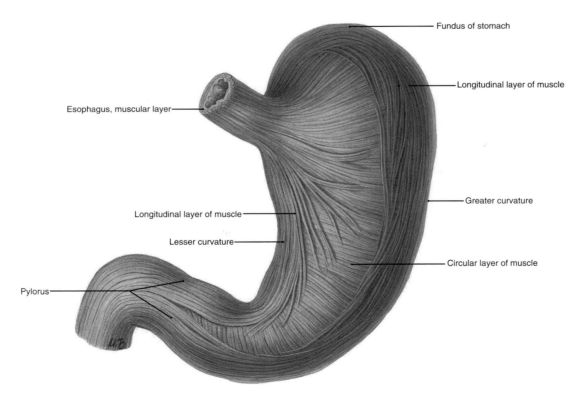

FIGURE 262.2 **The External Muscular Layers of the Stomach**

NOTE the longitudinal and circular muscle layers.

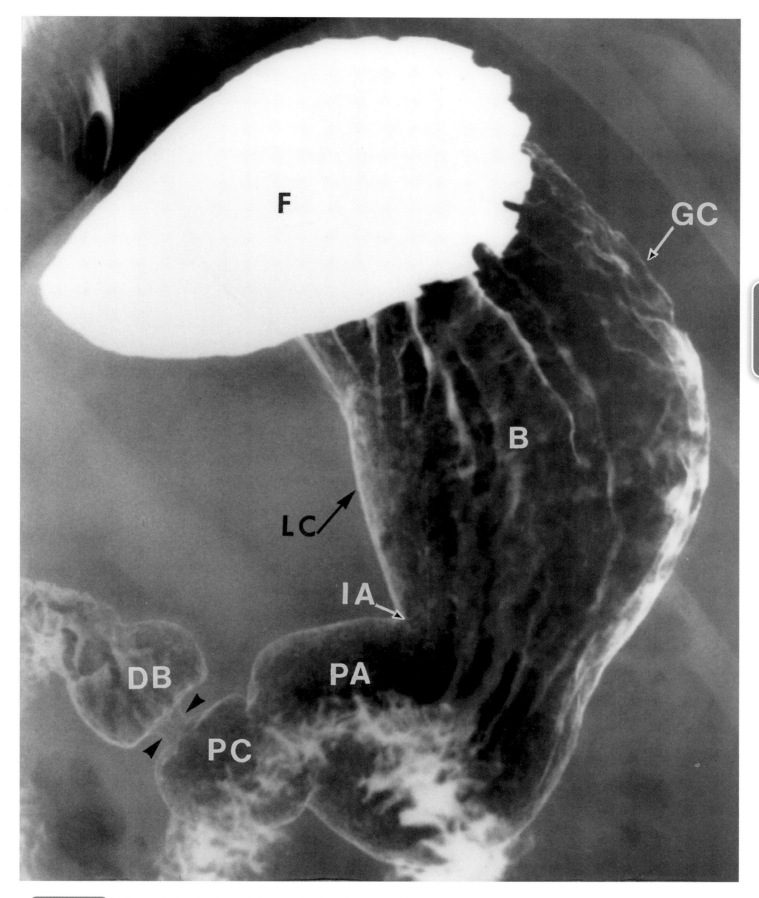

FIGURE 263 **X-Ray of the J-Shaped Stomach Showing Its Different Parts**

NOTE that the fundus is full of barium, explaining the solid white color. **F,** fundus; **GC,** greater curvature; **B,** body; **LC,** lesser curvature; **IA,** angular incisure; **PA,** pyloric antrum; **PC,** pyloric canal; **DB,** duodenal bulb.

(Contributed by Edward J.H. Nathanial, MD, PhD, Professor of Anatomy, University of Manitoba, Winnipeg, Canada.)

PLATE 264   Blood Supply to the Stomach; the Stomach and Greater Omentum

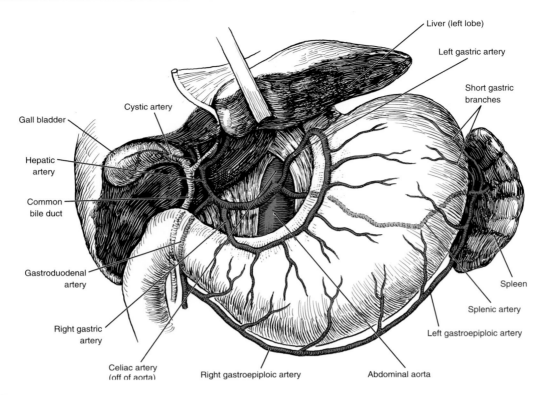

FIGURE 264.1   The Celiac Trunk (Artery) and Its Branches

NOTE: (1) The celiac trunk divides into the **splenic, left gastric,** and **hepatic arteries.**

(2) The **left** and **right gastric arteries** supply the lesser curvature of the stomach, while the **right** and **left gastroepiploic arteries** supply the greater curvature of the stomach.

(3) The **gastroduodenal artery** descends behind the duodenum and gives off the right gastroepiploic artery.

(From *Clemente's Anatomy Dissector,* 2nd Edition, Baltimore, Lippincott Williams & Wilkins, 2007.)

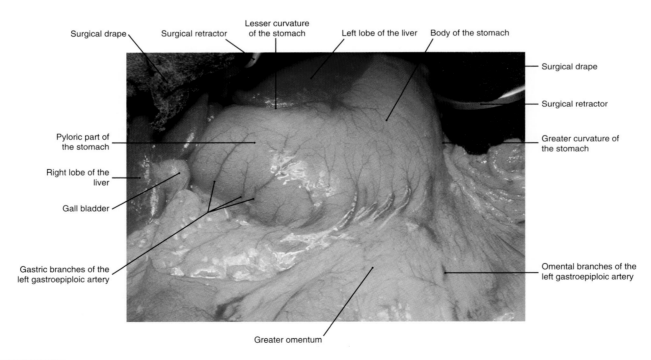

FIGURE 264.2   The Stomach and Greater Omentum

NOTE that the arteries supplying the stomach are gastric branches that ascend from the gastroepiploic arteries that course along the greater curvature.

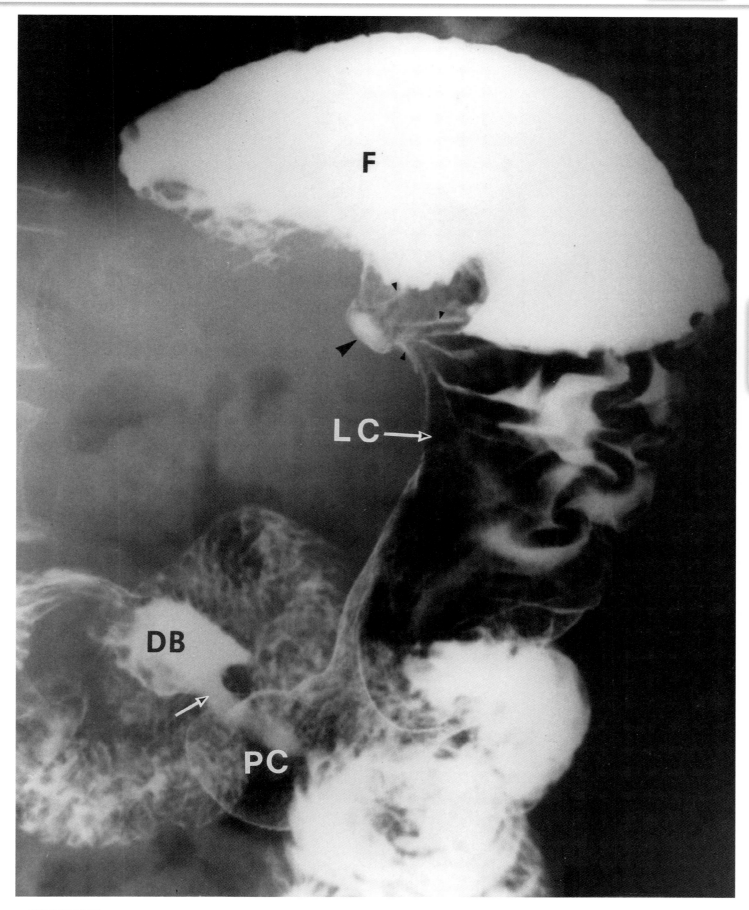

FIGURE 265 **An X-Ray of the Stomach Showing a Small Ulcer**

NOTE that a small ulcer (bold arrowhead) is located along the upper part of the lesser curvature (**LC**). Small arrowheads indicate the mucosal folds radiating from the ulcer center. The contrast medium has filled the fundus (**F**) and the pyloric canal (**PC**). The pyloric sphincter (arrow) separates the duodenal bulb (**DB**) from the pyloric canal (**PC**). Know that ulcers of the stomach are potentially malignant.

(Contributed by Edward J.H. Nathanial, MD, PhD, Professor of Anatomy, University of Manitoba, Winnipeg, Canada.)

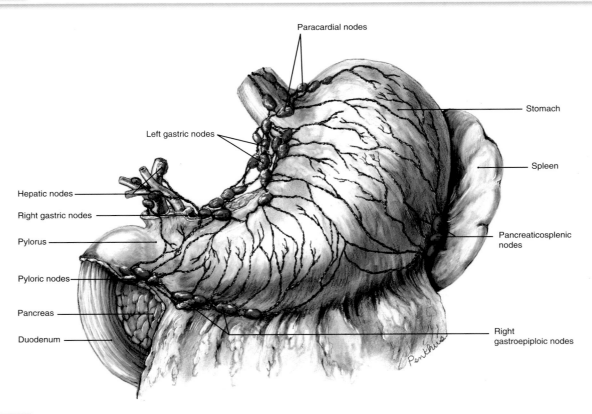

FIGURE 266.1 **Lymphatic Vessels and Nodes of the Stomach**

(From C.D. Clemente. *Gray's Anatomy*, 30th American Edition. Baltimore: Lea & Febiger, 1985.)

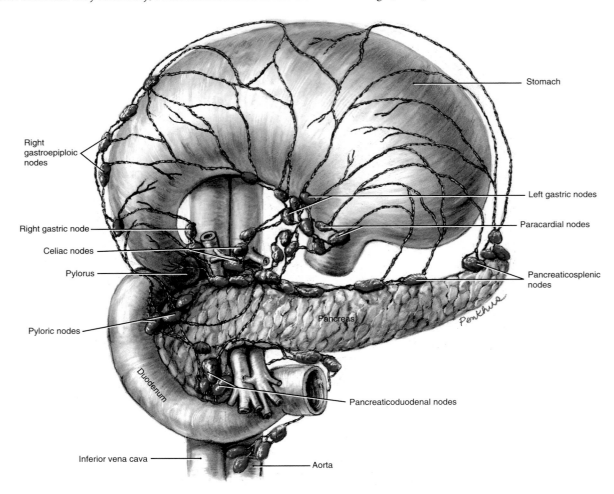

FIGURE 266.2 **Lymphatic Vessels and Nodes of the Stomach, Pancreas, and Duodenum**

(From C.D. Clemente. *Gray's Anatomy*, 30th American Edition. Baltimore: Lea & Febiger, 1985.)

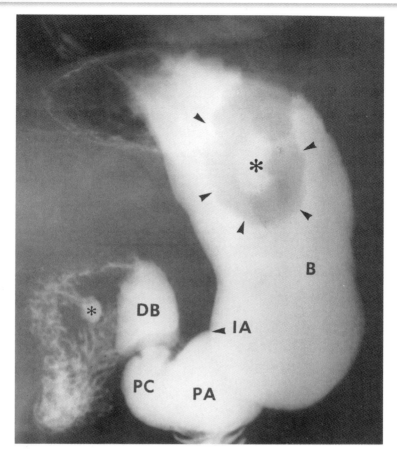

FIGURE 267.1 **X-Ray of the Stomach Showing a Large Ulcer on the Posterior Wall**

NOTE: (1) This is an X-ray of the stomach (filled with contrast medium) showing a large ulcer (outlined by arrows) on the posterior wall located at the junction of the fundus and body of the stomach. An asterisk indicates the central part of the ulcer.
(2) Perforations of ulcers on the posterior wall often allow stomach contents to enter the omental bursa. Since ulcers of the stomach have a greater propensity to become malignant, they are treated more aggressively and with greater care.
(3) A small diverticulum (small asterisk) filled with contrast medium is seen in the ascending part of the duodenum.
B, body of stomach; **PA,** pyloric antrum; **PC,** pyloric canal; **DB,** duodenal bulb; **IA,** angular incisure.

(Contributed by Edward J.H. Nathanial, MD, PhD, Professor of Anatomy, University of Manitoba, Winnipeg, Canada.)

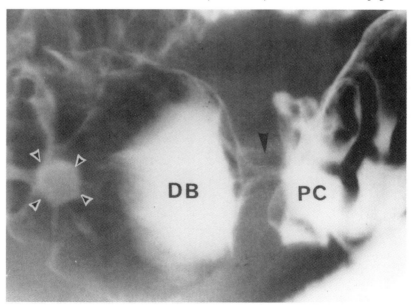

FIGURE 267.2 **X-Ray of the Pyloroduodenal Junction Showing a Duodenal Ulcer**

NOTE: (1) The anatomy of the pyloroduodenal junction is shown in this X-ray. The pyloric sphincter (black arrowhead) marks the junction of the pyloric canal (**PC**) with the duodenal bulb (**DB**). Observe that a duodenal ulcer is outlined by the white arrowheads.
(2) Duodenal ulcers are generally benign and, hence, treated conservatively or less aggressively. The pyloric sphincter is located at the narrow site between the pyloric canal and the duodenal bulb.

(Contributed by Edward J.H. Nathanial, MD, PhD, Professor of Anatomy, University of Manitoba, Winnipeg, Canada.)

PLATE 268 | The Duodenum: Anterior View and Longitudinal Section

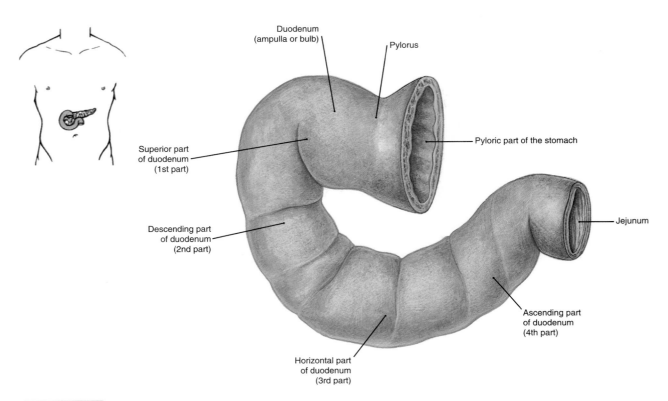

Duodenum
(ampulla or bulb)

Pylorus

Superior part
of duodenum
(1st part)

Pyloric part of the stomach

Descending part
of duodenum
(2nd part)

Jejunum

Ascending part
of duodenum
(4th part)

Horizontal part
of duodenum
(3rd part)

FIGURE 268.1 **The Duodenum: Anterior View**

NOTE the superior (1st part), descending (2nd part), transverse (3rd part), and ascending (4th part) parts of the duodenum. The duodenum is 10 in. in length (25 cm) and leads into the jejunum.

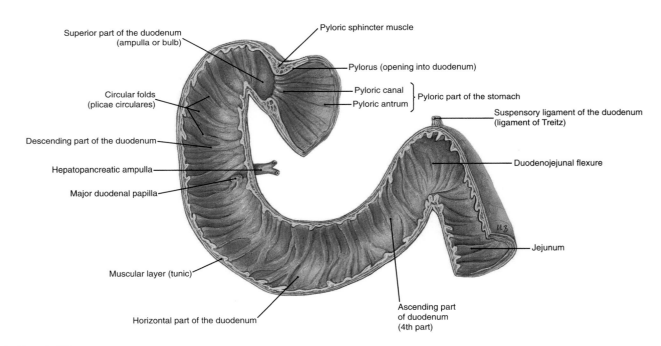

Superior part of the duodenum
(ampulla or bulb)

Pyloric sphincter muscle

Pylorus (opening into duodenum)

Circular folds
(plicae circulares)

Pyloric canal

Pyloric antrum

Pyloric part of the stomach

Descending part of the duodenum

Suspensory ligament of the duodenum
(ligament of Treitz)

Hepatopancreatic ampulla

Duodenojejunal flexure

Major duodenal papilla

Muscular layer (tunic)

Jejunum

Horizontal part of the duodenum

Ascending part
of duodenum
(4th part)

FIGURE 268.2 **Longitudinal Section of the Duodenum**

NOTE: (1) The **major hepatopancreatic ampulla** and **papilla** (opening) where the combined common bile duct and pancreatic duct open into the duodenum.
(2) The **minor pancreatic ampulla** and **papilla** (not shown in this figure) open about 2 cm proximal to the major ampulla and papilla. It is the site where the accessory pancreatic duct opens into the duodenum.

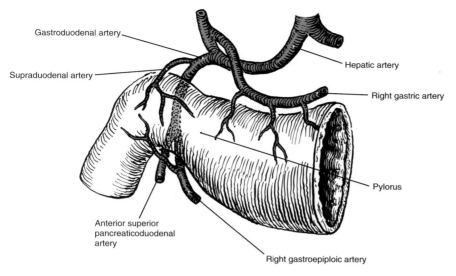

Gastroduodenal artery

Supraduodenal artery

Hepatic artery

Right gastric artery

Anterior superior pancreaticoduodenal artery

Pylorus

Right gastroepiploic artery

FIGURE 269.1 **Arteries to the Pyloric-Duodenal Region (Anterior View)**

NOTE the **gastroduodenal artery** and its **supraduodenal branch.**

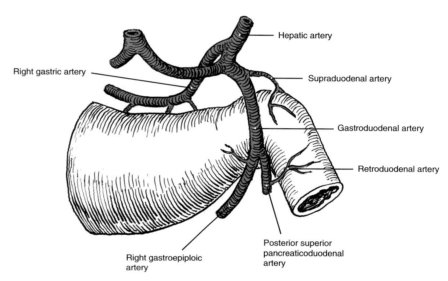

Hepatic artery

Right gastric artery

Supraduodenal artery

Gastroduodenal artery

Retroduodenal artery

Right gastroepiploic artery

Posterior superior pancreaticoduodenal artery

FIGURE 269.2 **Arteries to the Pyloric-Duodenal Region (Posterior View)**

NOTE the **gastroduodenal artery.** Also see its **supraduodenal** and **retroduodenal branches.**

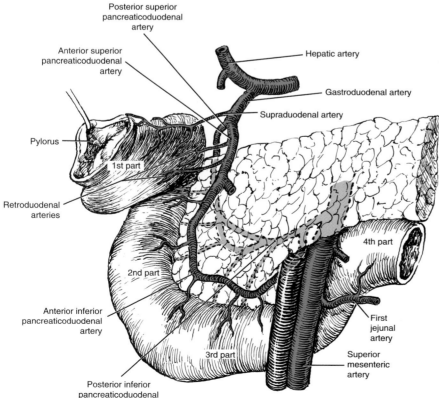

Posterior superior pancreaticoduodenal artery

Anterior superior pancreaticoduodenal artery

Hepatic artery

Gastroduodenal artery

Supraduodenal artery

Pylorus

1st part

Retroduodenal arteries

4th part

2nd part

Anterior inferior pancreaticoduodenal artery

First jejunal artery

3rd part

Superior mesenteric artery

Posterior inferior pancreaticoduodenal artery

FIGURE 269.3 **Gastroduodenal Artery and Its Pancreaticoduodenal Branch**

NOTE the superior mesenteric artery and vein. In persons who lose a lot of weight quickly, these vessels can obstruct the third part of the duodenum, giving rise to the **superior mesenteric syndrome.**

(From *Clemente's Anatomy Dissector,* 2nd Edition. Baltimore: Lippincott Williams & Wilkins, 2007.)

PLATE 270 Liver: Surface Projection (Dorsocranial View)

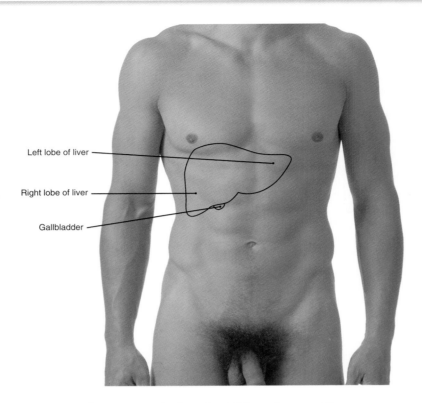

FIGURE 270.1 **Surface Projection of the Liver during the Midrespiratory Phase**

NOTE: (1) The position of the healthy liver is related to the various phases of the respiratory cycle. This figure demonstrates the position of the liver between inspiration and expiration (midrespiratory phase).

(2) During inspiration, the diaphragm descends and pushes the liver inferiorly. During expiration, the diaphragm elevates and with it also the liver. The dome of the right lobe of the liver during expiration rises to the level of the right fifth rib.

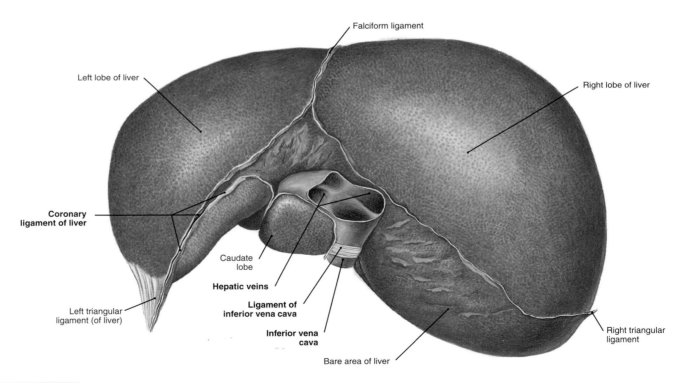

FIGURE 270.2 **Dorsocranial View of the Liver**

NOTE: (1) The visceral peritoneum closely adheres to the surface of the liver and is called the **coronary ligament.** Between its two leaves a portion of the liver, called the **bare area,** is devoid of peritoneum and is in contact with the abdominal surface of the diaphragm.

(2) The **hepatic veins** converge superiorly to empty into the superior vena cava.

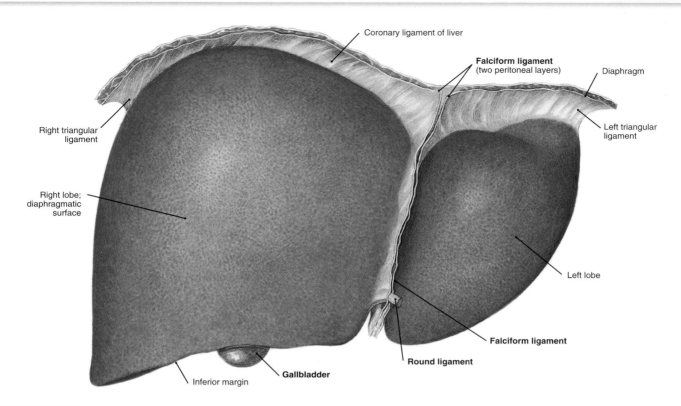

FIGURE 271.1 **Anterior Surface of the Liver (with Diaphragmatic Attachment)**

NOTE: The **falciform ligament** separates the right and left lobes of the liver. It contains a fibrous cord, the **round ligament of the liver,** which was the **umbilical vein** during fetal life. Also observe the fundus of the gall bladder below the inferior margin of the liver.

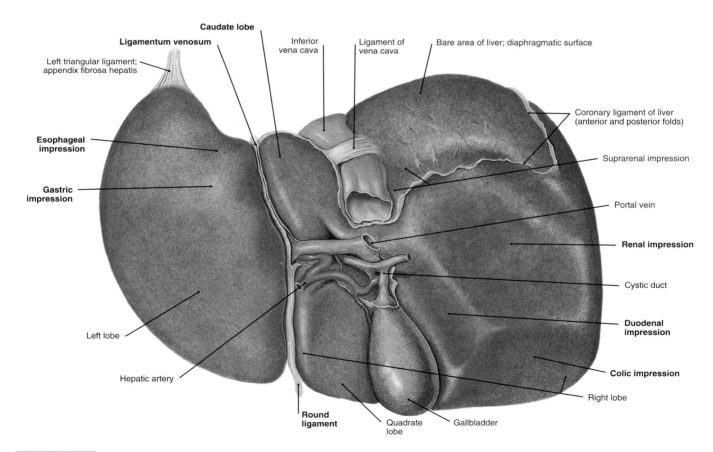

FIGURE 271.2 **Posterior (Visceral) Surface of the Liver and the Gallbladder**

NOTE the impressions made by the abdominal organs on the ventral surface of the liver, and the inferior vena cava, which separates the **caudate** and **right lobes.** The gallbladder, portal vein, hepatic artery, and common bile duct bound the **quadrate lobe,** and the **ligamentum venosus** (ductus venosus) extends from the round ligament (umbilical vein).

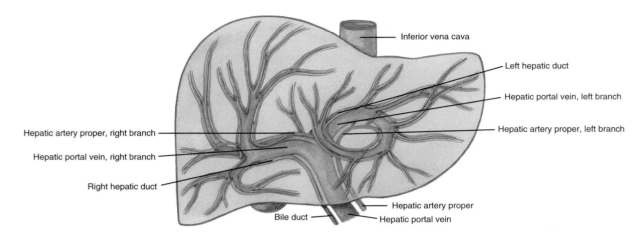

FIGURE 272.1 Branching of the Portal Vein, Hepatic Artery, and Bile Duct

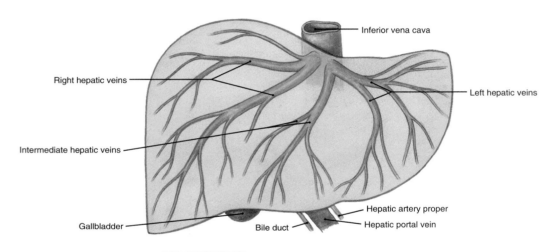

FIGURE 272.2 Draining Pattern of the Hepatic Veins

FIGURES 272.1 and 272.2 Branching Patterns of the Portal Vein, Hepatic Artery, and Tributaries of the Hepatic Vein

NOTE: (1) The portal vein and hepatic artery branch in such a way that segmental regions of the liver that receive their own arterial and venous branches.

(2) The portal vein and hepatic artery and veins divide the organ functionally and anatomically into a right and a left liver.

(3) The branching of these vessels forms the basis of the segmental anatomy of the liver, which is extremely important surgically, since they allow segmental resection of the liver when appropriate.

(4) The portal vein initially divides into right and left branches, as does the hepatic artery. The main fissure of this division is along a line that "passes from the tip of the gallbladder to the site where the falciform ligament disappears posteriorly." (From Launois B and Jamieson GG (eds). Surgical anatomy of the liver and associated structures. In: Modern operative techniques in liver surgery. Edinburgh: Churchill Livingstone, 1993.)

(5) There are eight liver **segments.** The right and left livers each divides into sectors that then divide into segments (four on the left and four on the right). Each segment receives a branch of the portal vein and the hepatic artery and drains into its own segmental hepatic vein.

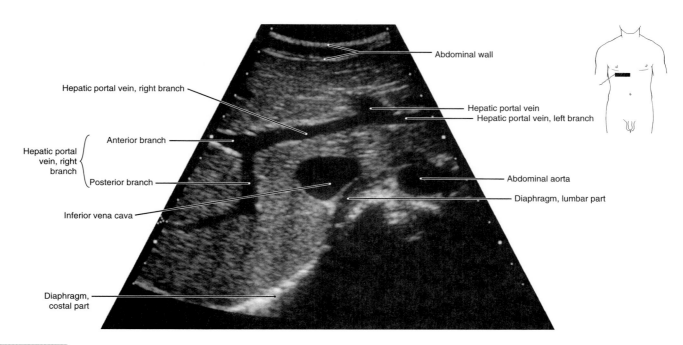

Abdominal wall

Hepatic portal vein, right branch

Hepatic portal vein
Hepatic portal vein, left branch

Anterior branch

Hepatic portal vein, right branch

Posterior branch

Abdominal aorta

Diaphragm, lumbar part

Inferior vena cava

Diaphragm, costal part

FIGURE 273.1 Ultrasound of Openings of the Hepatic Veins into the Inferior Vena Cava (Inferior Aspect)

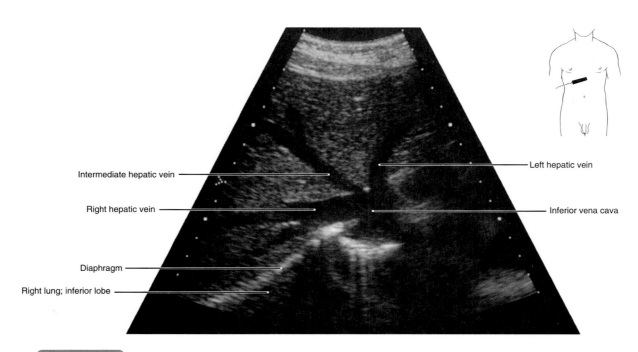

Intermediate hepatic vein

Right hepatic vein

Left hepatic vein

Inferior vena cava

Diaphragm

Right lung; inferior lobe

FIGURE 273.2 Ultrasound of the Portal Vein and Its Division into Right and Left Branches

PLATE 274 Segments of the Liver

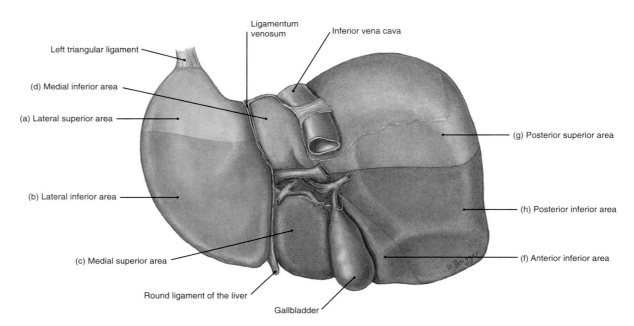

FIGURE 274.1 **Segments of the Liver: Anterior (Diaphragmatic) Surface**

FIGURE 274.2 **Segments of the Liver: Posterior (Visceral) Surface**

NOTE: (1) Topographically, there are four lobes of the liver: the right and left lobes (separated by the falciform ligament) and the **caudate** and **quadrate** lobes (best seen on the visceral surface).

(2) The caudate lobe is located between the **ligamentum venosum** and the **inferior vena cava** and the quadrate lobe lies between the **gallbladder** and the **round ligament of the liver** (see Fig. 271.2).

(3) Of considerable surgical importance is the division of the liver into **hepatic divisions and segments.** These have been determined in relationship to the divisions of the hepatic artery and the accompanying branching of the hepatic ducts and portal vein.

(4) There are **four hepatic divisions: anterior, posterior, medial,** and **lateral.** Each of these is divided into **superior** and **inferior areas,** making a total of **eight hepatic segments:**

  (a) Lateral superior segment
  (b) Lateral inferior segment
  (c) Medial superior segment
  (d) Medial inferior segment
  (e) Anterior superior segment
  (f) Anterior inferior segment
  (g) Posterior superior segment
  (h) Posterior inferior segment

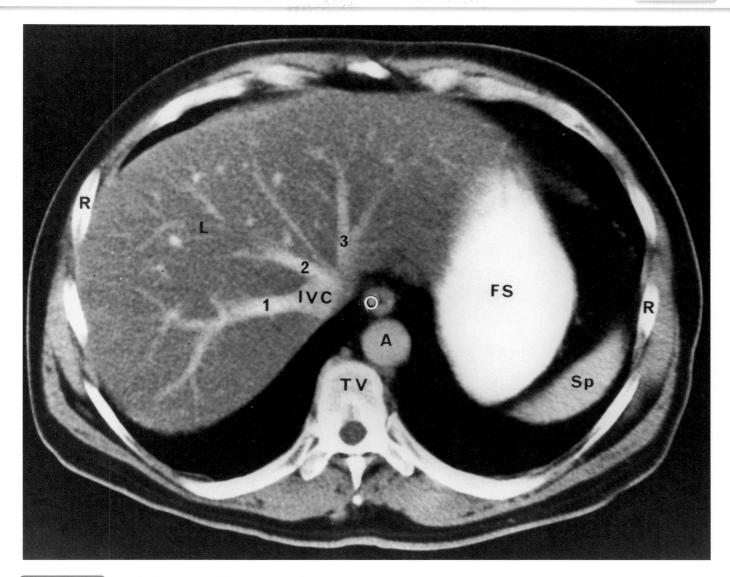

FIGURE 275.1 **CT of the Upper Abdomen at Thoracic Level T10–T11**

NOTE: (1) Three hepatic veins, labeled **1, 2,** and **3,** are draining blood from the **right lobe,** intermediate region (**caudate** and **quadrate lobes**), and the **left lobe** into the inferior vena cava (**IVC**).

(2) The distribution of hepatic veins provides lines of segmental demarcation for the abdominal surgeon performing hepatic resection. Observe that the fundus of the stomach (**FS**), which is filled with contract medium, and the spleen (**Sp**) are seen.

L, liver; **A,** aorta; **O,** esophagus; **TV,** thoracic vertebra (T10); **R,** ribs.

(Contributed by Edward J.H. Nathanial, MD, PhD, Professor of Anatomy, University of Manitoba, Winnipeg, Canada.)

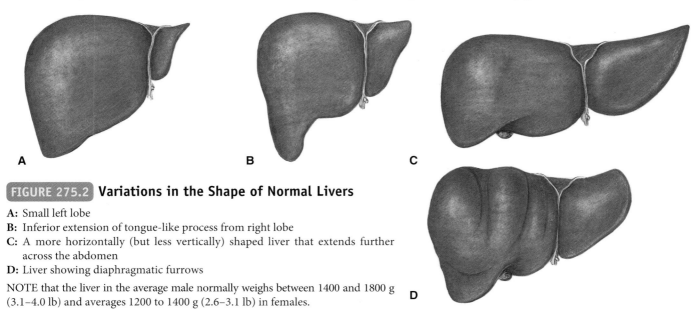

FIGURE 275.2 **Variations in the Shape of Normal Livers**

A: Small left lobe

B: Inferior extension of tongue-like process from right lobe

C: A more horizontally (but less vertically) shaped liver that extends further across the abdomen

D: Liver showing diaphragmatic furrows

NOTE that the liver in the average male normally weighs between 1400 and 1800 g (3.1–4.0 lb) and averages 1200 to 1400 g (2.6–3.1 lb) in females.

PLATE 276 CT of Upper Abdomen

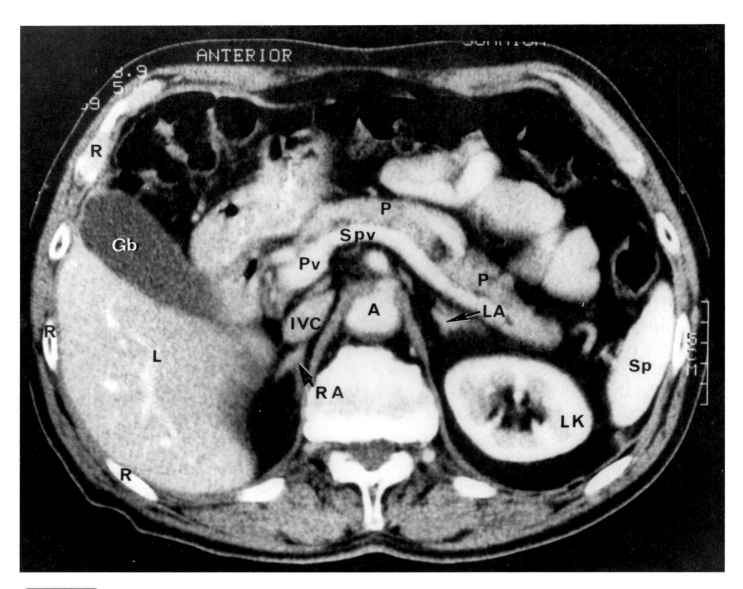

FIGURE 276 **CT of the Upper Abdomen Showing the Organs at the Level of About L1**

NOTE: (1) The splenic vein (**Spv**) flowing into the portal vein (**Pv**). Note also the aorta (**A**), the inferior vena cava (**IVC**), the right adrenal (suprarenal) gland (**RA**), and the left adrenal gland (**LA**); **see arrows.**

(2) The pancreas (**P**) is oriented across the abdomen and is directed toward the hilum of the spleen (**Sp**). Observe the gallbladder (**Gb**), the liver (**L**), the left kidney (**LK**), and the ribs (**R**).

(3) The aorta (**A**) anterior to the body of the vertebra and, to its right side, the inferior vena cava (**IVC**). Observe the bony rib cage affording protection for these important organs.

L, Liver; **P,** Pancreas; **IVC,** Inferior Vena Cava; **Gb,** Gall bladder; **LK,** Left Kidney; **A,** Aorta; **RA,** Right Adrenal (Suprarenal) Gland; **SpV,** Splenic Vein; **R,** Ribs; **LA,** Left Adrenal Gland; **Sp,** Spleen; **PR,** Portal Vein.

(Contributed by Edward J.H. Nathanial, MD, PhD, Professor of Anatomy, University of Manitoba, Winnipeg, Canada.)

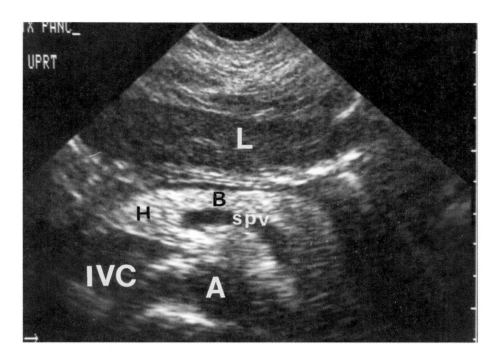

FIGURE 277.1 **Transverse Ultrasound of the Upper Abdomen**

NOTE that the normal pancreas is seen with splenic vein (**spv**) located just posterior to the pancreatic head (**H**) and pancreatic body (**B**) and is seen as a curved dark structure. Observe the locations of the aorta (**A**) and the inferior vena cava (**IVC**).

(Contributed by Edward J.H. Nathanial, MD, PhD, Professor of Anatomy, University of Manitoba, Winnipeg, Canada.)

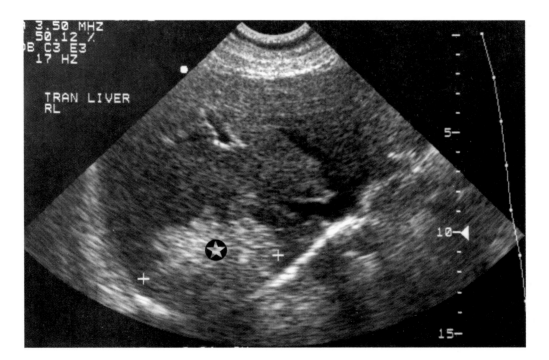

FIGURE 277.2 **Transverse Ultrasound of Abdomen Showing a Tumor Mass in the Liver**

NOTE that the tumor in this figure (**asterisk, star**), which measures 6.8 cm (indicated by the electronic calipers), is a metastatic mass, which in this patient, is secondary to a primary cancer in the transverse colon. The liver is a common site for metastases from cancers in the abdominal organs since the portal vein and hepatic veins have a capillary anastomosis system where metastatic cells can become attached and then continue to divide.

(Contributed by Edward J.H. Nathanial, MD, PhD, Professor of Anatomy, University of Manitoba, Winnipeg, Canada.)

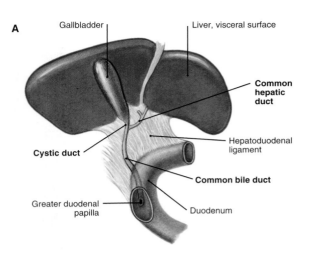

A

Gallbladder

Liver, visceral surface

Common hepatic duct

Hepatoduodenal ligament

Cystic duct

Common bile duct

Greater duodenal papilla

Duodenum

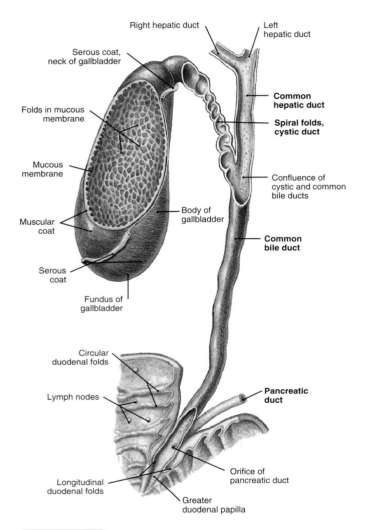

Right hepatic duct

Left hepatic duct

Serous coat, neck of gallbladder

Common hepatic duct

Folds in mucous membrane

Spiral folds, cystic duct

Mucous membrane

Confluence of cystic and common bile ducts

Muscular coat

Body of gallbladder

Serous coat

Common bile duct

Fundus of gallbladder

Circular duodenal folds

Lymph nodes

Pancreatic duct

Longitudinal duodenal folds

Orifice of pancreatic duct

Greater duodenal papilla

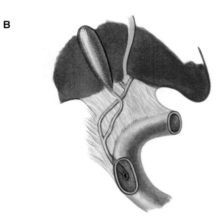

B

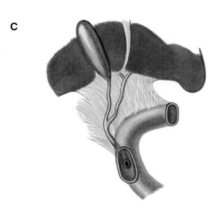

C

FIGURE 278.1 **Gallbladder and Biliary Duct System**

NOTE: (1) The wall of the gallbladder has been opened to reveal the meshwork characteristic of the surface of the mucosal layer. The pear-shaped gallbladder stores bile, which reaches it from the liver. Its capacity is about 35 ml.

(2) The spiral nature of the **cystic duct,** which emerges from the neck of the gallbladder. Normally, the cystic duct measures about 1½ in. in length and joins the **common hepatic duct** (which also is about 1½ in. long) to form the **common bile duct.**

(3) The common bile duct descends about 3 in. to open into the second or descending portion of the duodenum.

(4) At its point of entrance into the duodenum (greater duodenal papilla), the common bile duct is joined by the **main pancreatic duct** (duct of Wirsung).

FIGURE 278.2A–C **Variations in the Union of the Cystic and Common Hepatic Ducts**

NOTE: Usually the cystic duct lies to the right of the common hepatic duct at a point just superior to the level of the first part of the duodenum. Variations in this schema occur as indicated in the following three examples:

A: The union of the cystic and common hepatic ducts occurs close to the liver, resulting in short cystic and common hepatic ducts and a long common bile duct.

B: The cystic duct crosses to the left of the common hepatic duct and joins the hepatic duct low, resulting in a short common bile duct.

C: The cystic duct remains to the right of the common hepatic duct but still joins it close to the site of penetration of the duodenum, again resulting in a short common bile duct.

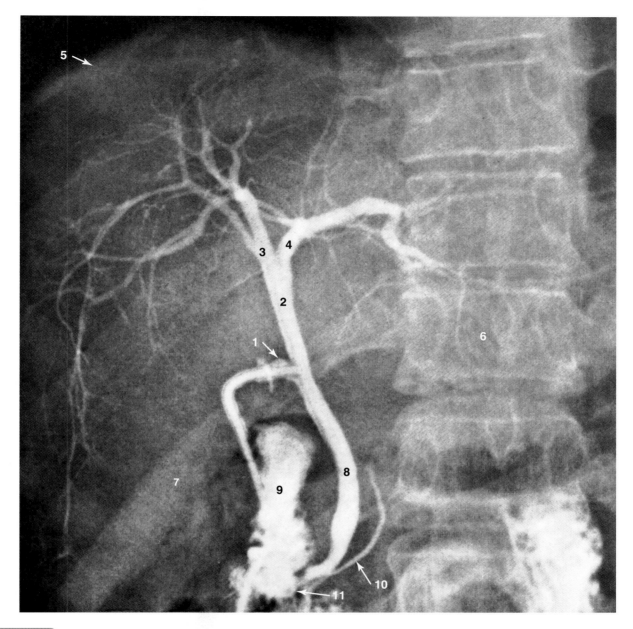

FIGURE 279.1 **Intraoperative Cholangiogram: Radiograph of Biliary Duct System**

NOTE: The gallbladder has been removed and a catheter and tube have been inserted through the stump of the cystic duct (**1**) into the common hepatic duct (**2**) and contrast medium injected into the biliary system. Other structures are numbered as follows:

3. Right hepatic duct
4. Left hepatic duct
5. Diaphragm
6. 11th thoracic vertebra
7. 11th rib
8. Common bile duct
9. Duodenum (second, descending part)
10. Main pancreatic duct
11. Greater duodenal papilla

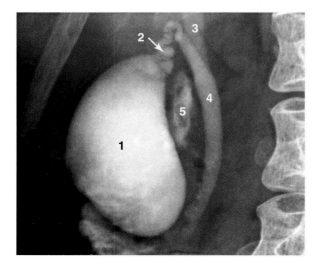

FIGURE 279.2 **Radiograph of Gallbladder and Biliary Ducts**

1. Body of the gallbladder
2. Cystic duct with spiral valves
3. Common hepatic duct
4. Union of common hepatic and cystic ducts to form common bile duct
5. Contrast medium in duodenum

PLATE 280 Blood Supply to the Gallbladder; Ultrasound of Gallbladder

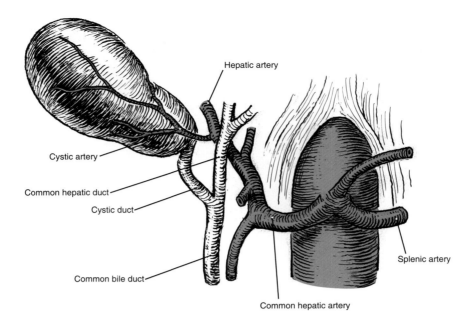

Hepatic artery

Cystic artery

Common hepatic duct

Cystic duct

Common bile duct

Splenic artery

Common hepatic artery

FIGURE 280.1 **The Cystic Artery and the Bile Ducts**

NOTE: (1) The cystic artery most often arises from the right hepatic artery to achieve the neck of the gallbladder. One or more accessory branches usually derive from the main cystic vessel.

(2) The origin of the cystic artery is important to the surgeon when performing gallbladder operations. In a large study, the following was found: **64%** derived from the right hepatic artery; **27%** from the hepatic trunk; **6%** from the left hepatic artery; and **2.5%** from the gastroduodenal artery and, in more rare cases, from the superior pancreaticoduodenal artery, right gastric artery, celiac trunk, or superior mesenteric artery.

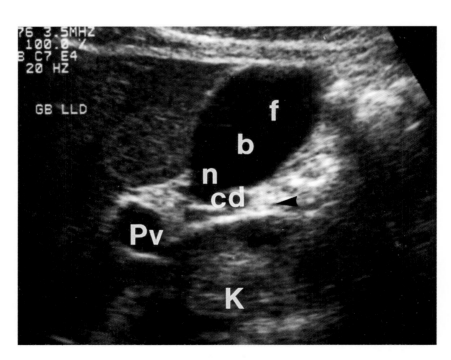

FIGURE 280.2 **Parasagittal Ultrasound of Abdomen Demonstrating the Parts of the Gallbladder**

NOTE: (1) This scan is of the right upper abdominal quadrant and shows the fundus (f), body (b), and neck (n) of the gallbladder.

(2) The other structures seen are the cystic duct, portal vein, and right kidney. The arrow points to a potential space known as the hepatorenal pouch of Morrison.

f, fundus of the gallbladder, **b;** body of the gallbladder; **n,** neck of the gallbladder; **cd,** cystic duct; **Pv,** portal vein; **K,** right kidney.

(Contributed by Edward J.H. Nathanial, MD, PhD, Professor of Anatomy, University of Manitoba, Winnipeg, Canada.)

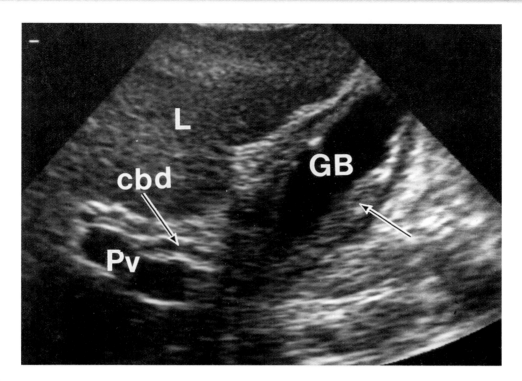

FIGURE 281.1 **Parasagittal Ultrasound of Abdomen Showing Inflammation of the Gallbladder**

NOTE that the wall of the gallbladder shows a thickening as the result of inflammation or **cholycystitis.** This condition often is caused by an impacted gallstone in the biliary tract, for example, within the cystic duct. This may lead to a stasis of bile within the gallbladder, causing an inflammation of its wall. In a case when bile cannot pass through the biliary tract, it then may become absorbed into the bloodstream and cause a yellowish skin discoloration called **jaundice.**

GB, gallbladder; **L,** liver; **Pv,** portal vein; **cbd,** common bile duct.

(Contributed by Edward J.H. Nathanial, MD, PhD, Professor of Anatomy, University of Manitoba, Winnipeg, Canada.)

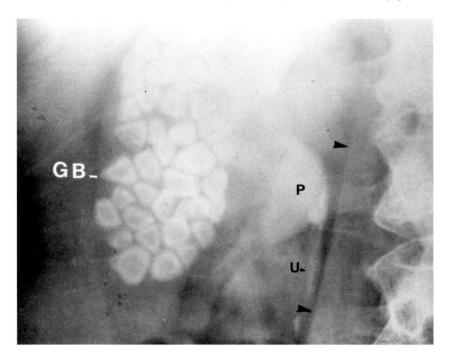

FIGURE 281.2 **X-Ray of the Gallbladder Showing the Presence of Numerous Gallstones**

NOTE: (1) The gallbladder in this X-ray is filled with gallstones. It is thought that gallstones form when there is a blockage for the release of bile into the duodenum along the biliary tract. This may be due to pressure of a tumor in the region or to a small stone in the biliary tract.

(2) The stasis of bile in the gallbladder, due to delayed emptying, appears to be one of the conditions that predispose a person to form gallstones. An increased secretion of cholesterol from the liver into the bile has long been considered a precipitating condition in the formation of gallstones. This may be related to dietary factors. There are also good twin studies that point to a genetic factor that may also be involved in gallstone formation.

(Contributed by Edward J.H. Nathanial, MD, PhD, Professor of Anatomy, University of Manitoba, Winnipeg, Canada.)

PLATE 282 Pancreas and Duodenum

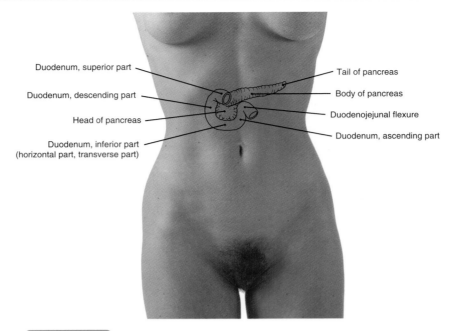

FIGURE 282.1 Surface Projection of the Duodenum and Pancreas

Duodenum, superior part

Duodenum, descending part

Head of pancreas

Duodenum, inferior part
(horizontal part, transverse part)

Tail of pancreas

Body of pancreas

Duodenojejunal flexure

Duodenum, ascending part

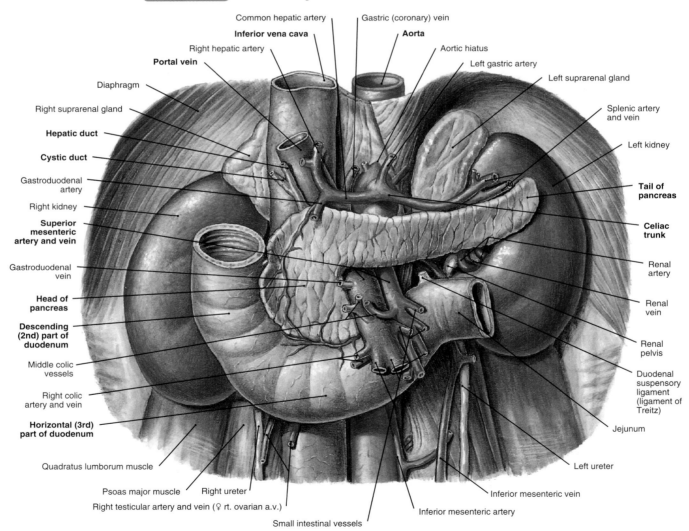

Common hepatic artery

Inferior vena cava

Right hepatic artery

Portal vein

Diaphragm

Right suprarenal gland

Hepatic duct

Cystic duct

Gastroduodenal artery

Right kidney

Superior mesenteric artery and vein

Gastroduodenal vein

Head of pancreas

Descending (2nd) part of duodenum

Middle colic vessels

Right colic artery and vein

Horizontal (3rd) part of duodenum

Quadratus lumborum muscle

Psoas major muscle   Right ureter

Right testicular artery and vein (♀ rt. ovarian a.v.)

Small intestinal vessels

Gastric (coronary) vein

Aorta

Aortic hiatus

Left gastric artery

Left suprarenal gland

Splenic artery and vein

Left kidney

Tail of pancreas

Celiac trunk

Renal artery

Renal vein

Renal pelvis

Duodenal suspensory ligament (ligament of Treitz)

Jejunum

Left ureter

Inferior mesenteric vein

Inferior mesenteric artery

FIGURE 282.2 Pancreas and Duodenum

NOTE: (1) The **head** of the pancreas lies to the right of the midline and is in contact with the inferior vena cava and the common bile duct dorsally and the transverse colon (not shown) ventrally.

(2) The **body** of the pancreas crosses the midline at the L1 level, and it is in contact posteriorly with the aorta, the superior mesenteric vessels, the left kidney, and the left adrenal gland.

(3) The **tail** of the pancreas is in contact with the spleen laterally, the left kidney posteriorly, and the splenic flexure of the colon anteriorly.

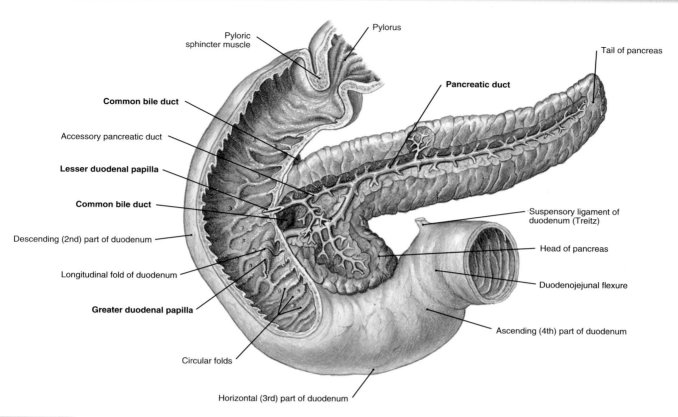

FIGURE 283.1 **Pancreatic Duct System**

NOTE: (1) The main pancreatic duct system has been dissected in this specimen. Observe how the accessory pancreatic duct extends straight into the duodenum through the lesser duodenal papilla. The main pancreatic duct, however, bends caudally to drain most of the head of the pancreas and then opens into the greater duodenal papilla with the common bile duct.

(2) From the pylorus to the duodenojejunal flexure, the duodenum measures about 10 in. At its termination, a suspensory ligament (of Treitz) marks the commencement of the jejunum. Here the small intestine becomes surrounded by peritoneum and is suspended from the posterior abdominal wall by the mesentery of the small intestine.

(3) The duodenum and pancreas are both retroperitoneal structures.

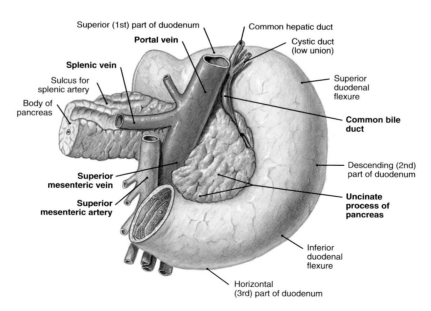

FIGURE 283.2 **Head of Pancreas and Duodenum (Dorsal View)**

NOTE: (1) This posterior view of the pancreatic head and its **uncinate process** shows the **common bile duct** embedded in the pancreas as the duct descends adjacent to the duodenum.

(2) Observe the **portal vein** as it ascends to the liver coursing posterior to the pancreatic head. Realize that the portal vein is the continuation superiorly beyond the junction of the **splenic vein** and the **superior mesenteric vein.**

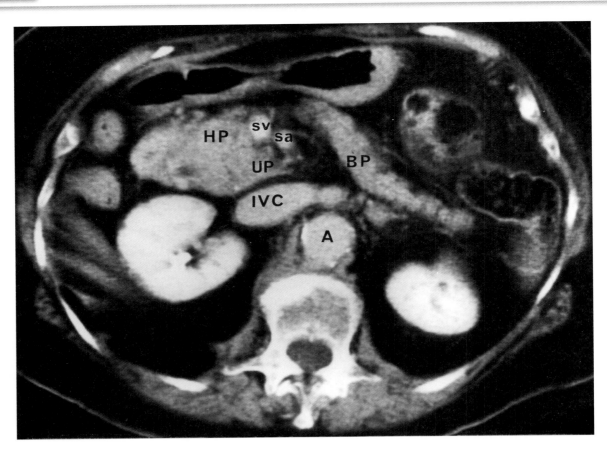

FIGURE 284.1 **CT Passing through the Level of the Second Lumbar Vertebra in a Normal Abdomen**

NOTE the head, body, and uncinate process of the pancreas.

HP, head of the pancreas; **BP,** body of the pancreas; **UP,** uncinate process of the pancreas; **A,** aorta; **IVC,** inferior vena cava; **sv,** superior mesenteric vein; **sa,** superior mesenteric artery.

(Contributed by Edward J.H. Nathanial, MD, PhD, Professor of Anatomy, University of Manitoba, Winnipeg, Canada.)

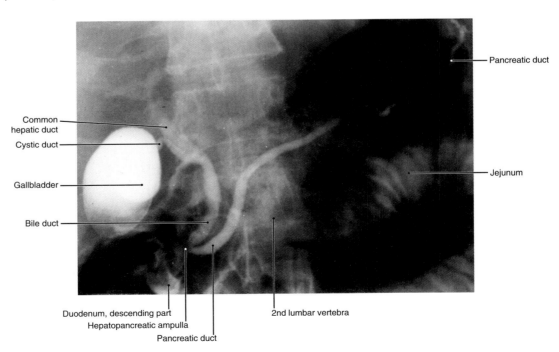

FIGURE 284.2 **Pancreatic Duct, Common Bile Duct, and Gallbladder**

NOTE: (1) This radiograph was taken following the injection of a contrast medium through a cannula placed in the common duct formed by junction of the main pancreatic duct and the common bile duct along the second part of the duodenum.

(2) The pancreatic duct is visible throughout its extent (i.e., from the splenic hilum to the hepatopancreatic ampulla). Also visible are the common hepatic duct and the common bile duct along with the gallbladder and a short part of the cystic duct.

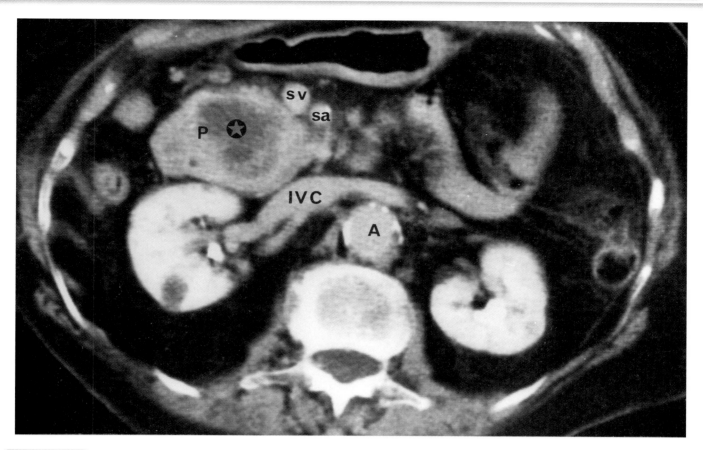

FIGURE 285.1 **Transaxial Image Showing a Tumor in the Head of the Pancreas**

NOTE: (1) A low-density tumor in the head of the pancreas. Tumors in the head of the pancreas are located in a deep-seated location. Because of this, they are often not diagnosed until very late when the prognosis is poor.

(2) A noninvasive technique such as a CT scan provides a valuable tool for an early diagnosis and for a more favorable outcome. Observe the inferior vena cava receiving the left and right renal veins.

P, pancreas; **sv,** superior mesenteric vein; **sa,** superior mesenteric artery; **A,** aorta; **IVC,** inferior vena cava.

(Contributed by Edward J.H. Nathanial, MD, PhD, Professor of Anatomy, University of Manitoba, Winnipeg, Canada.)

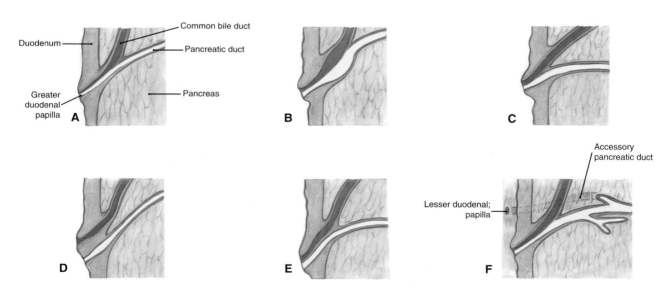

FIGURE 285.2A–F **Variations in Union of the Common Bile Duct and the Pancreatic Duct**

A: Pancreatic and common bile ducts join early, resulting in a long hepatopancreatic duct.
B: A long hepatopancreatic duct is modified by an expanded ampulla.
C: Pancreatic and common bile ducts join very close to the greater duodenal papilla, resulting in a short hepatopancreatic duct.
D: Both pancreatic and common bile ducts open separately on a somewhat larger duodenal papilla.
E: Pancreatic and common bile ducts drain through a single opening. The ducts are separated by a septum.
F: Long hepatopancreatic duct along with a well-developed accessory pancreatic duct (seen behind), which opens through the lesser duodenal papilla.

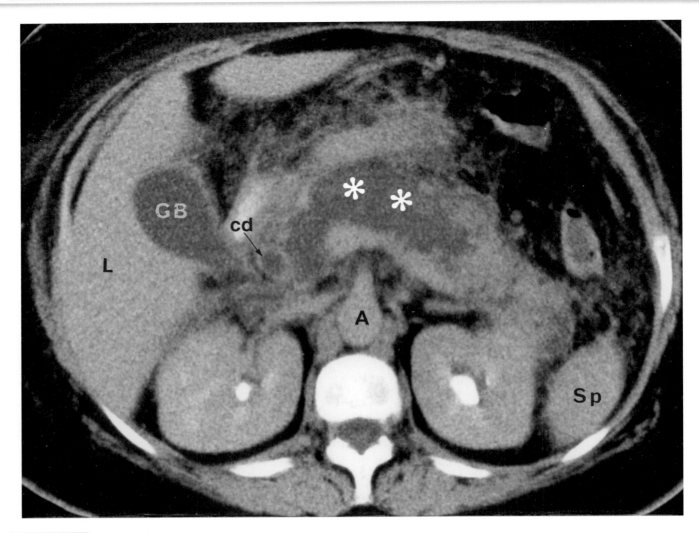

FIGURE 286.1 **CT Showing Diffuse Inflammation of the Pancreas**

NOTE: (1) Inflammation of the pancreas is called pancreatitis, which is an extremely painful condition. The darker area indicates regions of pancreatic necrosis (**asterisks**).

(2) Pancreatitis is frequently seen in alcoholics and in patients with gallstones that impact the ampulla of Vater.

(3) The dilated common bile duct (cd).

L, liver; **GB,** gallbladder; **Sp,** spleen; **A,** aorta; **cd,** common bile duct.

(Contributed by Edward J.H. Nathanial, MD, PhD, Professor of Anatomy, University of Manitoba, Winnipeg, Canada.)

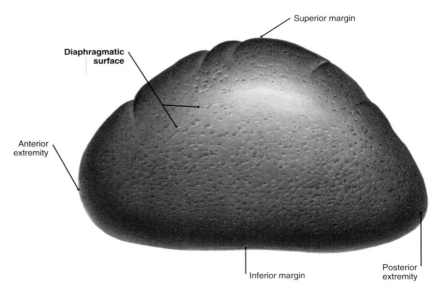

FIGURE 286.2 **Spleen (Diaphragmatic Surface)**

NOTE: The diaphragmatic surface of the spleen is directed posterolaterally. The normal spleen may vary in weight from 100 to 400 g. Its proximity to the 9th, 10th, and 11th ribs makes it vulnerable to rib fractures in this region.

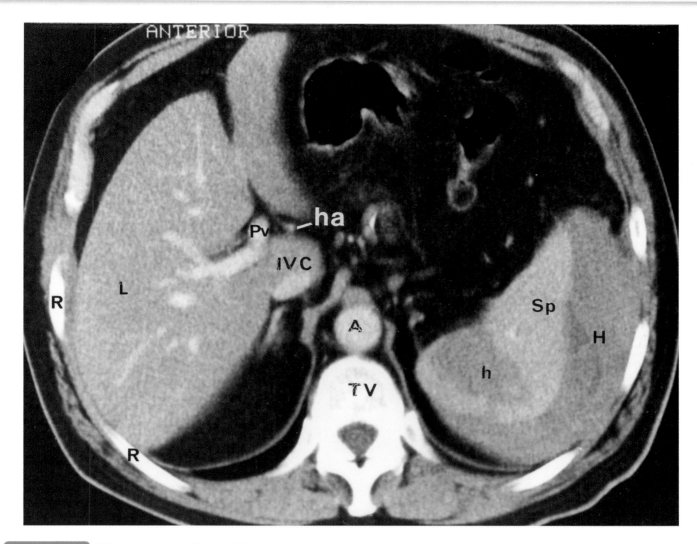

FIGURE 287.1 **CT through the Upper Abdomen**

NOTE: (1) The liver (**L**) and the portal vein (**Pv**) entering it. Observe the small diameter of the hepatic artery (**ha**) that supplies the liver in contrast
to the large portal vein emphasizing the amount of blood brought by these two vessels to the liver.

(2) The large subcapsular hemorrhage (**H**) in the spleen (**Sp**). Also observe the wedge-shaped hemorrhage (**h**). See the profiles of the ribs (**R**) and
realize how they protect the many important thoracic organs and some of the upper abdominal organs. **TV**, thoracic vertebrae; **A,** aorta; **IVC,**
inferior vena cava.

(Contributed by Edward J.H. Nathanial, MD, PhD, Professor of Anatomy, University of Manitoba, Winnipeg, Canada.)

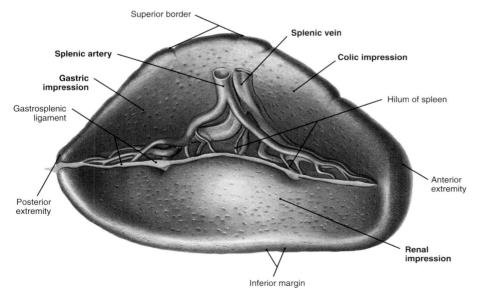

Superior border

Splenic vein

Splenic artery

Colic impression

Gastric
impression

Gastrosplenic
ligament

Hilum of spleen

Posterior
extremity

Anterior
extremity

Renal
impression

Inferior margin

FIGURE 287.2 **Spleen (Visceral Surface)**

NOTE: The spleen is situated in the left hypochondriac region between the fundus of the stomach and the diaphragm. Its visceral surface shows the gastric and renal impressions that conform to the shapes of the stomach and left kidney. In addition, the left colic flexure, the tail of the pancreas, and the left adrenal gland, which overlies the left kidney, are related to this visceral surface.

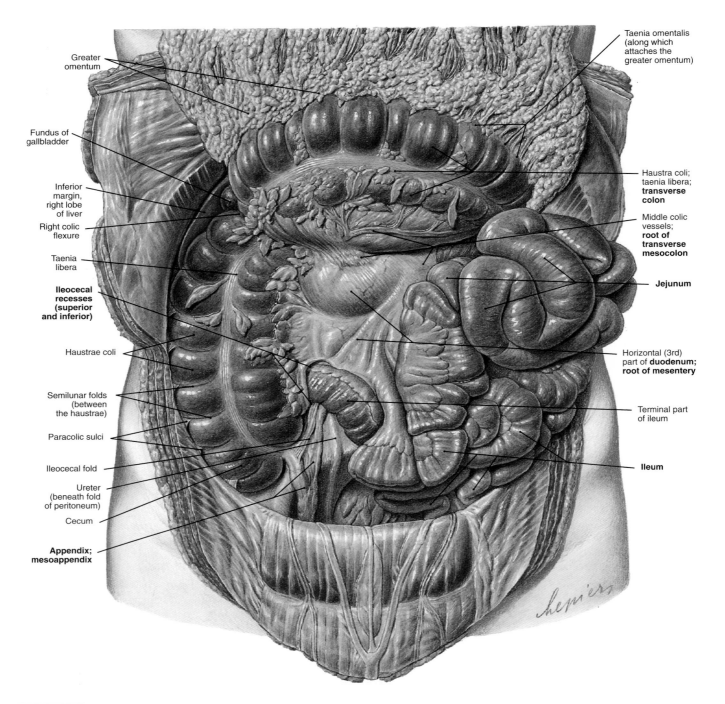

Greater
omentum

Fundus of
gallbladder

Inferior
margin,
right lobe
of liver

Right colic
flexure

Taenia
libera

**Ileocecal
recesses
(superior
and inferior)**

Haustrae coli

Semilunar folds
(between
the haustrae)

Paracolic sulci

Ileocecal fold

Ureter
(beneath fold
of peritoneum)

Cecum

**Appendix;
mesoappendix**

Taenia omentalis
(along which
attaches the
greater omentum)

Haustra coli;
taenia libera;
**transverse
colon**

Middle colic
vessels;
**root of
transverse
mesocolon**

Jejunum

Horizontal (3rd)
part of **duodenum;
root of mesentery**

Terminal part
of ileum

Ileum

FIGURE 288 Abdominal Cavity: Jejunum, Ileum, and Ascending and Transverse Colons

NOTE: (1) The greater omentum has been reflected superiorly, and the jejunum and ileum have been pulled to the left to expose the **root of the mesentery of the small intestine**.

(2) The horizontal (third) part of the duodenum, which is retroperitoneal and is covered by the smooth and glistening peritoneum.

(3) The junction of the distal portion of the ileum with the cecum. At this **ileocecal junction** the **ileocecal fold,** the **appendix,** and the **mesoappendix** can be identified. The appendix may extend cranially behind the cecum, toward the left and behind the ileum, or as demonstrated here, inferiorly over the pelvic brim.

(4) The transverse colon and the small intestine beyond the duodenal junction are more mobile than most other organs because they are attached to the transverse mesocolon and the mesentery.

(5) The retroperitoneal position of the **right ureter** as it descends over the pelvic brim on its course toward the urinary bladder in the pelvis.

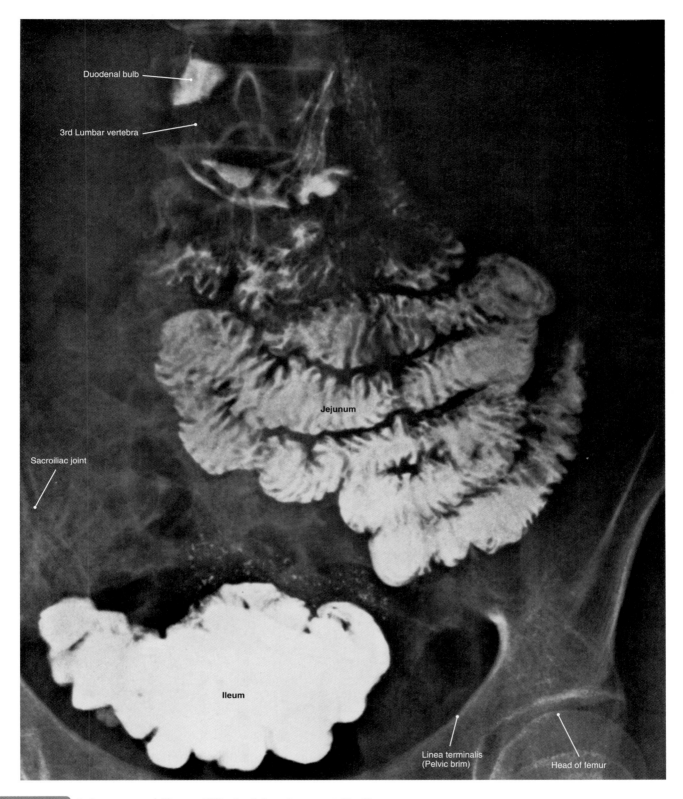

FIGURE 289 **Jejunum and Ileum Filled with a Contrast Medium**

NOTE: (1) The **jejunum** and **ileum** extend between the duodenojejunal junction and the ileocecal valve. This part of the small intestine is completely covered with peritoneum and can be seen to be arranged in a series of coils;

(2) The jejunum is about 1½ in. in diameter and about two-fifths of the small intestine beyond the duodenum, while the ileum is the distal three-fifths and is slightly smaller in diameter.

(From Wicke, 4th ed.)

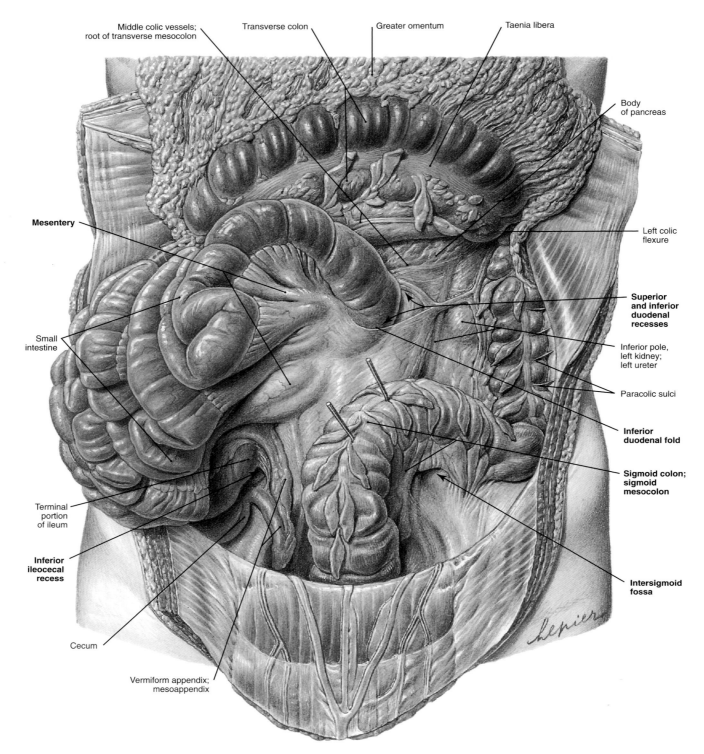

Middle colic vessels;
root of transverse mesocolon

Transverse colon

Greater omentum

Taenia libera

Body
of pancreas

Mesentery

Left colic
flexure

**Superior
and inferior
duodenal
recesses**

Small
intestine

Inferior pole,
left kidney;
left ureter

Paracolic sulci

**Inferior
duodenal fold**

**Sigmoid colon;
sigmoid
mesocolon**

Terminal
portion
of ileum

**Inferior
ileocecal
recess**

**Intersigmoid
fossa**

Cecum

Vermiform appendix;
mesoappendix

FIGURE 290   Abdominal Cavity: Descending and Sigmoid Colons and the Duodenojejunal Junction

NOTE: (1) The transverse colon and greater omentum have been reflected upward and the jejunum and ileum have been pulled to the right to reveal the **duodenojejunal junction** and the **descending** and **sigmoid colon.**

(2) At the duodenojejunal junction the small intestine acquires a mesentery. At this site, there are frequently found duodenal fossae or recesses located in relationship to the junction. Among these, the **superior** and **inferior duodenal recesses** are found in more than 50% of cases. These are of importance because they represent possible sites of herniation.

(3) The sigmoid colon is mobile (because of its mesocolic attachment), whereas the descending colon is fixed to the posterior wall of the abdomen.

(4) The **intersigmoid fossa** is located behind the sigmoid mesocolon and between that mesocolon and the peritoneum reflected over the external iliac vessels.

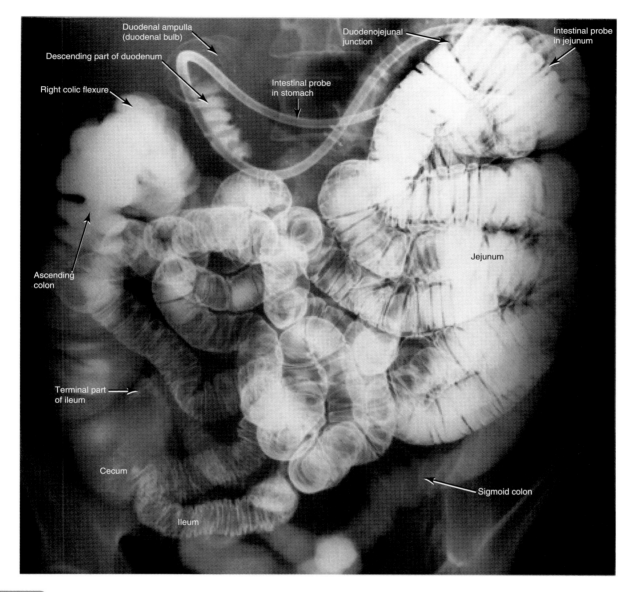

FIGURE 291 **Radiograph of the Jejunum, Ileum, Cecum, and Ascending Colon**

NOTE: (1) This radiograph of the small bowel was obtained following an injection of a contrast medium into the gastrointestinal tract. The intestinal probe in this case was introduced through the stomach and duodenum to the jejunum.

(2) The cecum, ascending colon, right colic flexure, and sigmoid colon are also recognizable.

(3) Some of the medium had entered the descending part of the duodenum also to be visualized.

(From Wicke, 4th ed.)

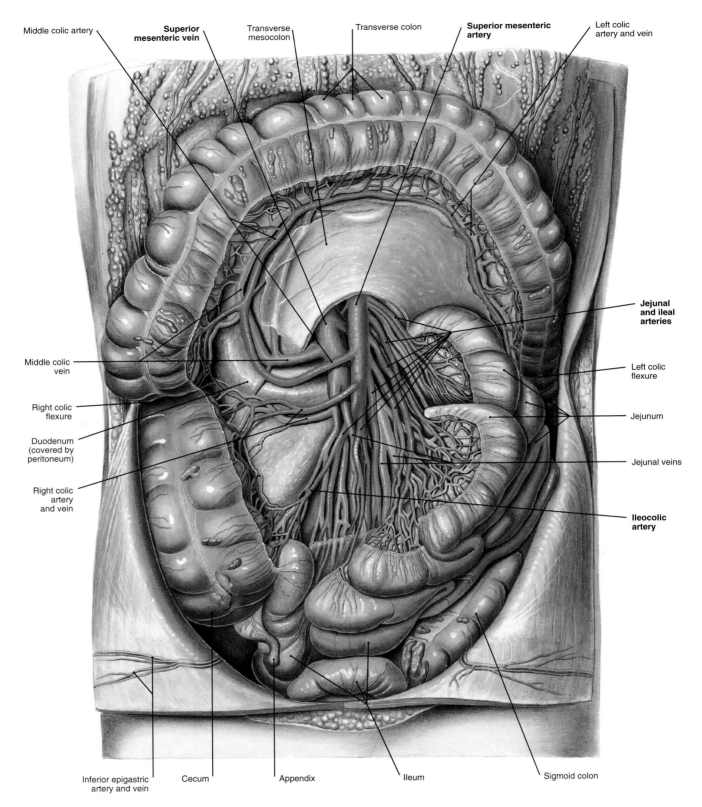

Middle colic artery

Superior mesenteric vein

Transverse mesocolon

Transverse colon

Superior mesenteric artery

Left colic artery and vein

Jejunal and ileal arteries

Left colic flexure

Jejunum

Jejunal veins

Ileocolic artery

Middle colic vein

Right colic flexure

Duodenum (covered by peritoneum)

Right colic artery and vein

Inferior epigastric artery and vein

Cecum

Appendix

Ileum

Sigmoid colon

FIGURE 292 **Abdominal Cavity: Superior Mesenteric Vessels and Branches**

NOTE: (1) The small intestine is pushed to the left and the loops of bowel have been dissected to expose the branches of the superior mesenteric vessels.

(2) The **jejunal and ileal arteries** branch from the left side of the mesenteric artery. There are about 15 of these vessels.

(3) Branching from the right side of the superior mesenteric artery are the **ileocolic, right colic,** and **middle colic arteries.** These vessels form rich anastomoses.

(4) The small intestine measures about 22 ft in length, commencing at the pyloric end of the stomach and extending to the ileocecal junction, where the large intestine starts.

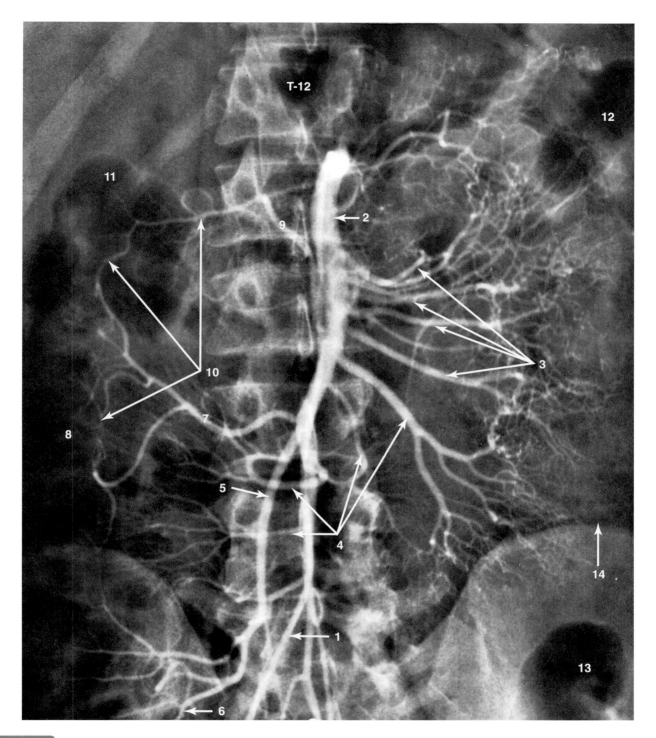

FIGURE 293 **Superior Mesenteric Arteriogram**

NOTE: (1) A catheter [1] has been inserted into the common iliac artery and through the abdominal aorta to the point of branching of the superior mesenteric artery [2]. Contrast medium was injected to visualize the principal branches of that vessel. The original radiograph is shown as a negative print.

(2) The jejunal [3] and ileal [4] arteries branching as a sequence of vessels (about 15 in number), which supply all of the small intestine beyond the duodenum.

(3) The ileocolic artery [5] and its appendicular branch [6], the right colic [7] and middle colic [9] arteries, which supply the cecum, ascending colon [8], and transverse colon. Anastomoses among these vessels along the margin of the colon contribute to the formation of the marginal artery [10].

(4) Other structures can be identified. These include the right colic flexure [11], the left colic flexure [12], the sigmoid colon [13], the body of the T12 vertebra, and the iliac crest [14].

(From Wicke, 3rd ed.)

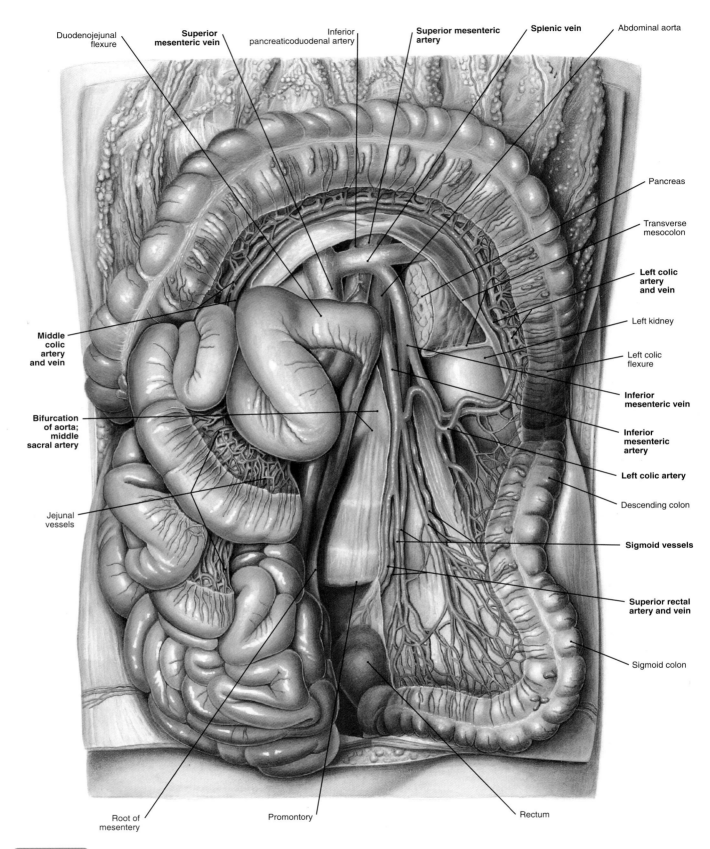

Duodenojejunal flexure

Superior mesenteric vein

Inferior pancreaticoduodenal artery

Superior mesenteric artery

Splenic vein

Abdominal aorta

Pancreas

Transverse mesocolon

Left colic artery and vein

Left kidney

Left colic flexure

Inferior mesenteric vein

Inferior mesenteric artery

Left colic artery

Descending colon

Sigmoid vessels

Superior rectal artery and vein

Sigmoid colon

Rectum

Middle colic artery and vein

Bifurcation of aorta; middle sacral artery

Jejunal vessels

Root of mesentery

Promontory

FIGURE 294 **Abdominal Cavity: Inferior Mesenteric Vessels and Branches**

NOTE: (1) The small intestine has been pushed to the right and parts of the pancreas and transverse mesocolon have been removed to expose the origin of the superior mesenteric artery from the aorta and the drainage of the superior mesenteric vein into the splenic vein.

(2) The inferior mesenteric artery supplies the descending colon via the **left colic artery** and the sigmoid colon and rectum via the **sigmoid** and **superior rectal arteries.**

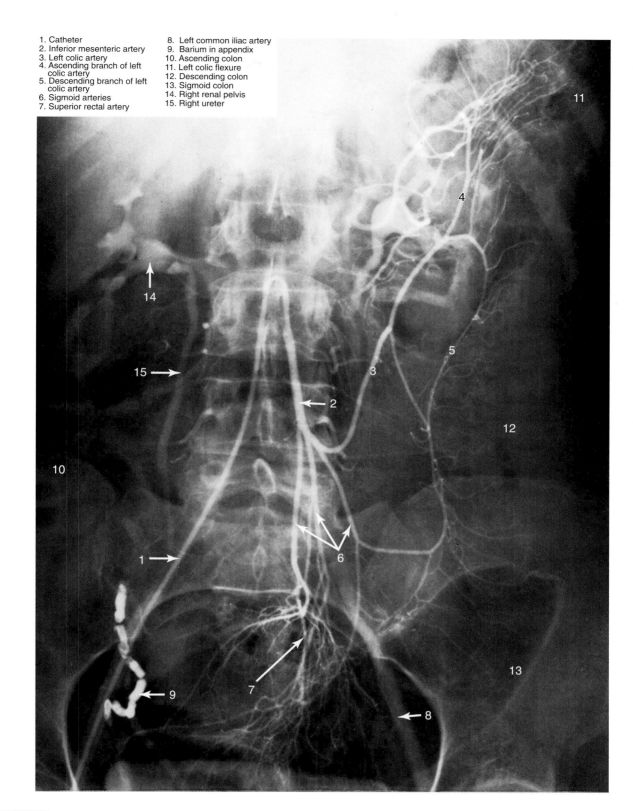

1. Catheter
2. Inferior mesenteric artery
3. Left colic artery
4. Ascending branch of left colic artery
5. Descending branch of left colic artery
6. Sigmoid arteries
7. Superior rectal artery
8. Left common iliac artery
9. Barium in appendix
10. Ascending colon
11. Left colic flexure
12. Descending colon
13. Sigmoid colon
14. Right renal pelvis
15. Right ureter

FIGURE 295 **Inferior Mesenteric Arteriogram**

NOTE: (1) A catheter [1] was inserted through the right internal iliac artery and directed upward into the abdominal aorta to the origin of the **inferior mesenteric artery** [2]. Contrast medium was injected into that artery to demonstrate its field of distribution.

(2) The branches of the inferior mesenteric artery shown above are normal. The **left colic artery** [3] shows both an ascending [4] and a descending [5] branch.

(3) Several **sigmoid arteries** [6] supply the sigmoid colon [13], and these anastomose above with branches of the left colic artery [3] and below with the **superior rectal artery** [7].

(From Wicke, 3rd ed.)

PLATE 296 The Abdominal Arteries

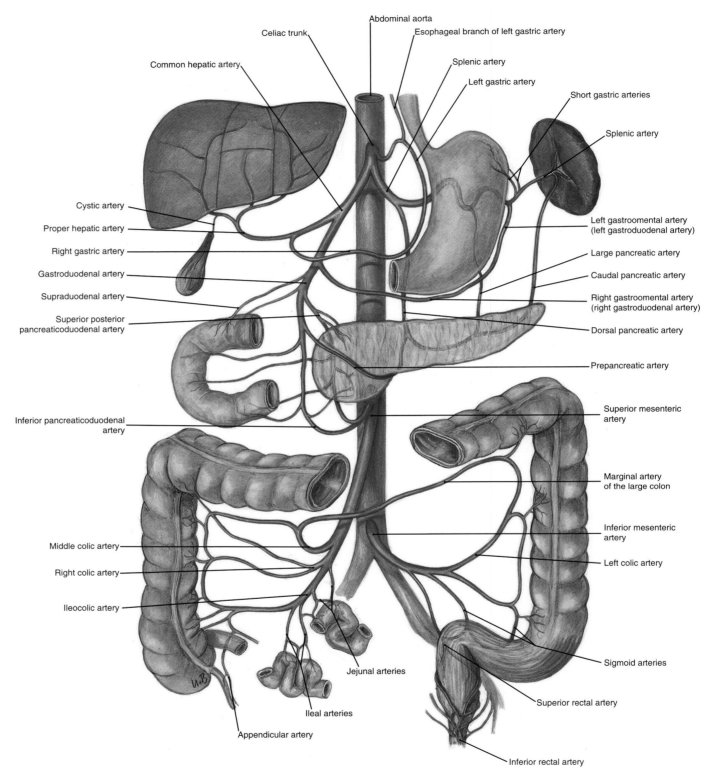

Abdominal aorta

Celiac trunk

Esophageal branch of left gastric artery

Common hepatic artery

Splenic artery

Left gastric artery

Short gastric arteries

Splenic artery

Cystic artery

Proper hepatic artery

Right gastric artery

Gastroduodenal artery

Supraduodenal artery

Superior posterior pancreaticoduodenal artery

Inferior pancreaticoduodenal artery

Middle colic artery

Right colic artery

Ileocolic artery

Left gastroomental artery (left gastroduodenal artery)

Large pancreatic artery

Caudal pancreatic artery

Right gastroomental artery (right gastroduodenal artery)

Dorsal pancreatic artery

Prepancreatic artery

Superior mesenteric artery

Marginal artery of the large colon

Inferior mesenteric artery

Left colic artery

Sigmoid arteries

Jejunal arteries

Ileal arteries

Appendicular artery

Superior rectal artery

Inferior rectal artery

FIGURE 296 **Arteries to the Abdominal Viscera**

NOTE that these abdominal arteries are branches from the **celiac trunk, superior mesenteric artery,** or **inferior mesenteric artery.**

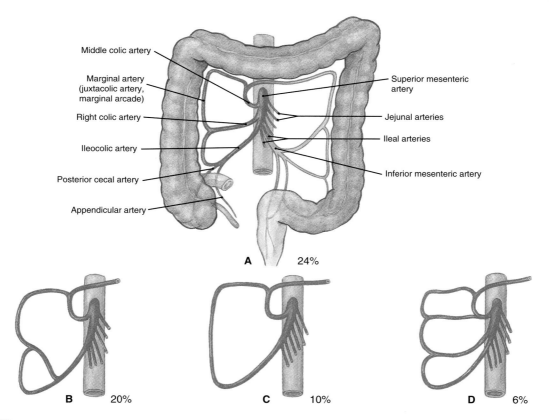

FIGURE 297.1 **Variations in the Branching of the Superior Mesenteric Artery**

NOTE: (1) Normal pattern: ascending and transverse colon supplied by three branches.
(2) Formation of an ileocolic and right colic trunk.
(3) Only two branches with the right colic artery absent.
(4) Two right colic arteries.

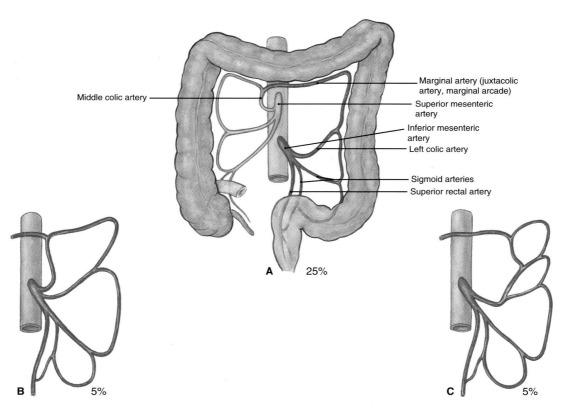

FIGURE 297.2 **Variations in the Branching of the Inferior Mesenteric Artery**

NOTE: (1) Single trunk that divides into three branches (for descending colon, sigmoid colon and rectum);
(2) An accessory middle colic artery branching from the inferior mesenteric artery;
(3) An accessory middle colic artery from the left colic artery. (For "normal pattern," see Fig. 294.)

PLATE 298 The Hepatic Portal Vein and Its Tributaries

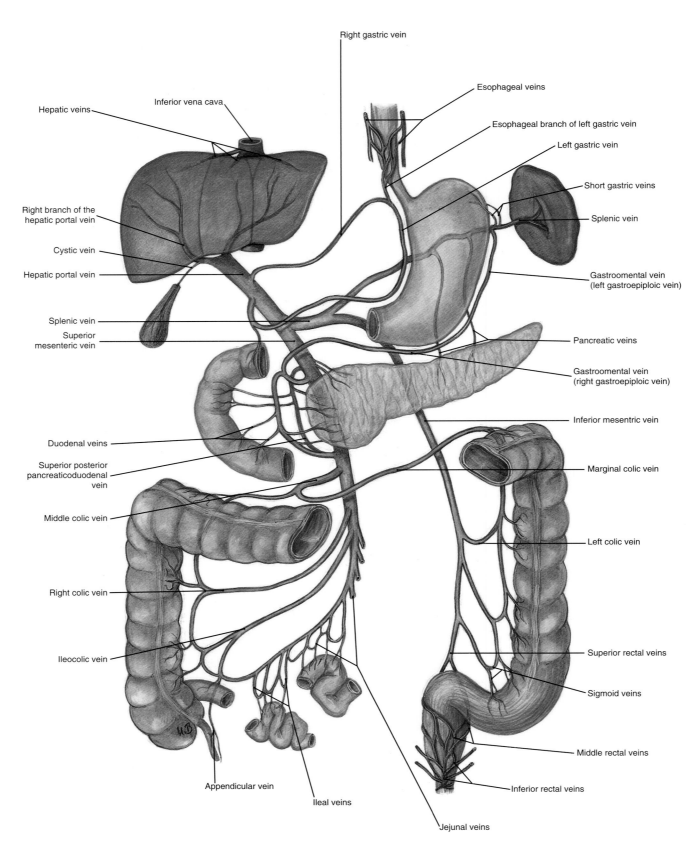

Right gastric vein

Esophageal veins

Esophageal branch of left gastric vein

Left gastric vein

Short gastric veins

Splenic vein

Hepatic veins

Inferior vena cava

Gastroomental vein
(left gastroepiploic vein)

Right branch of the
hepatic portal vein

Cystic vein

Hepatic portal vein

Pancreatic veins

Gastroomental vein
(right gastroepiploic vein)

Splenic vein

Superior
mesenteric vein

Inferior mesentric vein

Duodenal veins

Superior posterior
pancreaticoduodenal
vein

Marginal colic vein

Middle colic vein

Left colic vein

Right colic vein

Ileocolic vein

Superior rectal veins

Sigmoid veins

Middle rectal veins

Appendicular vein

Inferior rectal veins

Ileal veins

Jejunal veins

FIGURE 298 Venous Drainage of Abdominal Organs: Hepatic Portal Vein and Its Tributaries

NOTE: (1) The **inferior mesenteric vein** drains part of the transverse colon and the descending and sigmoid colons, and it flows into the splenic vein.

(2) The **superior mesenteric vein** drains the jejunum, ileum, ileocolic region, ascending colon, and part of the transverse colon. It ascends and receives pancreaticoduodenal branches, and **then** it is joined by the splenic vein to form the **portal vein.**

(3) The **splenic vein** not only receives venous blood from the inferior mesenteric vein but also drains the veins of the stomach. Esophageal veins draining the inferior part of the esophagus flow directly into the portal vein.

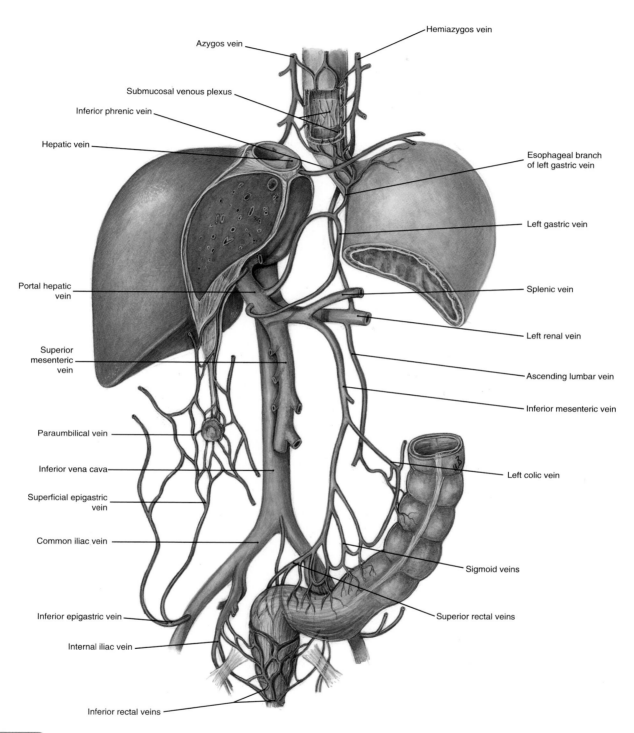

Hemiazygos vein

Azygos vein

Submucosal venous plexus

Inferior phrenic vein

Hepatic vein

Esophageal branch of left gastric vein

Left gastric vein

Portal hepatic vein

Splenic vein

Left renal vein

Superior mesenteric vein

Ascending lumbar vein

Inferior mesenteric vein

Paraumbilical vein

Inferior vena cava

Left colic vein

Superficial epigastric vein

Common iliac vein

Sigmoid veins

Inferior epigastric vein

Superior rectal veins

Internal iliac vein

Inferior rectal veins

FIGURE 299 **The Relationship of the Hepatic Portal Vein and the Inferior Vena Cava**

NOTE: (1) The **paraumbilical veins** allow an anastomosis between veins on the anterior thoracic wall (paraumbilical and inferior epigastric veins) and the hepatic portal system of veins.

(2) The superior vena cava ascends posterior to the liver, but it receives the hepatic veins just before it courses through the diaphragm on its way to the right atrium.

(3) The inferior mesenteric vein joins the splenic vein, which then joins the superior mesenteric vein to form the portal vein.

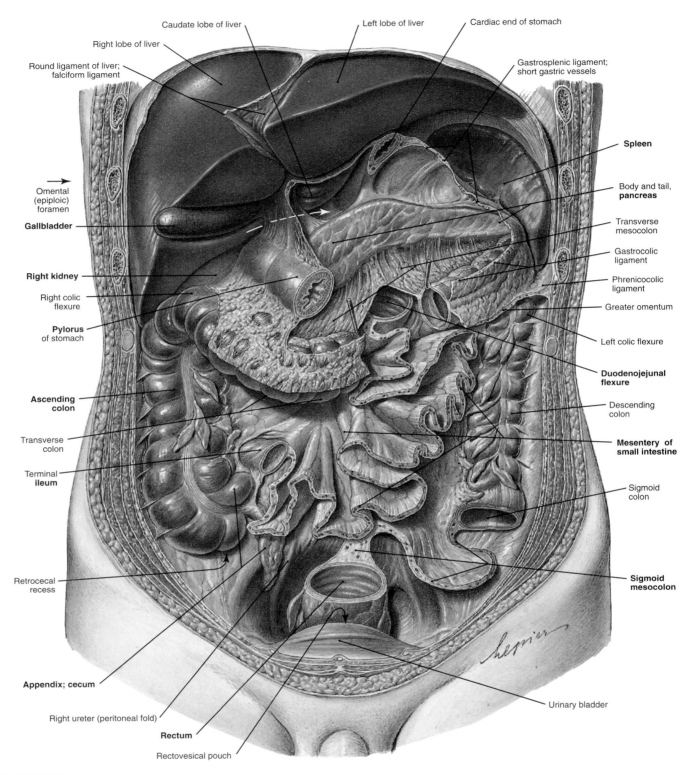

Caudate lobe of liver

Left lobe of liver

Cardiac end of stomach

Right lobe of liver

Round ligament of liver; falciform ligament

Gastrosplenic ligament; short gastric vessels

Spleen

Omental (epiploic) foramen

Gallbladder

Body and tail, **pancreas**

Transverse mesocolon

Gastrocolic ligament

Right kidney

Phrenicocolic ligament

Right colic flexure

Greater omentum

Pylorus of stomach

Left colic flexure

Duodenojejunal flexure

Ascending colon

Descending colon

Transverse colon

Mesentery of small intestine

Terminal **ileum**

Sigmoid colon

Retrocecal recess

Sigmoid mesocolon

Appendix; cecum

Urinary bladder

Right ureter (peritoneal fold)

Rectum

Rectovesical pouch

FIGURE 300 Abdominal Cavity: Large Intestine and Mesenteries

NOTE: (1) The stomach was cut just proximal to the pylorus and removed; the small intestine was severed at the duodenojejunal junction and at the distal ileum and also removed (by cutting the mesentery). A part of the transverse colon was resected along the greater omentum, and the sigmoid colon was removed to reveal its mesocolon.

(2) The **mesentery of the small intestine** extends obliquely across the posterior abdominal wall from the **duodenojejunal junction** to the **ileocecal junction.** In this 6 or 7 in., the mesenteric folds accommodate all of the loops of jejunum and ileum.

(3) The **ascending colon** and **descending colon** are fused to the posterior abdominal wall, whereas the **transverse colon** and **sigmoid colon** are suspended by their respective mesocolons.

(4) Vessels and nerves supplying the small intestine course between the layers of the mesentery to achieve the organ.

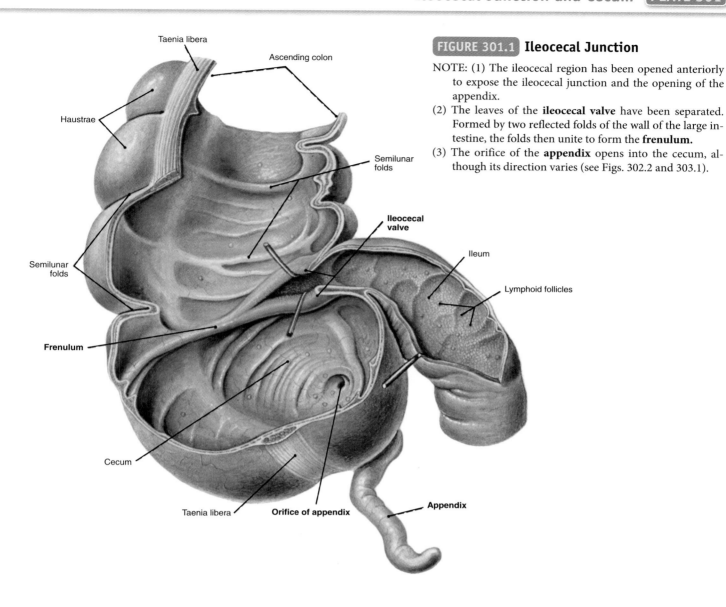

Taenia libera

Ascending colon

Haustrae

Semilunar folds

Semilunar folds

Ileocecal valve

Ileum

Lymphoid follicles

Frenulum

Cecum

Taenia libera

Orifice of appendix

Appendix

FIGURE 301.1 **Ileocecal Junction**

NOTE: (1) The ileocecal region has been opened anteriorly to expose the ileocecal junction and the opening of the appendix.

(2) The leaves of the **ileocecal valve** have been separated. Formed by two reflected folds of the wall of the large intestine, the folds then unite to form the **frenulum.**

(3) The orifice of the **appendix** opens into the cecum, although its direction varies (see Figs. 302.2 and 303.1).

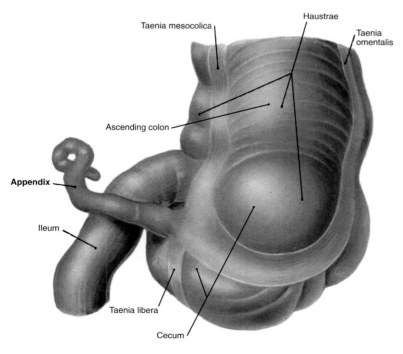

Haustrae

Taenia mesocolica

Taenia omentalis

Appendix

Ascending colon

Ileum

Taenia libera

Cecum

FIGURE 301.2 **Dorsal View of the Cecum and Appendix**

NOTE: (1) The attachments of the ileum and appendix to the cecum are clearly visualized with the peritoneum stripped away.

(2) The **taeniae coli** (three) are strips of longitudinal smooth muscle. The **taenia libera** is located anterior on the cecum, the **taenia mesocolica** is situated posteromedially, whereas the **taenia omentalis** is located posterolaterally on the cecum.

(3) The three taeniae come together at the origin of the appendix on the cecum.

PLATE 302 Vermiform Appendix

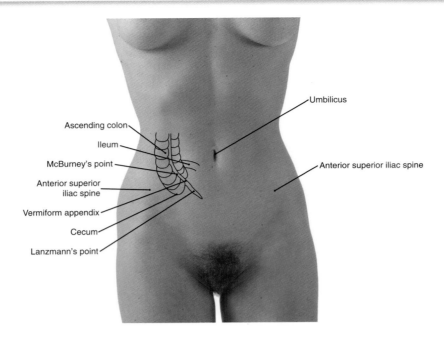

FIGURE 302.1 Surface Projection of the Cecum and the Vermiform Appendix

NOTE: (1) The vermiform appendix emerges from the posteromedial wall of the cecum slightly less than 1 in. (about 2 cm) distal to the end of the ileum.

(2) Inflammation of the appendix, called **appendicitis,** is indicated by severe abdominal pain. This often results from an obstruction of the lumen of the appendix that may be due to a proliferation of lymphatic nodules or by a fecalith (a hardened intestinal concretion that forms around a center of fecal matter). After a period of time, the walls of the appendix become inflamed, and pain is usually felt with or without pressure in the lower right quadrant.

(3) Another cause of appendicitis can be an interruption of the blood supply to the appendix.

*__Lanzmann's Point:__ A tender point in appendicitis situated on a line between the two anterior superior iliac spines, 5 to 6 cm from the right spine and 2 cm below McBurney's point.

**__McBurney's Point:__ A point of special tenderness in acute appendicitis situated about 2 in. (5 cm) from the right anterior superior iliac spine on a line between the spines and the umbilicus.

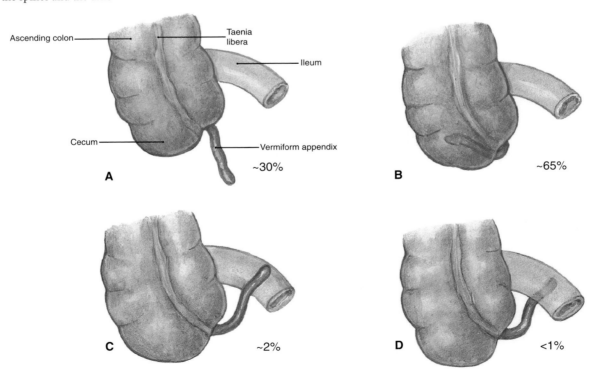

FIGURE 302.2 The Appendix: Variations in Location

A: Descending over the pelvic brim; **B:** retrocecal location; **C:** anterior to the ileum; **D:** posterior to the ileum.

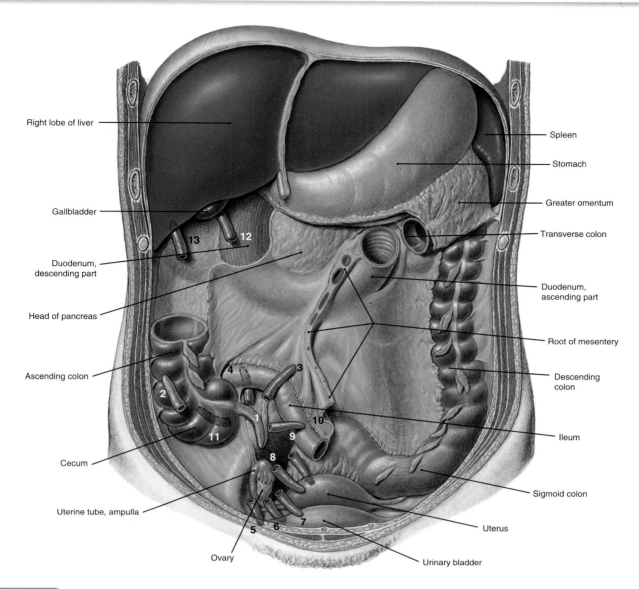

Right lobe of liver

Gallbladder

Duodenum, descending part

Head of pancreas

Ascending colon

Cecum

Uterine tube, ampulla

Ovary

Spleen

Stomach

Greater omentum

Transverse colon

Duodenum, ascending part

Root of mesentery

Descending colon

Ileum

Sigmoid colon

Uterus

Urinary bladder

FIGURE 303.1 Variations in the Location of the Appendix

NOTE that at least 13 sites for the appendix have been reported; most common are 11, 1, 3, 10, and 4, respectively.

1. Over the pelvic brim
2. Anterolaterally
3. Toward the root of the mesentery
4. Dorsal to the terminal ileum
5. Toward the deep inguinal ring
6. In the uterovesical pouch
7. Anterior to the bladder
8. On the uterus or uterine tube
9. In the rectouterine pouch
10. Medially, anterior to the ileum
11. Behind the cecum
12. Toward the gallbladder
13. Toward the liver

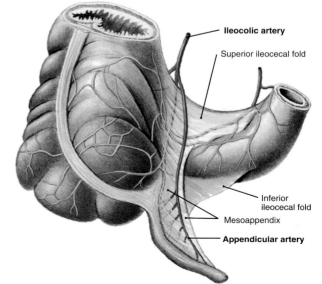

Ileocolic artery

Superior ileocecal fold

Inferior ileocecal fold

Mesoappendix

Appendicular artery

FIGURE 303.2 Blood Supply to the Vermiform Appendix

NOTE: The appendix usually receives its vascular supply by way of the **appendicular artery,** a branch of the ileocolic artery, and it descends either anterior to the ileocecal junction (as shown) or behind it.

PLATE 304 Large Intestine

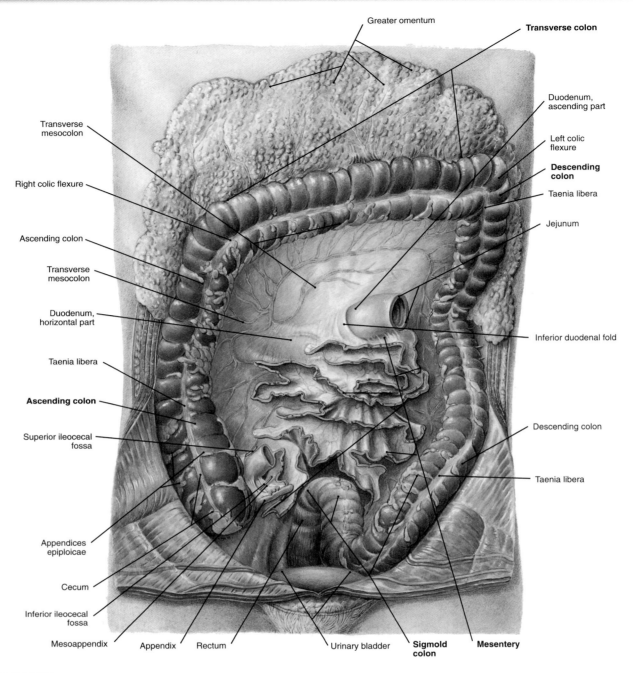

Greater omentum

Transverse colon

Duodenum, ascending part

Left colic flexure

Descending colon

Taenia libera

Jejunum

Inferior duodenal fold

Descending colon

Taenia libera

Descending colon

Mesentery

Sigmoid colon

Urinary bladder

Rectum

Appendix

Mesoappendix

Inferior ileocecal fossa

Cecum

Appendices epiploicae

Superior ileocecal fossa

Ascending colon

Taenia libera

Duodenum, horizontal part

Transverse mesocolon

Ascending colon

Right colic flexure

Transverse mesocolon

FIGURE 304.1 **Large Intestine from Cecum to Rectum ▲**

FIGURE 304.2 **Segment of Transverse Colon**

NOTE: (1) A cut was made along the **taenia libera** at the right of this segment of transverse colon, and its wall opened to show its inner surface.

(2) The greater omentum attaches along the **taenia omentalis,** the transverse mesocolon attaches along the **taenia mesocolica,** whereas the **taenia libera** is free from such attachments.

(3) The large intestine is about 5 ft long and its diameter (1.5–3 in.) varies, being widest at the cecum, then narrowing, and dilating again at the rectal ampulla.

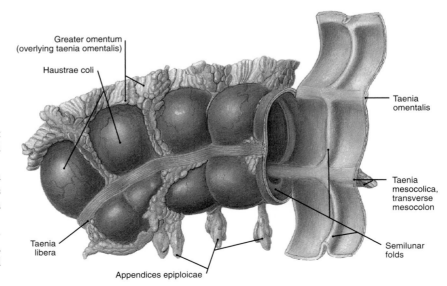

Greater omentum (overlying taenia omentalis)

Haustrae coli

Taenia omentalis

Taenia mesocolica, transverse mesocolon

Semilunar folds

Appendices epiploicae

Taenia libera

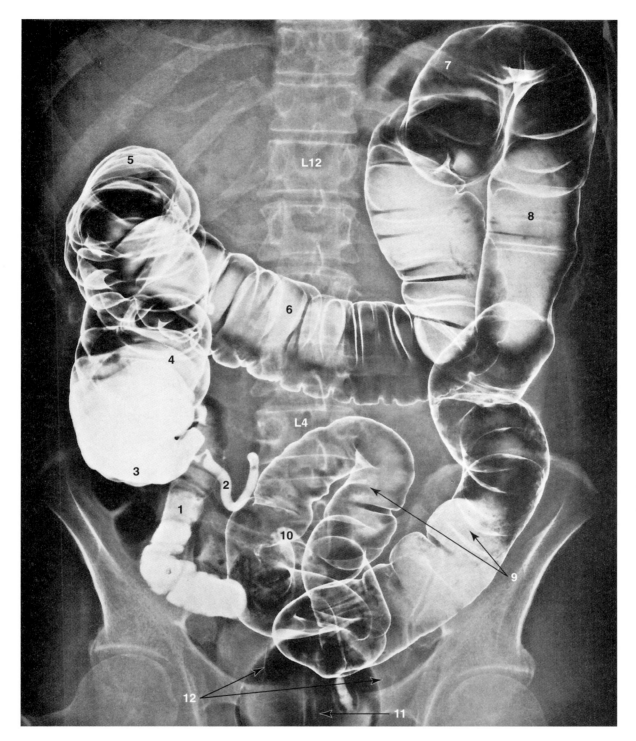

FIGURE 305 **Radiographic Anatomy of the Large Intestine (Double Contrast)**

NOTE: (1) In this patient, barium sulfate was administered as an enema and the mixture was then expelled and the colon insufflated with air (barium–air double contrast method).

(2) The cecum [3] is usually located in the iliac fossa of the lower right quadrant, and it forms a cul-de-sac that opens into the ascending colon [4]. The terminal ileum [1] most often joins the cecum on its medial or posterior surface. The appendix [2] extends from the cecum about 2 cm below the ileocecal opening. The right colic flexure [5] continues to the left to become the transverse colon [6].

(3) The transverse colon, suspended by its mesentery, crosses the abdomen. It turns inferiorly at the left colic flexure [7] as the descending colon [8].

(4) The descending colon becomes the sigmoid colon [9] at the inlet to the lesser pelvis. With its mesentery, the sigmoid colon leads into the rectum [10], within the true pelvis.

(5) The locations of the T12 and L4 vertebrae, the symphysis pubis [11], and an air-filled balloon [12].

(From Wicke, 3rd ed.)

PLATE 306 Abdominal Cavity 10: Roots of the Mesocolons and Mesentery

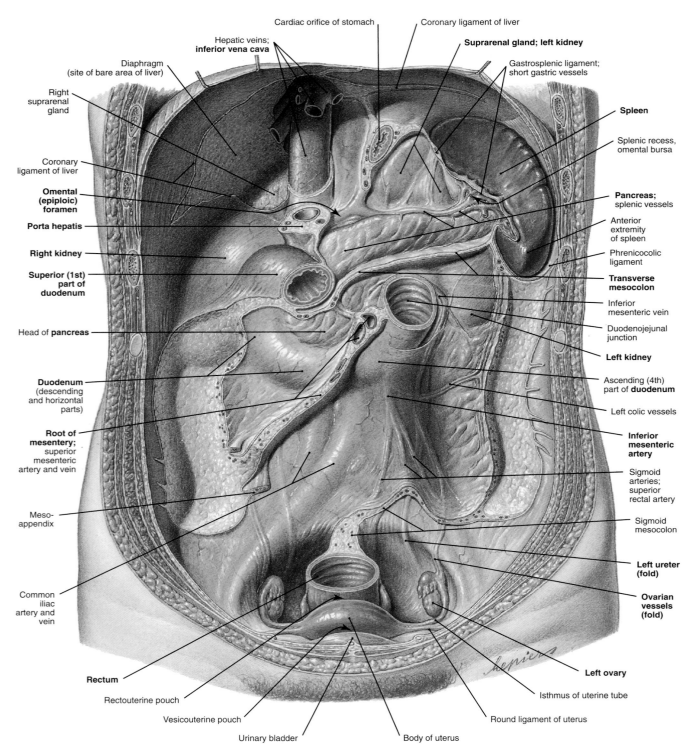

Cardiac orifice of stomach
Coronary ligament of liver
Hepatic veins;
inferior vena cava
Suprarenal gland; left kidney
Diaphragm
(site of bare area of liver)
Gastrosplenic ligament;
short gastric vessels
Right
suprarenal
gland
Spleen
Splenic recess,
omental bursa
Coronary
ligament of liver
Pancreas;
splenic vessels
**Omental
(epiploic)
foramen**
Anterior
extremity
of spleen
Porta hepatis
Phrenicocolic
ligament
Right kidney
**Transverse
mesocolon**
**Superior (1st)
part of
duodenum**
Inferior
mesenteric vein
Duodenojejunal
junction
Head of **pancreas**
Left kidney
Duodenum
(descending
and horizontal
parts)
Ascending (4th)
part of **duodenum**
Left colic vessels
**Root of
mesentery;**
superior
mesenteric
artery and vein
**Inferior
mesenteric
artery**
Sigmoid
arteries;
superior
rectal artery
Meso-
appendix
Sigmoid
mesocolon
**Left ureter
(fold)**
Common
iliac
artery and
vein
**Ovarian
vessels
(fold)**
Rectum
Left ovary
Isthmus of uterine tube
Rectouterine pouch
Vesicouterine pouch
Round ligament of uterus
Urinary bladder
Body of uterus

FIGURE 306 **Abdominal Cavity; Posterior Abdominal Peritoneum (Female)**

NOTE: (1) The stomach and the intestines (except for the duodenum and rectum) have been removed and their mesenteries cut close to their roots on the posterior abdominal wall. The liver and gallbladder were also removed, but the spleen and the retroperitoneal organs (duodenum, pancreas, adrenal glands, kidneys and ureters, aorta, and inferior vena cava) are intact.

(2) The ascending and descending portions of the large intestine are fused to the posterior abdominal wall with peritoneum covering their anterior surfaces.

(3) The course of the ureters and ovarian vessels descending over the pelvic brim. Observe the ovaries, uterine tubes, and uterus located in the pelvis and their relationship to the rectum and bladder.

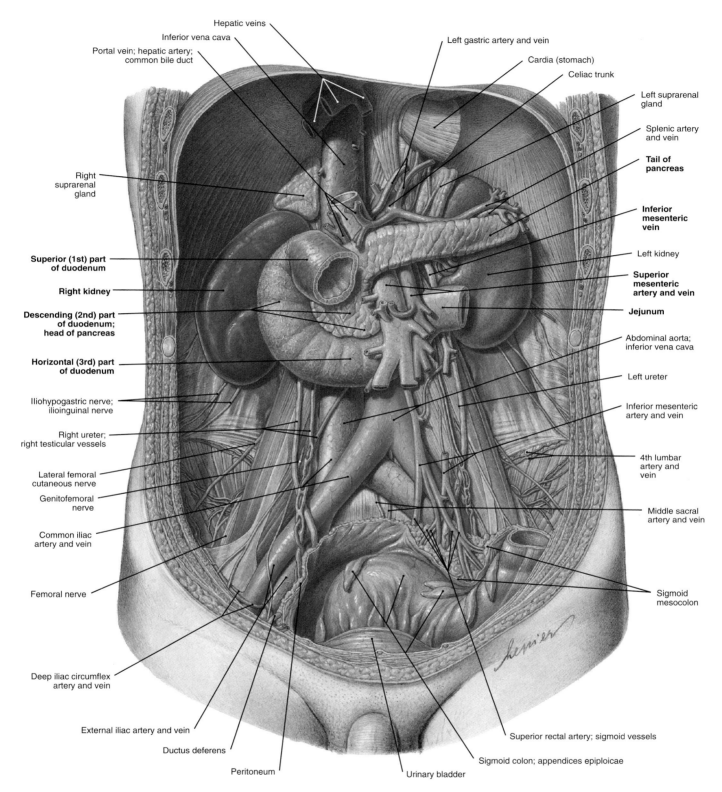

Hepatic veins
Inferior vena cava
Portal vein; hepatic artery; common bile duct
Left gastric artery and vein
Cardia (stomach)
Celiac trunk
Left suprarenal gland
Splenic artery and vein
Tail of pancreas
Right suprarenal gland
Inferior mesenteric vein
Left kidney
Superior (1st) part of duodenum
Superior mesenteric artery and vein
Right kidney
Jejunum
Descending (2nd) part of duodenum; head of pancreas
Abdominal aorta; inferior vena cava
Horizontal (3rd) part of duodenum
Left ureter
Iliohypogastric nerve; ilioinguinal nerve
Inferior mesenteric artery and vein
Right ureter; right testicular vessels
4th lumbar artery and vein
Lateral femoral cutaneous nerve
Genitofemoral nerve
Middle sacral artery and vein
Common iliac artery and vein
Femoral nerve
Sigmoid mesocolon
Deep iliac circumflex artery and vein
External iliac artery and vein
Superior rectal artery; sigmoid vessels
Ductus deferens
Sigmoid colon; appendices epiploicae
Peritoneum
Urinary bladder

FIGURE 307 **Abdominal Cavity: Retroperitoneal Organs (Male)**

NOTE: (1) The curvature of the duodenum lies ventral to the hilum of the right kidney, and the duodenojejunal junction is ventral to the lower medial border of the left kidney. The right kidney is slightly lower than the left.

(2) The head of the pancreas lies anterior to the inferior vena cava and within the curve of the duodenum. An extension of the pancreatic head, the uncinate process (see Fig. 283.2) lies behind the root of the superior mesenteric vessels.

(3) Upon crossing the midline at the L1 level, the posterior surface of the body and tail of the pancreas is in contact with the middle third of the left kidney.

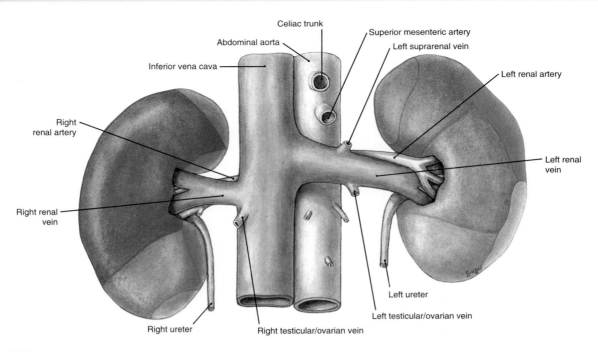

FIGURE 308.1 Anterior Surface Contact Relationships of the Kidneys

NOTE: (1) The relationships of abdominal organs to the anterior surface of the kidneys are characterized either by a peritoneal reflection (**serosal**) intervening between the overlying organ and the kidney or by a direct contact between the kidney and the overlying organ (**fibrous**).

(2) The structures in contact with the anterior surface of the **right kidney** are the right suprarenal gland, hepatorenal ligament, duodenum (second part), liver, right colic flexure and transverse colon, and a small area of the jejunum.

(3) The structures in contact with the anterior surface of the **left kidney** are the left suprarenal gland, stomach, spleen, pancreas, jejunum, and left colic flexure. (See **Color Code** below.)

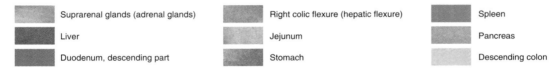

Suprarenal glands (adrenal glands)

Liver

Duodenum, descending part

Right colic flexure (hepatic flexure)

Jejunum

Stomach

Spleen

Pancreas

Descending colon

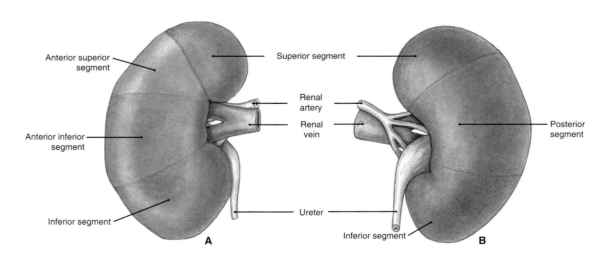

FIGURE 308.2 Segments of the Right Kidney

NOTE: **A:** Anterior surface of the renal segments.
B: Posterior surface of the renal segments.
Each segment has the same color on both anterior (**A**) and posterior (**B**) views of this right kidney.

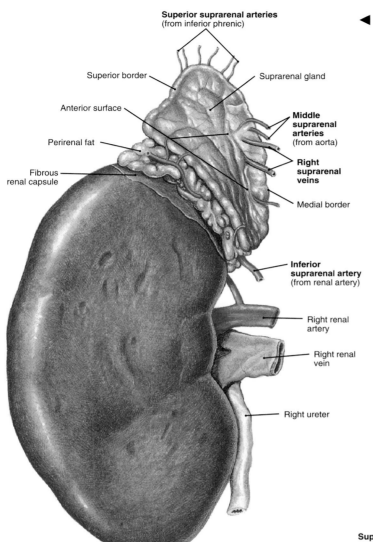

◄ FIGURE 309.1 **Right Kidney and Suprarenal Gland**

NOTE: (1) The suprarenal or adrenal gland is an endocrine gland whose secretions are vital for life. The glands are located in the posterior abdominal region and situated adjacent to the superior poles of the kidneys.

(2) The **right suprarenal gland** is pyramidal in shape, and its anterior surface lies behind the inferior vena cava and adjacent to the right lobe of the liver. Its posterior surface is in contact with the diaphragm and the right kidney.

(3) The suprarenal glands are highly vascular and receive arterial blood from branches directly off the aorta and others from the inferior phrenic and renal arteries. Venous blood is drained by a single vein or by a pair of veins that, on the right side, flow directly into the inferior vena cava, and on the left, into the renal vein.

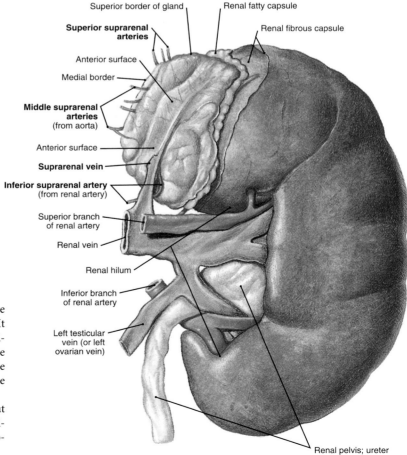

FIGURE 309.2 **Left Kidney and Suprarenal ►
Gland**

NOTE: (1) The **left suprarenal gland** is oriented onto the medial surface of the upper pole of the left kidney. It presents a crescentic shape with its concave surface adjacent to the kidney. Its anterior surface lies behind the cardiac end of the stomach and pancreas (behind the omental bursa), whereas its posterior surface rests on the crus of the diaphragm.

(2) The combined weight of the two glands averages about 10 g. The glands are each surrounded by an investing fibrous capsule, around which is a certain amount of areolar tissue.

PLATE 310 Suprarenal Vessels; Renal Arteriogram

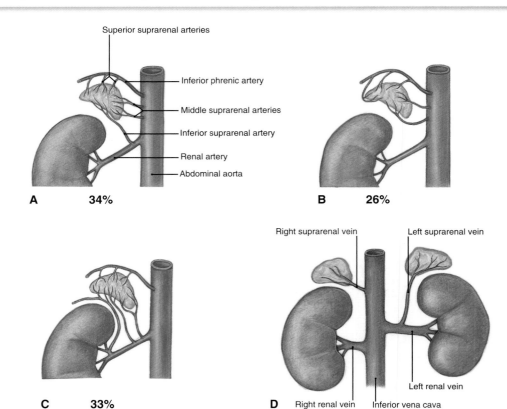

FIGURE 310.1A–D **Variations of the Arteries to the Suprarenal Gland; Suprarenal Veins**

NOTE that the suprarenal glands receive blood directly from the aorta and/or the renal arteries. Drainage of the veins differs on the two sides of the body.

A: Four arteries supplying the suprarenal gland (textbook case). **B:** Arterial supply only from the aorta. **C:** Arterial supply from the aorta and multiple vessels from the renal artery. **D:** Drainage from the renal veins.

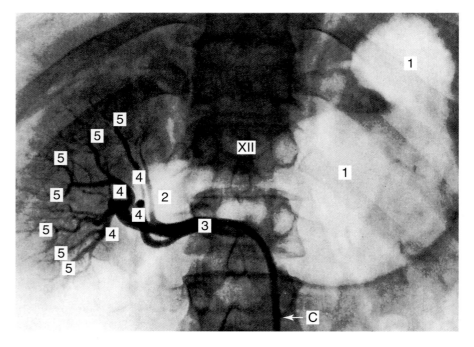

1. Stomach
2. Superior (1st) part of duodenum
3. Right renal artery
4. Interlobar arteries
5. Interlobular arteries
C. Catheter
XII. 12th thoracic vertebra

FIGURE 310.2 **Arteriogram of Right Renal Artery and Its Branches**

NOTE: (1) An arterial catheter [C] has beeen inserted into the femoral artery and passed through the abdominal aorta and then the **right renal artery.** Observe the division of the renal artery successively into **interlobar arteries.**

(2) As the interlobar arteries reach the junction of the renal cortex and medulla, they arch over the bases of the pyramids, forming **arcuate arteries** (not numbered in this figure). From the arcuate arteries branch a series of **interlobular arteries** [5], which extend through the afferent arterioles entering the renal glomeruli.

(3) The stomach [1] and superior part of the duodenum [2], which are filled with air.

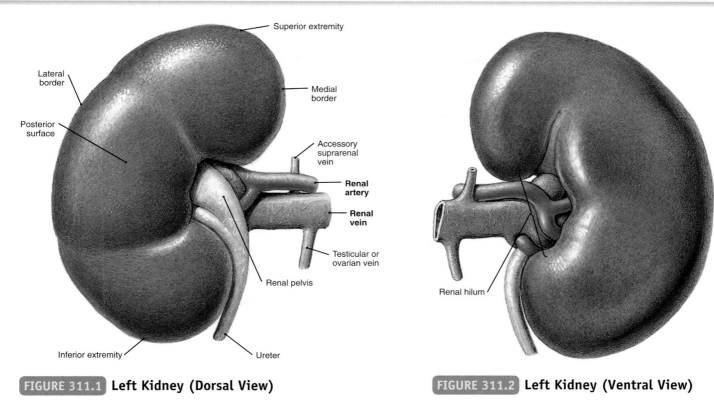

FIGURE 311.1 **Left Kidney (Dorsal View)**

FIGURE 311.2 **Left Kidney (Ventral View)**

NOTE: (1) The kidneys are paired, bean-shaped organs, and normally weigh about 125 to 150 g each. Their lateral borders are convex and their medial borders concave, the latter being interrupted by the renal vessels and the ureter.

(2) The **ureter** is the most posterior structure at the hilum (see Fig. 311.1). The **renal vein** is the most anterior structure at the hilum, but the **renal artery** frequently divides into anterior and posterior branches (or divisions), and the anterior branch often enters the kidney ventral to the renal vein, as shown in Figure 311.2.

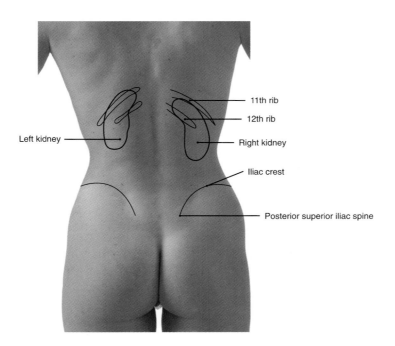

FIGURE 311.3 **Surface Anatomy of the Back, Showing the Projection of the Kidney**

NOTE: (1) The right kidney is more caudal than the left. Note that hle large sright lobe of the liver lies just superior to the right kidney.

(2) The inferior poles of the two kidneys are oriented more laterally than the superior poles. Observe the relationship of the kidneys to the 11th and 12th ribs on the two sides.

PLATE 312 Kidneys: Internal Structure, Longitudinal Section

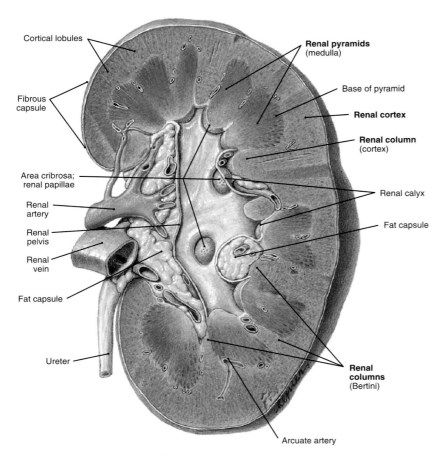

Cortical lobules

Fibrous capsule

Area cribrosa; renal papillae

Renal artery

Renal pelvis

Renal vein

Fat capsule

Ureter

Renal pyramids (medulla)

Base of pyramid

Renal cortex

Renal column (cortex)

Renal calyx

Fat capsule

Renal columns (Bertini)

Arcuate artery

FIGURE 312.1 **Left Kidney: Frontal Section through Renal Vessels**

NOTE: (1) The **cortex** of the kidney consists of an outer layer of somewhat lighter and granular-looking tissue, which is also seen to dip as **renal columns** (of Bertini) toward the pelvis of the kidney, thereby separating the conical **renal pyramids** of the **medulla.**

(2) Within the cortex are found the tufted glomeruli and convoluted tubules, whereas the renal pyramids principally contain the loops of Henle and the collecting tubes.

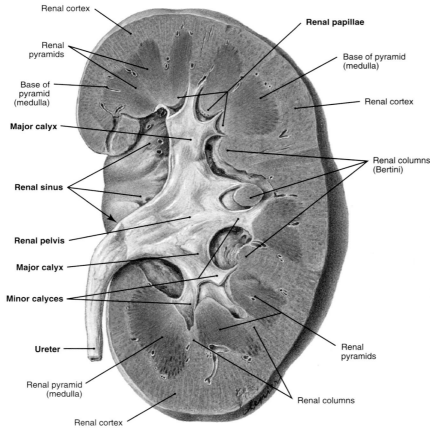

Renal cortex

Renal pyramids

Base of pyramid (medulla)

Major calyx

Renal sinus

Renal pelvis

Major calyx

Minor calyces

Ureter

Renal pyramid (medulla)

Renal cortex

Renal papillae

Base of pyramid (medulla)

Renal cortex

Renal columns (Bertini)

Renal pyramids

Renal columns

FIGURE 312.2 **Left Kidney: Frontal Section through Renal Pelvis**

NOTE: (1) This frontal section cuts through the renal pelvis and ureter. The **renal papillae** are cupped by small collecting tubes, the **minor calyces.**

(2) Several minor calyces unite to form a **major calyx,** whereas the **renal pelvis** is formed by the union of two or three major calyces. Leading from the renal pelvis is the somewhat more narrowed **ureter.**

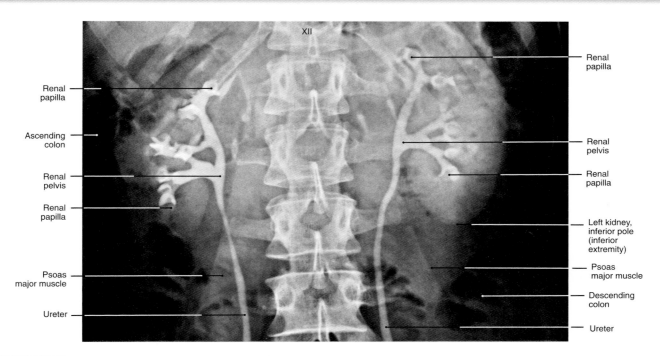

Renal papilla
Ascending colon
Renal pelvis
Renal papilla
Psoas major muscle
Ureter

XII

Renal papilla
Renal pelvis
Renal papilla
Left kidney, inferior pole (inferior extremity)
Psoas major muscle
Descending colon
Ureter

FIGURE 313.1 **Retrograde Pyelogram**

NOTE: (1) A radiopaque substance has been introduced into each ureter and forced into the renal pelvis, major calyces, and minor calyces of each side. Observe that into the minor calyces project the renal papillae, resulting in radiolucent invaginations into the radiopaque minor calyces.

(2) The shadow of the superior extremity of the left kidney extending to top of the body of the T12 vertebra, while the right kidney is somewhat more inferior.

(3) The lateral margins of the psoas major muscles. The ureters course toward the pelvis along their anterior surfaces.

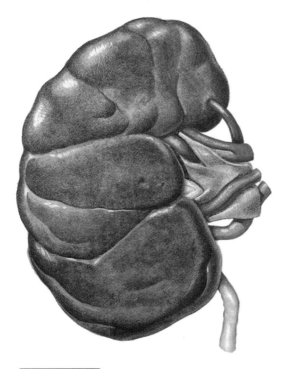

FIGURE 313.2 **Fetal Lobulation May Persist in the Adult Kidney**

NOTE: The kidney of the fetus is divided into small lobules that are separated by interlacing grooves on the renal surface. This lobulation usually disappears during the first postnatal year but may persist in the adult but with **no functional impairment.**

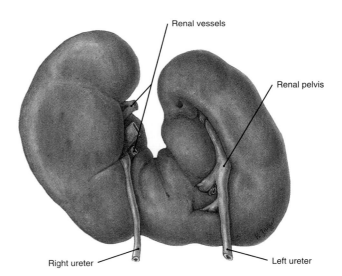

Renal vessels
Renal pelvis
Right ureter
Left ureter

FIGURE 313.3 **Horseshoe Kidney (Anterior View)**

NOTE: (1) **Horseshoe kidney** is a common anomaly (1 in 500 persons) in which the lower poles of the kidneys are fused.

(2) The fusion crosses the midline and is often found at the level of the aortic bifurcation. The ureters in the horseshoe kidney lie ventral to the renal vessels.

PLATE 314 Diaphragm and Other Muscles of the Posterior Abdominal Wall

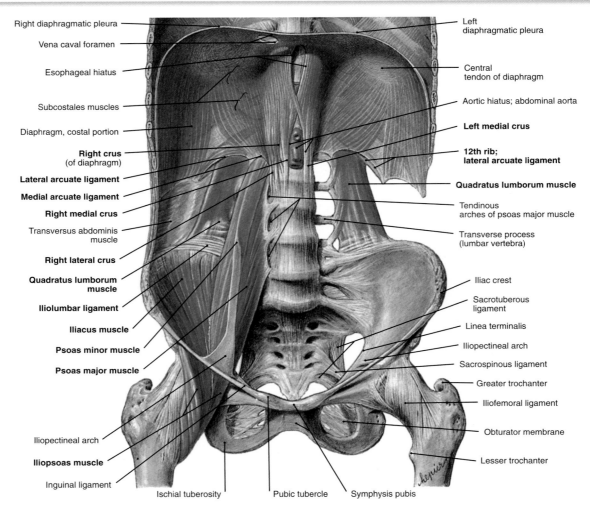

Right diaphragmatic pleura — Vena caval foramen — Esophageal hiatus — Subcostales muscles — Diaphragm, costal portion — **Right crus** (of diaphragm) — **Lateral arcuate ligament** — **Medial arcuate ligament** — **Right medial crus** — Transversus abdominis muscle — **Right lateral crus** — **Quadratus lumborum muscle** — **Iliolumbar ligament** — **Iliacus muscle** — **Psoas minor muscle** — **Psoas major muscle** — Iliopectineal arch — **Iliopsoas muscle** — Inguinal ligament — Ischial tuberosity — Pubic tubercle — Symphysis pubis

Left diaphragmatic pleura — Central tendon of diaphragm — Aortic hiatus; abdominal aorta — **Left medial crus** — **12th rib; lateral arcuate ligament** — **Quadratus lumborum muscle** — Tendinous arches of psoas major muscle — Transverse process (lumbar vertebra) — Iliac crest — Sacrotuberous ligament — Linea terminalis — Iliopectineal arch — Sacrospinous ligament — Greater trochanter — Iliofemoral ligament — Obturator membrane — Lesser trochanter

FIGURE 314 **Diaphragm and Posterior Abdominal Wall Structures**

NOTE: (1) The posterior attachments of the **diaphragm**: (a) the **right and left crura** arising from the bodies of the upper three or four lumbar vertebrae; (b) the **right and left medial arcuate ligaments** (thickenings in the psoas fascia); (c) the **lateral arcuate ligaments** along the 12th rib that lie superior to the quadratus lumborum muscle.

Muscle	Origin	Insertion	Innervation	Action
Diaphragm	**Sternal part:** Dorsum of xiphoid process. **Costal part:** Inner surfaces of cartilages and adjacent parts of lower six ribs. **Lumbar part:** Medial and lateral arcuate ligaments; crura from bodies of upper two or three lumbar vertebrae.	Central tendon of diaphragm	Phrenic nerve C3, C4, C5	Active during inspiration; assists in increasing intra-abdominal pressure
Quadratus lumborum	Iliolumbar ligament and the adjacent iliac crest	Medial half of the 12th rib and into the transverse processes of upper four lumbar vertebrae	Branches from T12, L1, L2, L3 (L4) nerves	Flexes vertebral column to the same side; fixes 12th rib in breathing; both muscles together extend lumbar vertebrae
Psoas major	Transverse process and body of T12 and upper four lumbar vertebrae; intervertebral disks between T12 and L5	Lesser trochanter of femur (also receives the fibers of iliacus muscle)	Branches from upper four lumbar nerves	Powerful flexor of thigh at hip; when femurs are fixed, they flex the trunk, as in sitting up from a supine position
Psoas minor (muscle present in about 40% of cadavers)	Lateral surface of bodies of T12 and L1 vertebrae	Pectineal line and iliopectineal eminence and the iliac fascia (often merges with psoas major tendon)	Branch from L1 nerve	Weak flexor of the thigh at the hip joint
Iliacus	Iliac fossa; anterior inferior iliac spine	Lesser trochanter of femur in common with tendon of psoas major muscle	Femoral nerve (L2, L3)	Powerful flexor of thigh at the hip joint

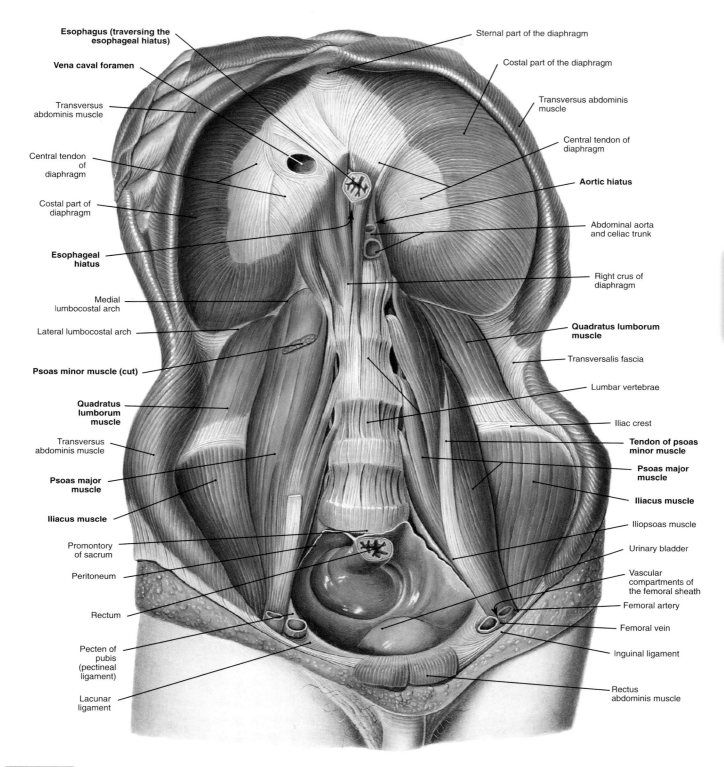

Esophagus (traversing the esophageal hiatus)

Vena caval foramen

Transversus abdominis muscle

Central tendon of diaphragm

Costal part of diaphragm

Esophageal hiatus

Medial lumbocostal arch

Lateral lumbocostal arch

Psoas minor muscle (cut)

Quadratus lumborum muscle

Transversus abdominis muscle

Psoas major muscle

Iliacus muscle

Promontory of sacrum

Peritoneum

Rectum

Pecten of pubis (pectineal ligament)

Lacunar ligament

Sternal part of the diaphragm

Costal part of the diaphragm

Transversus abdominis muscle

Central tendon of diaphragm

Aortic hiatus

Abdominal aorta and celiac trunk

Right crus of diaphragm

Quadratus lumborum muscle

Transversalis fascia

Lumbar vertebrae

Iliac crest

Tendon of psoas minor muscle

Psoas major muscle

Iliacus muscle

Iliopsoas muscle

Urinary bladder

Vascular compartments of the femoral sheath

Femoral artery

Femoral vein

Inguinal ligament

Rectus abdominis muscle

FIGURE 315 **Psoas Minor, Psoas Major, Iliacus, and Quadratus Lumborum Muscles and Diaphragm**

NOTE: (1) The **psoas minor muscle** lies anterior to the psoas major, and it merges with the lower part of the psoas major above the inguinal ligament.

(2) The **psoas major muscle** descends deep to the inguinal ligament and is joined by the iliacus muscle.

(3) The **iliacus muscle** arises from the iliac fossa, converges with the psoas major, and their joint tendon inserts onto the lesser trochanter of the femur.

(4) The **quadratus lumborum muscle** is a four-sided muscle on the dorsal wall of the abdomen, and it is located between the 12th rib, the iliac crest, and the transverse processes of the upper four lumbar vertebrae.

PLATE 316 Lumbar and Sacral Plexuses within Abdominopelvic Cavity

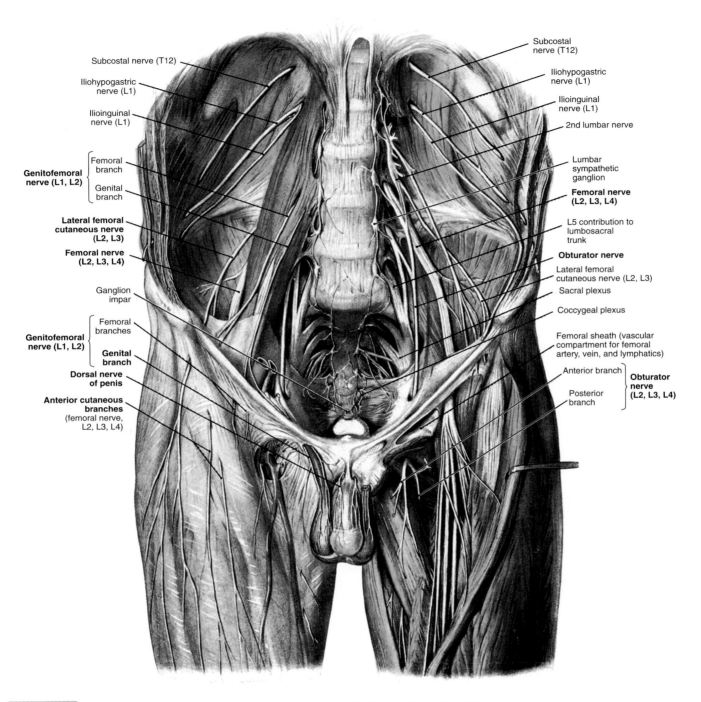

Subcostal nerve (T12)

Iliohypogastric nerve (L1)

Ilioinguinal nerve (L1)

Genitofemoral nerve (L1, L2) {Femoral branch / Genital branch

Lateral femoral cutaneous nerve (L2, L3)

Femoral nerve (L2, L3, L4)

Ganglion impar

Genitofemoral nerve (L1, L2) {Femoral branches / **Genital branch**

Dorsal nerve of penis

Anterior cutaneous branches (femoral nerve, L2, L3, L4)

Subcostal nerve (T12)

Iliohypogastric nerve (L1)

Ilioinguinal nerve (L1)

2nd lumbar nerve

Lumbar sympathetic ganglion

Femoral nerve (L2, L3, L4)

L5 contribution to lumbosacral trunk

Obturator nerve

Lateral femoral cutaneous nerve (L2, L3)

Sacral plexus

Coccygeal plexus

Femoral sheath (vascular compartment for femoral artery, vein, and lymphatics)

Anterior branch

Posterior branch

Obturator nerve (L2, L3, L4)

FIGURE 316 Lumbosacral Plexus: Posterior Abdominal Wall and Anterior Thigh

NOTE: (1) On the left side, the psoas muscles have been removed to reveal the **lumbar plexus** more completely. The lumbar nerves emerge from the spinal cord and descend along the posterior abdominal wall within the substance of the psoas muscles. The **12th thoracic** (subcostal) **nerve** courses around the abdominal wall below the 12th rib.

(2) The **first lumbar nerve** divides into **iliohypogastric** and **ilioinguinal branches.** The ilioinguinal nerve descends obliquely toward the iliac crest and penetrates the transversus and internal oblique muscles to join the spermatic cord, becoming cutaneous at the superficial inguinal ring.

(3) The **genitofemoral nerve** courses superficially on the surface of the psoas major muscle. It divides into a **genital branch** (which supplies the cremaster muscle and the skin of the scrotum) and a **femoral branch** (which is sensory to the upper anterior thigh).

(4) The **femoral** and **obturator nerves** derived from the posterior and anterior divisions of **L2, L3,** and **L4,** respectively, descend to innervate the anterior and medial groups of the femoral muscles.

(5) The femoral nerve enters the thigh beneath the inguinal ligament and Advides into both sensory and motor branches, whereas the obturator nerve courses more medially through the obturator foramen to innervate the adductor muscle group.

(6) L4 and L5 nerve roots (**lumbosacral trunk**) join with the upper three sacral nerves to form the **sacral plexus,** from which is derived, among other nerves, the large **sciatic nerve,** which reaches the gluteal region through the greater sciatic foramen.

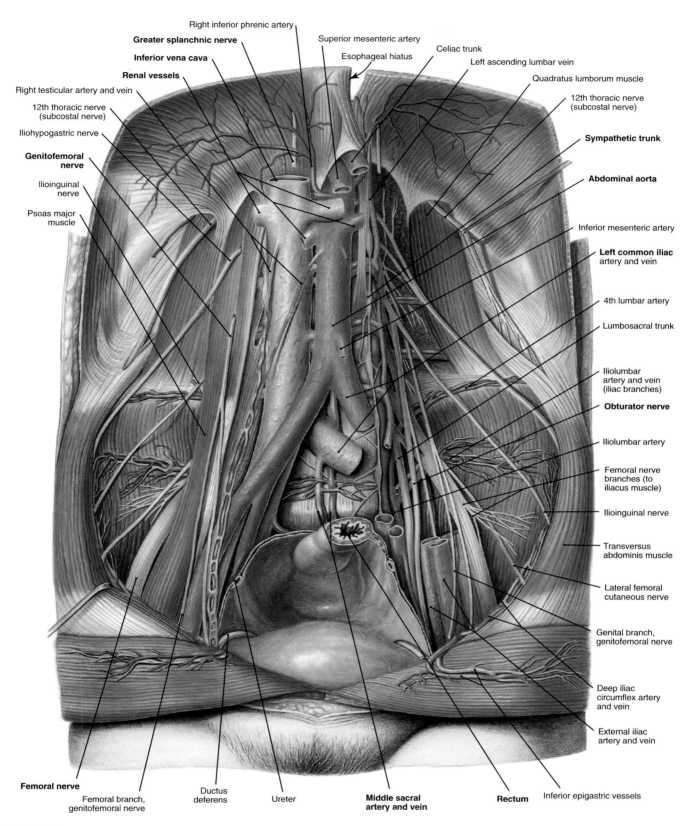

Right inferior phrenic artery

Greater splanchnic nerve

Inferior vena cava

Renal vessels

Right testicular artery and vein

12th thoracic nerve
(subcostal nerve)

Iliohypogastric nerve

Genitofemoral
nerve

Ilioinguinal
nerve

Psoas major
muscle

Superior mesenteric artery

Esophageal hiatus

Celiac trunk

Left ascending lumbar vein

Quadratus lumborum muscle

12th thoracic nerve
(subcostal nerve)

Sympathetic trunk

Abdominal aorta

Inferior mesenteric artery

Left common iliac
artery and vein

4th lumbar artery

Lumbosacral trunk

Iliolumbar
artery and vein
(iliac branches)

Obturator nerve

Iliolumbar artery

Femoral nerve
branches (to
iliacus muscle)

Ilioinguinal nerve

Transversus
abdominis muscle

Lateral femoral
cutaneous nerve

Genital branch,
genitofemoral nerve

Deep iliac
circumflex artery
and vein

External iliac
artery and vein

Femoral nerve

Femoral branch,
genitofemoral nerve

Ductus
deferens

Ureter

Middle sacral
artery and vein

Rectum

Inferior epigastric vessels

FIGURE 317 **Posterior Abdominal Vessels and Nerves**

NOTE: (1) The abdominal organs and the left psoas muscle have been removed. See the **greater splanchnic nerves** enter the abdomen through
the diaphragmatic crura. Identify the **inferior phrenic arteries** and the **abdominal sympathetic chain.**

(2) The **testicular arteries** arising from the aorta below the renal arteries. Inferiorly, the testicular artery and vein join the **ductus deferens** to
enter the inguinal canal through the abdominal inguinal ring just lateral to the inferior epigastric vessels. Observe the **middle sacral vessels**
descending into the pelvis in the midline.

PLATE 318 CT (T10) and Transverse Section (T11) of Abdomen

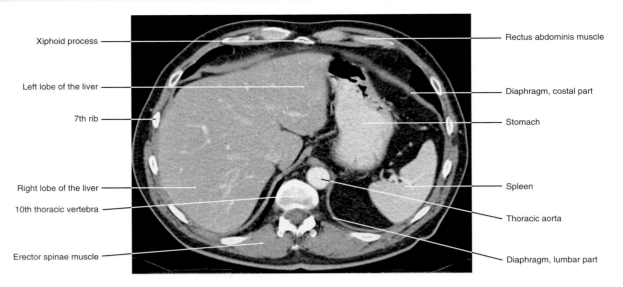

Xiphoid process

Left lobe of the liver

7th rib

Right lobe of the liver

10th thoracic vertebra

Erector spinae muscle

Rectus abdominis muscle

Diaphragm, costal part

Stomach

Spleen

Thoracic aorta

Diaphragm, lumbar part

FIGURE 318.1 **CT Transverse Section of the Abdomen at the Level of T10**

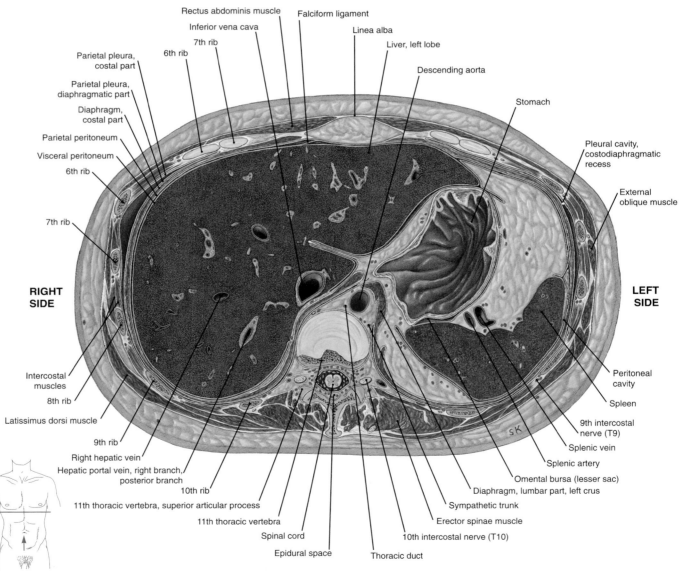

Rectus abdominis muscle Falciform ligament
Inferior vena cava
7th rib Linea alba
Parietal pleura, 6th rib Liver, left lobe
costal part
Descending aorta
Parietal pleura,
diaphragmatic part
Diaphragm,
costal part Stomach
Parietal peritoneum
Visceral peritoneum Pleural cavity,
costodiaphragmatic
6th rib recess

7th rib External
oblique muscle

RIGHT LEFT
SIDE SIDE

Peritoneal
cavity
Intercostal
muscles
8th rib Spleen
Latissimus dorsi muscle 9th intercostal
9th rib nerve (T9)
Right hepatic vein Splenic vein
Hepatic portal vein, right branch, Splenic artery
posterior branch Omental bursa (lesser sac)
10th rib Diaphragm, lumbar part, left crus
11th thoracic vertebra, superior articular process Sympathetic trunk
11th thoracic vertebra Erector spinae muscle
Spinal cord 10th intercostal nerve (T10)
Epidural space Thoracic duct

FIGURE 318.2 **Transverse Section of the Abdomen at the Level of T11 (Caudal Aspect)**

NOTE: (1) The aorta is seen to the left of the bodies of the thoracic vertebrae above the diaphragm. Observe the thoracic duct slightly to the right of the aorta.

(2) Below the diaphragm, the liver is mostly to the right and the spleen is to the left of the midline. Observe the location of the inferior vena cava posterior to the liver and to the right of the midline.

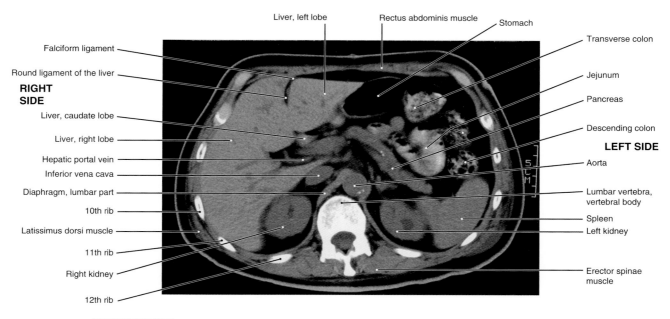

FIGURE 319.1 CT of Transverse Section of the Abdomen at L1 (Caudal Aspect)

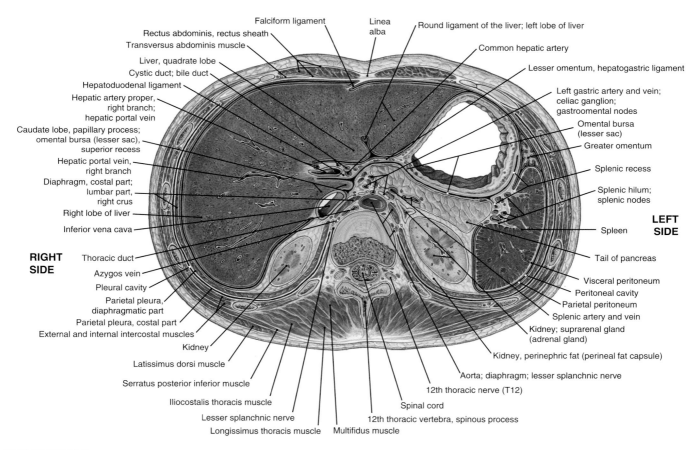

FIGURE 319.2 Transverse Section of the Abdomen between T12 and L1 (Caudal Aspect)

NOTE: (1) Both the parietal and the visceral layers of the peritoneum of the greater peritoneal sac (cavity) are shown in blue, while surrounding the lesser sac, the peritoneum is shown in blue–green.

(2) The kidneys, located anterior to the posterior abdominal wall, have been sectioned transversely. Also observe the perirenal fat surrounding them.

(3) The abdominal aorta is near or at the midline and the inferior vena cava to the right of the midline.

PLATE 320 Transverse Section of the Abdomen at L1; CT of Abdomen at L1

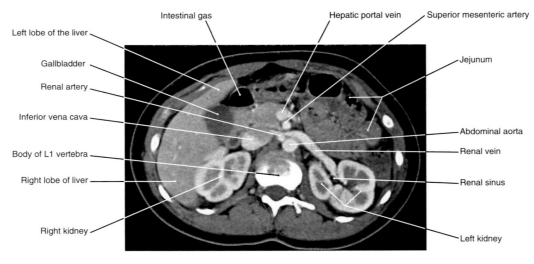

Liver, left lobe
Stomach
Gallbladder
Hepatic portal vein
Splenic vein
9th rib
Round
Transverse colon
ligament of
the liver
8th rib
Rectus abdominis muscle
Parietal peritoneum
Superior mesenteric artery
Peritoneal cavity
Pancreas
Diaphragm, costal part
Costodiaphragmatic
Pancreatic node
recess
Parietal pleura,
diaphragmatic part
Jejunum
Parietal pleura,
costal part
8th rib
9th rib
Liver,
right
lobe
Descending
colon
10th rib
Renal
artery
RIGHT
SIDE
LEFT
SIDE
11th rib
Latissimus
dorsi muscle
Inferior vena cava
Renal pelvis
Diaphragm, lumbar part
12th rib
Renal medulla
Sympathetic trunk
Minor calyx
Kidney
Renal sinus
Erector spinae muscle
1st lumbar vertebra
Renal cortex
Cauda equina
Renal vein
Inferior mesenteric artery
Abdominal aorta

FIGURE 320.1 Transverse Section through the Upper Abdomen at the Level of L1

NOTE: (1) This section goes through the hilum of the left kidney and shows the left renal vein crossing the vertebral column to then enter the inferior vena cava.

(2) The loops of jejunum on the left and the pancreas forming a bed for the posterior aspect of the stomach.

Intestinal gas
Hepatic portal vein
Superior mesenteric artery
Left lobe of the liver
Jejunum
Gallbladder
Renal artery
Inferior vena cava
Abdominal aorta
Body of L1 vertebra
Renal vein
Right lobe of liver
Renal sinus
Right kidney
Left kidney

FIGURE 320.2 CT of the Abdomen at the Level of L1

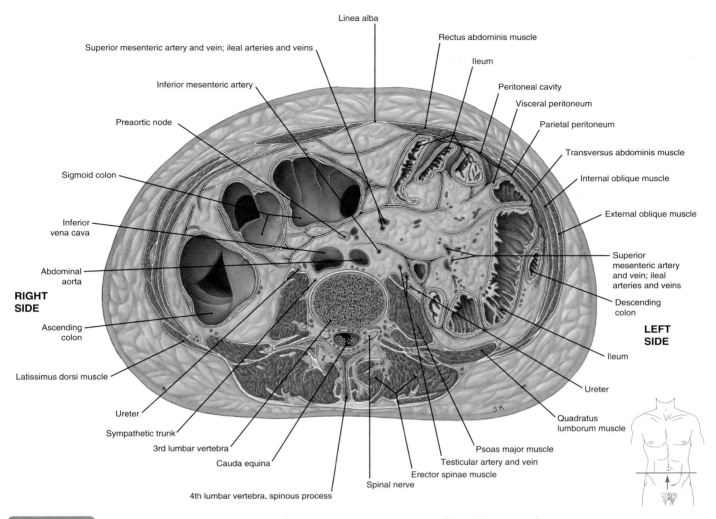

FIGURE 321.1 **Transverse Section of the Abdomen at the Level of L3 (Caudal Aspect)**

NOTE: (1) This section is through the lower abdomen and visualized from the caudal aspect.
(2) A loop of sigmoid colon extends far superiorly in the abdomen, and two parts of it are sectioned in this specimen.
(3) The inferior vena cava to the right of the midline and the aorta directly anterior to the body of the L3 vertebra.
(4) The spinal cord at this level shows the cauda equina. These are the roots of the lower lumbar and sacral nerves.

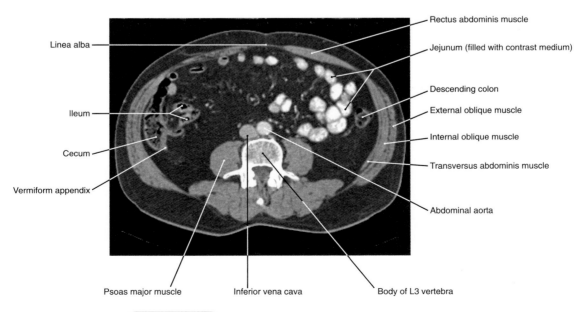

FIGURE 321.2 **CT of the Abdomen at the Level of L3**

PLATE 322 Cross Section and CT of Abdomen at L5 Level

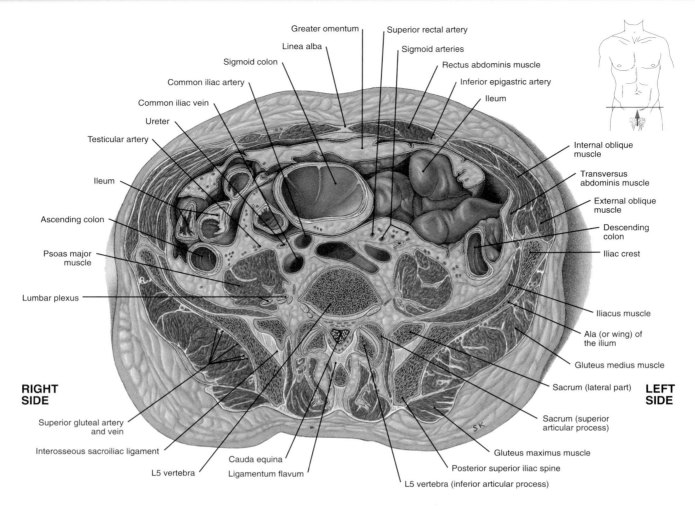

Greater omentum

Superior rectal artery

Linea alba

Sigmoid arteries

Sigmoid colon

Rectus abdominis muscle

Common iliac artery

Inferior epigastric artery

Common iliac vein

Ileum

Ureter

Testicular artery

Internal oblique muscle

Ileum

Transversus abdominis muscle

External oblique muscle

Ascending colon

Descending colon

Psoas major muscle

Iliac crest

Lumbar plexus

Iliacus muscle

Ala (or wing) of the ilium

Gluteus medius muscle

Sacrum (lateral part)

Superior gluteal artery and vein

Sacrum (superior articular process)

Interosseous sacroiliac ligament

Gluteus maximus muscle

Cauda equina

Posterior superior iliac spine

L5 vertebra

Ligamentum flavum

L5 vertebra (inferior articular process)

RIGHT SIDE

LEFT SIDE

FIGURE 322.1 Transverse Section through the Abdomen at the Fifth Lumbar Level (Sacroiliac Joint)

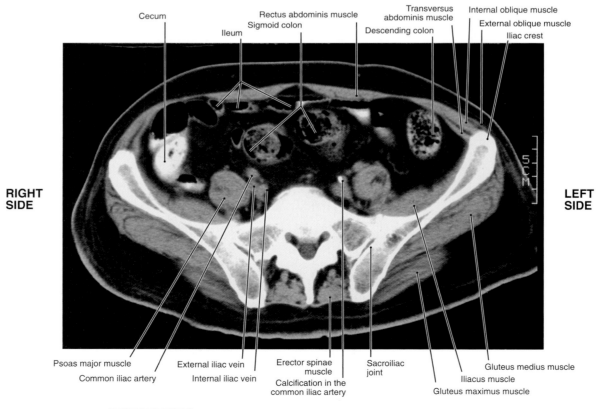

Cecum

Rectus abdominis muscle

Transversus abdominis muscle

Internal oblique muscle

Sigmoid colon

External oblique muscle

Ileum

Descending colon

Iliac crest

RIGHT SIDE

LEFT SIDE

Psoas major muscle

External iliac vein

Erector spinae muscle

Sacroiliac joint

Gluteus medius muscle

Common iliac artery

Internal iliac vein

Calcification in the common iliac artery

Iliacus muscle

Gluteus maximus muscle

FIGURE 322.2 CT at the Fifth Lumbar Level (Sacroiliac Joint)

CHAPTER 4   The Pelvis and Perineum

Plates

323 Bones of the Pelvis: Lateral View of Adult and Child

324 Bones of the Pelvis: Medial and Anterior Views

325 Radiograph of the Pelvis (A-P Projection); Diagram of the Male Pelvis

326 Bones and Ligaments of the Female Pelvis

327 Bones and Ligaments of the Male Pelvis

328 Female Pelvis: Viewed from Below; Hemisected Pelvis

329 Bones and Ligaments of the Female Pelvis: Posterior View; Sacroiliac Joint

330 Female Pelvis: Viewed from Above; Uterosalpingogram

331 Female Genitourinary Organs (Diagram)

332 Interior of the Uterus; Angles and Positions of the Uterus in the Pelvis

333 Female Pelvis: Peritoneal Reflections and Peritoneal Ligaments

334 Female Pelvis Reproductive Organs; CT of Female Pelvis

335 Female Pelvis: Blood Supply to Ovary, Uterus, and Vagina

336 Pregnant Uterus (Midsagittal View): Growth of Pregnant Uterus

337 Pregnant Uterus: Fetal X-Ray

338 Pregnant Uterus: Fetal Sonograms

339 Female Pelvis: Iliac Arteriogram

340 Female Pelvis: Branches of the Internal Iliac Artery

341 Female Pelvis: Pelvis Organs, Arteries, and Veins

342 Female Pelvis (Midsagittal View)

343 Female Pelvic Floor: Just Superior to the Perineum; Uterine Ligaments

344 Female External Genitalia

345 Female Perineum, Inferior View: Pelvic and Urogenital Diaphragms

346 Chart of the Muscles of the Anal and Urogenital Regions

347 Female Perineum: Muscles

348 Female Perineum: Vessels and Nerves

349 Superficial Urogenital Muscle Chart; Inner Surface of the Vagina

350 Female Urogenital Triangle: Surface Anatomy of Anal Region

351 Male Pelvis: Branches of Internal Iliac Artery to Bladder and Rectum

352 Posterior Abdominal Wall and Pelvis: Lymph Nodes and Channels

353 Male Pelvic Organs and Peritoneal Reflections

354 Male Bladder, Prostate, Seminal Vesicles, and Ductus Deferens

355 Male Pelvis and Perineum (Midsagittal Section)

356 Urethra, Seminal Vesicles, and Deferent and Ejaculatory Ducts

357 Diagram of Male Genitourinary Organs

358 Male Urogenital Diaphragm; Nerves in the Male Perineum

359 Rectum: Internal and External Surfaces (Frontal Section of Rectum)

360 Rectum: Arterial Supply; Median Section

361 Rectum: Venous Drainage (Diagrammatic Frontal Section)

362 Male Pelvis: Visceral Innervation; Pelvic Diaphragm

363 Female Pelvis: Cross Section and CT Image

364 Male Pelvis: Cross Section and CT Image

365 Male Perineum: Surface Anatomy; Muscles

366 Male Perineum: Vessels and Nerves

367 Male Perineum: Penis, Surface Anatomy; Dorsal Vessels and Nerves

368 Penis (Ventral Aspect): Corpus Spongiosum and Corpora Cavernosa

369 Spermatic Cord; Vascular Circulation of the Penis

370 Cross Sections through the Shaft of the Penis; Glans Penis

PLATE 323 Bones of the Pelvis: Lateral View of Adult and Child

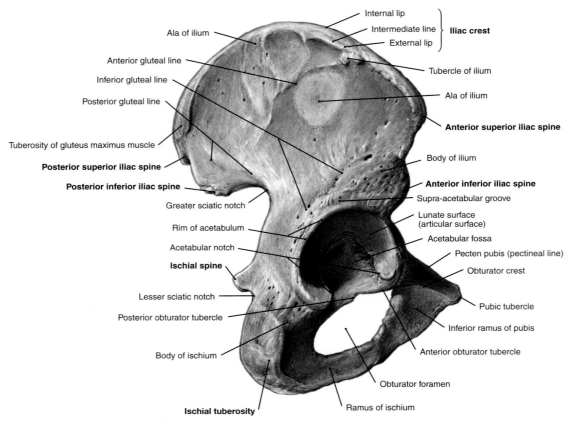

Ala of ilium

Anterior gluteal line

Inferior gluteal line

Posterior gluteal line

Tuberosity of gluteus maximus muscle

Posterior superior iliac spine

Posterior inferior iliac spine

Greater sciatic notch

Rim of acetabulum

Acetabular notch

Ischial spine

Lesser sciatic notch

Posterior obturator tubercle

Body of ischium

Ischial tuberosity

Internal lip

Intermediate line } **Iliac crest**

External lip

Tubercle of ilium

Ala of ilium

Anterior superior iliac spine

Body of ilium

Anterior inferior iliac spine

Supra-acetabular groove

Lunate surface (articular surface)

Acetabular fossa

Pecten pubis (pectineal line)

Obturator crest

Pubic tubercle

Inferior ramus of pubis

Anterior obturator tubercle

Obturator foramen

Ramus of ischium

FIGURE 323.1 **Lateral View of the Adult Right Hip Bone**

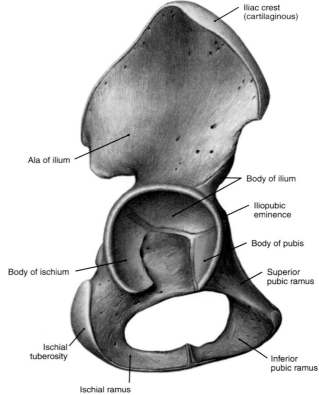

Iliac crest (cartilaginous)

Ala of ilium

Body of ilium

Iliopubic eminence

Body of pubis

Body of ischium

Superior pubic ramus

Ischial tuberosity

Inferior pubic ramus

Ischial ramus

FIGURE 323.2 **Hip Bone of 5-Year-Old Child (Lateral View)**

NOTE: The hipbone is formed by a fusion of the **ilium** (yellow), **ischium** (green), and **pubis** (orange). Although ossification of the inferior pubic ra-mus occurs during the 7th or 8th year, complete fusion of the three bones at the **acetabulum** occurs sometime between the 15th and 20th years.

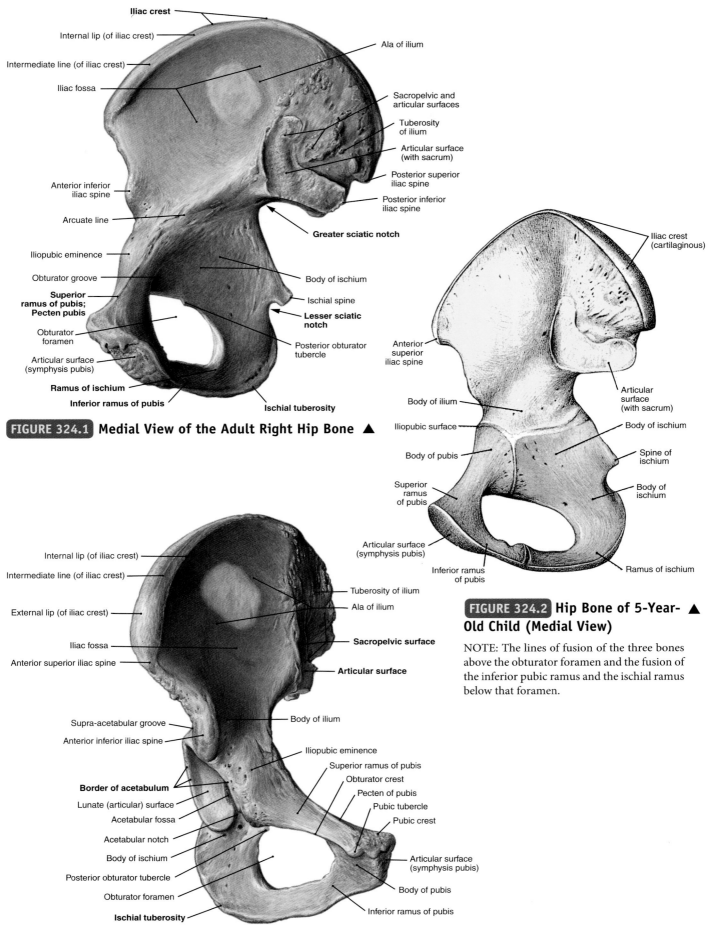

FIGURE 324.1 Medial View of the Adult Right Hip Bone ▲

Labels (Figure 324.1):
- Iliac crest
- Internal lip (of iliac crest)
- Intermediate line (of iliac crest)
- Iliac fossa
- Ala of ilium
- Sacropelvic and articular surfaces
- Tuberosity of ilium
- Articular surface (with sacrum)
- Posterior superior iliac spine
- Posterior inferior iliac spine
- Anterior inferior iliac spine
- Arcuate line
- Greater sciatic notch
- Iliopubic eminence
- Obturator groove
- Body of ischium
- Superior ramus of pubis; Pecten pubis
- Ischial spine
- Lesser sciatic notch
- Obturator foramen
- Articular surface (symphysis pubis)
- Posterior obturator tubercle
- Ramus of ischium
- Inferior ramus of pubis
- Ischial tuberosity

FIGURE 324.2 Hip Bone of 5-Year- ▲ Old Child (Medial View)

Labels (Figure 324.2):
- Iliac crest (cartilaginous)
- Anterior superior iliac spine
- Articular surface (with sacrum)
- Body of ischium
- Spine of ischium
- Body of ilium
- Iliopubic surface
- Body of pubis
- Body of ischium
- Superior ramus of pubis
- Articular surface (symphysis pubis)
- Inferior ramus of pubis
- Ramus of ischium

NOTE: The lines of fusion of the three bones above the obturator foramen and the fusion of the inferior pubic ramus and the ischial ramus below that foramen.

FIGURE 324.3 Anterior View of the Adult Right Hip Bone

Labels (Figure 324.3):
- Internal lip (of iliac crest)
- Intermediate line (of iliac crest)
- External lip (of iliac crest)
- Iliac fossa
- Anterior superior iliac spine
- Tuberosity of ilium
- Ala of ilium
- Sacropelvic surface
- Articular surface
- Supra-acetabular groove
- Anterior inferior iliac spine
- Body of ilium
- Iliopubic eminence
- Superior ramus of pubis
- Obturator crest
- Pecten of pubis
- Pubic tubercle
- Pubic crest
- Border of acetabulum
- Lunate (articular) surface
- Acetabular fossa
- Acetabular notch
- Body of ischium
- Posterior obturator tubercle
- Obturator foramen
- Articular surface (symphysis pubis)
- Body of pubis
- Inferior ramus of pubis
- Ischial tuberosity

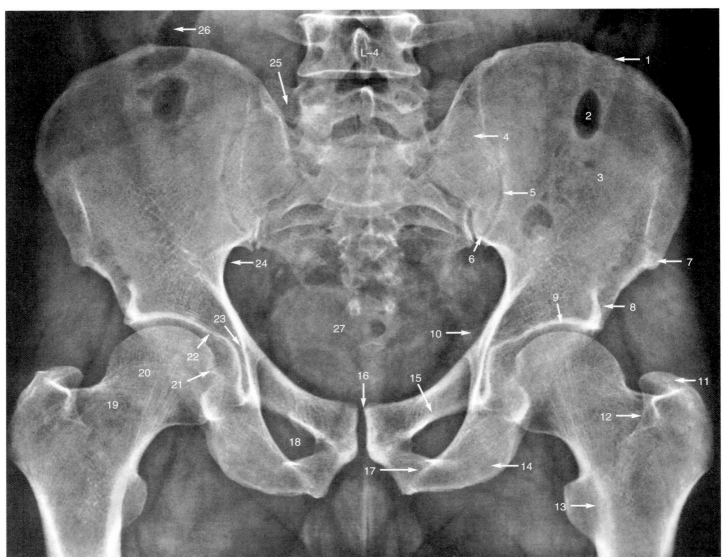

FIGURE 325.1 Radiograph of the Pelvis and the Sacroiliac and Hip Joints ▲

(From Wicke, 6th ed.)

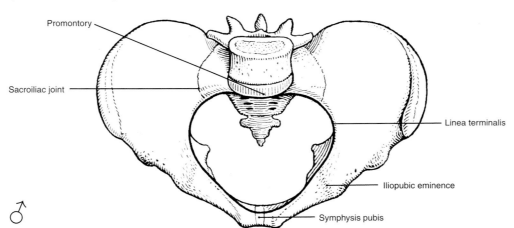

FIGURE 325.2 Diagram of the Male Pelvis

NOTE the following differences between the female and male pelvis
(1) The **pubic arch (subpubic angle)** is greater in females and, therefore, the **ischial tuberosities** are farther apart than in males.
(2) The **obturator foramen** is usually oval in shape in women but more rounded in men.
(3) The female **pelvic bones** are more delicate and lighter than the male pelvic bones.
(4) The **sacrum** is shorter and wider in females, and it is usually less curved than in males.
(5) The **ischial spines** project less in females, and the **sciatic notches** are usually wider and more shallow than in males.

Chapter 4 The Pelvis and Perineum

1. Iliac crest
2. Gas bubble in colon
3. Ala of ilium
4. Lateral part of sacrum
5. Sacroiliac joint
6. Posterior inferior iliac spine
7. Anterior superior iliac spine
8. Anterior inferior iliac spine
9. Lunate surface of acetabulum
10. Spine of ischium
11. Greater trochanter
12. Intertrochanteric crest
13. Lesser trochanter
14. Ischial tuberosity
15. Superior ramus of pubis
16. Symphysis pubis
17. Inferior ramus of pubis
18. Obturator foramen
19. Neck of femur
20. Head of femur
21. Fovea on head of femur
22. Acetabular fossa
23. Iliopubic eminence
24. Greater sciatic notch
25. Transverse process, L5 vertebra
26. Gas bubble in colon
27. Urinary bladder

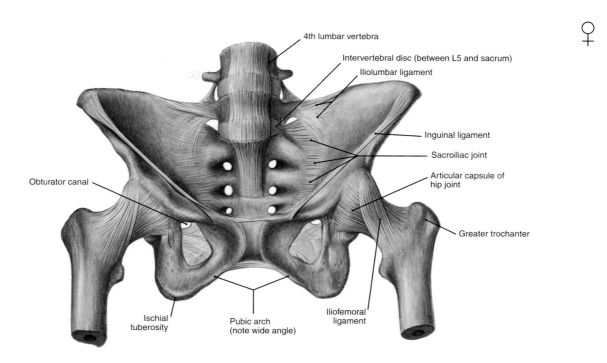

♀

4th lumbar vertebra

Intervertebral disc (between L5 and sacrum)

Iliolumbar ligament

Inguinal ligament

Sacroiliac joint

Articular capsule of
hip joint

Obturator canal

Greater trochanter

Ischial
tuberosity

Pubic arch
(note wide angle)

Iliofemoral
ligament

FIGURE 326.1 Female Pelvis and Ligaments: Articulations of the Pelvic Girdle and Hip Joints (Anteroinferior View)

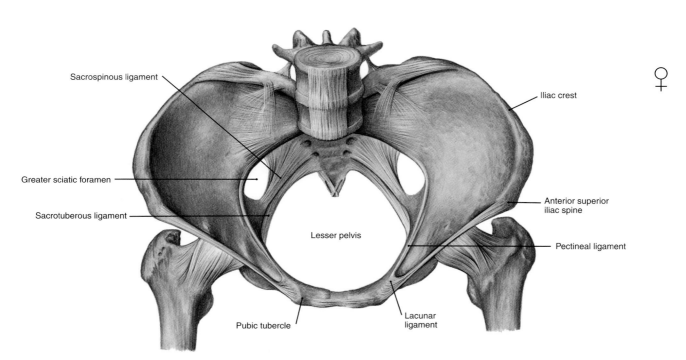

♀

Sacrospinous ligament

Iliac crest

Greater sciatic foramen

Sacrotuberous ligament

Anterior superior
iliac spine

Lesser pelvis

Pectineal ligament

Pubic tubercle

Lacunar
ligament

FIGURE 326.2 Female Pelvis and Ligaments Viewed from Front

NOTE: (1) The forward inclination of the pelvis shown here corresponds to the position of the pelvis while the person is standing upright.

(2) In addition to having wider diameters both at the pelvic inlet and outlet, the female lesser pelvis is more circular in shape than that in the male (compare with Fig. 327.2).

(3) The larger capacity of the lesser or true pelvis in the female, and the fact that the female hormones of pregnancy tend to relax the pelvic ligaments, serve to facilitate the function of childbearing.

PLATE 327 Bones and Ligaments of the Male Pelvis

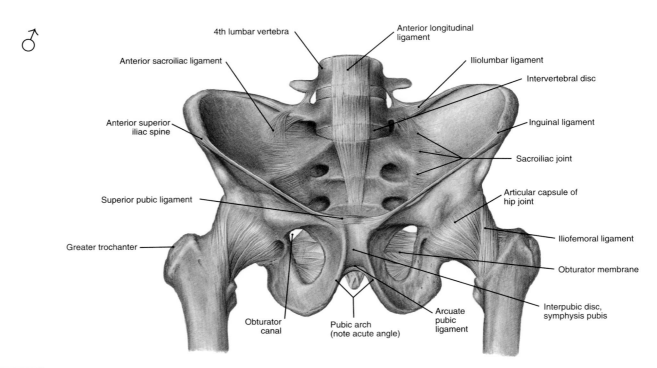

FIGURE 327.1 Male Pelvis and Associated Ligaments (Anteroinferior Aspect)

NOTE: (1) The pelvis is formed by the articulations of the left and right hip bones anteriorly at the **symphysis pubis** and posteriorly with the sacrum, coccyx, and fifth lumbar vertebra of the vertebral column.

(2) The articulations inferiorly of the pelvis with the two femora allow the weight of the head, trunk, and upper extremities to be transmitted to the lower limbs, thereby maintaining the upright posture characteristic of the human.

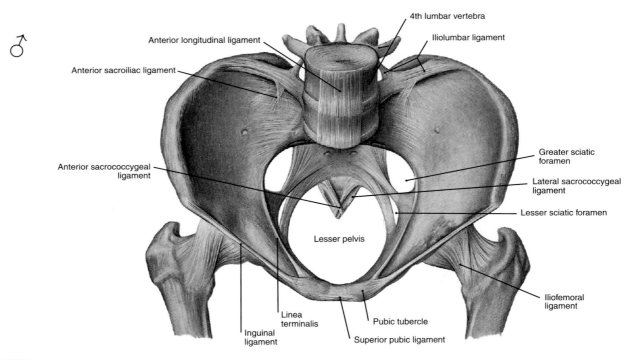

FIGURE 327.2 Male Pelvis and Ligaments Viewed from Above

NOTE: The size of the **pelvic inlet** (superior aperture of the **lesser pelvis**) and **inferior outlet** of the male pelvis is smaller than that in the female (see Fig. 326.2). Thus, the **lesser pelvis** is deeper and more narrow in the male, and its cavity has a smaller capacity than that seen in the female. In the male, the pelvic bones are thicker and heavier, and generally, the **major pelvis** (above the pelvic brim) is larger than that in the female.

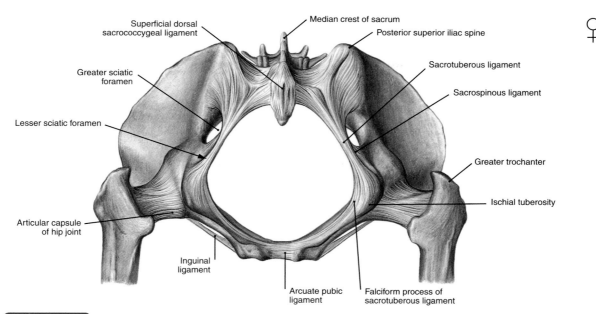

Superficial dorsal
sacrococcygeal ligament

Median crest of sacrum

Posterior superior iliac spine

Greater sciatic
foramen

Sacrotuberous ligament

Sacrospinous ligament

Lesser sciatic foramen

Greater trochanter

Ischial tuberosity

Articular capsule
of hip joint

Inguinal
ligament

Arcuate pubic
ligament

Falciform process of
sacrotuberous ligament

FIGURE 328.1 **Female Pelvic Outlet Showing the Pelvic Ligaments; Posteroinferior View**

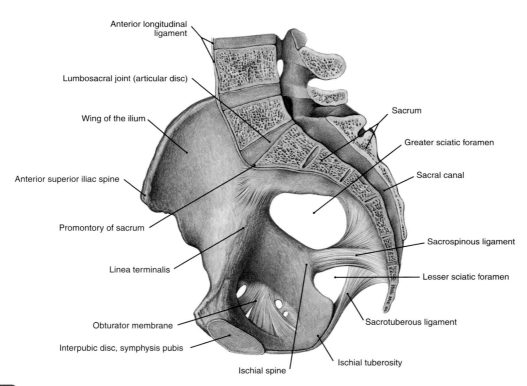

Anterior longitudinal
ligament

Lumbosacral joint (articular disc)

Wing of the ilium

Sacrum

Greater sciatic foramen

Anterior superior iliac spine

Sacral canal

Promontory of sacrum

Sacrospinous ligament

Linea terminalis

Lesser sciatic foramen

Obturator membrane

Sacrotuberous ligament

Interpubic disc, symphysis pubis

Ischial spine

Ischial tuberosity

FIGURE 328.2 **Articulations and Ligaments of the Female Hemisected Pelvis**

NOTE: (1) The **sacrospinous ligament** courses between the **sacrum** and the **ischial spine** and forms the lower border of the **greater sciatic foramen.**
(2) The **lesser sciatic foramen** is bounded above by the **sacrospinous ligament** and below by the **sacrotuberous ligament**. The latter extends between the **sacrum** and the **ischial tuberosity**.
(3) These two foramina allow the emergence of muscles, nerves, and arteries from the pelvis to the gluteal region and the entrance of veins from the gluteal region to the pelvis.
(4) Because the sacrum lies beneath the remainder of the vertebral column, considerable weight is transmitted to it from above. This tends to rotate the upper end of the sacrum forward and downward and its lower end and the coccyx backward and upward. The sacrotuberous and sacrospinous ligaments add stability to the sacroiliac joint by resisting these forces.

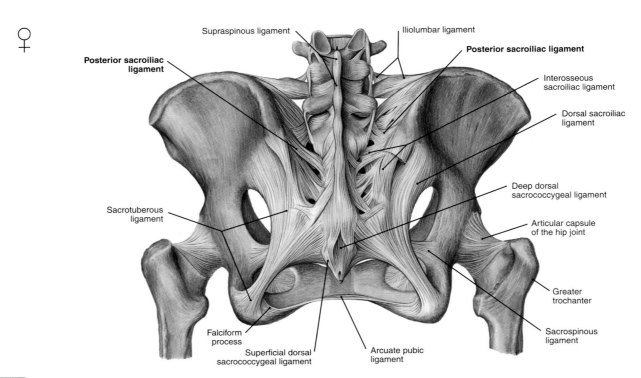

♀

Supraspinous ligament

Iliolumbar ligament

Posterior sacroiliac ligament

Posterior sacroiliac ligament

Interosseous sacroiliac ligament

Dorsal sacroiliac ligament

Deep dorsal sacrococcygeal ligament

Articular capsule of the hip joint

Sacrotuberous ligament

Greater trochanter

Falciform process

Superficial dorsal sacrococcygeal ligament

Arcuate pubic ligament

Sacrospinous ligament

FIGURE 329.1 Female Pelvis with Joints and Ligaments (Posterior Aspect)

NOTE: (1) Broad ligamentous bands articulate the two hip bones posteriorly with the sacrum and coccyx. Observe the strong **posterior (dorsal) sacroiliac ligament.**
(2) The posterior sacroiliac ligament is composed of short **transverse fibers** that interconnect the ilium with the upper part of the lateral crest of the sacrum, whereas the longer **vertical fibers** attach the third and fourth transverse tubercles of the sacrum to the superior and inferior posterior iliac spines, many blending with fibers of the sacrotuberous ligament.

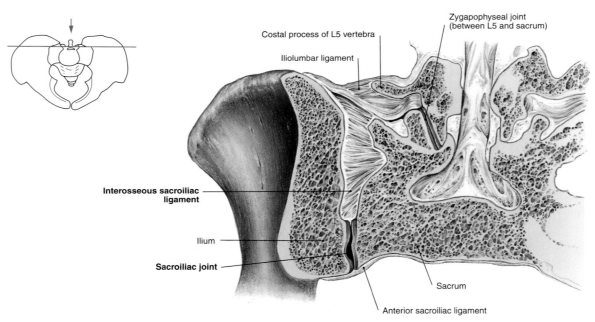

Costal process of L5 vertebra

Zygapophyseal joint (between L5 and sacrum)

Iliolumbar ligament

Interosseous sacroiliac ligament

Ilium

Sacroiliac joint

Sacrum

Anterior sacroiliac ligament

FIGURE 329.2 Frontal Section through the Sacroiliac Joint

NOTE: (1) The **sacroiliac joint** is a synovial joint connecting the **auricular surface** of the sacrum with the reciprocally curved **auricular surface** of the ilium.
(2) This joint is bound by the **anterior** and **interosseous sacroiliac ligaments** (shown in this figure) as well as the **posterior** (dorsal) **sacroiliac ligament** (shown in Fig. 329.1).
(3) The interosseous sacroiliac ligament is the strongest ligament between the sacrum and the ilium, and it stretches above and behind the synovial joint.

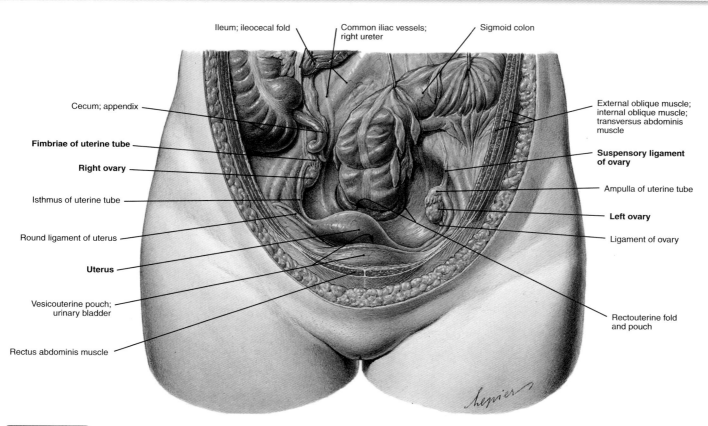

Ileum; ileocecal fold

Common iliac vessels; right ureter

Sigmoid colon

Cecum; appendix

Fimbriae of uterine tube

Right ovary

Isthmus of uterine tube

Round ligament of uterus

Uterus

Vesicouterine pouch; urinary bladder

Rectus abdominis muscle

External oblique muscle; internal oblique muscle; transversus abdominis muscle

Suspensory ligament of ovary

Ampulla of uterine tube

Left ovary

Ligament of ovary

Rectouterine fold and pouch

FIGURE 330.1 **Pelvic Viscera of an Adult Female (Anterior View)**

NOTE: (1) The ovaries are situated on the posterolateral aspect of the true pelvis on each side. Having descended from the posterior abdominal wall to their location just below the pelvic brim, the ovaries are held in position by peritoneal ligamentous attachments. The suspensory ligament of the ovary transmits the ovarian vessels and ovarian autonomic nerves.

(2) The uterus is positioned between the bladder and the rectum, and frequently it is located somewhat to one or the other side of the midline.

(3) The fimbriae of the uterine tubes extend from the ampullae of the tubes to encircle the upper medial surface of the ovaries. The uterine tubes vary from 3 to 6 in. in length, and they convey the ova to the uterus. It is within the uterine tube that fertilization of the ovum usually occurs.

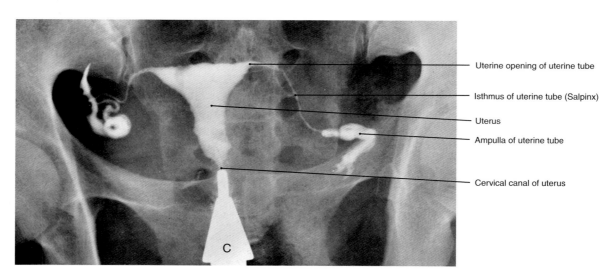

Uterine opening of uterine tube

Isthmus of uterine tube (Salpinx)

Uterus

Ampulla of uterine tube

Cervical canal of uterus

FIGURE 330.2 **Uterosalpingogram**

NOTE: (1) A cannula (C) was placed in the vagina, and radiopaque material was injected into the uterus and uterine tube. Observe the narrow lumen of the isthmus of the uterine tubes and how the tubes enlarge at the ampullae.

(2) On the specimen's left side (reader's right), even the fimbriated end of the tube is discernible, whereas on the specimen's right side (reader's left) a small portion of the radiopaque material has been forced into the pelvis through the opening in the uterine tube.

PLATE 331 Female Genitourinary Organs (Diagram)

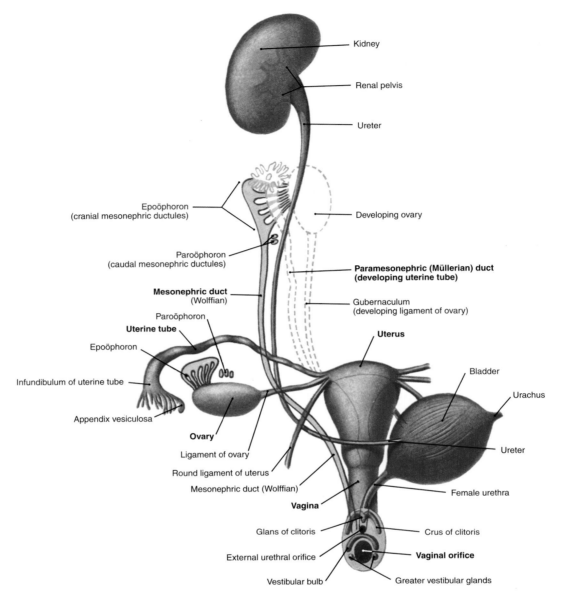

Kidney

Renal pelvis

Ureter

Epoöphoron
(cranial mesonephric ductules)

Developing ovary

Paroöphoron
(caudal mesonephric ductules)

**Paramesonephric (Müllerian) duct
(developing uterine tube)**

Mesonephric duct
(Wolffian)

Gubernaculum
(developing ligament of ovary)

Paroöphoron

Uterine tube

Epoöphoron

Uterus

Infundibulum of uterine tube

Bladder

Urachus

Appendix vesiculosa

Ovary

Ligament of ovary

Ureter

Round ligament of uterus

Mesonephric duct (Wolffian)

Vagina

Female urethra

Glans of clitoris

Crus of clitoris

External urethral orifice

Vaginal orifice

Vestibular bulb

Greater vestibular glands

FIGURE 331 **Diagram of the Female Genitourinary Organs and Their Embryologic Precursors**

NOTE: (1) This figure shows:
   (a) All of the organs of the adult female genitourinary system (dark red-brown).
   (b) The structures and relevant positions of the female genital organs (gonad and ligament of the ovary and uterine tube) prior to their descent into the pelvis (interrupted lines).
   (c) The structures that become atrophic during development (pink with red outline).
(2) The urinary system of females (as in males) includes the kidney, which produces urine from the blood; and the ureter, which conveys the urine to the bladder, where it is stored. Leading from the bladder is the urethra, through which urine passes to the external urethral orifice during micturition.
(3) The adult female genital system includes the **ovary, uterine tube, uterus,** and **vagina,** plus the associated glands and external genital organs.
(4) At one time during development, structures capable of developing into both male and female genital systems existed. In the female, the Müllerian, or paramesonephric, duct becomes vestigial. Also, the developing gonads become ovaries, while their attachments become the ligaments of the ovaries.
(5) The ovaries produce ova that are discharged periodically between adolescence and menopause. The ova are captured by the uterine tube, where fertilization may occur. If this happens, the fertilized ovum is transported to the uterus, and about a week after fertilization, implantation occurs in the wall of the uterus.

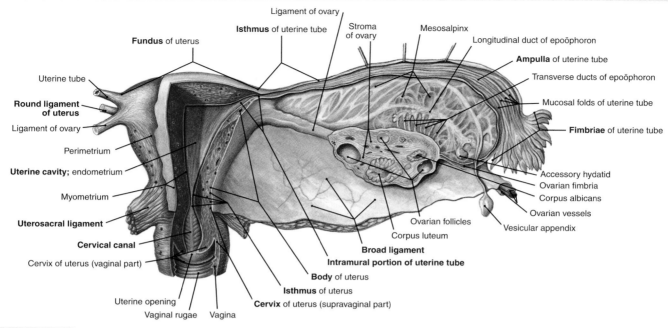

FIGURE 332.1 Frontal Section of Uterus, Uterine Tube, and Ovary

NOTE: (1) The vagina communicates with the pelvic cavity through the uterus and the uterine tube. The lumen of this pathway varies in diameter, and its most narrow sites are the isthmus of the uterus and the intrauterine (intramural) part of the uterine tube.
(2) The uterus consists of the **cervix** (vaginal and supravaginal portions), the **body,** and the **fundus.** The cervix and the body are interconnected by the **isthmus.**
(3) The attachments of the uterus include:
    (a) The **broad ligaments** that attach to the lateral margins of the uterus.
    (b) The fibrous **round ligaments** and the **ligaments of the ovaries** attached just below the uterine tubes.
    (c) The **uterosacral ligaments.**
    (d) The **cardinal ligaments (of Mackenrodt)** that attach along the lateral border of the uterus and vagina. With the pelvic diaphragm, the cardinal ligaments offer important support to the uterus and vagina.

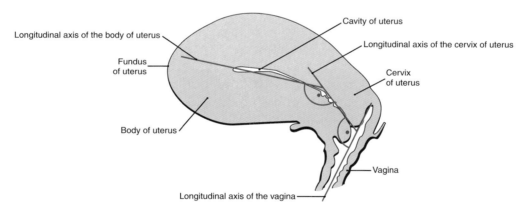

FIGURE 332.2 Normal Angles between the Vagina, Cervix, and Body of Uterus

NOTE that the uterus is in a normal anteverted, anteflexed position.

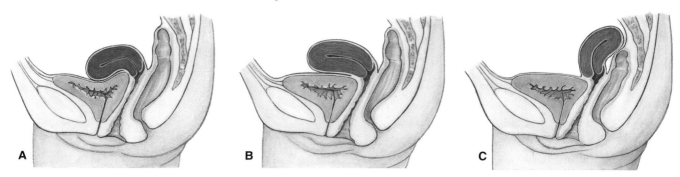

FIGURE 332.3A–C Variations in the Position of the Uterus in the Pelvis

A: Anteverted, anteflexed position. **B:** Anteverted but no anteflexion. **C:** Retroverted, retroflexed position.

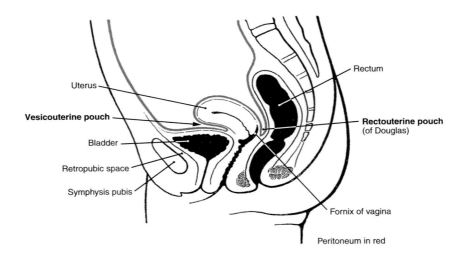

FIGURE 333.1 Diagram of Peritoneal Reflections over Female Pelvic Organs (Midsagittal Section)

NOTE: (1) The parietal peritoneum is reflected over the free abdominal surface of the pelvic organs. Observe that as the uterus and vagina are interposed between the bladder and the rectum, peritoneal pouches are formed between the bladder and the uterus (vesicouterine) and between the rectum and the uterus (rectouterine pouch of Douglas).

(2) The **vesicouterine pouch** is shallow. The forward tilt, or inclination, of the uterus (anteversion) toward the superior surface of the bladder reduces the potential size of the vesicouterine pouch.

(3) The vesicouterine pouch does not extend as far inferiorly as the vagina, whereas the deeper **rectouterine pouch** dips to the level of the posterior fornix of the vagina. This important anatomical relationship stresses the fact that the posterior fornix is separated from the peritoneal cavity only by the thin vaginal wall and the peritoneum.

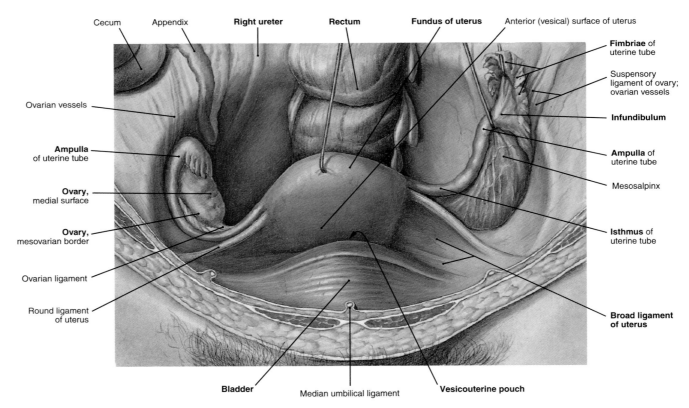

FIGURE 333.2 Female Pelvic Organs (Anterosuperior View)

NOTE: The body of the uterus has been elevated, thereby exposing the **vesicouterine pouch** and demonstrating the **broad ligaments.**

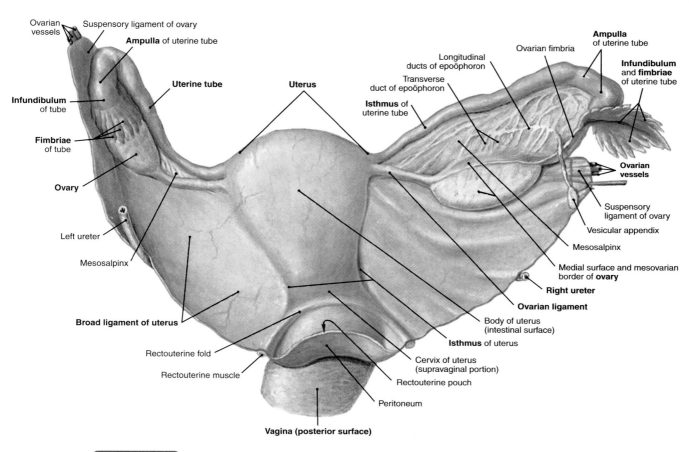

Ovarian vessels
Suspensory ligament of ovary
Ampulla of uterine tube
Uterine tube
Uterus
Longitudinal ducts of epoöphoron
Transverse duct of epoöphoron
Ovarian fimbria
Ampulla of uterine tube
Infundibulum and **fimbriae** of uterine tube
Infundibulum of tube
Isthmus of uterine tube
Fimbriae of tube
Ovary
Ovarian vessels
Suspensory ligament of ovary
Vesicular appendix
Left ureter
Mesosalpinx
Mesosalpinx
Medial surface and mesovarian border of **ovary**
Right ureter
Ovarian ligament
Body of uterus (intestinal surface)
Broad ligament of uterus
Isthmus of uterus
Rectouterine fold
Cervix of uterus (supravaginal portion)
Rectouterine muscle
Rectouterine pouch
Peritoneum
Vagina (posterior surface)

FIGURE 334.1 **Pelvic Reproductive Organs of an Immature Girl (Posterior View)**

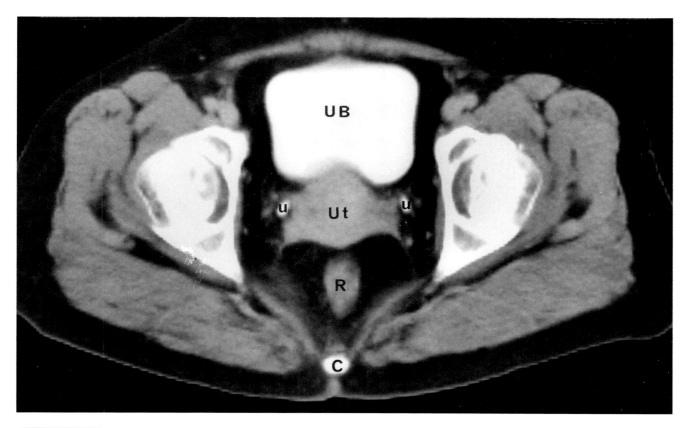

FIGURE 334.2 **CT of the Female Pelvis**

UB, urinary bladder; **u**, ureter; **Ut**, uterus; **R**, rectum; **C**, coccyx.

(Contributed by Edward J.H. Nathanial, MD, PhD, Professor of Anatomy, University of Manitoba, Winnipeg, Canada.)

PLATE 335 Female Pelvis: Blood Supply to Ovary, Uterus, and Vagina

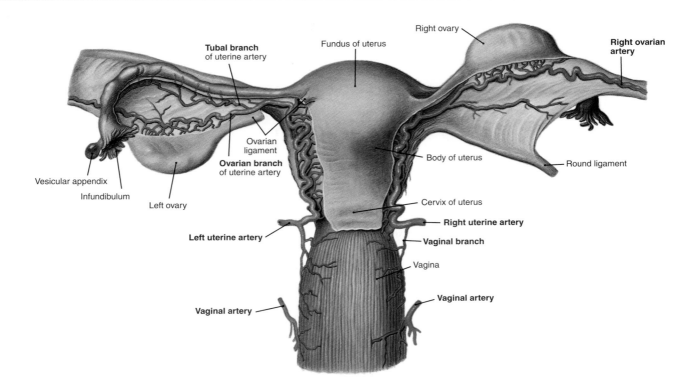

FIGURE 335.1 Arterial Supply to Female Pelvic Genital Organs

NOTE: (1) The vessels supplying the female pelvic genital organs are the **uterine arteries** from the internal iliac and the **ovarian arteries** that stem from the aorta. They anastomose freely along both lateral borders of the uterus.

(2) The uterine artery also anastomoses with the arterial supply to the vagina. Often the **vaginal arteries** arise from the uterine arteries, but they may branch from the inferior vesical artery or even directly from the internal iliac artery.

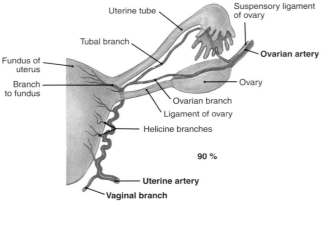

◀ **FIGURE 335.2** Diagram of Uterine and Ovarian Arteries

NOTE: This arterial pattern (similar to that shown in Fig. 335.1) is seen in about 90% of humans.

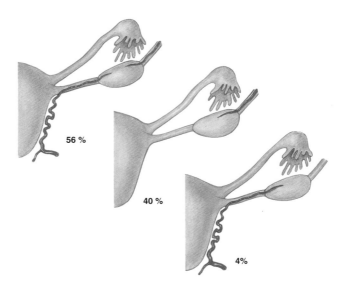

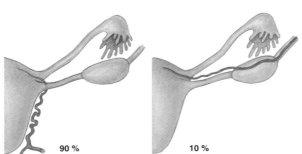

FIGURE 335.3 Arterial Supply to the Fundus of the Uterus

NOTE: In 90% of cases the fundus gets blood from the uterine artery, whereas in 10% it comes from the ovarian artery.

FIGURE 335.4 Arterial Supply to the Ovary

NOTE: In 56% of cases, blood to the ovary comes from both the ovarian and uterine arteries, in 40% from the ovarian artery only, and in 4% from the uterine artery only.

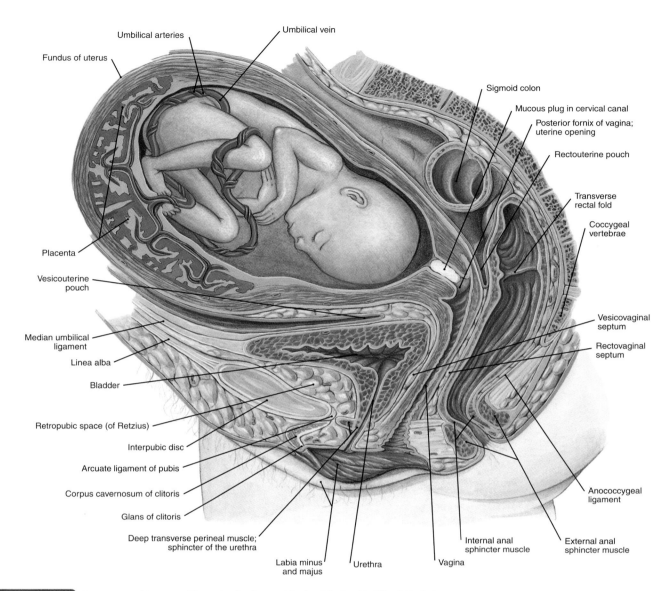

Umbilical arteries

Umbilical vein

Fundus of uterus

Sigmoid colon

Mucous plug in cervical canal

Posterior fornix of vagina; uterine opening

Rectouterine pouch

Transverse rectal fold

Coccygeal vertebrae

Placenta

Vesicouterine pouch

Vesicovaginal septum

Rectovaginal septum

Median umbilical ligament

Linea alba

Bladder

Retropubic space (of Retzius)

Interpubic disc

Arcuate ligament of pubis

Corpus cavernosum of clitoris

Glans of clitoris

Anococcygeal ligament

Deep transverse perineal muscle; sphincter of the urethra

Labia minus and majus

Urethra

Vagina

Internal anal sphincter muscle

External anal sphincter muscle

FIGURE 336.1 **Pregnant Uterus Shortly before Birth, Right Half of Pelvis**

NOTE: (1) The pelvis, including the uterus, has been hemisected, while the newborn fetus is shown intact.

(2) In this cephalic longitudinal presentation of the fetus, the placenta is oriented toward the maternal anterior abdominal wall, in contrast to the longitudinal presentation shown in Figure 337, which shows the back **positioned to the left side of the pelvis.**

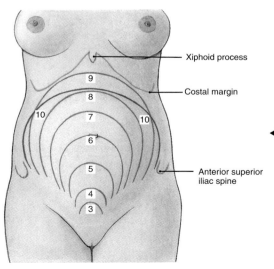

Xiphoid process

Costal margin

Anterior superior iliac spine

◀ **FIGURE 336.2** **Diagrammatic Representation of Uterine Growth during Pregnancy (Anterior View)**

NOTE: (1) Growth of the uterus is shown in 28-day **lunar months,** hence 10 months rather than 9 calendar months.

(2) By the end of the fourth lunar month, the uterus occupies most of the pelvis. Near the end of pregnancy, it occupies most of the abdomen and extends to the costal margin.

(3) During the last lunar month, the fetus (and fundus of the uterus) descends somewhat, in preparation for the birth process.

PLATE 337 **Pregnant Uterus: Fetal X-Ray**

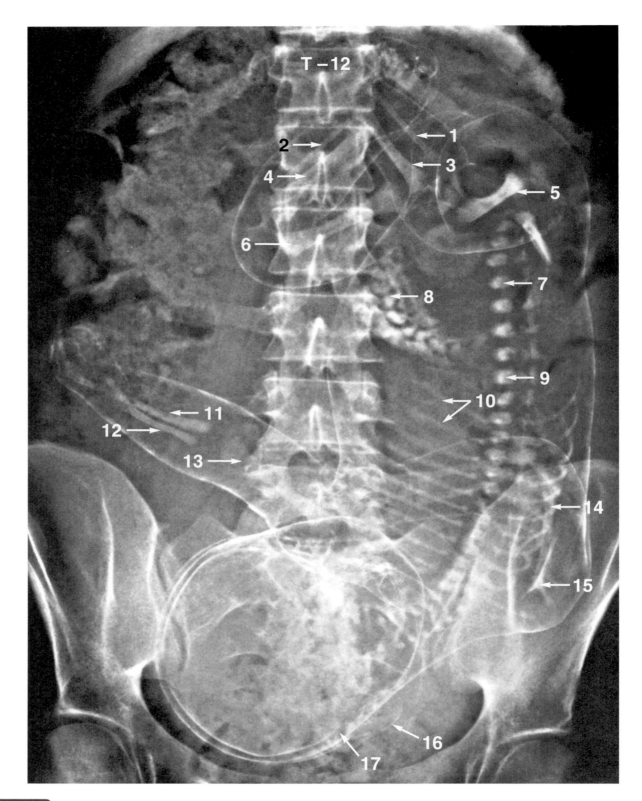

FIGURE 337 **Fetal Roentgenogram**

NOTE: The body contours of the near-term fetus in utero and a number of the ossifying bones. Observe that the uterus extends to the maternal T12 vertebral body level.

(From Wicke, 6th ed.)

1. Right fibula
2. Left fibula
3. Right tibia
4. Left tibia
5. Right femur
6. Left femur
7. L5 vertebra (fetal)
8. Small intestine (fetal)
9. L1 vertebra (fetal)
10. Ribs
11. Left ulna
12. Left radius
13. Left humerus
14. Right humerus
15. Right scapula
16. External ear
17. Fetal head

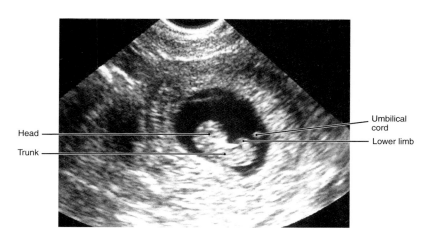

FIGURE 338.1 **Sonogram of Uterus during the 10th Week of Pregnancy**

NOTE: The embryo is oriented longitudinally within the chorionic cavity: head to the left, trunk, and lower limbs to the right.

(The figures on this plate are from Dr. H. Schillinger, Professor of Anatomy, University of Freiburg im Breisgau, Germany.)

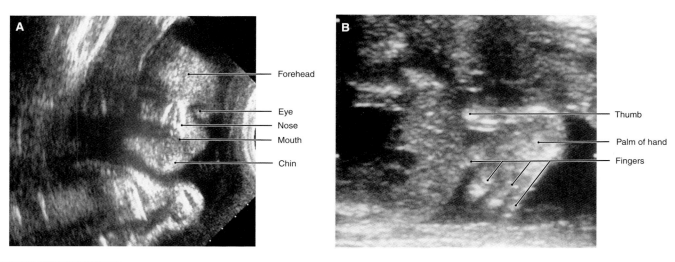

FIGURE 338.2A and B **Sonogram of Uterus during the 24th Week of Pregnancy**

NOTE: (1) In **A,** a frontal section through the face shows the facial features of the fetus, presenting the fetal "portrait."
(2) In **B,** the sonogram shows the fetal hand, clearly demonstrating all of the fingers and the thumb.

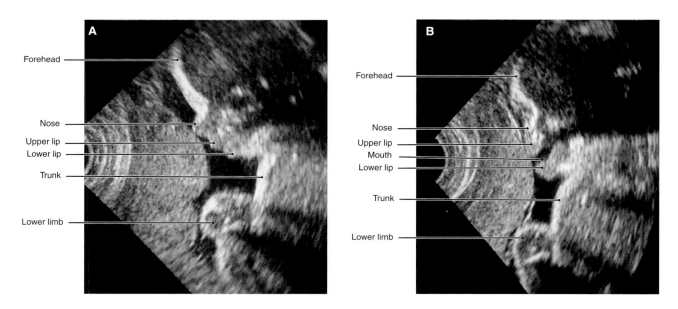

FIGURE 338.3A and B **Sonogram of Uterus during 28th Week of Pregnancy**

NOTE: (1) In **A,** the longitudinal section shows the fetal head and body in profile.
(2) In **B,** the fetus has opened its mouth and expanded its trunk, indicating the sporadic diaphragmatic and swallowing movements that occur during the latter part of fetal life, when large amounts of amniotic fluid are ingested.

PLATE 339 Female Pelvis: Iliac Arteriogram

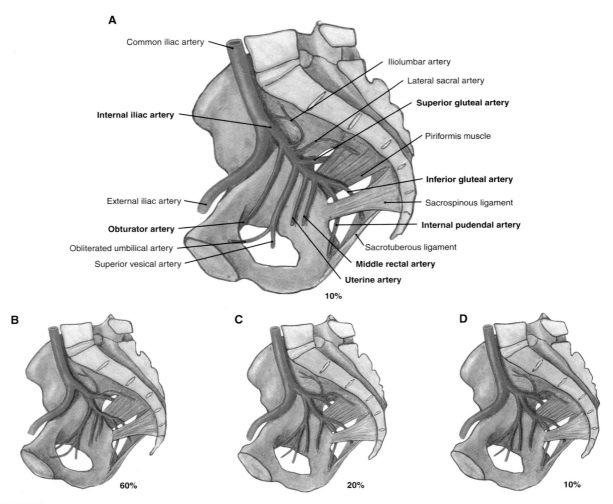

A

Common iliac artery

Iliolumbar artery

Lateral sacral artery

Superior gluteal artery

Internal iliac artery

Piriformis muscle

Inferior gluteal artery

External iliac artery

Sacrospinous ligament

Internal pudendal artery

Obturator artery

Obliterated umbilical artery

Sacrotuberous ligament

Superior vesical artery

Middle rectal artery

Uterine artery

10%

B   **C**   **D**

60%   20%   10%

FIGURE 339.1 Variations in the Divisions of the Internal Iliac Artery

NOTE: (1) In 10% of specimens (shown in **A**) the internal iliac artery itself gives off all branches.
(2) In 60% of specimens (shown in **B**) the internal iliac artery divides into two main branches—an anterior and a posterior trunk.
(3) In 20% of specimens (shown in **C**) the internal iliac artery divides into three branches.
(4) In 10% of specimens (shown in **D**) the internal iliac artery divides into more than three branches.

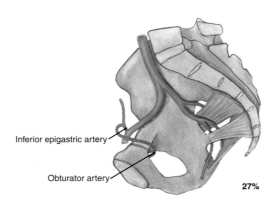

Inferior epigastric artery

Obturator artery

27%

FIGURE 339.2 Aberrant Origin of the Obturator Artery

NOTE: (1) The obturator artery arises from the internal iliac artery or one of its branches in nearly 70% of bodies, but in 27% of cases the obturator artery arises from the **inferior epigastric artery,** as shown in this figure.
(2) If the course of the aberrant obturator artery is lateral to the lacunar ligament, then repair of a femoral hernia is relatively safe, but if it curves along the free margin of the lacunar ligament, the vessel could easily be injured during hernia repair.

(From Picks, J.W., Anson, B.J., and Ashley, F.H. *Am J Anat.* 70:317–344, 1942.)

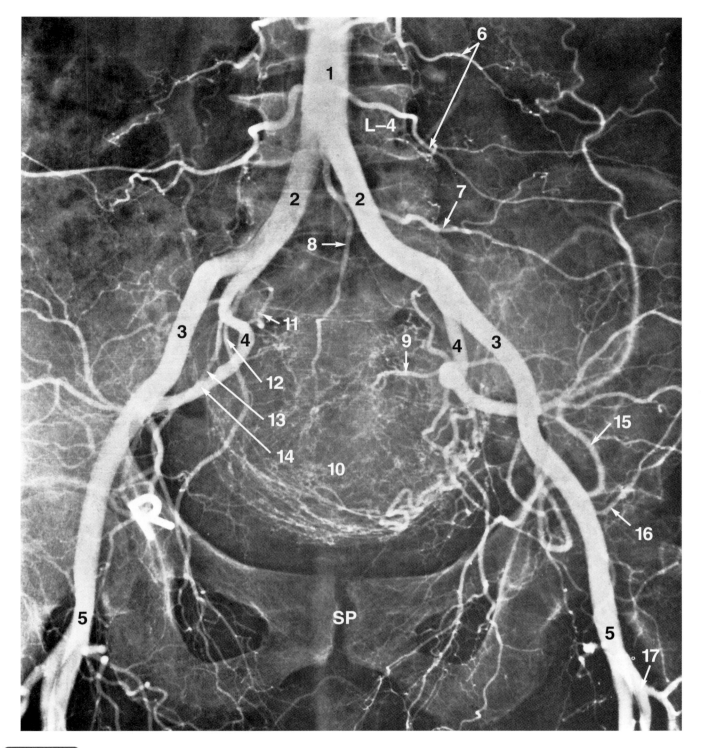

FIGURE 340 **Arteriogram of the Iliac Arteries and Their Branches in a Female**

NOTE: The bifurcation of the aorta (1) into the two common iliac arteries (2) occurs at the lower border of the body of the L4 vertebra. The common iliac vessels branch into external (3) and internal (4) iliac arteries. The internal iliac artery (4) on each side serves a number of branches to the pelvis, perineum, and gluteal region, whereas the external iliac artery (3), after giving off the inferior epigastric (15) and deep circumflex iliac (16) arteries, becomes the femoral artery below the inguinal ligament.

(From Wicke, 6th ed.)

1. Abdominal aorta
2. Common iliac artery
3. External iliac artery
4. Internal iliac artery
5. Femoral artery
6. Lumbar arteries
7. Iliolumbar artery
8. Median sacral artery
9. Uterine artery
10. Uterus
11. Lateral sacral artery
12. Obturator artery
13. Internal pudendal artery
14. Superior gluteal artery
15. Inferior epigastric artery
16. Deep circumflex iliac artery
17. Deep femoral artery
SP = Symphysis pubis
L4 = 4th lumbar vertebra

PLATE 341 Female Pelvis: Pelvis Organs, Arteries, and Veins

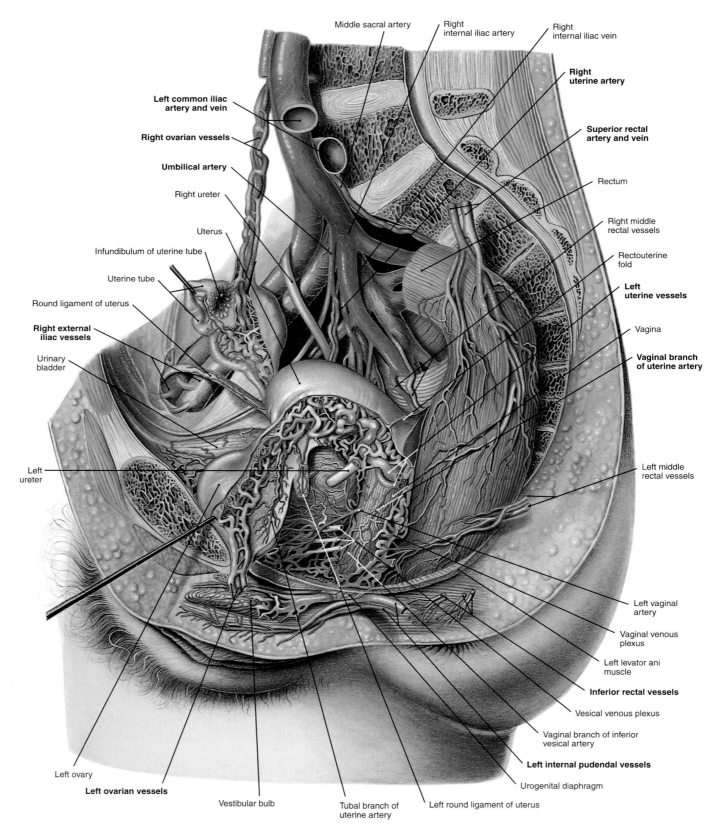

Middle sacral artery

Right internal iliac artery

Right internal iliac vein

Right uterine artery

Left common iliac artery and vein

Right ovarian vessels

Umbilical artery

Right ureter

Uterus

Infundibulum of uterine tube

Uterine tube

Round ligament of uterus

Right external iliac vessels

Urinary bladder

Left ureter

Superior rectal artery and vein

Rectum

Right middle rectal vessels

Rectouterine fold

Left uterine vessels

Vagina

Vaginal branch of uterine artery

Left middle rectal vessels

Left vaginal artery

Vaginal venous plexus

Left levator ani muscle

Inferior rectal vessels

Vesical venous plexus

Vaginal branch of inferior vesical artery

Left internal pudendal vessels

Urogenital diaphragm

Left ovary

Left ovarian vessels

Vestibular bulb

Tubal branch of uterine artery

Left round ligament of uterus

FIGURE 341 **Blood Vessels of the Female Pelvis and Genital System**

NOTE: (1) The left half of the pelvis has been removed to expose the pelvic organs and their dense plexuses of veins (**ovarian, vaginal, uterine,** and **vesical**), which accompany their respective arteries.

(2) With the exception of the **ovarian artery** (from the aorta) and the **superior rectal artery** (from the inferior mesenteric) all other arteries to the pelvic organs, perineum, and genital tract are derived from the **internal iliac artery** or its branches.

(3) The course of the **ureter** is a descending one, crossing the external iliac vessels over the pelvic brim. The ureter then courses **under the uterine vessels** before entering the bladder.

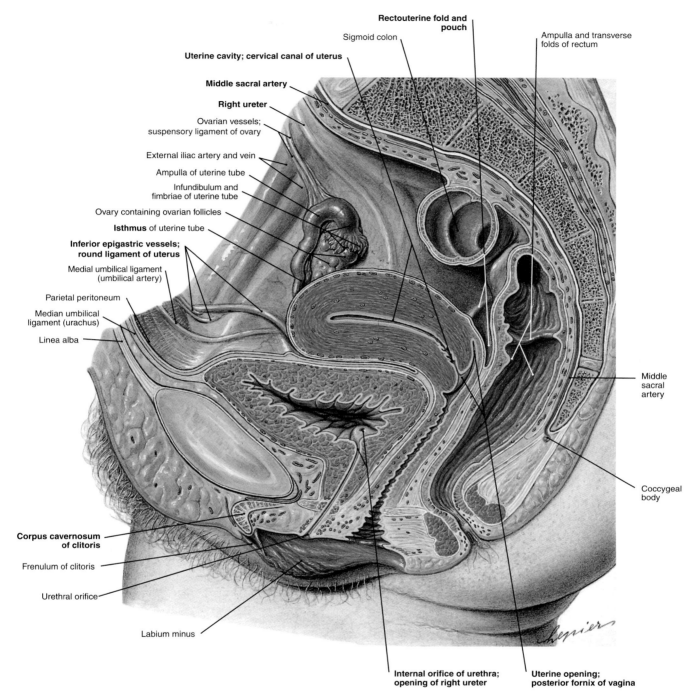

Rectouterine fold and pouch

Sigmoid colon

Ampulla and transverse folds of rectum

Uterine cavity; cervical canal of uterus

Middle sacral artery

Right ureter

Ovarian vessels; suspensory ligament of ovary

External iliac artery and vein

Ampulla of uterine tube

Infundibulum and fimbriae of uterine tube

Ovary containing ovarian follicles

Isthmus of uterine tube

Inferior epigastric vessels; round ligament of uterus

Medial umbilical ligament (umbilical artery)

Parietal peritoneum

Median umbilical ligament (urachus)

Linea alba

Middle sacral artery

Coccygeal body

Corpus cavernosum of clitoris

Frenulum of clitoris

Urethral orifice

Labium minus

Internal orifice of urethra; opening of right ureter

Uterine opening; posterior fornix of vagina

FIGURE 342 Adult Female Pelvis (Median Sagittal Section)

NOTE: (1) This medial view of the hemisected female pelvis shows the relationships of the **bladder, uterus, vagina, rectum, ovary,** and **uterine tube.** Observe the retropubic position of the empty bladder and the short course of the female urethra, leading from the bladder through the **urogenital diaphragm** to open in the midline, anterior to the vagina.

(2) The **posterior fornix** of the vagina reaches superiorly to lie in front of the **rectouterine pouch (of Douglas)**, being separated from it only by the vaginal wall. Observe that the vagina and uterus are interposed between the bladder and the rectum.

(3) The **round ligament of the uterus** is directed laterally and anteriorly to enter the deep inguinal ring, and note the course of the **inferior epigastric vessels** in relation to this ligament. Observe the **ovarian vessels** within the **suspensory ligament of the ovary** and the **ureter** along the posterolateral wall of the pelvis.

(4) Shown are the **large bowel** and the direct course of the **rectum** toward the **anal canal.** The peritoneum is reflected over the anterior surface of the rectum, thereby lining the rectouterine pouch.

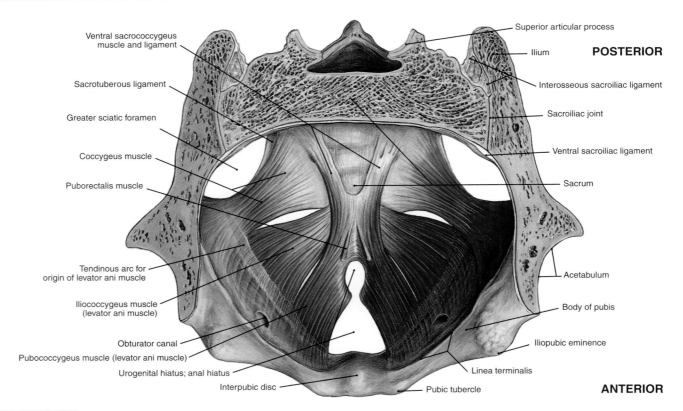

FIGURE 343.1 Muscular Floor of the Female Pelvis Viewed from Above

NOTE: (1) The muscular floor of the pelvis is formed anteriorly by the **pubococcygeus** and anterolaterally by the **iliococcygeus** portions of the **levator ani muscle** and posterolaterally by the **coccygeus muscle,** which lies above the sacrotuberous ligament.

(2) At the **urogenital hiatus** is located the **urogenital (UG) diaphragm,** which is formed by the deep transverse perineal muscles and the membranous sphincter of the urethra, which lie between two layers of fascia (see Fig. 345.2). The urethra and vagina penetrate through the UG diaphragm in the female.

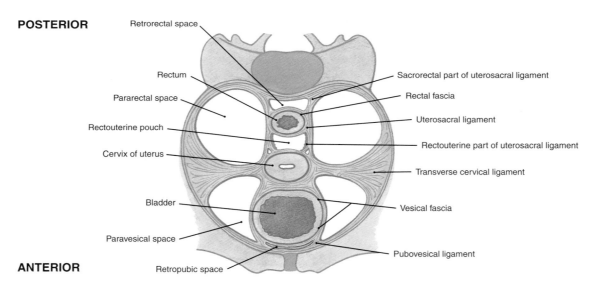

FIGURE 343.2 Uterine Ligaments at the Cervix Just above the Pelvic Floor (Diagram)

NOTE: (1) Just above the floor of the pelvis (formed by the levator ani and coccygeus muscles) is located the cervix of the uterus in women. Extending laterally from the uterine cervix and from the upper vagina to the fascia covering the levator ani muscles are the **transverse cervical ligaments** (also called **lateral cervical, cardinal, or Mackenrodt's ligaments**).

(2) The transverse cervical ligaments are located at the base of the broad ligaments and below the uterine vessels. Observe that the **uterosacral ligaments** also attach to the cervix and upper vagina but course backward around the rectum to the front of the sacrum.

(3) The uterus is supported in position by (a) its attachment to the bladder and rectum, (b) the transverse cervical and uterosacral ligaments, and (c) the musculature that forms the pelvic floor and urogenital diaphragm.

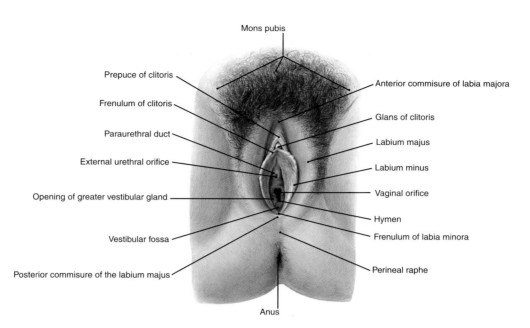

Mons pubis

Prepuce of clitoris

Frenulum of clitoris

Paraurethral duct

External urethral orifice

Opening of greater vestibular gland

Vestibular fossa

Posterior commisure of the labium majus

Anterior commisure of labia majora

Glans of clitoris

Labium majus

Labium minus

Vaginal orifice

Hymen

Frenulum of labia minora

Perineal raphe

Anus

FIGURE 344.1 **External Genitalia of an 18-Year-Old Virgin**

NOTE: (1) The female **external genitalia** are (a) the mons pubis, (b) the labia majora, (c) the labia minora, (d) the clitoris, and (e) the vestibule of the vagina. The **orifices** of the female perineum include the openings of the (a) urethra, (b) vagina, (c) ducts of the two greater vestibular glands, (d) small paraurethral ducts (of Skene), and (e) anus.

(2) The **mons pubis** is a rounded mound of skin and adipose tissue anterior to the symphysis pubis; in the adult it is covered with genital hair.

(3) The **labia majora** are two elongated folds of skin and fat extending from the mons pubis toward the anus. They vary in size and thickness depending on age and obesity, and their anterior ends receive the fibrous round ligaments of the uterus. The labia majora are the female structures homologous to the male scrotum.

(4) The **labia minora** are two thin folds of skin situated between the labia majora. They commence at the glans clitoris, and small extensions pass over the dorsum of the clitoris to form the **prepuce.** Posteriorly, they meet in the midline to form the **frenulum.**

(5) The **clitoris** is the homologue of the male penis. It is an erectile organ that measures 1 in. or less in length and consists of two corpora cavernosa attached by crura to the pubic rami. It is suspended by a fibrous ligament and capped by the **glans.**

(6) The **vestibule** of the vagina is the region between the two labia minora. Into it open the **urethra,** the **ducts of the greater vestibular glands,** and the **vagina.** In the virgin, the vaginal orifice is partially closed by a thin membrane, the **hymen,** which usually is ruptured at first copulation. Since its form and extent are quite variable, virginity cannot be absolutely determined by its absence.

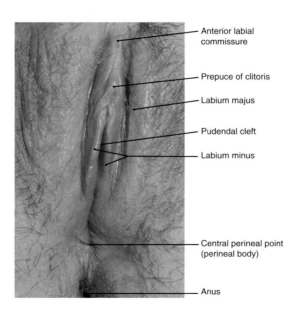

Anterior labial commissure

Prepuce of clitoris

Labium majus

Pudendal cleft

Labium minus

Central perineal point (perineal body)

Anus

FIGURE 344.2 **Perineal Structures in a 26-Year-Old Woman**

NOTE: In this photograph the labia minora are approximated so that the vaginal and urethral orifices are not visible.

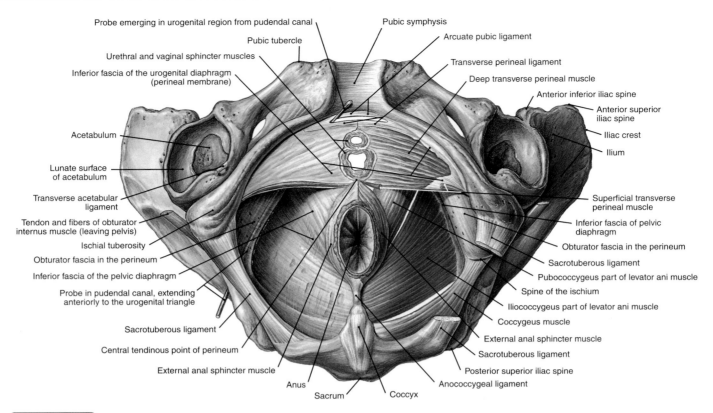

Probe emerging in urogenital region from pudendal canal
Pubic tubercle
Urethral and vaginal sphincter muscles
Inferior fascia of the urogenital diaphragm (perineal membrane)
Acetabulum
Lunate surface of acetabulum
Transverse acetabular ligament
Tendon and fibers of obturator internus muscle (leaving pelvis)
Ischial tuberosity
Obturator fascia in the perineum
Inferior fascia of the pelvic diaphragm
Probe in pudendal canal, extending anteriorly to the urogenital triangle
Sacrotuberous ligament
Central tendinous point of perineum
External anal sphincter muscle
Anus
Sacrum

Pubic symphysis
Arcuate pubic ligament
Transverse perineal ligament
Deep transverse perineal muscle
Anterior inferior iliac spine
Anterior superior iliac spine
Iliac crest
Ilium
Superficial transverse perineal muscle
Inferior fascia of pelvic diaphragm
Obturator fascia in the perineum
Sacrotuberous ligament
Pubococcygeus part of levator ani muscle
Spine of the ischium
Iliococcygeus part of levator ani muscle
Coccygeus muscle
External anal sphincter muscle
Sacrotuberous ligament
Posterior superior iliac spine
Anococcygeal ligament
Coccyx

FIGURE 345.1 Musculature of the Floor of the Female Pelvis, Viewed from the Inferior, or Perineal, Aspect

NOTE: (1) On the left side (reader's right) the inferior fascias of the pelvic and urogenital diaphragms have been removed.
(2) The musculature of the urogenital diaphragm completes the anterior part of the female pelvic floor but allows the urethra and vagina to traverse the urogenital hiatus.
(3) The **central point of the perineum** interposed in the midline between the urogenital diaphragm and the anterior end of the raphe formed by the two external anal sphincters.
(4) The anal hiatus is surrounded by the **pubococcygeus** parts of the levator ani muscles. These are reinforced above by the puborectalis muscle and below by the external sphincter. Observe that the **iliococcygeus** sweeps medially to the coccyx, but some fibers also insert into the short midline **anococcygeal raphe** and **ligament.**

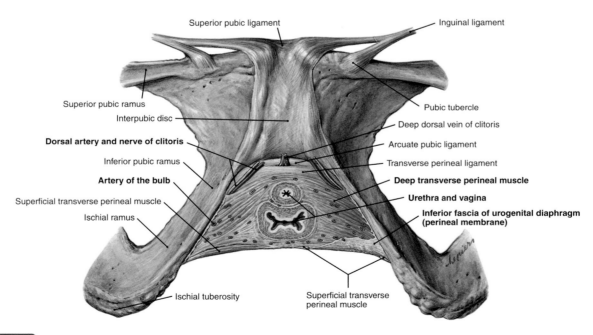

Superior pubic ligament
Inguinal ligament
Superior pubic ramus
Interpubic disc
Dorsal artery and nerve of clitoris
Inferior pubic ramus
Artery of the bulb
Superficial transverse perineal muscle
Ischial ramus
Pubic tubercle
Deep dorsal vein of clitoris
Arcuate pubic ligament
Transverse perineal ligament
Deep transverse perineal muscle
Urethra and vagina
Inferior fascia of urogenital diaphragm (perineal membrane)
Ischial tuberosity
Superficial transverse perineal muscle

FIGURE 345.2 Urogenital Diaphragm in the Female

NOTE: The female **urethra** and **vagina** both pass through the **urogenital diaphragm.** Observe the circular **sphincter** surrounding the membranous urethra and the **deep transverse perineal muscles** that are covered by deep fascia on both their superior and inferior surfaces.

MUSCLES RELATED TO THE PELVIC DIAPHRAGM

Muscle	Origin	Insertion	Innervation	Action
Levator ani consisting of: pubococcygeus iliococcygeus pubovaginalis levator of prostate puborectalis	From a tendinous arch (along the fascia of the obturator internus muscle). The arch extends from the symphysis pubis to the ischial spine	Into the coccyx; the anococcygeal raphe and ligament; the external anal sphincter, central tendinous point of the perineum	Pudendal nerve (S3, S4, S5)	Supports and slightly raises the floor of the pelvis; it resists intra-abdominal pressure, as in forced expiration
Coccygeus	Spine of the ischium; sacrospinous ligament	Lateral margin of coccyx and sacrum	Pudendal plexus (S4, S5 nerves)	Draws coccyx forward during parturition or defecation Supports pelvic floor
External anal sphincter: Subcutaneous part (a band of fibers just deep to the skin)	Attached anteriorly to the perineal body or central tendinous point and posteriorly to the anococcygeal ligament			
Superficial part (lies deep to the subcutaneous part; main part of muscle)	From the anococcygeal ligament	Into the perineal body or central tendinous point	Pudendal nerve, rectal branch (S4)	Anal sphincter is in a state of tonic contraction; upon defecation, the muscle relaxes
Deep part (forms a complete sphincter of the anal canal)	Fibers surround the anal canal and are applied closely to the internal anal sphincter			

DEEP MUSCLES OF THE UROGENITAL REGION

Muscle	Origin	Insertion	Innervation	Action
Deep transverse perineal muscle (female)	Inferior ramus of the ischium	To the side of the vagina, meeting fibers of the muscle from the other side	Perineal branch of the pudendal nerve (S2, S3, S4)	Helps fix the perineal body and assists the urethrovaginal sphincter
Deep transverse perineal muscle (male)	Inferior ramus of the ischium	Fibers course to the median line, where they interlace in a tendinous raphe with fibers from the other side	Perineal branch of the pudendal nerve (S2, S3, S4)	Helps fix the perineal body and assists the urethral sphincter
Urethrovaginal sphincter (female)	Inferior fibers: From the transverse perineal ligament Superior fibers: From the inner surface of the pubic ramus	Course backward on both sides of the urethra Encircle the lower end of the urethra	Perineal branch of the pudendal nerve (S2, 3, 4)	Acts as a voluntary constrictor of the urethra and vagina
Sphincter of the urethra (male) (surrounds the membranous part of the urethra)	Superficial part: From the transverse perineal ligament Deep part: From the ramus of the pubis	Most fibers form a circular sphincter that invests the membranous urethra; some fibers join the perineal body	Perineal branch of the pudendal nerve (S2, S3, S4)	Acts as the voluntary constrictor of the membranous urethra

PLATE 347 Female Perineum: Muscles

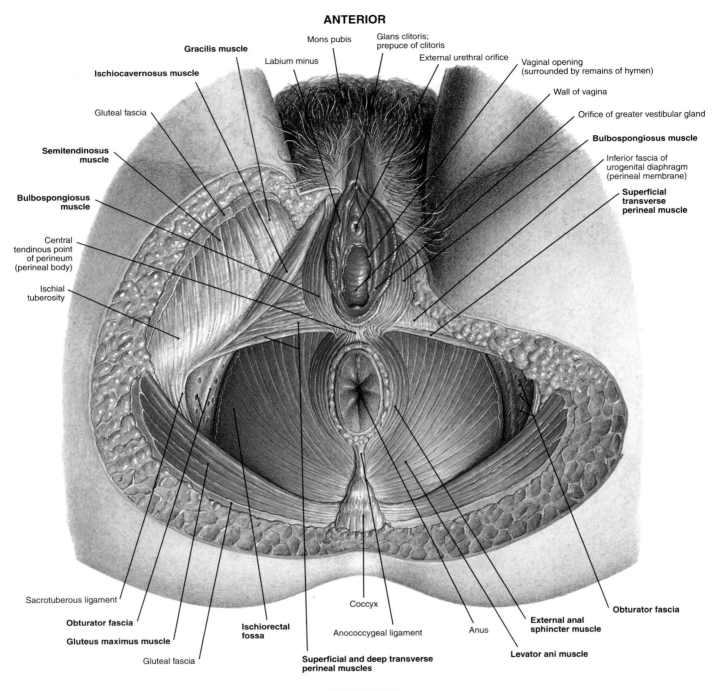

ANTERIOR

Gracilis muscle

Ischiocavernosus muscle

Gluteal fascia

Semitendinosus muscle

Bulbospongiosus muscle

Central tendinous point of perineum (perineal body)

Ischial tuberosity

Mons pubis

Labium minus

Glans clitoris; prepuce of clitoris

External urethral orifice

Vaginal opening (surrounded by remains of hymen)

Wall of vagina

Orifice of greater vestibular gland

Bulbospongiosus muscle

Inferior fascia of urogenital diaphragm (perineal membrane)

Superficial transverse perineal muscle

Sacrotuberous ligament

Obturator fascia

Gluteus maximus muscle

Gluteal fascia

Coccyx

Anococcygeal ligament

Superficial and deep transverse perineal muscles

Ischiorectal fossa

Anus

External anal sphincter muscle

Levator ani muscle

Obturator fascia

POSTERIOR

FIGURE 347 Muscles of the Female Perineum

NOTE: (1) The perineum is a diamond-shaped region located below the pelvis and separated from it by the muscular pelvic diaphragm. The perineum is bounded by the **symphysis pubis** anteriorly, the **coccyx** posteriorly, and the two **ischial tuberosities** laterally. A line drawn across the perineum anterior to the anus between the two ischial tuberosities divides the perineum into an anterior **urogenital region** and a posterior **anal region.**

(2) The *urogenital region* contains the external genitalia and the associated muscles and glands. Often books refer to *superficial and deep perineal compartments* (spaces or pouches). The **superficial perineal compartment** lies superficial to the inferior layer of fascia of the urogenital diaphragm, and it contains the ischiocavernosus, bulbocavernosus, and superficial transverse perineal muscles and the perineal vessels and nerves. It is limited superficially by a layer of deep fascia (the external perineal fascia) just deep to **Colles' fascia.**

(3) The **deep perineal compartment** is the space enclosed between the two layers of the urogenital diaphragm. It contains the deep transverse perineal and urethral sphincter muscles and is traversed by the urethra and the vagina in the female.

(4) The *anal region* is situated posterior to the urogenital region; it contains the anus surrounded by the external anal sphincter muscle. A large portion of the anal region is occupied by the two fat-filled **ischiorectal fossae.**

ANTERIOR

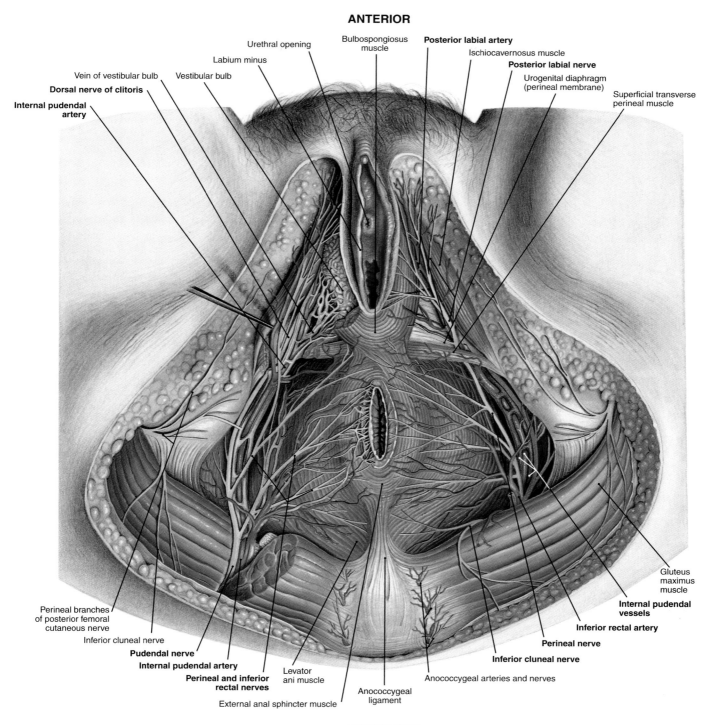

POSTERIOR

FIGURE 348 **Nerves and Blood Vessels of the Female Perineum**

NOTE: (1)   The branches of the **pudendal nerve** supply most of the perineal structures. This nerve arises from the second, third, and fourth sacral segments of the spinal cord. Within the pelvis it is joined by the **internal pudendal artery and vein.** The vessels and nerve leave the pelvis through the greater sciatic foramen along the lower border of the piriformis muscle and cross the ischial spine to reenter the pelvis through the lesser sciatic foramen.

(2)   The pudendal structures reach the perineum by way of the **pudendal canal** (of Alcock) deep to the fascia of the obturator internus muscle. Their branches, the **inferior rectal vessels** and **nerves,** cross the ischiorectal fossa toward the midline to supply the levator ani and external anal sphincter muscles as well as other structures in the anal region.

(3)   The pudendal vessels and nerve then continue anteriorly as the **perineal vessels** and **nerve** and enter the urogenital region by penetrating the urogenital diaphragm. They branch again into superficial and deep branches to supply structures in the superficial and deep compartments. The superficial branches supply the labia majora and the external genital structures, whereas the deep branches supply the muscles, vestibular bulb, and clitoris.

SUPERFICIAL MUSCLES OF THE UROGENITAL REGION

Muscle	Origin	Insertion	Innervation	Action
Superficial transverse perineal muscle (male and female)	Medial and anterior part of the ischial tuberosity	Into the perineal body (female) or central tendinous point (male) in front of the anus	Perineal branch of the pudendal nerve (S2, S3, S4)	Simultaneous contraction of the two muscles helps fix the central tendinous point of the perineum
Ischiocavernosus muscle (female)	Inner surface of the ischial tuberosity behind the crus clitoris and from the adjacent part of the ramus of the ischium	Fibers end in an aponeurosis, which inserts onto the sides and under the surface of the crus clitoris	Perineal branch of the pudendal nerve (S2, S3, S4)	Compresses the crus clitoris, retarding the return of blood and therapy helping to maintain erection of the clitoris
Ischiocavernosus muscle (male)	Inner surface of the ischial tuberosity behind the crus penis and from the ramus of the ischium on each side of the crus	Fibers end in an aponeurosis attached to the sides and under surface of the corpus cavernosum on each side as they join to form the body of the penis	Perineal branch of the pudendal nerve (S2, S3, S4)	Compresses the crus penis and thereby helps maintain erection
Bulbospongiosus muscle (female)	Fibers attached posteriorly to the perineal body	Fibers pass anteriorly around the vagina and are inserted into the corpora cavernosa clitoris	Perineal branch of the pudendal nerve (S2, S3, S4)	Decreases the orifice of the vagina; anterior fibers assist erection of the clitoris by compressing the deep dorsal vein of the clitoris
Bulbospongiosus muscle (male)	From the central tendinous point and the ventral extension of the median raphe between the two bulbospongiosus muscles	**Posterior fibers:** end in connective tissue of the fascia of UG diaphragm **Middle fibers:** encircle the bulb of the penis and the corpus spongiosum **Anterior fibers:** spread over the side of the corpus cavernosum and extend anteriorly as a tendinous expansion over the dorsal vessels	Perineal branch of the pudendal nerve (S2, S3, S4)	Aids in emptying the urethra at end of urination; by compressing the dorsal vein, it also helps maintain penile erection; contracts during ejaculation

FIGURE 349 **Internal Anatomy of the Vaginal Wall**

NOTE: (1) The uterus, external female genitalia, and opened vaginal wall are viewed from above.

(2) The vaginal rugae that characterize the inner vaginal wall. Also note the slit-like external os of the uterus and a mucous plug between its anterior and posterior lips.

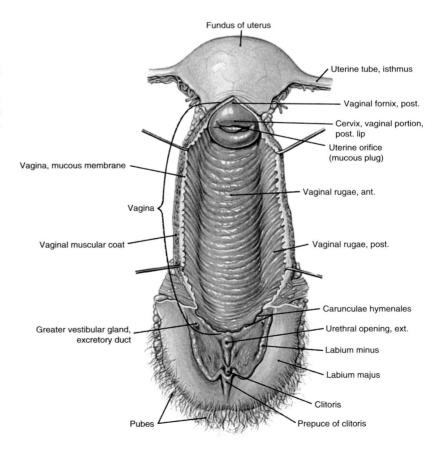

Fundus of uterus

Uterine tube, isthmus

Vaginal fornix, post.

Cervix, vaginal portion, post. lip

Uterine orifice (mucous plug)

Vagina, mucous membrane

Vaginal rugae, ant.

Vagina

Vaginal muscular coat

Vaginal rugae, post.

Carunculae hymenales

Greater vestibular gland, excretory duct

Urethral opening, ext.

Labium minus

Labium majus

Clitoris

Pubes

Prepuce of clitoris

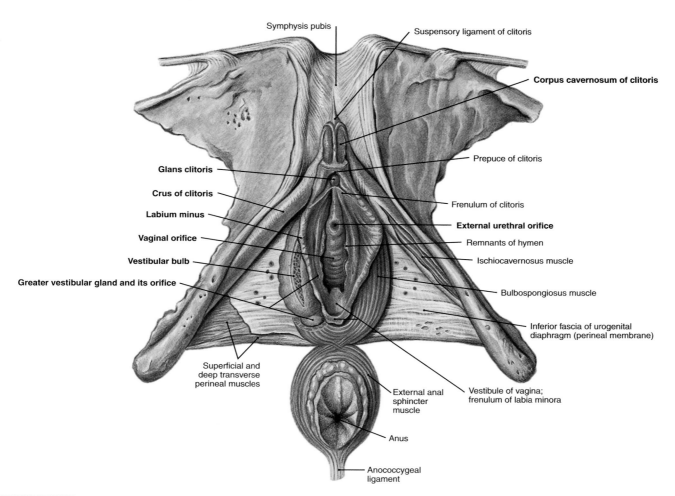

Symphysis pubis

Suspensory ligament of clitoris

Corpus cavernosum of clitoris

Prepuce of clitoris

Glans clitoris

Crus of clitoris

Labium minus

Vaginal orifice

Vestibular bulb

Greater vestibular gland and its orifice

Frenulum of clitoris

External urethral orifice

Remnants of hymen

Ischiocavernosus muscle

Bulbospongiosus muscle

Inferior fascia of urogenital diaphragm (perineal membrane)

Superficial and deep transverse perineal muscles

External anal sphincter muscle

Vestibule of vagina; frenulum of labia minora

Anus

Anococcygeal ligament

FIGURE 350.1 **Dissected Female External Genitalia**

NOTE: (1) The skin and fascia of the labia majora have been removed. Observe the **crura, body** and **glans clitoris,** the **vestibular bulbs,** and the location of the **greater vestibular glands.**

(2) Each crus of the clitoris is covered by an **ischiocavernosus muscle,** and the vestibular bulbs are surrounded by the **bulbospongiosus muscles.**

(3) The **greater vestibular glands** (of Bartholin) are found just behind the vestibular bulbs. During sexual stimulation, they secrete a viscous fluid that lubricates the vagina.

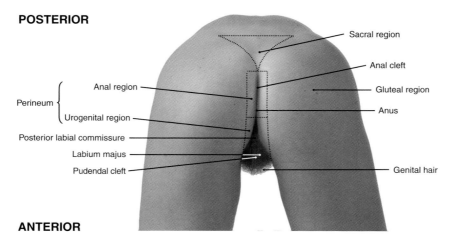

POSTERIOR

Sacral region

Anal cleft

Anal region

Gluteal region

Perineum

Anus

Urogenital region

Posterior labial commissure

Labium majus

Pudendal cleft

Genital hair

ANTERIOR

FIGURE 350.2 **Surface Anatomy of the Female Sacral, Gluteal, and Perineal Regions (Posteroinferior View)**

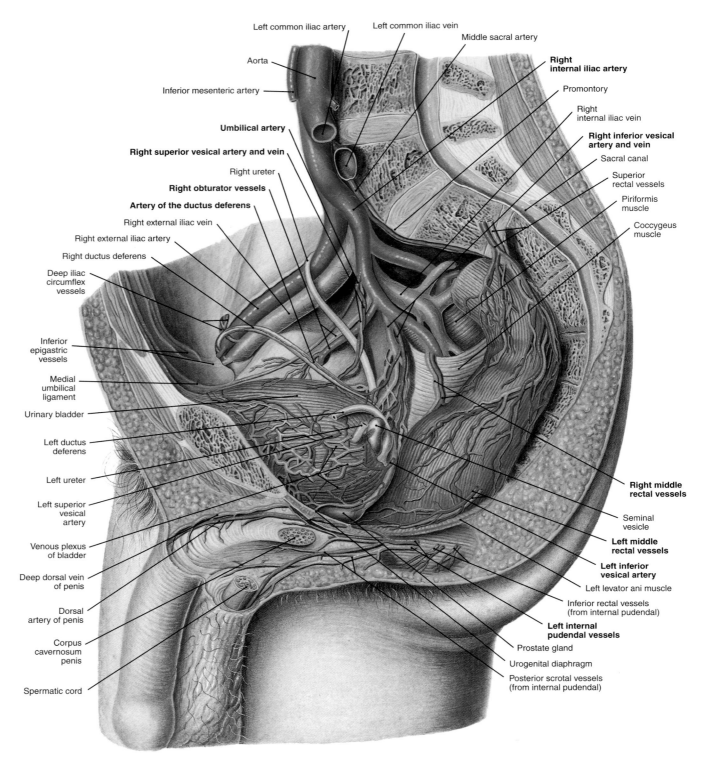

Left common iliac artery

Left common iliac vein

Middle sacral artery

Aorta

Right internal iliac artery

Inferior mesenteric artery

Promontory

Right internal iliac vein

Umbilical artery

Right inferior vesical artery and vein

Right superior vesical artery and vein

Sacral canal

Right ureter

Superior rectal vessels

Right obturator vessels

Piriformis muscle

Artery of the ductus deferens

Coccygeus muscle

Right external iliac vein

Right external iliac artery

Right ductus deferens

Deep iliac circumflex vessels

Inferior epigastric vessels

Medial umbilical ligament

Urinary bladder

Left ductus deferens

Left ureter

Right middle rectal vessels

Left superior vesical artery

Seminal vesicle

Left middle rectal vessels

Left inferior vesical artery

Venous plexus of bladder

Left levator ani muscle

Deep dorsal vein of penis

Inferior rectal vessels (from internal pudendal)

Left internal pudendal vessels

Dorsal artery of penis

Prostate gland

Corpus cavernosum penis

Urogenital diaphragm

Posterior scrotal vessels (from internal pudendal)

Spermatic cord

FIGURE 351 **Blood Vessels of the Male Pelvis, Perineum, and External Genitalia**

NOTE: (1) The aorta bifurcates into the **common iliac arteries,** which then divide into the **external** and **internal iliac arteries.** The external iliac becomes the principal arterial trunk of the lower extremity, whereas the internal iliac artery supplies the organs of the pelvis and perineum.

(2) The **visceral branches** of the internal iliac are: (a) the umbilical (from which is derived the superior vesical artery), (b) the inferior vesical, (c) the artery of the vas deferens (uterine artery in females), and (d) the middle rectal.

(3) The **parietal branches** include: (a) the iliolumbar, (b) lateral sacral, (c) superior gluteal, (d) inferior gluteal, (e) obturator, and (f) internal pudendal.

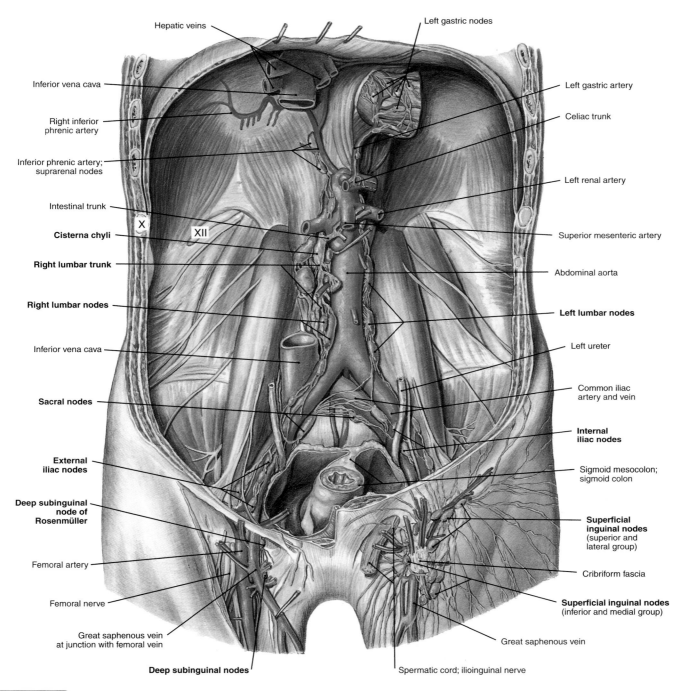

Hepatic veins

Left gastric nodes

Inferior vena cava

Left gastric artery

Right inferior phrenic artery

Celiac trunk

Inferior phrenic artery; suprarenal nodes

Left renal artery

Intestinal trunk

Cisterna chyli

X

XII

Right lumbar trunk

Superior mesenteric artery

Abdominal aorta

Right lumbar nodes

Left lumbar nodes

Inferior vena cava

Left ureter

Sacral nodes

Common iliac artery and vein

Internal iliac nodes

External iliac nodes

Sigmoid mesocolon; sigmoid colon

Deep subinguinal node of Rosenmüller

Superficial inguinal nodes (superior and lateral group)

Femoral artery

Cribriform fascia

Femoral nerve

Superficial inguinal nodes (inferior and medial group)

Great saphenous vein at junction with femoral vein

Great saphenous vein

Deep subinguinal nodes

Spermatic cord; ilioinguinal nerve

FIGURE 352 Inguinal, Pelvic, and Lumbar (Aortic) Lymph Nodes

NOTE: (1) Chains of lymph nodes and lymphatic vessels lie along the paths of major blood vessels from the inguinal region to the diaphragm. The **superficial inguinal nodes** lie just distal to the inguinal ligament within the superficial fascia.

(2) There are 10 to 20 superficial inguinal nodes, and they receive drainage from the genitalia, perineum, gluteal region, and anterior abdominal wall. More deeply, **subinguinal nodes** drain the lower extremity, one of which lies in the femoral ring (Rosenmüller's or Cloquet's node).

(3) Within the pelvis, visceral lymph nodes lie close to the organs that they drain and they channel lymph along the paths of major blood vessels, such as the **external, internal,** and **common iliac nodes** located along these vessels in the pelvis.

(4) On the posterior abdominal wall are located the **right** and **left lumbar** chains coursing along the abdominal aorta, while **preaortic nodes** are arranged around the roots of the major unpaired aortic branches, forming the **celiac** and **superior** and **inferior mesenteric nodes.**

(5) At the level of the L2 vertebra, there is a confluence of lymph channels that forms a dilated sac, the **cisterna chyli.** This is located somewhat posterior and to the right of the aorta, and it marks the commencement of the **thoracic duct.**

PLATE 353 Male Pelvic Organs and Peritoneal Reflections

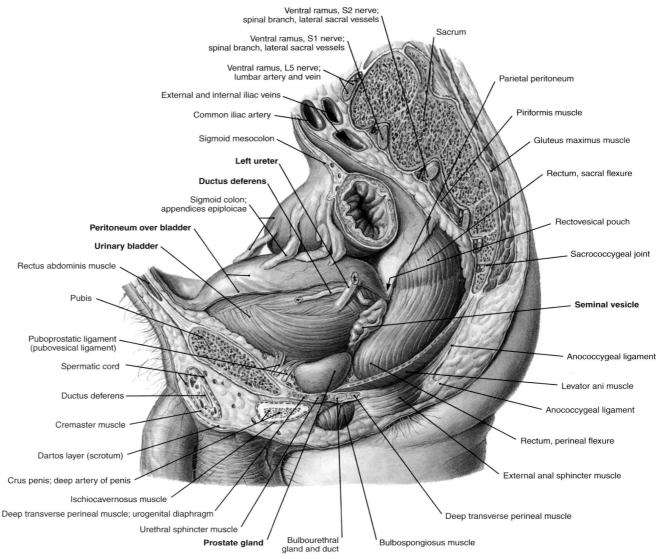

Ventral ramus, S2 nerve;
spinal branch, lateral sacral vessels

Ventral ramus, S1 nerve;
spinal branch, lateral sacral vessels

Ventral ramus, L5 nerve;
lumbar artery and vein

External and internal iliac veins

Common iliac artery

Sigmoid mesocolon

Left ureter

Ductus deferens

Sigmoid colon;
appendices epiploicae

Peritoneum over bladder

Urinary bladder

Rectus abdominis muscle

Pubis

Puboprostatic ligament
(pubovesical ligament)

Spermatic cord

Ductus deferens

Cremaster muscle

Dartos layer (scrotum)

Crus penis; deep artery of penis

Ischiocavernosus muscle

Deep transverse perineal muscle; urogenital diaphragm

Urethral sphincter muscle

Prostate gland

Bulbourethral
gland and duct

Bulbospongiosus muscle

Sacrum

Parietal peritoneum

Piriformis muscle

Gluteus maximus muscle

Rectum, sacral flexure

Rectovesical pouch

Sacrococcygeal joint

Seminal vesicle

Anococcygeal ligament

Levator ani muscle

Anococcygeal ligament

Rectum, perineal flexure

External anal sphincter muscle

Deep transverse perineal muscle

FIGURE 353.1 Male Pelvic Organs Viewed from the Left Side

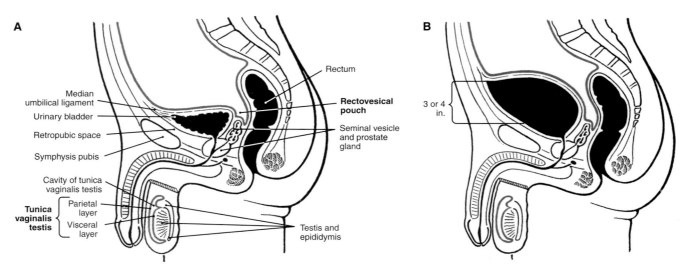

A

Median
umbilical ligament

Urinary bladder

Retropubic space

Symphysis pubis

Cavity of tunica
vaginalis testis

**Tunica
vaginalis
testis** { Parietal layer / Visceral layer

Rectum

**Rectovesical
pouch**

Seminal vesicle
and prostate
gland

Testis and
epididymis

B

3 or 4
in.

FIGURE 353.2A and B Peritoneal Reflection over the Pelvic Organs: Empty and Full Bladder

NOTE: (1) When the bladder is empty **(A),** the peritoneum extends down to the level of the symphysis pubis, but when the bladder is full **(B),** the peritoneum is elevated 3 or 4 in.

(2) The prostate and bladder may be reached **without entering the peritoneal cavity** anteriorly above the pubis and through the perineum by ascending in front of the rectum.

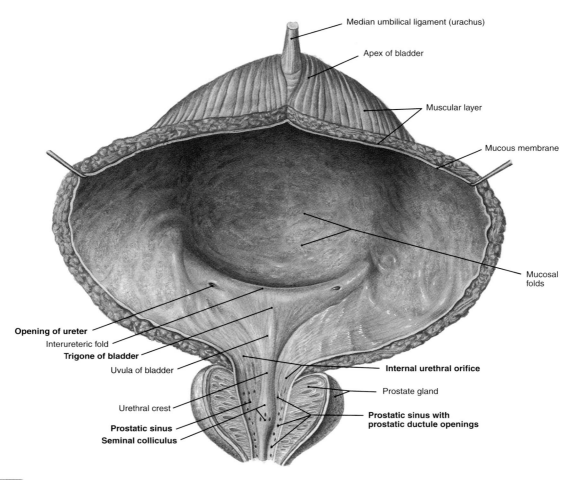

Median umbilical ligament (urachus)

Apex of bladder

Muscular layer

Mucous membrane

Mucosal folds

Opening of ureter
Interureteric fold
Trigone of bladder
Uvula of bladder

Internal urethral orifice

Prostate gland

Urethral crest

Prostatic sinus with prostatic ductule openings

Prostatic sinus
Seminal colliculus

FIGURE 354.1 **Bladder and Prostatic Urethra Incised Anteriorly**

NOTE: (1) The smooth triangular area at the base of the bladder called the **trigone,** which is bounded by the two orifices of the ureters and the opening of the prostatic urethra.

(2) The **seminal colliculus** is a mound on the posterior wall of the prostatic urethra, on both sides of which lie the **prostatic sinuses.** Into these open the ducts of the prostate gland. In the center of the colliculus is a small blind pouch, the **prostatic utricle;** on both sides of the utricle are the single orifices of the **ejaculatory ducts** (openings not labeled).

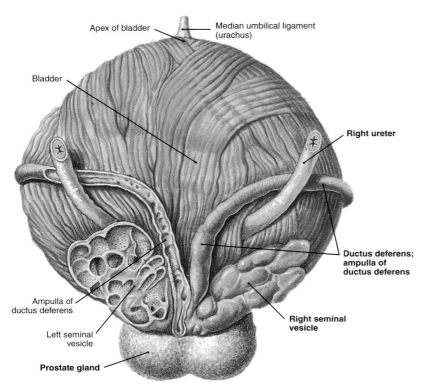

Apex of bladder

Median umbilical ligament (urachus)

Bladder

Right ureter

Ductus deferens; ampulla of ductus deferens

Ampulla of ductus deferens

Right seminal vesicle

Left seminal vesicle

Prostate gland

FIGURE 354.2 **Posterior Surface of the Bladder: Seminal Vesicles, Ureters, and Deferent Ducts**

NOTE: (1) The ureters, deferent ducts, seminal vesicles, and prostate gland are all in contact with the inferior aspect of the posterior surface of the bladder.

(2) The **ureters** penetrate the bladder diagonally at points about 2 in. apart. Upon entering the bladder, each ureter is crossed anteriorly by the ductus deferens.

(3) The deferent ducts join the ducts of the lobulated seminal vesicles to form the two ejaculatory ducts.

(4) The prostate hugs the bladder at its outlet, surrounding the prostatic urethra.

(5) All of these organs lie directly in front of the rectum and can be palpated during a rectal examination.

PLATE 355 Male Pelvis and Perineum (Midsagittal Section)

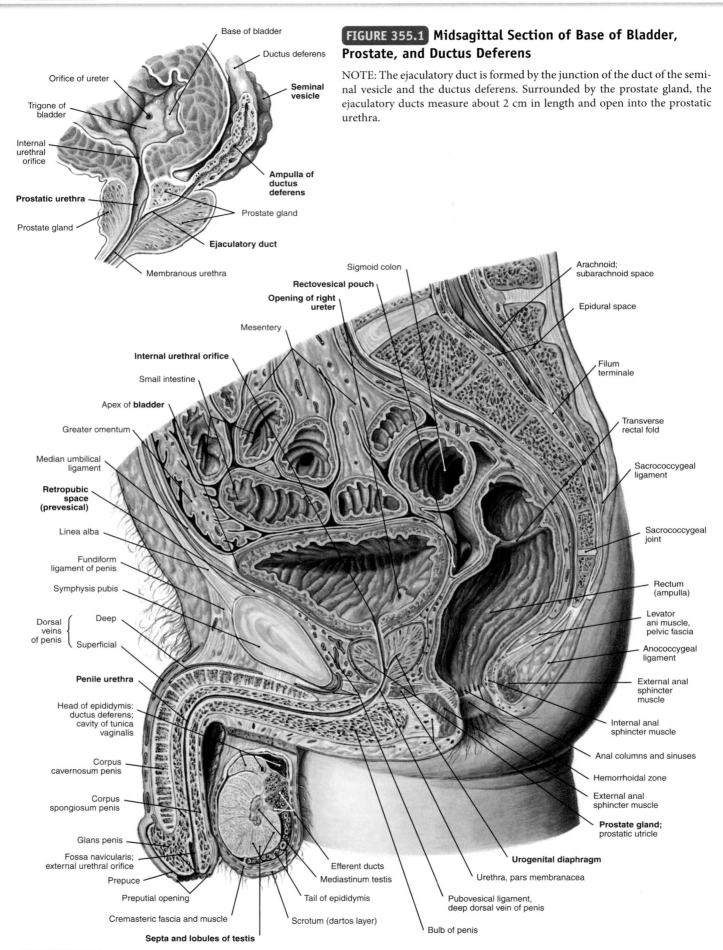

FIGURE 355.1 **Midsagittal Section of Base of Bladder, Prostate, and Ductus Deferens**

NOTE: The ejaculatory duct is formed by the junction of the duct of the seminal vesicle and the ductus deferens. Surrounded by the prostate gland, the ejaculatory ducts measure about 2 cm in length and open into the prostatic urethra.

Base of bladder

Ductus deferens

Orifice of ureter

Seminal vesicle

Trigone of bladder

Internal urethral orifice

Ampulla of ductus deferens

Prostatic urethra

Prostate gland

Prostate gland

Ejaculatory duct

Membranous urethra

Sigmoid colon

Rectovesical pouch

Opening of right ureter

Mesentery

Arachnoid; subarachnoid space

Epidural space

Internal urethral orifice

Small intestine

Filum terminale

Apex of **bladder**

Greater omentum

Transverse rectal fold

Median umbilical ligament

Sacrococcygeal ligament

Retropubic space (prevesical)

Linea alba

Sacrococcygeal joint

Fundiform ligament of penis

Rectum (ampulla)

Symphysis pubis

Levator ani muscle, pelvic fascia

Dorsal veins of penis — Deep

Superficial

Anococcygeal ligament

Penile urethra

External anal sphincter muscle

Head of epididymis: ductus deferens; cavity of tunica vaginalis

Internal anal sphincter muscle

Anal columns and sinuses

Corpus cavernosum penis

Hemorrhoidal zone

Corpus spongiosum penis

External anal sphincter muscle

Glans penis

Prostate gland; prostatic utricle

Fossa navicularis; external urethral orifice

Urogenital diaphragm

Prepuce

Efferent ducts

Urethra, pars membranacea

Preputial opening

Mediastinum testis

Cremasteric fascia and muscle

Tail of epididymis

Pubovesical ligament, deep dorsal vein of penis

Scrotum (dartos layer)

Septa and lobules of testis

Bulb of penis

FIGURE 355.2 **Median Sagittal Section of the Male Pelvis and Perineum Showing the Pelvic Viscera and the External Genitalia**

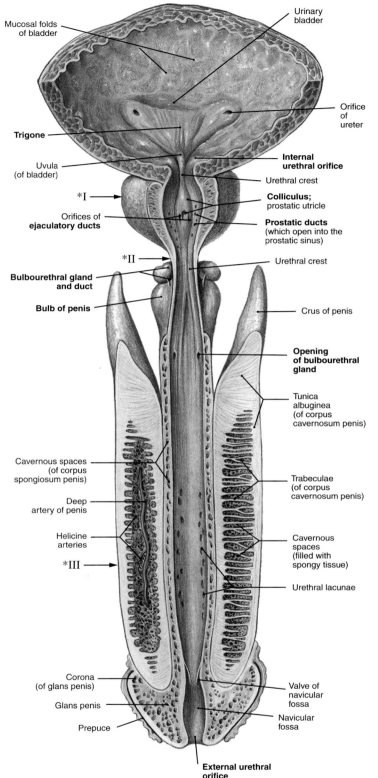

Figure 356.1 labels (left diagram):

Mucosal folds of bladder

Urinary bladder

Trigone

Uvula (of bladder)

*I

Orifices of ejaculatory ducts

Orifice of ureter

Internal urethral orifice

Urethral crest

Colliculus; prostatic utricle

Prostatic ducts (which open into the prostatic sinus)

*II

Urethral crest

Bulbourethral gland and duct

Bulb of penis

Crus of penis

Opening of bulbourethral gland

Tunica albuginea (of corpus cavernosum penis)

Cavernous spaces (of corpus spongiosum penis)

Deep artery of penis

Helicine arteries

*III

Trabeculae (of corpus cavernosum penis)

Cavernous spaces (filled with spongy tissue)

Urethral lacunae

Corona (of glans penis)

Glans penis

Prepuce

Valve of navicular fossa

Navicular fossa

External urethral orifice

* Parts of urethra
I = Prostatic part
II = Membranous part
III = Penile part

◄ **FIGURE 356.1** **Male Urethra and Its Associated Orifices**

NOTE: (1) The male urethra extends from the internal urethral orifice at the bladder to the external urethral orifice at the end of the glans penis. In males, it traverses the prostate gland, the urogenital diaphragm (membrane), and penis, and is, therefore, divided into **prostatic, membranous,** and **penile** parts.

(2) Before ejaculation, a viscous fluid from the **bulbourethral glands** (of Cowper) lubricates the urethra. These glands are located in the urogenital diaphragm, but their ducts open 1 in. distally in the penile urethra.

(3) The total urethra measures between 7 and 8 in. in length, the prostatic part about 1½ in., the membranous part about ½ in., and the penile part 5 to 6 in. The **prostatic urethra** receives the secretions of the ejaculatory ducts along with those from the prostate. Enlargement of the prostate, often occurring in older men, tends to constrict the urethra at this site, resulting in difficulty in urination.

(4) The **membranous urethra** is short and narrow and it is completely surrounded by the circular fibers of the voluntary urethral sphincter muscle. Relaxation of this sphincter initiates urination, while its tonic contraction constricts the urethra and maintains urinary continence.

(5) The **penile urethra** is surrounded initially by the bulb of the penis and the bulbospongiosus muscle. It traverses the penile shaft within the corpus spongiosum penis. The internal surface of the distal half is marked by small recesses called the urethral lacunae.

FIGURE 356.2 **Radiograph of Bladder, Seminal ▶ Vesicles, Deferent Ducts, and Ejaculatory Ducts**

NOTE: The bladder has been filled with air and appears light, while the seminal vesicles, deferent ducts, and ejaculatory ducts stand out as dark because of an injected contrast medium.

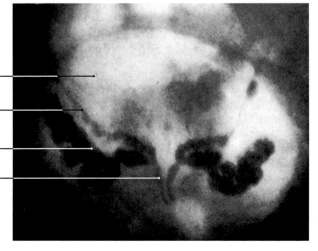

Bladder (air filled)

Ductus deferens

Seminal vesicle

Ejaculatory duct

PLATE 357 **Diagram of Male Genitourinary Organs**

FIGURE 357.1 **Diagram of the Male Genitourinary System** ▶

NOTE: (1) This figure shows: (a) the organs of the adult male genitourinary system (dark red-brown), (b) the structures of the genital system prior to the descent of the testis (interrupted blue lines), and (c) those structures that partially or entirely became atrophic and disappeared during development (pink structures with red outlines).

(2) The **urinary system** includes the *kidneys,* which produce urine by filtration of the blood, the *ureters,* which convey urine to the *bladder,* where it is stored, and the *urethra,* through which urine is discharged.

(3) The adult male genital system includes the *testis,* where sperm is generated, and the *epididymis* and *ductus deferens,* which transport sperm to the *ejaculatory duct,* where the *seminal vesicle* joins the genital system. The *prostate* and *bulbourethral glands,* along with the ejaculatory ducts, join the *urethra,* which then courses through the prostate and *penis.*

(4) Embryologically, structures capable of developing into either sex exist in all individuals. In the male the **mesonephric** (Wolffian) **duct** becomes the epididymis, ductus deferens, ejaculatory duct, and seminal vesicle along with the penis, while the **paramesonephric** (Müllerian) **duct** is suppressed.

(5) The testes are developed on the posterior abdominal wall, to which each is attached by a fibrous genital ligament called the **gubernaculum testis.** As development continues, each testis *migrates* from its site of formation so that by the fifth month it lies adjacent to the abdominal inguinal ring. The gubernaculum is still attached to anterior abdominal wall tissue, which by this time has evaginated as the developing scrotum. The testes then commence their descent through the inguinal canal so that by the eighth month they usually lie in the scrotum attached by a peritoneal reflection, the processus vaginalis testis, which becomes the **tunica vaginalis testis.**

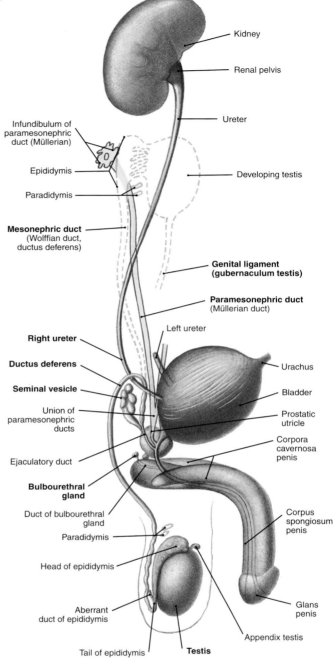

FIGURE 357.1 labels: Kidney; Renal pelvis; Ureter; Infundibulum of paramesonephric duct (Müllerian); Epididymis; Developing testis; Paradidymis; Mesonephric duct (Wolffian duct, ductus deferens); Genital ligament (gubernaculum testis); Paramesonephric duct (Müllerian duct); Left ureter; Right ureter; Urachus; Ductus deferens; Bladder; Seminal vesicle; Union of paramesonephric ducts; Prostatic utricle; Corpora cavernosa penis; Ejaculatory duct; Bulbourethral gland; Corpus spongiosum penis; Duct of bulbourethral gland; Paradidymis; Head of epididymis; Glans penis; Aberrant duct of epididymis; Appendix testis; Tail of epididymis; Testis

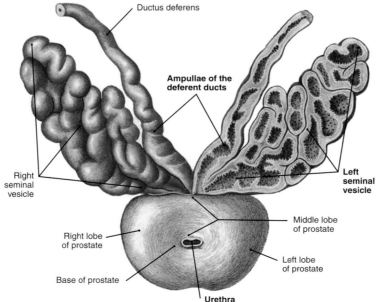

Labels: Ductus deferens; Ampullae of the deferent ducts; Right seminal vesicle; Left seminal vesicle; Right lobe of prostate; Middle lobe of prostate; Left lobe of prostate; Base of prostate; Urethra

◀ **FIGURE 357.2** **Prostate Gland, Seminal Vesicles, and Ampullae of the Deferent Ducts (Superior View)**

NOTE: (1) The left seminal vesicle and ductus deferens were cut longitudinally, while the urethra was cut transversely, distal to the bladder.

(2) The **prostate gland** is conical in shape and normally measures just over 1½ in. across, 1 in. in thickness, and slightly longer than 1 in. vertically. In the young adult, it weighs about 25 g and is formed by two lateral lobes surrounding a middle lobe.

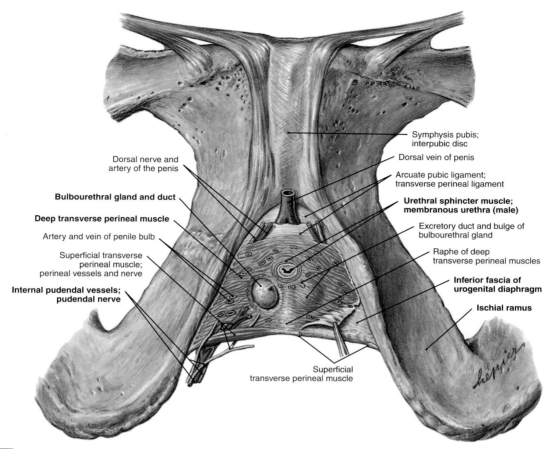

Dorsal nerve and
artery of the penis

Bulbourethral gland and duct

Deep transverse perineal muscle

Artery and vein of penile bulb

Superficial transverse
perineal muscle;
perineal vessels and nerve

**Internal pudendal vessels;
pudendal nerve**

Symphysis pubis;
interpubic disc

Dorsal vein of penis

Arcuate pubic ligament;
transverse perineal ligament

**Urethral sphincter muscle;
membranous urethra (male)**

Excretory duct and bulge of
bulbourethral gland

Raphe of deep
transverse perineal muscles

**Inferior fascia of
urogenital diaphragm**

Ischial ramus

Superficial
transverse perineal muscle

FIGURE 358.1 Urogenital Diaphragm; Deep Transverse Perineal Muscle (Male)

NOTE: (1) The **deep transverse perineal muscle** stretches between the ischial rami and is covered by fascia on both its internal (pelvic or superior) surface and its external (perineal or inferior) surface. These two fascias and the muscle form the **urogenital diaphragm.**

(2) The region between the two fascias is often referred to as the **deep perineal compartment** (pouch, cleft, or space). In the male it contains: (a) the deep transverse perineal muscle, (b) the sphincter of the urethra, (c) the bulbourethral glands, (d) the membranous urethra, and (e) branches of the internal pudendal vessels and nerve.

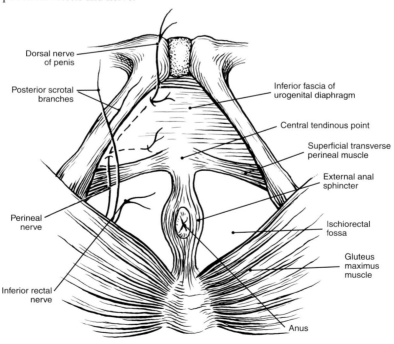

Dorsal nerve
of penis

Posterior scrotal
branches

Perineal
nerve

Inferior rectal
nerve

Inferior fascia of
urogenital diaphragm

Central tendinous point

Superficial transverse
perineal muscle

External anal
sphincter

Ischiorectal
fossa

Gluteus
maximus
muscle

Anus

FIGURE 358.2 Branches of the Pudendal Nerve in the Perineum

NOTE: (1) The perineal branches of the pudendal nerve emerge at the lateral aspect of the ischiorectal fossa.

(2) The inferior rectal nerve crosses the fossa to supply the levator ani and external anal sphincter muscles.

(3) The remaining branches course anteriorly into the urogenital triangle region and supply sensory innervation to all structures there and motor innervation to the urogenital muscles.

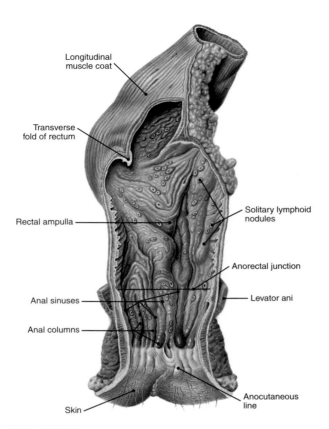

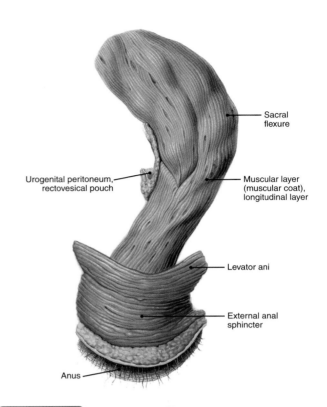

FIGURE 359.1 **Inner Surface of the Rectum and Anal Canal**

NOTE: (1) The sigmoid colon becomes the **rectum** at the level of the middle of the sacrum. The rectum, 5 in. in length, then becomes the **anal canal,** the terminal 1½ in. of the gastrointestinal tract. The rectum is dilated near its junction with the anal canal, giving rise to the **rectal ampulla.**

(2) The rectal mucosa is thrown into transverse folds, usually three in number, called **horizontal folds** or **valves of Houston.**

(3) Below the rectal ampulla is a series of vertical folds, called the **anal columns,** each containing an artery and a vein. Between the anal columns are the **anal sinuses.** If the veins in this region become varicosed, a condition called hemorrhoids, or piles, results.

(4) Distal to the anal columns is a zone, **Hilton's line,** where the epithelium changes from columnar to stratified squamous.

FIGURE 359.2 **External Surface of the Rectum (Lateral View)**

NOTE: (1) The rectum shows a dorsally directed **sacral flexure** proximally and a less pronounced **perineal flexure** distally. Peritoneum ensheathes the rectum ventrally almost as far as the ampulla (to the bladder in the male and the uterus in the female).

(2) The fibers of the **levator ani muscle** (which form the floor of the pelvis) surround the rectum and are continued distally as the **external anal sphincter muscle.**

(3) The **internal anal sphincter muscle** (seen in Figs. 359.1 and 359.3) is composed of smooth muscle and really represents a thickening of the muscular layer in the wall of the rectum.

FIGURE 359.3 **Frontal Section through the Rectum (Diagrammatic)**

NOTE: The **external anal sphincter** consists of **subcutaneous, superficial,** and **deep** parts. Compare this diagram with Figure 359.1.

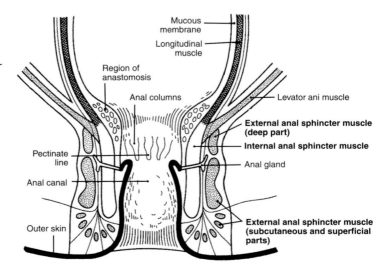

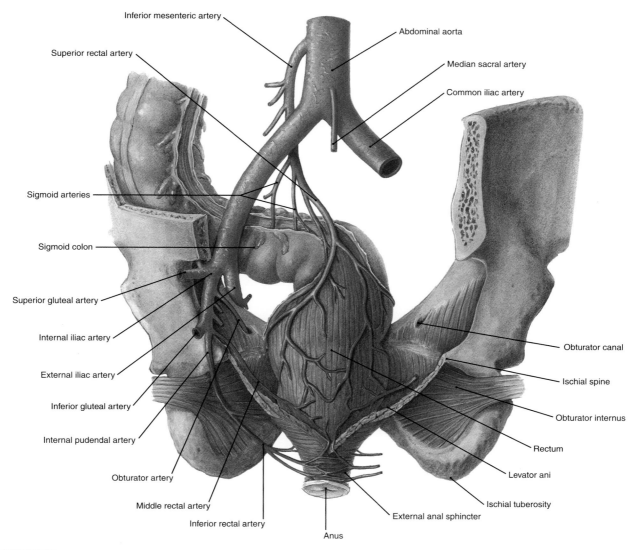

Inferior mesenteric artery

Superior rectal artery

Abdominal aorta

Median sacral artery

Common iliac artery

Sigmoid arteries

Sigmoid colon

Superior gluteal artery

Internal iliac artery

External iliac artery

Inferior gluteal artery

Internal pudendal artery

Obturator artery

Middle rectal artery

Inferior rectal artery

Anus

Obturator canal

Ischial spine

Obturator internus

Rectum

Levator ani

Ischial tuberosity

External anal sphincter

FIGURE 360.1 Arterial Blood Supply to the Rectum (Posterior View)

NOTE: (1) The superior, middle, and inferior rectal arteries form an anastomosis along the entire rectum.
(2) The **superior** rectal artery has an **abdominal source,** the **middle** rectal artery has a **pelvic source,** and the **inferior** rectal artery has a **perineal source.**

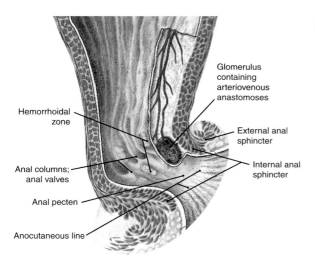

Glomerulus
containing
arteriovenous
anastomoses

Hemorrhoidal
zone

External anal
sphincter

Anal columns;
anal valves

Internal anal
sphincter

Anal pecten

Anocutaneous line

FIGURE 360.2 Rectum and Anal Canal: Median Section

NOTE: (1) The **anal canal** commences where the ampulla of the rectum narrows, and it ends at the anus.
(2) There are 6 to 11 vertical folds called **anal columns.** Each contains arteriovenous anastomoses. The anal columns are joined by folds of mucous membranes called **anal valves.**
(3) The anal valves are situated along a line called the **pectinate line** or **anal pectin.** The **anocutaneous line** is seen adjacent, where usually there is a transition to stratified squamous epithelium from the columnar epithelium of the gastrointestinal tract.

PLATE 361 Rectum: Venous Drainage (Diagrammatic Frontal Section)

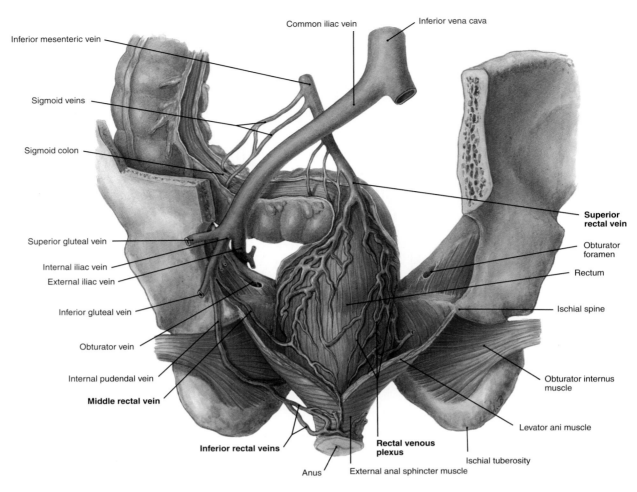

Inferior mesenteric vein

Common iliac vein

Inferior vena cava

Sigmoid veins

Sigmoid colon

Superior gluteal vein

Internal iliac vein

External iliac vein

Inferior gluteal vein

Obturator vein

Internal pudendal vein

Middle rectal vein

Inferior rectal veins

Anus

Rectal venous plexus

External anal sphincter muscle

Superior rectal vein

Obturator foramen

Rectum

Ischial spine

Obturator internus muscle

Levator ani muscle

Ischial tuberosity

FIGURE 361.1 **Venous Drainage of the Rectum (Posterior View)**

NOTE: Blood from the middle and inferior rectal veins eventually drains into the inferior vena cava, while blood returning from the superior rectal vein drains into the portal circulation by way of the inferior mesenteric vein. This allows a route of **collateral circulation** between these two venous systems.

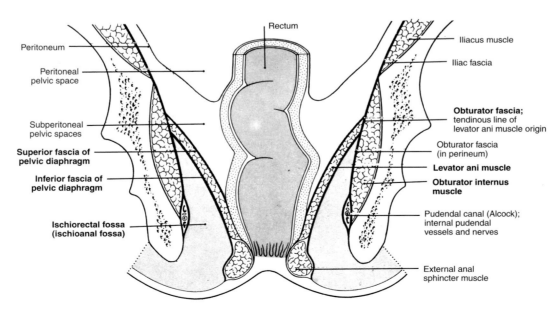

Rectum

Peritoneum

Peritoneal pelvic space

Subperitoneal pelvic spaces

Superior fascia of pelvic diaphragm

Inferior fascia of pelvic diaphragm

Ischiorectal fossa (ischioanal fossa)

Iliacus muscle

Iliac fascia

Obturator fascia; tendinous line of levator ani muscle origin

Obturator fascia (in perineum)

Levator ani muscle

Obturator internus muscle

Pudendal canal (Alcock); internal pudendal vessels and nerves

External anal sphincter muscle

FIGURE 361.2 **Diagram of Frontal Section through Pelvis and Perineum**

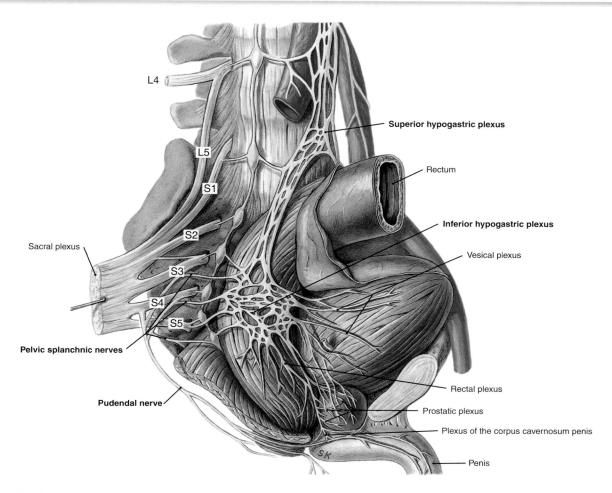

FIGURE 362.1 Autonomic and Visceral Afferent Innervation of the Pelvic Organs

NOTE: (1) *Postganglionic sympathetic fibers* course downward in the **superior hypogastric plexus** from lower lumbar ganglia and continue in the specific visceral plexuses (i.e., rectal, vesical, etc.) to supply pelvic organs with sympathetic innervation.

(2) *Preganglionic parasympathetic fibers* to the pelvic organs emerge from the S2, S3, and S4 spinal nerves to form the **pelvic splanchnic nerves.** They also course through the specific visceral plexuses and then synapse with postganglionic parasympathetic neurons within the walls of the viscera.

(3) **Visceral afferent fibers** from the pelvic organs course centrally along with these autonomic fibers. Their cell bodies lie in their respective dorsal-root ganglia, and they enter the spinal cord by way of the dorsal roots from these ganglia.

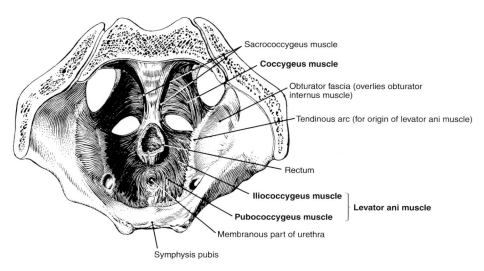

FIGURE 362.2 Muscular Floor of the Pelvis: Pelvic Diaphragm

NOTE: (1) The **pelvic diaphragm** consists of the **levator ani** (iliococcygeus and pubococcygeus parts) **muscle** and the **coccygeus muscle** along with two fascial layers, which cover the *pelvic* (supra-anal fascia) and *perineal* (infra-anal fascia) surfaces of these two muscles.

(2) The muscles composing the pelvic diaphragm stretch across the pelvic floor in a concave sling-like manner and separate the structures of the pelvis from those in the perineum below. In males, the pelvic diaphragm is perforated by the anal canal and the urethra.

PLATE 363 Female Pelvis: Cross Section and CT Image

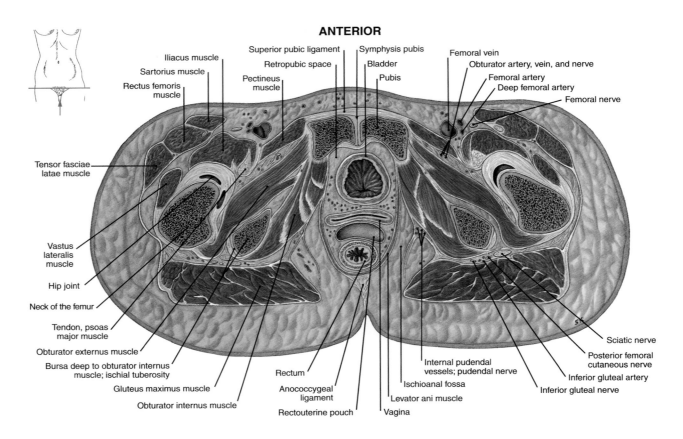

ANTERIOR

Iliacus muscle
Sartorius muscle
Rectus femoris muscle
Superior pubic ligament
Retropubic space
Pectineus muscle
Symphysis pubis
Bladder
Pubis
Femoral vein
Obturator artery, vein, and nerve
Femoral artery
Deep femoral artery
Femoral nerve

Tensor fasciae latae muscle
Vastus lateralis muscle
Hip joint
Neck of the femur
Tendon, psoas major muscle
Obturator externus muscle
Bursa deep to obturator internus muscle; ischial tuberosity
Gluteus maximus muscle
Obturator internus muscle

Rectum
Anococcygeal ligament
Rectouterine pouch
Vagina
Levator ani muscle
Ischioanal fossa
Internal pudendal vessels; pudendal nerve
Inferior gluteal nerve
Inferior gluteal artery
Posterior femoral cutaneous nerve
Sciatic nerve

FIGURE 363.1 Cross Section of the Female Pelvis at the Level of the Symphysis Pubis

NOTE: The viscera medially and the **obturator internus muscle** laterally in the pelvis. Also observe the attachment of the **levator ani muscle** from the fascia overlying the obturator internus muscle and how the levator separates the pelvis from the perineum below. Compare this figure with Figure 363.2.

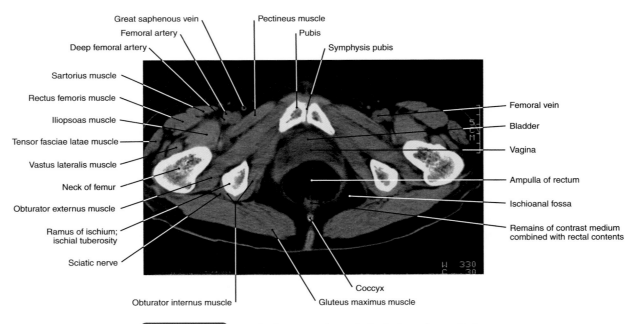

Great saphenous vein
Femoral artery
Deep femoral artery
Sartorius muscle
Rectus femoris muscle
Iliopsoas muscle
Tensor fasciae latae muscle
Vastus lateralis muscle
Neck of femur
Obturator externus muscle
Ramus of ischium; ischial tuberosity
Sciatic nerve

Pectineus muscle
Pubis
Symphysis pubis

Femoral vein
Bladder
Vagina
Ampulla of rectum
Ischioanal fossa
Remains of contrast medium combined with rectal contents

Obturator internus muscle
Coccyx
Gluteus maximus muscle

FIGURE 363.2 CT of the Female Pelvis Taken from Below

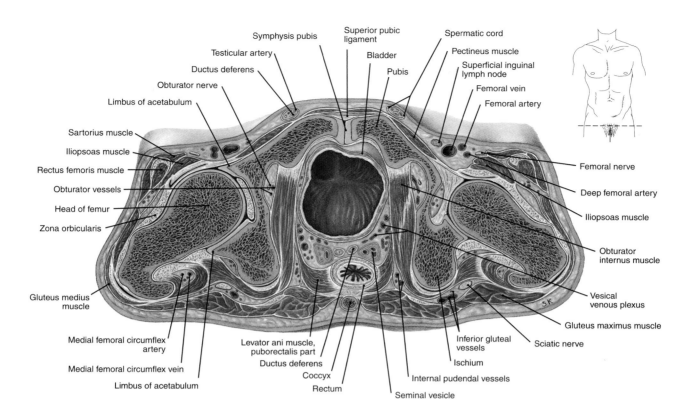

FIGURE 364.1 **Cross Section of the Male Pelvis at the Level of the Symphysis Pubis**

NOTE: (1) The **ductus deferens** and the **seminal vesicle** are located behind the **bladder** on both sides, and behind these, observe the position of the **rectum.**

(2) The **obturator internus muscle** forms the lateral wall of the true pelvis and the levator ani (in this figure, its puborectalis part) arises from the obturator fascia that covers its medial surface.

(3) The **vesical plexus of veins** surrounding the bladder. This plexus anastomoses with the prostatic plexus below, and both drain into the internal iliac vein. Thus, venous blood from the bladder and prostate usually enters the inferior vena cava and goes to the lungs, although anastomoses also exist with the rectal system of veins and with the vertebral system of veins.

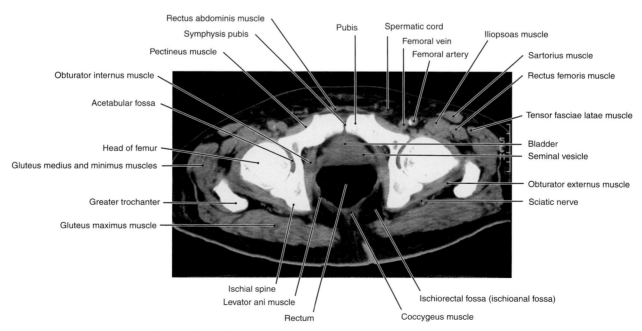

FIGURE 364.2 **CT of the Male Pelvis Taken from Below**

PLATE 365 Male Perineum: Surface Anatomy; Muscles

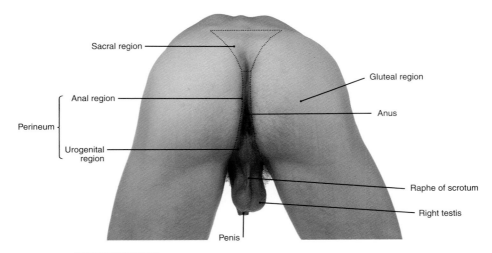

Sacral region

Gluteal region

Anal region

Anus

Perineum

Urogenital region

Raphe of scrotum

Right testis

Penis

FIGURE 365.1 Surface Anatomy of the Male Perineum

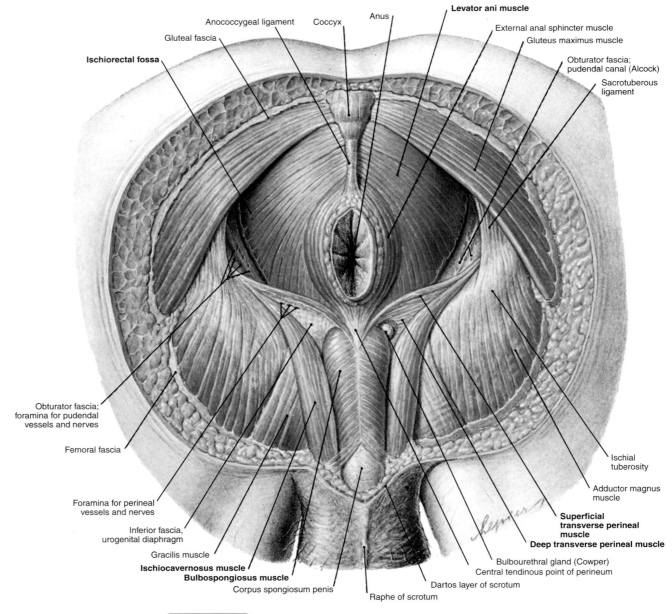

Anococcygeal ligament

Coccyx

Anus

Levator ani muscle

Gluteal fascia

External anal sphincter muscle

Gluteus maximus muscle

Ischiorectal fossa

Obturator fascia; pudendal canal (Alcock)

Sacrotuberous ligament

Obturator fascia; foramina for pudendal vessels and nerves

Femoral fascia

Ischial tuberosity

Adductor magnus muscle

Foramina for perineal vessels and nerves

Superficial transverse perineal muscle

Inferior fascia, urogenital diaphragm

Deep transverse perineal muscle

Gracilis muscle

Bulbourethral gland (Cowper)

Ischiocavernosus muscle

Central tendinous point of perineum

Bulbospongiosus muscle

Dartos layer of scrotum

Corpus spongiosum penis

Raphe of scrotum

FIGURE 365.2 Superficial Muscles of the Male Perineum

POSTERIOR

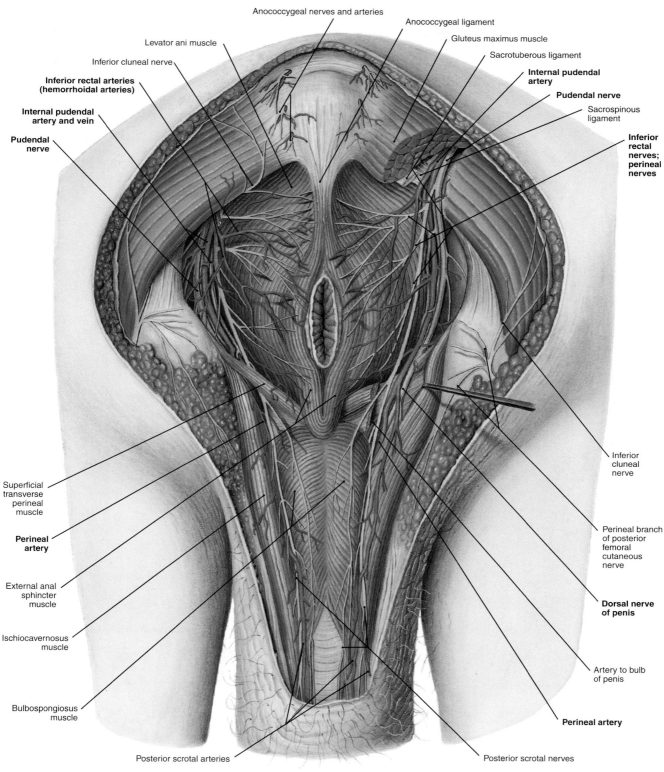

Anococcygeal nerves and arteries

Levator ani muscle

Inferior cluneal nerve

Inferior rectal arteries (hemorrhoidal arteries)

Internal pudendal artery and vein

Pudendal nerve

Anococcygeal ligament

Gluteus maximus muscle

Sacrotuberous ligament

Internal pudendal artery

Pudendal nerve

Sacrospinous ligament

Inferior rectal nerves; perineal nerves

Inferior cluneal nerve

Perineal branch of posterior femoral cutaneous nerve

Dorsal nerve of penis

Artery to bulb of penis

Perineal artery

Superficial transverse perineal muscle

Perineal artery

External anal sphincter muscle

Ischiocavernosus muscle

Bulbospongiosus muscle

Posterior scrotal arteries

Posterior scrotal nerves

ANTERIOR

FIGURE 366 **Nerves and Blood Vessels of the Male Perineum**

NOTE: (1) The skin of the perineum and the fat of the ischiorectal fossa have been removed to expose the muscles, vessels, and nerves of both the **anal** and **urogenital regions.**

(2) The **internal pudendal vessels** and **nerves** emerge from the pelvis to the gluteal region and vthen course to the perineum by way of the **pudendal canal** (of Alcock). At the lateral border of the **ischiorectal fossa** their branches, the **inferior rectal vessels** and **nerves,** cross the fossa transversely to supply the levator ani and external anal sphincter muscles.

(3) The main trunks of the vessels and nerve continue anteriorly, pierce the urogenital diaphragm, and become the **perineal vessels** and **nerve** and the **dorsal vessels** and **nerve of the penis.** The muscles of the urogenital triangle are innervated by the perineal nerve, while the dorsal nerve of the penis is the main sensory nerve of that organ.

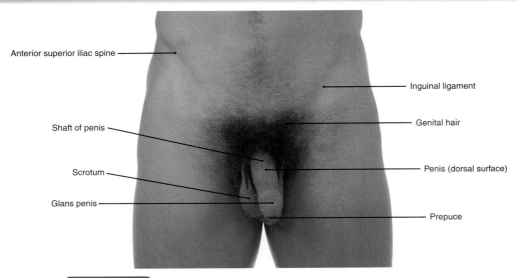

Anterior superior iliac spine

Shaft of penis

Scrotum

Glans penis

Inguinal ligament

Genital hair

Penis (dorsal surface)

Prepuce

FIGURE 367.1 Surface Anatomy of the Male External Genitalia

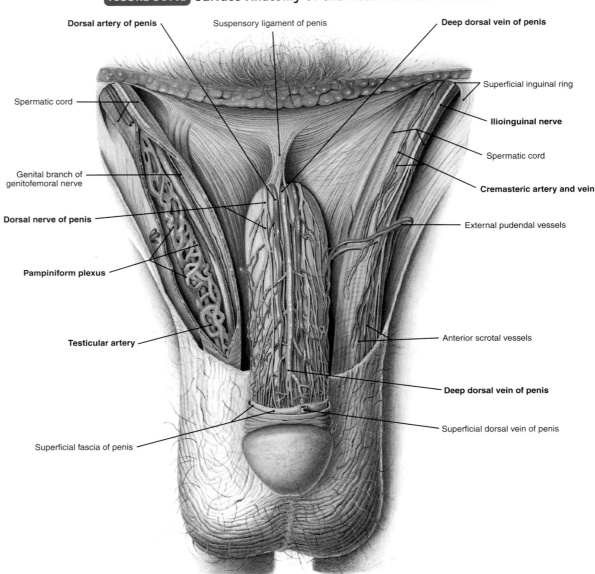

Dorsal artery of penis

Suspensory ligament of penis

Deep dorsal vein of penis

Spermatic cord

Superficial inguinal ring

Ilioinguinal nerve

Spermatic cord

Genital branch of genitofemoral nerve

Cremasteric artery and vein

Dorsal nerve of penis

External pudendal vessels

Pampiniform plexus

Testicular artery

Anterior scrotal vessels

Deep dorsal vein of penis

Superficial fascia of penis

Superficial dorsal vein of penis

FIGURE 367.2 Vessels and Nerves of the Penis and Spermatic Cord

NOTE: (1) The skin has been removed from the anterior pubic region and the penis, revealing the superficial vessels and nerves of the penis and left **spermatic cord.** The right spermatic cord has been slit open to show the deeper structures within (see Fig. 369.1).

(2) Along the surface of the spermatic cord course the **ilioinguinal nerve** and the **cremasteric artery** and **vein.** Within the cord are found the **ductus deferens** and **testicular artery** surrounded by the **pampiniform plexus of veins.**

(3) Beneath the fascia of the penis and in the midline, courses the unpaired **deep dorsal vein of the penis.** Along the sides of the vein, observe the paired **dorsal arteries** and **nerves of the penis.**

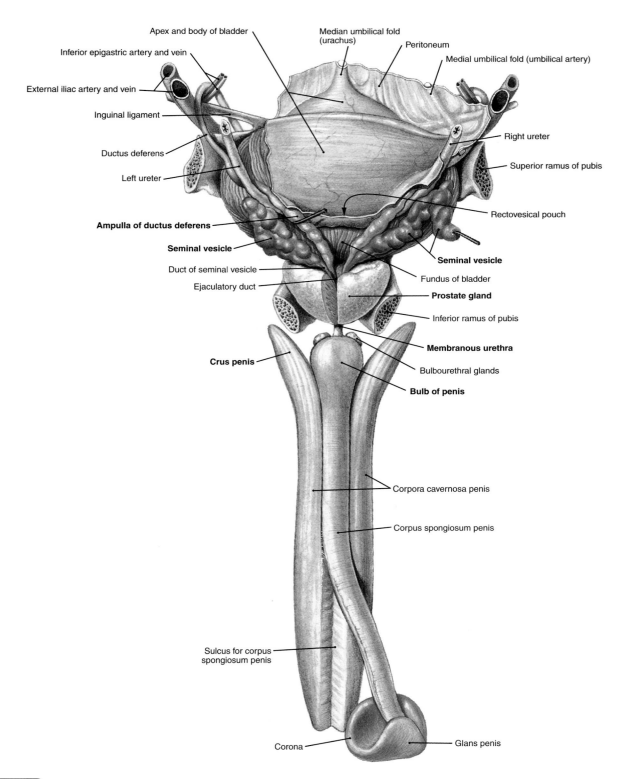

FIGURE 368 **Erectile Bodies of the Penis Attached to the Bladder and Other Organs by the Membranous Urethra**

NOTE: (1) The deep fascia, which closely invests the erectile bodies of the penis, has been removed, and the distal part of the **corpus spongiosum penis** (which contains the penile urethra) has been displaced from its position between the two **corpora cavernosa penis.**

(2) The posterior surface of the **bladder** and **prostate** and the associated **seminal vesicles, ductus deferens,** and **bulbourethral glands** are also demonstrated. These structures all communicate with the **urethra,** the membranous part of which is in continuity with the **penile urethra.**

(3) The tapered **crura** of the corpora cavernosa penis, which diverge laterally to become adherent to the ischial and pubic rami. They are surrounded by fibers of the ischiocavernosus muscles (see Fig. 366). The base of the corpus spongiosum penis is also expanded and is called the **bulb of the penis.** It is surrounded by the bulbocavernosus muscle (see Fig. 365.2).

PLATE 369 Spermatic Cord; Vascular Circulation of the Penis

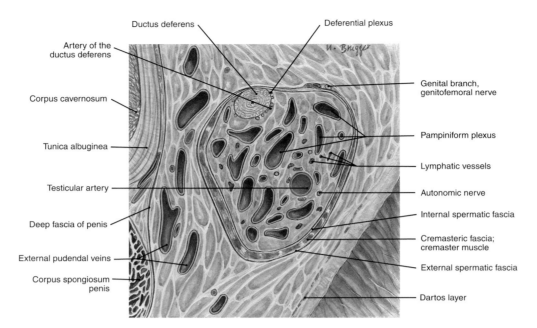

FIGURE 369.1 Transverse Section of the Spermatic Cord within the Scrotum

NOTE: (1) The spermatic cord contains the: (a) ductus deferens, (b) artery of the ductus deferens, (c) testicular artery, (d) cremasteric artery, (e) pampiniform plexus of veins, (f) lymphatic vessels, and (g) sympathetic and sensory nerve fibers and some fat. These are surrounded by the internal and external spermatic fascial layers and the cremaster muscle.
(2) The spermatic cord traverses the superficial inguinal ring, the inguinal canal, and the abdominal inguinal ring.
(3) The arteries and nerves descend to the testis from the abdomen, while the ductus deferens, the veins, and the lymphatics ascend to the abdomen from the scrotum.
(4) The spermatic cord is covered by the external spermatic fascia, the internal spermatic fascia, and the cremaster muscle.

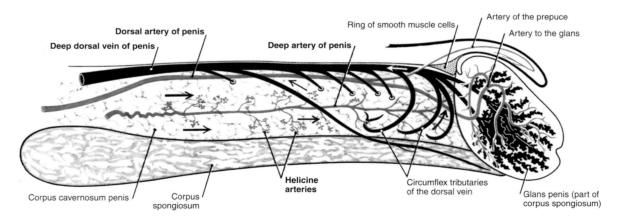

FIGURE 369.2 Longitudinal Section through the Penis, Showing Its Vascular Circulation

NOTE: (1) The dorsal and deep arteries of the penis supply blood principally to the corpora cavernosa but also to the glans penis of the corpus spongiosum.
(2) The **helicine branches** of the deep artery and the **circumflex tributaries** of the deep dorsal vein that return blood from the corpora and the glans.
(3) The venous drainage from the glans penis, the corpora cavernosa, and the corpus spongiosum is along the **deep dorsal vein of the penis,** while the superficial dorsal vein (not shown in this figure) drains the prepuce and skin of the penis.

FIGURE 370.1 Section through Middle of Penis ▶
(see Fig. 370.4)

NOTE: (1) The penis is composed of two corpora cavernosa penis containing erectile tissue and one corpus spongiosum penis seen ventrally and in the midline that contains the penile portion of the urethra.

(2) The three corpora are surrounded by a closely investing layer of deep fascia. In erection, blood fills the erectile tissue, causing the corpora to become rigid. The thin-walled veins are compressed between the corpora and the deep fascia. Erection is maintained by preventing venous blood from draining back into the general circulation.

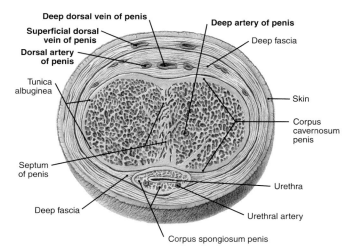

FIGURE 370.2 Section at Neck of the Glans Penis
(see Fig. 370.4)

NOTE: This section is taken from the proximal part of the glans penis. The corpora cavernosa penis become smaller distally, while the corona of the glans penis is formed by the spongy tissue of the corpus spongiosum penis.

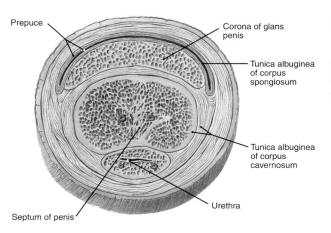

FIGURE 370.3 Section Midway along the Glans Penis ▶
(see Fig. 370.4)

NOTE: This cross section at the level of the middle of the glans penis shows that the corpora cavernosa penis are diminishing in size. At this site, the glans occupies a larger portion of the cross section.

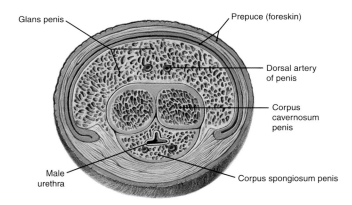

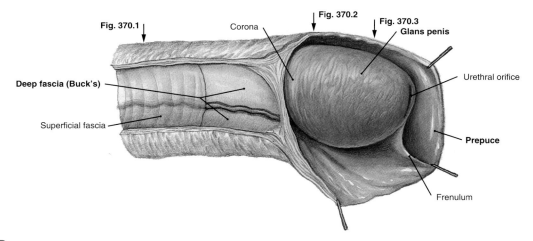

FIGURE 370.4 Distal End of Penis

NOTE: The distal end of the penis consists of the glans penis, which is attached by the frenulum to a duplicated fold of skin, the prepuce. Observe that the skin of the penis is thin and delicate and is loosely attached to the underlying deep fascia and corpora, accounting for its freely movable nature. (Arrows indicate cross sections seen above.)

CHAPTER 5 The Back, Vertebral Column, and Spinal Cord

Plates

371 Surface Anatomy and Skeletal Structures of the Back

372 The Back: Dermatomes and Cutaneous Nerves

373 Superficial Muscles of the Back; Muscle Chart

374 Intermediate Back Muscles and the Latissimus Dorsi

375 Erector Spinae and Semispinalis Muscles

376 The Back: Intermediate and Deep Back Muscles

377 The Back: Erector Spinae Muscle

378 The Back: Transversospinal Groups of Muscles

379 Chart of Intermediate and Deep Back Muscles

380 Semispinalis, Multifidus, and Rotator Deep Back Muscles: Chart; Figure

381 Posterior Neck Muscles; Suboccipital Triangle

382 The Back: Superficial Vessels and Nerves

383 The Back: Deep Vessels and Nerves; Suboccipital Region

384 Suboccipital Region: Muscles, Vessels, and Nerves

385 Suboccipital Region: Nerves and Muscle Chart

386 The Back: Primary Rami of Spinal Nerves; Cross Section of Back

387 Vertebral Column and the Pectoral and Pelvic Girdles

388 Cervical Vertebrae

389 Cervical Vertebrae and the Atlantooccipital Membranes

390 Craniovertebral Joints and Ligaments

391 Craniovertebral Joints and Ligaments; X-Ray of Atlas and Axis

392 Vertebral Column

393 Thoracic Vertebrae; Costovertebral Joints

394 Costovertebral Joints and Ligaments 1

395 Costovertebral Joints and Ligaments 2

396 Lumbar Vertebrae

397 Cervical and Lumbar Vertebrae: Intervertebral Disks and Ligaments

398 Intervertebral Disks

399 Sacrum and Coccyx

400 Radiographs: Cervical Spine (Lateral View); Thoracic Spine (Anteroposterior View)

401 Radiographs: Lumbar Spine (Anterior and Lateral Views)

402 Spinal Cord (Infant); Spinal Nerves (Adult, Diagram)

403 Spinal Cord (Dorsal and Ventral Views)

404 Spinal Cord: Arterial Supply and Spinal Roots

405 Spinal Cord: Cauda Equina

406 Spinal Cord: Cross Section; Spinal Arteries

407 Vertebral Veins; Cross Section, Third Lumbar Level

408 Lumbar and Sacral Puncture into the Spinal Cord

FIGURE 371.1 Surface Anatomy of the Back

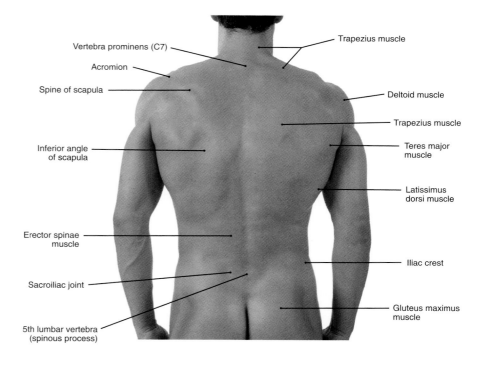

Vertebra prominens (C7)

Acromion

Spine of scapula

Inferior angle of scapula

Erector spinae muscle

Sacroiliac joint

5th lumbar vertebra (spinous process)

Trapezius muscle

Deltoid muscle

Trapezius muscle

Teres major muscle

Latissimus dorsi muscle

Iliac crest

Gluteus maximus muscle

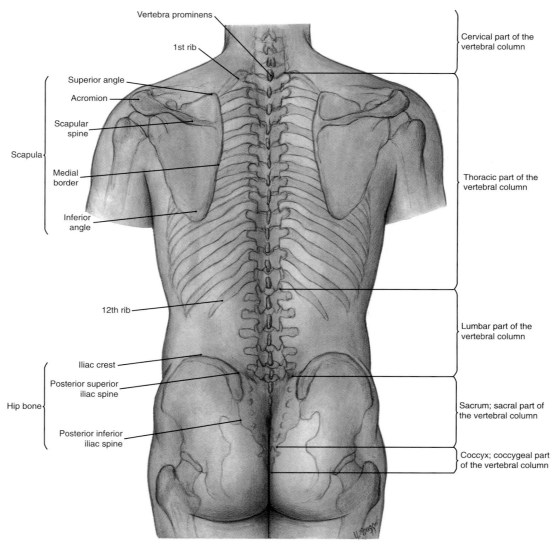

Vertebra prominens

1st rib

Superior angle

Acromion

Scapular spine

Scapula

Medial border

Inferior angle

12th rib

Iliac crest

Posterior superior iliac spine

Hip bone

Posterior inferior iliac spine

Cervical part of the vertebral column

Thoracic part of the vertebral column

Lumbar part of the vertebral column

Sacrum; sacral part of the vertebral column

Coccyx; coccygeal part of the vertebral column

FIGURE 371.2 Skeletal Structures in the Back of the Trunk

PLATE 372 **The Back: Dermatomes and Cutaneous Nerves**

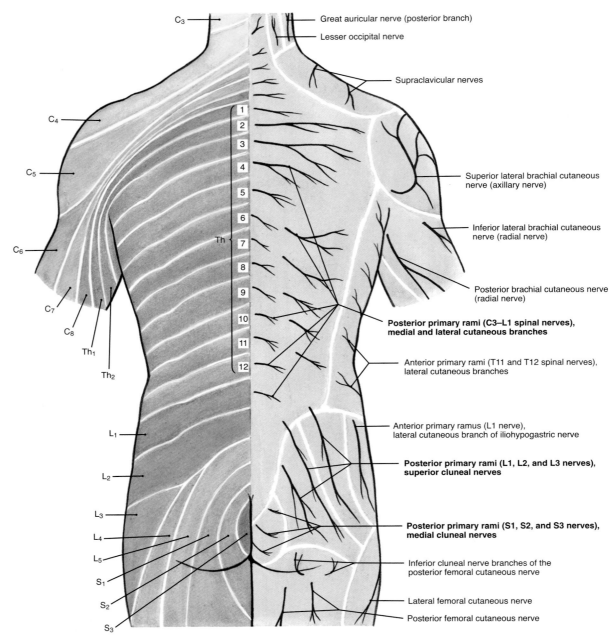

FIGURE 372 **Dermatomes and Cutaneous Nerve Distribution (Posterior Aspect of the Body)**

NOTE: (1) **Dermatomes** are shown on the left and the **cutaneous nerve** distribution and surface areas for the dorsum of the trunk are shown on the right.

(2) An area of skin supplied by the cutaneous branches of a single nerve is called a dermatome. There is considerable overlap between adjacent segmental nerves and, although the loss of a single spinal nerve produces an area of altered sensation, it does not result in total sensory loss.

(3) Destruction of at least three consecutive spinal nerves is required to produce a total sensory loss of the dermatome supplied by the middle nerve of the three.

(4) Mapping of skin areas affected by herpes zoster (shingles) has added to our knowledge of dermatome distribution. Another experimental procedure is that of "remaining sensibility." In the latter, dermatome areas are established in animals after severance of several roots above and below the intact root whose dermatome is being studied.

(5) The posterior primary rami of spinal nerves C3 through L1 (boldface) supply the posterior skin of the trunk, while the lateral neck, upper limb, and lateral trunk are supplied by anterior primary rami.

(6) The posterior primary rami (boldface) of L1, L2, and L3 (superior cluneal nerves) as well as the posterior primary rami (boldface) of S1, S2, and S3 (medial cluneal nerves) supply the gluteal and sacral regions. The remaining nerves of the posterior lower trunk and limbs are from anterior primary rami.

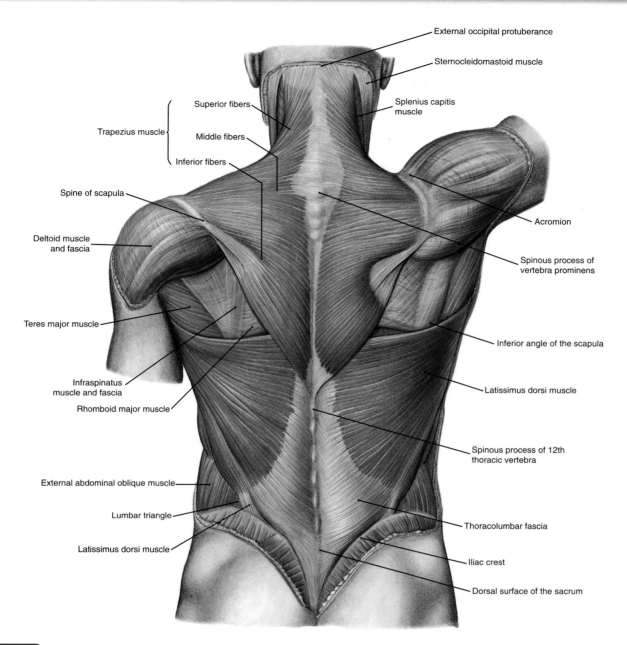

External occipital protuberance

Sternocleidomastoid muscle

Superior fibers

Splenius capitis muscle

Trapezius muscle — Middle fibers

Inferior fibers

Spine of scapula

Acromion

Deltoid muscle and fascia

Spinous process of vertebra prominens

Teres major muscle

Inferior angle of the scapula

Infraspinatus muscle and fascia

Latissimus dorsi muscle

Rhomboid major muscle

Spinous process of 12th thoracic vertebra

External abdominal oblique muscle

Lumbar triangle

Thoracolumbar fascia

Latissimus dorsi muscle

Iliac crest

Dorsal surface of the sacrum

FIGURE 373 **The Superficial Muscles of the Back: Trapezius and Latissimus Dorsi**

NOTE that although the trapezius and latissimus dorsi are superficial muscles of the back, they both insert onto pectoral girdle bones—that is, the scapula and the humerus.

SUPERFICIAL MUSCLES OF THE BACK				
Muscle	**Origin**	**Insertion**	**Innervation**	**Action**
Trapezius	Middle third of the superior nuchal line; external occipital protuberance; ligamentum nuchae; spinous processes of C7 and T1 to T12 vertebrae	Lateral third of the clavicle; medial margin of acromion; spine of the scapula	Motor fibers from spinal part of the accessory nerve (XI); sensory fibers from C3, C4	Assists serratus anterior in rotating the scapula during abduction of the humerus between 90 and 180 degrees; upper fibers elevate the scapula; lower fibers depress the scapula; middle fibers adduct the scapula; occipital fibers draw the head laterally
Latissimus dorsi	Thoracolumbar fascia; spinous processes of lower six thoracic vertebrae and five lumbar vertebrae and the sacrum; iliac crest; lower three or four ribs	Floor of the intertubercular sulcus of the humerus	Thoracodorsal nerve from the posterior cord of the brachial plexus (C6, C7, C8)	Extends, adducts, and medially rotates humerus; with insertion fixed, it elevates the trunk to the arms, as in climbing

PLATE 374 Intermediate Back Muscles and the Latissimus Dorsi

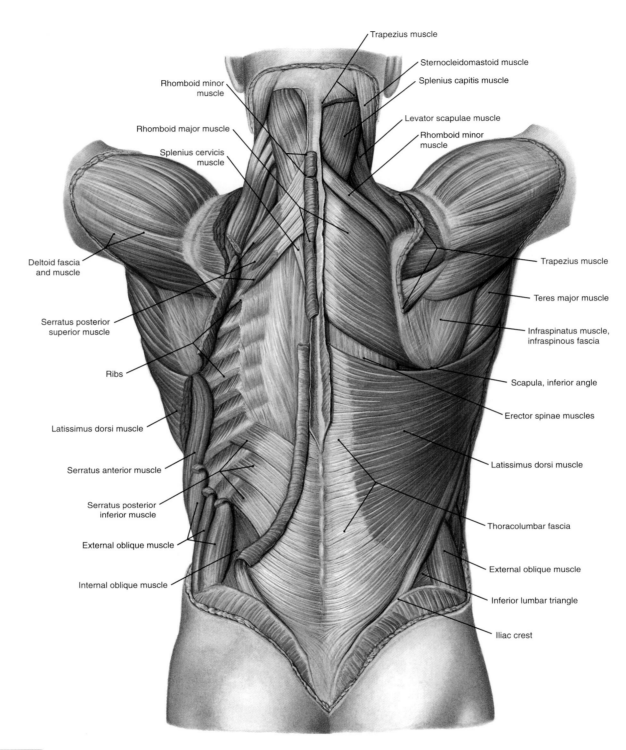

FIGURE 374 **Superficial and Intermediate Back Muscles (Posterior View)**

NOTE: (1) On the right side, the trapezius has been removed to reveal the rhomboid muscles, the levator scapulae, and the splenius capitis. The latissimus dorsi and the thoracolumbar fascia are still intact.

(2) On the left side, the trapezius, the latissimus dorsi, and the rhomboid muscles have been removed to expose the serratus posterior superior, the serratus posterior inferior, and several ribs.

(3) The erector spinae muscle and its overlying fascia (labeled on the right and shown extensively on the left but not labeled) extends longitudinally and considered the strongest and most important deep back muscle (see Fig. 375).

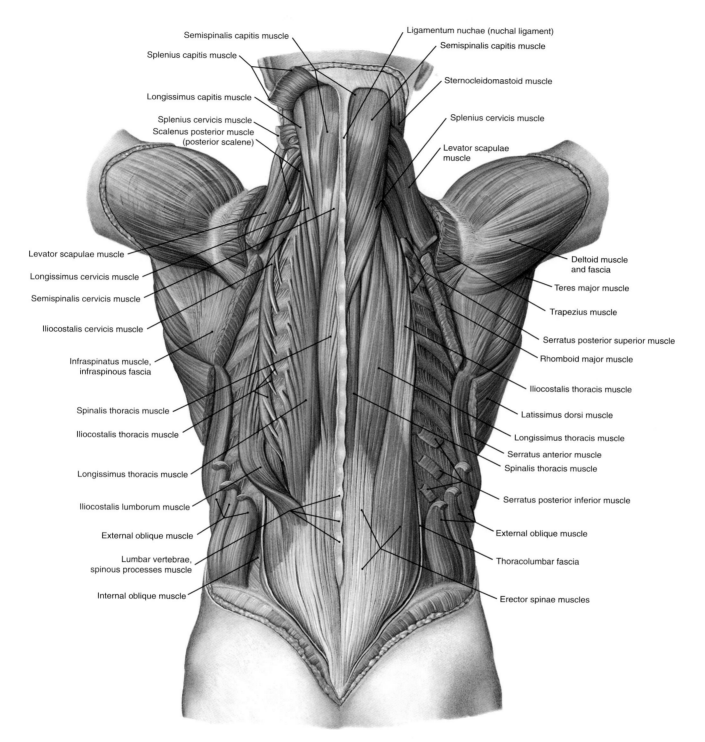

Semispinalis capitis muscle

Splenius capitis muscle

Longissimus capitis muscle

Splenius cervicis muscle
Scalenus posterior muscle
(posterior scalene)

Levator scapulae muscle

Longissimus cervicis muscle

Semispinalis cervicis muscle

Iliocostalis cervicis muscle

Infraspinatus muscle,
infraspinous fascia

Spinalis thoracis muscle

Iliocostalis thoracis muscle

Longissimus thoracis muscle

Iliocostalis lumborum muscle

External oblique muscle

Lumbar vertebrae,
spinous processes muscle

Internal oblique muscle

Ligamentum nuchae (nuchal ligament)
Semispinalis capitis muscle

Sternocleidomastoid muscle

Splenius cervicis muscle

Levator scapulae
muscle

Deltoid muscle
and fascia

Teres major muscle

Trapezius muscle

Serratus posterior superior muscle

Rhomboid major muscle

Iliocostalis thoracis muscle

Latissimus dorsi muscle

Longissimus thoracis muscle

Serratus anterior muscle

Spinalis thoracis muscle

Serratus posterior inferior muscle

External oblique muscle

Thoracolumbar fascia

Erector spinae muscles

FIGURE 375 **Erector Spinae Muscles and Semispinalis Capitis Muscles**

NOTE: (1) The trapezius and latissimus dorsi muscles have been removed, as have the rhomboid muscles and the serratus posterior (superior and inferior) muscles.

(2) The erector spinae muscle is seen intact on the right side, while its iliocostalis, longissimus, and spinalis columns have been separated on the left side. This muscle is a strong extensor and lateral flexor of the vertebral column (and head).

(3) The two semispinalis capitis muscles superiorly following the removal of the splenius capitis muscles. Observe the tendinous intersections that are characteristic of this muscle.

PLATE 376 **The Back: Intermediate and Deep Back Muscles**

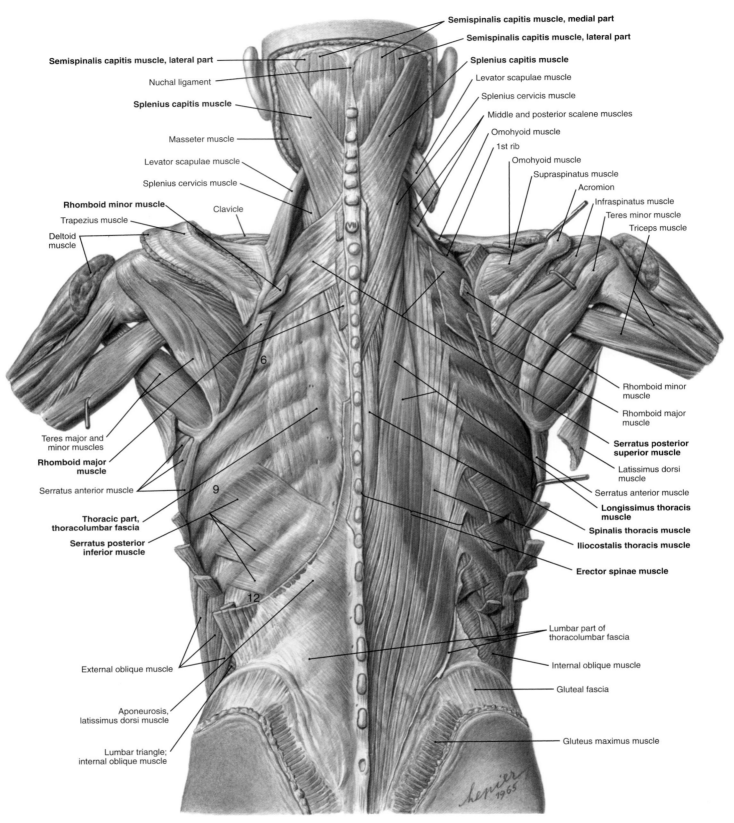

Semispinalis capitis muscle, medial part

Semispinalis capitis muscle, lateral part

Splenius capitis muscle

Levator scapulae muscle

Splenius cervicis muscle

Middle and posterior scalene muscles

Omohyoid muscle

1st rib

Omohyoid muscle

Supraspinatus muscle

Acromion

Infraspinatus muscle

Teres minor muscle

Triceps muscle

Semispinalis capitis muscle, lateral part

Nuchal ligament

Splenius capitis muscle

Masseter muscle

Levator scapulae muscle

Splenius cervicis muscle

Rhomboid minor muscle

Trapezius muscle

Clavicle

Deltoid muscle

Teres major and minor muscles

Rhomboid major muscle

Serratus anterior muscle

Thoracic part, thoracolumbar fascia

Serratus posterior inferior muscle

External oblique muscle

Aponeurosis, latissimus dorsi muscle

Lumbar triangle; internal oblique muscle

6

9

12

Rhomboid minor muscle

Rhomboid major muscle

Serratus posterior superior muscle

Latissimus dorsi muscle

Serratus anterior muscle

Longissimus thoracis muscle

Spinalis thoracis muscle

Iliocostalis thoracis muscle

Erector spinae muscle

Lumbar part of thoracolumbar fascia

Internal oblique muscle

Gluteal fascia

Gluteus maximus muscle

FIGURE 376 **Muscles of the Back: Intermediate Layer (Left), Deep Layer (Right)**

NOTE: (1) On the left side, the superficial back muscles (trapezius and latissimus dorsi) have been cut, as have the rhomboids, which attach the vertebral border of the scapula to the vertebral column. Observe the underlying serratus posterior superior and inferior muscles.

(2) On the right side, the serratus posterior muscles and the thoracolumbar fascia have been removed, exposing the erector spinae muscle (formerly called sacrospinalis muscle).

(3) In the neck, the splenius cervicis, splenius capitis, and semispinalis capitis underlie the trapezius.

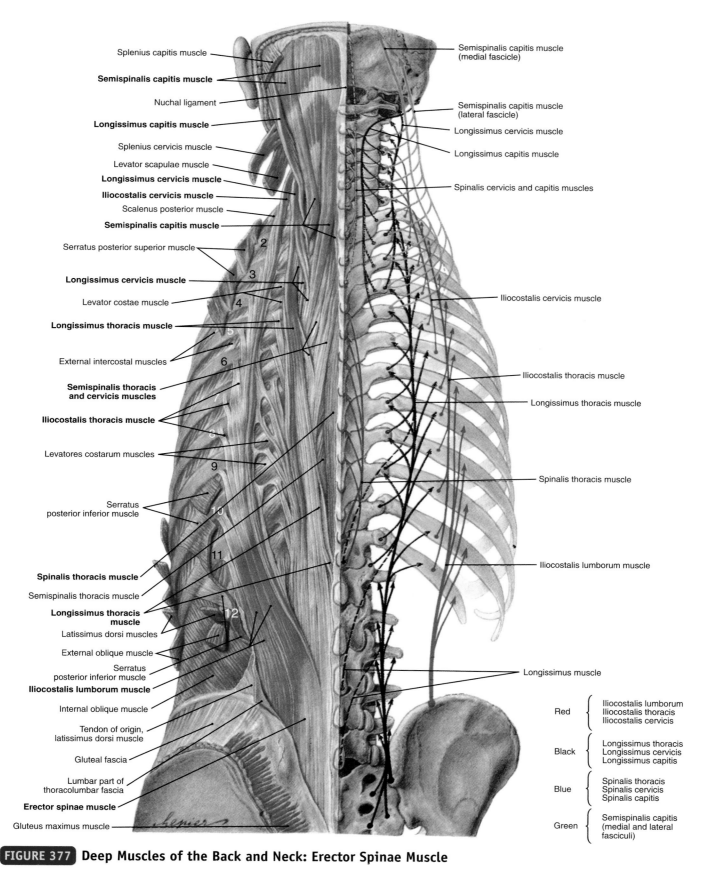

Splenius capitis muscle

Semispinalis capitis muscle

Nuchal ligament

Longissimus capitis muscle

Splenius cervicis muscle

Levator scapulae muscle

Longissimus cervicis muscle

Iliocostalis cervicis muscle

Scalenus posterior muscle

Semispinalis capitis muscle

Serratus posterior superior muscle

Longissimus cervicis muscle

Levator costae muscle

Longissimus thoracis muscle

External intercostal muscles

Semispinalis thoracis and cervicis muscles

Iliocostalis thoracis muscle

Levatores costarum muscles

Serratus posterior inferior muscle

Spinalis thoracis muscle

Semispinalis thoracis muscle

Longissimus thoracis muscle

Latissimus dorsi muscles

External oblique muscle

Serratus posterior inferior muscle

Iliocostalis lumborum muscle

Internal oblique muscle

Tendon of origin, latissimus dorsi muscle

Gluteal fascia

Lumbar part of thoracolumbar fascia

Erector spinae muscle

Gluteus maximus muscle

Semispinalis capitis muscle (medial fascicle)

Semispinalis capitis muscle (lateral fascicle)

Longissimus cervicis muscle

Longissimus capitis muscle

Spinalis cervicis and capitis muscles

Iliocostalis cervicis muscle

Iliocostalis thoracis muscle

Longissimus thoracis muscle

Spinalis thoracis muscle

Iliocostalis lumborum muscle

Longissimus muscle

Red	Iliocostalis lumborum Iliocostalis thoracis Iliocostalis cervicis
Black	Longissimus thoracis Longissimus cervicis Longissimus capitis
Blue	Spinalis thoracis Spinalis cervicis Spinalis capitis
Green	Semispinalis capitis (medial and lateral fasciculi)

FIGURE 377 **Deep Muscles of the Back and Neck: Erector Spinae Muscle**

NOTE: (1) **On the left,** the erector spinae (sacrospinalis) muscle is separated into iliocostalis, longissimus, and spinalis parts. In the neck, observe the semispinalis capitis, which has both medial and lateral fascicles. The semispinalis cervicis and thoracis extend inferiorly from above and lie deep to the sacrospinalis layer of musculature.

(2) **On the right,** all of the muscles have been removed and their attachments have been diagrammed by means of colored lines and arrows.

PLATE 378 The Back: Transversospinal Groups of Muscles

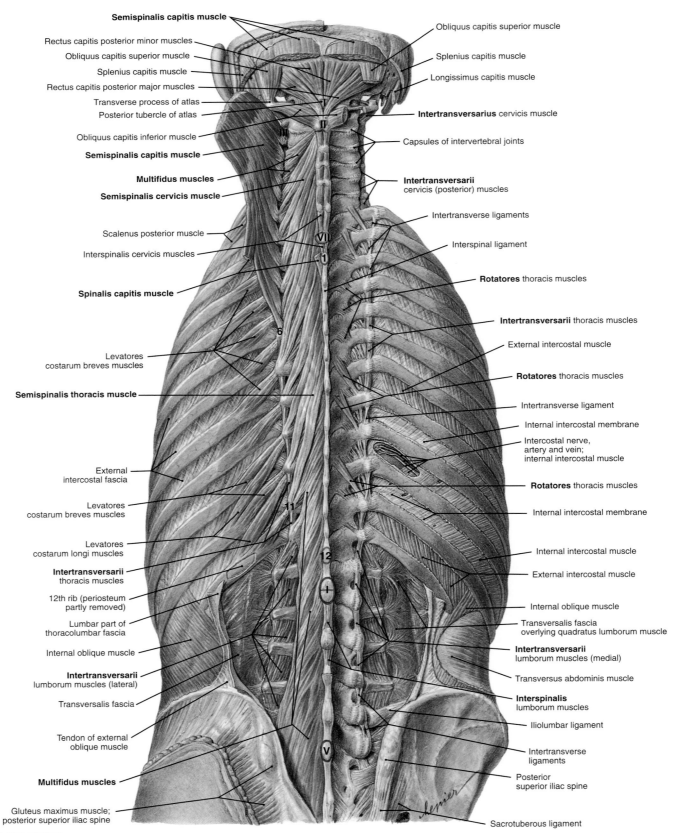

Semispinalis capitis muscle

Rectus capitis posterior minor muscles

Obliquus capitis superior muscle

Splenius capitis muscle

Rectus capitis posterior major muscles

Transverse process of atlas

Posterior tubercle of atlas

Obliquus capitis inferior muscle

Semispinalis capitis muscle

Multifidus muscles

Semispinalis cervicis muscle

Scalenus posterior muscle

Interspinalis cervicis muscles

Spinalis capitis muscle

Levatores costarum breves muscles

Semispinalis thoracis muscle

External intercostal fascia

Levatores costarum breves muscles

Levatores costarum longi muscles

Intertransversarii thoracis muscles

12th rib (periosteum partly removed)

Lumbar part of thoracolumbar fascia

Internal oblique muscle

Intertransversarii lumborum muscles (lateral)

Transversalis fascia

Tendon of external oblique muscle

Multifidus muscles

Gluteus maximus muscle; posterior superior iliac spine

Obliquus capitis superior muscle

Splenius capitis muscle

Longissimus capitis muscle

Intertransversarius cervicis muscle

Capsules of intervertebral joints

Intertransversarii cervicis (posterior) muscles

Intertransverse ligaments

Interspinal ligament

Rotatores thoracis muscles

Intertransversarii thoracis muscles

External intercostal muscle

Rotatores thoracis muscles

Intertransverse ligament

Internal intercostal membrane

Intercostal nerve, artery and vein; internal intercostal muscle

Rotatores thoracis muscles

Internal intercostal membrane

Internal intercostal muscle

External intercostal muscle

Internal oblique muscle

Transversalis fascia overlying quadratus lumborum muscle

Intertransversarii lumborum muscles (medial)

Transversus abdominis muscle

Interspinalis lumborum muscles

Iliolumbar ligament

Intertransverse ligaments

Posterior superior iliac spine

Sacrotuberous ligament

FIGURE 378 Deep Muscles of the Back and Neck: Transversospinal Group

NOTE: (1) **The transversospinal** groups of muscles lie deep to the **erector spinae,** and they extend between the transverse processes of the vertebrae and the spinous processes of higher vertebrae. These muscles are extensors of the vertebral column or acting individually and on one side, they bend and rotate the vertebrae of that side.

(2) Within this group of muscles are the **semispinalis** (thoracis, cervicis, and capitis), the **multifidus,** the **rotatores** (lumborum, thoracis, cervicis), the **interspinales** (lumborum, thoracis, cervicis), and the **intertransversarii.**

INTERMEDIATE MUSCLES OF THE BACK

Muscle	Origin	Insertion	Innervation	Action
Rhomboid major	Spinous processes of T2 to T5 thoracic vertebrae	Medial border of scapula between the scapular spine and inferior angle	Dorsal scapular nerve (C5)	Adducts the scapula by pulling it medially toward the vertebral column; rotates the scapula by depressing the lateral angle; helps fix scapula to thoracic wall
Rhomboid minor	Spinous process of C7 and T1 vertebrae	Medial border of scapula at the level of the spine of the scapula	Dorsal scapular nerve (C5)	Assists the rhomboid major muscle
Levator scapulae	Transverse processes of atlas and axis and the posterior tubercles of the transverse processes of C3 and C4 vertebrae	Superior angle and upper medial border of scapula	C3 and C4 nerves and the dorsal scapular nerve (C5)	Elevates superior border of scapula; rotates scapula laterally thereby tilting the glenoid cavity downward
Serratus posterior superior	Spinous processes of C7 and T1 to T3 thoracic vertebrae	Onto the upper borders of the second, third, fourth, and fifth ribs	Ventral primary rami of T1 to T4 spinal nerves	Elevates the second to fifth ribs
Serratus posterior inferior	Spinous processes of T11, T12, and upper three lumbar vertebrae	Onto the inferior border of the lower four ribs	Ventral primary rami of T9, T10, T11, and T12 spinal nerves	Draws the lower four ribs downward and backward

DEEP MUSCLES OF THE BACK

Muscle	Origin	Insertion	Innervation	Action
ERECTOR SPINAE MUSCLES				
ILIOCOSTALIS MUSCLE (Lateral Column)				
Iliocostalis lumborum	Posteromedial part of the iliac crest and from the most lateral part of the common tendon of the erector spinae muscle	By six or seven muscle fascicles onto the inferior borders of the lower six or seven ribs at their angles	Dorsal primary rami of lower thoracic and upper lumbar nerves	Extends, laterally flexes, and assists in rotation of the vertebral column; can depress the ribs
Iliocostalis thoracis	Upper borders of the lower six ribs at their angles	Upper borders of the first six ribs at their angles and on the transverse process of the seventh cervical vertebra	Dorsal primary rami of the C8 and upper six thoracic spinal nerves	Extends, laterally flexes, and assists in rotation of the thoracic vertebrae
Iliocostalis cervicis	Angles of the third, fourth, fifth, and sixth ribs	Posterior tubercles of transverse processes of fourth, fifth, and sixth cervical vertebrae	Dorsal primary rami of the lower cervical and upper thoracic spinal nerves	Extends, laterally flexes, and assists in rotation of lower cervical and upper thoracic vertebrae
LONGISSIMUS MUSCLE (Intermediate Column)				
Longissimus thoracis	Intermediate continuation of the erector spinae muscle; transverse processes of the lumbar vertebrae	Onto the tips of transverse processes of all thoracic vertebrae; onto the lower 9 or 10 ribs between their tubercles and angles	Dorsal primary rami of the thoracic and lumbar spinal nerves	Extends and laterally flexes the vertebral column; also able to depress the ribs
Longissimus cervicis muscle	Tips of transverse processes of upper four or five thoracic vertebrae	Posterior tubercles of transverse processes of C2 to C6 cervical vertebrae	Dorsal primary rami of upper thoracic and lower cervical spinal nerves	Extends vertebral column and bends it to one side
Longissimus capitis	From transverse processes of upper four or five thoracic vertebrae; articular processes of lower three or four cervical vertebrae	Posterior margin of the mastoid process of the temporal bone	Dorsal primary rami of middle and lower cervical spinal nerves	Extends the head; muscle of one side bends head to the same side and turns face to that side
SPINALIS MUSCLE (Medial Column)				
Spinalis thoracis	From spinous processes of T11, T12, L1, and L2 vertebrae	Spinous processes of upper four to eight thoracic vertebrae	Dorsal primary rami of thoracic spinal nerves	Extends vertebral column
Spinalis cervicis	Spinous processes of C7, T1, and T2 vertebrae and ligamentum nuchae	Spinous process of the axis and those of the C3 and C4	Dorsal primary rami of lower cervical spinal nerves	Extends the cervical vertebrae
Spinalis capitis	Spinous processes of lower cervical and upper thoracic vertebrae	Inserts with the semispinalis capitis muscle between the superior and inferior nuchal lines of the occipital bone	Dorsal primary rami of upper cervical spinal nerves	Extends the head

DEEP MUSCLES OF THE BACK (Continued) Muscle	Origin	Insertion	Innervation	Action
TRANSVERSOSPINALIS GROUP OF MUSCLES				
SEMISPINALIS MUSCLES				
Semispinalis thoracis	Transverse processes of the 6th to 10th thoracic vertebrae	Spinous processes of C7, C8, and upper four thoracic vertebrae	Dorsal primary rami of lower cervical and upper thoracic spinal nerves	Extends vertebral column and rotates it to the opposite side
Semispinalis cervicis	Transverse processes of upper five or six thoracic vertebrae	Spinous processes of the axis and third, fourth, and fifth cervical vertebrae	Dorsal primary rami of the middle cervical spinal nerves	Extends cervical spinal column; rotates vertebrae to opposite side
Semispinalis capitis	Tips of transverse processes of the C7 and upper six or seven thoracic vertebrae	Between the superior and inferior nuchal lines on the occipital bone	Dorsal primary rami of the cervical spinal nerves	Extends the head and rotates it such that the face is turned to the opposite side
MULTIFIDUS MUSCLES				
Lumborum thoracis cervicis	From the back of the sacrum; mamillary processes of lumbar vertebrae; transverse processes of all thoracic vertebrae; articular processes of lower four cervical vertebrae	Onto the spinous processes of higher vertebrae; each multifidus muscle spans two to four vertebrae	Supplied segmentally by dorsal primary rami of the lumbar, thoracic spinal nerves	Bends or laterally flexes the vertebral column and rotates it to the opposite side; both multifidi columns acting together extend the vertebral column
ROTATORES MUSCLES				
Rotatores thoracis	From transverse processes of thoracic vertebrae deep to the multifidus muscles	On the base of the spine of thoracic vertebra above the origin or the one above that	Dorsal primary rami of the thoracic spinal nerves	Extend the vertebral column and bend it toward the opposite side
Rotatores cervicis (These are less well defined.)	From the articular processes of the cervical vertebrae	To the base of the spines of the cervical vertebra immediately above	Dorsal primary rami of cervical spinal nerves	Extend cervical vertebrae and bend them to the opposite side
Rotatores lumborum (These are less well defined.)	From the mamillary processes of the lumbar vertebrae	To the base of the spines of the lumbar vertebra immediately above	Dorsal primary rami of lumbar spinal nerves	Extend lumbar vertebrae and bend them to the opposite side

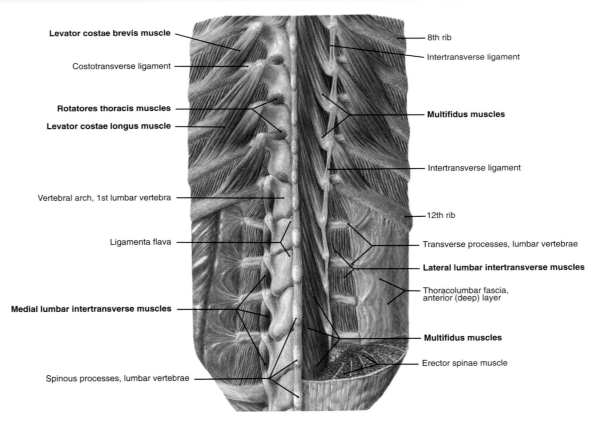

Levator costae brevis muscle
Costotransverse ligament
Rotatores thoracis muscles
Levator costae longus muscle
Vertebral arch, 1st lumbar vertebra
Ligamenta flava
Medial lumbar intertransverse muscles
Spinous processes, lumbar vertebrae

8th rib
Intertransverse ligament
Multifidus muscles
Intertransverse ligament
12th rib
Transverse processes, lumbar vertebrae
Lateral lumbar intertransverse muscles
Thoracolumbar fascia, anterior (deep) layer
Multifidus muscles
Erector spinae muscle

FIGURE 380 Multifidus, Rotator, Levator Costae, and Intertransverse Muscles of the Deep Back

NOTE: The erector spinae and semispinalis muscles have been removed.

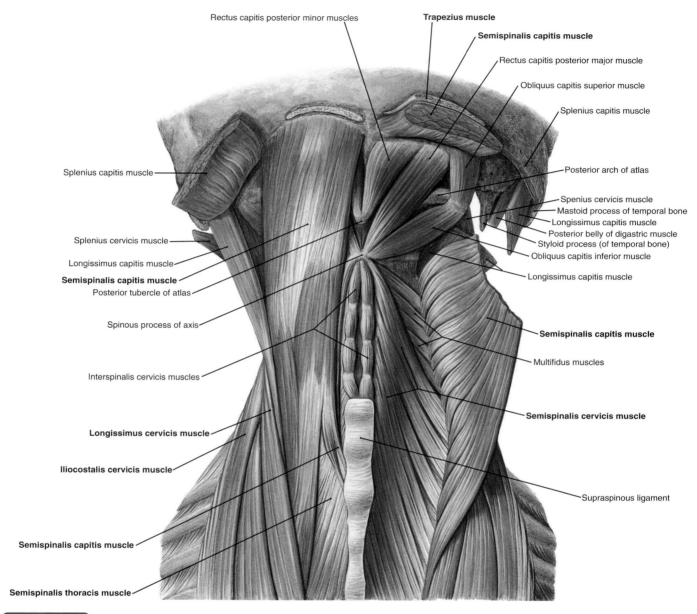

Rectus capitis posterior minor muscles

Trapezius muscle

Semispinalis capitis muscle

Rectus capitis posterior major muscle

Obliquus capitis superior muscle

Splenius capitis muscle

Splenius capitis muscle

Posterior arch of atlas

Spenius cervicis muscle

Mastoid process of temporal bone

Longissimus capitis muscle

Posterior belly of digastric muscle

Styloid process (of temporal bone)

Obliquus capitis inferior muscle

Splenius cervicis muscle

Longissimus capitis muscle

Semispinalis capitis muscle

Posterior tubercle of atlas

Longissimus capitis muscle

Spinous process of axis

Semispinalis capitis muscle

Multifidus muscles

Interspinalis cervicis muscles

Semispinalis cervicis muscle

Longissimus cervicis muscle

Iliocostalis cervicis muscle

Supraspinous ligament

Semispinalis capitis muscle

Semispinalis thoracis muscle

FIGURE 381.1 **The Semispinalis Capitis Muscle (Left) and Suboccipital Triangle (Right)**

NOTE that the semispinalis capitis is a strong extensor of the head, and at the same time, it rotates the head so that the face turns to the opposite side.

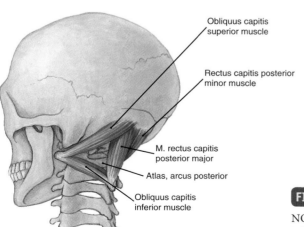

Obliquus capitis superior muscle

Rectus capitis posterior minor muscle

M. rectus capitis posterior major

Atlas, arcus posterior

Obliquus capitis inferior muscle

FIGURE 381.2 **Left Suboccipital Triangle**

NOTE that the suboccipital triangle is bounded by the obliquus capitis superior and inferior and the rectus capitis posterior major muscles.

PLATE 382 **The Back: Superficial Vessels and Nerves**

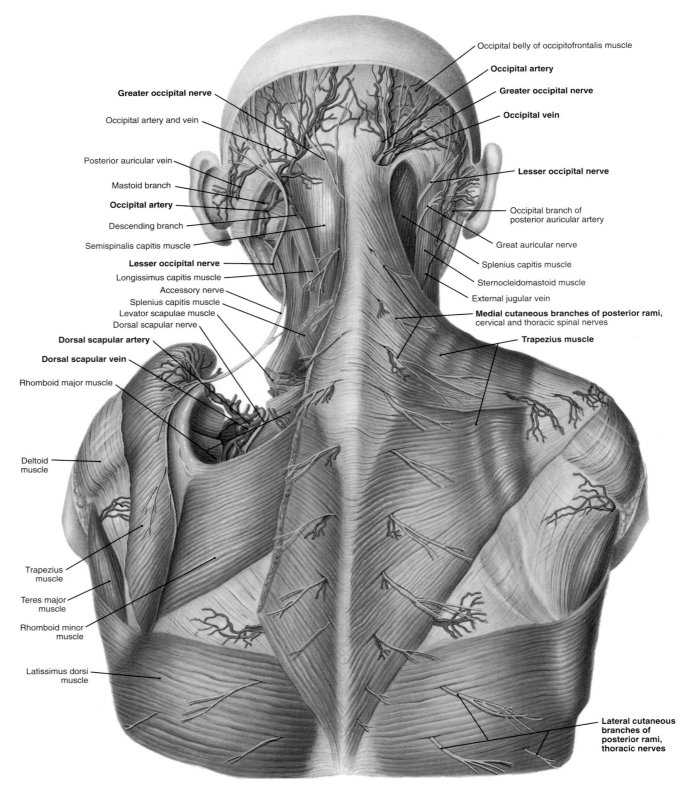

Occipital belly of occipitofrontalis muscle

Occipital artery

Greater occipital nerve

Occipital vein

Greater occipital nerve

Occipital artery and vein

Posterior auricular vein

Mastoid branch

Lesser occipital nerve

Occipital artery

Descending branch

Occipital branch of
posterior auricular artery

Semispinalis capitis muscle

Great auricular nerve

Lesser occipital nerve

Splenius capitis muscle

Longissimus capitis muscle

Sternocleidomastoid muscle

Accessory nerve

Splenius capitis muscle

External jugular vein

Levator scapulae muscle

Medial cutaneous branches of posterior rami,
cervical and thoracic spinal nerves

Dorsal scapular nerve

Dorsal scapular artery

Trapezius muscle

Dorsal scapular vein

Rhomboid major muscle

Deltoid
muscle

Trapezius
muscle

Teres major
muscle

Rhomboid minor
muscle

Latissimus dorsi
muscle

**Lateral cutaneous
branches of
posterior rami,
thoracic nerves**

FIGURE 382 **Nerves and Vessels of the Superficial and Intermediate Muscle Layers of the Upper Back and Posterior Neck**

NOTE: (1) The cutaneous branches of the **posterior primary rami** of the cervical and thoracic spinal nerves supplying the posterior neck and back segmentally. Observe the **accessory nerve (XI)** as it descends to supply the trapezius and sternocleidomastoid muscles.

(2) The **greater occipital nerve,** a sensory nerve from the posterior primary ramus of the C2 spinal nerve. It is accompanied by the occipital vessels. Also observe the **lesser occipital nerve,** which courses to the skin of the lateral posterior scalp and arises from the **anterior primary ramus** of C2.

(3) The **dorsal scapular nerve** and **vessels** that course beneath the **levator scapulae** and **rhomboid muscles.**

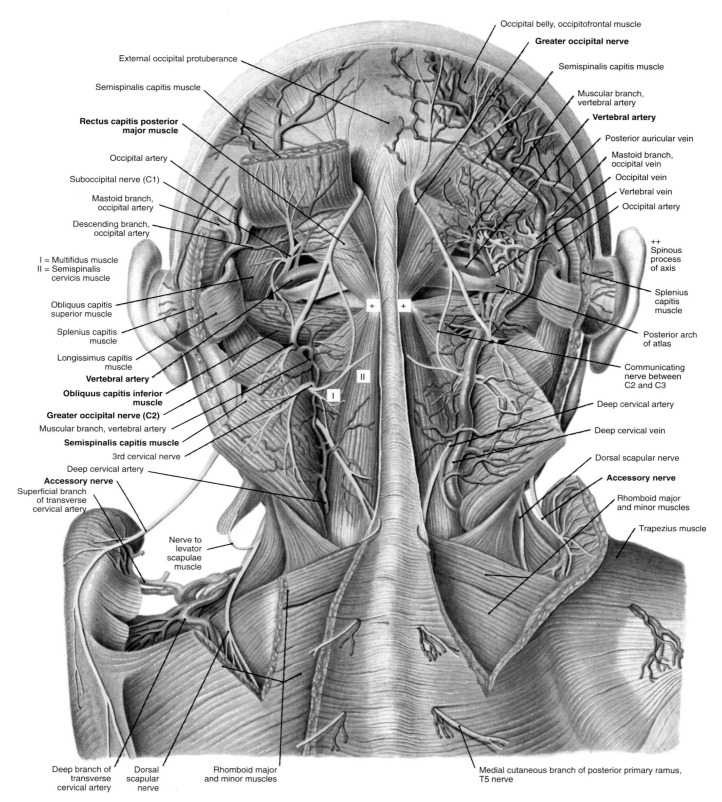

External occipital protuberance

Semispinalis capitis muscle

Rectus capitis posterior major muscle

Occipital artery

Suboccipital nerve (C1)

Mastoid branch, occipital artery

Descending branch, occipital artery

I = Multifidus muscle
II = Semispinalis cervicis muscle

Obliquus capitis superior muscle

Splenius capitis muscle

Longissimus capitis muscle

Vertebral artery

Obliquus capitis inferior muscle

Greater occipital nerve (C2)

Muscular branch, vertebral artery

Semispinalis capitis muscle

3rd cervical nerve

Deep cervical artery

Accessory nerve

Superficial branch of transverse cervical artery

Nerve to levator scapulae muscle

Occipital belly, occipitofrontal muscle

Greater occipital nerve

Semispinalis capitis muscle

Muscular branch, vertebral artery

Vertebral artery

Posterior auricular vein

Mastoid branch, occipital vein

Occipital vein

Vertebral vein

Occipital artery

++ Spinous process of axis

Splenius capitis muscle

Posterior arch of atlas

Communicating nerve between C2 and C3

Deep cervical artery

Deep cervical vein

Dorsal scapular nerve

Accessory nerve

Rhomboid major and minor muscles

Trapezius muscle

Deep branch of transverse cervical artery

Dorsal scapular nerve

Rhomboid major and minor muscles

Medial cutaneous branch of posterior primary ramus, T5 nerve

FIGURE 383 **Deep Vessels and Nerves of the Suboccipital Region and Upper Back; Suboccipital Triangle**

NOTE: (1) The **suboccipital triangle** lies deep to the semispinalis muscle and is bounded by the **rectus capitis posterior major, obliquus capitis superior,** and **obliquus capitis inferior.**

(2) The **vertebral artery** crosses the base of the suboccipital triangle, while the **suboccipital nerve** (posterior primary ramus of C1) courses *through* the triangle to supply motor innervation to the deep three muscles that bound the triangle as well as to the rectus capitis posterior minor and the overlying semispinalis capitis muscle.

(3) The **greater occipital nerve** (posterior primary ramus of C2), a sensory nerve, emerges below the obliquus capitis inferior and then courses medially and superiorly to become subcutaneous just lateral to and below the external occipital protuberance.

PLATE 384 Suboccipital Region: Muscles, Vessels, and Nerves

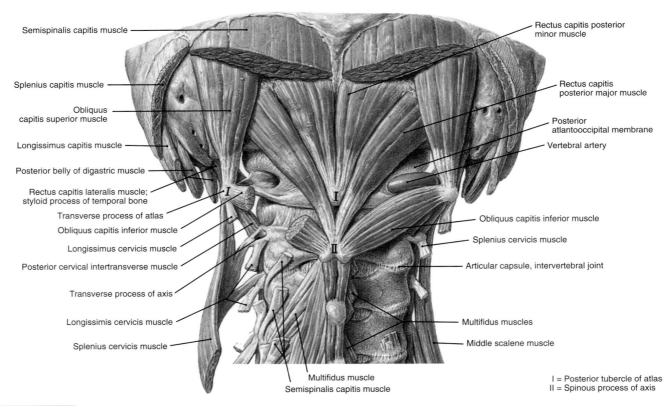

Semispinalis capitis muscle

Splenius capitis muscle

Obliquus capitis superior muscle

Longissimus capitis muscle

Posterior belly of digastric muscle

Rectus capitis lateralis muscle; styloid process of temporal bone

Transverse process of atlas

Obliquus capitis inferior muscle

Longissimus cervicis muscle

Posterior cervical intertransverse muscle

Transverse process of axis

Longissimis cervicis muscle

Splenius cervicis muscle

Rectus capitis posterior minor muscle

Rectus capitis posterior major muscle

Posterior atlantooccipital membrane

Vertebral artery

Obliquus capitis inferior muscle

Splenius cervicis muscle

Articular capsule, intervertebral joint

Multifidus muscles

Middle scalene muscle

Multifidus muscle

Semispinalis capitis muscle

I = Posterior tubercle of atlas
II = Spinous process of axis

FIGURE 384.1 Muscles of the Suboccipital Triangle

NOTE: (1) The **obliquus capitis inferior, obliquus capitis superior,** and **rectus capitis posterior major muscles** outline the **suboccipital triangle.**

(2) The **vertebral artery** crosses the floor of the triangle and penetrates the posterior atlantooccipital membrane to enter the foramen magnum. There the two vertebral arteries join to form the **basilar artery** on the ventral aspect of the brainstem.

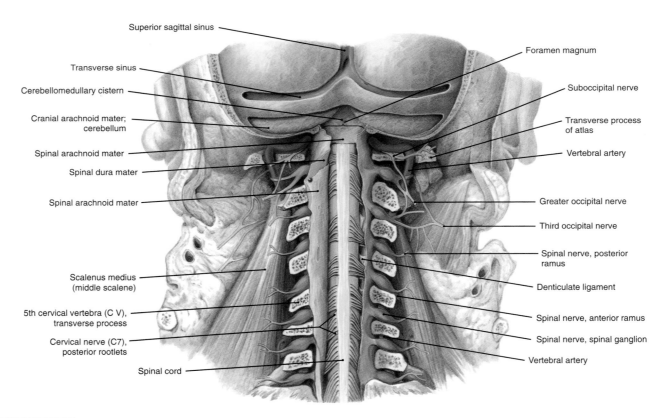

Superior sagittal sinus

Transverse sinus

Cerebellomedullary cistern

Cranial arachnoid mater; cerebellum

Spinal arachnoid mater

Spinal dura mater

Spinal arachnoid mater

Scalenus medius (middle scalene)

5th cervical vertebra (C V), transverse process

Cervical nerve (C7), posterior rootlets

Spinal cord

Foramen magnum

Suboccipital nerve

Transverse process of atlas

Vertebral artery

Greater occipital nerve

Third occipital nerve

Spinal nerve, posterior ramus

Denticulate ligament

Spinal nerve, anterior ramus

Spinal nerve, spinal ganglion

Vertebral artery

FIGURE 384.2 Suboccipital Region: Vertebral Artery and Occipital Nerves

NOTE: The assent and 90-degree turn medially taken by the vertebral arteries along the superior border of the atlas to achieve the ventral surface of the medulla oblongata.

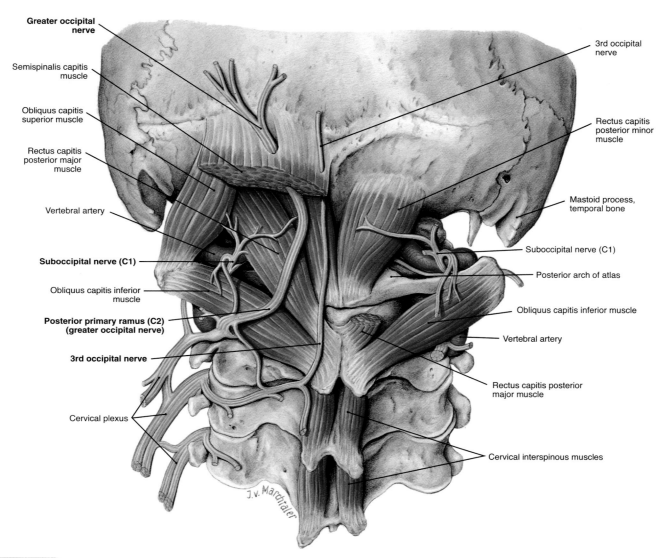

Greater occipital
nerve

Semispinalis capitis
muscle

Obliquus capitis
superior muscle

Rectus capitis
posterior major
muscle

Vertebral artery

Suboccipital nerve (C1)

Obliquus capitis inferior
muscle

**Posterior primary ramus (C2)
(greater occipital nerve)**

3rd occipital nerve

Cervical plexus

3rd occipital
nerve

Rectus capitis
posterior minor
muscle

Mastoid process,
temporal bone

Suboccipital nerve (C1)

Posterior arch of atlas

Obliquus capitis inferior muscle

Vertebral artery

Rectus capitis posterior
major muscle

Cervical interspinous muscles

J.v. Mardriater

FIGURE 385 **Nerves of the Suboccipital Region**

NOTE: (1) The **suboccipital nerve (C1),** primarily a motor nerve, emerges from the spinal cord above the atlas, courses through the suboccipital
triangle, and supplies motor innervation to all four suboccipital muscles.

(2) The **greater occipital (C2)** and **third occipital (C3) nerves** branch from the posterior primary rami of those segments. After passing through
the deep muscles of the back, they become purely sensory to supply the skin on the posterior scalp and neck.

MUSCLES OF THE SUBOCCIPITAL REGION				
Muscle	**Origin**	**Insertion**	**Innervation**	**Action**
Rectus capitis posterior major	Spinous process of axis	Lateral part of inferior nuchal line of occipital bone	Suboccipital nerve (dorsal ramus of C1)	Extends the head and rotates it to the same side
Rectus capitis posterior minor	Tubercle on the posterior arch of the atlas	Medial part of inferior nuchal line of occipital bone	Suboccipital nerve (dorsal ramus of C1)	Extends the head
Obliquus capitis superior	Upper surface of transverse process of the atlas	Onto occipital bone between superior and inferior nuchal lines	Suboccipital nerve (dorsal ramus of C1)	Extends the head and bends it laterally
Obliquus capitis inferior	Apex of spinous process of axis	Inferior and dorsal part of transverse process of the atlas	Suboccipital nerve (dorsal ramus of C1)	Rotates the atlas and thereby turns the face toward the same side

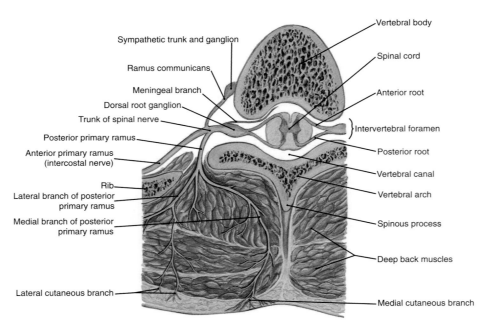

FIGURE 386.1 Branching of a Typical Spinal Nerve

NOTE: (1) Fibers from both **dorsal** and **ventral roots** join to form a **spinal nerve.** That nerve soon divides into a **posterior** and an **anterior primary ramus.** The posterior primary ramus courses dorsally to innervate the muscles and skin of the back. The anterior primary ramus courses anteriorly around the body to innervate the rest of the segment.

(2) The posterior primary rami of typical spinal nerves are smaller than the anterior rami, and each usually divides into medial and lateral branches, which contain both motor and sensory fibers innervating back structures.

(3) Unlike anterior primary rami, which join to form the cervical, brachial, and lumbosacral plexuses, the peripheral nerves derived from the posterior rami do not intercommunicate and form plexuses. There is, however, some segmental overlap of peripheral sensory fields, as seen with the anterior rami.

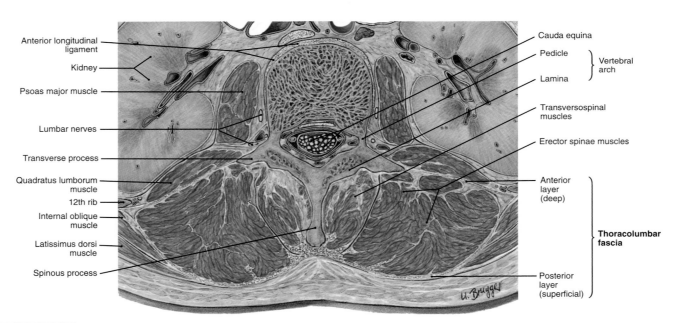

FIGURE 386.2 Cross Section at the L2 Vertebral Level: Deep Back Muscles and Thoracolumbar Fascia

NOTE: (1) This cross section of the deep back shows the lumbar part of the **thoracolumbar fascia** as it encloses the divisions of the erector spinae and transversospinal muscles. The fascia is formed by a posterior (superficial) layer and an anterior (deep) layer.

(2) Medially, the layers of the thoracolumbar fascia attach to the spinous and transverse processes of the lumbar vertebrae, and laterally, they become continuous with the aponeuroses and fascias of the latissimus dorsi and anterior abdominal muscles.

(3) The quadratus lumborum and psoas major muscles located deep to the erector spinae. Observe the relationship of the kidneys anterior to the quadratus lumborum muscles.

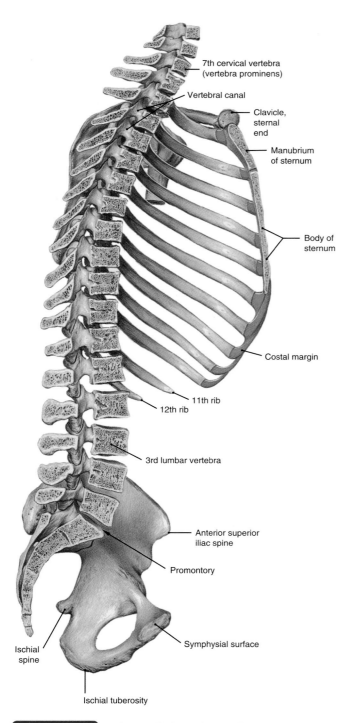

FIGURE 387.1 Left Medial Surface of the Vertebral Column Sectioned in the Median Plane

NOTE: (1) The sectioned vertebral column is shown from vertebra C5 inferiorly to the tip of the coccyx.

(2) The **vertebral canal** within which descends the spinal cord from the medulla oblongata of the brain.

(3) The C7 vertebra has a spinous process that is usually longer than the other cervical vertebrae and, therefore, is often called the **vertebra prominens.**

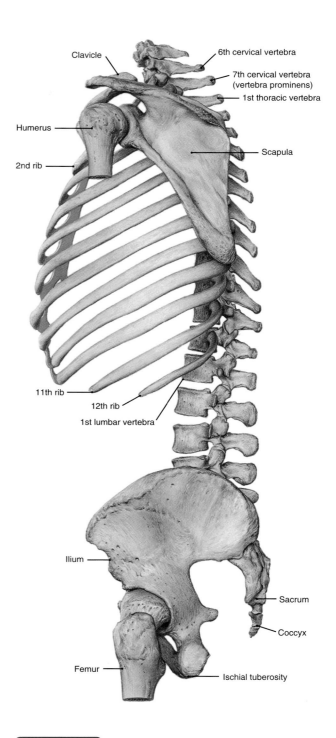

FIGURE 387.2 Left Lateral Surface of the Vertebral Column Sectioned in the Median Plane

NOTE: The scapula does not articulate with the vertebral column, whereas the pelvis articulates with the sacrum to form the **sacroiliac joint.**

PLATE 388 Cervical Vertebrae

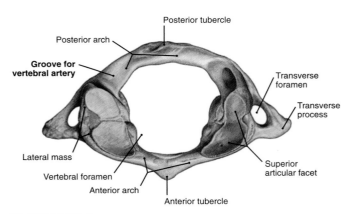

FIGURE 388.1 Atlas, Viewed from Above

NOTE: The superior articular facets are the sites of the occipito-atlantal joints behind which are the grooves for the vertebral arteries.

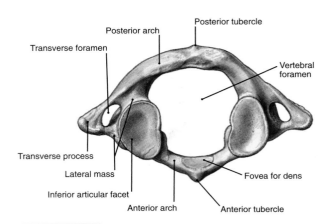

FIGURE 388.2 Atlas (Caudal View)

NOTE: The inferior articular facets on the inferior surface of the lateral mass articulate with the axis below.

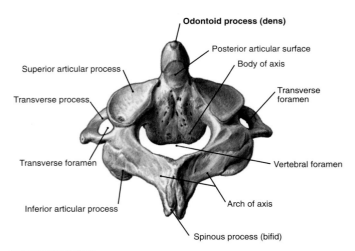

FIGURE 388.3 Posterior View of the Axis

NOTE: The large body and the odontoid process of the axis and the posterior articular facet articulates with the anterior arch of the atlas.

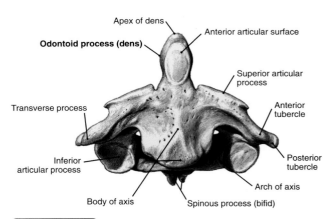

FIGURE 388.4 Anterior View of the Axis

NOTE: The articular facet on the anterior surface of the odontoid process behind (posterior) extends the transverse ligament of the atlas.

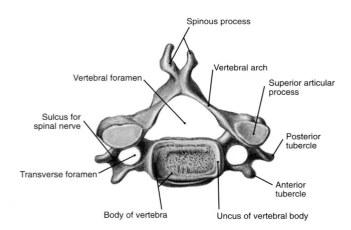

FIGURE 388.5 Fifth Cervical Vertebra (from Above)

NOTE: The fifth cervical vertebra is typical of third, fourth, and sixth cervical vertebrae, and different from the first (atlas), second (axis), and seventh, which present special features. Also note the delicate structure of this vertebra.

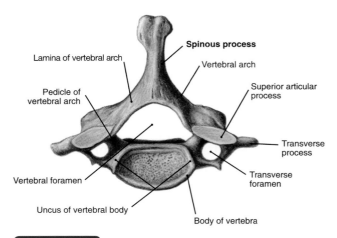

FIGURE 388.6 Seventh Cervical Vertebra (from Above)

NOTE: The seventh cervical vertebra, being transitional between cervical and thoracic vertebrae, has a transverse foramen similar to the cervical and a large spinous process similar to the thoracic. The latter gives it the name **vertebra prominens.**

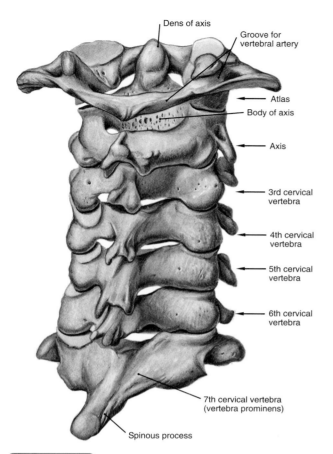

FIGURE 389.1 **Cervical Spinal Column (Dorsal)**

NOTE: While flexion and extension of the head are performed at the atlantooccipital joint, turning of the head to the left or right is the result of rotation of the atlas on the axis.

FIGURE 389.2 **Cervical Vertebrae (Ventral View)**

NOTE: Only a small part of the second to seventh cervical vertebrae is shown above and below the convex anterior surfaces of the bodies of the third to sixth vertebrae.

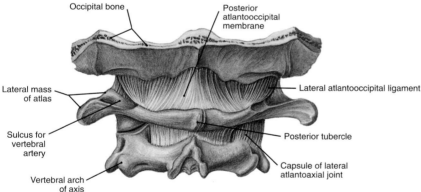

◄ **FIGURE 389.3** **Atlantooccipital and Atlantoaxial Joints (Posterior View)**

NOTE: From the posterior margin of the foramen magnum to the upper border of the posterior arch of the atlas stretches the posterior atlantooccipital membrane.

FIGURE 389.4 **Articulations of Occipital** ▶
Bone and First Three Vertebrae
(Anterior View)

NOTE: Extending between the occipital bone and the anterior arch of the atlas is the anterior atlantooccipital membrane, which continues laterally to join the articular capsules. Also observe the anterior longitudinal ligament.

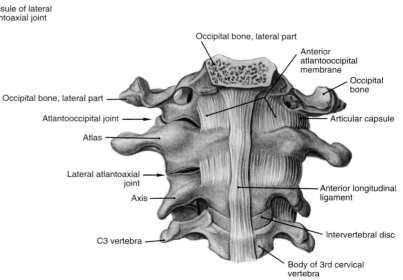

Chapter 5 The Back, Vertebral Column, and Spinal Cord

PLATE 390 **Craniovertebral Joints and Ligaments**

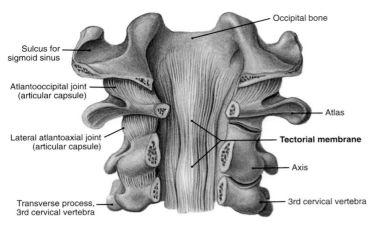

Occipital bone

Sulcus for sigmoid sinus

Atlantooccipital joint (articular capsule)

Lateral atlantoaxial joint (articular capsule)

Atlas

Tectorial membrane

Axis

Transverse process, 3rd cervical vertebra

3rd cervical vertebra

◀ **FIGURE 390.1** **Tectorial Membrane (Dorsal View)**

NOTE: The tectorial membrane is a broadened upward extension of the posterior longitudinal ligament and attaches the axis to the occipital bone (see also, Fig. 391.1). It covers the posterior surface of the odontoid process and lies dorsal to the cruciform ligament, covering it as well.

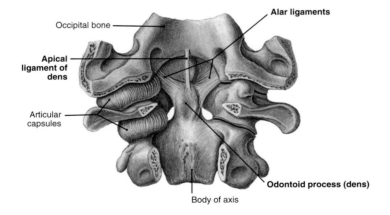

Cruciform ligament (superior longitudinal part)

Alar ligaments

Articular capsule

Cruciform ligament (transverse part)

Cruciform ligament (inferior longitudinal part)

Basilar part of occipital bone

Hypoglossal canal

Sulcus for sigmoid sinus

Atlantooccipital joint

Posterior arch of atlas

Lateral atlantoaxial joint

Axis

◀ **FIGURE 390.2** **Atlantooccipital and Atlantoaxial Joints Showing the Cruciform Ligament (Posterior View)**

NOTE: The posterior arches to the atlas and axis have been removed, and the cruciform ligament is seen from this posterior view. It consists of the transverse ligament (see Fig. 390.4) and the longitudinal fascicles that extend superiorly and inferiorly.

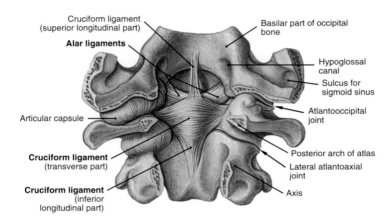

Alar ligaments

Occipital bone

Apical ligament of dens

Articular capsules

Odontoid process (dens)

Body of axis

◀ **FIGURE 390.3** **Alar and Apical Ligaments (Posterior View)**

NOTE: This figure is oriented the same as Figure 390.2. The cruciform ligament has been removed to reveal the odontoid process of the axis. This is attached superiorly to the occipital bone by the two alar ligaments and the apical ligament of the dens. These ligaments tend to limit lateral rotation of the skull.

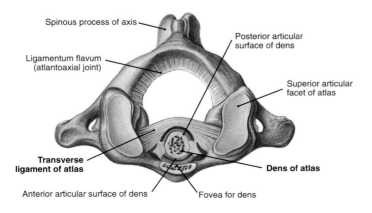

Spinous process of axis

Ligamentum flavum (atlantoaxial joint)

Posterior articular surface of dens

Superior articular facet of atlas

Transverse ligament of atlas

Dens of atlas

Anterior articular surface of dens

Fovea for dens

◀ **FIGURE 390.4** **Median Atlantoaxial Joint (from Above)**

NOTE: The odontoid process of the axis articulates with the anterior arch of the atlas, thereby forming the median atlantoaxial joint, and the thick and strong transverse ligament (part of the cruciform) of the atlas retains the dens on its posterior surface.

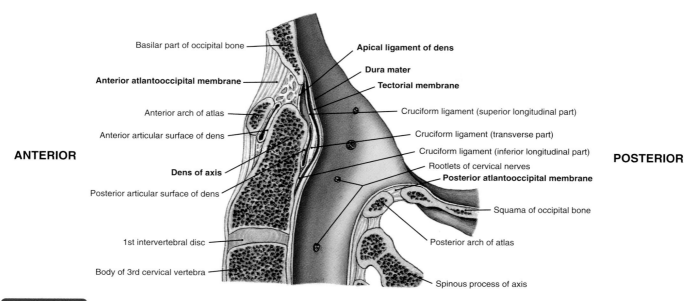

FIGURE 391.1 Median Sagittal Section of Atlantooccipital and Atlantoaxial Regions

NOTE: The relationships from anterior to posterior of the following structures: the anterior arch of the atlas, the joint between the atlas and the odontoid process (median atlantoaxial joint), the "joint" between the odontoid process and the transverse ligament of the atlas, the tectorial membrane, and finally, the dura mater covering the spinal cord.

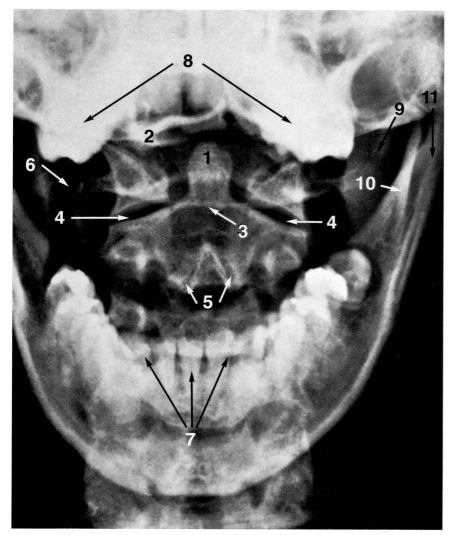

1. Odontoid process of axis
2. Anterior arch of atlas (inferior margin)
3. Posterior arch of atlas (inferior margin)
4. Lateral atlantoaxial joints
5. Spinous process of axis (bifid)
6. Transverse process of atlas
7. Inferior dental arch
8. Superior dental arch
9. Styloid process of temporal bone
10. Coronoid process of mandible
11. Condylar process of mandible

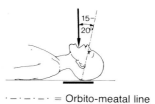

= Orbito-meatal line

FIGURE 391.2 Radiograph of the Odontoid Process and the Atlantoaxial Joints

NOTE: This is an anteroposterior projection taken through the oral cavity as shown in the diagram.

PLATE 392 **Vertebral Column**

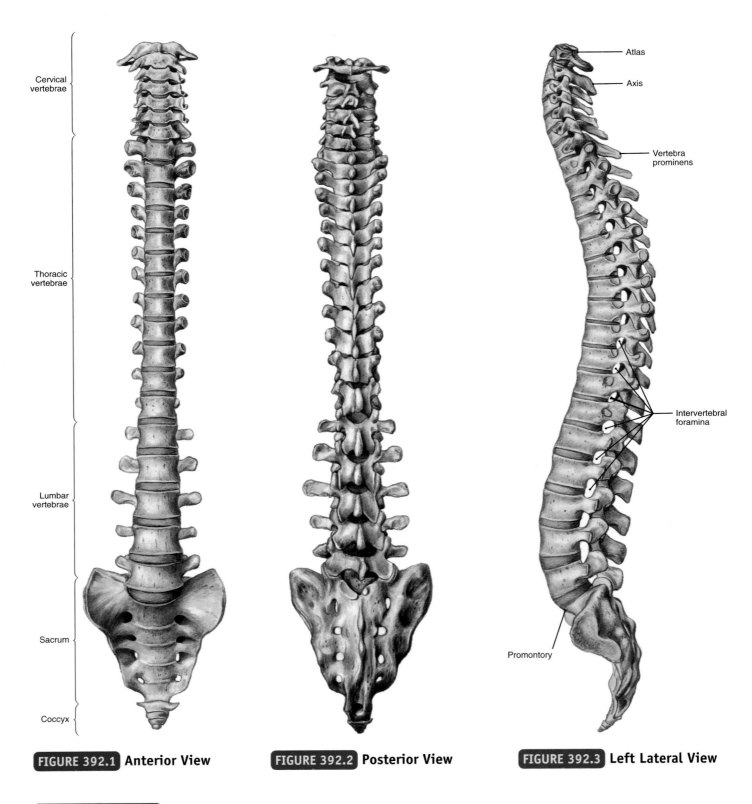

Cervical vertebrae

Thoracic vertebrae

Lumbar vertebrae

Sacrum

Coccyx

Atlas

Axis

Vertebra prominens

Intervertebral foramina

Promontory

FIGURE 392.1 **Anterior View**

FIGURE 392.2 **Posterior View**

FIGURE 392.3 **Left Lateral View**

FIGURE 392.1–392.3 **Vertebral Column, Including the Sacrum and Coccyx**

NOTE: (1) The vertebral column normally consists of 7 **cervical,** 12 **thoracic,** and 5 **lumbar** vertebrae and the **sacrum** and **coccyx.** Its principal functions are to assist in the maintenance of the erect posture in humans, to encase and protect the spinal cord, and to allow attachments of the musculature vertportant for covements of the head and trunk.

(2) From a dorsal or ventral view, the normal spinal column is straight. When viewed from the side, the vertebral column presents two ventrally convex curvatures (cervical and lumbar) and two dorsally convex curvatures (thoracic and sacral).

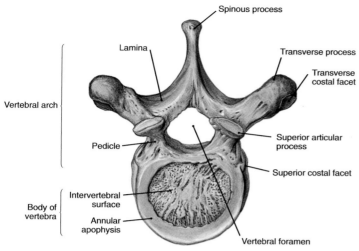

FIGURE 393.1 Sixth Thoracic Vertebra (from Above)

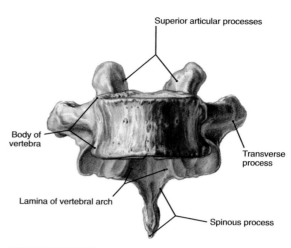

FIGURE 393.2 Tenth Thoracic Vertebra (Ventral View)

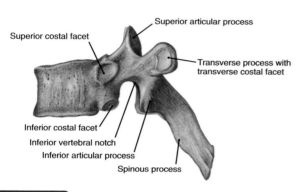

FIGURE 393.3 Sixth Thoracic Vertebra (from Left Lateral Side)

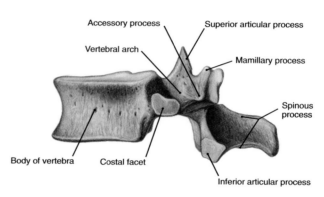

FIGURE 393.4 Twelfth Thoracic Vertebra (Lateral View)

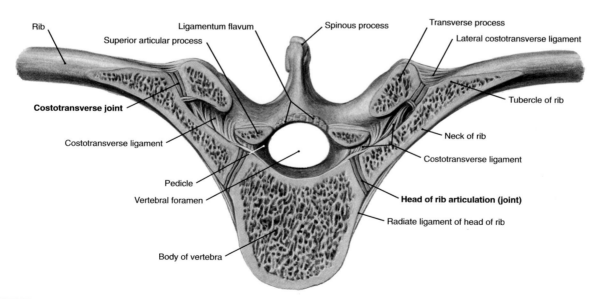

FIGURE 393.5 Costovertebral Joints, Transverse Section as Seen from Above

NOTE: Each rib articulates with the thoracic vertebrae at two places: (a) the **head of the rib** with the **vertebral body** and (b) the **tubercle** on the **neck of the rib** with the **transverse process** of the vertebra.

PLATE 394 Costovertebral Joints and Ligaments 1

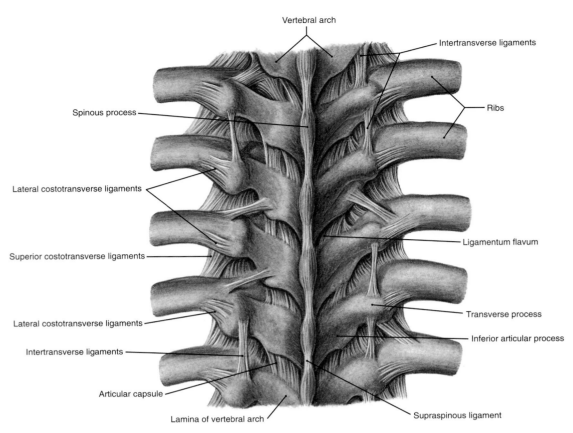

FIGURE 394.1 Lower Costovertebral Joints (Posterior View)

NOTE: (1) Five pairs of costovertebral joints, viewed from behind, show to advantage the articulations between the necks and the tubercles of the ribs and the transverse processes of the thoracic vertebrae.

(2) The ligaments that connect these gliding joints are the **costotransverse, lateral costotransverse,** and **superior costotransverse.**

(3) The costotransverse joints (neck of rib with transverse process) are not to be confused with the joints between the heads of the ribs and the bodies of the vertebrae.

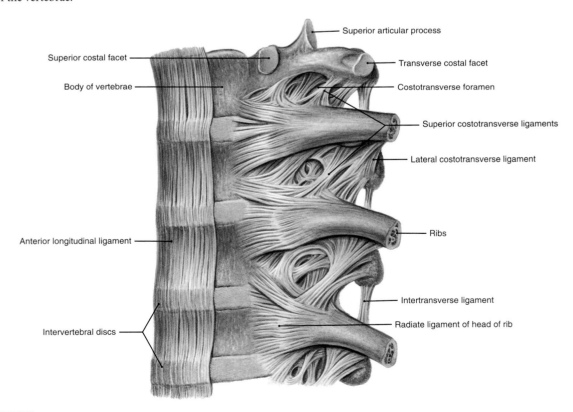

FIGURE 394.2 Costovertebral Joints (Lateral View Showing the Radiate Ligaments of the Heads of the Ribs)

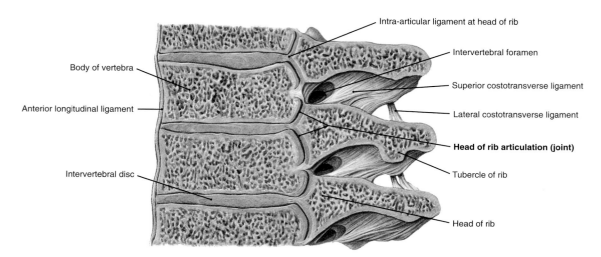

FIGURE 395.1 Sagittal Section through the Spinal Column Showing the Costovertebral Joints

NOTE: The following important structures are shown: the intervertebral disks, the intra-articular and costotransverse ligaments, and the intervertebral foramina, which transmit the spinal nerves and their accompanying vessels.

FIGURE 395.2 Anterior Longitudinal Ligament ▶ (Ventral View)

NOTE: The **anterior longitudinal ligament** extends from the axis to the sacrum along the anterior aspect of the bodies of the vertebrae and the intervertebral disks to which it is firmly attached. Its fibers are white and glistening and can readily be identified.

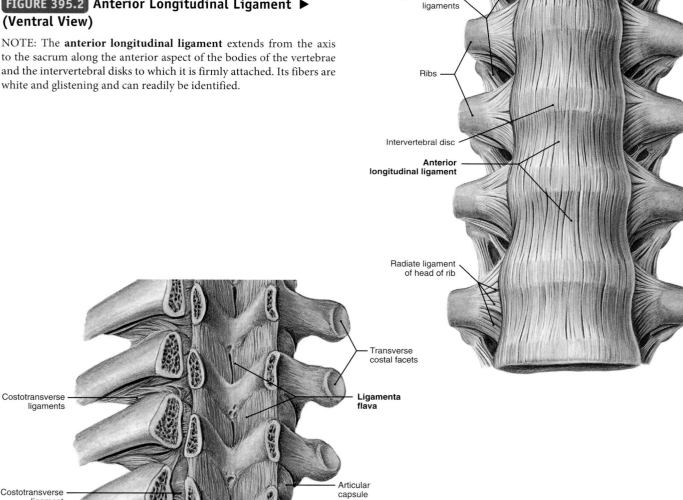

◀ **FIGURE 395.3** Ligamenta Flava (Anterior View)

NOTE: The bodies of the thoracic vertebrae have been removed, revealing from within the vertebral foramina the ligamenta flava interconnecting the laminae of the dorsal vertebral arches. The pedicles have been cut, and on the left, the ribs have been removed. The **ligamenta flava** are formed by yellow, elastic tissue.

PLATE 396 Lumbar Vertebrae

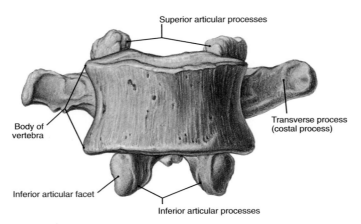

Spinous process

Vertebral arch (lamina)

Mamillary process

Accessory process

Vertebral foramen

Vertebral arch (lamina)

Superior articular process

Transverse process

Pedicle

Body of vertebra

FIGURE 396.1 Lumbar Vertebra (Cranial View)

Superior articular processes

Body of vertebra

Inferior articular facet

Transverse process (costal process)

Inferior articular processes

FIGURE 396.2 Lumbar Vertebra (Anterior View)

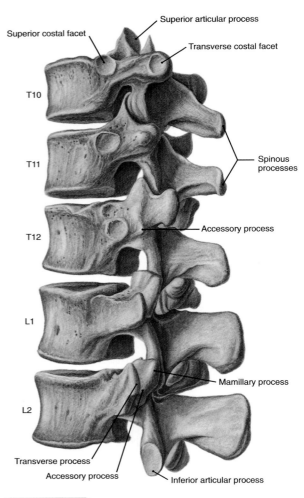

Superior costal facet

Superior articular process

Transverse costal facet

T10

T11

T12

L1

L2

Spinous processes

Accessory process

Mamillary process

Transverse process

Accessory process

Inferior articular process

FIGURE 396.3 Last Three Thoracic and First Two Lumbar Vertebrae (Lateral View)

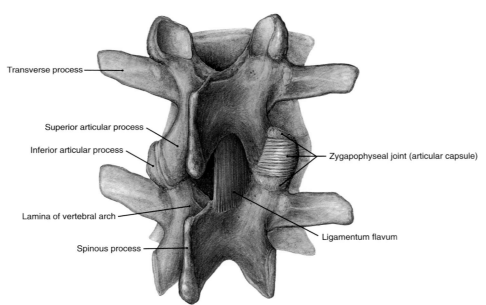

Transverse process

Superior articular process

Inferior articular process

Lamina of vertebral arch

Spinous process

Zygapophyseal joint (articular capsule)

Ligamentum flavum

FIGURE 396.4 Zygapophyseal Joints and Ligamenta Flava between Adjacent Lumbar Vertebrae

NOTE: (1) In this posterior view, the articular capsule of the zygapophyseal joint (between the articular processes) and the ligamentum flavum have been removed on the left side.

(2) Each ligamentum flavum is attached to the anterior surface of the lamina above and to the posterior surface of the lamina below. They are elastic and permit separation of the laminae during flexion of the spine, and they inhibit abrupt and extreme movements of the vertebral column, thus protecting the intervertebral disks (see also, Fig. 395.3).

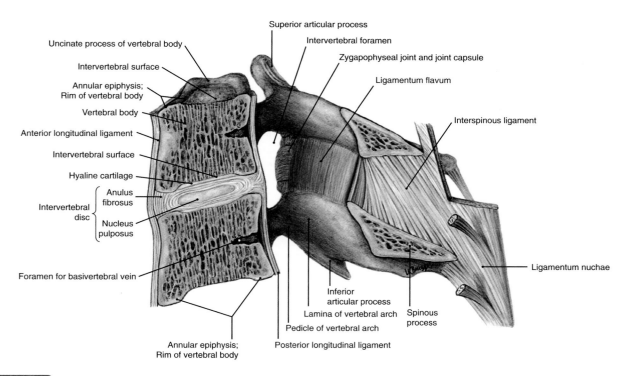

FIGURE 397.1 Cervical Intervertebral Joints: Median Sagittal Section

NOTE: (1) The long spinous processes of the cervical vertebrae and the strong interspinous ligaments. Observe the blending of fibers of the interspinous ligaments with the ligamentum nuchae of the dorsal cervical region.

(2) The intervertebral disk between the bodies of the two cervical vertebrae is shown; also note the nucleus pulposus surrounded by the annulus fibrosis.

(3) The anterior and posterior longitudinal ligaments and the foramina for the basivertebral veins.

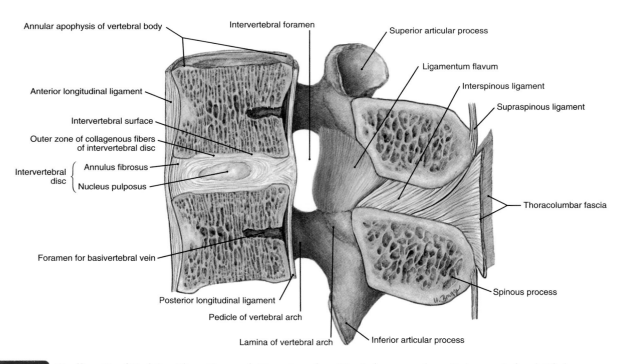

FIGURE 397.2 Median Sagittal Section through Two Lumbar Vertebrae and an Intervertebral Disk

NOTE: (1) The anterior and posterior longitudinal ligaments ventral and dorsal to the bodies of the lumbar vertebrae.

(2) The ligamentum flavum forms an important ligamentous connection between the laminae of adjacent vertebral arches on the dorsal aspect of the vertebral canal.

Chapter 5 The Back, Vertebral Column, and Spinal Cord

PLATE 398 Intervertebral Disks

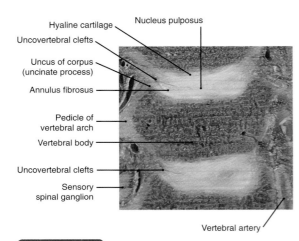

FIGURE 398.1 Two Cervical Intervertebral Disks: Frontal Section through the Centers of the Vertebral Bodies

NOTE: (1) The intervertebral disks are located between the bodies of adjacent vertebrae (in this case cervical vertebrae).

(2) Hyaline cartilage covers the end plates of the vertebral bodies and lies adjacent to the annulus fibrosus.

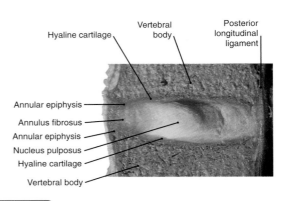

FIGURE 398.2 Median Sagittal Section through a Lumbar Intervertebral Disk

NOTE: (1) The **nucleus pulposus** that forms the inner core is soft and gelatinous in early years and consists of mucoid material and a few cells.

(2) After 10 or 12 years of age the mucoid material is gradually replaced by fibrocartilage, and the center of the disk becomes more like the annulus that surrounds it. (See notes for Fig. 398.3.)

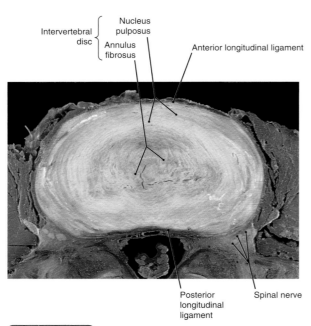

FIGURE 398.3 Photograph of a Lumbar Intervertebral Disk (Viewed from Above)

NOTE: (1) The annulus fibrosus consists of a thin band of collagenous fibers and a thicker band of fibrocartilage.

(2) In later adolescence and in the young adult, the intervertebral disks are strong and can withstand most vertical forces that impinge on the vertebral column, such as jumping or sitting upright.

(3) After several decades, some degeneration may occur that weakens the annulus fibrosus. These changes may account for the fact that in the elderly there may be a displacement of the nucleus pulposus (after even a mild strain) into or through the annulus, resulting in pain.

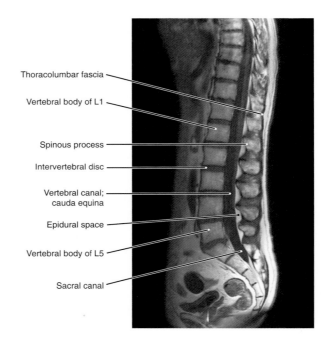

FIGURE 398.4 Magnetic Resonance Image of the Lumbar Vertebrae (Median Sagittal Section)

NOTE: (1) The spinous processes and the bodies of the lumbar vertebrae.

(2) The intervertebral disks arranged sequentially between the vertebral bodies.

(3) The so-called disk problem that results from displacement of disk material is most likely to occur in the cervical or lumbar regions and especially between the L4-L5 vertebral body.

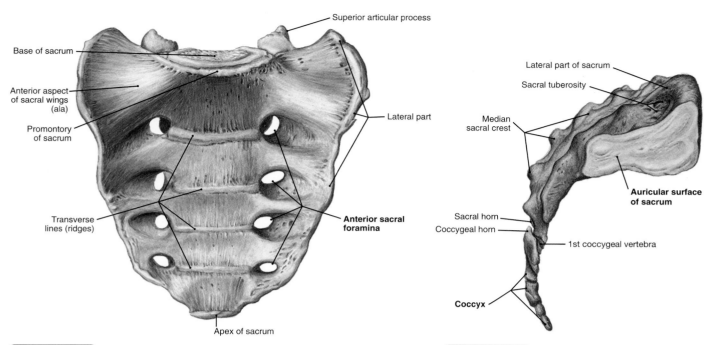

FIGURE 399.1 Sacrum, Anterior or Pelvic Surface

NOTE: (1) The sacrum is a large triangular bone formed by the fusion of five sacral vertebrae, and it is wedged between the two hip bones, with which it articulates laterally.

(2) Superiorly, the sacrum articulates with the fifth lumbar vertebra, and inferiorly with the coccyx.

(3) The anterior (pelvic) surface of the sacrum is concave and shows four pelvic foramina on each side. These transmit the ventral rami of the upper four sacral nerves.

FIGURE 399.2 Sacrum and Coccyx (Lateral View)

NOTE: The auricular (ear-shaped) surface of the sacrum articulates with the iliac portion of the pelvis. Inferiorly, the sacral apex joins the coccyx.

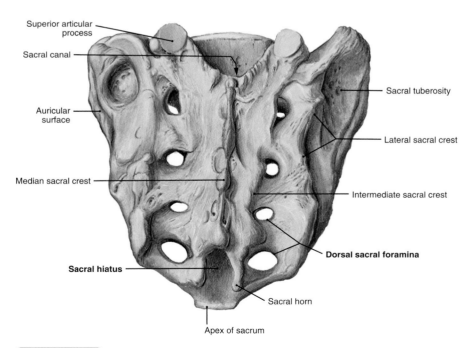

FIGURE 399.3 Sacrum (Posterior Surface)

NOTE: On the dorsal surface of the sacrum, the foramina transmit the dorsal rami of the sacral nerves. The dorsal laminae of the fifth sacral vertebra fail to fuse, thereby leaving a midline opening into the sacral canal called the sacral hiatus.

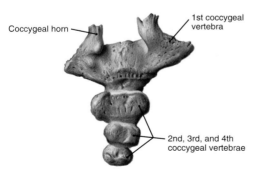

FIGURE 399.4 Coccyx (Dorsal View)

NOTE: This coccyx has four segments, but in many people there are three or five.

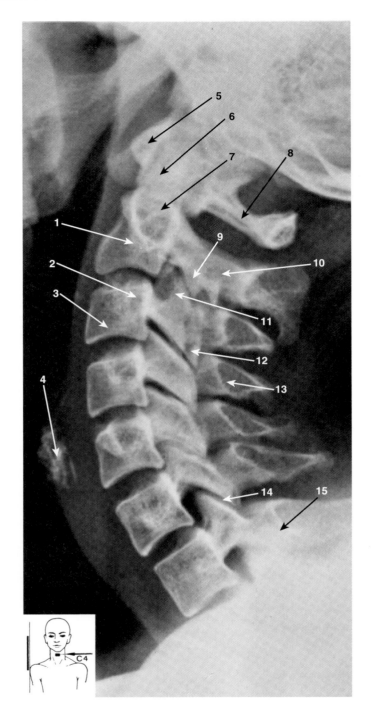

FIGURE 400.1 Cervical Spinal Column (Lateral View)

1. Body of axis
2. Transverse process of C3 vertebra
3. Body of C3 vertebra
4. Lamina of cricoid cartilage
5. Anterior arch of atlas
6. Odontoid process of axis
7. Transverse process of axis
8. Posterior arch of atlas
9. Inferior articular process
10. Spinous process
11. Superior articular process
12. Inferior articular process
13. Spinous process
14. Intervertebral articulation
15. Spinous process, vertebra prominens (C7)

(From Wicke, 6th ed.)

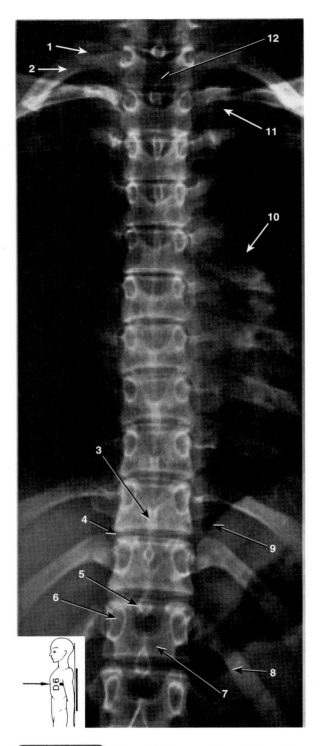

FIGURE 400.2 Spinal Column, Thoracic Region (Anteroposterior Projection)

1. Neck of first rib
2. First rib
3. Spinous process
4. Inferior articular process
5. Superior articular process
6. Pedicle of vertebral arch
7. Twelfth thoracic vertebra
8. Twelfth rib
9. Diaphragm
10. Left contour of the heart
11. Clavicle
12. T1 vertebra

(From Wicke, 6th ed.)

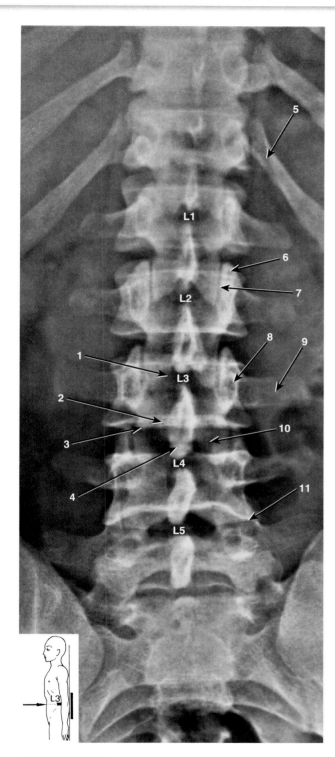

FIGURE 401.1 Spinal Column, Lumbar Region (Anteroposterior Projection)

1. Body of L3 vertebra
2. Posterior margin of L3 vertebra
3. Anterior margin of L4 vertebra
4. Spinous process of L3
5. Twelfth rib
6. Superior articular process
7. Intervertebral articulation (zygapophyseal joint)
8. Pedicle of vertebral arch
9. Costal process
10. Lamina of vertebral arch
11. Inferior articular process

(From Wicke, 6th ed.)

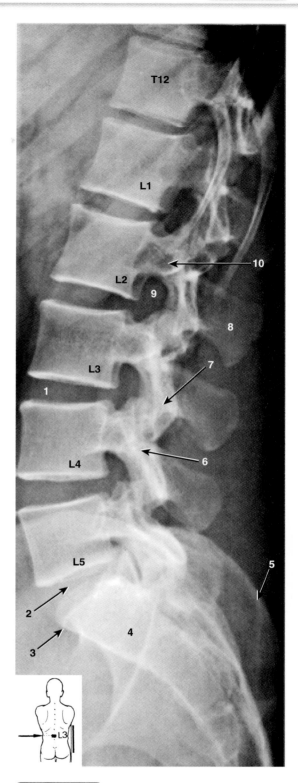

FIGURE 401.2 Spinal Column, Lumbar Region (Lateral Projection)

1. Intervertebral disk space
2. Lumbosacral joint
3. Promontory
4. Sacrum
5. Iliac crest
6. Superior articular process of L4 vertebra
7. Inferior articular process of L3 vertebra
8. Spinous process of L2 vertebra
9. Intervertebral foramen
10. Costal process

(From Wicke, 6th ed.)

Chapter 5 The Back, Vertebral Column, and Spinal Cord

PLATE 402 Spinal Cord (Infant); Spinal Nerves (Adult, Diagram)

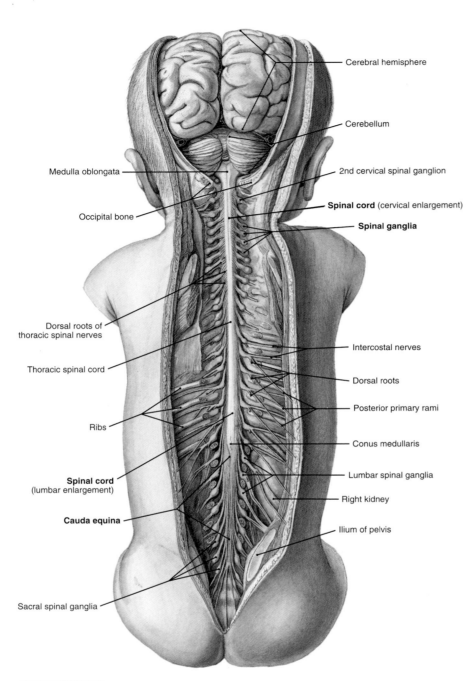

Cerebral hemisphere

Cerebellum

Medulla oblongata

2nd cervical spinal ganglion

Occipital bone

Spinal cord (cervical enlargement)

Spinal ganglia

Dorsal roots of
thoracic spinal nerves

Intercostal nerves

Thoracic spinal cord

Dorsal roots

Posterior primary rami

Ribs

Conus medullaris

Lumbar spinal ganglia

Spinal cord
(lumbar enlargement)

Right kidney

Cauda equina

Ilium of pelvis

Sacral spinal ganglia

FIGURE 402.1 Spinal Cord and Brain of a Newborn Child
(Posterior View)

NOTE: (1) The central nervous system has been exposed by the removal of the dorsal
part of the spinal column and of the dorsal cranium. The spinal ganglia have been
dissected, as have their corresponding spinal nerves.

(2) Although in this dissection it appears as though the substance of the spinal cord terminates at about L1, it is more usual in the newborn for the cord to end at about L3
or L4, thereby filling the spinal canal more completely than in the adult.

(3) The dorsal root ganglion of the first cervical nerve may be very small and often absent
(see small ganglion above that of C2). Both anterior and posterior primary rami of
C1 are principally motor, although from time to time C1 will have a small cutaneous
branch.

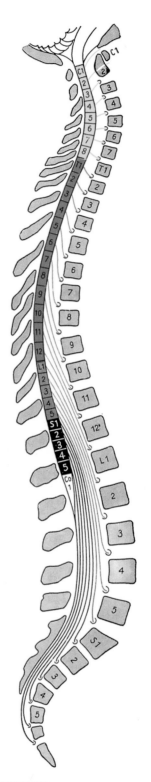

FIGURE 402.2 Emerging Spinal
Nerves and Segments in the Adult

Yellow: Cervical segments (C1–C8)
Red: Thoracic segments (T1–T12)
Blue: Lumbar segments (L1–L5)
Black: Sacral segments (S1–S5)
White: Coccygeal segments (C0)

NOTE: Many spinal nerves travel long dis-
tances before they leave the vertebral canal in
the adult.

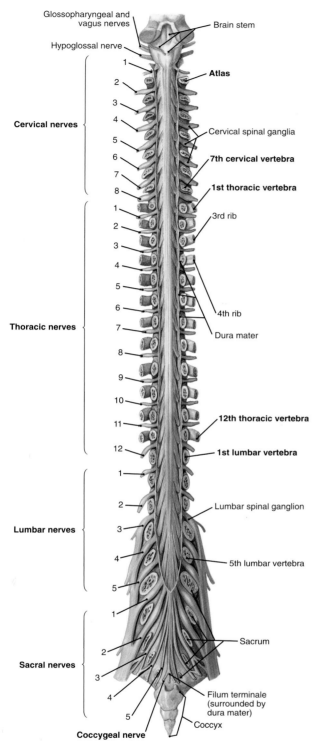

FIGURE 403.1 Spinal Cord within the Vertebral Canal (Dorsal View)

NOTE: (1) The first cervical nerve emerges above the first vertebra and the eighth cervical nerve emerges below the seventh vertebra.

(2) The cervical spinal cord is continuous above with the medulla oblongata of the brainstem.

(3) Each spinal nerve is formed by the union of the dorsal and ventral roots of that segment, and it emerges between the two adjacent vertebrae through the intervertebral foramen.

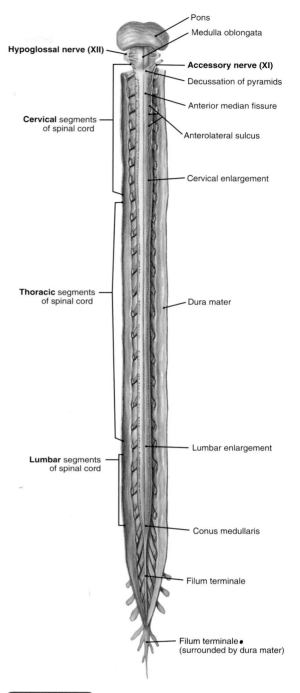

FIGURE 403.2 Spinal Cord (Ventral View)

NOTE: (1) The origin of the spinal portion of the accessory nerve (XI) arising from the cervical spinal cord and ascending to join the bulbar portion of that nerve.

(2) The alignment of the rootlets of the hypoglossal nerve (XII) with the ventral roots of the spinal cord.

(3) The anterior median fissure is located in the longitudinal midline of the spinal cord. Within this fissure courses the anterior spinal artery (see Fig. 404.1).

(4) The cervical and lumbar enlargements caused by the large numbers of sensory and motor neurons located in these regions that are required to supply innervation to the upper and lower limbs.

PLATE 404 Spinal Cord: Arterial Supply and Spinal Roots

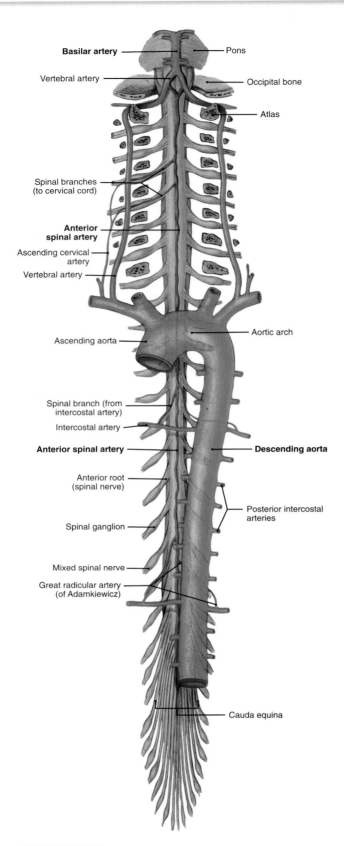

Basilar artery
Pons
Vertebral artery
Occipital bone
Atlas
Spinal branches
(to cervical cord)
**Anterior
spinal artery**
Ascending cervical
artery
Vertebral artery
Ascending aorta
Aortic arch
Spinal branch (from
intercostal artery)
Intercostal artery
Anterior spinal artery
Descending aorta
Anterior root
(spinal nerve)
Posterior intercostal
arteries
Spinal ganglion
Mixed spinal nerve
Great radicular artery
(of Adamkiewicz)
Cauda equina

FIGURE 404.1 Anterior Spinal Artery

NOTE: The anterior spinal artery is formed by vessels from the
vertebral arteries. It receives anastomotic branches from certain
cervical, thoracic, and lumbar segmental arteries along the spinal
roots. An especially large branch (artery of Adamkiewicz) arises
in the lower thoracic or upper lumbar region.

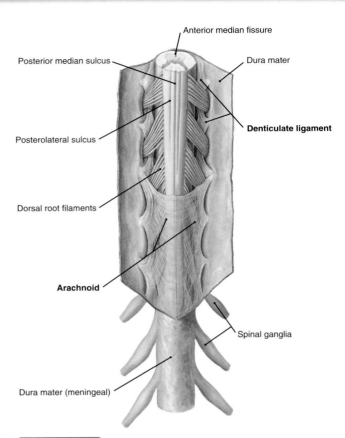

Anterior median fissure
Posterior median sulcus
Dura mater
Posterolateral sulcus
Denticulate ligament
Dorsal root filaments
Arachnoid
Spinal ganglia
Dura mater (meningeal)

FIGURE 404.2 Spinal Cord with Dura Mater
Dissected Open (Dorsal View)

NOTE: Extensions of the pia mater to the meningeal dura mater between the roots of the spinal nerves are called **denticulate ligaments.**
The arachnoid sends fine attachments to both the pia and the dura.

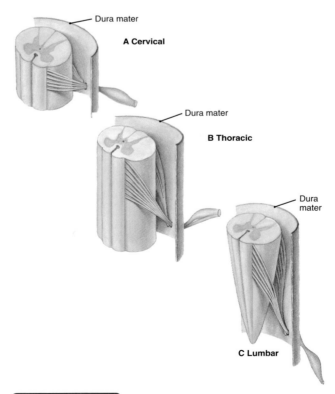

Dura mater
A Cervical
Dura mater
B Thoracic
Dura
mater
C Lumbar

FIGURE 404.3A–C Relationship of the Dorsal and
Ventral Roots to the Dura Mater (Various Spinal
Levels)

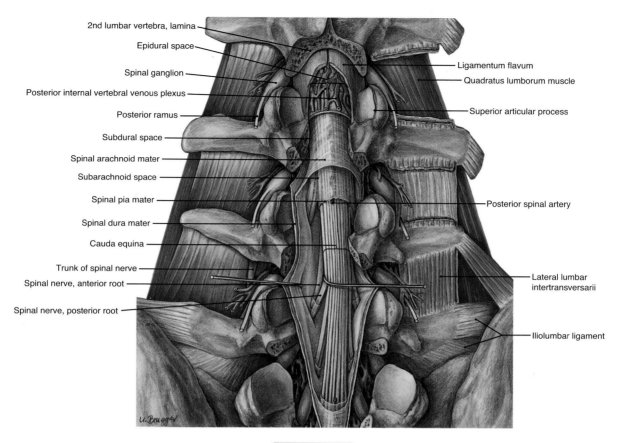

2nd lumbar vertebra, lamina
Epidural space
Spinal ganglion
Posterior internal vertebral venous plexus
Posterior ramus
Subdural space
Spinal arachnoid mater
Subarachnoid space
Spinal pia mater
Spinal dura mater
Cauda equina
Trunk of spinal nerve
Spinal nerve, anterior root
Spinal nerve, posterior root

Ligamentum flavum
Quadratus lumborum muscle
Superior articular process
Posterior spinal artery
Lateral lumbar intertransversarii
Iliolumbar ligament

▲ FIGURE 405.1 **Dorsal View of the Vertebral Canal from the Second to the Fifth Lumbar Vertebral Level**

NOTE: (1) The vertebral arches have been removed to show the vertebral canal below the conus medullaris.
(2) The anterior (ventral) and posterior (dorsal) roots coursing together through the intervertebral foramina in the lumbar region.
(3) The dorsal root ganglia at each segmental lumbar level.
(4) The formation of spinal roots below the conus medullaris (L2 level of the spinal cord) is often called the **cauda equina** (horse's tail).

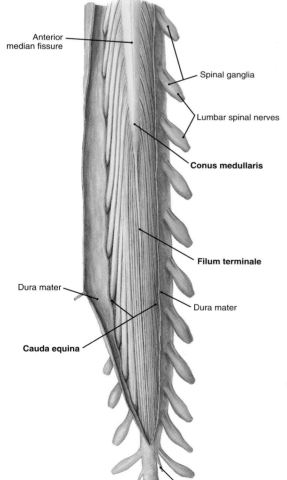

Anterior median fissure
Spinal ganglia
Lumbar spinal nerves
Conus medullaris
Filum terminale
Dura mater
Dura mater
Cauda equina
Coccygeal nerve

◄ FIGURE 405.2 **Conus Medullaris and Cauda Equina (Ventral)**

NOTE: (1) The termination of the neural part of the spinal cord at the conus medullaris. Its membranous continuation as the filum terminale measures about 20 cm and extends as far as the coccyx.
(2) The cauda equina refers to the roots of the spinal nerves below the conus, and these are seen to surround the filum.
(3) Prolongations of the dura continue to cover the spinal nerves for some distance as they enter the intervertebral foramen.

Chapter 5 The Back, Vertebral Column, and Spinal Cord

PLATE 406 Spinal Cord: Cross Section; Spinal Arteries

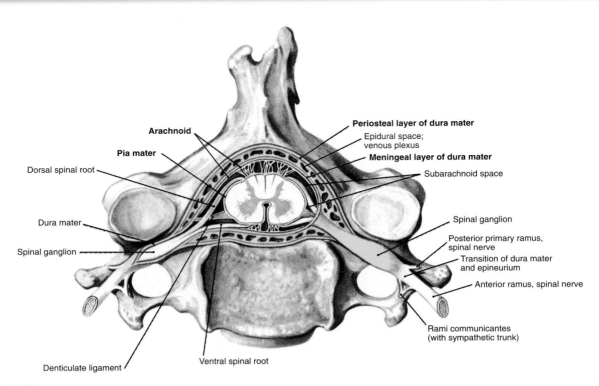

FIGURE 406.1 **Meninges of the Spinal Cord Shown at Cervical Level (Transverse Section)**

NOTE: (1) The meningeal dura mater (inner layer of yellow) surrounds the spinal cord and continues along the spinal nerve through the intervertebral foramen. Its outer periosteal layer is formed of connective tissue that closely adheres to the bone of the vertebrae forming the vertebral canal.

(2) The delicate filmlike arachnoid, which lies between the meningeal layer of the dura mater and the vascularized pia mater, which is closely applied to the cord.

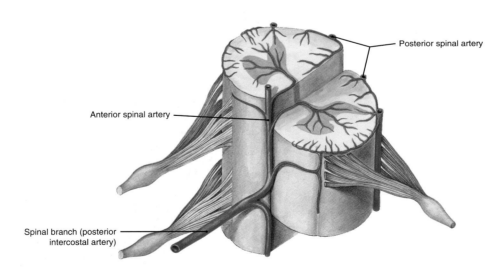

FIGURE 406.2 **Spinal Arteries and Their Sulcal Branches**

NOTE: (1) As the **anterior spinal artery** descends in the anterior median sulcus, it gives off **sulcal branches** that penetrate the spinal cord.

(2) These sulcal branches usually arise singly, and each turns to the right or left to supply that half of the spinal cord. When each branch is given off it *does not bifurcate* to supply both sides.

(3) Each sulcal branch turns to one side of the cord, and the next branch turns to the other. This alternating pattern (as shown in this figure) occurs along the length of the spinal cord.

(4) Each of the two **posterior spinal arteries** supplies its respective side of the cord.

(5) The spinal arteries anastomose with the spinal branches of the segmental arteries (especially those from the intercostal and lumbar arteries).

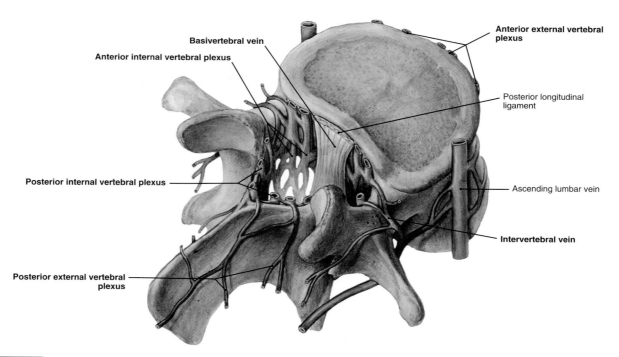

FIGURE 407.1 **Veins of the Vertebral Column**

NOTE: (1) The veins drain blood from the vertebrae, and the contents of the spinal canal form plexuses that extend the entire length of the spinal column (Batson's veins).

(2) The plexuses are grouped according to whether they lie external to or within the vertebral canal. Thus, they include **external vertebral, internal vertebral, basivertebral, intervertebral**, and **veins of the spinal cord**.

(3) The basivertebral veins drain the bodies of the vertebrae and may flow into anterior external or anterior internal vertebral plexuses.

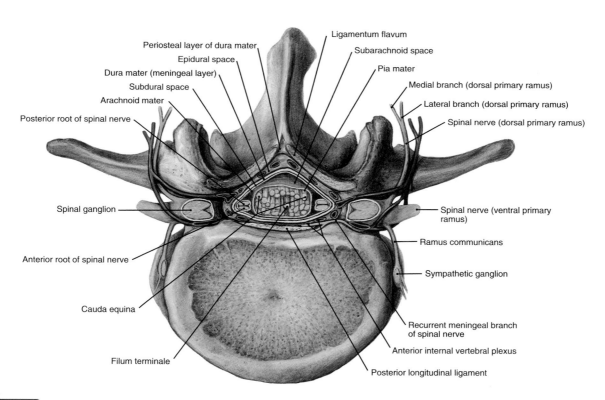

FIGURE 407.2 **Cross Section of the Cauda Equina within the Vertebral Canal**

NOTE: (1) This cross section is at the level of the third lumbar vertebra, one segment or more below the site where the spinal cord ends.

(2) Specimens of cerebrospinal fluid may be obtained by performing lumbar punctures between the laminae or spines of the third and fourth or fourth and fifth lumbar vertebrae.

PLATE 408 Lumbar and Sacral Puncture into the Spinal Cord

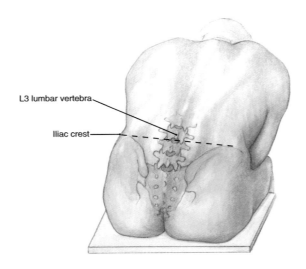

L3 lumbar vertebra

Iliac crest

FIGURE 408.1 **Position of Patient for Lumbar Puncture**

NOTE that the patient is sitting and bent forward as far as possible in order to increase the space between the vertebrae. For orientation, observe that the junction between the L3 and L4 vertebrae is at the level of the iliac crest.

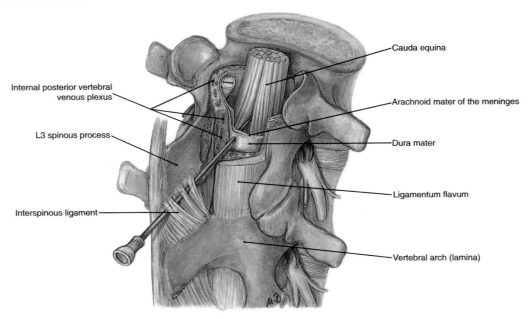

Cauda equina

Internal posterior vertebral venous plexus

Arachnoid mater of the meninges

L3 spinous process

Dura mater

Ligamentum flavum

Interspinous ligament

Vertebral arch (lamina)

FIGURE 408.2 **Lumbar Injection into the Cauda Equina**

NOTE that the needle is inserted just below the spinous process of the L3 vertebra, and realize that the spinal cord becomes the nonneural conus medularis just below the L2 vertebra.

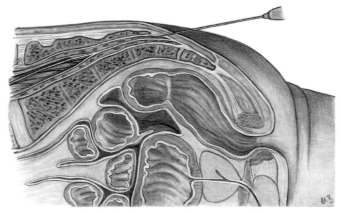

FIGURE 408.3 **Sacral Puncture into the Cauda Equina**

NOTE that the needle is inserted into the sacral hiatus in order to produce a caudal epidural anesthesia. This method can be used to anesthetize the lower sacral and coccygeal nerves.

Plates

409 Lower Limb: Photographs (Anterior and Posterior Views)

410 Lower Limb: Surface Anatomy and Peripheral Nerve Fields (Anterior View)

411 Lower Limb: Cutaneous Nerves (Anterior and Posterior Views)

412 Bones and Joints of the Lower Extremity

413 Lower Extremity: Arteries and Bones

414 Muscles and Fasciae on the Anterior Aspect of the Lower Limb

415 Muscles and Fasciae on the Posterior Aspect of the Lower Limb

416 Lower Limb: Anterior Thigh, Superficial Vessels and Nerves (Dissection 1)

417 Superficial and Deep Inguinal Lymph Nodes; Saphenous Opening

418 Lower Extremity: Anterior Thigh Muscles, Superficial View (Dissection 2)

419 Individual Muscles of the Anterior Thigh (Dissection 3)

420 Lower Extremity: Anterior Thigh Muscles (Dissection 4)

421 Anterior and Medial Thigh Muscles, Intermediate Layer (Dissection 5)

422 Arteries of the Hip Region; Deep Femoral and Circumflex Iliac Arteries

423 Lower Extremity: Femoral Vessels and Nerves; Adductor Canal (Dissection 6)

424 Anterior and Medial Thigh Muscles, Deep Layer (Dissection 7)

425 Anterior and Medial Thigh, Deep Vessels and Nerves (Dissection 8)

426 Lower Extremity: Anterior Thigh, Movements and Muscle Chart

427 Lower Extremity: Chart of Thigh Muscles

428 Gluteal Region and Thigh: Superficial Vessels and Nerves (Dissection 1)

429 Lower Extremity: Muscles of the Thigh (Lateral View)

430 Lower Extremity: Gluteus Maximus (Dissection 2)

431 Gluteal Region: Gluteal Muscles (Superficial and Deep)

432 Gluteal Region: Gluteus Medius and Lateral Rotators (Dissection 3)

433 Gluteal Region: Deep Vessels and Nerves (Dissection 4)

434 Chart of Gluteal Muscles; Safe Zone for Gluteal Injections

435 The Gluteal Muscles; Safe Gluteal Quadrant

436 Posterior Thigh: Sciatic Nerve and Popliteal Vessels (Dissection 1)

437 Lower Extremity: Posterior Thigh Muscles (Dissection 2)

438 Lower Extremity: Posterior Thigh, Deep Muscles (Dissection 3)

439 Posterior Thigh and Gluteal Region: Deep Vessels and Nerves (Dissection 4)

440 Anterior and Medial Nerves of the Lower Limb

441 Posterior Nerves of the Lower Limb

442 Popliteal Fossa, Vessels and Nerves (Dissections 1, 2)

443 Knee Region: Medial and Posterior Aspects (Dissection 3)

444 Lower Extremity: Popliteal Fossa, Deep Arteries (Dissection 4)

445 Lower Extremity: Popliteal Fossa, Femoral–Popliteal–Tibial Arteriogram

446 Anterior Leg, Superficial Vessels and Nerves (Dissection 1)

447 Anterior Leg, Investing Fascia and Muscles (Dissections 2, 3)

448 Compartments of Leg; Muscle Chart, Anterior and Lateral Compartments

449 Anterior Compartment of the Leg: Vessels, Lymphatics, and Muscles

450 Anterior and Lateral Leg: Deep Arteries and Nerves (Dissection 4)

451 Anterior and Lateral Compartments: Deep Muscles (Dissection 5)

452 Lower Extremity: Lateral Compartment of the Leg (Dissection 6)

453 Fibular Nerves; Ankle and Foot Movements

454 Dorsum of the Foot: Superficial Vessels and Nerves (Dissection 1)

455 Dorsum of the Foot: Superficial Muscles and Tendon Sheaths (Dissection 2)

456 Dorsum and Malleolar Regions of the Foot: Tendons and Tendon Sheaths

457 Dorsum of the Foot: Muscles and Tendons (Dissection 3)

458 Dorsum of the Foot: Muscles and Tendons (Dissection 4)

459 Dorsum of the Foot: Deep Vessels and Nerves (Dissection 5)

460 Posterior Leg; Superficial Vessels and Nerves (Dissection 1)

461 Posterior Leg, Crural Fascia; Superficial Muscles (Dissections 2, 3)

462 Knee, Calf, and Foot: Muscles and Tendons (Medial View)

463 Posterior Leg: Soleus and Plantaris Muscles (Dissection 4)

464 Posterior Compartment of the Leg: Soleus Muscle Level (Dissection 5)

465 Posterior Leg: Arteries and Nerves, Deep to Soleus Muscle (Dissection 6)

466 Posterior Compartment of the Leg: Deep Muscle Group (Dissection 7)

467 Posterior Compartment of the Leg: Deep Vessels and Nerves (Dissection 8)

468 Posterior Compartment of the Leg: Attachments of Muscles; Muscle Chart

469 Posterior Leg: Tibialis Posterior and Flexor Hallucis Longus (Dissection 9)

470 Plantar Foot: Aponeurosis, Vessels and Nerves (Dissections 1, 2)

471 Plantar Aspect of the Foot: First Layer of Muscles (Dissection 3)

472 Plantar Aspect of the Foot: Second Layer of Muscles (Dissection 4)

473 Plantar Aspect of the Foot: Plantar Arteries and Nerves (Dissection 5)

474 Plantar Aspect of the Foot: Deep Vessels and Nerves (Dissection 6)

475 Plantar Aspect of the Foot: Third Layer of Plantar Muscles (Dissection 7)

476 Plantar Aspect of the Foot: Diagram of Arteries; Interosseous Muscles

477 Plantar Aspect of the Foot: Chart of Plantar Muscles

478 Bones of Lower Limb: Muscle Attachments; Femur (Anterior View)

479 Bones of Lower Limb: Muscle Attachments; Femur (Posterior View)

480 Joints of Lower Limb: Hip Joint, Ligaments and Frontal Section

481 Joints of Lower Limb: Hip Joint, Frontal Section and Opened Socket

482 The Hip Joint and the Head of the Femur

483 Blood Supply to Upper Femur; Radiograph of Hip Joint

484 Joints of the Lower Limb: Knee Joint, Patellar Structures; Anteroposterior X-Ray

485 Knee Joint: Synovial Folds and Cruciate Ligaments (Anterior View)

486 Right Knee Joint (Frontal Section); Tibial Collateral Ligament

487 Knee Joint (Posterior Superficial View); Internal Ligaments

488 Knee Joint: Transverse and Sagittal Sections

489 Four Magnetic Resonance Images (MRIs) of the Knee Joint

490 Arthrogram of the Right Knee

491 Arthroscopic Images of the Knee Joint

492 Knee Joint: Synovial Cavity and Bursae

493 Radiographs of Knee Joint

494 Knee Joint: Synovial Membranes (Bursae): Movements at Joint

495 Joints of the Lower Limb: Knee Joint, the Menisci; Patella

496 Bones and Joints of the Lower Limb: Tibia and Tibiofibular Joints

497 Bones and Joints of the Lower Limb: Tibia and Fibula

498 Joints of Lower Limb: Talocrural (Ankle) Joint: X-Ray (Coronal Section)

499 Talocrural (Ankle) Joint: Articular Surface (Posterior View)

500 Bones of the Foot and Muscle Attachments (Dorsal View)

501 Bones of the Foot and Muscle Attachments (Plantar View)

502 Bones and Ligaments of the Right Foot (Lateral View)

503 Bones and Ligaments of the Right Foot (Medial View)

504 Talocrural Joint: Sagittal Section of the Foot; Medial Ligaments

505 Talocalcaneonavicular, Intertarsal, and Tarsometatarsal Joints

506 Joints of Lower Limb: Ligaments on the Plantar Surface of the Foot

507 Talocrural Joint: Sagittal Section; Tarsal and Metatarsal Joints

508 Radiograph and MRI of Ankle, Subtalar, and Talocalcaneonavicular Joints

509 Longitudinal Arches of the Foot

510 High Cross Section of the Right Thigh through the Neck of the Femur

511 Cross Section and MRI through the Middle of the Right Thigh

512 Cross Section and MRI through the Distal End of the Right Femur

513 Cross Section and MRI through the Middle of the Right Leg

514 Cross Sections: Lower Right Leg and Proximal Right Foot

515 Cross Section and MRI of the Foot through the Metatarsal Bones

516 Compartments of the Right Foot: Frontal Section, Midmetatarsal Level

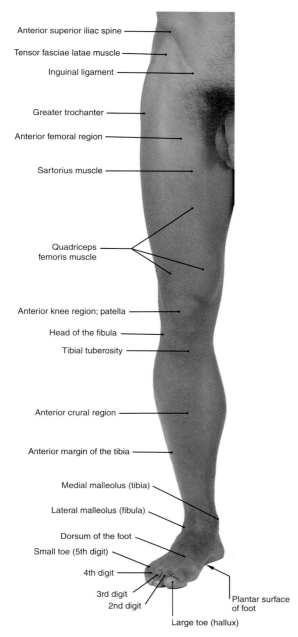

Anterior superior iliac spine

Tensor fasciae latae muscle

Inguinal ligament

Greater trochanter

Anterior femoral region

Sartorius muscle

Quadriceps femoris muscle

Anterior knee region; patella

Head of the fibula

Tibial tuberosity

Anterior crural region

Anterior margin of the tibia

Medial malleolus (tibia)

Lateral malleolus (fibula)

Dorsum of the foot

Small toe (5th digit)

4th digit

3rd digit

2nd digit

Plantar surface of foot

Large toe (hallux)

FIGURE 409.1 **Photograph of the Anterior Surface of the Lower Limb**

NOTE: (1) The following bony landmarks are shown:
   (a) Anterior superior iliac spine
   (b) Greater trochanter
   (c) Patella
   (d) Head of the fibula
   (e) Tibial tuberosity
   (f) Anterior margin of the tibia
   (g) Medial and lateral malleoli
(2) The inguinal ligament, which forms the lower anterior boundary of the abdominal wall, separating it from the anterior thigh inferiorly.
(3) Deep to the surface areas shown in this figure course branches of the cutaneous nerves that supply the anterior and lateral aspects of the thigh and leg and the dorsum of the foot. These branches are shown in Figure 411.1.

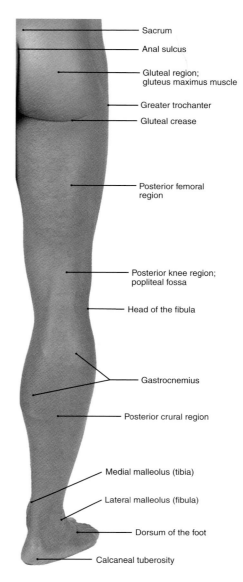

Sacrum

Anal sulcus

Gluteal region; gluteus maximus muscle

Greater trochanter

Gluteal crease

Posterior femoral region

Posterior knee region; popliteal fossa

Head of the fibula

Gastrocnemius

Posterior crural region

Medial malleolus (tibia)

Lateral malleolus (fibula)

Dorsum of the foot

Calcaneal tuberosity

FIGURE 409.2 **Photograph of the Posterior Surface of the Lower Limb**

NOTE: (1) The following bony landmarks are shown:
   (a) Sacrum
   (b) Greater trochanter
   (c) Head of the fibula
   (d) Medial and lateral malleoli
   (e) Calcaneal tuberosity
(2) The **gluteal crease.** Midway between the greater trochanter laterally and the ischial tuberosity medially and deep to this crease is found the large **sciatic nerve** descending in the posterior thigh. **The nerve is vulnerable at this site because only skin and superficial fascia overlie it.**
(3) The **popliteal fossa** located behind the knee joint. Deep to the skin at this site are found the tibial and fibular divisions of the sciatic nerve and the popliteal artery and vein.
(4) The **calcaneal tuberosity** into which inserts the calcaneus tendon formed as the common tendon of the gastrocnemius, soleus, and plantaris muscles.

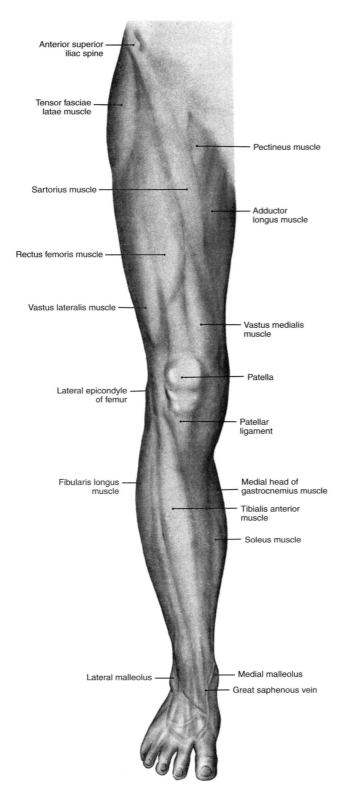

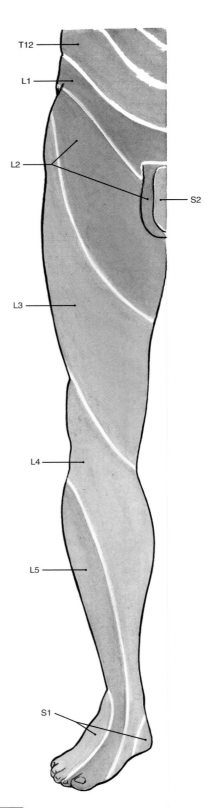

FIGURE 410.1 **Surface Anatomy of the Right Lower Limb (Anterior View)**

NOTE: (1) The pectineus and adductor longus muscles forming the floor of the femoral triangle. Also observe the sartorius muscle coursing inferomedially and the tensor fasciae latae that shapes the rounded upper lateral contour of the thigh.

(2) The leg is shaped laterally by the fibularis muscles, anteriorly by the tibialis anterior, and medially by the gastrocnemius and soleus muscles.

FIGURE 410.2 **Segmental Cutaneous Innervation of the Right Lower Extremity (Dermatomes: Anterior View)**

NOTE: (1) As a rule, the lumbar segments of the spinal cord supply cutaneous innervation to the anterior aspect of the lower limb, and the dermatomes are segmentally arranged in order from L1 to L5.

(2) The first sacral segment supplies the skin over the medial malleolus and the dorsolateral aspect of the foot.

Chapter 6 The Lower Limb

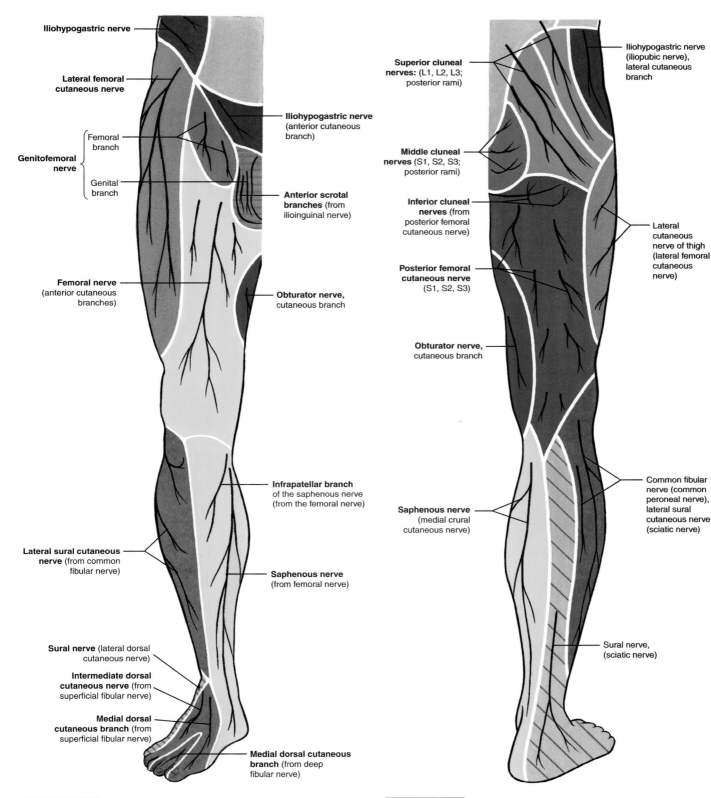

FIGURE 411.1 Cutaneous Nerve Branches (Anterior Surface)

NOTE: (1) Cutaneous branches of the femoral nerve supply the skin of the anteromedial thigh, and the **saphenous nerve** supplies the anteromedial and posteromedial leg.

(2) The **lateral sural branch** of the **common fibular nerve** supplies the anterolateral and posterolateral leg skin.

(3) The fields supplied by the **superficial and deep fibular nerves** on the anterior leg and foot dorsum.

(4) The knowledge of the course of these nerves is important in administering local anesthesia.

FIGURE 411.2 Cutaneous Nerve Branches (Posterior Surface)

NOTE: (1) Cutaneous innervation of the gluteal region:
  (a) Lateral branch of **iliohypogastric nerve** (anterior ramus: L1)
  (b) **Superior cluneal nerves** (posterior rami: L1–L3)
  (c) Middle cluneal nerves (posterior rami: S1–S3)
  (d) Inferior cluneal nerves (S1–S3)

(2) Skin of posterior thigh supplied by the **posterior and lateral femoral cutaneous nerves** and **obturator nerve.**

(3) Skin of posterior leg supplied the **saphenous, sural,** and **lateral sural nerves.**

Chapter 6 The Lower Limb

PLATE 412 Bones and Joints of the Lower Extremity

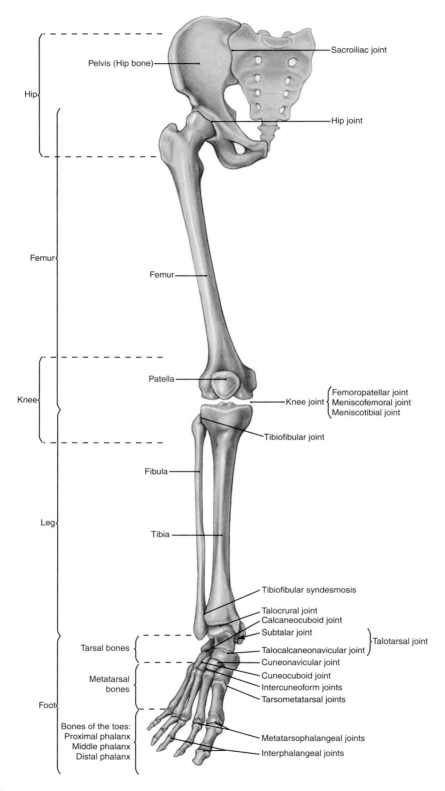

Sacroiliac joint

Pelvis (Hip bone)

Hip

Hip joint

Femur

Femur

Patella

Knee

Knee joint
- Femoropatellar joint
- Meniscofemoral joint
- Meniscotibial joint

Tibiofibular joint

Fibula

Leg

Tibia

Tibiofibular syndesmosis

Talocrural joint

Calcaneocuboid joint

Subtalar joint

Talotarsal joint

Tarsal bones

Talocalcaneonavicular joint

Cuneonavicular joint

Metatarsal bones

Cuneocuboid joint

Intercuneoform joints

Tarsometatarsal joints

Foot

Bones of the toes:
Proximal phalanx
Middle phalanx
Distal phalanx

Metatarsophalangeal joints

Interphalangeal joints

FIGURE 412 Bones and Joints of the Lower Limb

NOTE the following joints: **hip, knee, tibiofibular, ankle (talocrural), tarsal, tarsometatarsal, metatarsophalangeal, and interphalangeal joints.**

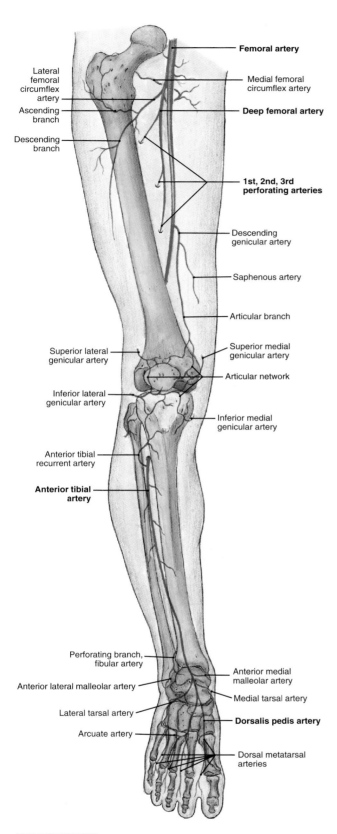

Femoral artery

Lateral femoral circumflex artery

Ascending branch

Descending branch

Medial femoral circumflex artery

Deep femoral artery

1st, 2nd, 3rd perforating arteries

Descending genicular artery

Saphenous artery

Articular branch

Superior lateral genicular artery

Superior medial genicular artery

Articular network

Inferior lateral genicular artery

Inferior medial genicular artery

Anterior tibial recurrent artery

Anterior tibial artery

Perforating branch, fibular artery

Anterior lateral malleolar artery

Anterior medial malleolar artery

Medial tarsal artery

Lateral tarsal artery

Dorsalis pedis artery

Arcuate artery

Dorsal metatarsal arteries

FIGURE 413.1 Arteries and Bones of the Lower Limb (Anterior View)

NOTE: The anastomoses in the hip and knee regions, and the **perforating branches** of the **deep femoral artery.** In the anterior leg, the **anterior tibial artery** descends between the tibia and the fibula to achieve the malleolar region and the foot dorsum.

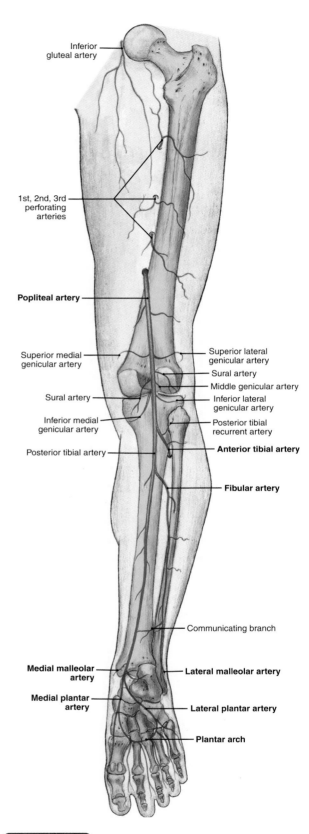

Inferior gluteal artery

1st, 2nd, 3rd perforating arteries

Popliteal artery

Superior medial genicular artery

Superior lateral genicular artery

Sural artery

Middle genicular artery

Sural artery

Inferior lateral genicular artery

Inferior medial genicular artery

Posterior tibial recurrent artery

Posterior tibial artery

Anterior tibial artery

Fibular artery

Communicating branch

Medial malleolar artery

Lateral malleolar artery

Medial plantar artery

Lateral plantar artery

Plantar arch

FIGURE 413.2 Arteries and Bones of the Lower Limb (Posterior View)

NOTE: The branches of the **popliteal artery** at the knee and its continuation as the **posterior tibial artery.** In the foot this vessel divides to form the **medial** and **lateral plantar arteries,** which then anastomose to form the **plantar arch.**

PLATE 414 Muscles and Fasciae on the Anterior Aspect of the Lower Limb

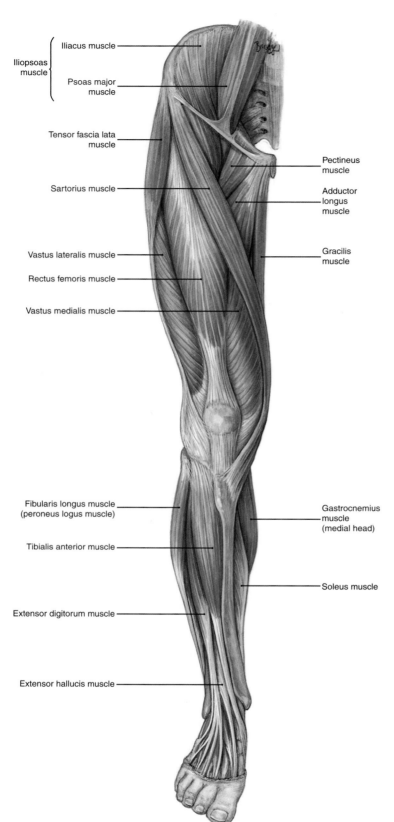

Iliopsoas muscle
- Iliacus muscle
- Psoas major muscle

Tensor fascia lata muscle

Sartorius muscle

Vastus lateralis muscle

Rectus femoris muscle

Vastus medialis muscle

Pectineus muscle

Adductor longus muscle

Gracilis muscle

Fibularis longus muscle (peroneus logus muscle)

Tibialis anterior muscle

Extensor digitorum muscle

Extensor hallucis muscle

Gastrocnemius muscle (medial head)

Soleus muscle

FIGURE 414.1 **Muscles of the Lower Limb**

NOTE the anterior and medial thigh muscles and also the anterior and lateral muscles of the leg.

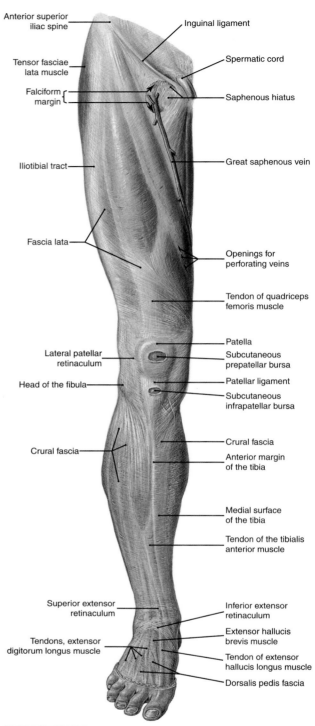

Anterior superior iliac spine

Tensor fasciae lata muscle

Falciform margin

Iliotibial tract

Fascia lata

Lateral patellar retinaculum

Head of the fibula

Crural fascia

Superior extensor retinaculum

Tendons, extensor digitorum longus muscle

Inguinal ligament

Spermatic cord

Saphenous hiatus

Great saphenous vein

Openings for perforating veins

Tendon of quadriceps femoris muscle

Patella

Subcutaneous prepatellar bursa

Patellar ligament

Subcutaneous infrapatellar bursa

Crural fascia

Anterior margin of the tibia

Medial surface of the tibia

Tendon of the tibialis anterior muscle

Inferior extensor retinaculum

Extensor hallucis brevis muscle

Tendon of extensor hallucis longus muscle

Dorsalis pedis fascia

FIGURE 414.2 **The Deep Fasciae of the Anterior and Medial Thigh (Fascia Lata) and the Crural Fascia of the Leg**

NOTE the great saphenous vein, the saphenous hiatus, and the fascia lata of the anterior thigh. Observe the closely investing crural fascia over the anterior and lateral compartment muscles of the leg.

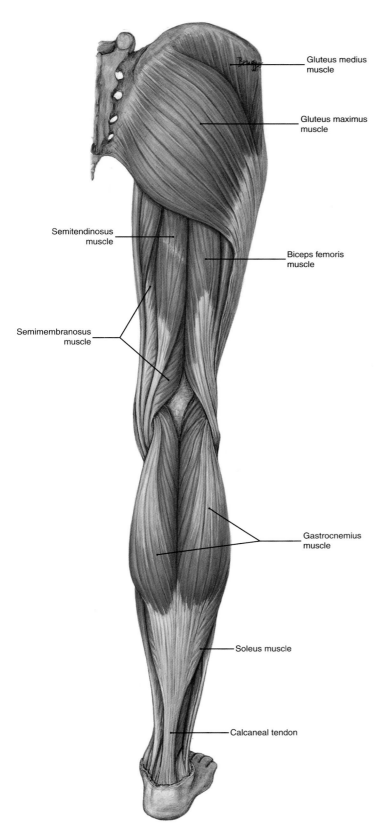

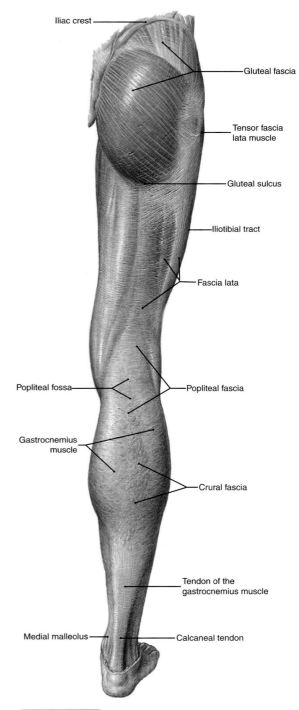

FIGURE 415.1 **Muscles of the Lower Limb: Posterior Aspect of Thigh and Leg**

NOTE the hamstring muscles of the posterior thigh and the gastrocnemius and soleus muscles of the posterior leg.

FIGURE 415.2 **Fascia of the Gluteal Region and the Fascia Lata of the Posterior Thigh and Crural Fascia of the Posterior Leg**

NOTE the iliac crest, gluteal sulcus, iliotibial band, and the crural fascia below the knee.

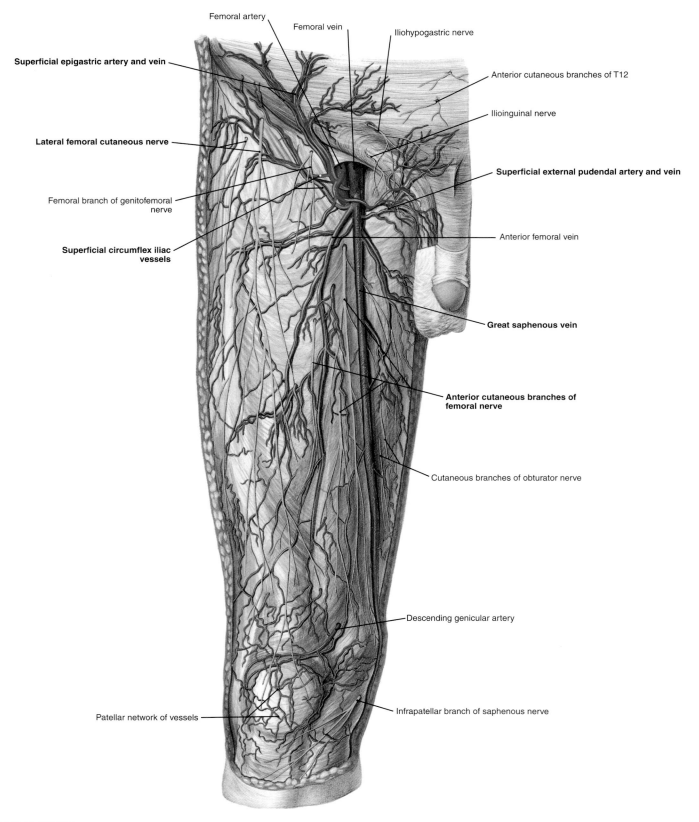

Femoral artery

Femoral vein

Iliohypogastric nerve

Superficial epigastric artery and vein

Anterior cutaneous branches of T12

Ilioinguinal nerve

Lateral femoral cutaneous nerve

Superficial external pudendal artery and vein

Femoral branch of genitofemoral nerve

Anterior femoral vein

Superficial circumflex iliac vessels

Great saphenous vein

Anterior cutaneous branches of femoral nerve

Cutaneous branches of obturator nerve

Descending genicular artery

Patellar network of vessels

Infrapatellar branch of saphenous nerve

FIGURE 416 Superficial Nerves and Blood Vessels of the Anterior Thigh

NOTE: (1) The **great saphenous vein** as it ascends the anterior and medial aspect of the thigh. Just below (1½ in.) the inguinal ligament, it penetrates the deep fascia through the **saphenous opening** to enter the **femoral vein.**

(2) The superficial branches of the **femoral artery** and the superficial veins drain into the **great saphenous vein.** These include the: (a) **superficial epigastric,** (b) **external pudendal,** and (c) **superficial circumflex iliac** arteries and veins.

(3) The principal cutaneous nerves of the anterior thigh. Compare these with those shown in Figure 411.1.

◄ **FIGURE 417.1** Superficial Inguinal Lymph Nodes

NOTE: (1) The superficial tissues of the genitalia, lower anterior abdominal wall, inguinal region, and anterior thigh drain into the **superficial inguinal lymphatic nodes.**

(2) These nodes are located around the femoral vessels just inferior to the inguinal ligament and usually number between 10 and 15. In turn, these nodes drain into the external iliac nodes within the pelvis.

Labels for top-left figure: Inguinal ligament, Superficial circumflex iliac vein, Great saphenous vein, Superficial epigastric vein, Superficial inguinal nodes, Spermatic cord, Superficial external pudendal veins, Accessory saphenous vein, Great saphenous vein, Adductor longus

FIGURE 417.2 Saphenous Opening in the ► Fascia Lata

NOTE: (1) The *femoral sheath* (dense connective tissue that surrounds the femoral artery and vein) has been removed in this dissection, revealing the sharply defined **falciform margin** of the **saphenous opening.**

(2) The great saphenous vein receives its superficial tributaries before it enters the saphenous opening.

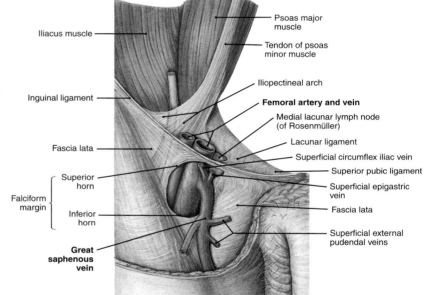

Labels: Iliacus muscle, Inguinal ligament, Fascia lata, Superior horn, Inferior horn, Falciform margin, **Great saphenous vein**, Psoas major muscle, Tendon of psoas minor muscle, Iliopectineal arch, **Femoral artery and vein**, Medial lacunar lymph node (of Rosenmüller), Lacunar ligament, Superficial circumflex iliac vein, Superior pubic ligament, Superficial epigastric vein, Fascia lata, Superficial external pudendal veins

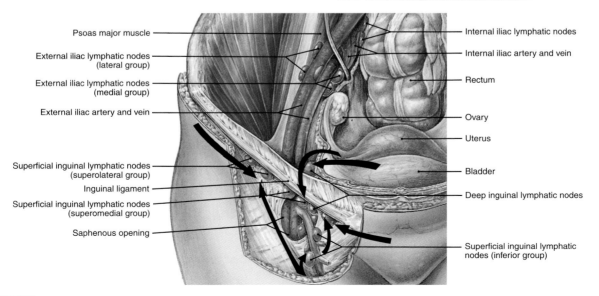

Labels: Psoas major muscle, External iliac lymphatic nodes (lateral group), External iliac lymphatic nodes (medial group), External iliac artery and vein, Superficial inguinal lymphatic nodes (superolateral group), Inguinal ligament, Superficial inguinal lymphatic nodes (superomedial group), Saphenous opening, Internal iliac lymphatic nodes, Internal iliac artery and vein, Rectum, Ovary, Uterus, Bladder, Deep inguinal lymphatic nodes, Superficial inguinal lymphatic nodes (inferior group)

FIGURE 417.3 Superficial and Deep Inguinal Lymphatic Nodes

NOTE: The directions of flow (arrows) of lymph from adjacent tissues into the superficial and deep inguinal nodes. The superficial nodes are divided into superolateral, superomedial, and inferomedial groups, while the deep nodes are closest to the femoral vessels.

Chapter 6 The Lower Limb

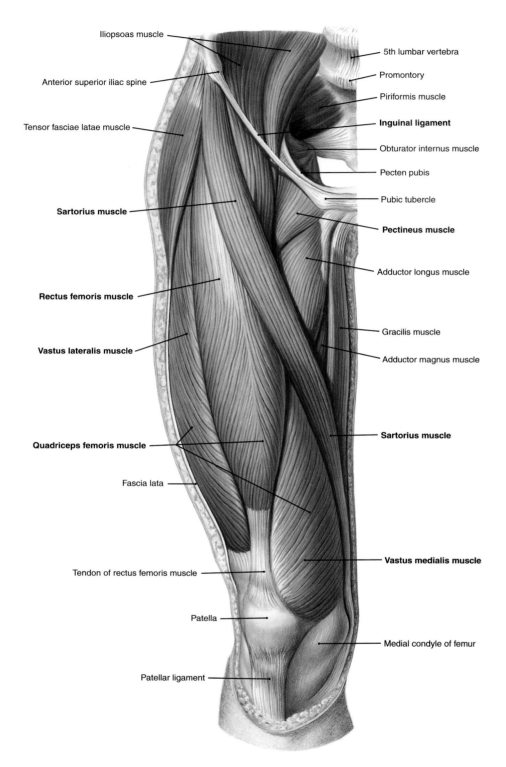

Iliopsoas muscle

Anterior superior iliac spine

Tensor fasciae latae muscle

Sartorius muscle

Rectus femoris muscle

Vastus lateralis muscle

Quadriceps femoris muscle

Fascia lata

Tendon of rectus femoris muscle

Patella

Patellar ligament

5th lumbar vertebra

Promontory

Piriformis muscle

Inguinal ligament

Obturator internus muscle

Pecten pubis

Pubic tubercle

Pectineus muscle

Adductor longus muscle

Gracilis muscle

Adductor magnus muscle

Sartorius muscle

Vastus medialis muscle

Medial condyle of femur

FIGURE 418 **Anterior Muscles of the Thigh: Superficial View (Right)**

NOTE: (1) The long narrow **sartorius muscle,** which arises on the anterior superior iliac spine and passes obliquely across the anterior femoral muscles to insert on the medial aspect of the body of the tibia. The sartorius flexes, abducts, and rotates the thigh laterally at the hip joint, and it flexes and rotates the leg medially at the knee joint.

(2) The **quadriceps femoris muscle** forms the bulk of the anterior femoral muscles, and both the sartorius and quadriceps muscles are innervated by the femoral nerve.

(3) Above and medial to the sartorius muscle are visible, in order, the iliopsoas, pectineus, adductor longus, adductor magnus, and gracilis muscles.

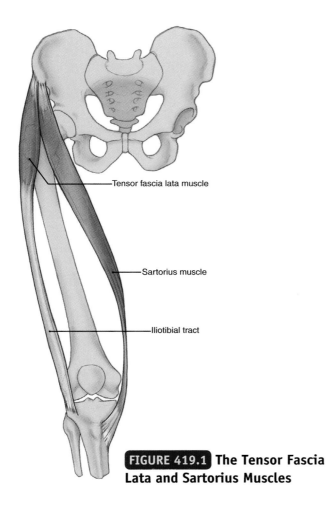

FIGURE 419.1 The Tensor Fascia Lata and Sartorius Muscles

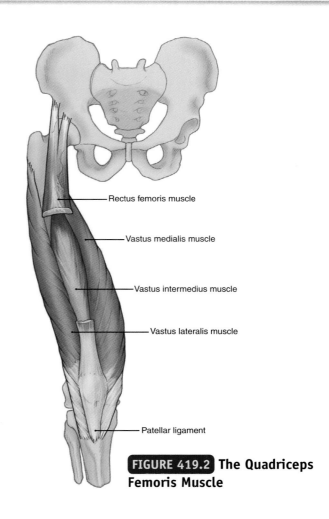

FIGURE 419.2 The Quadriceps Femoris Muscle

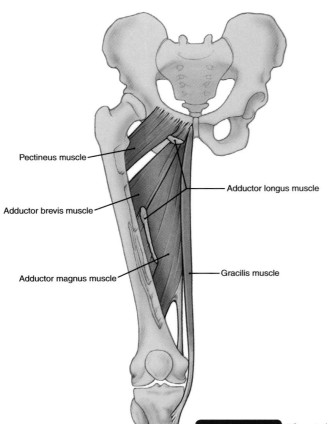

FIGURE 419.3 The Adductor Muscles and the Pectineus and Gracilis Muscles

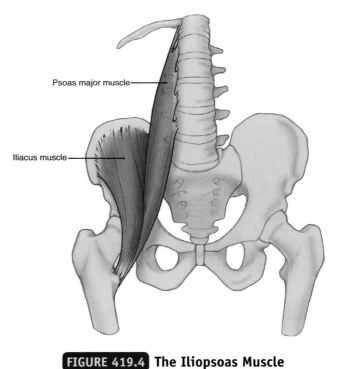

FIGURE 419.4 The Iliopsoas Muscle

PLATE 420 Lower Extremity: Anterior Thigh Muscles (Dissection 4)

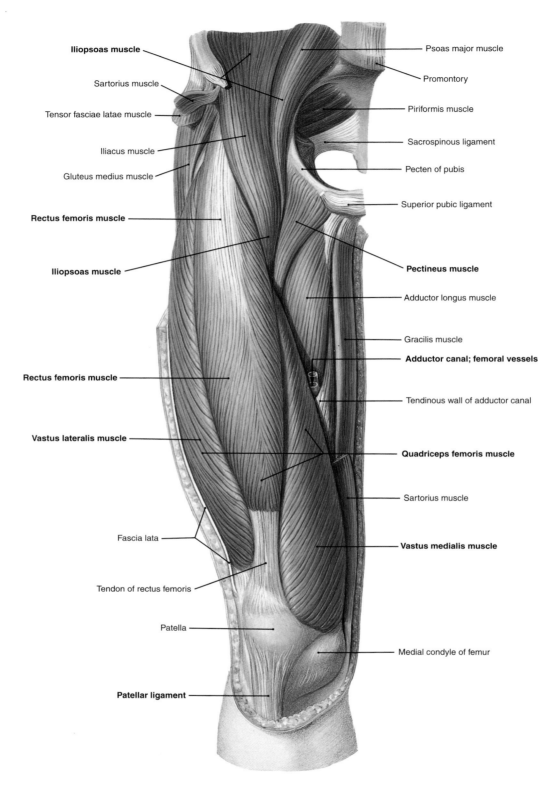

Iliopsoas muscle

Sartorius muscle

Tensor fasciae latae muscle

Iliacus muscle

Gluteus medius muscle

Rectus femoris muscle

Iliopsoas muscle

Rectus femoris muscle

Vastus lateralis muscle

Fascia lata

Tendon of rectus femoris

Patella

Patellar ligament

Psoas major muscle

Promontory

Piriformis muscle

Sacrospinous ligament

Pecten of pubis

Superior pubic ligament

Pectineus muscle

Adductor longus muscle

Gracilis muscle

Adductor canal; femoral vessels

Tendinous wall of adductor canal

Quadriceps femoris muscle

Sartorius muscle

Vastus medialis muscle

Medial condyle of femur

FIGURE 420 Quadriceps Femoris, Iliopsoas, and Pectineus Muscles

NOTE: (1) The **quadriceps femoris muscle** consists of the rectus femoris and the three vastus muscles (lateralis, intermedius, and medialis) as it converges inferiorly to form a powerful tendon that encases the patella and inserts onto the **tuberosity of the tibia.** The entire quadriceps extends the leg at the knee, while the rectus femoris also flexes the thigh at the hip.

(2) The **iliopsoas muscle** is the most powerful flexor of the thigh at the hip joint, and it inserts on the **lesser trochanter.**

(3) The quadrangular and flat **pectineus muscle** medial to the iliopsoas. Sometimes called the key to the femoral triangle, this muscle is normally supplied by the femoral nerve, but in slightly over 10% of cases it also receives a branch from one of the obturator nerves.

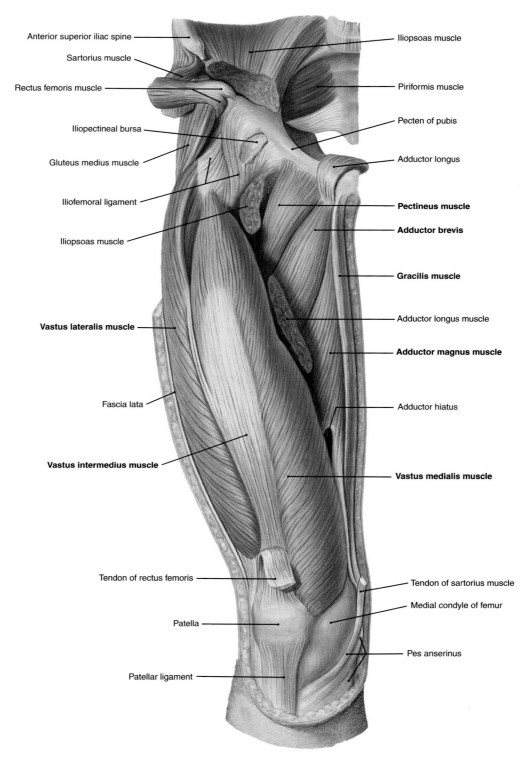

Anterior superior iliac spine

Sartorius muscle

Rectus femoris muscle

Iliopectineal bursa

Gluteus medius muscle

Iliofemoral ligament

Iliopsoas muscle

Vastus lateralis muscle

Fascia lata

Vastus intermedius muscle

Tendon of rectus femoris

Patella

Patellar ligament

Iliopsoas muscle

Piriformis muscle

Pecten of pubis

Adductor longus

Pectineus muscle

Adductor brevis

Gracilis muscle

Adductor longus muscle

Adductor magnus muscle

Adductor hiatus

Vastus medialis muscle

Tendon of sartorius muscle

Medial condyle of femur

Pes anserinus

[FIGURE 421] **Intermediate Layer of Anterior and Medial Thigh Muscles**

NOTE: (1) The **rectus femoris** and **iliopsoas muscles** are cut to expose the underlying **vastus intermedius,** situated between the **vastus lateralis** and the **vastus medialis.**

(2) The **adductor longus** has also been reflected. This displays the **pectineus, adductor brevis,** and **magnus muscles** and the long **gracilis muscle.**

(3) The quadriceps femoris is the most powerful extensor of the leg. During extension, however, there is a natural tendency to displace the patella laterally out of its groove on the patellar surface of the femur because of the natural angulation of the femur with respect to the bones of the leg.

(4) The muscle fibers of the **vastus medialis** descend further inferiorly than those of the vastus lateralis, and the lowest fibers insert directly along the medial border of the patella. The medial pull of these fibers is thought to be essential in maintaining the stability of the patella on the femur.

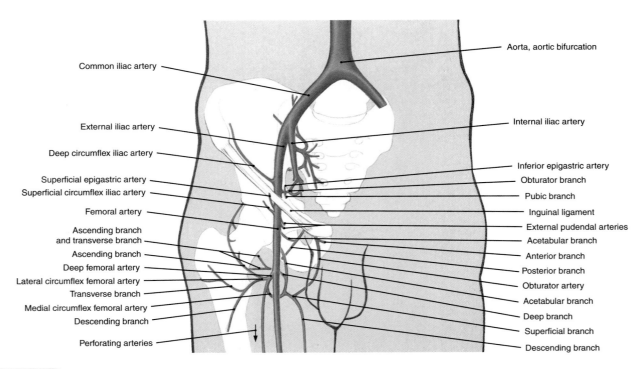

Common iliac artery

External iliac artery

Deep circumflex iliac artery

Superficial epigastric artery
Superficial circumflex iliac artery

Femoral artery

Ascending branch
and transverse branch

Ascending branch
Deep femoral artery
Lateral circumflex femoral artery
Transverse branch
Medial circumflex femoral artery
Descending branch

Perforating arteries

Aorta, aortic bifurcation

Internal iliac artery

Inferior epigastric artery
Obturator branch
Pubic branch
Inguinal ligament
External pudendal arteries
Acetabular branch
Anterior branch
Posterior branch
Obturator artery
Acetabular branch
Deep branch
Superficial branch
Descending branch

FIGURE 422.1 **Arteries of the Right Hip Region and the Thigh**

NOTE: (1) The branching pattern of the deep femoral artery (profundus femoris) shown in this drawing is observed in 55% to 60% of cases studied.
(2) A number of the branches of the internal iliac artery are not labeled in this figure, but these can be seen in Figures 339 and 340.

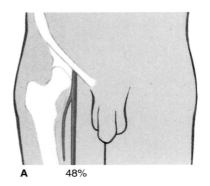 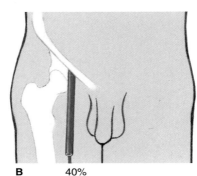 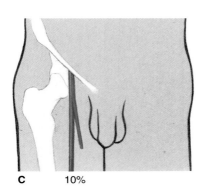

A   48%   B   40%   C   10%

FIGURE 422.2 **Variations in the Position of the Deep Femoral Artery**

NOTE: (1) In **A,** the vessel is lateral or lateral and dorsal to the femoral artery.
(2) In **B,** the vessel is posterior to the femoral artery.
(3) In **C,** the vessel is medial to the femoral artery.

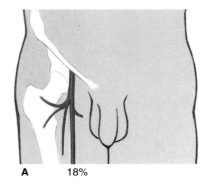 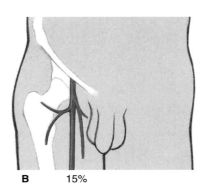

A   18%   B   15%

FIGURE 422.3 **Variations in the Origins of the Femoral Circumflex Arteries**

NOTE: (1) In **A,** the separate origin of the medial femoral circumflex artery is shown.
(2) In **B,** the separate origin of the lateral femoral circumflex artery is shown.

Chapter 6 The Lower Limb

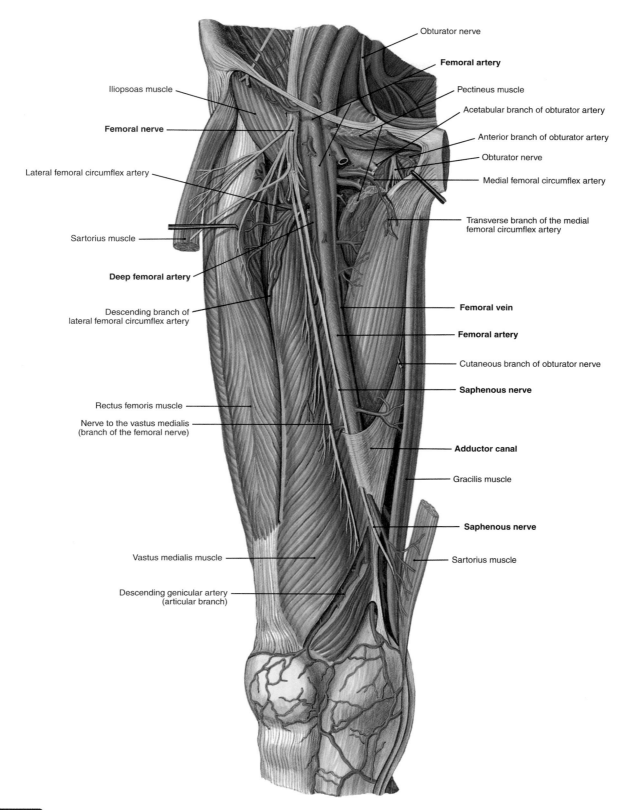

Obturator nerve

Femoral artery

Pectineus muscle

Acetabular branch of obturator artery

Anterior branch of obturator artery

Obturator nerve

Medial femoral circumflex artery

Transverse branch of the medial femoral circumflex artery

Femoral vein

Femoral artery

Cutaneous branch of obturator nerve

Saphenous nerve

Adductor canal

Gracilis muscle

Saphenous nerve

Sartorius muscle

Iliopsoas muscle

Femoral nerve

Lateral femoral circumflex artery

Sartorius muscle

Deep femoral artery

Descending branch of lateral femoral circumflex artery

Rectus femoris muscle

Nerve to the vastus medialis (branch of the femoral nerve)

Vastus medialis muscle

Descending genicular artery (articular branch)

FIGURE 423 **Femoral Vessels and Nerves**

NOTE: (1) The femoral vessels, the saphenous branch of the femoral nerve, and the nerve to the vastus medialis all enter the **adductor canal (of Hunter).**

(2) The **saphenous nerve,** after coursing some distance in the canal, penetrates the overlying fascia to reach the superficial leg region; the **nerve to the vastus medialis** traverses the more proximal part of the canal and then divides into muscular branches to supply the vastus medialis muscle.

(3) The **femoral artery and vein** course through the entire canal and then leave it by way of an opening in the adductor magnus muscle called the **adductor hiatus.** The vessels course to the back of the lower limb to become the **popliteal artery and vein.**

PLATE 424 Anterior and Medial Thigh Muscles, Deep Layer (Dissection 7)

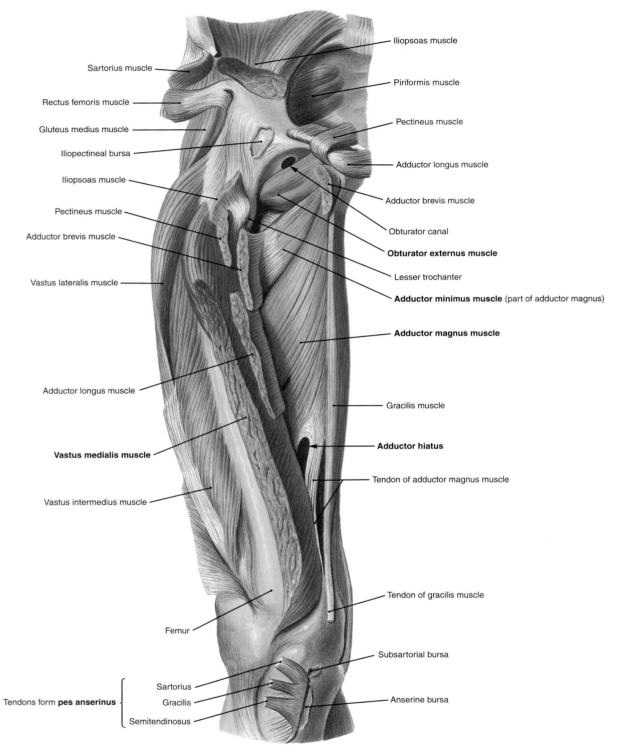

Sartorius muscle

Rectus femoris muscle

Gluteus medius muscle

Iliopectineal bursa

Iliopsoas muscle

Pectineus muscle

Adductor brevis muscle

Vastus lateralis muscle

Adductor longus muscle

Vastus medialis muscle

Vastus intermedius muscle

Femur

Tendons form **pes anserinus**
Sartorius
Gracilis
Semitendinosus

Iliopsoas muscle

Piriformis muscle

Pectineus muscle

Adductor longus muscle

Obturator canal

Obturator externus muscle

Lesser trochanter

Adductor minimus muscle (part of adductor magnus)

Adductor magnus muscle

Gracilis muscle

Adductor hiatus

Tendon of adductor magnus muscle

Tendon of gracilis muscle

Subsartorial bursa

Anserine bursa

FIGURE 424 **Deep Layer of Anterior and Medial Thigh Muscles (Right)**

NOTE: (1) The rectus femoris and vastus medialis have been removed, thereby exposing the shaft of the femur. Likewise, the adductor longus and brevis and the pectineus muscles have been reflected, exposing the **obturator externus,** the **adductor magnus,** and the **adductor minimus** (which usually is just the upper portion of the adductor magnus).

(2) The common insertion of the tendons of the **sartorius, gracilis,** and **semitendinosus muscles** on the medial aspect of the medial condyle of the tibia. The divergent nature of this insertion resembles a goose's foot (pes anserinus). This tendinous formation can be used by surgeons to strengthen the medial aspect of the capsule of the knee joint.

(3) The tendinous opening on the adductor magnus, called the **adductor hiatus,** through which the femoral vessels course to (or from) the popliteal fossa.

(4) The **obturator externus muscle** stretching across the inferior surface of the obturator membrane to insert laterally on the neck of the femur. This muscle rotates the femur laterally, and it is not part of the adductor group of muscles.

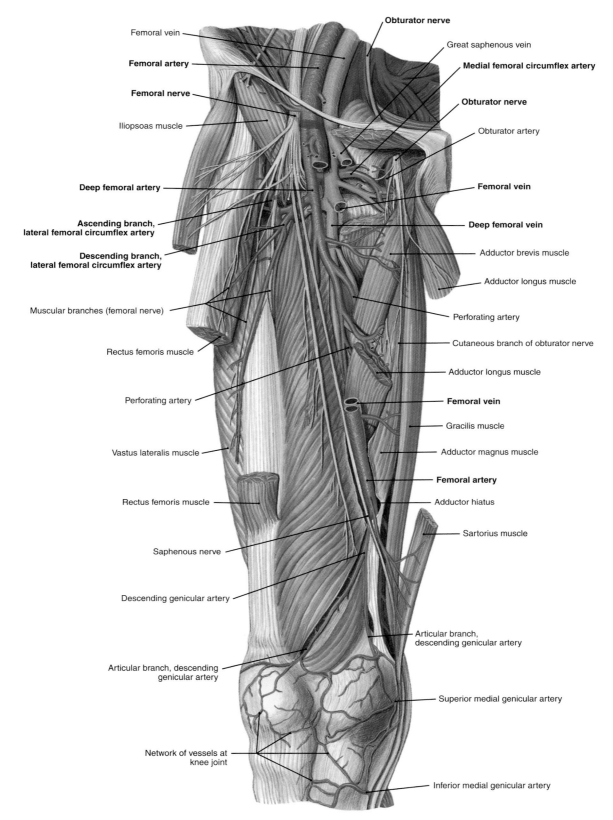

Obturator nerve

Femoral vein

Great saphenous vein

Femoral artery

Medial femoral circumflex artery

Femoral nerve

Obturator nerve

Iliopsoas muscle

Obturator artery

Deep femoral artery

Femoral vein

Ascending branch, lateral femoral circumflex artery

Deep femoral vein

Adductor brevis muscle

Descending branch, lateral femoral circumflex artery

Adductor longus muscle

Muscular branches (femoral nerve)

Perforating artery

Cutaneous branch of obturator nerve

Rectus femoris muscle

Adductor longus muscle

Perforating artery

Femoral vein

Gracilis muscle

Vastus lateralis muscle

Adductor magnus muscle

Femoral artery

Rectus femoris muscle

Adductor hiatus

Sartorius muscle

Saphenous nerve

Descending genicular artery

Articular branch, descending genicular artery

Articular branch, descending genicular artery

Superior medial genicular artery

Network of vessels at knee joint

Inferior medial genicular artery

FIGURE 425 Femoral and Obturator Nerves and Deep Femoral Artery

NOTE: (1) The **obturator nerve** supplies the adductor muscles, the gracilis, and the obturator externus while the femoral nerve innervates all the other anterior thigh muscles.

(2) The **deep femoral artery** is the largest branch of the femoral artery, and it gives off both the **medial** and **lateral femoral circumflex arteries**. Observe the femoral vessels traversing the femoral canal.

(3) In about 50% of cases, the deep femoral artery branches from the lateral side of the femoral artery; in 40%, it branches from the posterior aspect of the femoral artery and courses behind it; and in 10%, the deep femoral artery arises from the medial side of the femoral artery.

PLATE 426 Lower Extremity: Anterior Thigh, Movements and Muscle Chart

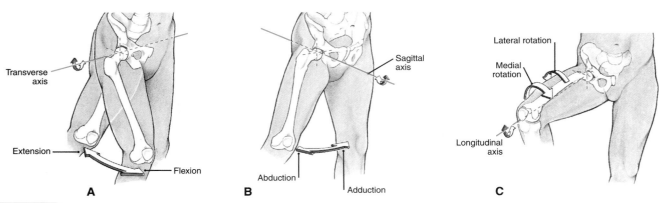

FIGURE 426 Movements of the Thigh at the Hip Joint

In **A, flexion** and **extension** occur through the transverse axis of the hip joint.
In **B, abduction** and **adduction** occur through the sagittal axis of the hip joint.
In **C, medial rotation** and **lateral rotation** occur around the longitudinal axis of the hip joint.

ANTERIOR MUSCLES OF THE HIP				
Muscle	**Origin**	**Insertion**	**Innervation**	**Action**
Rectus femoris head of the quadriceps femoris	Straight head: Anterior inferior iliac spine Reflected head: The groove above the acetabulum	With the other three parts of the quadriceps femoris, the rectus forms a common tendon that encases the patella and inserts onto the tibial tuberosity	Femoral nerve (L2, L3, L4)	All four parts extend the leg at the knee joint; the rectus femoris also helps flex the thigh at the hip joint
Psoas major	Transverse process and body of T12 and upper four lumbar vertebrae; intervertebral disks between T12 and L5	Lesser trochanter of femur (also receives the fibers of iliacus muscle)	Branches from upper four lumbar nerves	Powerful flexor of thigh at hip; when femurs are fixed, they flex the trunk, as in sitting up from a supine position
Psoas minor (muscle present in about 40% of cadavers)	Lateral surface of bodies of T12 and L1 vertebrae	Pectineal line and iliopectineal eminence and the iliac fascia (often merges with psoas major tendon)	Branch from L1 nerve	Weak flexor of the trunk
Iliacus	Iliac fossa; anterior inferior iliac spine	Lesser trochanter of femur in common with tendon of psoas major muscle	Femoral nerve (L2, L3)	Powerful flexor of thigh at the hip joint

ANTERIOR THIGH MUSCLES				
Muscle	**Origin**	**Insertion**	**Innervation**	**Action**
Sartorius	Anterior superior iliac spine	Superior part of the medial surface of the tibia	Femoral nerve (L2, L3)	Flexes, abducts, and laterally rotates the thigh at the hip joint; flexes and medially rotates the leg at the knee joint
Quadriceps femoris muscle **Rectus femoris**	Straight head: Anterior inferior iliac spine Reflected head: the groove above the acetabulum	All four parts of the quadriceps femoris form a common tendon that encases the patella and finally inserts onto the tibial tuberosity	Femoral nerve (L2, L3, L4)	All four parts extend the leg at the knee joint; the rectus femoris also helps flex the thigh at the hip joint
Vastus medialis	Intertrochanteric line and the medial lip of the linea aspera on the femur			
Vastus lateralis	Greater trochanter and the lateral lip of the linea aspera			
Vastus intermedius	Anterior and lateral surface of the body of the femur			
Articularis genu	Anterior surface of the lower part of the femur	Upper part of the synovial membrane of the knee joint	Femoral nerve (L2, L3, L4)	Draws the synovial membrane upward during extension of the leg to prevent its compression

MEDIAL THIGH MUSCLES

Muscle	Origin	Insertion	Innervation	Action
Pectineus	Pectineal line of the pubis	Along the pectineal line of the femur, between the lesser trochanter and the linea aspera	Femoral nerve (L2, L3); may also receive a branch from the obturator or the accessory obturator nerve when present	Flexes, adducts, and medially rotates the femur
Adductor longus	From the anterior pubis, where the pubic crest joins the symphysis pubis	Middle third of the femur along the linea aspera	Obturator nerve (L2, L3, L4)	Adducts, flexes, and medially rotates the femur
Adductor brevis	Outer surface of the inferior pubic ramus between the gracilis and the obturator externus	Along the pectineal line of the femur and the upper part of the linea aspera behind the pectineus	Obturator nerve (L2, L3, L4)	Adducts, flexes, and medially rotates the femur
Adductor magnus	Inferior ramus of pubis; ramus of the ischium and the ischial tuberosity	Medial lip of the upper two-thirds of the linea aspera; the medial supracondylar line and the adductor tubercle	Obturator nerve (L2, L3, L4): sciatic nerve (tibial division) for the hamstring part of the muscle	Powerful adductor of the thigh; upper part flexes and medially rotates the thigh; lower part extends and laterally rotates the thigh
Adductor minimus	The upper more horizontal part of the adductor magnus, which receives the name adductor minimus when it forms a distinct muscle			
Gracilis	From the body of the pubis and the adjacent inferior pubic ramus	Upper part of the medial surface of the tibia below the medial condyle	Obturator nerve (L2, L3)	Adducts the thigh; also flexes the leg at the knee and medially rotates the leg
Obturator externus	Medial part of the outer surface of obturator membrane and medial margin of obturator foramen	Trochanteric fossa of the femur	Obturator nerve (L3, L4)	Laterally rotates the thigh

LATERAL THIGH MUSCLE

Muscle	Origin	Insertion	Innervation	Action
Tensor fasciae latae	Outer lip of the iliac crest; also from the anterior superior iliac spine	Iliotibial tract, which then descends to attach to the lateral condyle of the tibia	Superior gluteal nerve (L4, L5)	Abducts, flexes, and medially rotates the thigh; tenses the iliotibial tract, thereby helping extend the leg at the knee

POSTERIOR THIGH MUSCLES

Muscle	Origin	Insertion	Innervation	Action
Biceps femoris	Long head: Ischial tuberosity in common with other hamstring muscles, Short head: Lateral lip of the linea aspera of the femur	Lateral surface of the head of the fibula and a small slip to lateral condyle of the tibia	Long head: Tibial part of sciatic nerve (S1, S2, S3) Short head: Common fibular part sciatic nerve (L5, S1, S2)	Flexes the leg and rotates the tibia laterally; long head also extends the thigh at the hip joint
Semitendinosus	Ischial tuberosity in common with other hamstring muscles	Medial surface of the upper part of the body of the tibia	Tibial part of the sciatic nerve (L5, S1, S2)	Flexes the leg and rotates the tibia medially; extends the thigh
Semimembranosus	Ischial tuberosity in common with other hamstring muscles	Posterior aspect of the medial condyle of the tibia	Tibial part of the sciatic nerve (L5, S1, S2)	Flexes the leg and rotates it medially; extends the thigh

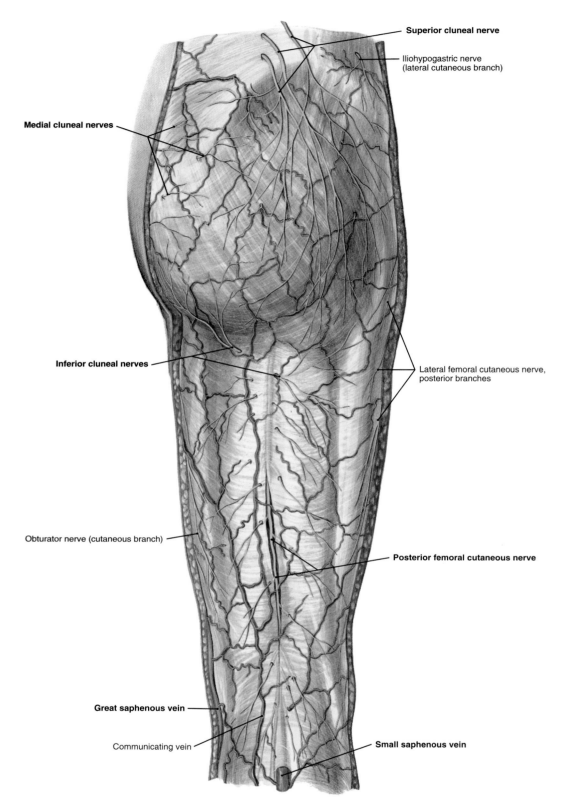

Superior cluneal nerve

Iliohypogastric nerve
(lateral cutaneous branch)

Medial cluneal nerves

Inferior cluneal nerves

Lateral femoral cutaneous nerve,
posterior branches

Obturator nerve (cutaneous branch)

Posterior femoral cutaneous nerve

Great saphenous vein

Communicating vein

Small saphenous vein

FIGURE 428 Superficial Veins and Nerves of the Gluteal Region and Posterior Thigh

NOTE: (1) The principal cutaneous nerves supplying the **gluteal region** are the:
    (a) **Superior cluneal nerves** (from the posterior primary rami of L1, L2, L3),
    (b) **Medial cluneal nerves** (from the posterior primary rami of S1, S2, S3), and
    (c) **Inferior cluneal nerves** (from the posterior femoral cutaneous nerve: anterior primary rami of S1, S2, S3).
(2) The skin of the **posterior thigh** is supplied primarily by the **posterior femoral cutaneous nerve (S1, S2, S3),** but posterolaterally it also
    receives branches from the lateral femoral cutaneous nerve, and posteromedially, cutaneous branches from the obturator nerve.

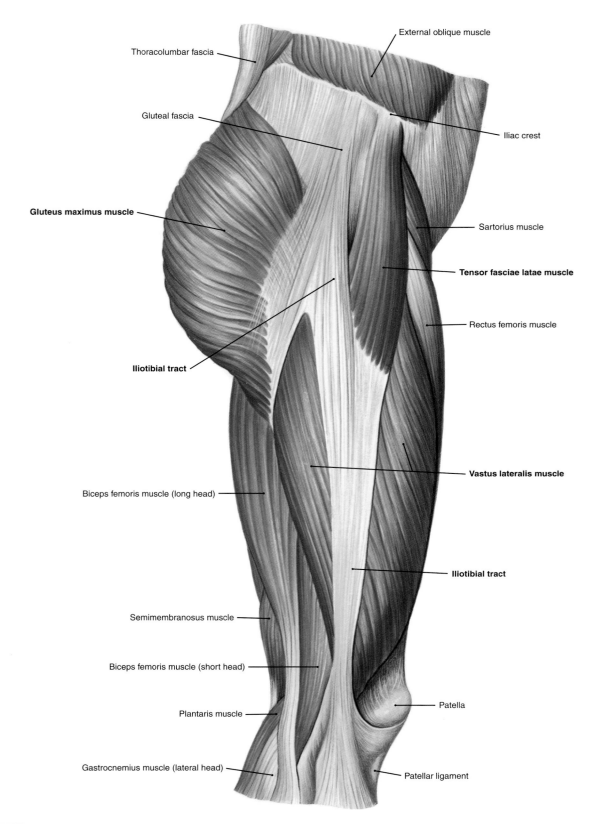

External oblique muscle

Thoracolumbar fascia

Gluteal fascia

Iliac crest

Gluteus maximus muscle

Sartorius muscle

Tensor fasciae latae muscle

Rectus femoris muscle

Iliotibial tract

Vastus lateralis muscle

Biceps femoris muscle (long head)

Iliotibial tract

Semimembranosus muscle

Biceps femoris muscle (short head)

Patella

Plantaris muscle

Gastrocnemius muscle (lateral head)

Patellar ligament

FIGURE 429 **Superficial Thigh and Gluteal Muscles (Lateral View)**

NOTE: (1) The massive size of the **vastus lateralis, biceps femoris,** and **gluteus maximus muscles** is seen from this lateral side.

(2) The **iliotibial tract** (or band) stretches, superficially, the length of the thigh. Its muscle, the **tensor fasciae latae,** helps keep the dense fascia lata taut.

(3) The fascia lata is a very tight layer of deep fascia that surrounds the thigh muscles (see Fig. 414.2). Because of this, the tensor fasciae latae assists in extension of the leg at the knee joint and in helping maintain an erect posture.

Chapter 6 The Lower Limb

PLATE 430 Lower Extremity: Gluteus Maximus (Dissection 2)

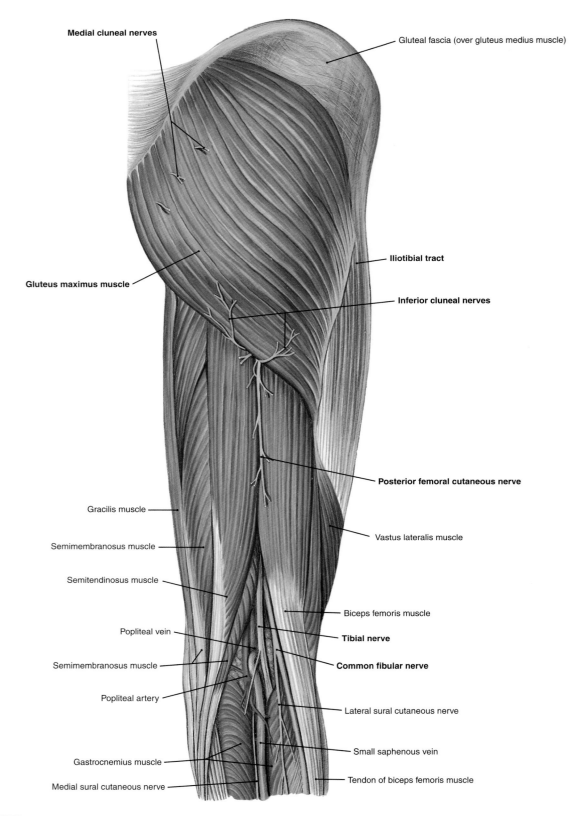

Medial cluneal nerves

Gluteal fascia (over gluteus medius muscle)

Gluteus maximus muscle

Iliotibial tract

Inferior cluneal nerves

Posterior femoral cutaneous nerve

Gracilis muscle

Vastus lateralis muscle

Semimembranosus muscle

Semitendinosus muscle

Biceps femoris muscle

Popliteal vein

Tibial nerve

Semimembranosus muscle

Common fibular nerve

Popliteal artery

Lateral sural cutaneous nerve

Small saphenous vein

Gastrocnemius muscle

Tendon of biceps femoris muscle

Medial sural cutaneous nerve

FIGURE 430 **Hamstring Muscles of Posterior Thigh and Gluteus Maximus (Superficial Dissection)**

NOTE: (1) The emergence of the posterior femoral cutaneous nerve below the inferior border of the gluteus maximus muscle, and its descent down the middle of the thigh.

(2) The appearance of the major vessels (popliteal artery and vein) and the sciatic nerve (tibial and common fibular nerves) in the popliteal fossa.

(3) The posterior thigh contains the **hamstring muscles.** These include four muscles, the **long head of the biceps femoris,** the **semitendinosus muscle,** the **semimembranosus muscle,** and the ischiocondylar part of the **adductor magnus muscle.**

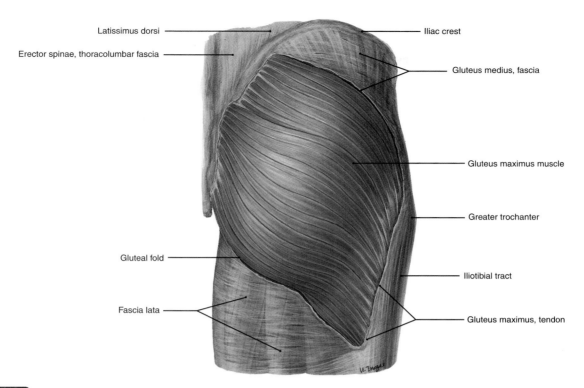

Latissimus dorsi

Erector spinae, thoracolumbar fascia

Iliac crest

Gluteus medius, fascia

Gluteus maximus muscle

Greater trochanter

Gluteal fold

Iliotibial tract

Fascia lata

Gluteus maximus, tendon

FIGURE 431.1 **Right Gluteus Maximus Muscle (Posterior View)**

NOTE: (1) The gluteus maximus muscle forms the contour of the buttocks. It arises from the posterior gluteal line of the ilium and the posterior surfaces of the sacrum, coccyx, and sacrotuberous ligament.

(2) The muscle fibers extend inferolaterally and end in a broad tendon that crosses the greater trochanter to insert on the iliotibial band of the fascia lata and the gluteal tuberosity of the femur.

(3) While the gluteus maximus is a powerful extensor and lateral rotator of the thigh, its upper fibers abduct the thigh and its lower fibers adduct the thigh.

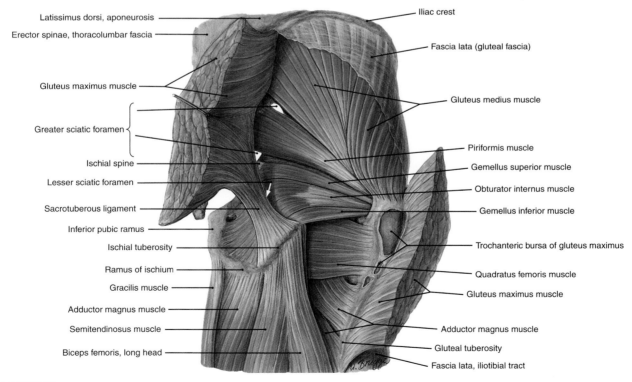

Latissimus dorsi, aponeurosis

Erector spinae, thoracolumbar fascia

Iliac crest

Fascia lata (gluteal fascia)

Gluteus maximus muscle

Gluteus medius muscle

Greater sciatic foramen

Piriformis muscle

Ischial spine

Gemellus superior muscle

Lesser sciatic foramen

Obturator internus muscle

Sacrotuberous ligament

Gemellus inferior muscle

Inferior pubic ramus

Trochanteric bursa of gluteus maximus

Ischial tuberosity

Ramus of ischium

Quadratus femoris muscle

Gracilis muscle

Gluteus maximus muscle

Adductor magnus muscle

Semitendinosus muscle

Adductor magnus muscle

Gluteal tuberosity

Biceps femoris, long head

Fascia lata, iliotibial tract

FIGURE 431.2 **Deep Muscles of the Gluteal and Hip Regions (Posterior View)**

NOTE: (1) Deep to the gluteus maximus are found the gluteus medius, gluteus minimus, piriformis, the two gemellus muscles (superior and inferior), the obturator internus, and the quadratus femoris.

(2) The gluteus medius (and the gluteus minimus deep to the medius) are abductors and **medial** rotators, while the other gluteal muscles are also abductors, but they are **lateral** rotators of the thigh. The piriformis also helps abduct the flexed thigh.

Chapter 6 The Lower Limb

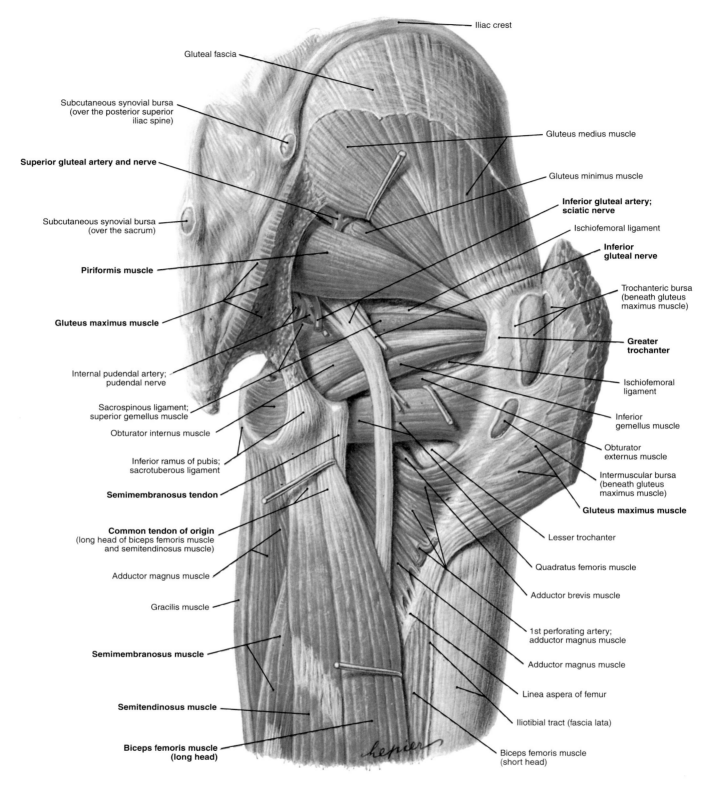

Iliac crest

Gluteal fascia

Subcutaneous synovial bursa
(over the posterior superior
iliac spine)

Superior gluteal artery and nerve

Subcutaneous synovial bursa
(over the sacrum)

Piriformis muscle

Gluteus maximus muscle

Internal pudendal artery;
pudendal nerve

Sacrospinous ligament;
superior gemellus muscle

Obturator internus muscle

Inferior ramus of pubis;
sacrotuberous ligament

Semimembranosus tendon

Common tendon of origin
(long head of biceps femoris muscle
and semitendinosus muscle)

Adductor magnus muscle

Gracilis muscle

Semimembranosus muscle

Semitendinosus muscle

**Biceps femoris muscle
(long head)**

Gluteus medius muscle

Gluteus minimus muscle

**Inferior gluteal artery;
sciatic nerve**

Ischiofemoral ligament

**Inferior
gluteal nerve**

Trochanteric bursa
(beneath gluteus
maximus muscle)

**Greater
trochanter**

Ischiofemoral
ligament

Inferior
gemellus muscle

Obturator
externus muscle

Intermuscular bursa
(beneath gluteus
maximus muscle)

Gluteus maximus muscle

Lesser trochanter

Quadratus femoris muscle

Adductor brevis muscle

1st perforating artery;
adductor magnus muscle

Adductor magnus muscle

Linea aspera of femur

Iliotibial tract (fascia lata)

Biceps femoris muscle
(short head)

FIGURE 432 Middle and Deep Gluteal Muscles and the Sciatic Nerve

NOTE: (1) The gluteus maximus has been reflected to show the centrally located **piriformis muscle,** which is the key structure in understanding the anatomy of this region.

(2) The piriformis muscle, as do most other structures that leave the pelvis to enter the gluteal region, passes through the **greater sciatic foramen.** The nerves and vessels enter the gluteal region from the pelvis either above or below the piriformis muscle. The important **sciatic nerve** enters the gluteal region **below** the piriformis.

(3) In addition to the piriformis, observe the **gluteus medius, the obturator internus,** with two **gemelli** above and below it, and the **quadratus femoris** muscles. The gluteus medius and minimus muscles are abductors and medial rotators of the thigh and all the other muscles are lateral rotators.

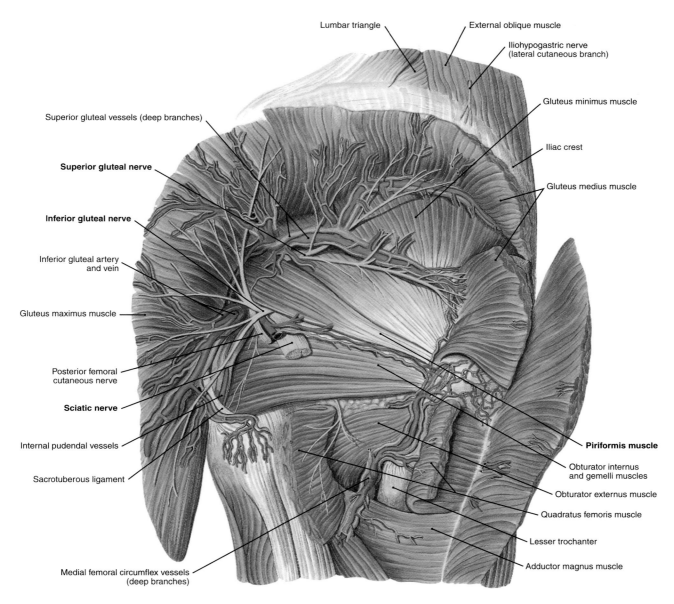

Lumbar triangle

External oblique muscle

Iliohypogastric nerve
(lateral cutaneous branch)

Gluteus minimus muscle

Superior gluteal vessels (deep branches)

Iliac crest

Superior gluteal nerve

Gluteus medius muscle

Inferior gluteal nerve

Inferior gluteal artery
and vein

Gluteus maximus muscle

Posterior femoral
cutaneous nerve

Sciatic nerve

Piriformis muscle

Obturator internus
and gemelli muscles

Internal pudendal vessels

Obturator externus muscle

Sacrotuberous ligament

Quadratus femoris muscle

Lesser trochanter

Adductor magnus muscle

Medial femoral circumflex vessels
(deep branches)

FIGURE 433 **Deep Vessels and Nerves of the Gluteal Region**

NOTE: (1) The gluteus maximus and gluteus medius muscles and the sciatic nerve have been cut to expose the short lateral rotators and the **gluteus minimus muscle**.

(2) **Above the piriformis** the **superior gluteal artery, vein,** and **nerve** enter the gluteal region through the greater sciatic foramen; **below the piriformis** the following structures enter the gluteal region by way of the greater sciatic foramen: the **inferior gluteal vessels** and **nerve,** the **sciatic nerve,** the **nerve to the obturator internus muscle,** the **posterior femoral cutaneous nerve,** the **nerve to the quadratus femoris muscle,** and the **internal pudendal vessels** and **pudendal nerve.**

(3) The internal pudendal artery and vein and the pudendal nerve, after entering the gluteal region through the greater sciatic foramen, cross the sacrospinous ligament and reenter the pelvis through the **lesser sciatic foramen** and course in the pudendal canal to get to the perineum. The other structure that passes through the lesser sciatic foramen is the **tendon of the obturator internus muscle.**

(4) To separate the gluteus medius muscle from the gluteus minimus muscle as shown in this figure, dissect along the course of the superior gluteal vessels and nerve, since these structures lie in the plane between the medius and minimus.

PLATE 434 Chart of Gluteal Muscles; Safe Zone for Gluteal Injections

MUSCLES OF THE GLUTEAL REGION

Muscle	Origin	Insertion	Innervation	Action
Gluteus maximus	Outer surface of the ilium and iliac crest; dorsal surface of the sacrum; lateral side of coccyx and the sacrotuberous ligament	Into the iliotibial band, which then descends to attach to the lateral condyle of tibia; also onto the gluteal tuberosity of the femur	Inferior gluteal nerve (L5, S1, S2)	Powerful extensor of the thigh; lateral rotator of the thigh; helps steady the extended leg; extends the trunk when distal end is fixed
Gluteus medius	External surface of the ilium between the anterior and posterior gluteal lines	Lateral surface of greater trochanter of the femur	Superior gluteal nerve (L4, L5, S1)	Abducts and medially rotates the thigh; helps steady the pelvis
Gluteus minimus	Outer surface of ilium between the anterior and inferior gluteal lines	Anterior border of greater trochanter and on the fibrous capsule of the hip joint	Superior gluteal nerve (L4, L5, S1)	Abducts and medially rotates the thigh; helps steady the pelvis
Piriformis	Anterior (pelvic) surface of the sacrum and the inner surface of sacrotuberous ligament	Upper border of the greater trochanter of the femur	Muscular branches from the S1 and S2 nerves	Laterally rotates the extended thigh; when the thigh is flexed, it abducts the femur
Obturator internus	Pelvic surface of obturator membrane and from the bone surrounding the obturator foramen	Medial surface of greater trochanter proximal to the trochanteric fossa	Nerve to the obturator internus (L5, S1)	Laterally rotates the extended thigh and abducts the flexed thigh
Superior gemellus	Outer surface of the ischial spine	Medial surface of greater trochanter with tendon of the obturator interius	Nerve to the obturator internus (L5, S1)	Laterally rotates the extended thigh and abducts the flexed thigh
Inferior gemellus	From the ischial tuberosity	Medial surface of greater trochanter with tendon of the obturator internus	Nerve to the quadratus femoris (L5, S1)	Laterally rotates the extended thigh and abducts the flexed thigh
Quadratus femoris	Lateral border of the ischial tuberosity	Quadrate tubercle on the posterior surface of the femur; also onto the intertrochanteric crest of the femur	Nerve to the quadratus femoris (L5, S1)	Laterally rotates the thigh

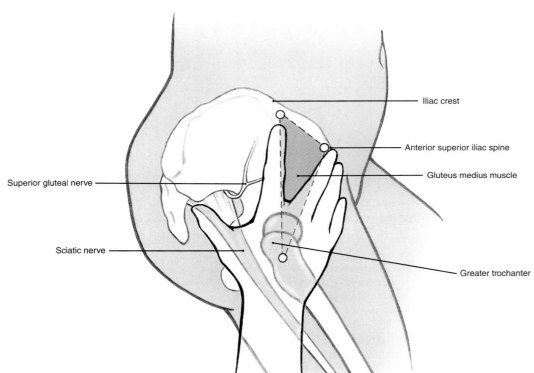

FIGURE 434 **Quick Method of Determining the Safe Zone for Intramuscular Gluteal Injection**

NOTE: The safe zone can be visualized quickly by:
(1) Placing the palm of the right hand over the right greater trochanter (or left hand over the left greater trochanter),
(2) Directing the index finger vertically to the iliac crest and spreading the middle finger to the anterior superior iliac spine,
(3) The colored region shown in this diagram between the index and middle fingers is the safe zone and avoids the superior gluteal vessels and nerve as well as the sciatic nerve and other important gluteal structures.

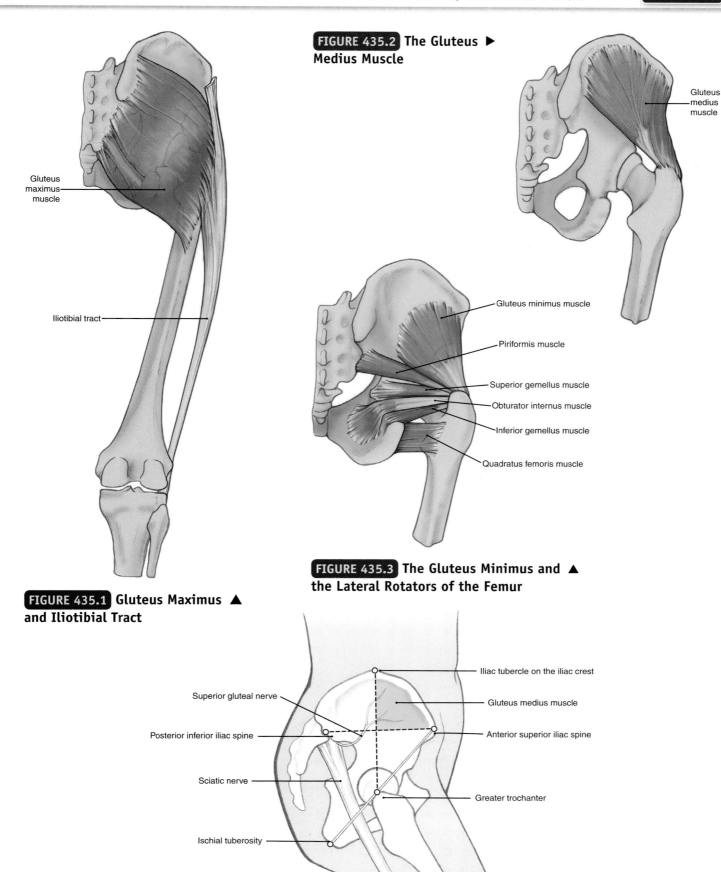

FIGURE 435.2 The Gluteus ▶
Medius Muscle

Gluteus medius muscle

Gluteus maximus muscle

Iliotibial tract

Gluteus minimus muscle

Piriformis muscle

Superior gemellus muscle

Obturator internus muscle

Inferior gemellus muscle

Quadratus femoris muscle

FIGURE 435.3 The Gluteus Minimus and ▲
the Lateral Rotators of the Femur

FIGURE 435.1 Gluteus Maximus ▲
and Iliotibial Tract

Iliac tubercle on the iliac crest

Superior gluteal nerve

Gluteus medius muscle

Posterior inferior iliac spine

Anterior superior iliac spine

Sciatic nerve

Greater trochanter

Ischial tuberosity

FIGURE 435.4 Safe Quadrant for Injections into the Gluteal Region

NOTE: In this figure the four quadrants of the gluteal region are determined by a **transverse line** between the **anterior superior iliac spine** anteriorly and the **posterior inferior iliac spine** posteriorly that intersects a **vertical line** between the **greater trochanter** inferiorly and the **iliac crest** superiorly. The colored upper lateral quadrant is the safe zone for intramuscular injection.

Chapter 6 The Lower Limb

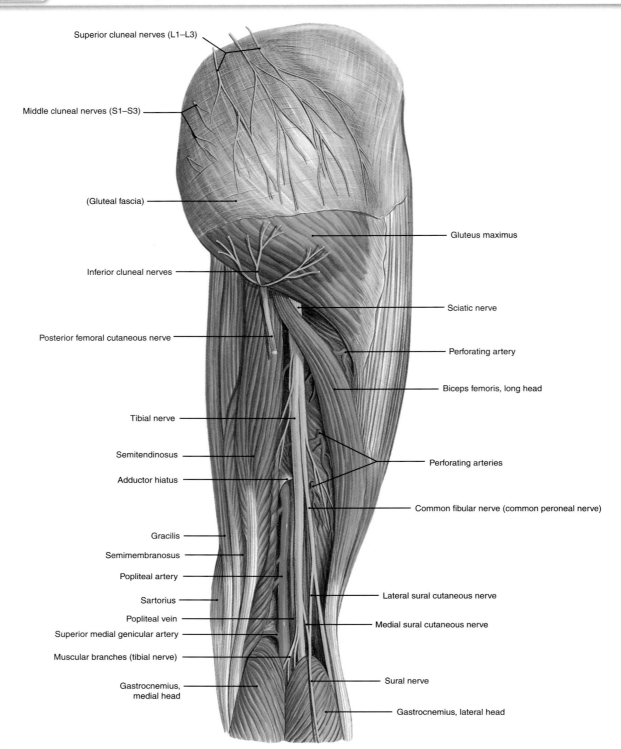

Superior cluneal nerves (L1–L3)

Middle cluneal nerves (S1–S3)

(Gluteal fascia)

Gluteus maximus

Inferior cluneal nerves

Sciatic nerve

Posterior femoral cutaneous nerve

Perforating artery

Biceps femoris, long head

Tibial nerve

Semitendinosus

Perforating arteries

Adductor hiatus

Common fibular nerve (common peroneal nerve)

Gracilis

Semimembranosus

Popliteal artery

Lateral sural cutaneous nerve

Sartorius

Popliteal vein

Medial sural cutaneous nerve

Superior medial genicular artery

Muscular branches (tibial nerve)

Sural nerve

Gastrocnemius, medial head

Gastrocnemius, lateral head

FIGURE 436 Descent of the Sciatic Nerve from the Gluteus Maximus to the Popliteal Fossa; the Popliteal Vessels

POSTERIOR THIGH MUSCLES				
Muscle	**Origin**	**Insertion**	**Innervation**	**Function**
Biceps femoris	Long head: Ischial tuberosity in common with other hamstring muscles	Lateral surface of the head of the fibula and a small slip to lateral condyle of tibia	Long head: Tibial part of sciatic nerve (S1, S2, S3)	Flexes the leg and rotates the tibia laterally; long head also extends the thigh at the hip joint
	Short head: Lateral lip of the linea aspera of the femur		Short head: Peroneal part of the sciatic nerve (L5, S1, S2)	
Semitendinosus	Ischial tuberosity in common with other hamstring muscles	Medial surface of the upper part of the body of the tibia	Tibial part of the sciatic nerve (L5, S1, S2)	Flexes the leg and rotates the tibia medially; extends the thigh
Semimembranosus	Ischial tuberosity in common with other hamstring muscles	Posterior aspect of the medial condyle of the tibia	Tibial part of the sciatic nerve (L5, S1, S2)	Flexes the leg and rotates it medially; extends the thigh

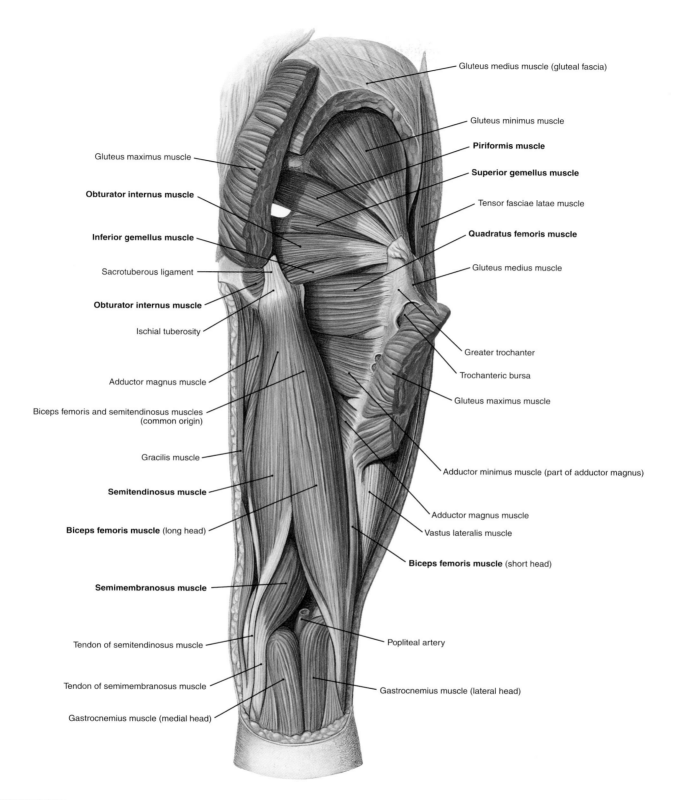

Gluteus medius muscle (gluteal fascia)

Gluteus minimus muscle

Piriformis muscle

Superior gemellus muscle

Tensor fasciae latae muscle

Quadratus femoris muscle

Gluteus medius muscle

Greater trochanter

Trochanteric bursa

Gluteus maximus muscle

Adductor minimus muscle (part of adductor magnus)

Adductor magnus muscle

Vastus lateralis muscle

Biceps femoris muscle (short head)

Popliteal artery

Gastrocnemius muscle (lateral head)

Gluteus maximus muscle

Obturator internus muscle

Inferior gemellus muscle

Sacrotuberous ligament

Obturator internus muscle

Ischial tuberosity

Adductor magnus muscle

Biceps femoris and semitendinosus muscles (common origin)

Gracilis muscle

Semitendinosus muscle

Biceps femoris muscle (long head)

Semimembranosus muscle

Tendon of semitendinosus muscle

Tendon of semimembranosus muscle

Gastrocnemius muscle (medial head)

FIGURE 437 **Hamstring Muscles of Posterior Thigh and Deep Muscles of Gluteal Region**

NOTE: (1) For a muscle to be considered a **hamstring muscle,** it must:
  (a) arise from the **ischial tuberosity,**
  (b) receive innervation from the **tibial division of the sciatic nerve,** and
  (c) cross **both** the hip and knee joints.
(2) The long head of the biceps is a hamstring, but the short head is not, because it arises from the femur and is supplied by the common fibular division of the sciatic nerve.
(3) The **ischiocondylar part** of the adductor magnus meets two criteria as a hamstring but crosses only the hip joint. Its insertion, however, on the adductor tubercle is embryologically continuous with the tibial collateral ligament, which does attach below on the tibia.

PLATE 438 Lower Extremity: Posterior Thigh, Deep Muscles (Dissection 3)

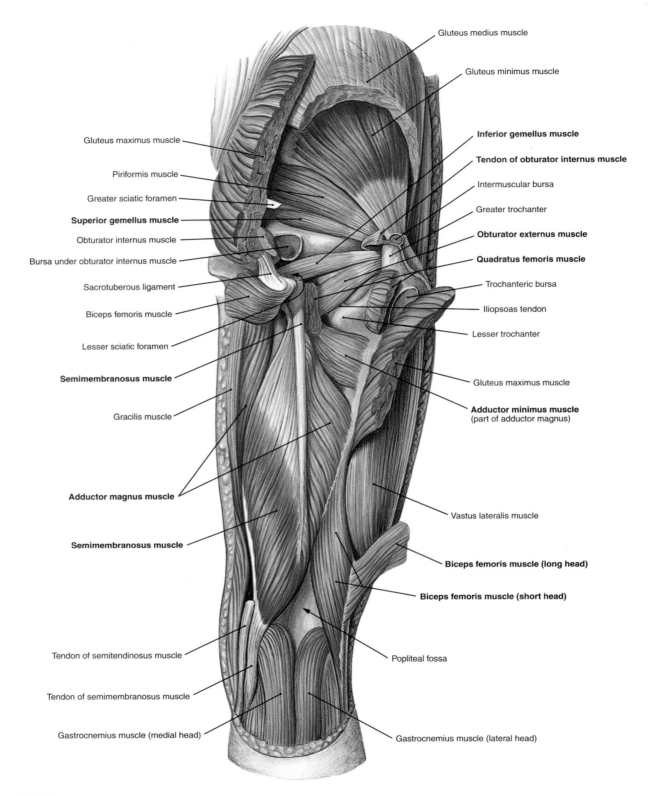

Gluteus medius muscle

Gluteus minimus muscle

Inferior gemellus muscle

Tendon of obturator internus muscle

Intermuscular bursa

Greater trochanter

Obturator externus muscle

Quadratus femoris muscle

Trochanteric bursa

Iliopsoas tendon

Lesser trochanter

Gluteus maximus muscle

Adductor minimus muscle
(part of adductor magnus)

Vastus lateralis muscle

Biceps femoris muscle (long head)

Biceps femoris muscle (short head)

Popliteal fossa

Gastrocnemius muscle (lateral head)

Gluteus maximus muscle

Piriformis muscle

Greater sciatic foramen

Superior gemellus muscle

Obturator internus muscle

Bursa under obturator internus muscle

Sacrotuberous ligament

Biceps femoris muscle

Lesser sciatic foramen

Semimembranosus muscle

Gracilis muscle

Adductor magnus muscle

Semimembranosus muscle

Tendon of semitendinosus muscle

Tendon of semimembranosus muscle

Gastrocnemius muscle (medial head)

FIGURE 438 **Hamstring Muscles of Posterior Thigh (Deep Dissection) and Deep Gluteal Muscles**

NOTE: (1) The common tendon of the long head of the biceps femoris and semitendinosus muscles has been cut in the thigh close to the ischial tuberosity. This exposes the origin of the **semimembranosus muscle,** the breadth of the **adductor magnus muscle,** and the **short head of the biceps femoris muscle.**
(2) The **short head of the biceps femoris muscle** arising from the lateral lip of the linea aspera of the femur, between the attachments of the vastus lateralis and the adductor magnus muscles. It descends to join the tendon of the long head before insertion.
(3) In the gluteal region, the quadratus femoris muscle has been severed and reflected, thereby revealing the **obturator externus muscle** beneath. Also, the tendon of the obturator internus muscle has been cut (between the gemelli) exposing the bursa deep to that tendon.

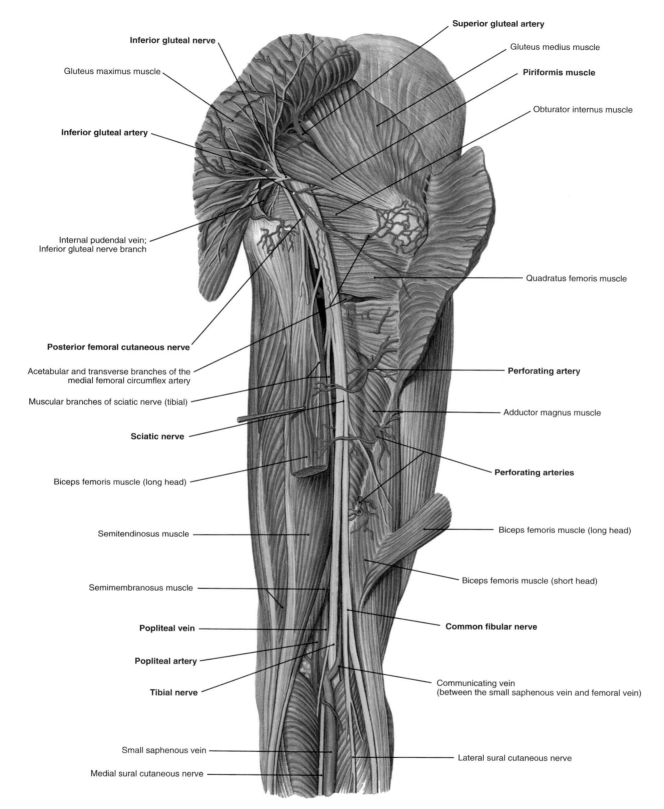

Superior gluteal artery

Gluteus medius muscle

Piriformis muscle

Obturator internus muscle

Inferior gluteal nerve

Gluteus maximus muscle

Inferior gluteal artery

Internal pudendal vein;
Inferior gluteal nerve branch

Quadratus femoris muscle

Posterior femoral cutaneous nerve

Acetabular and transverse branches of the
medial femoral circumflex artery

Perforating artery

Muscular branches of sciatic nerve (tibial)

Adductor magnus muscle

Sciatic nerve

Perforating arteries

Biceps femoris muscle (long head)

Biceps femoris muscle (long head)

Semitendinosus muscle

Biceps femoris muscle (short head)

Semimembranosus muscle

Common fibular nerve

Popliteal vein

Popliteal artery

Communicating vein
(between the small saphenous vein and femoral vein)

Tibial nerve

Small saphenous vein

Lateral sural cutaneous nerve

Medial sural cutaneous nerve

FIGURE 439 **Vessels and Nerves of the Posterior Thigh and Gluteal Region (Deep Dissection)**

NOTE: (1) The course of the **sciatic nerve** as it passes through the greater sciatic foramen in the gluteal region, inferior to the piriformis muscle, lateral to the ischial tuberosity and under cover of the gluteus maximus muscle. It enters the thigh nearly midway between the ischial tuberosity and the greater trochanter.

(2) The **superior and inferior gluteal arteries** and the **posterior femoral cutaneous nerve** in the gluteal region. In the thigh, observe the **perforating arteries,** branches of the **deep femoral artery,** and the fact that the sciatic nerve splits to become the **tibial and common fibular nerves.**

PLATE 440 Anterior and Medial Nerves of the Lower Limb

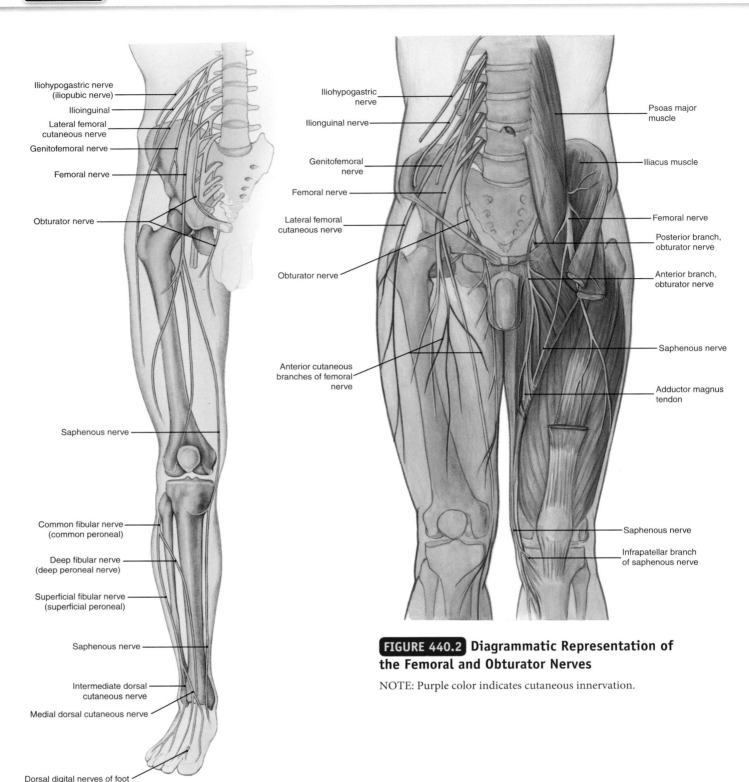

Iliohypogastric nerve
(iliopubic nerve)

Ilioinguinal

Lateral femoral
cutaneous nerve

Genitofemoral nerve

Femoral nerve

Obturator nerve

Saphenous nerve

Common fibular nerve
(common peroneal)

Deep fibular nerve
(deep peroneal nerve)

Superficial fibular nerve
(superficial peroneal)

Saphenous nerve

Intermediate dorsal
cutaneous nerve

Medial dorsal cutaneous nerve

Dorsal digital nerves of foot

Iliohypogastric
nerve

Ilionguinal nerve

Genitofemoral
nerve

Femoral nerve

Lateral femoral
cutaneous nerve

Obturator nerve

Anterior cutaneous
branches of femoral
nerve

Psoas major
muscle

Iliacus muscle

Femoral nerve

Posterior branch,
obturator nerve

Anterior branch,
obturator nerve

Saphenous nerve

Adductor magnus
tendon

Saphenous nerve

Infrapatellar branch
of saphenous nerve

FIGURE 440.2 Diagrammatic Representation of the Femoral and Obturator Nerves

NOTE: Purple color indicates cutaneous innervation.

FIGURE 440.1 Nerves of the Lower Limb (Anterior Aspect)

NOTE: (1) The **femoral nerve** is the principal nerve of the anterior thigh, but the **obturator nerve** supplies muscles of the medial thigh.

(2) The **lateral femoral cutaneous nerve** (L2, L3) supplies the skin of the lateral thigh.

(3) The **saphenous nerve** (a sensory branch of the femoral nerve) supplies the skin of the medial leg.

(4) All **other branches** below the knee are derived from the **sciatic nerve.**

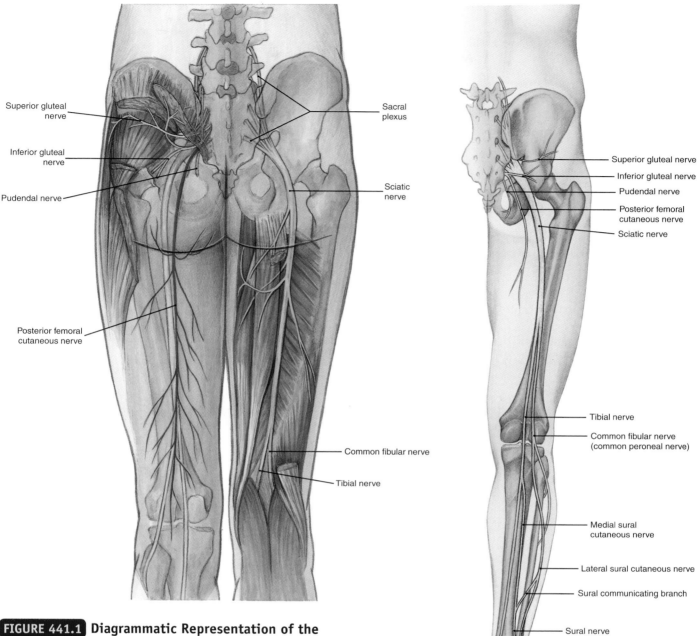

Superior gluteal nerve

Inferior gluteal nerve

Pudendal nerve

Posterior femoral cutaneous nerve

Sacral plexus

Sciatic nerve

Common fibular nerve

Tibial nerve

Superior gluteal nerve

Inferior gluteal nerve

Pudendal nerve

Posterior femoral cutaneous nerve

Sciatic nerve

Tibial nerve

Common fibular nerve (common peroneal nerve)

Medial sural cutaneous nerve

Lateral sural cutaneous nerve

Sural communicating branch

Sural nerve

Lateral dorsal cutaneous nerve

Lateral plantar nerve

Medial plantar nerve

FIGURE 441.1 Diagrammatic Representation of the Sciatic and Posterior Femoral Cutaneous Nerves

NOTE: Purple color indicates cutaneous innervation.

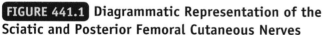

FIGURE 441.2 Nerves of the Lower Limb (Posterior Aspect)

NOTE: (1) The **sciatic nerve** supplies the posterior thigh and all other structures below the knee *EXCEPT* the skin of the medial leg, which is supplied by the **saphenous nerve,** a branch of the **femoral nerve.**

(2) The **fibular nerves (superficial** and **deep)** supply all of the muscles of the leg and foot and the skin of the dorsal and plantar surfaces of the foot.

(3) The **common fibular nerve** divides into superficial and deep fibular branches as it courses around the head of the fibula (see Fig. 440.1).

PLATE 442 Popliteal Fossa, Vessels and Nerves (Dissections 1, 2)

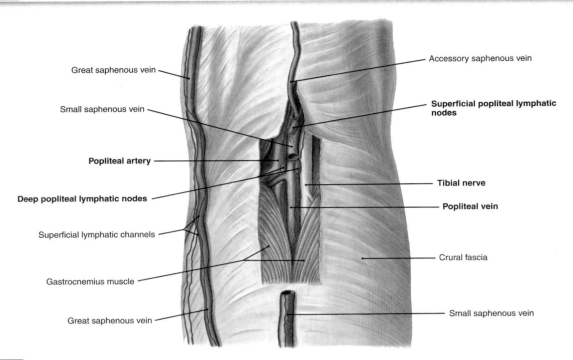

FIGURE 442.1 Subcutaneous Dissection of the Popliteal Fossa

NOTE: The skin and crural fascia have been removed over the popliteal fossa and a part of the small saphenous vein has been resected. Observe the popliteal vessels and nerves and the **popliteal lymphatic nodes** and **channels** deeper in the fossa.

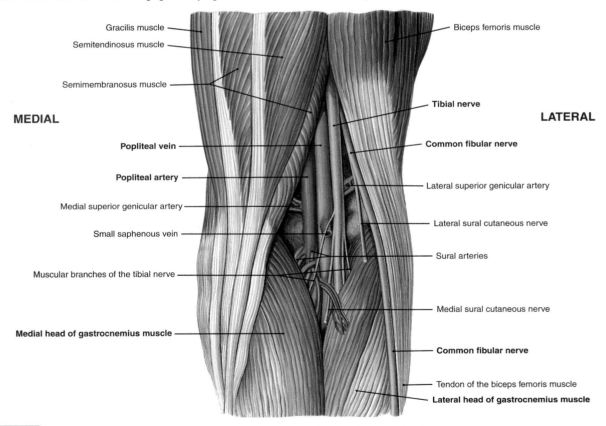

FIGURE 442.2 Nerves and Vessels of the Popliteal Fossa (Superficial View)

NOTE: (1) The relationships of the **popliteal vessels** and **nerve** within the popliteal fossa. The **sciatic nerve** has already divided into the laterally directed **common fibular nerve** and the **tibial nerve,** which continues directly into the calf. Both the common fibular and the tibial nerves lie superficial to the vessels in the popliteal fossa.

(2) The popliteal vein is located between the tibial nerve and popliteal artery, while the artery is the deepest (most anterior) and most medial of three structures.

(3) The two muscular branches of the tibial nerve innervating the two heads of the gastrocnemius muscle, and a descending sensory branch, the **medial sural cutaneous nerve,** to the calf. Also note the **lateral sural cutaneous nerve** from the common fibular nerve.

(4) The popliteal fossa is about 2.5 cm (1 in.) wide at its maximum, and in the undissected specimen, the fossa is filled with fat, and the vessels and nerves are initially difficult to see.

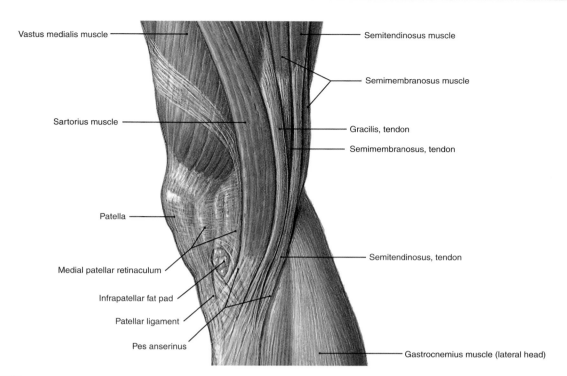

FIGURE 443.1 Medial Surface of the Knee Region

NOTE: The tendons of the sartorius, gracilis, and semitendinosus form the so-called pes anserinus (goose's foot). This formation of tendons strengthens the medial aspect of the knee joint.

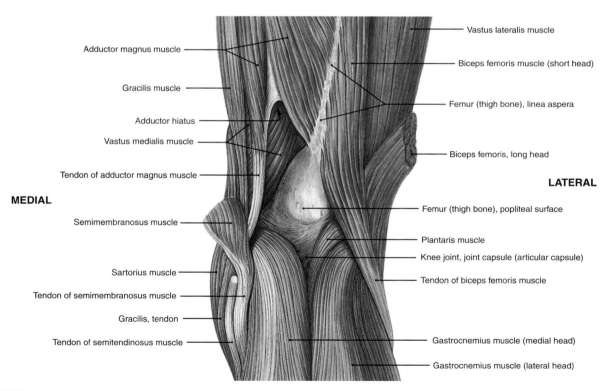

FIGURE 443.2 Deep Muscles That Bound the Popliteal Fossa

NOTE: (1) The **popliteal fossa** is a diamond-shaped space behind the knee joint. Its *superior boundaries* are the **long head of the biceps femoris muscle** laterally and the **semimembranosus** and **semitendinosus muscles** medially (see Fig. 442.2). All three of these muscles have been cut in this dissection, exposing the more deeply located **adductor magnus** and **vastus medialis** medially and the **short head of the biceps femoris** laterally.

(2) The *inferior boundaries* of the fossa are the **medial** and **lateral heads of the gastrocnemius muscle,** which arise from the medial and lateral condyles of the femur.

(3) The inferior opening of the **adductor canal** (the adductor hiatus), which transmits the **femoral artery** and **vein** from and to the anterior aspect of the thigh.

Chapter 6 The Lower Limb

PLATE 444 Lower Extremity: Popliteal Fossa, Deep Arteries (Dissection 4)

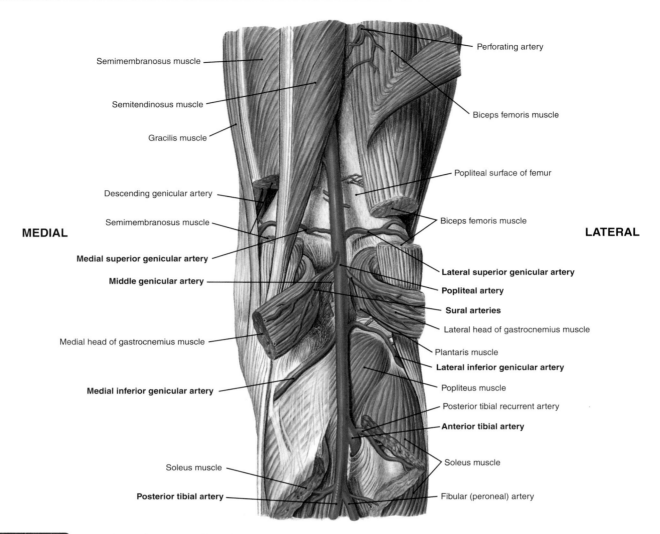

Semimembranosus muscle

Semitendinosus muscle

Gracilis muscle

Descending genicular artery

Semimembranosus muscle

MEDIAL

Medial superior genicular artery

Middle genicular artery

Medial head of gastrocnemius muscle

Medial inferior genicular artery

Soleus muscle

Posterior tibial artery

Perforating artery

Biceps femoris muscle

Popliteal surface of femur

Biceps femoris muscle

LATERAL

Lateral superior genicular artery

Popliteal artery

Sural arteries

Lateral head of gastrocnemius muscle

Plantaris muscle

Lateral inferior genicular artery

Popliteus muscle

Posterior tibial recurrent artery

Anterior tibial artery

Soleus muscle

Fibular (peroneal) artery

FIGURE 444.1 Branches of the Popliteal Artery

NOTE: (1) Within the popliteal fossa, the popliteal artery most frequently gives rise to two **superior (lateral** and **medial) genicular,** one **middle genicular,** and two **inferior (lateral** and **medial) genicular arteries.**

(2) The **popliteal artery** bifurcates into the **posterior tibial** and the **anterior tibial.** The latter penetrates an aperture above the interosseous membrane to reach the anterior compartment. Somewhat lower, the **fibular artery** branches from the posterior tibial. The pattern shown here occurs in about **90% of cases.** Variations in this pattern are shown in Figure 444.2.

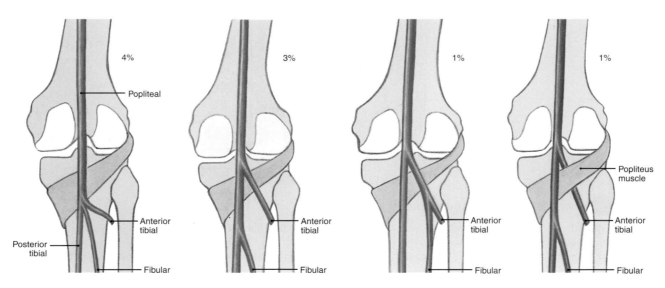

4%

Popliteal

3%

1%

1%

Popliteus muscle

Anterior tibial

Anterior tibial

Anterior tibial

Anterior tibial

Posterior tibial

Fibular

Fibular

Fibular

Fibular

FIGURE 444.2 Variations in the Branching Pattern of the Anterior Tibial and Fibular Arteries

See NOTE 2 under Figure 444.1.

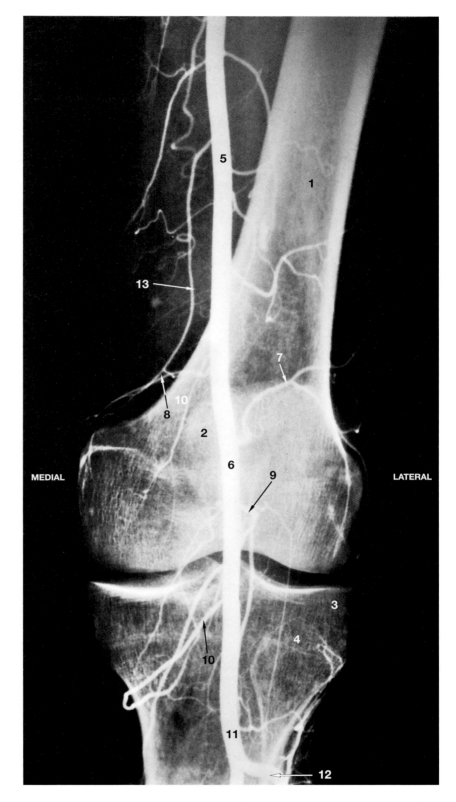

1. Femur
2. Patella
3. Tibia
4. Head of fibula
5. Femoral artery
6. Popliteal artery
7. Lateral superior genicular artery
8. Medial superior genicular artery
9. Middle genicular artery
10. Inferior genicular artery
11. Popliteal artery
12. Anterior tibial artery
13. Descending genicular artery

FIGURE 445 **Arteriogram of the Left Femoral–Popliteal–Tibial Arterial Tree (Anteroposterior Projection)**

NOTE: (1) This arteriogram shows the branches from the femoral, popliteal, and tibial arteries in the lower third of the thigh and the upper part of the calf. Observe the following bony structures: **femur** [1], **patella** [2], **tibia** [3], and **fibula** [4].

(2) The course of the **femoral artery** [5] as it becomes the **popliteal artery** [6] just above the popliteal fossa. Observe the following branches from the popliteal artery: **superior genicular** [7, 8], **middle genicular** [9], and single **inferior genicular** [10] in this patient.

(3) Below the popliteal fossa the **popliteal artery** [11] can be seen giving off the **anterior and posterior tibial arteries** just above the lower edge of the angiogram.

(4) The **descending genicular artery** [13], a branch of the femoral above the popliteal fossa, as it courses downward to participate in the anastomosis around the knee joint.

(From Wicke, 6th ed.)

PLATE 446 Anterior Leg, Superficial Vessels and Nerves (Dissection 1)

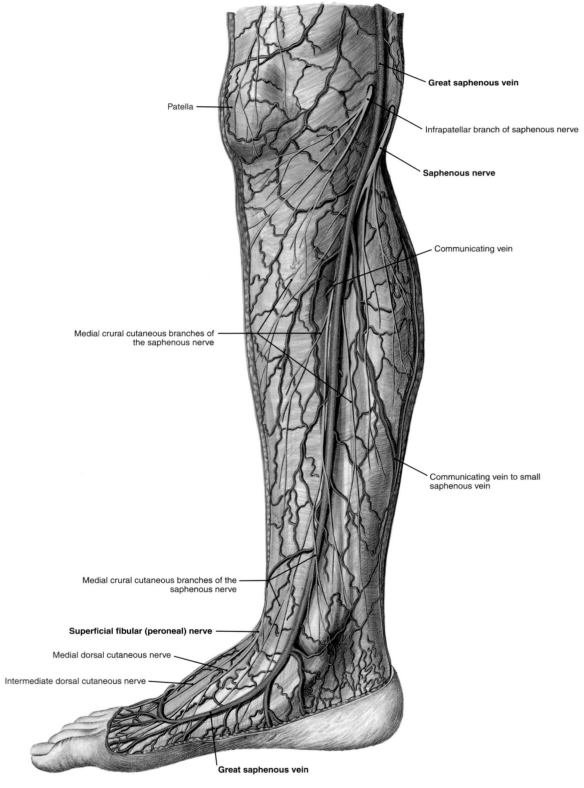

Great saphenous vein

Patella

Infrapatellar branch of saphenous nerve

Saphenous nerve

Communicating vein

Medial crural cutaneous branches of the saphenous nerve

Communicating vein to small saphenous vein

Medial crural cutaneous branches of the saphenous nerve

Superficial fibular (peroneal) nerve

Medial dorsal cutaneous nerve

Intermediate dorsal cutaneous nerve

Great saphenous vein

FIGURE 446 Superficial Veins and Nerves on the Anterior and Medial Aspects of the Leg and Foot

NOTE: (1) The **great saphenous vein** is formed on the medial aspect of the foot, courses anterior to the medial malleolus, and ascends along the medial side of the leg.

(2) Branches of the **saphenous nerve** accompany the great saphenous vein below the knee. This nerve becomes superficial medially just below the knee and is the largest branch of the femoral nerve. It functions as the sensory nerve that supplies the skin over most of the medial half of the leg region (i.e., between the knee and the ankle).

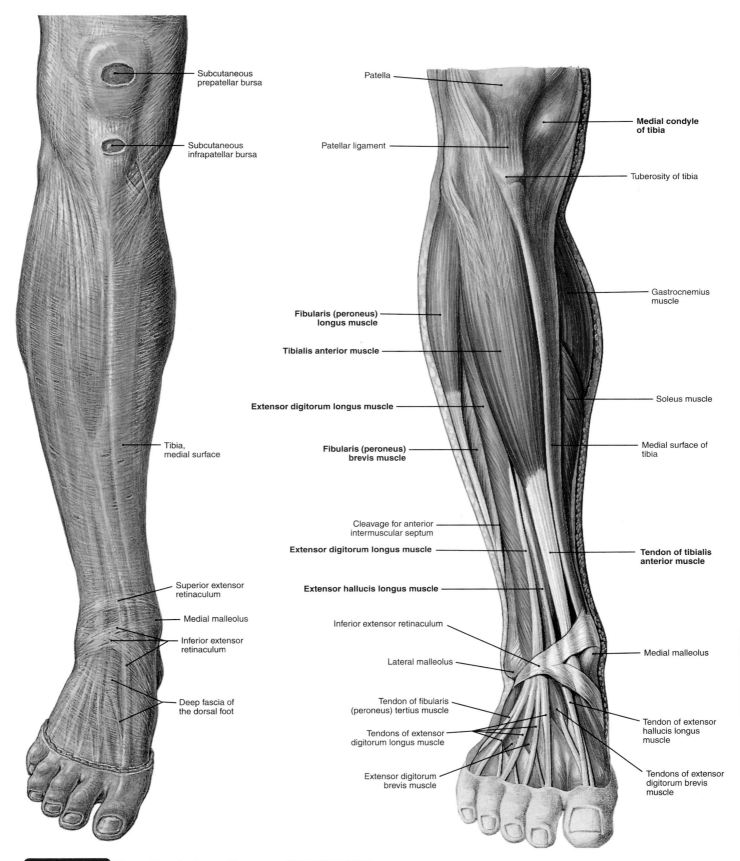

Subcutaneous prepatellar bursa

Subcutaneous infrapatellar bursa

Tibia, medial surface

Superior extensor retinaculum

Medial malleolus

Inferior extensor retinaculum

Deep fascia of the dorsal foot

Patella

Medial condyle of tibia

Patellar ligament

Tuberosity of tibia

Gastrocnemius muscle

Fibularis (peroneus) longus muscle

Tibialis anterior muscle

Extensor digitorum longus muscle

Soleus muscle

Fibularis (peroneus) brevis muscle

Medial surface of tibia

Cleavage for anterior intermuscular septum

Extensor digitorum longus muscle

Tendon of tibialis anterior muscle

Extensor hallucis longus muscle

Inferior extensor retinaculum

Lateral malleolus

Medial malleolus

Tendon of fibularis (peroneus) tertius muscle

Tendons of extensor digitorum longus muscle

Tendon of extensor hallucis longus muscle

Extensor digitorum brevis muscle

Tendons of extensor digitorum brevis muscle

FIGURE 447.1 Deep Fascia Investing the Leg and Dorsal Foot

NOTE: The deep fascia binds the muscles and the **superior and inferior extensor retinacula** bind the tendons of the anterior and lateral leg muscles.

FIGURE 447.2 Muscles of Anterior Compartment of Leg

NOTE: (1) The medial surface of the tibia separates muscles in the anterior compartment from those of the calf, posteriorly.

(2) The anterior compartment muscles include the **tibialis anterior, extensor hallucis longus, extensor digitorum,** and **fibularis tertius,** which dorsiflex the foot. The long extensors also extend the toes (Plate 449).

Chapter 6 The Lower Limb

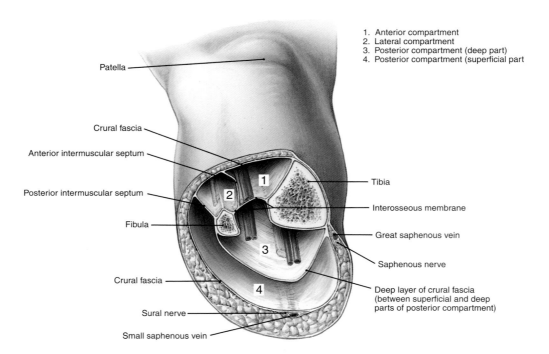

1. Anterior compartment
2. Lateral compartment
3. Posterior compartment (deep part)
4. Posterior compartment (superficial part

Patella

Crural fascia

Anterior intermuscular septum

Posterior intermuscular septum

Fibula

Crural fascia

Sural nerve

Small saphenous vein

Tibia

Interosseous membrane

Great saphenous vein

Saphenous nerve

Deep layer of crural fascia
(between superficial and deep
parts of posterior compartment)

FIGURE 448 Compartments of the Leg, Diagrammatic Representation: Cross Section

NOTE: This figure shows the compartments of the **left leg** viewed upward from below.

MUSCLES OF THE ANTERIOR COMPARTMENT OF THE LEG

Muscle	Origin	Insertion	Innervation	Action
Tibialis anterior	Lateral condyle and lateral surface of upper half of the tibia; the interosseous membrane and crural fascia	On the medial and plantar surfaces of the 1st metatarsal bone and the medial cuneiform bone	Deep fibular (peroneal) nerve (L4, L5)	Dorsiflexes the foot at the ankle joint; inverts and adducts the foot at the subtalar and midtarsal joints
Extensor hallucis longus	Medial surface of the fibula; the anterior part of the interosseous membrane and the crural fascia	Dorsal surface of the base of the distal phalanx of the great toe (or hallux)	Deep fibular (peroneal) nerve (L5, S1)	Extends the great toe; dorsiflexes the foot and tends to invert (supinate) the foot
Extensor digitorum longus	Lateral condyle of the tibia; upper three-fourths of anterior surface of the fibula and the interosseous membrane	On the distal phalanges of the four lateral toes	Deep fibular (peroneal) nerve (L5, S1)	Extends the lateral four digits; dorsiflexes the foot and tends to evert (pronate) the foot
Fibularis tertius	Distal third of the anterior surface of the fibula and the interosseous membrane	Dorsal surface of the base of the fifth metatarsal bone	Deep fibular (peroneal) nerve (L5, S1)	Dorsiflexes the foot and assists in everting (i.e., pronating) the foot

MUSCLES OF THE LATERAL COMPARTMENT OF THE LEG

Muscle	Origin	Insertion	Innervation	Action
Fibularis longus	Head and upper two-thirds of the lateral surface of the body of the fibula	Lateral aspect of the base of the first metatarsal bone and the medial cuneiform bone (on the plantar surface of the foot)	Superficial fibular (peroneal) nerve (L4, S1, S2)	Everts the foot (i.e., tends to pronate the foot); it also is a weak plantar flexor of the foot
Fibularis brevis	Distal two-thirds of the lateral surface of the fibula and the intermuscular septum	Lateral surface and base of the fifth metatarsal bone	Superficial fibular (peroneal) nerve (L4, L5, S1)	Everts the foot (i.e., tends to pronate the foot); also acts as a weak plantar flexor of the foot

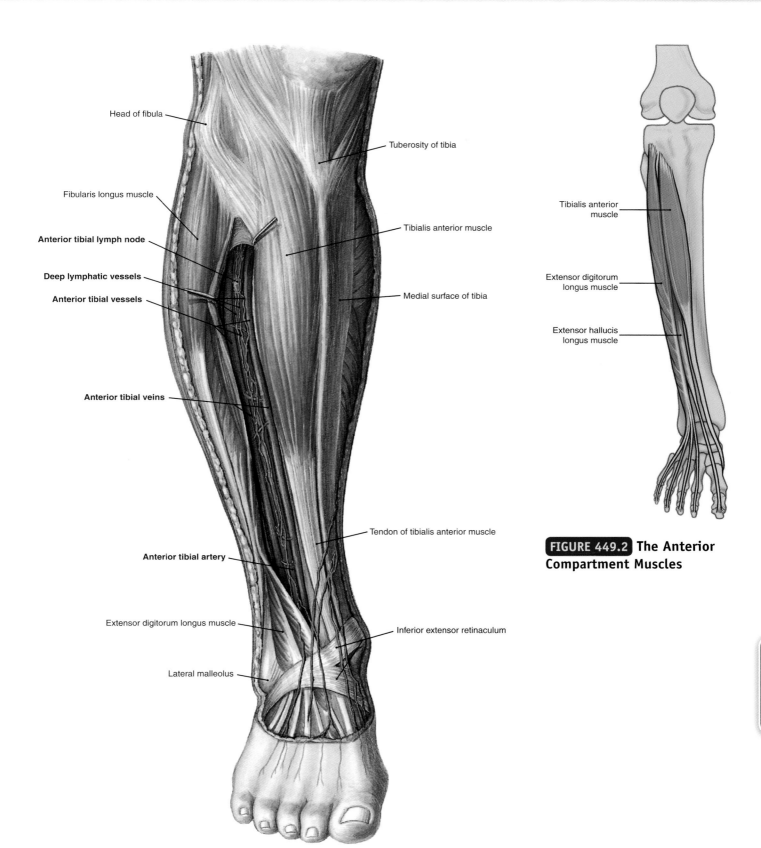

Head of fibula

Fibularis longus muscle

Anterior tibial lymph node

Deep lymphatic vessels

Anterior tibial vessels

Anterior tibial veins

Anterior tibial artery

Extensor digitorum longus muscle

Lateral malleolus

Tuberosity of tibia

Tibialis anterior muscle

Medial surface of tibia

Tendon of tibialis anterior muscle

Inferior extensor retinaculum

Tibialis anterior muscle

Extensor digitorum longus muscle

Extensor hallucis longus muscle

FIGURE 449.2 **The Anterior Compartment Muscles**

FIGURE 449.1 **Anterior Tibial Compartment: Vessels and Lymphatic Channels**

NOTE: (1) By separating the **tibialis anterior muscle** from the other muscles in the anterior compartment, the **anterior tibial artery** is exposed descending to the dorsum of the foot.

(2) The artery is accompanied by a pair of **anterior tibial veins (venae comitantes),** which ascend to join the posterior tibial vein to help form the popliteal vein.

(3) Lymphatic channels from the dorsum of the foot course superiorly along the path of these vessels, and at times, a lymph node can be found just below the knee.

Chapter 6 The Lower Limb

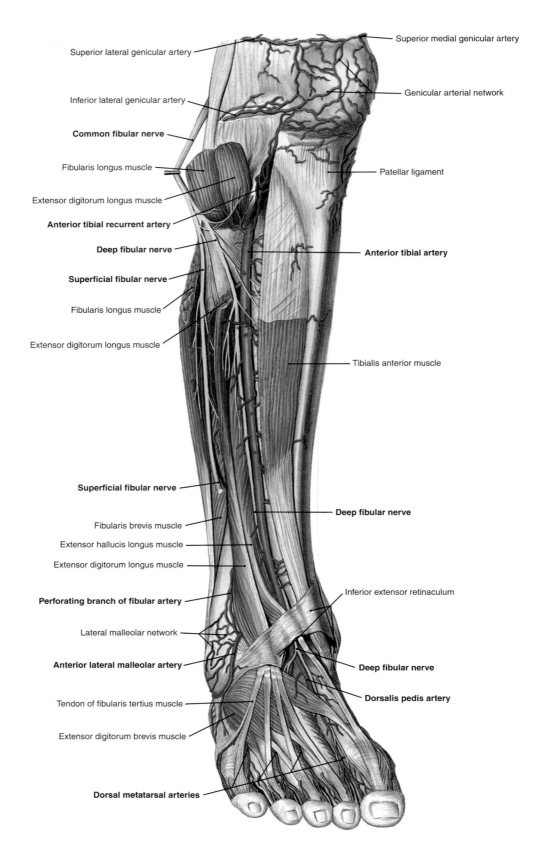

Superior lateral genicular artery

Inferior lateral genicular artery

Common fibular nerve

Fibularis longus muscle

Extensor digitorum longus muscle

Anterior tibial recurrent artery

Deep fibular nerve

Superficial fibular nerve

Fibularis longus muscle

Extensor digitorum longus muscle

Superficial fibular nerve

Fibularis brevis muscle

Extensor hallucis longus muscle

Extensor digitorum longus muscle

Perforating branch of fibular artery

Lateral malleolar network

Anterior lateral malleolar artery

Tendon of fibularis tertius muscle

Extensor digitorum brevis muscle

Dorsal metatarsal arteries

Superior medial genicular artery

Genicular arterial network

Patellar ligament

Anterior tibial artery

Tibialis anterior muscle

Deep fibular nerve

Inferior extensor retinaculum

Deep fibular nerve

Dorsalis pedis artery

FIGURE 450 Deep Dissection of the Anterior and Lateral Compartments: Nerves and Arteries

NOTE: (1) As the **common fibular nerve** courses laterally around the head of the fibula, it divides into the **superficial** and **deep fibular nerves,** which innervate the muscles of the lateral and anterior compartments.

(2) The deep fibular nerve is joined by the **anterior tibial artery,** which descends toward the foot, where it becomes the **dorsalis pedis artery.**

(3) The superficial fibular nerve becomes cutaneous about 7 in. above the lateral malleolus, while the deep fibular nerve becomes cutaneous between the large and second toes.

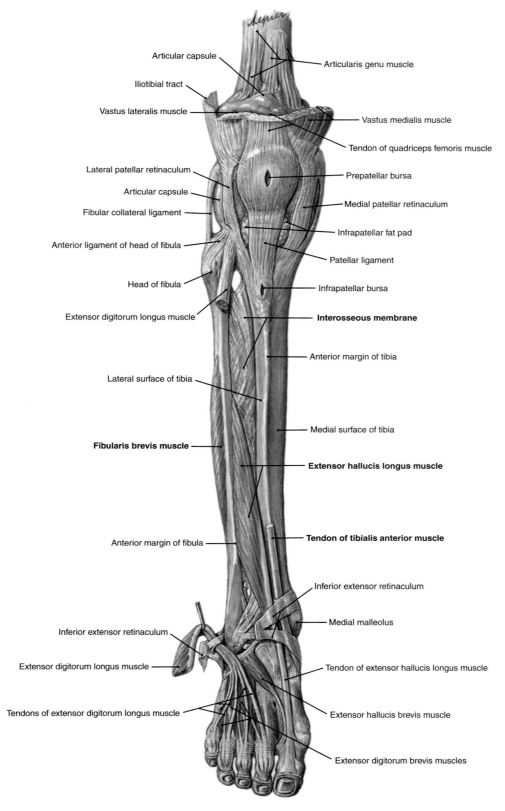

Articular capsule

Articularis genu muscle

Iliotibial tract

Vastus lateralis muscle

Vastus medialis muscle

Tendon of quadriceps femoris muscle

Lateral patellar retinaculum

Prepatellar bursa

Articular capsule

Medial patellar retinaculum

Fibular collateral ligament

Infrapatellar fat pad

Anterior ligament of head of fibula

Patellar ligament

Head of fibula

Infrapatellar bursa

Extensor digitorum longus muscle

Interosseous membrane

Anterior margin of tibia

Lateral surface of tibia

Medial surface of tibia

Fibularis brevis muscle

Extensor hallucis longus muscle

Tendon of tibialis anterior muscle

Anterior margin of fibula

Inferior extensor retinaculum

Medial malleolus

Inferior extensor retinaculum

Extensor digitorum longus muscle

Tendon of extensor hallucis longus muscle

Tendons of extensor digitorum longus muscle

Extensor hallucis brevis muscle

Extensor digitorum brevis muscles

FIGURE 451 **Deep Dissection of the Anterior and Lateral Compartments: Muscles**

NOTE: (1) The bellies of the tibialis anterior and fibularis longus muscles have been removed and the extensor digitorum longus muscle has been reflected. Observe the full extent of the **extensor hallucis longus** and the belly of the **fibularis brevis muscle**.

(2) The interosseous membrane between the tibia and the fibula and the opening above its upper border through which course the anterior tibial vessels.

PLATE 452 Lower Extremity: Lateral Compartment of the Leg (Dissection 6)

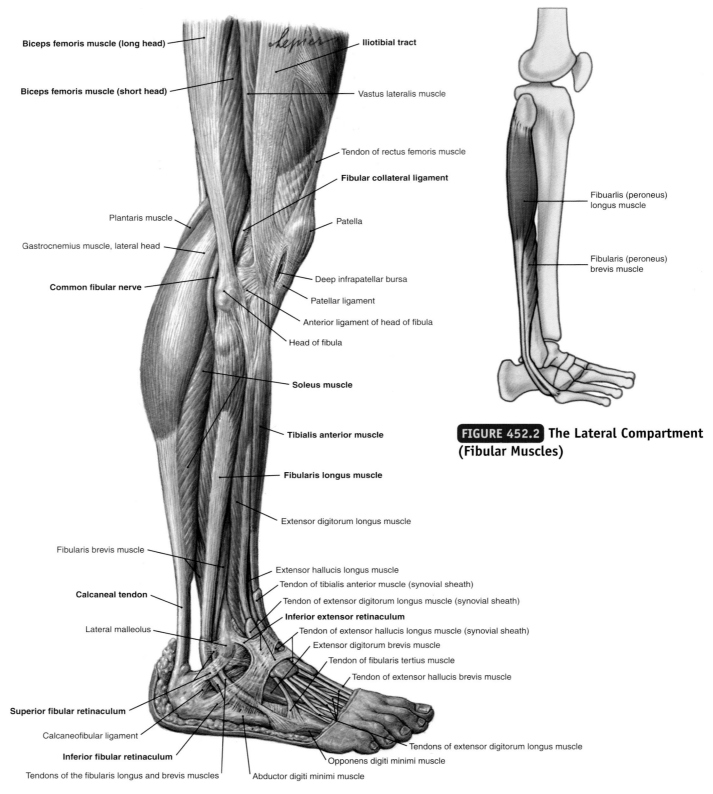

Biceps femoris muscle (long head)

Biceps femoris muscle (short head)

Plantaris muscle

Gastrocnemius muscle, lateral head

Common fibular nerve

Fibularis brevis muscle

Calcaneal tendon

Lateral malleolus

Superior fibular retinaculum

Calcaneofibular ligament

Inferior fibular retinaculum

Tendons of the fibularis longus and brevis muscles

Iliotibial tract

Vastus lateralis muscle

Tendon of rectus femoris muscle

Fibular collateral ligament

Patella

Deep infrapatellar bursa

Patellar ligament

Anterior ligament of head of fibula

Head of fibula

Soleus muscle

Tibialis anterior muscle

Fibularis longus muscle

Extensor digitorum longus muscle

Extensor hallucis longus muscle

Tendon of tibialis anterior muscle (synovial sheath)

Tendon of extensor digitorum longus muscle (synovial sheath)

Inferior extensor retinaculum

Tendon of extensor hallucis longus muscle (synovial sheath)

Extensor digitorum brevis muscle

Tendon of fibularis tertius muscle

Tendon of extensor hallucis brevis muscle

Tendons of extensor digitorum longus muscle

Opponens digiti minimi muscle

Abductor digiti minimi muscle

Fibuarlis (peroneus) longus muscle

Fibularis (peroneus) brevis muscle

FIGURE 452.2 The Lateral Compartment (Fibular Muscles)

FIGURE 452.1 Lateral Compartment Muscles and Tendons of the Right Leg (Lateral View)

NOTE: (1) The **fibularis longus** and **brevis** occupy the lateral compartment of the leg, and their tendons descend into the foot behind the lateral malleolus. The fibularis longus tendon crosses the sole of the foot to insert on the base of the first metatarsal bone, while the fibularis brevis inserts directly onto the base of the fifth metatarsal bone.

(2) The superficial location of the **head of the fibula** and its relationship to the **common fibular nerve**. Trauma to the lateral side of the leg could cause injury to this nerve, resulting in a condition called foot drop, because the dorsiflexors would be denervated and the action of the plantar flexors in the posterior compartment would no longer be opposed.

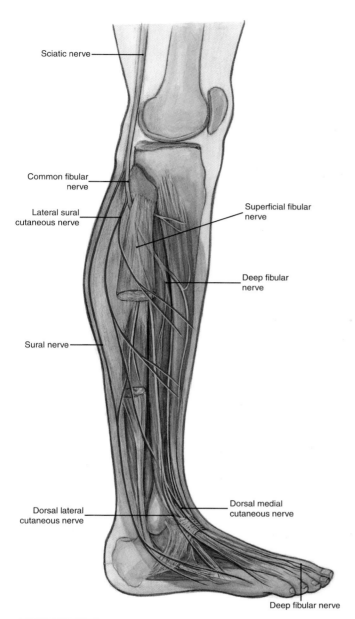

FIGURE 453.1 **Superficial and Deep Fibular Nerves**

NOTE: The cutaneous nerves are in purple.

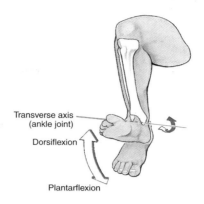

FIGURE 453.2 **Dorsiflexion and Plantar Flexion of the Foot (at Ankle Joint)**

NOTE: that (1) **Dorsiflexion:**
(a) Attempts to approximate the dorsum of the foot to the anterior leg surface.
(b) Is considered as extension at ankle joint.
(c) Is performed by muscles in the anterior compartment of the leg.

(2) **Plantar flexion:**
(a) Reverses dorsiflexion and also occurs when one stands on one's toes.
(b) Is considered as flexion at ankle joint.
(c) Is performed by muscles in the posterior compartment of the leg.

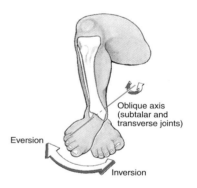

FIGURE 453.3 **Inversion and Eversion of the Foot (at Subtalar and Transverse Joint)**

NOTE: that (1) **Inversion:**
(a) Attempts to supinate the foot, that is, to turn the sole medially or inward.
(b) Is performed by muscles in the leg that attach medially on the foot (tibialis anterior *and* posterior; extensor *and* flexor hallucis longus).

(2) **Eversion:**
(a) Attempts to pronate the foot, that is, to turn the sole laterally or outward.
(b) Is performed by muscles in the leg that attach laterally on the foot such as fibularis longus, brevis, and tertius.

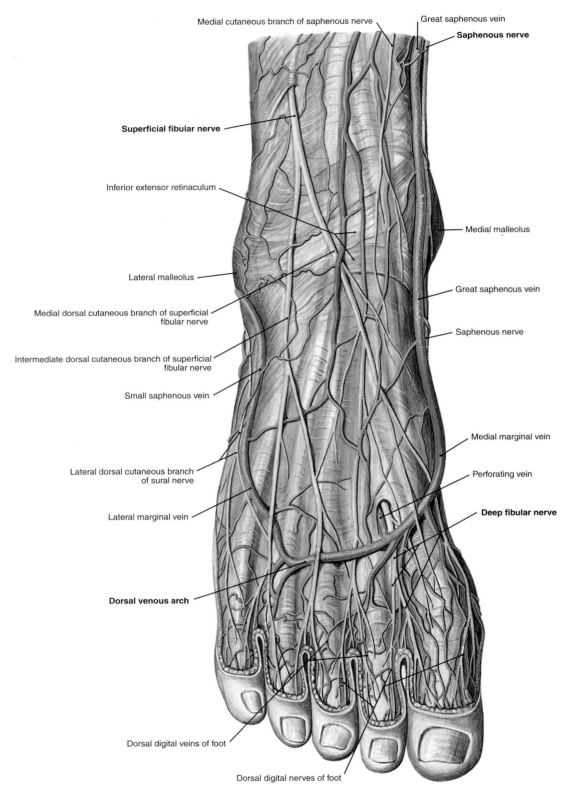

Medial cutaneous branch of saphenous nerve

Great saphenous vein

Saphenous nerve

Superficial fibular nerve

Inferior extensor retinaculum

Medial malleolus

Lateral malleolus

Great saphenous vein

Medial dorsal cutaneous branch of superficial fibular nerve

Saphenous nerve

Intermediate dorsal cutaneous branch of superficial fibular nerve

Small saphenous vein

Medial marginal vein

Perforating vein

Lateral dorsal cutaneous branch of sural nerve

Deep fibular nerve

Lateral marginal vein

Dorsal venous arch

Dorsal digital veins of foot

Dorsal digital nerves of foot

FIGURE 454 Superficial Nerves and Veins of the Dorsal Right Foot

NOTE: (1) Cutaneous innervation of the dorsal foot is supplied principally by the **superficial fibular nerve** (L4, L5, S1). In addition, the **deep fibular nerve** (L4, L5) supplies the adjacent sides of the first and second toes, while the **lateral dorsal cutaneous nerve** (S1, S2; terminal branch of the sural nerve in the foot) supplies the lateral and dorsal aspects of the fifth digit.

(2) The digital and metatarsal veins drain back from the toes to form the dorsal venous arch of the foot. From this arch, the **great saphenous vein** ascends medially and the **small saphenous vein** laterally on the foot dorsum.

(3) The cutaneous branch of the **saphenous nerve** extends downward as far as the ankle joint anteriorly. Medially, the main trunk of the saphenous nerve can extend inferiorly as far as the metatarsophalangeal joint of the large toe.

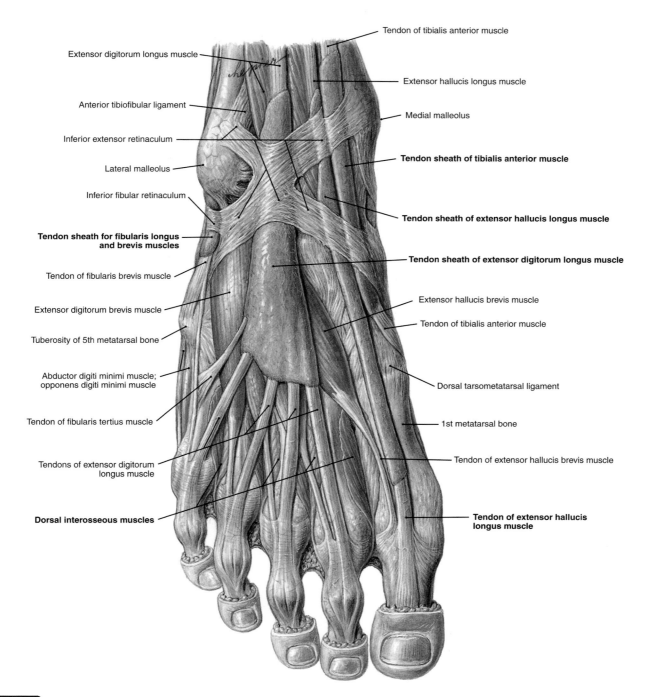

Tendon of tibialis anterior muscle

Extensor digitorum longus muscle

Anterior tibiofibular ligament

Inferior extensor retinaculum

Extensor hallucis longus muscle

Medial malleolus

Lateral malleolus

Tendon sheath of tibialis anterior muscle

Inferior fibular retinaculum

Tendon sheath for fibularis longus and brevis muscles

Tendon sheath of extensor hallucis longus muscle

Tendon of fibularis brevis muscle

Tendon sheath of extensor digitorum longus muscle

Extensor digitorum brevis muscle

Extensor hallucis brevis muscle

Tuberosity of 5th metatarsal bone

Tendon of tibialis anterior muscle

Abductor digiti minimi muscle; opponens digiti minimi muscle

Dorsal tarsometatarsal ligament

Tendon of fibularis tertius muscle

1st metatarsal bone

Tendons of extensor digitorum longus muscle

Tendon of extensor hallucis brevis muscle

Dorsal interosseous muscles

Tendon of extensor hallucis longus muscle

FIGURE 455 **Muscles, Tendons, and Tendon Sheaths of the Dorsal Right Foot (Superficial View)**

NOTE: (1) The tendons of the tibialis anterior, extensor hallucis longus, and extensor digitorum longus are bound by the Y-shaped (or X-shaped) inferior extensor retinaculum as they enter the dorsum of the foot at the level of the ankle joint.

(2) The extensor tendons insert onto the dorsal aspect of the distal phalanx of each toe. In addition, the tendons of the extensor digitorum longus also insert onto the dorsum of the middle phalanx of the four lateral toes.

(3) The tendon of the fibularis tertius inserts on the base of the fifth metatarsal bone (and at times the fourth also).

(4) Separate synovial sheaths (shown in blue) surround the tendons of the tibialis anterior and extensor hallucis longus. Also note the common synovial sheath for the main tendon and the individual digital tendons of the extensor digitorum longus.

(5) The tendon sheaths laterally and medially under the two malleoli are shown in Figures 456.1 and 456.2.

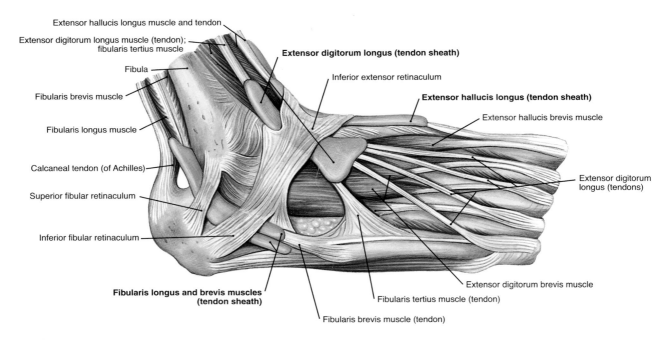

FIGURE 456.1 Tendons and Synovial Sheaths: Right Dorsum of Foot and Ankle Region (Lateral View)

NOTE: (1) Similar to the wrist, tendons at the ankle region passing from the leg into the foot are bound by closely investing **retinacula** and are surrounded by **synovial sheaths**, which are indicated in blue in this figure and in Figure 456.2.

(2) Anterior to the ankle joint and on the dorsum of the foot are three separate synovial sheaths, one that includes the extensor digitorum longus and the fibularis tertius, a second for the extensor hallucis longus, and a third for the tibialis anterior (see Figs. 452.1 and 455).

(3) Behind the lateral malleolus is a single tendon sheath for the fibularis longus and brevis muscles, which then splits distally to continue along each individual tendon for some distance.

(4) The inferior extensor retinaculum and the superior and inferior fibular retinacula, which bind the tendons and their sheaths close to the bone.

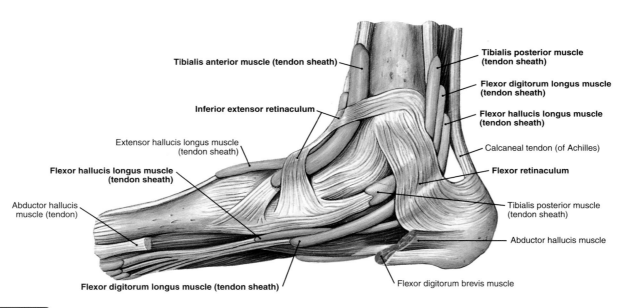

FIGURE 456.2 Tendons and Synovial Sheaths: Right Dorsum of Foot and Ankle Region (Medial View)

NOTE: (1) From this medial view can be seen the synovial sheaths and tendons of the tibialis anterior and extensor hallucis longus on the dorsum of the foot as well as the three tendons that course beneath the medial malleolus into the plantar aspect of the foot from the posterior compartment: the tibialis posterior, the flexor digitorum longus, and the flexor hallucis longus.

(2) The bifurcating nature of the inferior extensor retinaculum, and the manner in which the flexor retinaculum secures the structures beneath the medial malleolus.

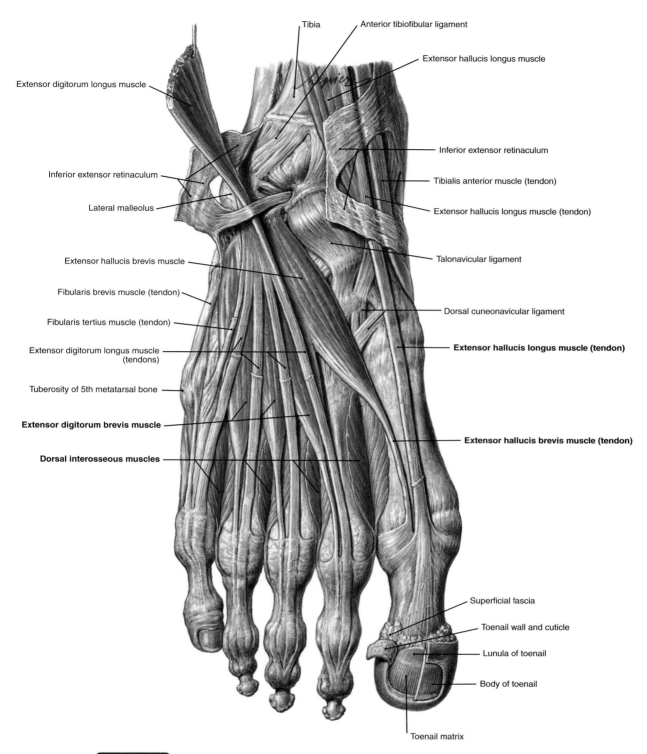

Tibia

Anterior tibiofibular ligament

Extensor hallucis longus muscle

Extensor digitorum longus muscle

Inferior extensor retinaculum

Tibialis anterior muscle (tendon)

Inferior extensor retinaculum

Lateral malleolus

Extensor hallucis longus muscle (tendon)

Extensor hallucis brevis muscle

Talonavicular ligament

Fibularis brevis muscle (tendon)

Fibularis tertius muscle (tendon)

Dorsal cuneonavicular ligament

Extensor digitorum longus muscle (tendons)

Extensor hallucis longus muscle (tendon)

Tuberosity of 5th metatarsal bone

Extensor digitorum brevis muscle

Extensor hallucis brevis muscle (tendon)

Dorsal interosseous muscles

Superficial fascia

Toenail wall and cuticle

Lunula of toenail

Body of toenail

Toenail matrix

FIGURE 457 Muscles and Tendons on the Dorsal Aspect of the Right Foot

| MUSCLES ON THE DORSUM OF THE FOOT | | | | |
Muscle	Origin	Insertion	Innervation	Function
Extensor hallucis brevis	Dorsal aspect of the calcaneus bone	Lateral side of the base of the proximal phalanx of the great toe	Deep fibular nerve (L5, S1)	Helps extend the proximal phalanx of the great toe
Extensor digitorum brevis	Dorsal and lateral aspect of the calcaneus bone	Lateral side of the tendons of the extensor digitorum longus muscle for the second, third, and fourth toes	Deep fibular nerve (L5, S1)	Helps extend the proximal phalanges of the second, third, and fourth toes

PLATE 458 Dorsum of the Foot: Muscles and Tendons (Dissection 4)

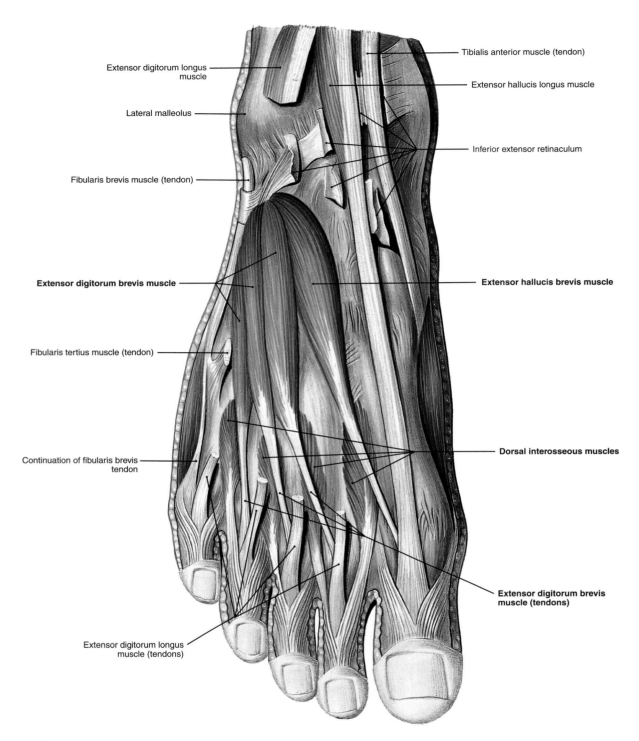

Extensor digitorum longus muscle

Lateral malleolus

Fibularis brevis muscle (tendon)

Extensor digitorum brevis muscle

Fibularis tertius muscle (tendon)

Continuation of fibularis brevis tendon

Extensor digitorum longus muscle (tendons)

Tibialis anterior muscle (tendon)

Extensor hallucis longus muscle

Inferior extensor retinaculum

Extensor hallucis brevis muscle

Dorsal interosseous muscles

Extensor digitorum brevis muscle (tendons)

FIGURE 458 Intrinsic Muscles of the Dorsal Foot (Right)

NOTE: (1) The inferior extensor retinaculum has been opened and the tendons of the extensor digitorum longus and fibularis tertius muscles have been severed.

(2) The **extensor hallucis brevis muscle** and the three small bellies of the **extensor digitorum brevis.** The delicate tendons of these muscles insert on the proximal phalanx of the medial four toes.

(3) The four **dorsal interosseous muscles.** These muscles abduct the toes from the longitudinal axis of the foot (down the middle of the second toe). The first dorsal interosseous muscle inserts on the medial side of the second toe, while the remaining three insert on the lateral side of the second, third, and fourth toes.

(4) Although the dorsal interosseous muscles are usually designated as the deepest layer of muscles on the **plantar** aspect of the foot, they can best be seen on the dorsal surface following reflection of the tendons of the extensor digitorum longus and brevis muscles.

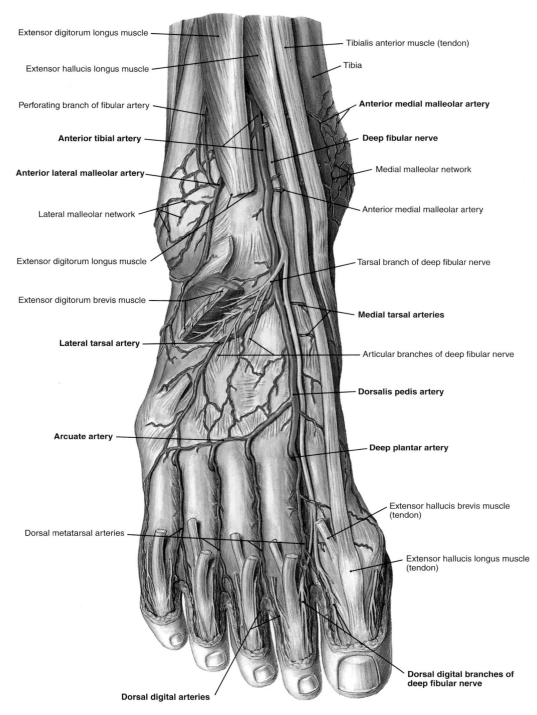

Extensor digitorum longus muscle

Extensor hallucis longus muscle

Perforating branch of fibular artery

Anterior tibial artery

Anterior lateral malleolar artery

Lateral malleolar network

Extensor digitorum longus muscle

Extensor digitorum brevis muscle

Lateral tarsal artery

Arcuate artery

Dorsal metatarsal arteries

Dorsal digital arteries

Tibialis anterior muscle (tendon)

Tibia

Anterior medial malleolar artery

Deep fibular nerve

Medial malleolar network

Anterior medial malleolar artery

Tarsal branch of deep fibular nerve

Medial tarsal arteries

Articular branches of deep fibular nerve

Dorsalis pedis artery

Deep plantar artery

Extensor hallucis brevis muscle (tendon)

Extensor hallucis longus muscle (tendon)

Dorsal digital branches of deep fibular nerve

FIGURE 459 **Deep Nerves and Arteries of the Dorsal Foot**

NOTE: (1) The deeply coursing **anterior tibial artery** and **deep fibular nerve** and their branches have been exposed. They enter the foot between tendons of the extensor hallucis longus and extensor digitorum longus muscles.

(2) The anterior tibial artery becomes the **dorsalis pedis artery** below the ankle joint. The **deep plantar artery** branches from the dorsalis pedis and perforates the tissue between the first two metatarsal bones to enter the plantar foot. Also note the **malleolar, tarsal, arcuate, dorsal metatarsal,** and **digital arteries.**

(3) The **deep fibular nerve** supplies the extensor hallucis and extensor digitorum brevis muscles in the foot and continues distally to terminate as two dorsal digital nerves, which supply sensory innervation to the adjacent sides of the great toe and the second toe. Sensory innervation on the dorsal aspect of the other toes is derived from the **superficial fibular nerve.**

PLATE 460 **Posterior Leg; Superficial Vessels and Nerves (Dissection 1)**

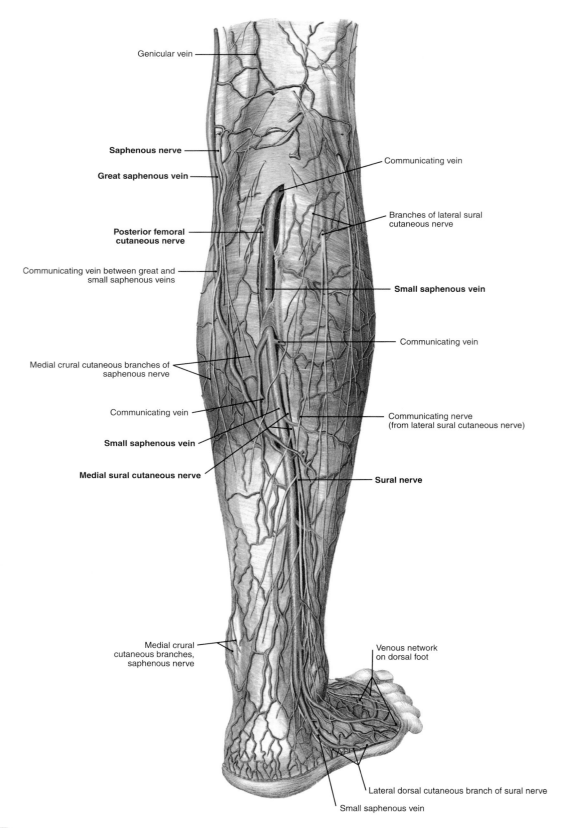

Genicular vein

Saphenous nerve

Great saphenous vein

Communicating vein

Posterior femoral
cutaneous nerve

Branches of lateral sural
cutaneous nerve

Communicating vein between great and
small saphenous veins

Small saphenous vein

Communicating vein

Medial crural cutaneous branches of
saphenous nerve

Communicating vein

Communicating nerve
(from lateral sural cutaneous nerve)

Small saphenous vein

Medial sural cutaneous nerve

Sural nerve

Medial crural
cutaneous branches,
saphenous nerve

Venous network
on dorsal foot

Lateral dorsal cutaneous branch of sural nerve

Small saphenous vein

FIGURE 460 Superficial Veins and Cutaneous Nerves of the Posterior Leg and Dorsal Foot

NOTE: (1) The **small saphenous vein** forms on the dorsolateral aspect of the foot and ascends to the popliteal fossa, and superficial communicating branches interconnect it to the great saphenous vein.

(2) The **sural nerve** is formed by the junction of a large branch, the medial sural cutaneous nerve (from the tibial nerve), and the lateral sural cutaneous branches from the common fibular nerve. This nerve supplies most of the posterolateral part of the leg, and medial crural cutaneous branches of the **saphenous nerve** supply the posteromedial leg.

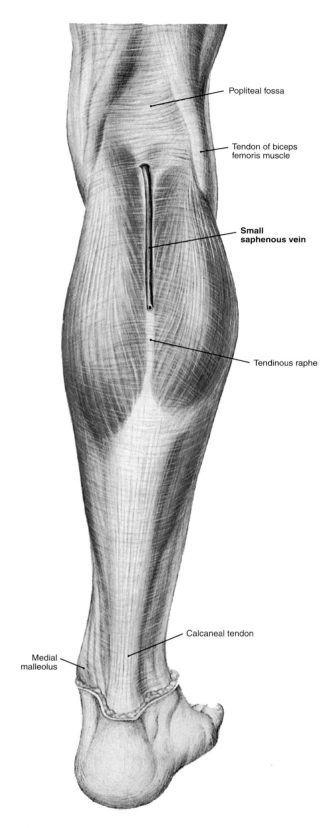

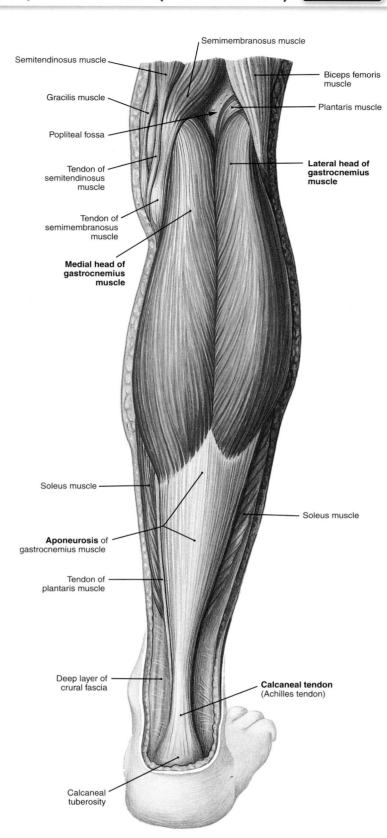

FIGURE 461.1 Deep Fascia of the Leg (the Crural Fascia) (Posterior View)

NOTE: The deep fascia of the leg closely invests all the muscles between the knee and the ankle and forms the fascial covering over the popliteal fossa. It is continuous above with the fascia lata of the thigh and below with the retinacula that bind the tendons close to the bones in the ankle region.

FIGURE 461.2 Muscles of the Posterior Leg: Superficial Calf Muscles

NOTE: (1) The **gastrocnemius muscle** arises by two heads from the condyles and posterior surface of the femur. It inserts by means of the strong **calcaneal tendon** onto the tuberosity of the calcaneus.

(2) The gastrocnemius is a strong plantar flexor of the foot, and its continued action also flexes the leg at the knee.

PLATE 462 Knee, Calf, and Foot: Muscles and Tendons (Medial View)

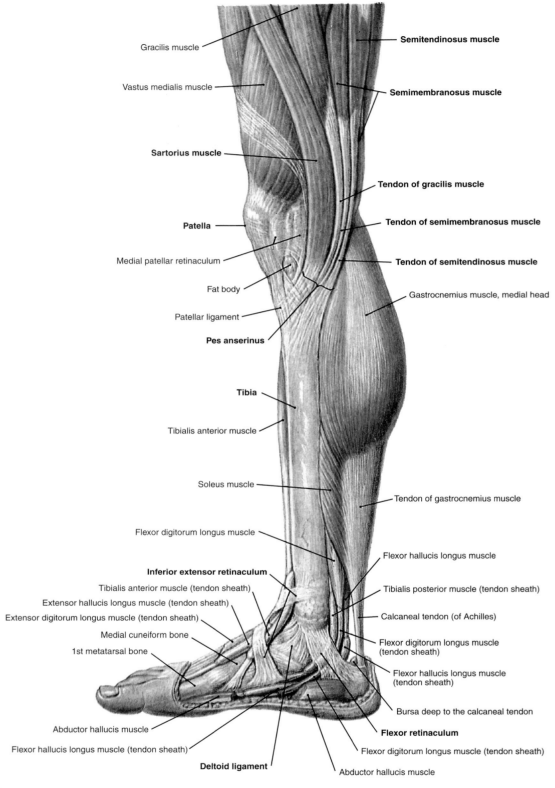

Gracilis muscle

Vastus medialis muscle

Sartorius muscle

Patella

Medial patellar retinaculum

Fat body

Patellar ligament

Pes anserinus

Tibia

Tibialis anterior muscle

Soleus muscle

Flexor digitorum longus muscle

Inferior extensor retinaculum

Tibialis anterior muscle (tendon sheath)

Extensor hallucis longus muscle (tendon sheath)

Extensor digitorum longus muscle (tendon sheath)

Medial cuneiform bone

1st metatarsal bone

Abductor hallucis muscle

Flexor hallucis longus muscle (tendon sheath)

Deltoid ligament

Semitendinosus muscle

Semimembranosus muscle

Tendon of gracilis muscle

Tendon of semimembranosus muscle

Tendon of semitendinosus muscle

Gastrocnemius muscle, medial head

Tendon of gastrocnemius muscle

Flexor hallucis longus muscle

Tibialis posterior muscle (tendon sheath)

Calcaneal tendon (of Achilles)

Flexor digitorum longus muscle (tendon sheath)

Flexor hallucis longus muscle (tendon sheath)

Bursa deep to the calcaneal tendon

Flexor retinaculum

Flexor digitorum longus muscle (tendon sheath)

Abductor hallucis muscle

FIGURE 462 Medial View of the Leg: Knee, Posterior Compartment, Ankle and Foot Regions

NOTE: (1) The medial head of the gastrocnemius muscle. Observe how its tendon inserts onto the tuberosity of the calcaneus, while the tendons of the tibialis posterior, flexor digitorum longus, and flexor hallucis longus enter the plantar surface of the foot.

(2) The flexor retinaculum holds these deep posterior compartment muscles close to the bone, thereby increasing their efficiency when they contract. Without these retinacula, muscular contraction would result in a bowing of the tendons and a loss of power.

(3) The tendons of the sartorius, gracilis, and semitendinosus form the so-called pes anserinus (goose's foot). This tendinous formation helps protect the medial aspect of the knee, while the tendon of the semimembranosus helps reinforce the capsule of the knee joint posteriorly.

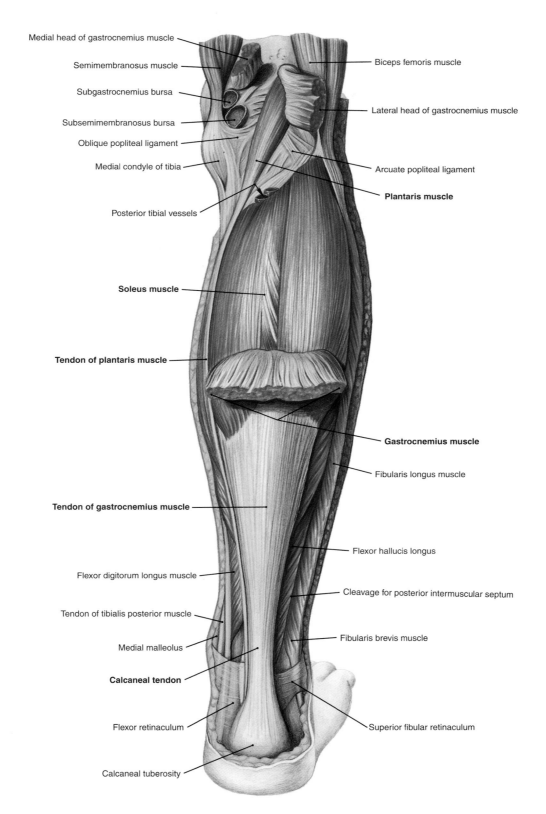

Medial head of gastrocnemius muscle

Semimembranosus muscle

Subgastrocnemius bursa

Subsemimembranosus bursa

Oblique popliteal ligament

Medial condyle of tibia

Posterior tibial vessels

Soleus muscle

Tendon of plantaris muscle

Tendon of gastrocnemius muscle

Flexor digitorum longus muscle

Tendon of tibialis posterior muscle

Medial malleolus

Calcaneal tendon

Flexor retinaculum

Calcaneal tuberosity

Biceps femoris muscle

Lateral head of gastrocnemius muscle

Arcuate popliteal ligament

Plantaris muscle

Gastrocnemius muscle

Fibularis longus muscle

Flexor hallucis longus

Cleavage for posterior intermuscular septum

Fibularis brevis muscle

Superior fibular retinaculum

FIGURE 463 **Muscles of the Posterior Leg: Soleus and Plantaris Muscles**

NOTE: (1) Both heads of the gastrocnemius muscle have been severed. Observe the stumps of their origins from the femur above and the lower flap reflected downward to uncover the **soleus** and **plantaris muscles**.

(2) The soleus muscle is broad and thick and arises from the posterior surface of the fibula, the intermuscular septum, and the dorsal aspect of the tibia. Its fibers join the calcaneal tendon and insert in common with the gastrocnemius muscle.

(3) The small plantaris muscle has a long thin tendon that also joins the calcaneal tendon. Although the function of the plantaris is of little significance, its long tendon can be used by surgeons when that type of tissue is required.

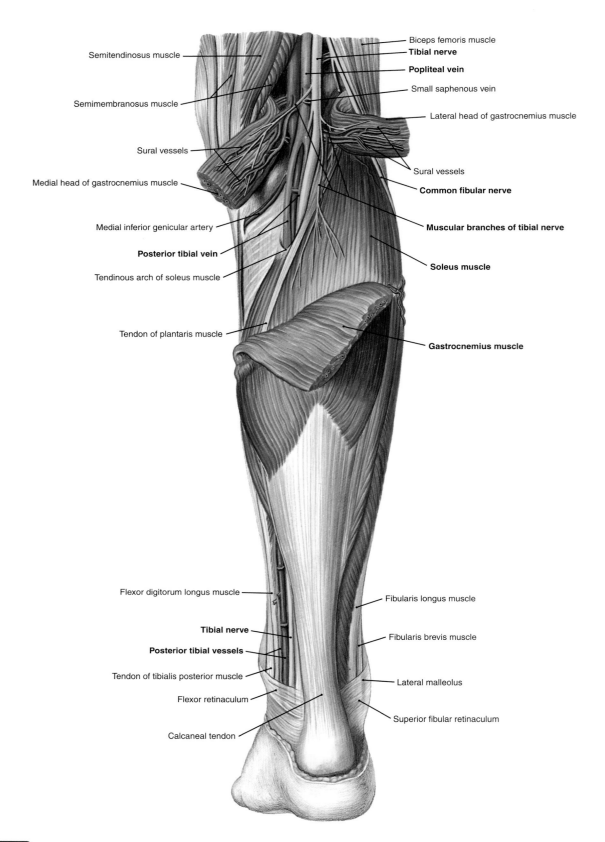

Semitendinosus muscle

Semimembranosus muscle

Sural vessels

Medial head of gastrocnemius muscle

Medial inferior genicular artery

Posterior tibial vein

Tendinous arch of soleus muscle

Tendon of plantaris muscle

Flexor digitorum longus muscle

Tibial nerve

Posterior tibial vessels

Tendon of tibialis posterior muscle

Flexor retinaculum

Calcaneal tendon

Biceps femoris muscle

Tibial nerve

Popliteal vein

Small saphenous vein

Lateral head of gastrocnemius muscle

Sural vessels

Common fibular nerve

Muscular branches of tibial nerve

Soleus muscle

Gastrocnemius muscle

Fibularis longus muscle

Fibularis brevis muscle

Lateral malleolus

Superior fibular retinaculum

FIGURE 464 **Nerves and Vessels of the Posterior Leg above and below the Soleus Muscle**

NOTE: (1) The popliteal vessels and tibial nerve, descending from the popliteal fossa into the posterior compartment and the leg, commence to course medially in a gradual manner so that at the ankle they lie behind the medial malleolus.

(2) From the popliteal fossa, sural branches of the popliteal artery and muscular branches of the tibial nerve descend to supply the gastrocnemius and soleus muscles. These neurovascular structures course through a tendinous arch in the soleus muscle and descend deep to the soleus and become superficial again several inches above the medial malleolus.

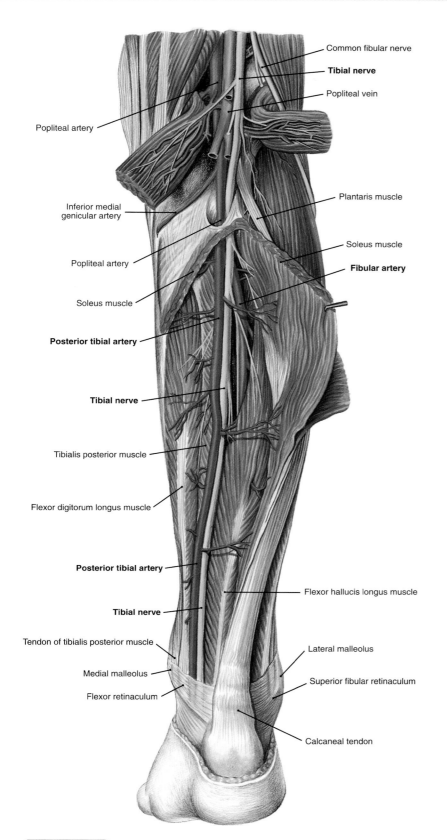

Common fibular nerve

Tibial nerve

Popliteal vein

Popliteal artery

Plantaris muscle

Inferior medial genicular artery

Soleus muscle

Popliteal artery

Fibular artery

Soleus muscle

Posterior tibial artery

Tibial nerve

Tibialis posterior muscle

Flexor digitorum longus muscle

Posterior tibial artery

Flexor hallucis longus muscle

Tibial nerve

Tendon of tibialis posterior muscle

Lateral malleolus

Medial malleolus

Superior fibular retinaculum

Flexor retinaculum

Calcaneal tendon

FIGURE 465.1 Nerves and Vessels of the Right Posterior Leg: Intermediate Dissection

NOTE: (1) The soleus muscle was severed and reflected laterally to expose the course of the tibial nerve and posterior tibial artery.

(2) This vessel and nerve descend in the leg between the superficial and deep muscles of the posterior compartment, between the flexor hallucis longus and flexor digitorum longus.

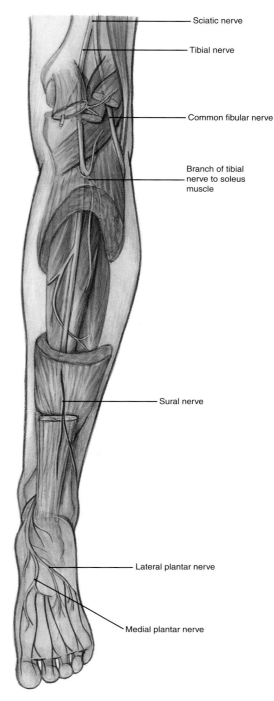

Sciatic nerve

Tibial nerve

Common fibular nerve

Branch of tibial nerve to soleus muscle

Sural nerve

Lateral plantar nerve

Medial plantar nerve

FIGURE 465.2 The Tibial Nerve in the Posterior Compartment of the Leg

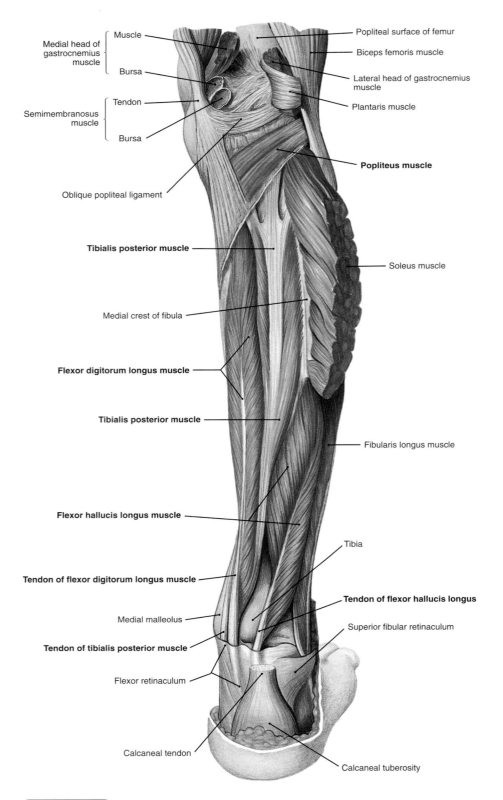

Muscle

Medial head of gastrocnemius muscle

Bursa

Tendon

Semimembranosus muscle

Bursa

Oblique popliteal ligament

Tibialis posterior muscle

Medial crest of fibula

Flexor digitorum longus muscle

Tibialis posterior muscle

Flexor hallucis longus muscle

Tendon of flexor digitorum longus muscle

Medial malleolus

Tendon of tibialis posterior muscle

Flexor retinaculum

Calcaneal tendon

Popliteal surface of femur

Biceps femoris muscle

Lateral head of gastrocnemius muscle

Plantaris muscle

Popliteus muscle

Soleus muscle

Fibularis longus muscle

Tibia

Tendon of flexor hallucis longus

Superior fibular retinaculum

Calcaneal tuberosity

FIGURE 466.1 Deep Muscles of the Posterior Compartment of the Leg

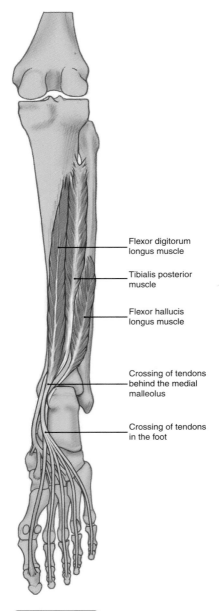

Flexor digitorum longus muscle

Tibialis posterior muscle

Flexor hallucis longus muscle

Crossing of tendons behind the medial malleolus

Crossing of tendons in the foot

FIGURE 466.2 Deep Muscles of the Posterior Leg

NOTE: (1) The four deep posterior compartment muscles are: (a) the **popliteus,** (b) the **flexor digitorum longus,** (c) the **tibialis posterior,** and (d) the **flexor hallucis longus.**

(2) The **popliteus** is a femorotibial muscle and it tends to rotate the leg medially; however, when the tibia is fixed and the knee joint is **locked,** this muscle rotates the femur laterally on the tibia and thereby it "**unlocks**" the knee joint.

(3) The other three muscles are cruropedal muscles, and as a group, they invert the foot, flex the toes, and assist in plantar flexion at the ankle joint.

(4) The tibialis posterior is closest to bone behind the medial malleolus, the flexor hallucis longus is most lateral, and the flexor digitorum is in between the two.

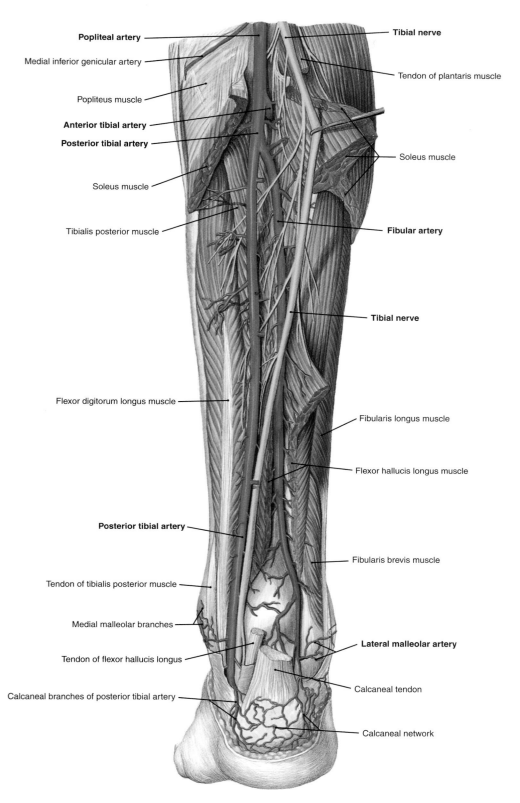

Popliteal artery

Medial inferior genicular artery

Popliteus muscle

Anterior tibial artery

Posterior tibial artery

Soleus muscle

Tibialis posterior muscle

Flexor digitorum longus muscle

Posterior tibial artery

Tendon of tibialis posterior muscle

Medial malleolar branches

Tendon of flexor hallucis longus

Calcaneal branches of posterior tibial artery

Tibial nerve

Tendon of plantaris muscle

Soleus muscle

Fibular artery

Tibial nerve

Fibularis longus muscle

Flexor hallucis longus muscle

Fibularis brevis muscle

Lateral malleolar artery

Calcaneal tendon

Calcaneal network

FIGURE 467 **Deep Nerves and Arteries of the Posterior Compartment of the Leg**

NOTE: (1) The soleus muscle was resected and the tibial nerve pulled laterally. Observe the branching of the **fibular artery** from the posterior tibial and its descending course toward the lateral malleolus.

(2) In the popliteal fossa, the tibial nerve courses superficially to the popliteal artery, whereas at the ankle, the posterior tibial artery is superficial to the tibial nerve.

(3) Behind the medial malleolus, the neurovascular structures are located between the tendons of the flexor digitorum longus and flexor hallucis longus.

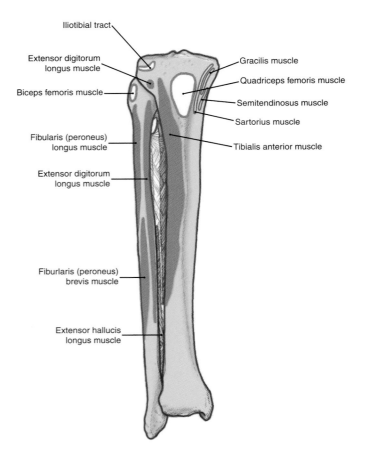

FIGURE 468.1 Attachments of the Anterior and Lateral Compartment Muscles on the Anterior Surfaces of the Fibula and Tibia

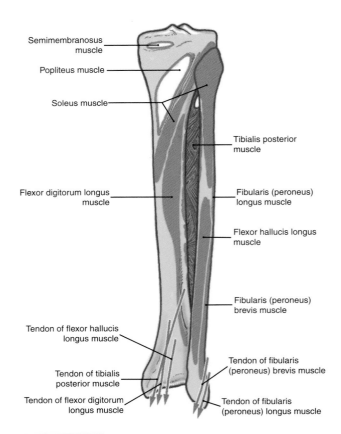

FIGURE 468.2 Attachments of the Lateral and Deep Posterior Compartment Muscles on the Posterior Surfaces of the Fibula and Tibia

MUSCLES OF THE POSTERIOR COMPARTMENT OF THE LEG

Muscle	Origin	Insertion	Innervation	Action
SUPERFICIAL GROUP				
Gastrocnemius	Medial head: Medial epicondyle of the femur Lateral head: Lateral epicondyle of the femur	Posterior surface of the calcaneus by means of the calcaneal tendon	Tibial nerve (S1, S2)	Plantar flexes the foot; flexes the leg at knee joint, tends to supinate the foot
Soleus	Posterior surface of head and upper third or body of fibula; soleal line and medial border of tibia	Joins the tendon of the gastrocnemius to insert on the calcaneus by means of the calcaneal tendon	Tibial nerve (S1, S2)	Plantar flexes the foot; important as a postural muscle during ordinary standing
Plantaris	Posterior aspect of lateral epicondyle of femur and from the oblique popliteal ligament	Into the calcaneal tendon with the gastrocnemius and soleus muscles	Tibial nerve (S1, S2)	Assists the gastrocnemius in plantar flexion of the foot and flexing the leg (weak action)
DEEP GROUP				
Popliteus	Lateral epicondyle of the femur; the lateral meniscus of the knee joint	Posterior surface of the body of the tibia proximal to the soleal line	Tibial nerve (L4, L5, S1)	Flexes and medially rotates the tibia when femur is fixed; laterally rotates the femur to unlock the knee joint when the tibia is fixed
Tibialis posterior	Posterior surface of interosseous membrane; posterior surface of tibia and medial surface of the fibula	Tuberosity of the navicular bone; slips to calcaneus, the three cuneiforms, the cuboid, and the second, third, and fourth metatarsal bones	Tibial nerve (L5, S1)	Plantar flexes the foot; inverts and adducts the foot (tends to supinate the foot)

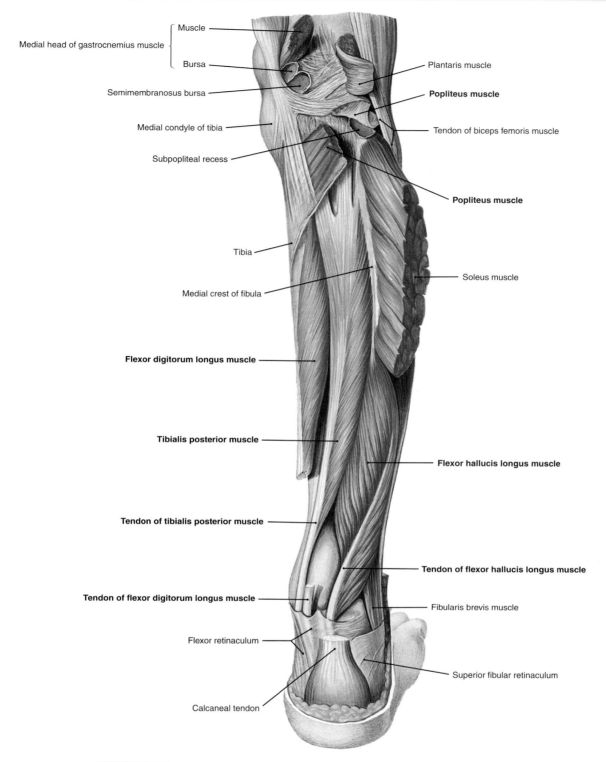

Muscle

Medial head of gastrocnemius muscle

Bursa

Semimembranosus bursa

Medial condyle of tibia

Subpopliteal recess

Tibia

Medial crest of fibula

Flexor digitorum longus muscle

Tibialis posterior muscle

Tendon of tibialis posterior muscle

Tendon of flexor digitorum longus muscle

Flexor retinaculum

Calcaneal tendon

Plantaris muscle

Popliteus muscle

Tendon of biceps femoris muscle

Popliteus muscle

Soleus muscle

Flexor hallucis longus muscle

Tendon of flexor hallucis longus muscle

Fibularis brevis muscle

Superior fibular retinaculum

FIGURE 469 Tibialis Posterior and Flexor Hallucis Longus Muscles

MUSCLES OF THE POSTERIOR COMPARTMENT OF THE LEG (Continued)				
Muscle	**Origin**	**Insertion**	**Innervation**	**Action**
Flexor digitorum longus	Posterior surface of tibia and fascia over tibialis posterior	Bases of the distal phalanx of the four lateral toes	Tibial nerve (S1, S2)	Flexes distal phalanx of lateral four toes; plantar flexes and supinates the foot
Flexor hallucis longus	Lower two-thirds of the posterior fibula and lower part of the interosseous membrane	Base of the distal phalanx of the large toe (hallux)	Tibial nerve (S1, S2)	Flexes distal phalanx of large toe; plantar flexes and supinates the foot

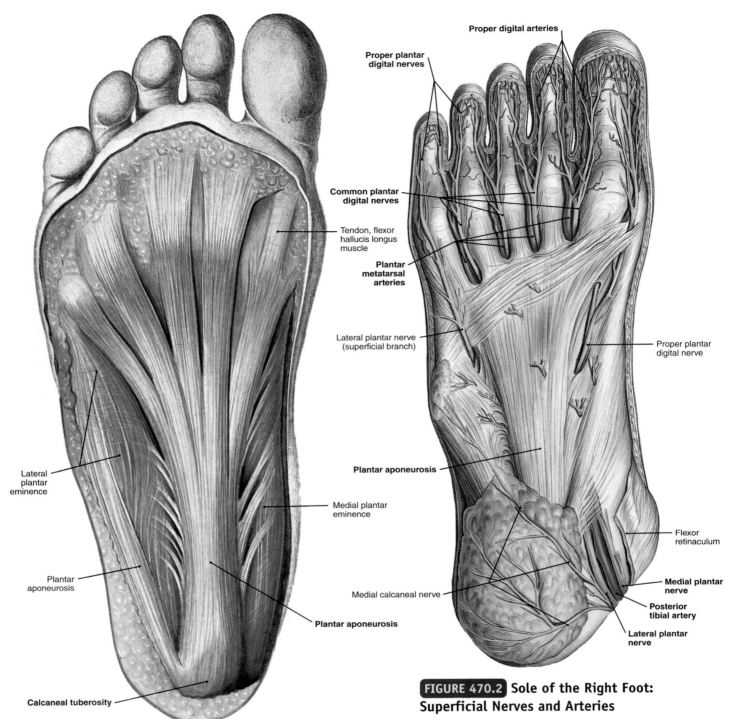

FIGURE 470.1 Sole of the Right Foot: Plantar Aponeurosis

NOTE: (1) The **plantar aponeurosis** stretching along the sole of the foot. Similar to the palmar aponeurosis in the hand, the plantar aponeurosis is a thickened layer of deep fascia serving a protective function to underlying muscles, vessels, and nerves.

(2) The longitudinal orientation of the plantar aponeurosis and its attachment behind to the calcaneal tuberosity. The aponeurosis divides distally into digital slips, one to each toe. At the margins, fibers partially cover the medial and lateral plantar eminences.

FIGURE 470.2 Sole of the Right Foot: Superficial Nerves and Arteries

NOTE: (1) The **medial** and **lateral plantar nerves** and **posterior tibial artery** as they enter the foot behind the medial malleolus and then immediately course beneath the plantar aponeurosis toward the digits. Cutaneous branches of the nerves penetrate the aponeurosis to supply the overlying skin and fascia.

(2) Between digital slips of the plantar aponeurosis, the vessels and nerves course superficially toward the toes. **Metatarsal arteries** and **common plantar digital nerves** divide to supply adjacent portions of the toes as **proper plantar digital arteries** and **nerves**.

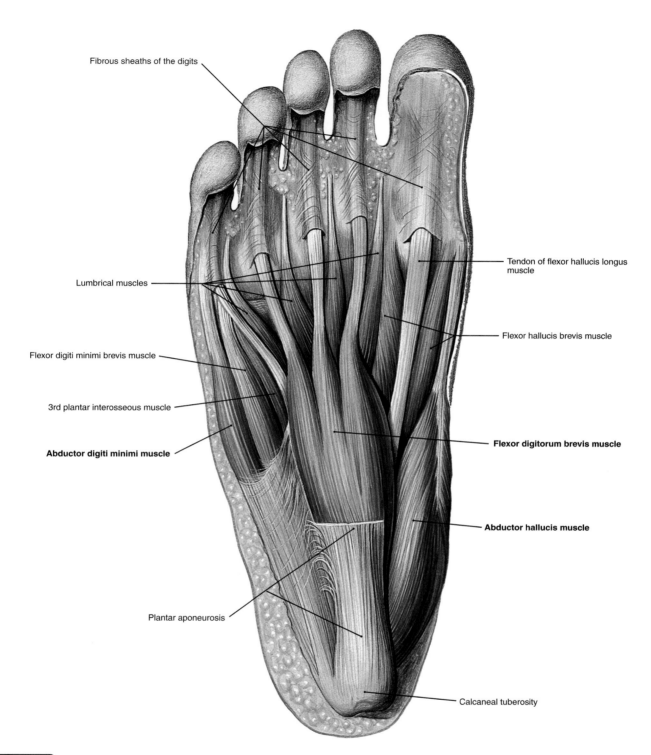

Fibrous sheaths of the digits

Lumbrical muscles

Flexor digiti minimi brevis muscle

3rd plantar interosseous muscle

Abductor digiti minimi muscle

Plantar aponeurosis

Tendon of flexor hallucis longus muscle

Flexor hallucis brevis muscle

Flexor digitorum brevis muscle

Abductor hallucis muscle

Calcaneal tuberosity

FIGURE 471 **Sole of the Foot: First Layer of Plantar Muscles**

NOTE: (1) With most of the plantar aponeurosis removed, three muscles comprising the first layer of plantar muscles are exposed. These are the **abductor hallucis,** the **flexor digitorum brevis,** and the **abductor digiti minimi.**

(2) All three muscles of the first layer arise from the tuberosity of the calcaneus. The abductor hallucis inserts on the proximal phalanx of the large toe. The flexor digitorum brevis separates into four tendons that insert onto the middle phalanges of the four lateral toes. The abductor digiti minimi inserts on the proximal phalanx of the small toe.

(3) The terminal parts of the tendons of the short and long flexors of the toes course within osseous–aponeurotic canals to their insertions on bone.

(4) These canals are covered inferiorly by **digital fibrous sheaths** that arch over the tendons and attach to the sides of the phalanges. Within the canals, **synovial sheaths** are closely reflected around the tendons, allowing for their movement upon muscular contraction.

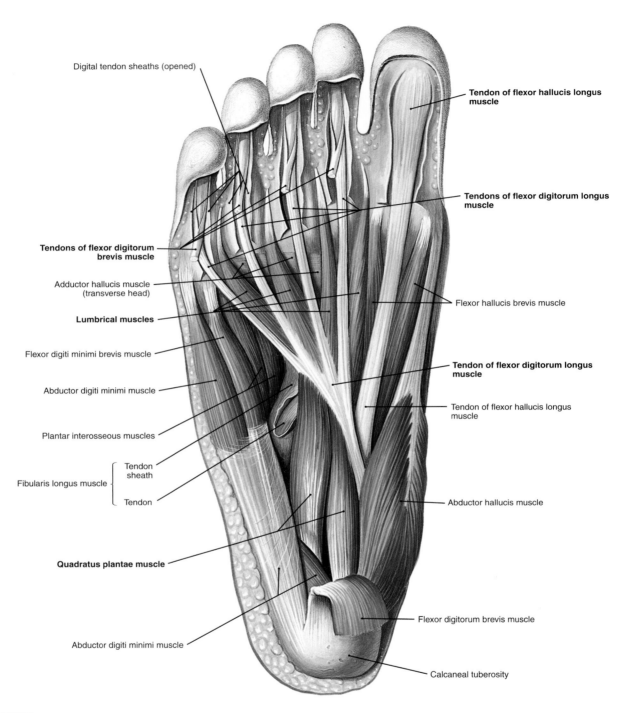

Digital tendon sheaths (opened)

Tendon of flexor hallucis longus muscle

Tendons of flexor digitorum longus muscle

Tendons of flexor digitorum brevis muscle

Adductor hallucis muscle (transverse head)

Flexor hallucis brevis muscle

Lumbrical muscles

Flexor digiti minimi brevis muscle

Tendon of flexor digitorum longus muscle

Abductor digiti minimi muscle

Tendon of flexor hallucis longus muscle

Plantar interosseous muscles

Tendon sheath

Fibularis longus muscle

Abductor hallucis muscle

Tendon

Quadratus plantae muscle

Flexor digitorum brevis muscle

Abductor digiti minimi muscle

Calcaneal tuberosity

FIGURE 472 Sole of the Right Foot: Second Layer of Plantar Muscles

NOTE: (1) The tendons of the flexor digitorum brevis muscle were severed and removed, thereby exposing the underlying tendons of the **flexor digitorum longus muscle.**

(2) The muscles of the **second layer** in the plantar foot include the **quadratus plantae muscle** and the four **lumbrical muscles.** The quadratus plantae arises by two heads from the calcaneus and inserts into the tendon of the flexor digitorum longus muscle.

(3) The four lumbrical muscles arise from the tendons of the flexor digitorum longus muscle. They insert on the medial aspect of the first phalanx of the lateral four toes as well as on the dorsal extensor hoods of the toes.

(4) The quadratus plantae muscle helps align the pull of the tendons of the flexor digitorum longus by distraightening the diagonal vector of the long tendon.

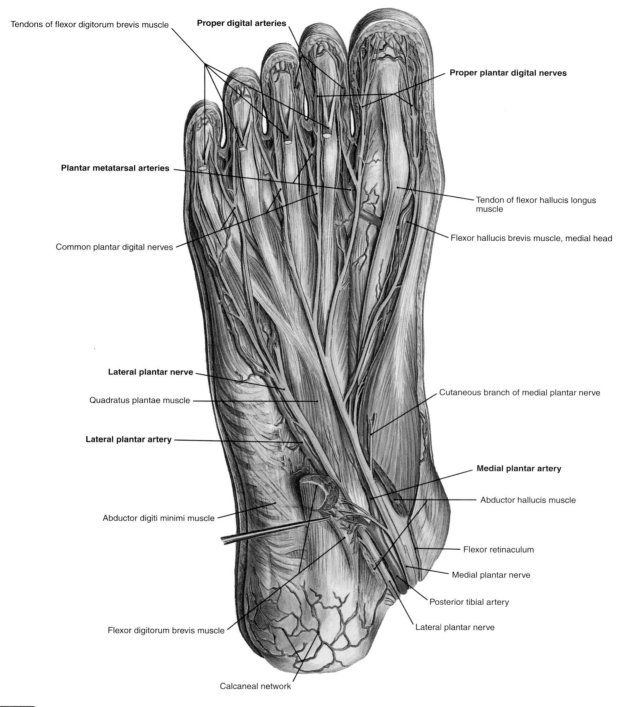

Tendons of flexor digitorum brevis muscle

Proper digital arteries

Proper plantar digital nerves

Plantar metatarsal arteries

Tendon of flexor hallucis longus muscle

Flexor hallucis brevis muscle, medial head

Common plantar digital nerves

Lateral plantar nerve

Quadratus plantae muscle

Cutaneous branch of medial plantar nerve

Lateral plantar artery

Medial plantar artery

Abductor hallucis muscle

Abductor digiti minimi muscle

Flexor retinaculum

Medial plantar nerve

Posterior tibial artery

Lateral plantar nerve

Flexor digitorum brevis muscle

Calcaneal network

FIGURE 473 **Sole of the Right Foot: The Plantar Nerves and Arteries**

NOTE: (1) While the tibial nerve divides into **medial** and **lateral plantar nerves** just below the medial malleolus, the posterior tibial artery enters the plantar surface of the foot as a single vessel and then divides into **medial** and **lateral plantar arteries** beneath or at the medial border of the abductor hallucis muscle.

(2) The lateral plantar nerve supplies the lateral 1½ digits with cutaneous innervation, while the medial plantar nerve supplies the medial 3½ digits. Observe the formation of the **common plantar digital nerves**, which then divide into the **proper plantar digital nerves**.

(3) The main trunks of the plantar vessels and nerves cross the sole of the foot from medial to lateral deep to the flexor digitorum brevis and abductor hallucis muscles (first layer) but superficial to the quadratus plantae and lumbrical muscles (second layer).

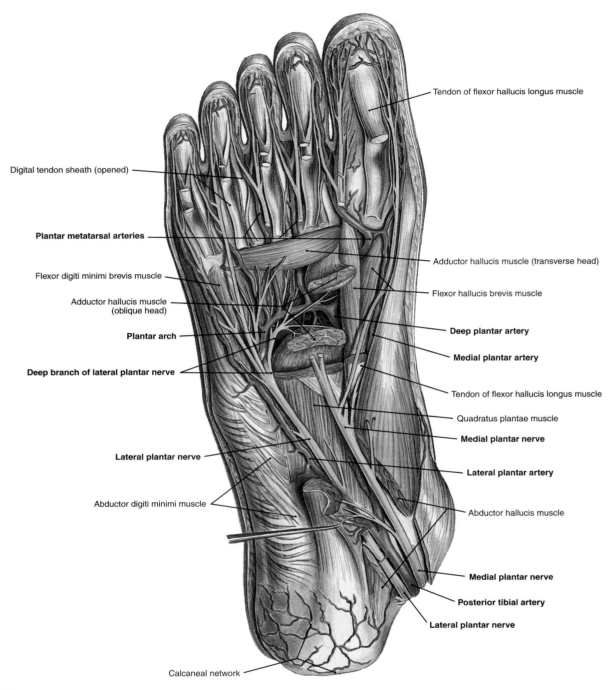

Tendon of flexor hallucis longus muscle

Digital tendon sheath (opened)

Plantar metatarsal arteries

Flexor digiti minimi brevis muscle

Adductor hallucis muscle (oblique head)

Plantar arch

Deep branch of lateral plantar nerve

Lateral plantar nerve

Abductor digiti minimi muscle

Adductor hallucis muscle (transverse head)

Flexor hallucis brevis muscle

Deep plantar artery

Medial plantar artery

Tendon of flexor hallucis longus muscle

Quadratus plantae muscle

Medial plantar nerve

Lateral plantar artery

Abductor hallucis muscle

Medial plantar nerve

Posterior tibial artery

Lateral plantar nerve

Calcaneal network

FIGURE 474 Sole of the Right Foot: Plantar Arch and Deep Vessels and Nerves

NOTE: (1) The formation of the **deep plantar arch** principally from the lateral plantar artery and the junction of the deep plantar arch with the deep plantar artery from the foot dorsum (see Fig. 459). From the plantar arch branch **plantar metatarsal arteries,** which divide into **proper original arteries.**

(2) The muscles of the foot are innervated in the following manner:

	Medial plantar nerve	Lateral plantar nerve
First layer	Abductor hallucis; flexor digitorum brevis	Abductor digiti minimi
Second layer	First lumbrical	Quadratus plantae; second, third, and fourth lumbrical
Third layer	Flexor hallucis brevis	Adductor hallucis; flexor digiti minimi brevis
Fourth layer		Plantar interossei; dorsal interossei

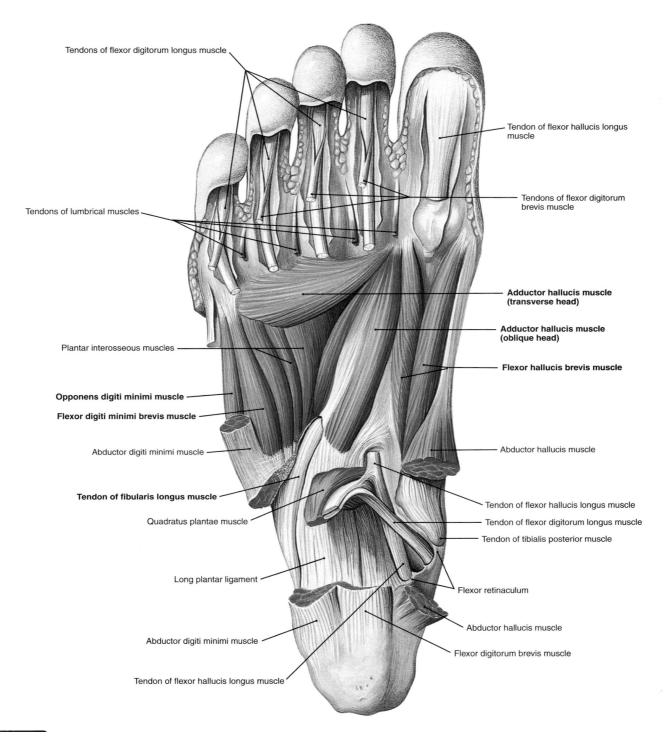

Tendons of flexor digitorum longus muscle

Tendon of flexor hallucis longus muscle

Tendons of lumbrical muscles

Tendons of flexor digitorum brevis muscle

Plantar interosseous muscles

Adductor hallucis muscle (transverse head)

Adductor hallucis muscle (oblique head)

Flexor hallucis brevis muscle

Opponens digiti minimi muscle

Flexor digiti minimi brevis muscle

Abductor digiti minimi muscle

Abductor hallucis muscle

Tendon of fibularis longus muscle

Tendon of flexor hallucis longus muscle

Quadratus plantae muscle

Tendon of flexor digitorum longus muscle

Tendon of tibialis posterior muscle

Long plantar ligament

Flexor retinaculum

Abductor digiti minimi muscle

Abductor hallucis muscle

Flexor digitorum brevis muscle

Tendon of flexor hallucis longus muscle

FIGURE 475 **Sole of the Right Foot: Third Layer of Plantar Muscles**

NOTE: (1) The third layer of plantar muscles consists of two flexors and an *ad*ductor (with two heads), in contrast to the first layer, which contains one flexor and two *ab*ductors. Thus, the **flexor hallucis brevis, the flexor digiti minimi brevis,** and the **oblique** and **transverse heads** of the **adductor hallucis** form the third layer of plantar muscles.

(2) At times, the fibers of the flexor digiti minimi brevis that insert on the lateral side of the first phalanx of the fifth toe are referred to as a separate muscle: the **opponens digiti minimi**.

(3) The tendon of the **fibularis longus muscles**, which crosses the plantar aspect of the foot obliquely to insert on the lateral side of the base of the first metatarsal and the first (medial) cuneiform bone.

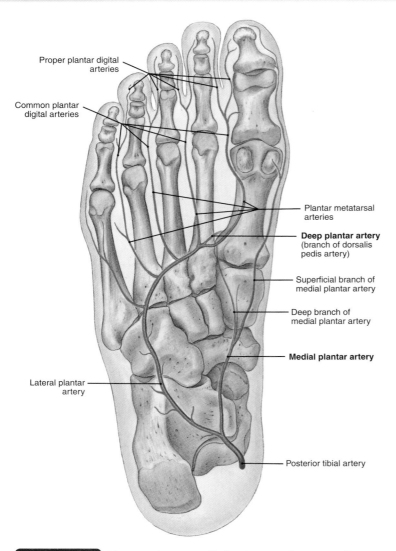

Proper plantar digital arteries

Common plantar digital arteries

Plantar metatarsal arteries

Deep plantar artery (branch of dorsalis pedis artery)

Superficial branch of medial plantar artery

Deep branch of medial plantar artery

Medial plantar artery

Lateral plantar artery

Posterior tibial artery

FIGURE 476.1 **Plantar Aspect of the Foot: Diagram of Arteries and Bones**

NOTE: The **posterior tibial artery** enters the foot medially behind the medial malleolus, divides into **medial** and **lateral plantar arteries**, and anastomoses with the deep plantar branch of the **dorsalis pedis artery** between the first and second digits.

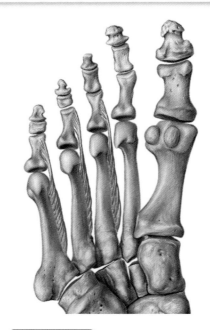

FIGURE 476.2 **Plantar Interossei**

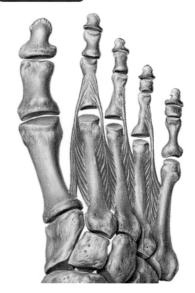

FIGURE 476.3 **Dorsal Interossei**

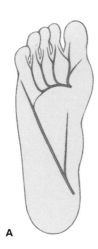

A

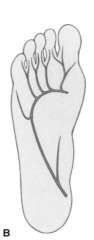

B

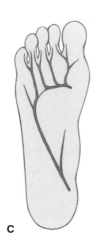

C

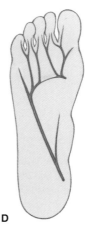

D

FIGURE 476.4 **Variations in the Arteries on the Plantar Aspect of the Foot**

NOTE: **A:** Deep plantar arch principally from the dorsalis pedis artery (from the foot dorsum).
B: Deep plantar arch supplied mainly from the lateral plantar branch of the posterior tibial artery.
C: Fifth and part of fourth toes by lateral plantar artery, medial toes by dorsalis pedis artery.
D: Fifth, fourth, and lateral part of third toe by lateral plantar artery, medial toes by dorsalis pedis artery.

MUSCLES OF THE SOLE OF THE FOOT

Muscle	Origin	Insertion	Innervation	Action
FIRST LAYER OF MUSCLES				
Abductor hallucis	Flexor retinaculum; medial process of calcaneal tuberosity; plantar aponeurosis	Medial side of the base of the proximal phalanx of the large toe	Medial plantar nerve (L5, S1)	Abducts and flexes the large toe; helps maintain the medial longitudinal arch
Flexor digitorum brevis	Medial process of calcaneal tuberosity; plantar aponeurosis	By four tendons onto the middle phalanx of the lateral four toes	Medial plantar nerve (L5, S1)	Flexes the lateral four toes
Abductor digiti minimi	Medial and lateral processes of the calcaneal tuberosity; plantar aponeurosis	Lateral side of the base of the proximal phalanx of the small toe	Lateral planter nerve (S2, S3)	Abducts and flexes the little toe
SECOND LAYER OF MUSCLES				
Quadratus plantae	By two heads from the plantar surface of the calcaneus; long plantar ligament	Lateral and deep surfaces of the tendons of the flexor digitorum longus muscle	Lateral plantar nerve (S2, S3)	Assists the flexor digitorum longus; straightens the pull of flexor digitorum longus along longitudinal axis of foot
First lumbrical	Medial side of the first tendon (to second toe) of the flexor digitorum longus	Passes along the medial side of second toe and inserts on its dorsal digital expansion	Medial plantar nerve (L5, S1)	Flexes the proximal phalanx at the metatarsophalangeal joint; extends the interphalangeal joints
Second, third, and fourth lumbrical	Each muscle by two heads from the adjacent surfaces of the second, third, and fourth tendons (to the third, fourth, and fifth toes) of the flexor digitorum longus muscle	Course along the medial sides of the third, fourth, and fifth toes and insert on their respective dorsal digital expansions	Lateral plantar nerve (S2, S3)	Action same as the first lumbrical
THIRD LAYER OF MUSCLES				
Flexor hallucis brevis	Plantar surface of cuboid and lateral (third) cuneiform bones; tendon of the tibialis posterior	By two tendons onto the sides of the base of the proximal phalanx of the large toe	Medial plantar nerve (L5, S1)	Flexes the proximal phalanx of the large toe at the metatarsophalangeal joint
Flexor digiti minimi	Base of the fifth metatarsal bone; the sheath of the tendon of the fibularis longus	Lateral side of the base of the proximal phalanx of the small toe	Lateral plantar nerve (S2, S3)	Flexes the proximal phalanx of the small toe at the metatarsophalangeal joint
Adductor hallucis Transverse head	Plantar metatarsophalangeal ligaments of third, fourth, and fifth toes; deep transverse metatarsal ligaments between the toes	By a common tendon to lateral aspect of the base of the proximal phalanx of the large toe	Lateral plantar nerve (S2, S3)	Adducts large toe; flexes large toe at metatarsophalangeal joint
Oblique head	Bases of the second, third, and fourth metatarsal bones; sheath of the tendon of fibularis longus muscle			
FOURTH LAYER OF MUSCLES				
Plantar interossei (three muscles)	Bases and medial sides of third, fourth, and fifth metatarsal bones	Bases of proximal phalanx of third, fourth, and fifth toes (medial side); onto the dorsal digital expansions	Lateral plantar nerve (S2, S3)	Adduct third, fourth, and fifth toes; flex metatarsophalangeal joints; extend interphalangeal joints
Dorsal interossei (four muscles)	Each by two heads from adjacent sides of metatarsal bones	Proximal phalanx and dorsal digital expansions of second, third, and fourth toes	Lateral plantar nerve (S2, S3)	Abduct second, third, and fourth toes; flex metatarsophalangeal joints and extend interphalangeal joints

PLATE 478 **Bones of Lower Limb: Muscle Attachments; Femur (Anterior View)**

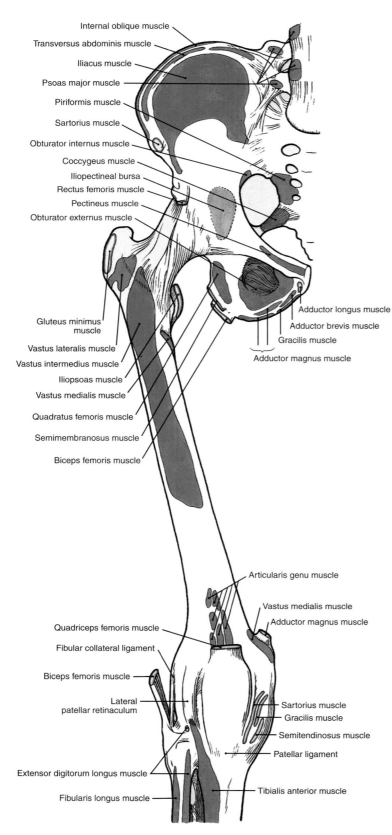

Internal oblique muscle
Transversus abdominis muscle
Iliacus muscle
Psoas major muscle
Piriformis muscle
Sartorius muscle
Obturator internus muscle
Coccygeus muscle
Iliopectineal bursa
Rectus femoris muscle
Pectineus muscle
Obturator externus muscle

Gluteus minimus muscle
Vastus lateralis muscle
Vastus intermedius muscle
Iliopsoas muscle
Vastus medialis muscle
Quadratus femoris muscle
Semimembranosus muscle
Biceps femoris muscle

Adductor longus muscle
Adductor brevis muscle
Gracilis muscle
Adductor magnus muscle

Articularis genu muscle
Vastus medialis muscle
Adductor magnus muscle

Quadriceps femoris muscle
Fibular collateral ligament
Biceps femoris muscle
Lateral patellar retinaculum
Extensor digitorum longus muscle
Fibularis longus muscle

Sartorius muscle
Gracilis muscle
Semitendinosus muscle
Patellar ligament
Tibialis anterior muscle

FIGURE 478.1 **Anterior View of Right Pelvis and Femur Showing Muscle Attachments**

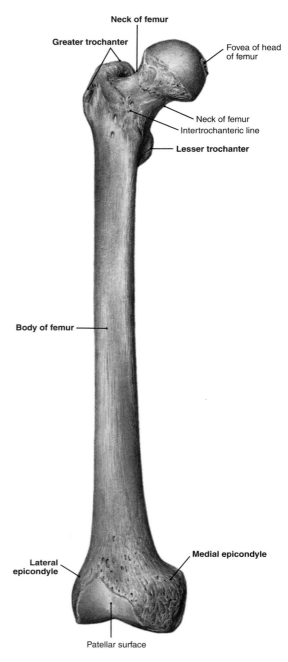

Neck of femur
Greater trochanter
Fovea of head of femur
Neck of femur
Intertrochanteric line
Lesser trochanter

Body of femur

Lateral epicondyle
Medial epicondyle

Patellar surface

FIGURE 478.2 **Right Femur (Anterior View)**

NOTE: (1) The femur is the longest and strongest bone in the body and it transmits to the tibia and feet the weight of the body above the hip joints. It consists of an upper extremity, the **head,** the **body** or **shaft,** and a **distal extremity** enlarged by two **condyles.**

(2) The spherical head of the femur fits into the **acetabulum** of the pelvis. Below the head of the femur is the somewhat narrowed femoral **neck** and two prominent tubercles, the **greater** and **lesser trochanters.**

(3) The anterior surface of the body of the femur is smooth and its proximal two-thirds gives origin to the vastus intermedius muscle.

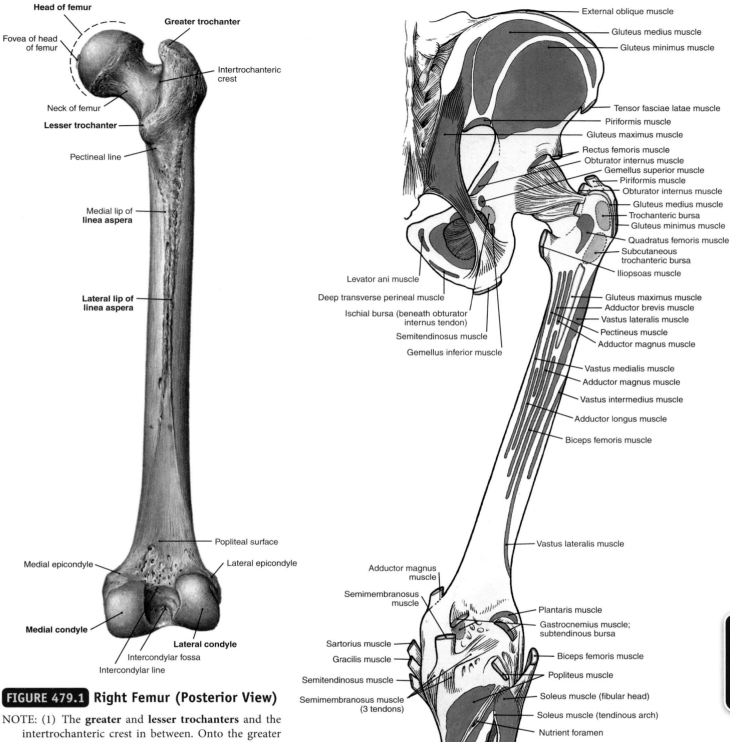

Head of femur

Fovea of head of femur

Greater trochanter

Intertrochanteric crest

Neck of femur

Lesser trochanter

Pectineal line

Medial lip of **linea aspera**

Lateral lip of **linea aspera**

Popliteal surface

Medial epicondyle

Lateral epicondyle

Medial condyle

Lateral condyle

Intercondylar fossa

Intercondylar line

External oblique muscle

Gluteus medius muscle

Gluteus minimus muscle

Tensor fasciae latae muscle

Piriformis muscle

Gluteus maximus muscle

Rectus femoris muscle

Obturator internus muscle

Gemellus superior muscle

Piriformis muscle

Obturator internus muscle

Gluteus medius muscle

Trochanteric bursa

Gluteus minimus muscle

Quadratus femoris muscle

Subcutaneous trochanteric bursa

Iliopsoas muscle

Levator ani muscle

Deep transverse perineal muscle

Ischial bursa (beneath obturator internus tendon)

Semitendinosus muscle

Gemellus inferior muscle

Gluteus maximus muscle

Adductor brevis muscle

Vastus lateralis muscle

Pectineus muscle

Adductor magnus muscle

Vastus medialis muscle

Adductor magnus muscle

Vastus intermedius muscle

Adductor longus muscle

Biceps femoris muscle

Vastus lateralis muscle

Adductor magnus muscle

Semimembranosus muscle

Sartorius muscle

Gracilis muscle

Semitendinosus muscle

Semimembranosus muscle (3 tendons)

Plantaris muscle

Gastrocnemius muscle; subtendinous bursa

Biceps femoris muscle

Popliteus muscle

Soleus muscle (fibular head)

Soleus muscle (tendinous arch)

Nutrient foramen

Tibialis posterior muscle

Soleus muscle (tibial head)

Soleus muscle (fibular head)

Flexor digitorum longus muscle

FIGURE 479.1 **Right Femur (Posterior View)**

NOTE: (1) The **greater** and **lesser trochanters** and the intertrochanteric crest in between. Onto the greater trochanter insert the gluteus medius and minimus, the piriformis, and the obturator internus. On the lesser trochanter inserts the iliopsoas, while the quadratus femoris attaches along the intertrochanteric crest.

(2) The thick, longitudinally oriented ridge, the **linea aspera,** along the posterior surface of the body of the femur. It also serves for muscle attachments.

(3) The **medial** and **lateral condyles** and **epicondyles** inferiorly. The condyles articulate with the tibia and the intercondyloid fossa affords attachment for the cruciate ligaments.

FIGURE 479.2 **Posterior View of Right Pelvis and Femur Showing Muscle Attachments**

Chapter 6 The Lower Limb

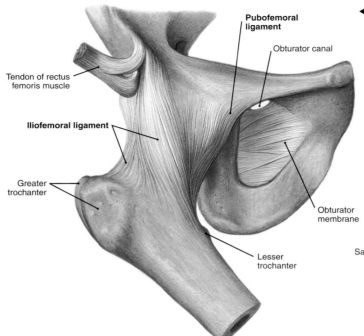

Pubofemoral ligament

Obturator canal

Tendon of rectus femoris muscle

Iliofemoral ligament

Greater trochanter

Lesser trochanter

Obturator membrane

◄ FIGURE 480.1 Right Hip Joint (Anterior View)

NOTE: (1) The hip joint is a typical ball-and-socket joint and consists of the **head of the femur,** which fits snugly in a deepened cavity, the **acetabular fossa.** The bones are held in position by a series of extremely strong ligaments.

(2) The **articular capsule** of the hip joint is reinforced by the **iliofemoral, pubofemoral,** and **ischiofemoral ligaments,** the **acetabular labrum,** the **transverse acetabular ligament,** and the **ligament of the head of the femur.**

(3) The longitudinally oriented fibers of the iliofemoral and pubofemoral ligaments seen anteriorly on the capsule.

FIGURE 480.2 Right Hip Joint (Posterior View) ▶

NOTE: Fibers of the **ischiofemoral ligament** are directed almost horizontally across the capsule of the hip joint. Whereas anteriorly (Fig. 478.2) the capsule attaches along the intertrochanteric line of the femur, posteriorly it encircles the femoral neck. The capsule is thinnest and weaker posteriorly.

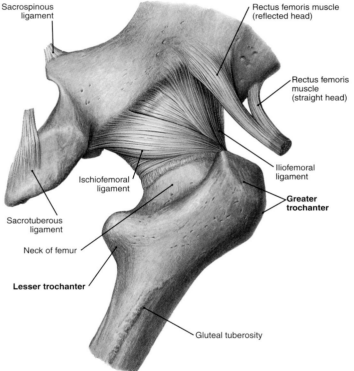

Sacrospinous ligament

Rectus femoris muscle (reflected head)

Rectus femoris muscle (straight head)

Iliofemoral ligament

Ischiofemoral ligament

Greater trochanter

Sacrotuberous ligament

Neck of femur

Lesser trochanter

Gluteal tuberosity

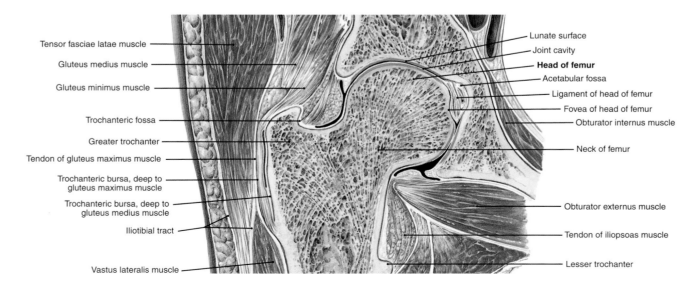

Tensor fasciae latae muscle

Gluteus medius muscle

Gluteus minimus muscle

Trochanteric fossa

Greater trochanter

Tendon of gluteus maximus muscle

Trochanteric bursa, deep to gluteus maximus muscle

Trochanteric bursa, deep to gluteus medius muscle

Iliotibial tract

Vastus lateralis muscle

Lunate surface

Joint cavity

Head of femur

Acetabular fossa

Ligament of head of femur

Fovea of head of femur

Obturator internus muscle

Neck of femur

Obturator externus muscle

Tendon of iliopsoas muscle

Lesser trochanter

FIGURE 480.3 Frontal Section through the Right Hip Joint and Some Surrounding Soft Tissues

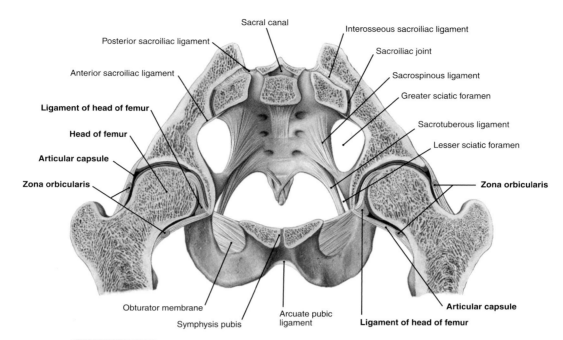

FIGURE 481.1 Frontal Section of the Pelvis Showing Both Hip Joints

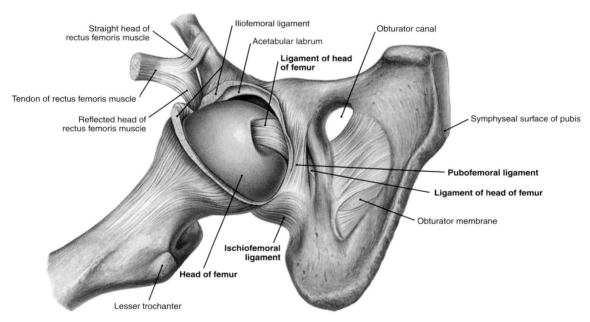

FIGURE 481.2 Anterior Exposure of the Right Hip Joint

NOTE: The articular capsule of the hip joint has been opened near the acetabular labrum. This exposes the cartilage-covered head of the femur within the joint cavity. Observe the ligament of the femoral head attached to the femur where cartilage is lacking.

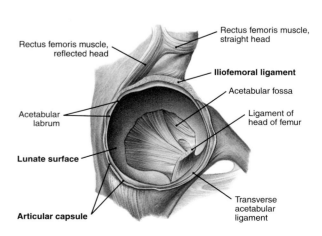

FIGURE 481.3 Socket of the Right Hip Joint ▶

NOTE: (1) The acetabulum is surrounded by a fibrocartilaginous rim, the **acetabular labrum.** This deepens the joint cavity and accommodates enough of the distal head of the femur so that it cannot be pulled from its socket without injuring the acetabular labrum.

(2) The bony acetabulum is incomplete below. Here the acetabular notch is partially covered by the **transverse acetabular ligament.** Through the free portion of the acetabular notch course vessels and nerves that supply the head of the **femur.**

(3) The **ligament of the head of the femur** attaches the femoral head by two bands to either side of the acetabular notch.

PLATE 482 **The Hip Joint and the Head of the Femur**

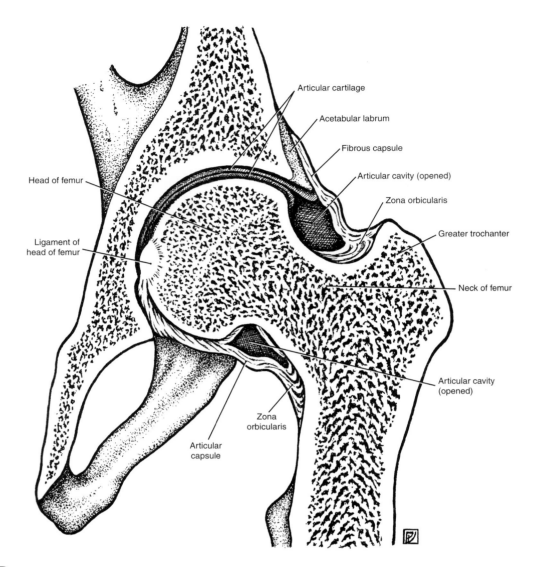

Articular cartilage

Acetabular labrum

Fibrous capsule

Articular cavity (opened)

Zona orbicularis

Greater trochanter

Head of femur

Neck of femur

Ligament of head of femur

Articular cavity (opened)

Zona orbicularis

Articular capsule

FIGURE 482.1 **Frontal Section through the Hip Joint**

(From *Clemente's Anatomy Dissector,* 2nd Edition, Lippincott Williams & Wilkins, Baltimore, 2007.)

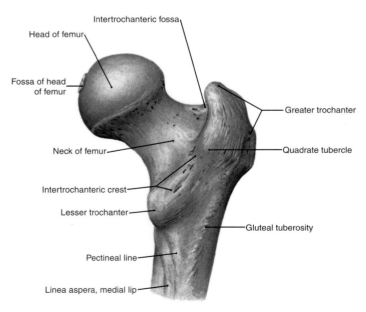

Intertrochanteric fossa

Head of femur

Fossa of head of femur

Greater trochanter

Neck of femur

Quadrate tubercle

Intertrochanteric crest

Lesser trochanter

Gluteal tuberosity

Pectineal line

Linea aspera, medial lip

FIGURE 482.2 **Superior End of the Femur**

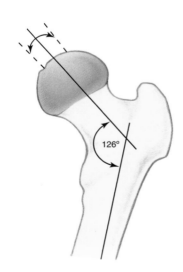

126°

FIGURE 482.3 **Variation in the Angle between the Femoral Neck and the Shaft**

NOTE that this angle is about 150 degrees in infancy and about 126 degrees in the adult.

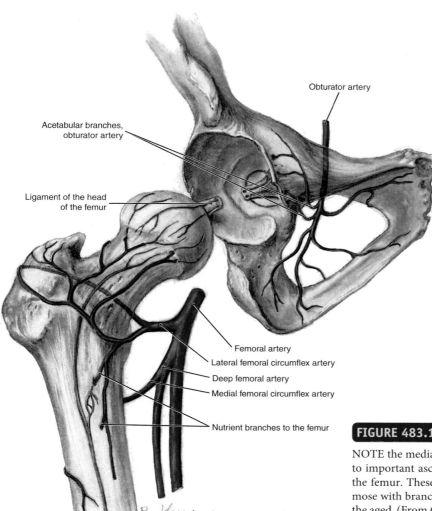

Obturator artery

Acetabular branches, obturator artery

Ligament of the head of the femur

Femoral artery

Lateral femoral circumflex artery

Deep femoral artery

Medial femoral circumflex artery

Nutrient branches to the femur

`FIGURE 483.1` **Arterial Supply to the Hip Joint**

NOTE the medial and lateral femoral circumflex arteries that give rise to important ascending branches of the femoral artery to the neck of the femur. These supply the neck and head of the femur and anastomose with branches above in the young. These connections are lost in the aged. (From *Clemente's Anatomy Dissector,* 2nd Edition, Lippincott Williams & Wilkins, Baltimore, 2007.)

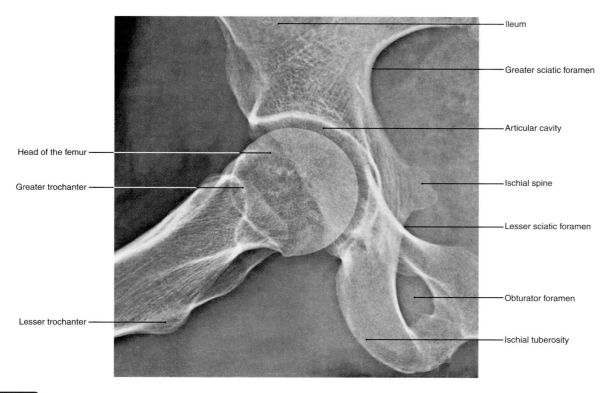

Ileum

Greater sciatic foramen

Articular cavity

Head of the femur

Greater trochanter

Ischial spine

Lesser sciatic foramen

Obturator foramen

Lesser trochanter

Ischial tuberosity

`FIGURE 483.2` **Radiograph of the Hip Joint**

NOTE that the thigh is abducted and flexed and the subject is in the supine position.

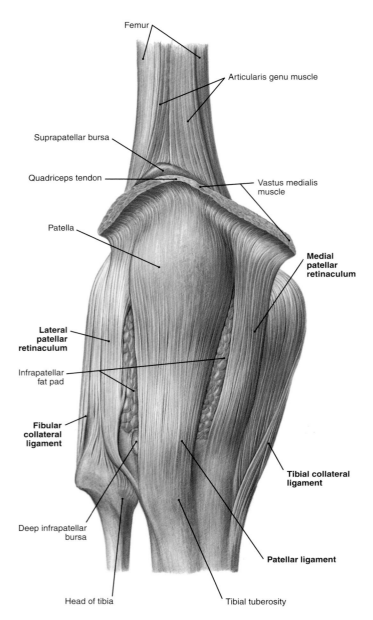

FIGURE 484.1 **Right Knee Joint (Anterior View)**

NOTE: (1) The deep fascia has been removed, and the bellies of the four heads of the quadriceps femoris muscle have been cut to expose the quadriceps tendon, the patella, and the patellar ligament.

(2) The **patellar ligament** inserts onto the tibial tuberosity located on the proximal aspect of the anterior tibial surface.

(3) The **medial** and **lateral patellar retinacula.** These structures reinforce the anteromedial and anterolateral parts of the fibrous capsule of the knee joint and often (but not shown in this figure) they are attached to the borders of the patellar ligament and patella.

(4) The **tibial** and **fibular collateral ligaments** and the location of the **deep infrapatellar bursa.**

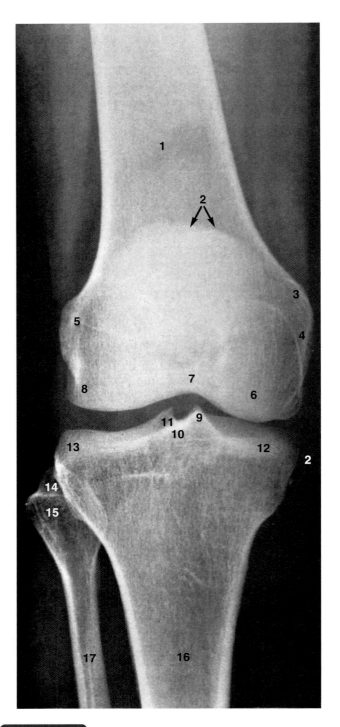

FIGURE 484.2 **Radiograph of the Right Knee (Anteroposterior Projection)**

NOTE: The following bony structures on the femur, tibia, and fibula in the region of the knee.

1. Body of femur
2. Margin of patella
3. Adductor tubercle
4. Medial epicondyle
5. Lateral epicondyle
6. Medial condyle of femur
7. Intercondylar fossa
8. Lateral condyle of femur
9. Medial intercondylar tubercle
10. Anterior intercondylar area
11. Lateral intercondylar tubercle
12. Medial condyle of tibia
13. Lateral condyle of tibia
14. Apex of head of fibula
15. Head of fibula
16. Body of tibia
17. Body of fibula

(From Wicke, 6th ed.)

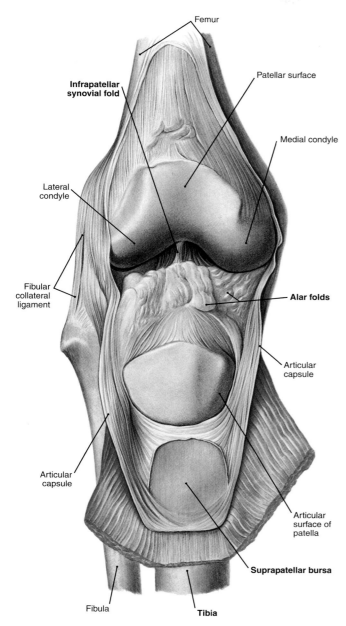

FIGURE 485.1 **Knee Joint Opened Anteriorly**

NOTE: (1) In this dissection, the anterior part of the articular capsule and the quadriceps tendon have been cut and reflected downward along with the **suprapatellar bursa.** The articular surface of the **patella** has also been pulled inferiorly away from its normal position on the femur.

(2) From the medial and lateral borders of the patella, the synovial membrane projects as fringe-like **alar folds** on each side. These converge in the midline to form the **infrapatellar synovial fold,** which attaches above to the intercondylar fossa of the femur.

(3) Upon removal of the infrapatellar synovial fold and any fat in the region, the anterior cruciate ligament and the menisci become exposed, as seen in Figure 485.2.

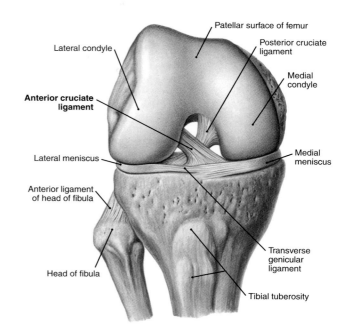

FIGURE 485.2 **Flexed Right Knee Joint (Anterior View) Showing the Cruciate Ligaments**

NOTE: (1) The **anterior cruciate ligament** is best exposed from this frontal approach. It extends from the posterior part of the medial surface of the lateral femoral condyle to the anterior surface of the tibial plateau.

(2) The anterior cruciate ligament helps prevent the posterior, or backward, displacement of the femur on the upper tibial plateau.

(3) More importantly, however, the anterior cruciate ligament limits extension of the lateral condyle to which it is attached. When it becomes taut, it causes medial rotation of the femur. This allows the medial condyle, which has a longer and more curved articular surface than the lateral condyle, to reach its full extension, placing the knee joint in a "locked position."

(4) Thus, the "locked" knee joint is achieved because:

   (a) The medial condyle has a longer articular surface and a greater curvature than that of the lateral condyle.

   (b) After the anterior cruciate ligament becomes taut, the lateral condyle can rotate around the "radius of the ligament" and forces the medial condyle to glide backward into its full extension.

   (c) Medial rotation of the femur at the same time causes the oblique popliteal ligament and the medial and lateral collateral ligaments to tighten as well. (From Last RJ. Anatomy, Regional and Applied. Edinburgh: Churchill Livingstone, 1978.)

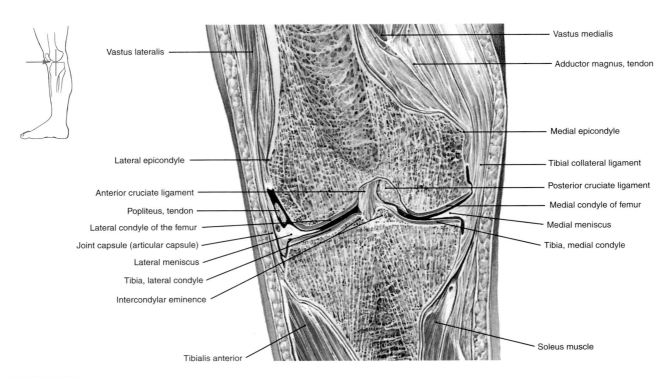

FIGURE 486.1 Frontal Section through the Right Knee Joint

NOTE: (1) The anterior and posterior cruciate ligaments and the medial and lateral menisci.

(2) The tendon of the popliteus muscle adjacent to the lateral meniscus and lateral condyle. It attaches to both of these structures, and during the first phase of flexion of the knee in taking a step, this muscle retracts the meniscus in order not to have it crushed between the lateral condyles of the tibia and femur (see Fig. 466.1).

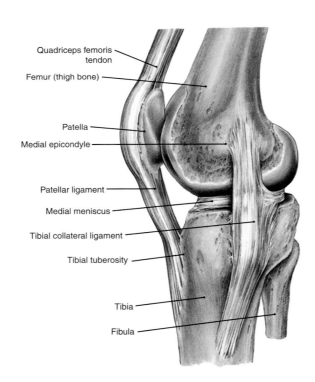

FIGURE 486.2 Right Knee Joint and the Tibial Collateral Ligament in Full Extension

NOTE: Only the posterior fibers of the tibial collateral ligament attach to the medial meniscus, while all the other fibers attach to the medial condyles of both the femur and the tibia.

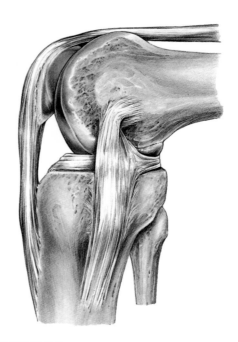

FIGURE 486.3 Right Knee Joint and the Tibial Collateral Ligament in Flexion

NOTE: During flexion, the posterior fibers of the tibial collateral ligament and those attaching to the femur become twisted and, thus, help stabilize the medial meniscus to which the ligament is attached.

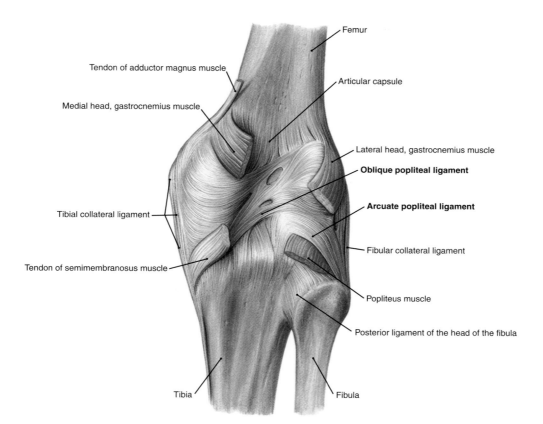

FIGURE 487.1 **Knee Joint (Posterior View, Superficial Dissection)**

NOTE: (1) The posterior aspect of the articular capsule is reinforced by the oblique and arcuate popliteal ligaments, and, to some extent, by the tendons of origin and insertion of muscles.

(2) From its insertion, the tendon of the semimembranosus muscle expands upward and laterally across the posterior surface of the articular capsule of the knee joint as the **oblique popliteal ligament.**

(3) The **arcuate popliteal ligament** is a band of fibers attached to the head of the fibula and courses superficially to the popliteus muscle to blend with the oblique popliteal ligament and the fibular collateral ligament.

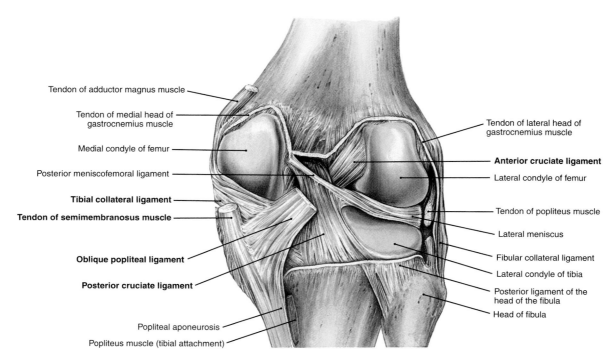

FIGURE 487.2 **Posterior View of the Knee Joint with the Articular Capsule Opened**

NOTE: This more diagrammatic figure should be compared with the dissection in Figure 487.1.

PLATE 488 Knee Joint: Transverse and Sagittal Sections

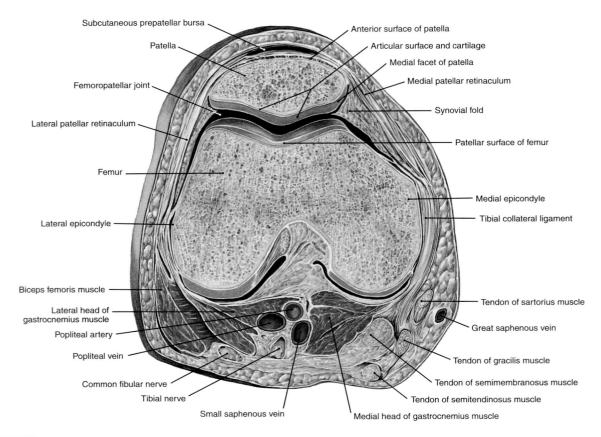

FIGURE 488.1 Transverse Section through the Knee Joint and the Popliteal Fossa

NOTE: The relationship of the muscles, vessels, and nerves in the popliteus fossa to the bony structures of the knee joint.

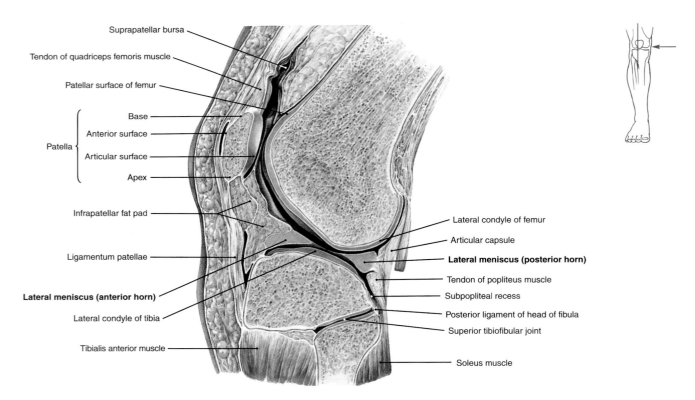

FIGURE 488.2 Sagittal Section through the Lateral Part of the Knee Joint

NOTE: The horns of the lateral meniscus, the tendon of the popliteus muscle, and the superior tibiofibular joint. Compare these structures in this drawing with those in the MRI section seen in Figure 489.2.

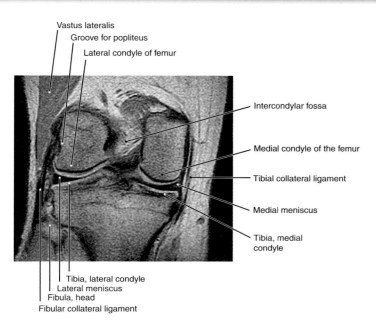

Vastus lateralis
Groove for popliteus
Lateral condyle of femur

Intercondylar fossa

Medial condyle of the femur

Tibial collateral ligament

Medial meniscus

Tibia, medial condyle

Tibia, lateral condyle
Lateral meniscus
Fibula, head
Fibular collateral ligament

FIGURE 489.1 MRI of the Knee Joint (Frontal Section) ◄

NOTE: This MRI frontal section cuts through the intercondylar eminence of the tibia (not labeled) and the intercondylar fossa of the femur. Observe the menisci, which in this frontal section, have a triangular shape.

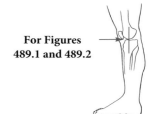

For Figures 489.1 and 489.2

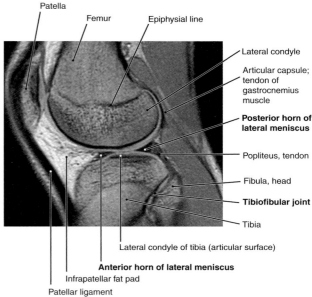

Patella
Femur
Epiphysial line

Lateral condyle

Articular capsule; tendon of gastrocnemius muscle

Posterior horn of lateral meniscus

Popliteus, tendon

Fibula, head

Tibiofibular joint

Tibia

Lateral condyle of tibia (articular surface)

Anterior horn of lateral meniscus
Infrapatellar fat pad
Patellar ligament

FIGURE 489.2 MRI of the Knee Joint (Sagittal Section) ►

NOTE: This sagittal section cuts through the lateral part of the knee joint and shows the **horns of the lateral meniscus,** the **tendon of the popliteus muscle,** and the **superior tibiofibular joint.** Compare this image with Figure 488.2.

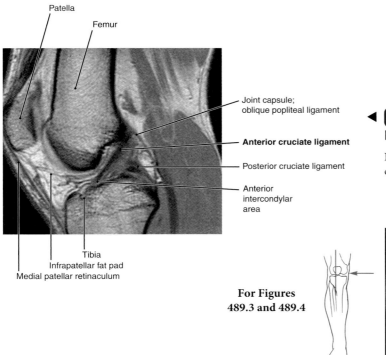

Patella
Femur

Joint capsule; oblique popliteal ligament

Anterior cruciate ligament

Posterior cruciate ligament

Anterior intercondylar area

Tibia
Infrapatellar fat pad
Medial patellar retinaculum

For Figures 489.3 and 489.4

FIGURE 489.3 MRI of the Knee Joint in Extension A ◄

NOTE: This sagittal section shows both the anterior and posterior cruciate ligaments.

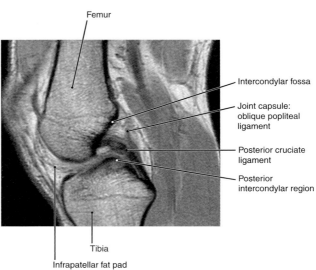

Femur

Intercondylar fossa

Joint capsule: oblique popliteal ligament

Posterior cruciate ligament

Posterior intercondylar region

Tibia
Infrapatellar fat pad

FIGURE 489.4 MRI of the Knee Joint in Extension B ►

NOTE: This sagittal section shows the posterior cruciate ligament to good advantage.

PLATE 490 Arthrogram of the Right Knee

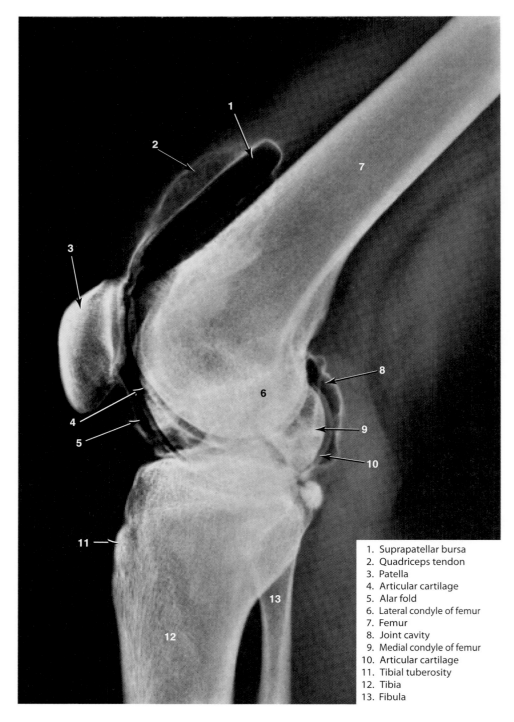

1. Suprapatellar bursa
2. Quadriceps tendon
3. Patella
4. Articular cartilage
5. Alar fold
6. Lateral condyle of femur
7. Femur
8. Joint cavity
9. Medial condyle of femur
10. Articular cartilage
11. Tibial tuberosity
12. Tibia
13. Fibula

FIGURE 490 Arthrogram of the Knee Joint

NOTE: (1) An arthrogram is a radiograph of a joint taken during arthrography, which is an examination of a joint following the injection into the joint of a radiopaque agent (or gas).

(2) An arthroscope is an instrument that uses fiber optics and permits visualization of the inside of a joint. This is achieved by puncturing the joint through a small incision in the joint capsule (see Plate 491).

(3) The large **suprapatellar bursa.** The **patella** is a bony structure within the tendon of the quadriceps femoris muscle. The tendon then continues inferiorly to the knee and inserts onto the **tibial tuberosity** as the patellar ligament.

(4) During development, the fibers of the quadriceps tendon and the patellar ligament that attaches to the **tibial tuberosity** were continuous, but upon further development the central part of the tendon becomes ossified to form the **patella.**

(5) People who kneel a lot may have inflammation of the bursae anterior to the patella and superior to the **patella.** This is sometimes called house-maid's knee.

(From Wicke, 6th ed.)

FIGURE 491.1 Arthroscopic Approaches to the Knee ▶

1. Arthroscope
2. Inlet and outlet for rinsing solution
3. Cold light source
4. Ocular or connector for visual system
5. Anterolateral approach
6. Anteromedial approach
7. Supplementary instrument

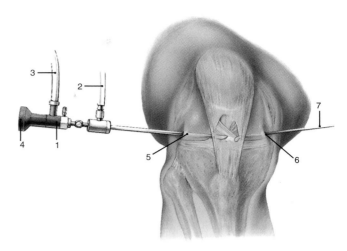

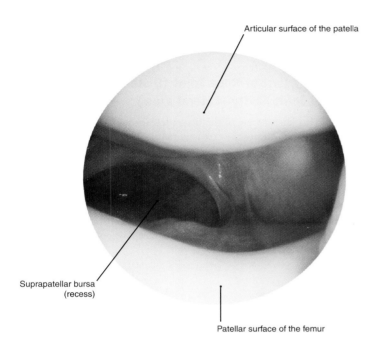

Articular surface of the patella

Suprapatellar bursa (recess)

Patellar surface of the femur

FIGURE 491.2 Knee Joint Arthroscopy A

NOTE: This is an inferior view of the femoropatellar joint.

FIGURE 491.3 Knee Joint Arthroscopy B ▶

NOTE: This image shows the medial free border of the lateral meniscus; the anterior part of the meniscus is being depressed by a probe.

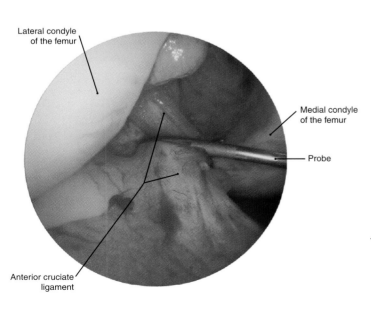

Lateral condyle of the femur

Medial condyle of the femur

Probe

Anterior cruciate ligament

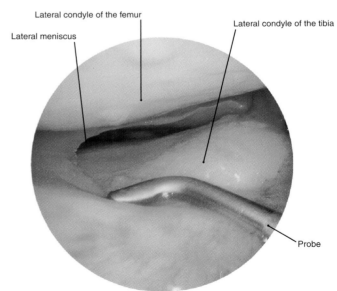

Lateral condyle of the femur

Lateral meniscus

Lateral condyle of the tibia

Probe

FIGURE 491.4 Knee Joint Arthroscopy C

NOTE: The distal part of the right anterior cruciate ligament is visible, and the highly vascular synovial membrane is being retracted by a probe.

PLATE 492 **Knee Joint: Synovial Cavity and Bursae**

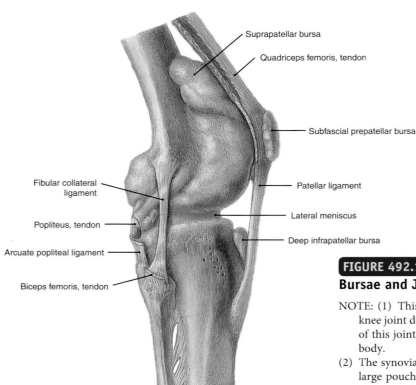

Suprapatellar bursa

Quadriceps femoris, tendon

Subfascial prepatellar bursa

Fibular collateral ligament

Patellar ligament

Lateral meniscus

Popliteus, tendon

Deep infrapatellar bursa

Arcuate popliteal ligament

Biceps femoris, tendon

FIGURE 492.1 Cast of Knee Joint (Distended) Showing Bursae and Joint Cavity (Lateral View)

NOTE: (1) This lateral view of the distended synovial cavity of the right knee joint demonstrates the extensive nature of the synovial membrane of this joint. It is more extensive in this joint than in any other in the body.

(2) The synovial membrane reaches *superiorly* above the patella to form a large pouch called the **suprapatellar bursa. Laterally,** it courses deep to the popliteal tendon and fibular collateral ligament. **Posteriorly,** it extends above the menisci as high as the origins of the gastrocnemius muscle. **Inferiorly,** the joint cavity descends below both the lateral and medial menisci.

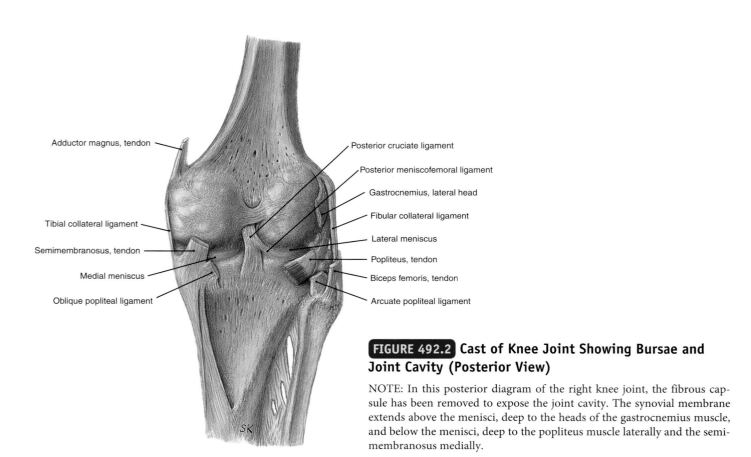

Adductor magnus, tendon

Posterior cruciate ligament

Posterior meniscofemoral ligament

Gastrocnemius, lateral head

Tibial collateral ligament

Fibular collateral ligament

Lateral meniscus

Semimembranosus, tendon

Popliteus, tendon

Medial meniscus

Biceps femoris, tendon

Oblique popliteal ligament

Arcuate popliteal ligament

FIGURE 492.2 Cast of Knee Joint Showing Bursae and Joint Cavity (Posterior View)

NOTE: In this posterior diagram of the right knee joint, the fibrous capsule has been removed to expose the joint cavity. The synovial membrane extends above the menisci, deep to the heads of the gastrocnemius muscle, and below the menisci, deep to the popliteus muscle laterally and the semimembranosus medially.

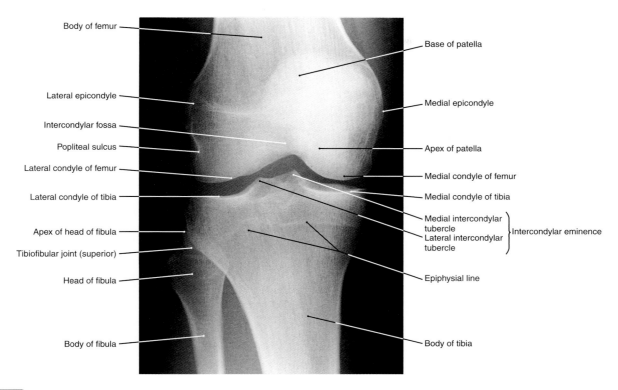

Body of femur

Lateral epicondyle

Intercondylar fossa

Popliteal sulcus

Lateral condyle of femur

Lateral condyle of tibia

Apex of head of fibula

Tibiofibular joint (superior)

Head of fibula

Body of fibula

Base of patella

Medial epicondyle

Apex of patella

Medial condyle of femur

Medial condyle of tibia

Medial intercondylar tubercle

Lateral intercondylar tubercle

}Intercondylar eminence

Epiphysial line

Body of tibia

FIGURE 493.1 Anterior–Posterior Radiograph of the Knee Joint

NOTE: This X-ray was made while the subject was reclined and the central beam was directed to the middle of the joint.

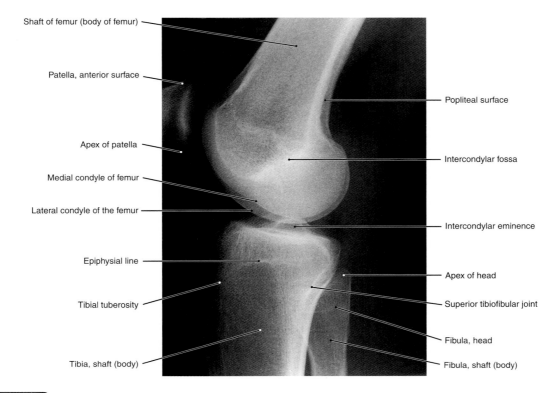

Shaft of femur (body of femur)

Patella, anterior surface

Apex of patella

Medial condyle of femur

Lateral condyle of the femur

Epiphysial line

Tibial tuberosity

Tibia, shaft (body)

Popliteal surface

Intercondylar fossa

Intercondylar eminence

Apex of head

Superior tibiofibular joint

Fibula, head

Fibula, shaft (body)

FIGURE 493.2 Lateral Radiograph of the Knee Joint

NOTE: This X-ray was made while the subject was reclined and the central beam was directed to the middle of the joint.

Chapter 6 The Lower Limb

PLATE 494 **Knee Joint: Synovial Membranes (Bursae): Movements at Joint**

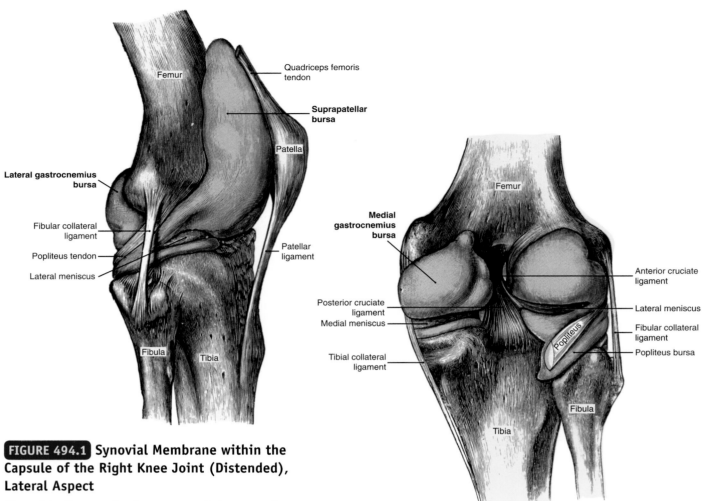

FIGURE 494.1 Synovial Membrane within the Capsule of the Right Knee Joint (Distended), Lateral Aspect

(From C.D. Clemente. *Gray's Anatomy,* 30th American Edition. Baltimore: Lea & Febiger, 1985.)

FIGURE 494.2 Synovial Membrane within the Capsule of the Right Knee Joint (Distended), Posterior Aspect

(From C.D. Clemente. *Gray's Anatomy,* 30th American Edition. Baltimore: Lea & Febiger, 1985.)

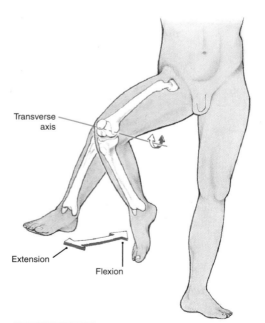

FIGURE 494.3 Knee Joint Movement (Sagittal Plane)

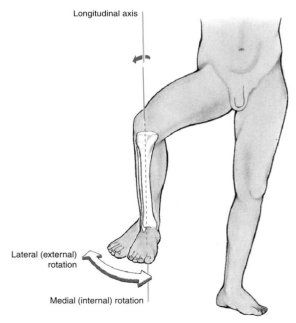

FIGURE 494.4 Knee Joint Movement (Transverse Plane)

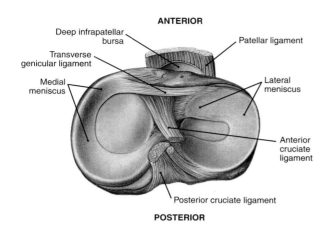

FIGURE 495.1 Condyles of the Right Tibia, Viewed from Above: Showing the Menisci and the Attachments on the Tibia of the Cruciate Ligaments

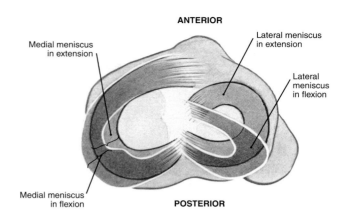

FIGURE 495.2 Superior Surface of the Right Tibial Surface Showing the Locations of the Menisci during Extension (Light Blue) and Their Changes in Position during Flexion (Purple)

NOTE: (1) The C-shaped menisci lie above the condyles of the tibia; they are triangular in cross section and composed of fibrous connective tissue and NOT of cartilage.

(2) The **medial meniscus** is larger and has a more open curve than that of the **lateral meniscus.** Both menisci are attached at their anterior and posterior horns to the tibial surface.

(3) The **lateral meniscus** receives a flat tendon of insertion from the upper fibers of the **popliteus muscle,** and this muscle comes into action during "unlocking" of the knee joint by slightly rotating the femur laterally in preparation to take a step. In addition, these fibers draw the posterior convexity of the lateral meniscus backward "out of harm's way" during flexion of the tibia at the knee joint.

(4) In addition to its attachment on the tibia, the **medial meniscus** is securely attached to the tibial collateral ligament and is frequently injured in athletes when:

  (a) The foot of the victim is planted firmly on the ground and the knee is semiflexed, and

  (b) The victim is hit from behind ("clipping in football"), causing the weight of the body to severely rotate the femur medially. Thus, the leg is abducted and the tibial collateral ligament and the medial meniscus can be torn.

FIGURE 495.3 Arterial Supply of the Menisci, Right Knee ▶

NOTE: The **medial** and **lateral genicular** arteries encircle the tibia and supply the menisci. The **middle genicular artery** supplies the cruciate ligaments.

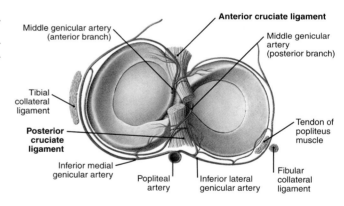

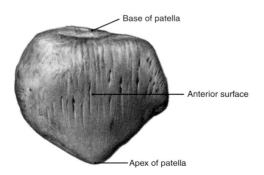

FIGURE 495.4 Anterior Aspect of the Right Patella

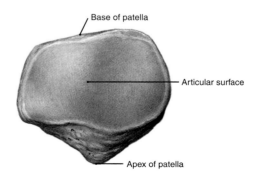

FIGURE 495.5 Posterior Aspect of the Right Patella

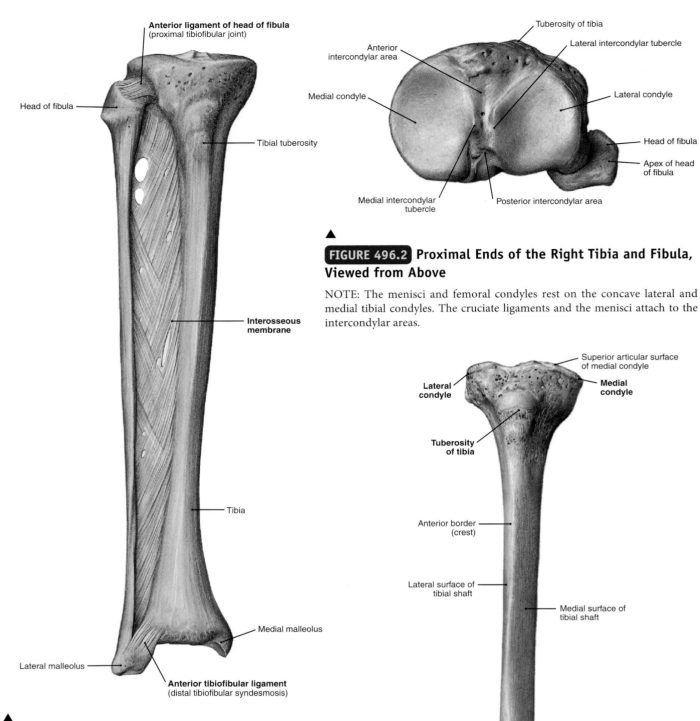

Anterior ligament of head of fibula
(proximal tibiofibular joint)

Head of fibula

Tibial tuberosity

Interosseous
membrane

Tibia

Medial malleolus

Lateral malleolus

Anterior tibiofibular ligament
(distal tibiofibular syndesmosis)

Tuberosity of tibia

Anterior
intercondylar area

Lateral intercondylar tubercle

Medial condyle

Lateral condyle

Head of fibula

Apex of head
of fibula

Medial intercondylar
tubercle

Posterior intercondylar area

▲

FIGURE 496.2 **Proximal Ends of the Right Tibia and Fibula,
Viewed from Above**

NOTE: The menisci and femoral condyles rest on the concave lateral and
medial tibial condyles. The cruciate ligaments and the menisci attach to the
intercondylar areas.

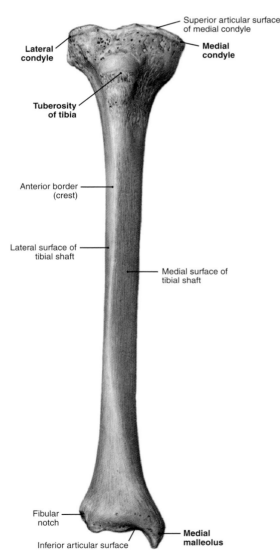

Superior articular surface
of medial condyle

Lateral
condyle

**Medial
condyle**

**Tuberosity
of tibia**

Anterior border
(crest)

Lateral surface of
tibial shaft

Medial surface of
tibial shaft

Fibular
notch

**Medial
malleolus**

Inferior articular surface

▲

FIGURE 496.1 **Tibiofibular Unions and the
Interosseous Membrane (Right Leg)**

NOTE: (1) From this anterior view the shafts of the fibula and tibia are
connected from the knee to the ankle by the **interosseous membrane.** In addition, the two bones are joined proximally (the tibiofibular joint) and distally (the tibiofibular syndesmosis).
(2) The head of the fibula articulates with the inferolateral aspect of
the lateral condyle of the tibia. This is a gliding joint whose fibrous
capsule is strengthened by **anterior** and **posterior ligaments of
the head of the fibula.**
(3) The syndesmosis between the distal ends of the fibula and the tibia
is bound by anterior and posterior tibiofibular ligaments.

FIGURE 496.3 **Right Tibia (Anterior View)** ▲

NOTE: The proximal extremity is marked by the tibial condyles
and the tibial tuberosity. The medial aspect of the distal extremity forms the medial malleolus.

FIGURES 497.1 and 497.2 Right Fibula ▶
(Medial and Lateral Views)

NOTE: (1) The fibula is a long slender bone situated lateral to the tibia, to which it articulates proximally and distally. The fibula expands inferiorly to form the **lateral malleolus.** The medial aspect of its inferior articular surface articulates with the tibia to form the **talocrural joint (ankle joint).**

(2) Although the fibula does not bear any weight of the trunk (not participating in the knee joint), it is important, since numerous muscles attach to its surface (see Figs. 468.1 and 468.2) and because it helps form the ankle joint.

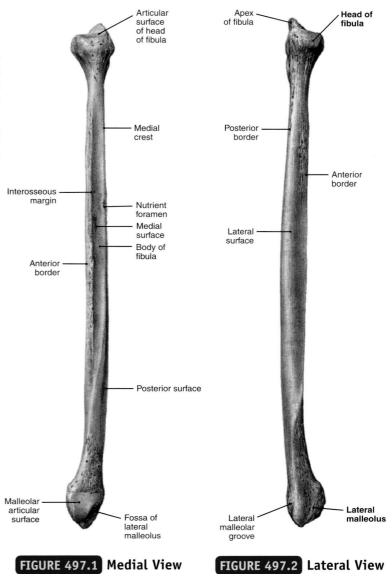

FIGURE 497.1 Medial View   **FIGURE 497.2** Lateral View

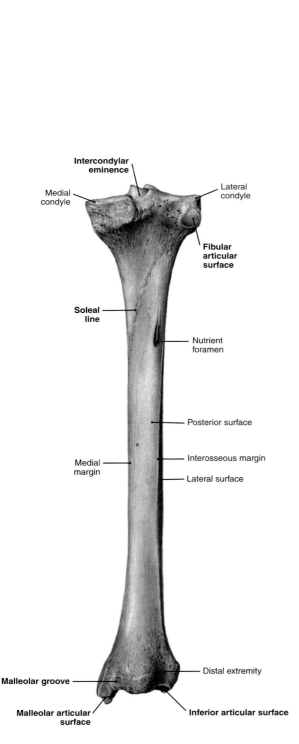

◀ **FIGURE 497.3** Right Tibia (Posterior View)

NOTE: (1) The smooth posterior surface of the shaft of the tibia is marked by a prominent ridge, the **soleal line,** and a large oblong **nutrient foramen.** The tibial shaft tapers toward a larger proximal extremity and a somewhat less pronounced distal extremity.

(2) Proximally, the medial and lateral condyles are separated by the intercondylar eminence, anterior and posterior to which attach the cruciate ligaments. Distally, the tibia articulates with the **talus,** and on this posterior surface, presents grooves for the passage of the tendons of the tibialis posterior, flexor digitorum longus, and flexor hallucis longus.

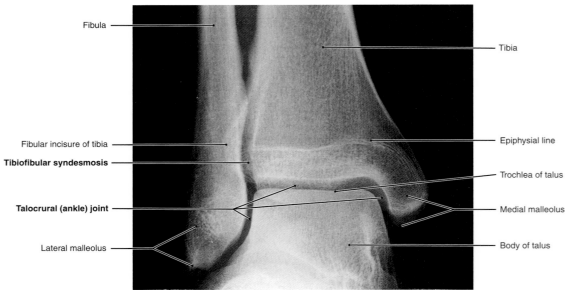

FIGURE 498.1 X-Ray of the Talocrural (Ankle) Joint and the Inferior Tibiofibular Syndesmosis

NOTE: (1) This is an anteroposterior radiograph showing both the ankle joint and the tibiofibular syndesmosis.

(2) The ankle joint is a ginglymus, or hinge, joint. The bony structures participating in this joint superiorly are the distal end of the **tibia** and its **medial malleolus** and the distal **fibula** and its **lateral malleolus.** Together these structures form a concave receptacle for the convex proximal surface of the **talus.**

(3) The inferior tibiofibular joint connects the convex or medial side of the lower part of the fibula with the concavity of the fibular notch of the tibia. These surfaces are separated by the upward prolongation (4–5 mm) of the synovial membrane of the talocrural joint. The part of the articulation that is fibrous is called **tibiofibular syndesmosis.**

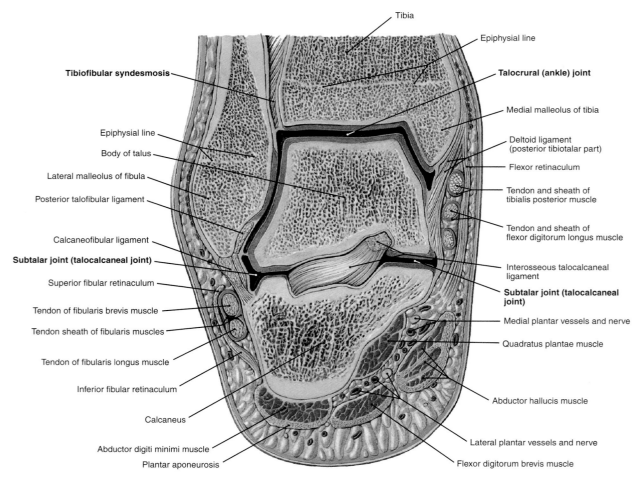

FIGURE 498.2 Coronal Section through the Talocrural (Ankle) and Subtalar Joints and the Tibiofibular Syndesmosis

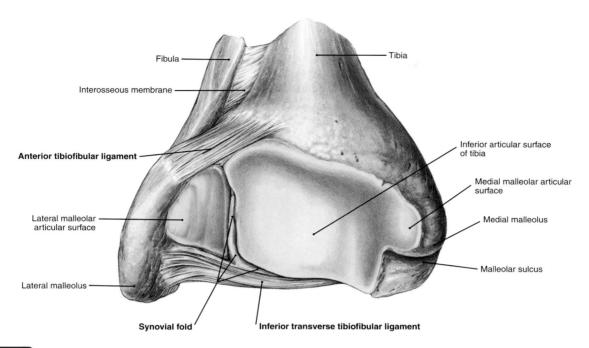

FIGURE 499.1 Inferior Articular Surface of the Tibia and Fibula at the Talocrural (Ankle) Joint

NOTE: (1) The medial and lateral sides of the upper part of the talocrural (ankle) joint are formed by the articular surfaces of the medial malleolus (tibia) and lateral malleolus (fibula). These grasp the sides of the talus.

(2) The inferior articular surface of the tibia is wider anteriorly than posteriorly to accommodate the broader anterior surface of the talus. In full dorsiflexion, the ankle joint is very stable and does not allow any side-to-side movement, but in full plantar flexion, a degree of side-to-side movement can occur.

(3) The synovial fold of the ankle joint that extends upward between the inferior surfaces of the fibula and tibia.

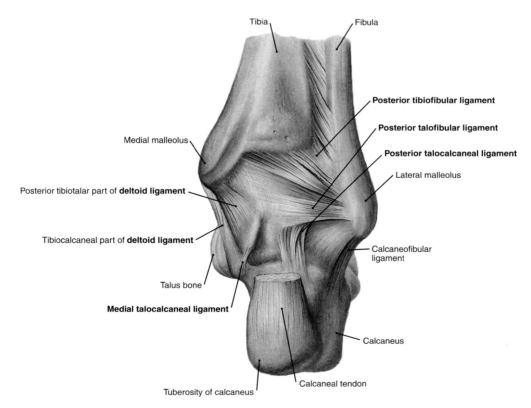

FIGURE 499.2 Ankle Joint (Talocrural) Viewed from Behind (Right Foot)

NOTE: (1) The posterior aspect of the articular capsule is somewhat strengthened by the posterior talofibular and posterior tibiofibular ligaments. The calcaneofibular ligament laterally and the strong deltoid ligament medially assist in protecting this joint.

(2) The ligamentous bands that help stabilize the talocalcaneal articulation posteriorly: the posterior and medial talocalcaneal ligaments.

Chapter 6 The Lower Limb

PLATE 500 Bones of the Foot and Muscle Attachments (Dorsal View)

FIGURE 500.1 Dorsal Aspect of the Bones of the ▶
Right Foot Showing the Attachments of Muscles

Red = origin; Blue = insertion

NOTE: (1) The insertion of the **calcaneal tendon** (of Achilles) on the posterior surface of the calcaneus. This tendon is the strongest in the body, and a bursa is interposed between the bone and the tendon.

(2) The only other muscle that attaches to the tarsal bones on this dorsal aspect is the **extensor digitorum brevis,** which arises from the dorsolateral surface of the calcaneus, distal to its articulation with the talus. Its medial part inserts on the proximal phalanx of the large toe, while its other three tendons insert on the middle phalanx of the second, third, and fourth toes.

(3) The insertions of the **fibularis brevis** and **tertius** onto the base of the fifth metatarsal.

(4) The four dorsal interosseous muscles, two of which insert on the second toe and the third and fourth insert on the dorsolateral aspect of the third and fourth toes.

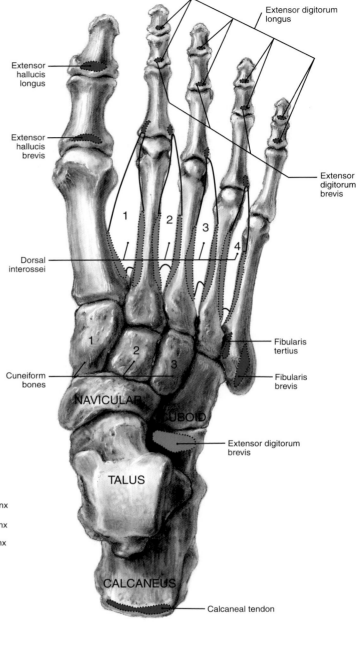

Extensor digitorum longus

Extensor hallucis longus

Extensor hallucis brevis

Extensor digitorum brevis

Dorsal interossei

Cuneiform bones

NAVICULAR

CUBOID

Fibularis tertius

Fibularis brevis

Extensor digitorum brevis

TALUS

CALCANEUS

Calcaneal tendon

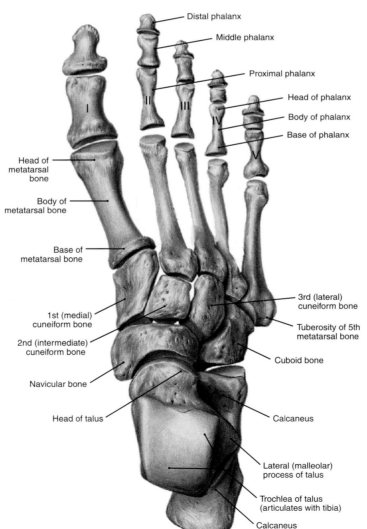

Distal phalanx

Middle phalanx

Proximal phalanx

Head of phalanx

Body of phalanx

Base of phalanx

Head of metatarsal bone

Body of metatarsal bone

Base of metatarsal bone

1st (medial) cuneiform bone

2nd (intermediate) cuneiform bone

Navicular bone

Head of talus

3rd (lateral) cuneiform bone

Tuberosity of 5th metatarsal bone

Cuboid bone

Calcaneus

Lateral (malleolar) process of talus

Trochlea of talus (articulates with tibia)

Calcaneus

◀ **FIGURE 500.2** Bones of the Right Foot (Dorsal View)

NOTE: (1) The skeleton of the foot consists of 7 **tarsal bones,** 5 **metatarsal bones,** and 14 **phalanges.** The toes are numbered in order from medial to lateral: the large toe is the first digit, while the small toe is the fifth digit.

(2) The weight of the body is transmitted by the tibia to the **talus,** which then redistributes this weight to the **calcaneus** inferiorly (the heel of the foot) and the **navicular bone** distally (toward the heads of the metatarsals and the "ball" of the foot).

(3) Distal to the navicular and calcaneus are the three **cuneiform bones** and the **cuboid;** these articulate with the individual metatarsal bones of the digits.

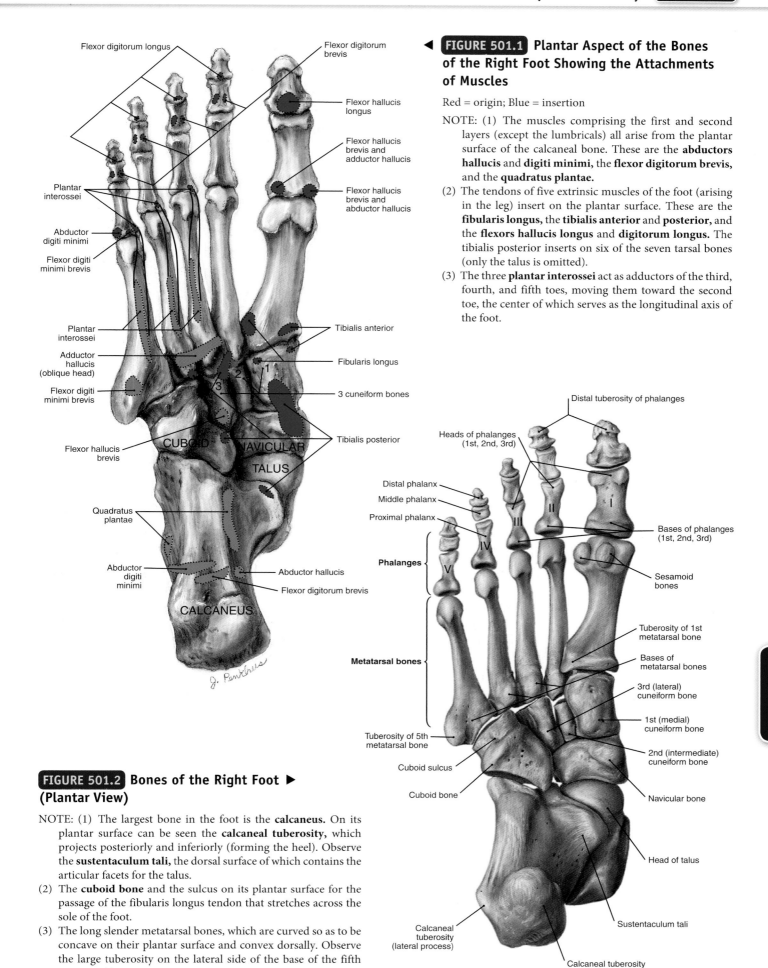

◄ FIGURE 501.1 Plantar Aspect of the Bones of the Right Foot Showing the Attachments of Muscles

Red = origin; Blue = insertion

NOTE: (1) The muscles comprising the first and second layers (except the lumbricals) all arise from the plantar surface of the calcaneal bone. These are the **abductors hallucis** and **digiti minimi,** the **flexor digitorum brevis,** and the **quadratus plantae.**

(2) The tendons of five extrinsic muscles of the foot (arising in the leg) insert on the plantar surface. These are the **fibularis longus,** the **tibialis anterior** and **posterior,** and the **flexors hallucis longus** and **digitorum longus.** The tibialis posterior inserts on six of the seven tarsal bones (only the talus is omitted).

(3) The three **plantar interossei** act as adductors of the third, fourth, and fifth toes, moving them toward the second toe, the center of which serves as the longitudinal axis of the foot.

**FIGURE 501.2 Bones of the Right Foot ►
(Plantar View)**

NOTE: (1) The largest bone in the foot is the **calcaneus.** On its plantar surface can be seen the **calcaneal tuberosity,** which projects posteriorly and inferiorly (forming the heel). Observe the **sustentaculum tali,** the dorsal surface of which contains the articular facets for the talus.

(2) The **cuboid bone** and the sulcus on its plantar surface for the passage of the fibularis longus tendon that stretches across the sole of the foot.

(3) The long slender metatarsal bones, which are curved so as to be concave on their plantar surface and convex dorsally. Observe the large tuberosity on the lateral side of the base of the fifth metatarsal bone.

Chapter 6 The Lower Limb

PLATE 502 Bones and Ligaments of the Right Foot (Lateral View)

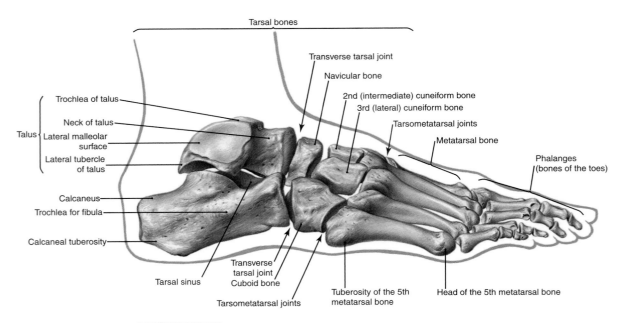

FIGURE 502.1 Skeleton of the Right Foot (Lateral View)

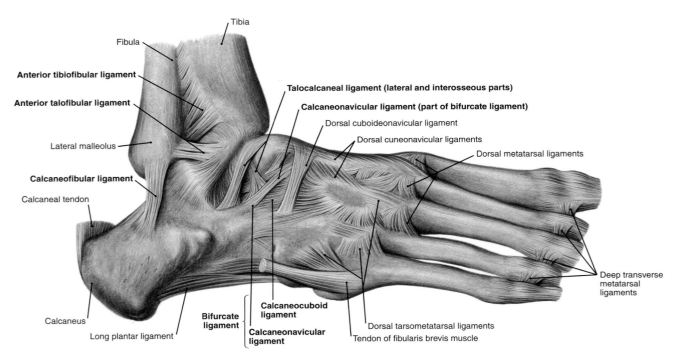

FIGURE 502.2 Lateral Ligaments of the Ankle Joint and of the Dorsolateral Foot (Right)

NOTE: (1) The fibula is attached to the tibia distally by the **anterior (inferior) tibiofibular ligament.** In addition, the lateral malleolus of the fibula is attached to the talus by the relatively weak **anterior talofibular ligament** and the much stronger **posterior talofibular ligament** (Fig. 499.2). The fibula is attached to the calcaneus by the **calcaneofibular ligament.** Together these latter three bands constitute the lateral ligament of the ankle.

(2) The **interosseous talocalcaneal ligament** is the principal ligament that strengthens the **subtalar joint** (between talus and calcaneus); the **lateral talocalcaneal ligament** also helps strengthen this joint as does the **medial talocalcaneal ligament,** which blends with the deltoid ligament (not shown).

(3) The (dorsal) **calcaneonavicular ligament,** part of the **bifurcate ligament,** attaches the dorsolateral aspect of the navicular bone with the calcaneus. Along with this (dorsal) calcaneonavicular ligament, the (dorsal) calcaneocuboid ligament constitutes the **"bifurcate" ligament.**

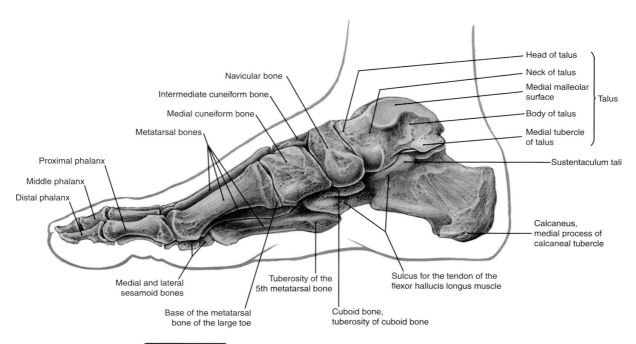

FIGURE 503.1 Skeleton of the Right Foot (Medial View)

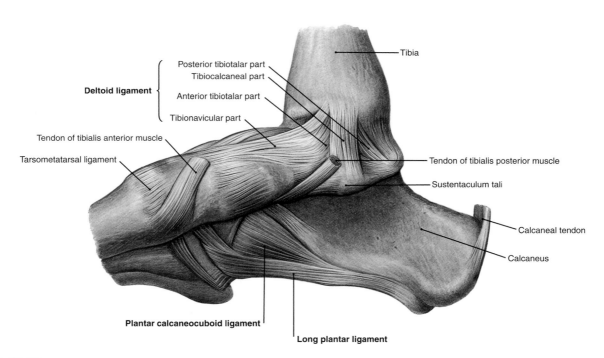

FIGURE 503.2 Ligaments of the Ankle and Foot: Medial View (Right Foot)

NOTE: (1) The medial aspect of the ankle joint is protected by the triangular **deltoid ligament,** which connects the tibia to the navicular, calcaneus, and talus. The deltoid ligament has four parts: (a) an **anterior tibionavicular** part that attaches the medial malleolus to the navicular, (b) a superficial **tibiocalcaneal part** attaching the malleolus to the sustentaculum tali of the calcaneus, and (c and d) the **anterior** and **posterior tibiotalar parts** that lie more deeply and attach the malleolus to the adjacent talus.

(2) The insertions of the tendons of the tibialis anterior and posterior muscles attach on this medial aspect of the foot. Also observe the **long plantar** and **plantar calcaneocuboid ligaments** on the plantar surface.

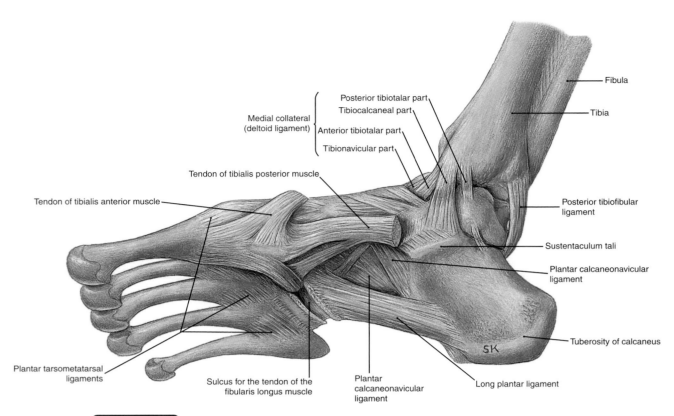

Fibula

Tibia

Posterior tibiotalar part

Tibiocalcaneal part

Medial collateral (deltoid ligament)

Anterior tibiotalar part

Tibionavicular part

Tendon of tibialis posterior muscle

Tendon of tibialis anterior muscle

Posterior tibiofibular ligament

Sustentaculum tali

Plantar calcaneonavicular ligament

Tuberosity of calcaneus

SK

Plantar tarsometatarsal ligaments

Sulcus for the tendon of the fibularis longus muscle

Plantar calcaneonavicular ligament

Long plantar ligament

FIGURE 504.1 Ligaments on the Medial Aspect of the Ankle Joint and Foot

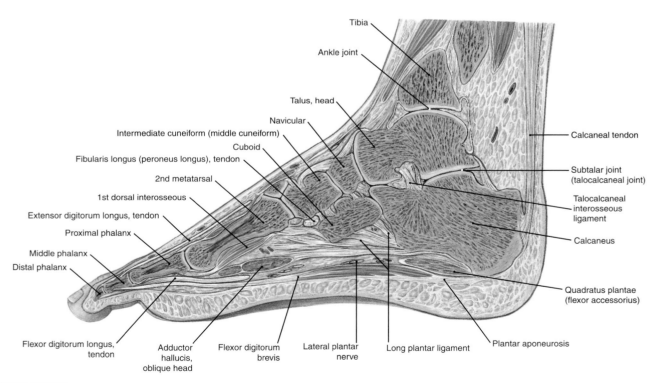

Tibia

Ankle joint

Talus, head

Navicular

Intermediate cuneiform (middle cuneiform)

Cuboid

Fibularis longus (peroneus longus), tendon

2nd metatarsal

1st dorsal interosseous

Extensor digitorum longus, tendon

Proximal phalanx

Middle phalanx

Distal phalanx

Calcaneal tendon

Subtalar joint (talocalcaneal joint)

Talocalcaneal interosseous ligament

Calcaneus

Quadratus plantae (flexor accessorius)

Flexor digitorum longus, tendon

Adductor hallucis, oblique head

Flexor digitorum brevis

Lateral plantar nerve

Long plantar ligament

Plantar aponeurosis

FIGURE 504.2 Sagittal Section through the Foot, Viewed from the Medial Aspect

NOTE: (1) This longitudinal section goes through the second toe.
(2) The relationship between the head of the talus proximally and the **navicular bone** distally, and the subtalar joint between the talus superiorly and the calcaneus inferiorly.
(3) The long plantar ligament. Observe this ligament also in Figure 506.1.

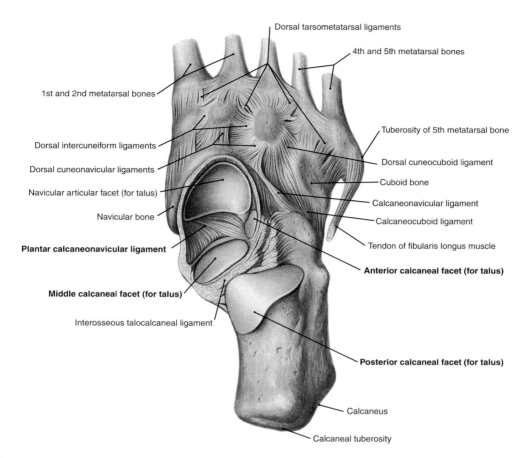

Dorsal tarsometatarsal ligaments

4th and 5th metatarsal bones

1st and 2nd metatarsal bones

Tuberosity of 5th metatarsal bone

Dorsal intercuneiform ligaments

Dorsal cuneocuboid ligament

Dorsal cuneonavicular ligaments

Cuboid bone

Navicular articular facet (for talus)

Calcaneonavicular ligament

Navicular bone

Calcaneocuboid ligament

Plantar calcaneonavicular ligament

Tendon of fibularis longus muscle

Anterior calcaneal facet (for talus)

Middle calcaneal facet (for talus)

Interosseous talocalcaneal ligament

Posterior calcaneal facet (for talus)

Calcaneus

Calcaneal tuberosity

FIGURE 505.1 Right Talocalcaneonavicular Joint (Viewed from Above)

NOTE: (1) The talus has been removed, which exposes the three articulations it makes inferiorly with the **calcaneus** and the one articulation it makes anteriorly with the **navicular bone.**

(2) The plantar **calcaneonavicular (spring) ligament** stretches across the plantar aspect of the talocalcaneonavicular joint.

(3) The stability of this joint is assisted dorsally by the calcaneonavicular part of the **bifurcate ligament;** however, the plantar calcaneonavicular (or spring) ligament is the principal support of the longitudinal arch of the foot.

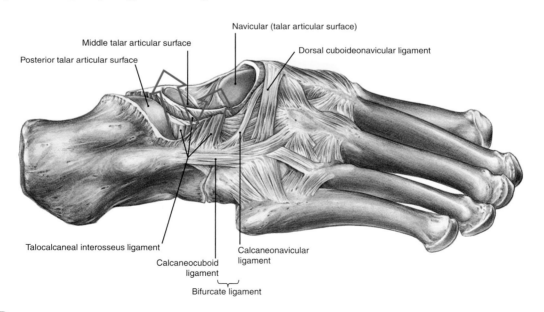

Navicular (talar articular surface)

Middle talar articular surface

Posterior talar articular surface

Dorsal cuboideonavicular ligament

Talocalcaneal interosseus ligament

Calcaneonavicular ligament

Calcaneocuboid ligament

Bifurcate ligament

FIGURE 505.2 Articular Surfaces of the Right Talocalcaneonavicular Joint

NOTE: (1) The posterior and middle articular surfaces of the talus articulate with the underlying calcaneus, while the anterior articular surface articulates with the navicular bone anteriorly.

(2) The **bifurcate ligament** is a strong band that attaches posteriorly to the superior surface of the calcaneus. Anteriorly, it bifurcates into the calcaneocuboid and calcaneonavicular ligaments and forms a lateral ligament of the talocalcaneonavicular joint.

(3) The two green arrows indicate the torsion of the talocalcaneal ligament.

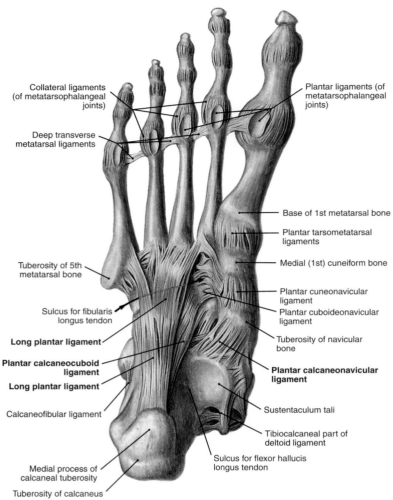

Collateral ligaments
(of metatarsophalangeal
joints)

Deep transverse
metatarsal ligaments

Tuberosity of 5th
metatarsal bone

Sulcus for fibularis
longus tendon

Long plantar ligament

**Plantar calcaneocuboid
ligament**

Long plantar ligament

Calcaneofibular ligament

Medial process of
calcaneal tuberosity

Tuberosity of calcaneus

Plantar ligaments (of
metatarsophalangeal
joints)

Base of 1st metatarsal bone

Plantar tarsometatarsal
ligaments

Medial (1st) cuneiform bone

Plantar cuneonavicular
ligament

Plantar cuboideonavicular
ligament

Tuberosity of navicular
bone

**Plantar calcaneonavicular
ligament**

Sustentaculum tali

Tibiocalcaneal part of
deltoid ligament

Sulcus for flexor hallucis
longus tendon

◄ **FIGURE 506.1** Ligaments on the Plantar Surface of the Right Foot (Superficial)

NOTE: (1) The **long plantar ligament** is the longest and most superficial of the plantar tarsal ligaments. It stretches from the calcaneus posteriorly to an oblique ridge on the plantar surface of the cuboid, where most of its fibers terminate.

(2) The superficial fibers of the long plantar ligament pass over the cuboid to insert on the bases of the lateral three metatarsal bones, thereby forming a tunnel for the **fibularis longus tendon**.

(3) The **plantar calcaneocuboid** or **short plantar ligament** is very strong and lies deep to the long plantar ligament and closer to the bones.

(4) Identify the **plantar calcaneonavicular (spring) ligament** medially. It is attached to the sustentaculum tali of the calcaneus and extends along the entire inferior surface of the navicular bone. It is important for the support of the medial arch of the foot.

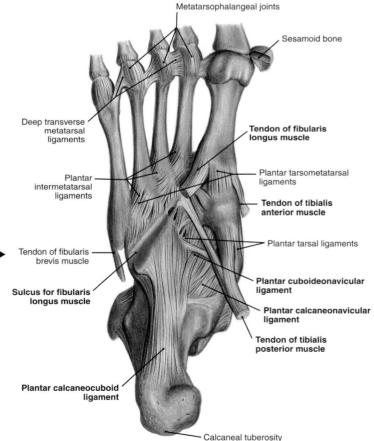

Metatarsophalangeal joints

Sesamoid bone

Deep transverse
metatarsal
ligaments

Plantar
intermetatarsal
ligaments

Tendon of fibularis
brevis muscle

Sulcus for fibularis
longus muscle

**Plantar calcaneocuboid
ligament**

**Tendon of fibularis
longus muscle**

Plantar tarsometatarsal
ligaments

**Tendon of tibialis
anterior muscle**

Plantar tarsal ligaments

**Plantar cuboideonavicular
ligament**

**Plantar calcaneonavicular
ligament**

**Tendon of tibialis
posterior muscle**

Calcaneal tuberosity

FIGURE 506.2 Plantar Calcaneonavicular Ligament ▶ and the Insertions of Three Tendons (Right Foot)

NOTE: (1) The metatarsal extensions of the long plantar ligament have been cut away to reveal the groove for the tendon of the fibularis longus muscle. This tendon inserts onto the base of the first metatarsal bone and the first (medial) cuneiform bone.

(2) Two other tendons insert on the medial side of the plantar surface: the tibialis anterior and posterior tendons.

(3) The fibers of the calcaneocuboid (short plantar) and calcaneonavicular (spring) ligaments all stem from the calcaneus and then diverge in a radial manner toward the medial side of the foot.

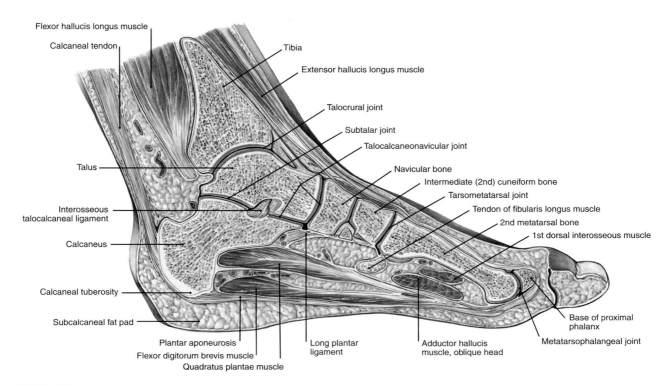

Flexor hallucis longus muscle

Calcaneal tendon

Tibia

Extensor hallucis longus muscle

Talocrural joint

Subtalar joint

Talocalcaneonavicular joint

Talus

Navicular bone

Intermediate (2nd) cuneiform bone

Tarsometatarsal joint

Tendon of fibularis longus muscle

Interosseous talocalcaneal ligament

2nd metatarsal bone

1st dorsal interosseous muscle

Calcaneus

Calcaneal tuberosity

Base of proximal phalanx

Subcalcaneal fat pad

Metatarsophalangeal joint

Plantar aponeurosis

Long plantar ligament

Adductor hallucis muscle, oblique head

Flexor digitorum brevis muscle

Quadratus plantae muscle

FIGURE 507.1 Sagittal Section of Foot Showing Talocrural, Subtalar, and Talocalcaneonavicular Joints

NOTE: (1) This sagittal section, viewed from the medial aspect, cuts through the trochlea, neck, and head of the talus.

(2) The **talocalcaneonavicular joint** anteriorly is of clinical significance because the weight of the body tends to push the head of the talus downward between the navicular and the calcaneus. This results in flat feet.

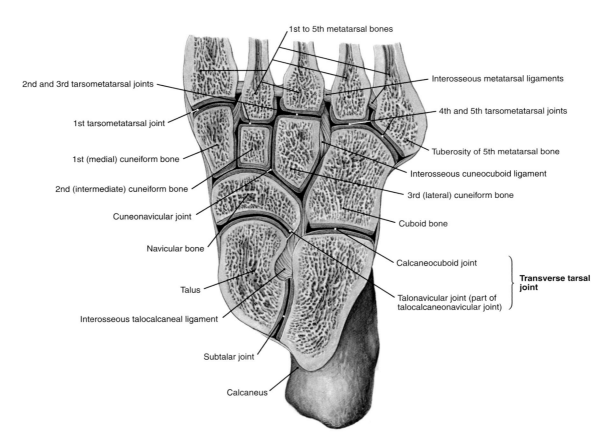

1st to 5th metatarsal bones

2nd and 3rd tarsometatarsal joints

Interosseous metatarsal ligaments

1st tarsometatarsal joint

4th and 5th tarsometatarsal joints

1st (medial) cuneiform bone

Tuberosity of 5th metatarsal bone

2nd (intermediate) cuneiform bone

Interosseous cuneocuboid ligament

Cuneonavicular joint

3rd (lateral) cuneiform bone

Navicular bone

Cuboid bone

Calcaneocuboid joint

Talus

Talonavicular joint (part of talocalcaneonavicular joint)

Transverse tarsal joint

Interosseous talocalcaneal ligament

Subtalar joint

Calcaneus

FIGURE 507.2 Intertarsal and Tarsometatarsal Joints (Horizontal Section of the Right Foot)

NOTE: The **transverse tarsal (midtarsal) joint** extends across the foot and actually is formed by two separate joint cavities, the **calcaneocuboid joint** laterally and the **talonavicular** part of the talcalcaneonavicular joint medially. These two joints allow some eversion and inversion movements of the foot.

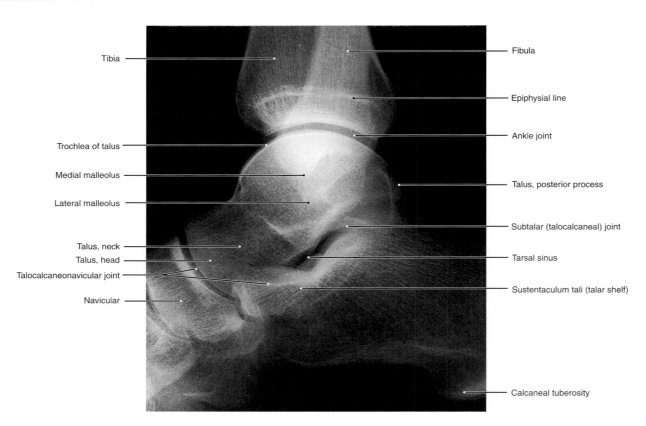

Tibia

Trochlea of talus

Medial malleolus

Lateral malleolus

Talus, neck
Talus, head
Talocalcaneonavicular joint

Navicular

Fibula

Epiphysial line

Ankle joint

Talus, posterior process

Subtalar (talocalcaneal) joint

Tarsal sinus

Sustentaculum tali (talar shelf)

Calcaneal tuberosity

FIGURE 508.1 Lateral Radiograph of the Subtalar and Talocalcaneonavicular Joints

NOTE: The convex head of the talus articulates with the oval, concave posterior **surface** of the navicular bone.

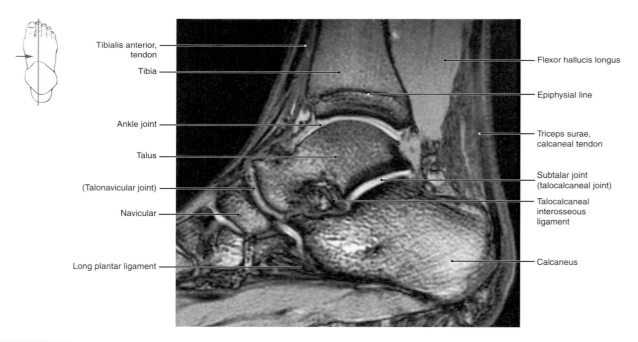

Tibialis anterior, tendon

Tibia

Ankle joint

Talus

(Talonavicular joint)

Navicular

Long plantar ligament

Flexor hallucis longus

Epiphysial line

Triceps surae, calcaneal tendon

Subtalar joint (talocalcaneal joint)

Talocalcaneal interosseous ligament

Calcaneus

FIGURE 508.2 MRI Showing the Ankle, Subtalar, and Talonavicular Joints

NOTE: This image is taken through the longitudinal axis of the foot.

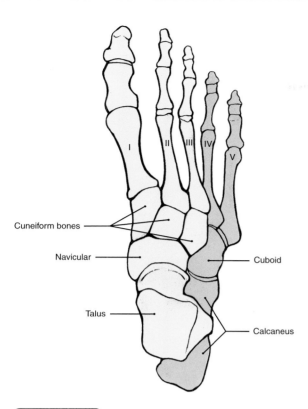

FIGURE 509.1 Longitudinal Arches of the Foot (Dorsal View)

NOTE: The **medial longitudinal arch** consists of the talus, navicular, three cuneiform bones, three medial metatarsal bones, and the phalanges of the large toe and those of the second and third toes.

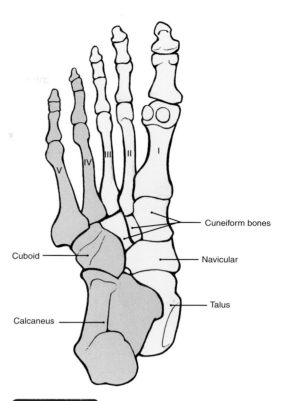

FIGURE 509.2 Longitudinal Arches of the Foot (Plantar View)

NOTE: The **lateral longitudinal arch consists** of the calcaneus and cuboid bones, the two lateral metatarsal bones, and the phalanges of the fourth and fifth toes.

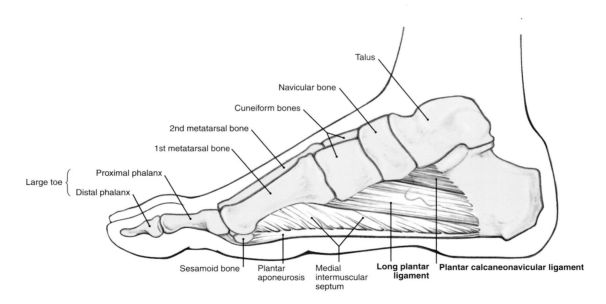

FIGURE 509.3 Longitudinal Arch of the Foot: Underlying Support Structures

NOTE: (1) The medial longitudinal arch of the foot is formed by the calcaneus, talus, navicular, three cuneiform, and the medial three metatarsal bones. Observe the arched nature of the medial margin of the foot.
(2) The integrity of the medial longitudinal arch depends on structures underlying the talocalcaneonavicular septum, but much more important are the **long plantar ligament** and especially the **plantar calcaneonavicular ligament.**

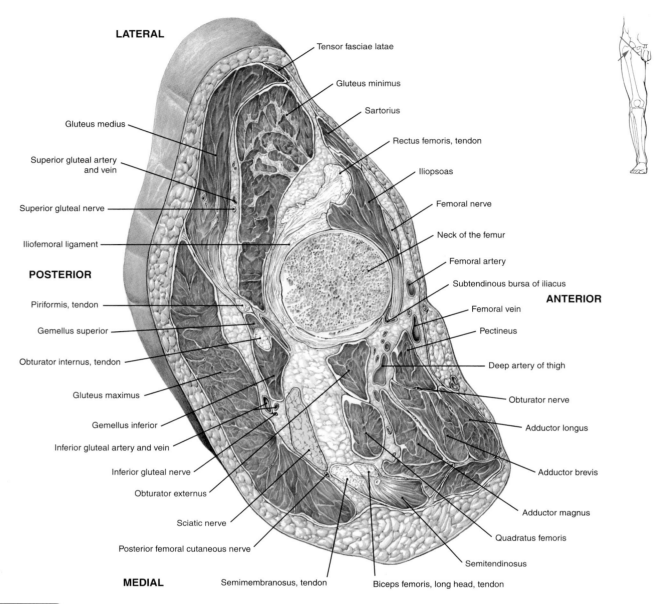

LATERAL

Tensor fasciae latae

Gluteus minimus

Sartorius

Gluteus medius

Rectus femoris, tendon

Superior gluteal artery and vein

Iliopsoas

Femoral nerve

Superior gluteal nerve

Neck of the femur

Iliofemoral ligament

Femoral artery

POSTERIOR

Subtendinous bursa of iliacus

ANTERIOR

Piriformis, tendon

Femoral vein

Gemellus superior

Pectineus

Obturator internus, tendon

Deep artery of thigh

Gluteus maximus

Obturator nerve

Gemellus inferior

Adductor longus

Inferior gluteal artery and vein

Inferior gluteal nerve

Adductor brevis

Obturator externus

Adductor magnus

Sciatic nerve

Quadratus femoris

Posterior femoral cutaneous nerve

Semitendinosus

MEDIAL   Semimembranosus, tendon   Biceps femoris, long head, tendon

FIGURE 510 **Cross Section through the Superior Aspect of the Right Thigh**

NOTE: (1) This section is through the femoral neck. See the tendon of the rectus femoris and the iliofemoral ligament. Observe the gluteus maximus, gluteus medius, and gluteus minimus along with the tendon of the obturator internus and the gemellus superior and gemellus inferior in the **gluteal region.**

(2) The sartorius, iliopsoas, pectineus, and femoral vessels and nerves in the **anterior thigh.** Observe the obturator externus located deep to the quadratus femoris, and note the adductor magnus, longus, and brevis in the **medial thigh.**

(3) The biceps femoris, semimembranosus, tendon of the semitendinosus, and the **sciatic nerve** in the **posterior thigh.**

CLINICAL NOTES from Professor Constantine P. Karakousis, Professor of Surgery, University of Buffalo, Buffalo, N.Y, (by personal communication):

(4) "In a medial compartment resection of the thigh due to sarcoma, resection of the adductor magnus may be required, and it should be kept in mind that as soon as the insertion of the adductor magnus to the linea aspera is divided, directly behind the medial portion of the adductor magnus lies the **sciatic nerve,** which is subject to injury unless some care is exercised."

(5) "The **sciatic nerve** lies between the ischial tuberosity and the greater trochanter, being lateral to the hamstring muscles. As it descends to the midthigh, the sciatic nerve assumes a position between the biceps femoris (long head) and the semitendinosus–semimembranosus muscles. For sarcomas in the buttocks, a longitudinal or slightly oblique incision is preferable to an incision along the fibers of the gluteus maximus. Such an incision can extend from the crest of the ilium to midway between the ischial tuberosity and the greater trochanter into the upper thigh. This provides an early exposure of the sciatic nerve below the lowermost fibers of the gluteus maximus and, therefore, resection of the gluteus maximus and any other gluteal muscles can be done safely by visualizing the sciatic nerve from this more distal point to the site where the nerve leaves the pelvis below the piriformis."

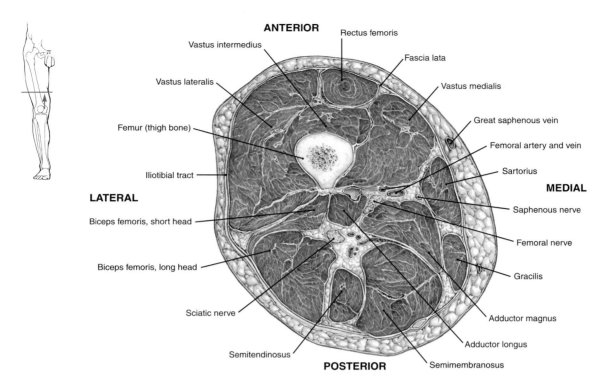

ANTERIOR

Vastus intermedius
Rectus femoris
Fascia lata
Vastus lateralis
Vastus medialis
Femur (thigh bone)
Great saphenous vein
Femoral artery and vein
Iliotibial tract
Sartorius
MEDIAL
LATERAL
Saphenous nerve
Biceps femoris, short head
Femoral nerve
Biceps femoris, long head
Gracilis
Sciatic nerve
Adductor magnus
Adductor longus
Semitendinosus
Semimembranosus
POSTERIOR

FIGURE 511.1 Cross Section through the Middle of the Right Thigh Viewed From the Distal Aspect

NOTE: (1) Compare this figure with the MRI seen in Figure 511.2.

(2) The **posterior** group of structures: biceps femoris, semitendinosus, semimembranosus, and the **sciatic nerve**.

(3) The **medial** structures: gracilis, adductor magnus, and adductor longus (the adductor brevis is more superior to this section).

(4) The **anterior** structures: four heads of the quadriceps muscle: rectus femoris, vastus lateralis, vastus intermedius, and vastus medialis.

CLINICAL NOTES from Professor Constantine P. Karakousis, Professor of Surgery, University of Buffalo, Buffalo, N.Y. (personal communication):

(5) "The bulk of the motor branches of the femoral nerve in the proximal groin deviate in an inferolateral direction along the branches of the lateral femoral circumflex artery and vein in a course between the rectus femoris, vastus intermedius, and vastus lateralis. A slender branch of the femoral nerve, however, remains outside the musculature until it reaches the middle of the vastus medialis, where it enters the muscle to provide its motor supply."

(6) "The difference in the course of the branch to vastus medialis as compared to the branches to the other heads of the quadriceps is useful in performing a modified anterior compartment resection of the anterior thigh for suitable cases of sarcoma, providing the tumor can adequately be resected, since it could potentially preserve the extensor action at the knee."

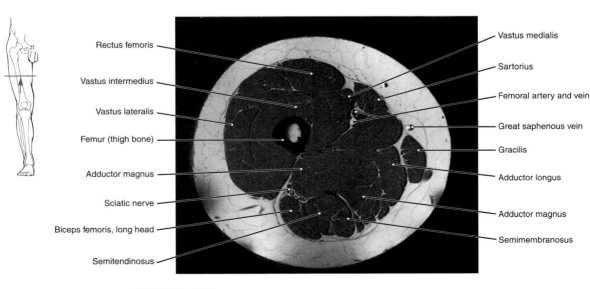

Rectus femoris
Vastus medialis
Sartorius
Vastus intermedius
Femoral artery and vein
Vastus lateralis
Great saphenous vein
Femur (thigh bone)
Gracilis
Adductor magnus
Adductor longus
Sciatic nerve
Adductor magnus
Biceps femoris, long head
Semimembranosus
Semitendinosus

FIGURE 511.2 MRI Near the Middle of the Right Thigh

Chapter 6 The Lower Limb

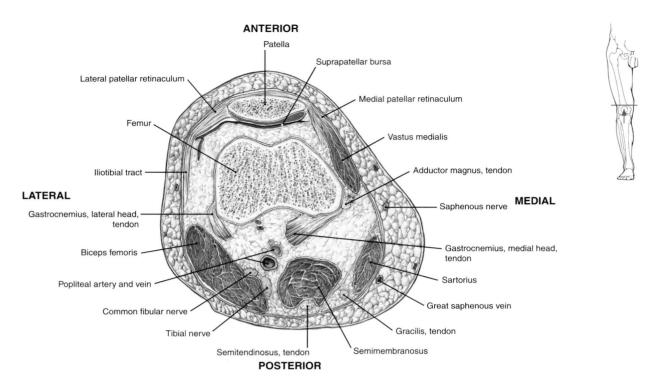

FIGURE 512.1 Cross Section of the Inferior Thigh at the Level of the Popliteal Fossa Viewed from the Distal Aspect

NOTE: (1) Compare this figure with the MRI in Figure 512.2.

(2) In this cross section through the inferior aspect of the right femur, see the **popliteal vessels, tibial nerve,** and **common fibular** (common peroneal) **nerve** in the popliteal fossa posterior to the femur. Observe that the nerves are superficial (i.e., more posterior) to the vessels and that the artery is most deeply located and the vein is between the nerves and the artery.

(3) The patella and the suprapatellar bursa are anterior to the femur and the lateral patellar retinaculum and the iliotibial tract are lateral to the femur.

(4) Posteriorly, identify the two heads of the gastrocnemius muscle, the inferior parts of the "hamstring muscles" (biceps femoris, tendon of the semitendinosus and semimembranosus muscles), the two superior ends of the gastrocnemius muscle, and the sartorius muscle (that has coursed around the thigh to the medial aspect of the knee at this level).

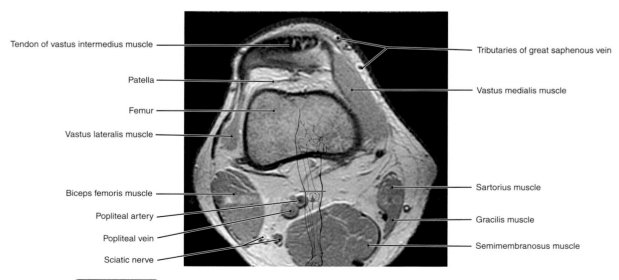

FIGURE 512.2 MRI: Cross Section through the Distal Part of the Right Thigh

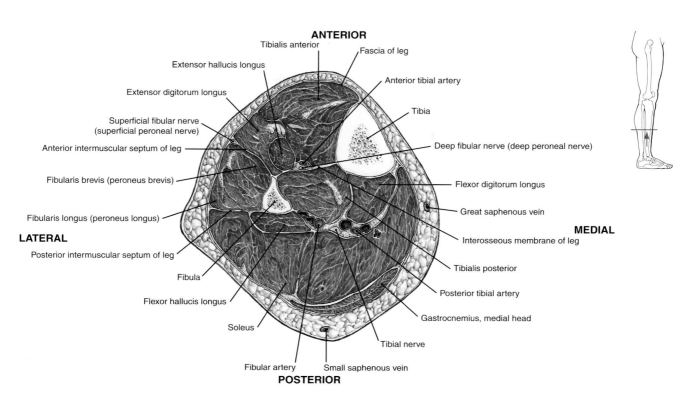

ANTERIOR

Tibialis anterior · Fascia of leg · Anterior tibial artery · Tibia · Deep fibular nerve (deep peroneal nerve) · Flexor digitorum longus · Great saphenous vein · Interosseous membrane of leg · Tibialis posterior · Posterior tibial artery · Gastrocnemius, medial head · Tibial nerve · Small saphenous vein

Extensor hallucis longus · Extensor digitorum longus · Superficial fibular nerve (superficial peroneal nerve) · Anterior intermuscular septum of leg · Fibularis brevis (peroneus brevis) · Fibularis longus (peroneus longus) · Posterior intermuscular septum of leg · Fibula · Flexor hallucis longus · Soleus · Fibular artery

LATERAL · MEDIAL · POSTERIOR

FIGURE 513.1 Cross Section through the Middle of the Right Leg

NOTE: (1) The tibia, fibula, and interosseous membrane (that interconnects the bones) and the intermuscular septa divide the leg into **anterior, lateral,** and **posterior compartments.**

(2) The **tibialis anterior, extensor hallucis longus, extensor digitorum longus, deep fibular nerve** (from the common fibular nerve), and **anterior tibial artery** are all located in the **anterior compartment.**

(3) The **fibularis longus, fibularis brevis** (peroneal longus and brevis), and **superficial fibular nerve** (from the common fibular nerve) that supply the two muscles are all located in the lateral compartment.

(4) The **posterior compartment** contains **superficial and deep parts.**

(5) The **superficial part** of the posterior compartment contains the **gastrocnemius muscle,** the **soleus muscle,** and the **tendon of the plantaris muscle** (this latter structure is not shown in this figure; see Fig. 464).

(6) The **deep part** of the posterior compartment contains the **flexor digitorum longus, tibialis posterior,** and **flexor hallucis longus** muscles.

(7) The **posterior tibial artery** (and **vein**), the **fibular artery** (a branch of the posterior tibial) and **vein,** and the **posterior tibial nerve** course in the plane between the superficial and deep posterior compartment structures.

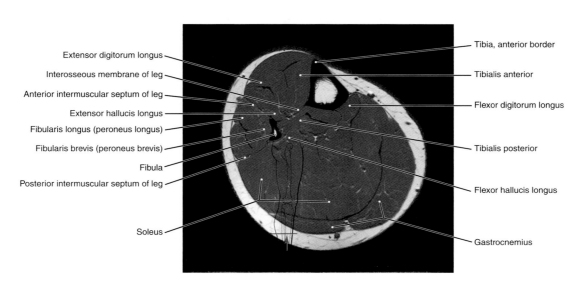

Extensor digitorum longus · Interosseous membrane of leg · Anterior intermuscular septum of leg · Extensor hallucis longus · Fibularis longus (peroneus longus) · Fibularis brevis (peroneus brevis) · Fibula · Posterior intermuscular septum of leg · Soleus

Tibia, anterior border · Tibialis anterior · Flexor digitorum longus · Tibialis posterior · Flexor hallucis longus · Gastrocnemius

FIGURE 513.2 MRI: Cross Section through the Middle of the Right Leg

PLATE 514 **Cross Sections: Lower Right Leg and Proximal Right Foot**

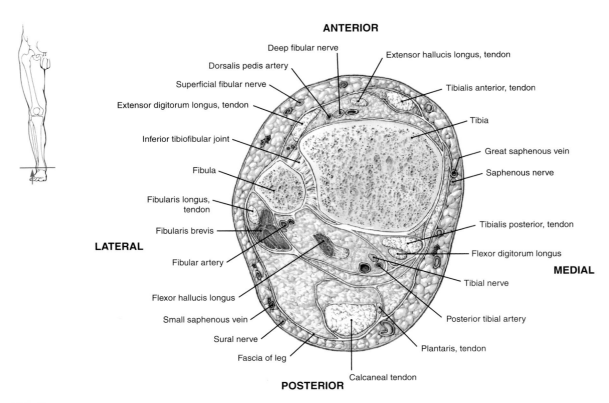

FIGURE 514.1 **Cross Section through the Right Leg Just Proximal to the Malleoli**

NOTE: (1) The **anterior compartment** tendons, the superficial and deep fibular nerves, and the dorsalis pedis artery anterior to the tibia.
(2) The fibula, tendon of the fibularis longus, and the fibularis brevis muscle in the **lateral compartment.**
(3) The flexor hallucis longus, tendons of the tibialis posterior and flexor digitorum longus, the tibial nerve, the posterior tibial artery and its branch, and the fibular artery are all in the **deep part** of the **posterior compartment.**
(4) The calcaneal tendon and the small tendon of the plantaris muscle in the superficial part of the posterior compartment.

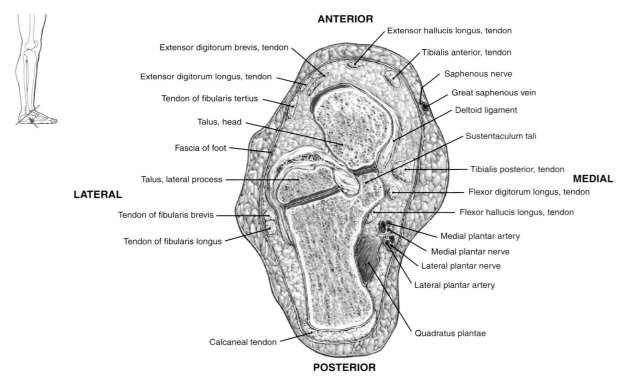

FIGURE 514.2 **Oblique Section through the Calcaneus and Talus of the Right Foot**

NOTE: The sustentaculum tali deep to the talus and the tendons of the leg descending anterior, lateral, and medial to the bony structures.

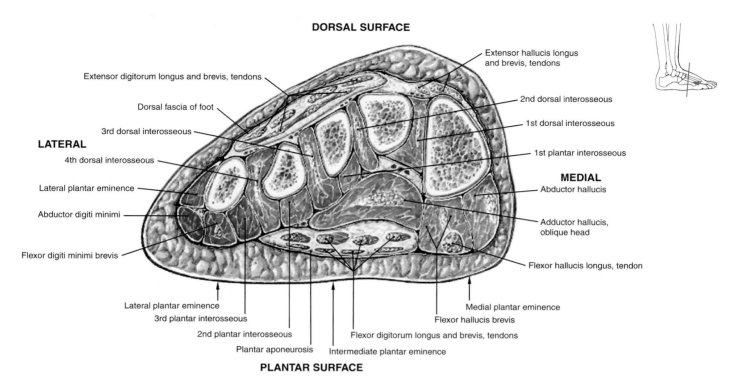

DORSAL SURFACE

Extensor digitorum longus and brevis, tendons

Dorsal fascia of foot

3rd dorsal interosseous

LATERAL

4th dorsal interosseous

Lateral plantar eminence

Abductor digiti minimi

Flexor digiti minimi brevis

Extensor hallucis longus and brevis, tendons

2nd dorsal interosseous

1st dorsal interosseous

1st plantar interosseous

MEDIAL

Abductor hallucis

Adductor hallucis, oblique head

Flexor hallucis longus, tendon

Lateral plantar eminence

3rd plantar interosseous

2nd plantar interosseous

Plantar aponeurosis

Intermediate plantar eminence

Medial plantar eminence

Flexor hallucis brevis

Flexor digitorum longus and brevis, tendons

PLANTAR SURFACE

FIGURE 515.1 **Frontal Section through the Metatarsal Bones of the Right Foot**

NOTE: (1) Compare this figure with Figure 515.2 and identify the metatarsal bones and the plantar and dorsal interosseous muscles.
(2) The abductor hallucis, flexor hallucis brevis, and tendon of the flexor hallucis longus on the medial side of plantar aspect of the foot.
(3) The tendons of the extensor digitorum longus and brevis muscles on the dorsum of the foot.
(4) The plantar aponeurosis and the tendons of the flexors digitorum longus and brevis on the plantar aspect of the foot; just dorsal to these is located the adductor hallucis.

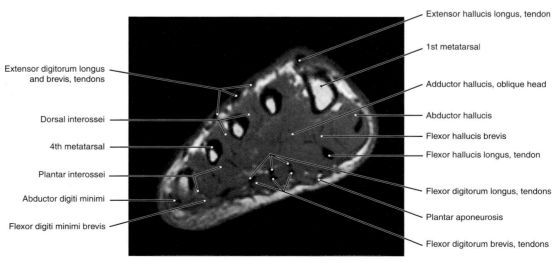

Extensor digitorum longus and brevis, tendons

Dorsal interossei

4th metatarsal

Plantar interossei

Abductor digiti minimi

Flexor digiti minimi brevis

Extensor hallucis longus, tendon

1st metatarsal

Adductor hallucis, oblique head

Abductor hallucis

Flexor hallucis brevis

Flexor hallucis longus, tendon

Flexor digitorum longus, tendons

Plantar aponeurosis

Flexor digitorum brevis, tendons

FIGURE 515.2 **MRI through the Metatarsal Bones of the Right Foot**

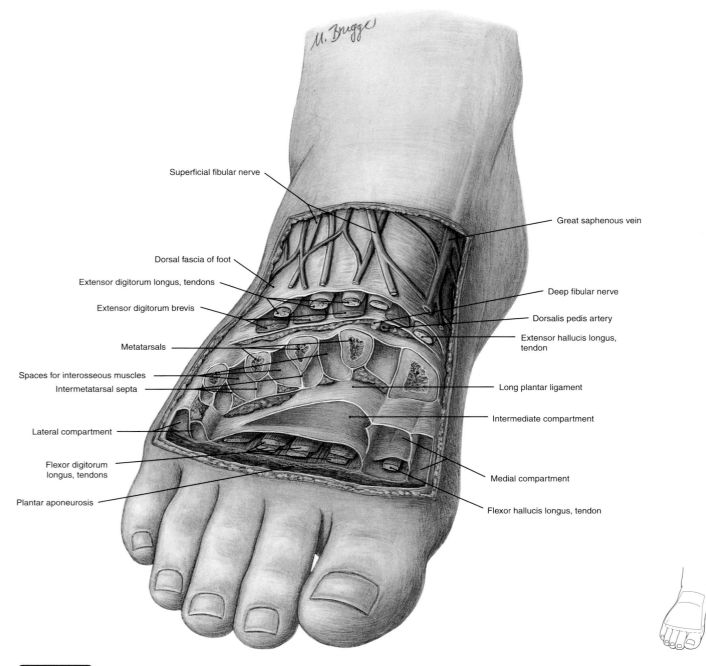

FIGURE 516 Compartments of the Foot Shown by a Frontal Section at the Midmetatarsal Level

NOTE compartments sequentially from dorsal to plantar sides:

(1) The superficial fibular nerve and superficial veins at the subcutaneous level on the foot dorsum.

(2) The extensor digitorum longus and extensor hallucis longus tendons and the bellies of the **extensor** digitorum brevis muscle of the foot dorsum. On the plantar aspect of these, observe the deep fibular nerve and dorsalis pedis artery.

(3) The metatarsal bones and the spaces for the dorsal and plantar interosseous muscles.

(4) On the plantar aspect of the metatarsal bones and interosseous muscles are the lateral, intermediate, and medial compartments that contain the intrinsic muscles on the plantar aspect of the foot (see Fig. 472).

The muscles of the **medial compartment** include the abductor hallucis and the flexor hallucis brevis, and just deep to these is the tendon of the flexor hallucis longus muscle.

The muscles of the **intermediate compartment** include the transverse and oblique heads of the adductor hallucis, and just on the plantar aspect of these are the quadratus plantae muscle, the tendons of the flexor digitorum longus muscle, and the lumbrical muscles.

The muscles of the **lateral compartment** are the opponens, flexor, and abductor digiti minimi muscles.

CHAPTER 7 The Neck and Head

Plates

517 Regions of the Neck and Head

518 Surface Anatomy of the Face; Tension Lines of Skin: Face and Neck

519 Neck: Sternocleidomastoid and Other Anterior Muscles

520 Diagrams: Triangles of the Neck; Coniotomy and Tracheotomy

521 Neck: Platysma Muscle

522 Superficial Vessels and Nerves of the Lateral Neck and Head

523 Neck: Anterior and Posterior Triangles

524 Nerves of the Lateral Neck, Scalp, and Face

525 Drainage Patterns of Lymphatic Channels in the Head and Neck

526 Lymph Nodes of the Head and Neck

527 Neck: Cervical Fascial Layers

528 Muscles of Posterior Neck, Including Scalene Muscles (Muscle Chart)

529 Neck: Vessels and Nerves, Platysma Level (Dissection 1)

530 Neck: Vessels and Nerves, Sternocleidomastoid Level (Dissection 2)

531 Neck: Vessels and Nerves, Investing Fascia Removed (Dissection 3)

532 Neck: Vessels and Nerves, Carotid Sheath Opened (Dissection 4)

533 Neck: Vessels and Nerves, Subclavian Artery (Dissection 5)

534 Neck: Vessels and Nerves, Brachial Plexus (Dissection 6)

535 Neck: Jugular System of Veins

536 Neck: Deep Veins, Arteries, and Thyroid Gland

537 Neck: Thyroid and Parathyroid Glands; Cross Section of the Anterior Neck

538 Scintiscan and Ultrasonogram of the Thyroid Gland; Goiter

539 Patterns of Lymph Drainage (Adult) and Chains of Nodes (Child)

540 Lymph Nodes in the Posterior Neck and Axilla; Carotid Arteries

541 Neck: Anterior Vertebral Muscles

542 Neck: Cross Section at C5; Anterior Vertebral Muscle Chart

543 Neck: Carotid and Vertebral Arteries; Variations of Vertebral Arteries

544 Neck: Subclavian Artery; Variations of Carotid and Vertebral Arteries

545 Neck: Suprahyoid Submandibular Region (Dissection Stages 1 and 2)

546 Neck: Suprahyoid Submandibular Region (Dissection Stages 3 and 4)

547 Face: Superficial Muscles (Anterior View)

548 Face: Superficial Muscles (Lateral View)

549 Muscle Chart: Suprahyoid Muscles; Muscles of Scalp, Ear, and Eyelids

550 Muscle Chart: Muscles of Nose and Mouth

551 Face: Muscles of Mastication; Parotid Gland

552 Face: Muscles of Mastication; Dermatomes of Head and Neck

553 Face: Superficial Vessels and Nerves (Dissection 1)

554 Face: Superficial Vessels and Nerves (Dissection 2)

555 Muscles of Mastication

556 Pterygoid Muscles and Other Deep Head Muscles (Seen from Below)

557 Temporomandibular Joint and Mandibular Ligaments

558 Temporomandibular Joint (Sagittal and Arthrographic Views)

559 Face: Superficial and Deep Arteries

560 Maxillary Artery and Its Variations

561 Superficial Veins of the Face and Skull

562 Internal Jugular Vein and Its Tributaries in the Superior Neck

563 Face: Deep Vessels and Nerves (Dissection 1)

564 Face: Deep Vessels and Nerves (Dissection 2)

565 Face: Infratemporal Fossa, Deep Vessels, and Nerves (Dissection 3)

566 Face: Infratemporal Fossa, Deep Vessels, and Nerves (Dissection 4)

567 Skull and Orbital Cavity (Anterior View)

568 Skull and Infratemporal Region (Lateral View)

569 Calvaria from Above; Occipital Bone (Posterior View)

570 Calvaria, Inner Surface; Skull Types

571 Newborn Skull (Anterior and Lateral Views)

572 Newborn Skull (Superior and Inferior Views)

573 Scalp and Frontal Section of Scalp, Skull, and Meninges

574 Skull: Diploic Veins; Radiograph of Internal Carotid Artery

575 Dura Mater and Meningeal Vessels from Above

576 Arteries and Veins on the External Surface of the Brain

577 Dura Mater and Dural Venous Sinuses (Lateral View)

578 Dural Venous Sinuses: Skull Base (Superior View)

579 Internal Carotid and Vertebral Arteries

580 Internal Carotid Artery: In the Cavernous Sinus; at the Skull Base

581 Cavernous Sinus; Arteries at the Base of the Brain; Circle of Willis

582 Circle of Willis: Normal and Variations

583 Carotid Arteriogram (Lateral View)

584 Vertebral Arteriogram (Posterior View)

585 Paramedian Section of the Skull

586 Base of the Skull: Foramina and Markings

587 Bony Floor of the Cranial Cavity; The Pituitary Gland

588 Base of the Skull (Inner Surface): Cranial Nerves and Vessels

589 Inferior Surface of the Brain: Cranial Nerves

590 Inferior Surface of the Brain: Dura Mater Removed, Arachnoid Intact

591 Base of Skull: Inferior Surface, Foramina, and Markings

592 Inferior Surface of the Bony Skull

593 Eye: Surface Anatomy (Anterior View)

594 Eye: Superficial Nerves and Muscles (Anterior View)

595 Bony Orbit (Anterior View and Frontal Section)

596 Bony Orbit: Medial and Lateral Walls

597 Orbital Septum, Eyelids, and Tarsal Plates

598 Lacrimal Gland and Lacrimal Apparatus

599 Lacrimal Apparatus

600 Orbit (Sagittal and Horizontal Sections)

601 Orbit from Above: Ophthalmic Nerve and Artery (Dissection 1)

602 Orbit from Above: Trochlear and Abducens Nerves (Dissection 2)

603 Orbit from Above: Optic Nerve; Ciliary Ganglion (Dissection 3)

604 Orbit from Above: Oculomotor Nerve and Eyeball (Dissection 4)

605 Extraocular Muscles: Superior and Left Lateral Views; MRI of Orbits

606 Orbit: Extraocular Muscles (Superior and Lateral Views)

607 Orbit: Extraocular Muscles, Insertions and Actions

608 Origins of Ocular Muscles; Ophthalmic Artery

609 Eyeball: Horizontal Section; Iris

610 Optic Disk; MRI of the Orbit; Lens

611 Arteries and Veins within the Orbital Cavity

612 Horizontal Section of the Eyeball; Select Orbital Nerves

613 External Nose; Lateral Wall of the Nasal Cavity

614 Nasal Cavity: Bones of the Lateral Wall

615 Nasal Septum: Skeletal Parts; Lateral Nasal Wall

616 Pterygopalatine Ganglion; Maxillary, Petrosal, and Facial Nerves

617 Paranasal Sinuses

618 Ethmoid Bone and Growth of the Frontal and Maxillary Sinuses

619 Oral Cavity: Palate and Tongue (Anterior View); Oral Muscles

620 Oral Cavity: Dissected Palate; Anterior View of Tongue and Oropharynx

621 Oral Cavity: Sublingual Region and Parotid Duct Orifice

622 Oral Cavity: Mouth (Anterior View); Muscular Floor (Sagittal Section)

623 Floor of the Oral Cavity Viewed from the Neck: Intact and Dissected

624 Floor of the Oral Cavity (Inferior and Superior Views)

625 Oral Cavity: Salivary Glands

626 Oral Cavity: Salivary Glands (Continued)

627 Oral Cavity: Midsagittal Section, the Tongue

628 Oral Cavity: Dorsum of Tongue; Taste Follicles and Nerves of Taste

629 Muscles of the Tongue and Pharynx; Lingual and Palatine Tonsils

630 Muscles of the Tongue and Pharynx (Continued)

631 Posterior Tongue and Palate; Transverse Sections of the Tongue

632 Nerves and Artery to the Tongue; Muscle Chart

633 Teeth: Innervation of Upper and Lower Teeth; Mandible

634 Teeth: Mandible, Mandibular Arch, and Lower Teeth

635 Upper Teeth and Palate from Below

636 Teeth, Upper and Lower: Deciduous and Permanent

637 Left Adult Permanent Teeth (Vestibular and Medial Aspects)

638 Left Adult Permanent Teeth (Oral and Distal Aspects)

639 Teeth: Longitudinal Section; Occlusal Surfaces; Impacted Molars

640 Teeth: Radiograph of Mandible and Maxilla

641 Pharynx: External Muscles (Lateral View)

642 Pharynx and Oral Cavity: Internal Midsagittal View

643 Pharynx from Behind: Muscles

644 Pharynx from Behind: Vessels and Nerves

645 Pharynx, Opened from Behind; Lymphatic Ring

646 Pharynx, Opened from Behind, Muscles; Soft Palate

647 Pharynx and Soft Palate from Behind: Vessels and Nerves

648 Muscle Chart: Muscles of the Palate and Pharynx

649 Larynx: Anterior Relationships, Vessels and Nerves

650 Larynx: Posterior Relationships, Vessels and Nerves

651 Larynx: Cartilages and Membranes

652 Larynx: Cartilages and Membranes (Continued)

653 Larynx: Muscles

654 Larynx: Muscles (Continued)

655 Larynx (Frontal and Midsagittal Sections)

656 Larynx in Cross Section; Laryngoscopic Views of the Larynx

657 External Ear: Surface Anatomy, Cartilage, and Muscles

658 Temporal Bone (Lateral View); Dissected Tympanic Cavity

659 Ear: External and Middle Ear (Frontal Sections)

660 Ear: Tympanic Membrane, External and Internal Surfaces

661 Ear: Lateral Wall of Tympanic Cavity; Middle Ear Ossicles

662 Middle and Internal Ear; Middle Ear Ossicles

663 Ear: Lateral Wall of Tympanic Cavity; Chorda Tympani Nerve

664 Ear: Medial Wall of the Tympanic Cavity

665 Ear: Facial Canal; Nerves of External and Middle Ear

666 Facial Canal: Temporal Bone Dissection; Course of Facial Nerve

667 Internal Ear Projected onto the Bony Base of the Skull

668 Right Membranous Labyrinth of the Inner Ear

PLATE 517 Regions of the Neck and Head

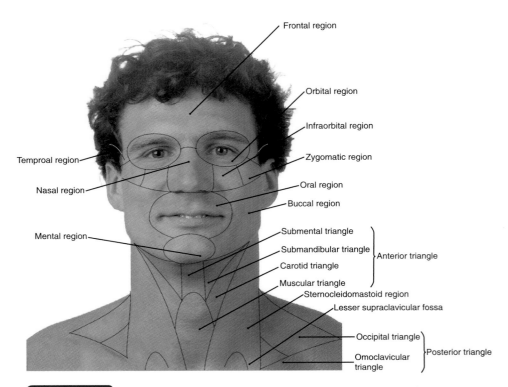

FIGURE 517.1 Regions of the Head and Neck (Anterior Aspect)

Frontal region

Orbital region

Infraorbital region

Zygomatic region

Temproal region

Oral region

Nasal region

Buccal region

Submental triangle

Submandibular triangle — Anterior triangle

Mental region

Carotid triangle

Muscular triangle

Sternocleidomastoid region

Lesser supraclavicular fossa

Occipital triangle — Posterior triangle

Omoclavicular triangle

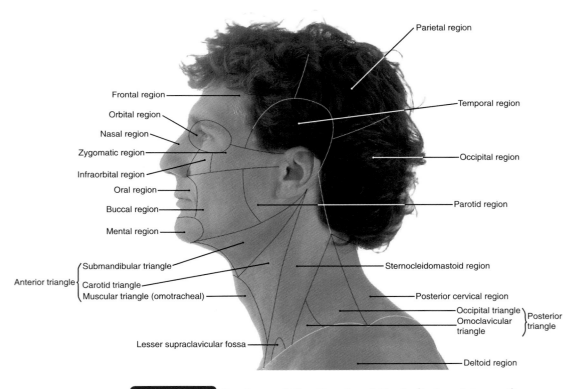

FIGURE 517.2 Regions of the Head and Neck (Lateral Aspect)

Parietal region

Frontal region

Temporal region

Orbital region

Nasal region

Zygomatic region

Occipital region

Infraorbital region

Oral region

Buccal region

Parotid region

Mental region

Submandibular triangle

Anterior triangle — Carotid triangle

Muscular triangle (omotracheal)

Sternocleidomastoid region

Posterior cervical region

Occipital triangle — Posterior triangle

Omoclavicular triangle

Lesser supraclavicular fossa

Deltoid region

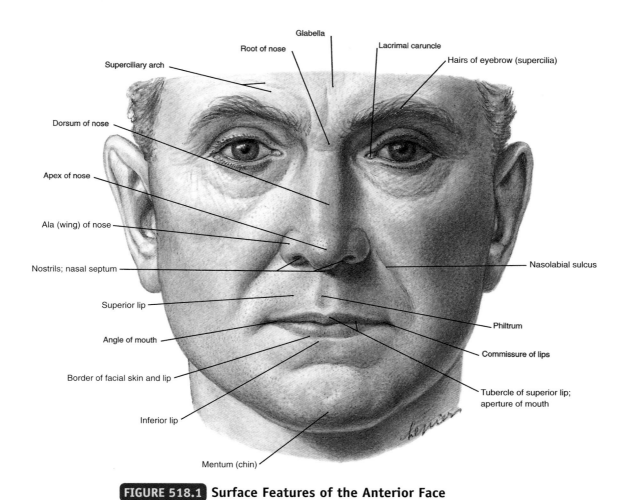

Glabella

Root of nose

Superciliary arch

Lacrimal caruncle

Hairs of eyebrow (supercilia)

Dorsum of nose

Apex of nose

Ala (wing) of nose

Nostrils; nasal septum

Nasolabial sulcus

Superior lip

Angle of mouth

Philtrum

Commissure of lips

Border of facial skin and lip

Tubercle of superior lip; aperture of mouth

Inferior lip

Mentum (chin)

FIGURE 518.1 **Surface Features of the Anterior Face**

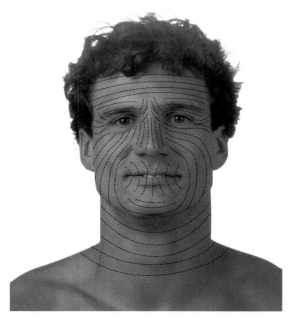

FIGURE 518.2 **Tension Lines of the Skin of the Head and Neck (Anterior Aspect)**

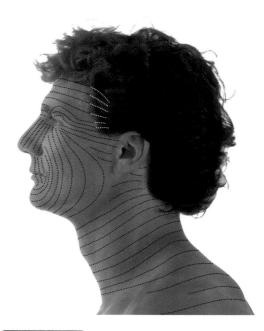

FIGURE 518.3 **Tension Lines of the Skin of the Head and Neck (Lateral Aspect)**

NOTE: For optimal healing, incision lines in the skin should be made along the lines of tension (Langer's lines).

PLATE 519 Neck: Sternocleidomastoid and Other Anterior Muscles

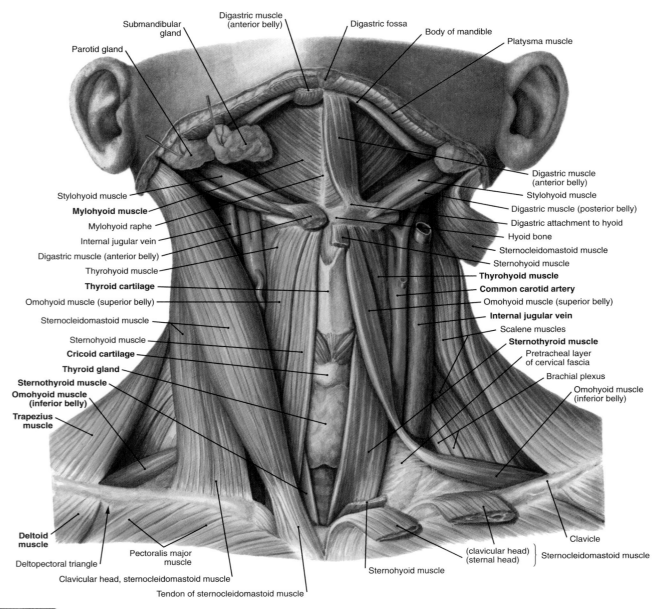

FIGURE 519 Anterior View of the Musculature of the Neck

NOTE: (1) The right superior belly of the digastric muscle was removed and the submandibular gland elevated to show the mylohyoid muscle. On the left side (reader's right), the sternocleidomastoid and sternohyoid muscles have been transected and the submandibular gland removed.

(2) Observe the relationship of the strap muscles to the thyroid gland and realize that below the thyroid gland and above the suprasternal notch, the trachea lies immediately under the skin.

INFRAHYOID MUSCLES OF THE NECK				
Muscle	**Origin**	**Insertion**	**Innervation**	**Action**
Sternohyoid	Manubrium of sternum and the medial end of the clavicle	Body of hyoid bone	Ansa cervicalis (C1, C2, C3)	Depresses the hyoid bone after food is swallowed
Sternothyroid	Posterior surface of the manubrium of the sternum	Oblique line on the lamina of the thyroid cartilage	Ansa cervicalis (C1, C2, C3)	Depresses the hyoid bone and the larynx
Thyrohyoid	Oblique line on the lamina of the thyroid cartilage	Lower border of the greater horn of the hyoid bone	Fibers from the C1 spinal nerve that course for a short distance with the hypoglossal nerve XII	Depresses the hyoid bone or elevates the larynx
Omohyoid	Upper border of the scapula near the suprascapular notch	Lower border of the body of the hyoid bone	Ansa cervicalis (C1, C2, C3)	Depresses and helps stabilize the hyoid bone

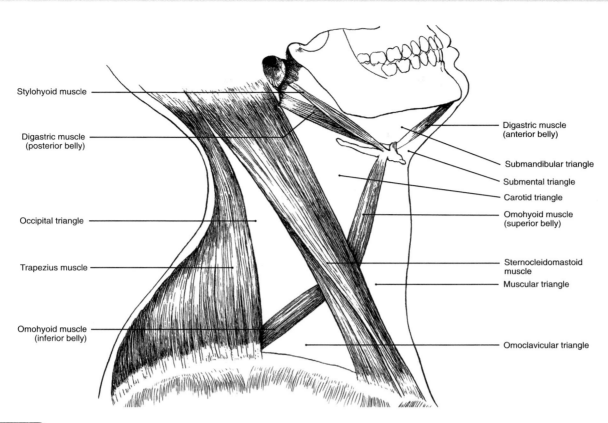

Stylohyoid muscle

Digastric muscle (posterior belly)

Occipital triangle

Trapezius muscle

Omohyoid muscle (inferior belly)

Digastric muscle (anterior belly)

Submandibular triangle

Submental triangle

Carotid triangle

Omohyoid muscle (superior belly)

Sternocleidomastoid muscle

Muscular triangle

Omoclavicular triangle

FIGURE 520.1 **Triangles of the Neck (Lateral View)**

NOTE: The triangles of the neck are useful in describing the location of cervical organs and other structures. The entire area anterior to the sternocleidomastoid muscle is called the **anterior triangle**, whereas the area posterior to this muscle is the **posterior triangle.**

Muscle	Origin	Insertion	Innervation	Action
Sternocleidomastoid	**Sternal head:** Upper part of the ventral surface of the manubrium of the sternum **Clavicular head:** Upper border and anterior surface of the medial third of the clavicle	Lateral surface of the mastoid process and the lateral half of the superior nuchal line	Motor fibers: Accessory nerve Sensory fibers: Anterior rami of C2 and C3 nerves	When one side acts: Bends the head laterally toward the shoulder of the same side; rotates the head, turning the face upward, directing it to the opposite side When both sides act: Flexes the head and neck

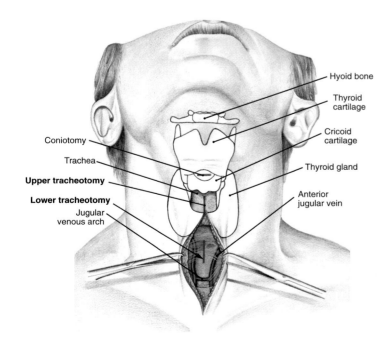

Coniotomy

Trachea

Upper tracheotomy

Lower tracheotomy

Jugular venous arch

Hyoid bone

Thyroid cartilage

Cricoid cartilage

Thyroid gland

Anterior jugular vein

FIGURE 520.2 **Projection of Larynx and Trachea Showing Sites for Entry into the Respiratory Pathway**

NOTE: (1) The hyoid bone, laryngeal cartilages (thyroid and cricoid), thyroid gland, and tracheal region of the anterior neck are projected to the surface, as are three sites where entrance into the respiratory tract may be achieved readily (in red).

(2) The upper transverse incision cuts through the cricothyroid ligament and conus elasticus and can be called a **cricothyrotomy** or **coniotomy**, while the **upper tracheotomy** and **lower tracheotomy** can be made in the trachea above or below the thyroid gland.

PLATE 521 Neck: Platysma Muscle

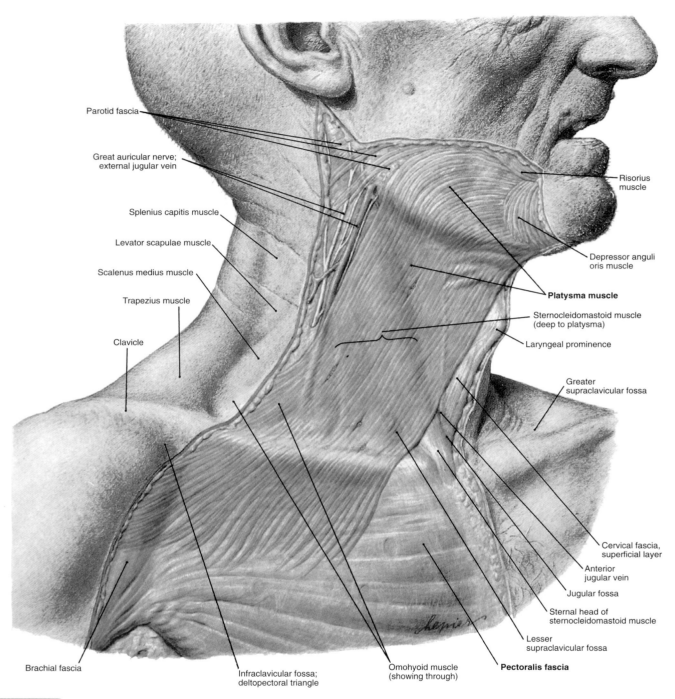

Parotid fascia

Great auricular nerve;
external jugular vein

Splenius capitis muscle

Levator scapulae muscle

Scalenus medius muscle

Trapezius muscle

Clavicle

Brachial fascia

Infraclavicular fossa;
deltopectoral triangle

Omohyoid muscle
(showing through)

Risorius
muscle

Depressor anguli
oris muscle

Platysma muscle

Sternocleidomastoid muscle
(deep to platysma)

Laryngeal prominence

Greater
supraclavicular fossa

Cervical fascia,
superficial layer

Anterior
jugular vein

Jugular fossa

Sternal head of
sternocleidomastoid muscle

Lesser
supraclavicular fossa

Pectoralis fascia

FIGURE 521 Right Platysma Muscle and Pectoral Fascia

NOTE: (1) The **platysma muscle** is a broad, thin quadrangular muscle located in the superficial fascia; it extends from the angle of the mouth and chin downward across the clavicle to the upper part of the thorax and anterior shoulder.

(2) The platysma is considered one of the muscles of facial expression, many of which do not attach to bony structures but arise and insert within the superficial fascia.

(3) Upon concentration, the platysma tends to depress the angle of the mouth and wrinkle the skin of the neck, thereby participating in the formation of facial expressions of anxiety, sadness, dissatisfaction, and suffering.

(4) Similar to other muscles of facial expression, the platysma is innervated by the **facial nerve (cervical branch)**, the seventh cranial nerve (VII).

(5) Overlying the pectoralis major is the well-developed pectoralis fascia, which extends from the midline in the thorax laterally to the axilla. Observe the external jugular vein and great auricular nerve exposed in the upper lateral aspect of the neck.

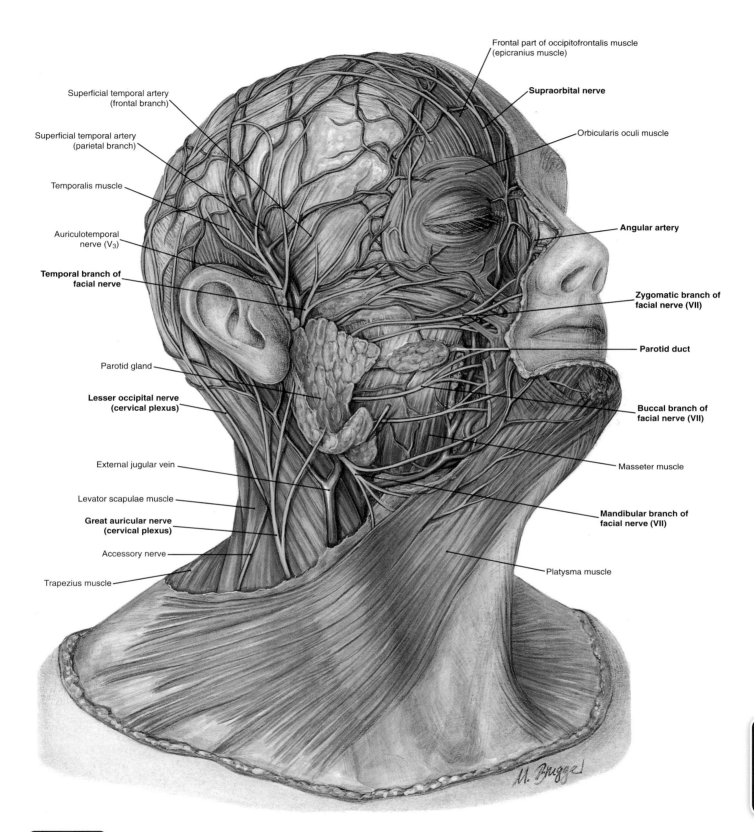

Frontal part of occipitofrontalis muscle
(epicranius muscle)

Supraorbital nerve

Orbicularis oculi muscle

Superficial temporal artery
(frontal branch)

Superficial temporal artery
(parietal branch)

Temporalis muscle

Auriculotemporal
nerve (V₃)

**Temporal branch of
facial nerve**

Parotid gland

**Lesser occipital nerve
(cervical plexus)**

External jugular vein

Levator scapulae muscle

**Great auricular nerve
(cervical plexus)**

Accessory nerve

Trapezius muscle

Angular artery

**Zygomatic branch of
facial nerve (VII)**

Parotid duct

**Buccal branch of
facial nerve (VII)**

Masseter muscle

**Mandibular branch of
facial nerve (VII)**

Platysma muscle

FIGURE 522 Superficial Lateral Vessels and Nerves of the Neck and Temporal and Facial Regions of the Head

NOTE: (1) The superficial temporal vessels, the branches of the facial nerve, and two branches of the cervical plexus of nerves (great auricular and lesser occipital).

(2) Also observe the supraorbital nerve, angular artery, and parotid duct.

PLATE 523 Neck: Anterior and Posterior Triangles

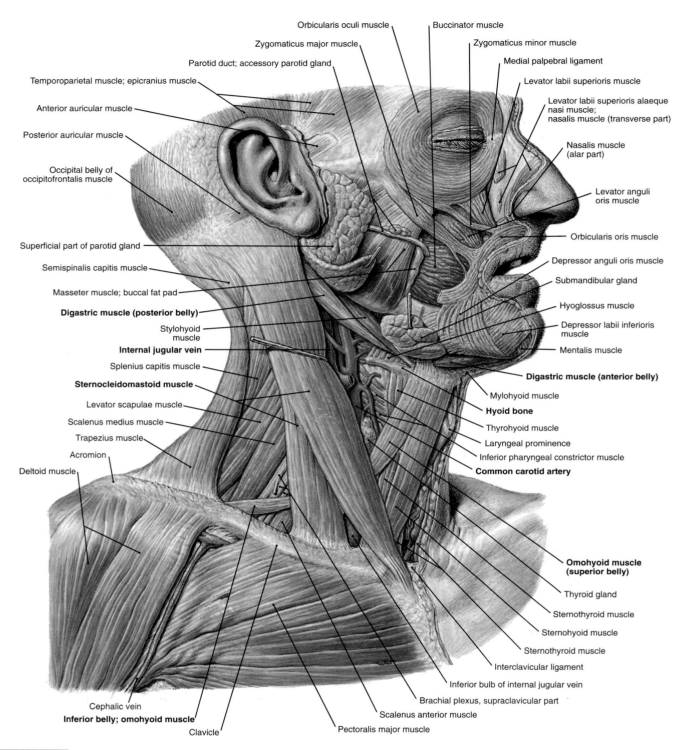

Orbicularis oculi muscle

Buccinator muscle

Zygomaticus major muscle

Zygomaticus minor muscle

Parotid duct; accessory parotid gland

Medial palpebral ligament

Temporoparietal muscle; epicranius muscle

Levator labii superioris muscle

Anterior auricular muscle

Levator labii superioris alaeque nasi muscle; nasalis muscle (transverse part)

Posterior auricular muscle

Nasalis muscle (alar part)

Occipital belly of occipitofrontalis muscle

Levator anguli oris muscle

Superficial part of parotid gland

Orbicularis oris muscle

Semispinalis capitis muscle

Depressor anguli oris muscle

Masseter muscle; buccal fat pad

Submandibular gland

Digastric muscle (posterior belly)

Hyoglossus muscle

Stylohyoid muscle

Depressor labii inferioris muscle

Internal jugular vein

Mentalis muscle

Splenius capitis muscle

Digastric muscle (anterior belly)

Sternocleidomastoid muscle

Mylohyoid muscle

Levator scapulae muscle

Hyoid bone

Scalenus medius muscle

Thyrohyoid muscle

Trapezius muscle

Laryngeal prominence

Acromion

Inferior pharyngeal constrictor muscle

Deltoid muscle

Common carotid artery

Omohyoid muscle (superior belly)

Thyroid gland

Sternothyroid muscle

Sternohyoid muscle

Sternothyroid muscle

Interclavicular ligament

Inferior bulb of internal jugular vein

Brachial plexus, supraclavicular part

Cephalic vein

Scalenus anterior muscle

Inferior belly; omohyoid muscle

Pectoralis major muscle

Clavicle

FIGURE 523 Anterior and Posterior Triangles of the Neck

NOTE: (1) The **anterior triangle** of the neck is bounded by the midline of the neck, the anterior border of the sternocleidomastoid muscle, and the mandible. This area is further subdivided by the superior belly of the omohyoid muscle and the two bellies of the digastric into:
  (a) **Muscular triangle** (midline, superior belly of omohyoid, and sternocleidomastoid).
  (b) **Carotid triangle** (superior belly of omohyoid, sternocleidomastoid muscle, and posterior belly of digastric).
  (c) **Submandibular triangle** (anterior and posterior bellies of digastric, and the inferior margin of the mandible).
  (d) **Submental triangle** (midline, anterior belly of digastric, and hyoid bone).
(2) The **posterior triangle** of the neck is bounded by the posterior border of the sternocleidomastoid muscle, the trapezius, and the clavicle. This area is further subdivided into the **occipital triangle** above and the **omoclavicular triangle** below by the inferior belly of the omohyoid.

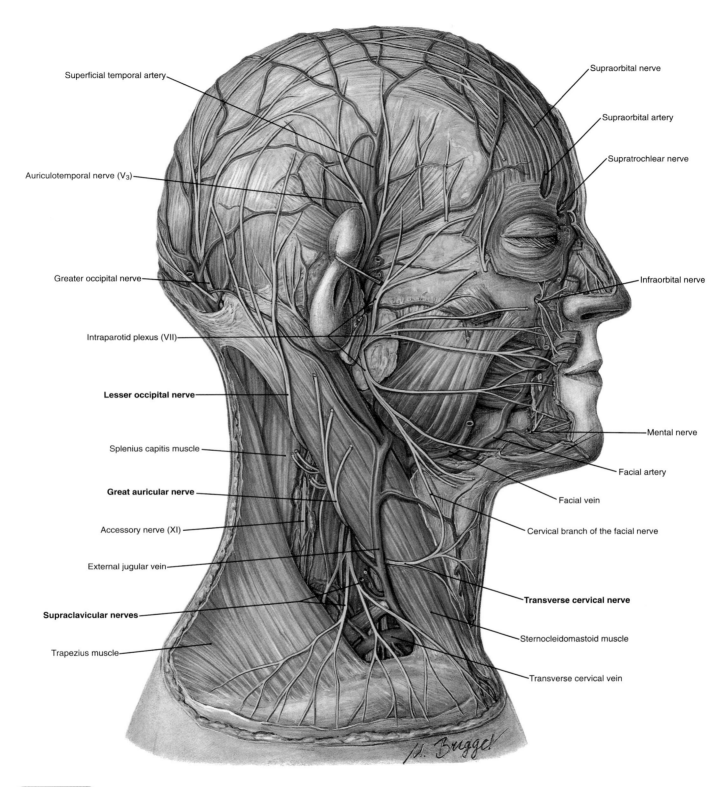

Superficial temporal artery

Auriculotemporal nerve (V₃)

Greater occipital nerve

Intraparotid plexus (VII)

Lesser occipital nerve

Splenius capitis muscle

Great auricular nerve

Accessory nerve (XI)

External jugular vein

Supraclavicular nerves

Trapezius muscle

Supraorbital nerve

Supraorbital artery

Supratrochlear nerve

Infraorbital nerve

Mental nerve

Facial artery

Facial vein

Cervical branch of the facial nerve

Transverse cervical nerve

Sternocleidomastoid muscle

Transverse cervical vein

FIGURE 524 **Nerves of the Face, Scalp, and Lateral Neck**

NOTE: (1) The great auricular, lesser occipital, transverse cervical, and supraclavicular branches of the cervical plexus.

(2) Observe the auriculotemporal branch of the mandibular division of the trigeminal nerve ascending in the temporal region anterior to the external ear.

(3) See the branches (not labeled) of the facial nerve as they emerge from the intraparotid plexus. These would include the temporal, zygomatic, buccal, mandibular, and cervical branches (see Fig. 522).

PLATE 525 Drainage Patterns of Lymphatic Channels in the Head and Neck

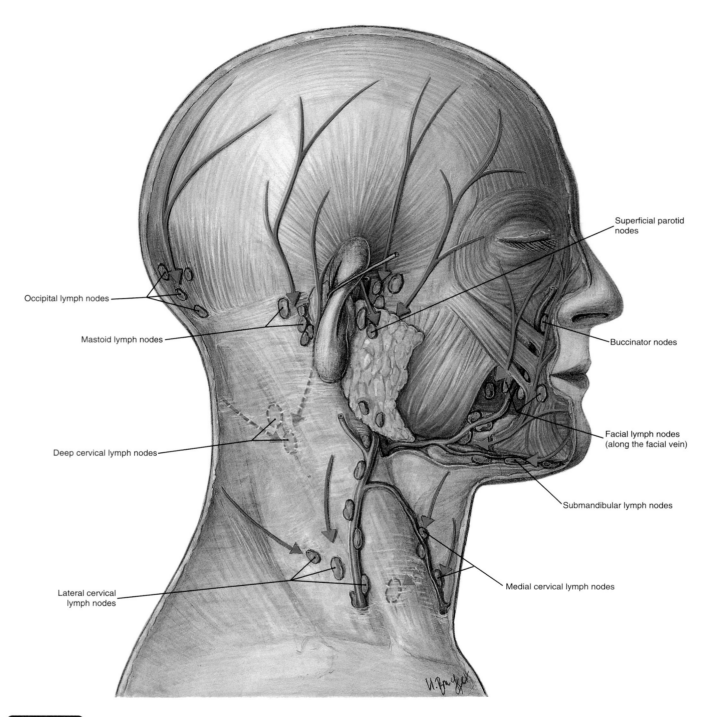

Superficial parotid nodes

Occipital lymph nodes

Mastoid lymph nodes

Buccinator nodes

Deep cervical lymph nodes

Facial lymph nodes (along the facial vein)

Submandibular lymph nodes

Medial cervical lymph nodes

Lateral cervical lymph nodes

FIGURE 525 Drainage Patterns of Lymph nodes on the Lateral Scalp and Face

NOTE: (1) The drainage patterns of lymph from the lateral scalp descend to mastoid nodes posterior to the external ear, and then this lymph continues inferiorly to deep cervical nodes. Lymph from the anterolateral scalp drains inferiorly toward parotid nodes anterior to the ear, and then it descends to lateral cervical nodes.

(2) Lymph from the anterior face (lateral to the nose and mouth) descends to submandibular nodes and then courses along veins in the anterior and lateral neck.

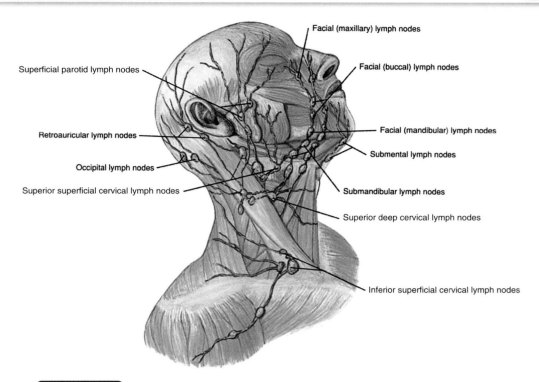

FIGURE 526.1 Superficial Lymph Nodes and Vessels of the Head and Neck

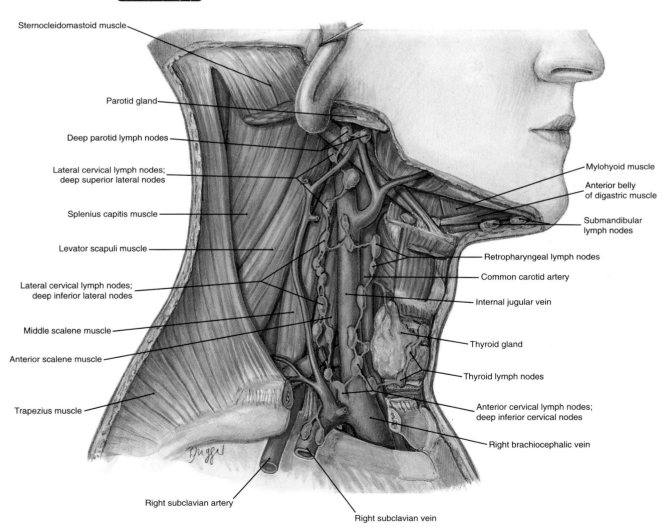

FIGURE 526.2 Chains of Lymph Nodes in the Lateral Neck

NOTE that in the lateral neck, there are chains of nodes that are collected along major veins such as the internal jugular vein and the external jugular vein (which are not labeled in this figure).

PLATE 527 **Neck: Cervical Fascial Layers**

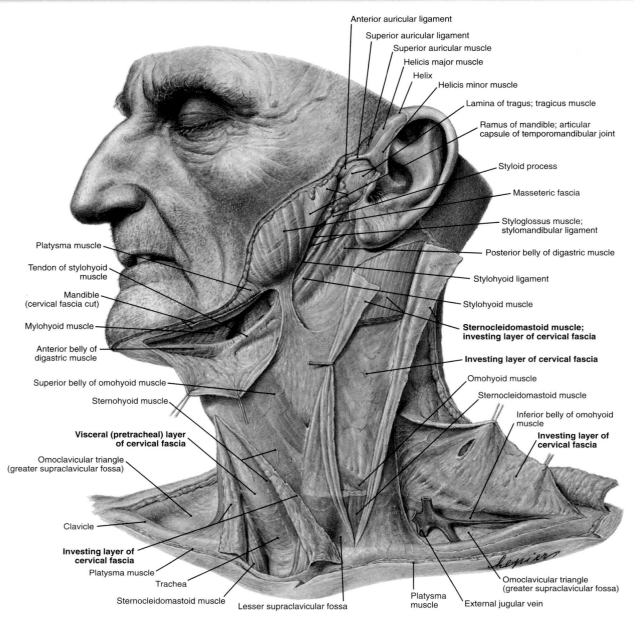

Anterior auricular ligament
Superior auricular ligament
Superior auricular muscle
Helicis major muscle
Helix
Helicis minor muscle
Lamina of tragus; tragicus muscle
Ramus of mandible; articular capsule of temporomandibular joint
Styloid process
Masseteric fascia
Styloglossus muscle; stylomandibular ligament
Posterior belly of digastric muscle
Stylohyoid ligament
Stylohyoid muscle
Sternocleidomastoid muscle; investing layer of cervical fascia
Investing layer of cervical fascia
Omohyoid muscle
Sternocleidomastoid muscle
Inferior belly of omohyoid muscle
Investing layer of cervical fascia

Platysma muscle
Tendon of stylohyoid muscle
Mandible (cervical fascia cut)
Mylohyoid muscle
Anterior belly of digastric muscle
Superior belly of omohyoid muscle
Sternohyoid muscle
Visceral (pretracheal) layer of cervical fascia
Omoclavicular triangle (greater supraclavicular fossa)
Clavicle
Investing layer of cervical fascia
Platysma muscle
Trachea
Sternocleidomastoid muscle
Lesser supraclavicular fossa
Platysma muscle
External jugular vein
Omoclavicular triangle (greater supraclavicular fossa)

FIGURE 527.1 **External Investing and Pretracheal Fascial Layers of the Neck**

NOTE: The **external investing layer** of deep fascia surrounds the sternocleidomastoid muscle, whereas the **pretracheal layer** of deep fascia is located deep to the investing layer and encloses the strap muscles.

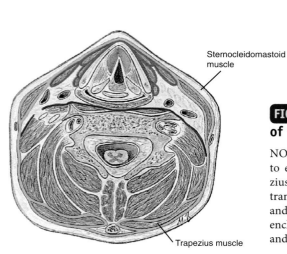

Sternocleidomastoid muscle

Trapezius muscle

A Transverse section

Cervical fascia

Investing layer (superficial layer)

Pretracheal layer

Prevertebral layer

FIGURE 527.2A and B **Fascial Planes of the Neck**

NOTE: The **external investing fascia** splits to encase the sternocleidomastoid and trapezius muscles. The **prevertebral fascia** courses transversely anterior to the vertebral column and its muscles, whereas the **pretracheal fascia** encloses the esophagus, trachea, thyroid gland, and strap muscles.

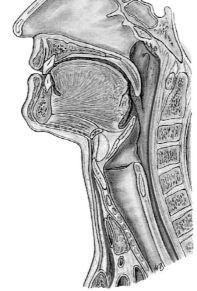

B Median section

Chapter 7 The Neck and Head

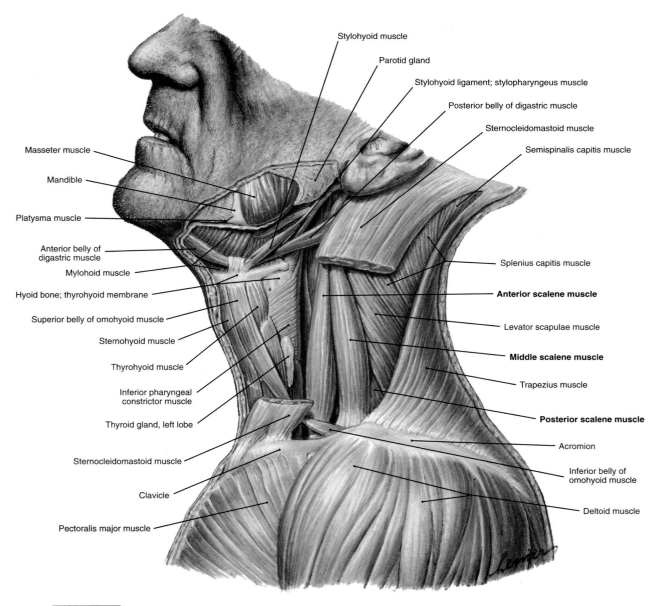

FIGURE 528 Muscular Floor of the Posterior Triangle of the Neck and the Scalene Muscles

MUSCLES OF THE POSTERIOR TRIANGLE OF THE NECK*

Muscle	Origin	Insertion	Innervation	Action
Anterior scalene	By four tendons, each one from the transverse processes of the third, fourth, fifth, and sixth cervical vertebrae	Onto the scalene tubercle of the first rib	Anterior rami of the fourth, fifth, and sixth cervical spinal nerves	When neck is fixed: elevates the first rib. When first rib is fixed: Bends neck forward and laterally, and rotates it to the opposite side
Middle scalene	Transverse processes of C2 to C7 vertebrae (often also from the atlas)	Superior surface of first rib between the tubercle and the groove for subclavian artery	Anterior rami of the third through the eighth cervical nerves	Same as anterior scalene muscle
Posterior scalene	Transverse processes of fourth, fifth, and sixth cervical vertebrae	Outer surface of the second rib	Anterior rami of the C6, C7, and C8 spinal nerves	Raises the second rib; or, bends and rotates the neck
Splenius capitis	Caudal half of the ligamentum nuchae; spinous processes of C7, and upper four thoracic vertebrae	Lateral third of the superior nuchal line and onto the mastoid process of the temporal bone	Dorsal rami of the middle cervical spinal nerves	Laterally flexes head; rotates head and neck to same side; when both muscles act they extend head and neck

*Levator scapulae and semispinalis capitis are described on Plate 379.

PLATE 529 Neck: Vessels and Nerves, Platysma Level (Dissection 1)

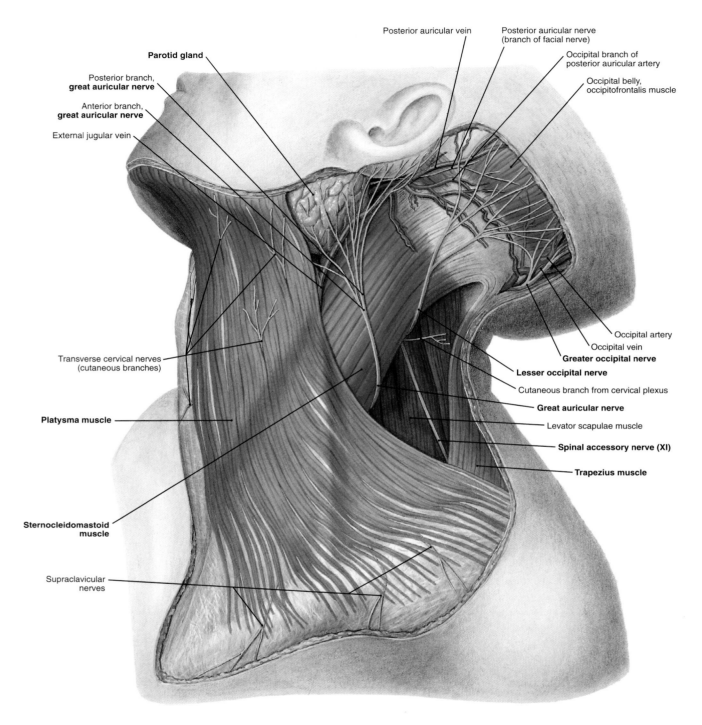

Posterior auricular vein

Posterior auricular nerve (branch of facial nerve)

Occipital branch of posterior auricular artery

Parotid gland

Occipital belly, occipitofrontalis muscle

Posterior branch, **great auricular nerve**

Anterior branch, **great auricular nerve**

External jugular vein

Occipital artery

Occipital vein

Greater occipital nerve

Transverse cervical nerves (cutaneous branches)

Lesser occipital nerve

Cutaneous branch from cervical plexus

Great auricular nerve

Levator scapulae muscle

Platysma muscle

Spinal accessory nerve (XI)

Trapezius muscle

Sternocleidomastoid muscle

Supraclavicular nerves

FIGURE 529 Nerves and Blood Vessels of the Neck, Stage 1: Platysma Layer

NOTE: (1) The skin has been removed from both the anterior and posterior triangle areas to reveal the platysma muscle. Observe the cutaneous branches of the **transverse cervical nerves**, derived from the cervical plexus and penetrating through the platysma and superficial fascia to reach the skin of the anterolateral aspect of the neck.

(2) Four other nerves: the **great auricular (C2, C3);** the **lesser occipital (C2);** the **greater occipital (C2);** and the **accessory (XI).**

(3) After it has supplied the sternocleidomastoid muscle, the accessory nerve (XI) descends in the posterior triangle to reach the trapezius muscle, which it also supplies.

(4) The **supraclavicular nerves**. These descend in the neck under cover of the deep fascia and platysma muscle. They become superficial just above the clavicle nend then cross that bone as the medial, intermediate, and lateral supraclavicular nerves (see also Fig. 530). They derive from the third and fourth cervical nerves and supply skin over the clavicle, the upper trunk (down to the second rib), and the shoulder from the acromion laterally to the midline anteriorly.

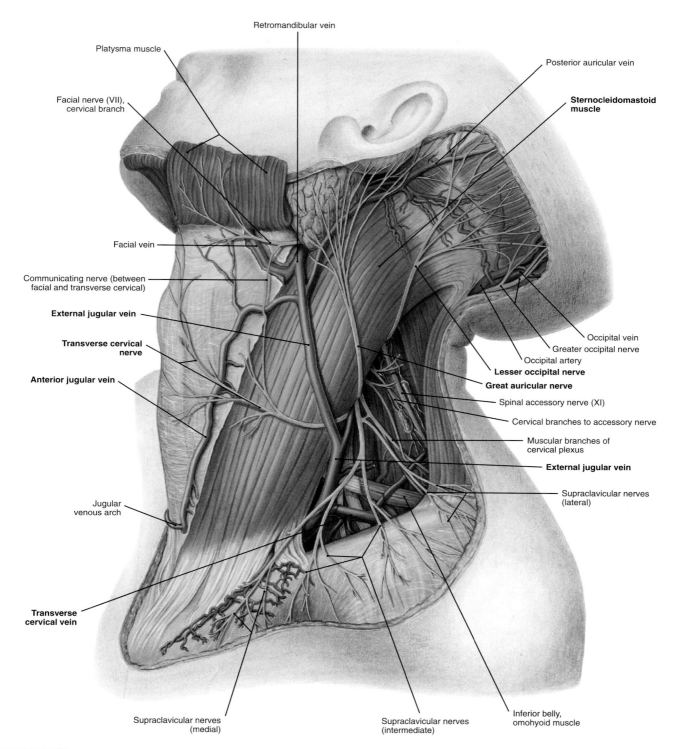

Retromandibular vein

Platysma muscle

Facial nerve (VII), cervical branch

Posterior auricular vein

Sternocleidomastoid muscle

Facial vein

Communicating nerve (between facial and transverse cervical)

External jugular vein

Transverse cervical nerve

Anterior jugular vein

Occipital vein

Greater occipital nerve

Occipital artery

Lesser occipital nerve

Great auricular nerve

Spinal accessory nerve (XI)

Cervical branches to accessory nerve

Muscular branches of cervical plexus

External jugular vein

Supraclavicular nerves (lateral)

Jugular venous arch

Transverse cervical vein

Supraclavicular nerves (medial)

Supraclavicular nerves (intermediate)

Inferior belly, omohyoid muscle

FIGURE 530 **Nerves and Blood Vessels of the Neck, Stage 2: Sternocleidomastoid Layer**

NOTE: (1) With the platysma muscle reflected upward, the full extent of the sternocleidomastoid muscle is exposed.

(2) The nerves of the cervical plexus diverge at the posterior border of the sternocleidomastoid muscle: the **great auricular** and **lesser occipital** ascend to the head, the **transverse cervical** (transverse colli) course across the neck, while the **supraclavicular nerves** descend over the clavicle.

(3) The **external jugular vein**, formed by the junction of the **retromandibular** and **posterior auricular veins**. The external jugular vein crosses the sternocleidomastoid muscle obliquely and receives tributaries from the anterior jugular, posterior external jugular (not shown), transverse cervical, and suprascapular vein (not shown) before it ends in the subclavian vein.

(4) The cervical branch of the **facial (VII) nerve** supplying the inner surface of the platysma muscle with motor innervation.

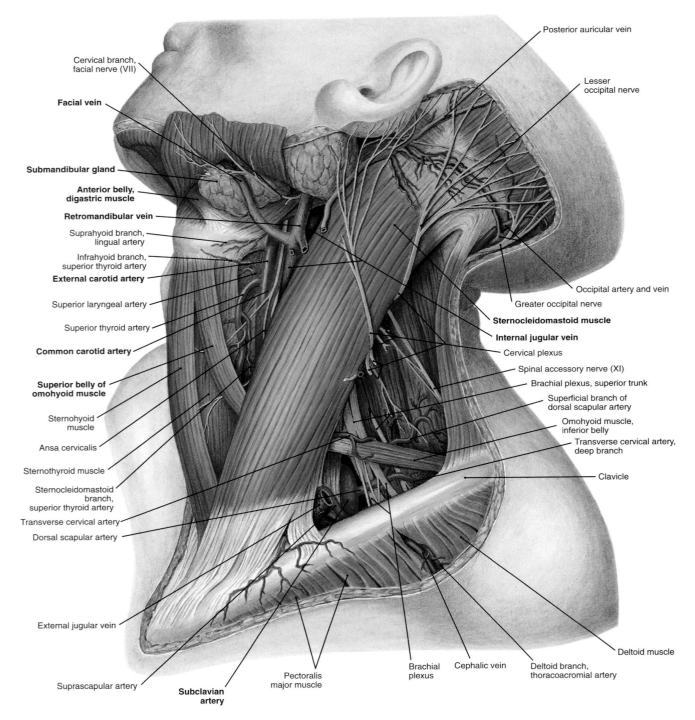

Posterior auricular vein

Cervical branch, facial nerve (VII)

Facial vein

Lesser occipital nerve

Submandibular gland

Anterior belly, digastric muscle

Retromandibular vein

Suprahyoid branch, lingual artery

Infrahyoid branch, superior thyroid artery

External carotid artery

Superior laryngeal artery

Occipital artery and vein

Greater occipital nerve

Superior thyroid artery

Sternocleidomastoid muscle

Common carotid artery

Internal jugular vein

Cervical plexus

Spinal accessory nerve (XI)

Superior belly of omohyoid muscle

Brachial plexus, superior trunk

Superficial branch of dorsal scapular artery

Sternohyoid muscle

Ansa cervicalis

Omohyoid muscle, inferior belly

Sternothyroid muscle

Transverse cervical artery, deep branch

Sternocleidomastoid branch, superior thyroid artery

Clavicle

Transverse cervical artery

Dorsal scapular artery

External jugular vein

Deltoid muscle

Suprascapular artery

Subclavian artery

Pectoralis major muscle

Brachial plexus

Cephalic vein

Deltoid branch, thoracoacromial artery

FIGURE 531 Nerves and Blood Vessels of the Neck, Stage 3: The Anterior Triangle

NOTE: (1) With the investing layer of fascia removed, the outlines of the muscular, carotid, and submandibular triangles within the anterior region of the neck are revealed.

(2) The infrahyoid (strap) muscles, which cover the thyroid gland and the lateral aspect of the larynx in the **muscular triangle.** This is bounded by the sternocleidomastoid, the midline, and the superior belly of the digastric muscle.

(3) The carotid vessels and internal jugular vein can be seen in the **carotid triangle,** which is bounded by the superior belly of the omohyoid, posterior belly of the digastric (not labeled), and the sternocleidomastoid.

(4) With the platysma muscle cut and reflected upward, the submandibular gland is seen in the **submandibular triangle,** between the anterior and posterior bellies of the digastric and the inferior border of the mandible.

(5) The spinal accessory nerve descending in the posterior triangle from beneath the sternocleidomastoid, which it supplies, to reach the trapezius muscle (not labeled), which it also supplies with motor innervation.

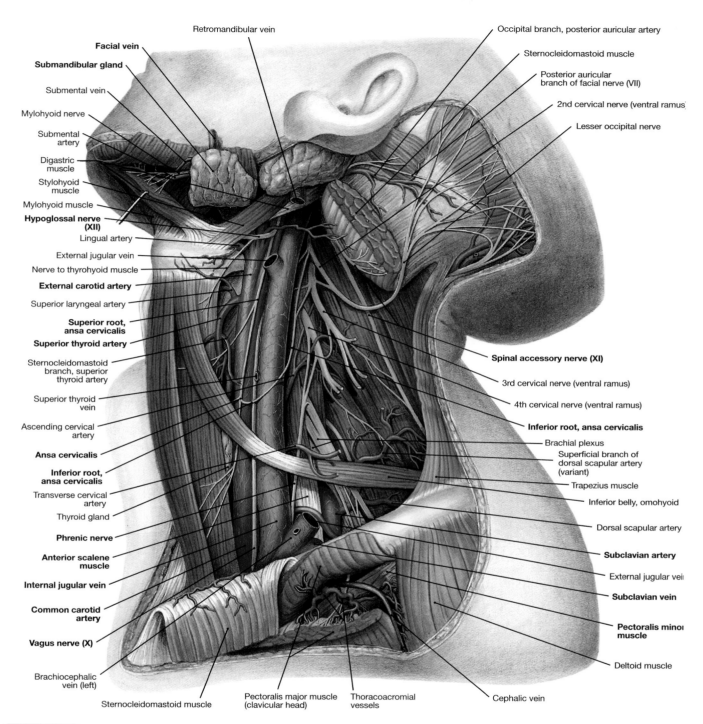

FIGURE 532 Nerves and Blood Vessels of the Neck, Stage 4: Large Vessels

NOTE: (1) The sternocleidomastoid and the superficial veins and nerves have been removed to expose the **carotid arteries, internal jugular vein, omohyoid muscle, vagus nerve,** and **ansa cervicalis**.

(2) Superiorly, the facial vein has been cut and the submandibular gland has been elevated, thereby exposing the **hypoglossal nerve (XII)**.

(3) Nerve fibers, originating from C1 and traveling for a short distance with the hypoglossal nerve, leave that nerve to descend in the neck. They form the **superior root of the ansa cervicalis** and are joined by other descending fibers from C2 and C3, which are called the **inferior root of the ansa cervicalis.** The ansa cervicalis supplies motor innervation for a number of strap muscles.

(4) The **common carotid artery, internal jugular vein,** and **vagus nerve**. These form a vertically oriented neurovascular bundle in the neck that is normally surrounded by the carotid sheath of deep fascia. The common carotid artery bifurcates at about the level of the hyoid bone to form the **external** and **internal carotid arteries**.

PLATE 533 Neck: Vessels and Nerves, Subclavian Artery (Dissection 5)

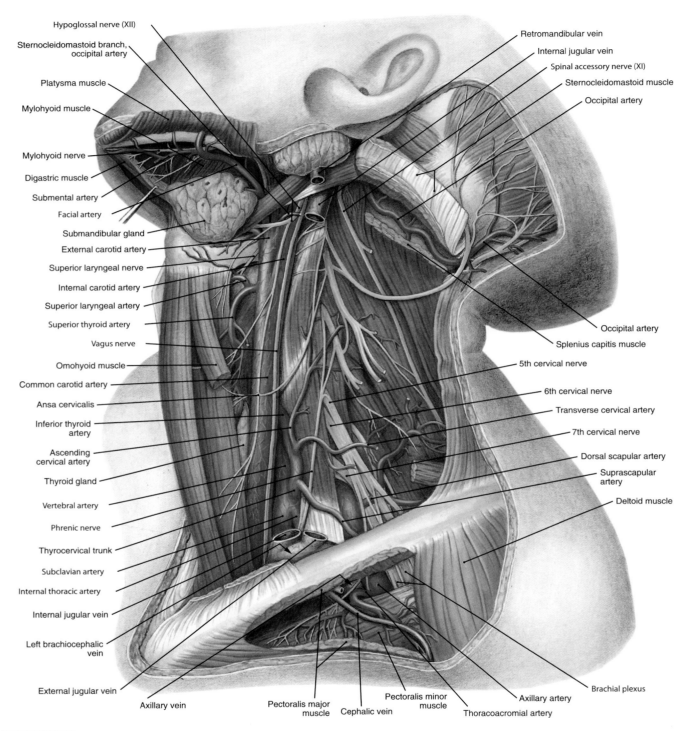

Hypoglossal nerve (XII)
Sternocleidomastoid branch, occipital artery
Platysma muscle
Mylohyoid muscle
Mylohyoid nerve
Digastric muscle
Submental artery
Facial artery
Submandibular gland
External carotid artery
Superior laryngeal nerve
Internal carotid artery
Superior laryngeal artery
Superior thyroid artery
Vagus nerve
Omohyoid muscle
Common carotid artery
Ansa cervicalis
Inferior thyroid artery
Ascending cervical artery
Thyroid gland
Vertebral artery
Phrenic nerve
Thyrocervical trunk
Subclavian artery
Internal thoracic artery
Internal jugular vein
Left brachiocephalic vein
External jugular vein
Axillary vein
Pectoralis major muscle
Cephalic vein
Pectoralis minor muscle
Thoracoacromial artery
Axillary artery
Brachial plexus
Deltoid muscle
Suprascapular artery
Dorsal scapular artery
7th cervical nerve
Transverse cervical artery
6th cervical nerve
5th cervical nerve
Splenius capitis muscle
Occipital artery
Occipital artery
Sternocleidomastoid muscle
Spinal accessory nerve (XI)
Internal jugular vein
Retromandibular vein

FIGURE 533 Nerves and Blood Vessels of the Neck, Stage 5: Subclavian Artery

NOTE: (1) With the internal and external jugular veins removed, the subclavian artery is exposed as it ascends from the thorax and loops within the subclavian triangle of the neck to descend beneath the clavicle into the axilla. Observe its **vertebral, thyrocervical,** and **internal thoracic** branches.

(2) The **transverse cervical artery** is a branch of the thyrocervical trunk from the subclavian.

(3) The **vagus nerve** coursing with the internal and common carotid arteries, and the **phrenic nerve** descending in the neck along the surface of the anterior scalene muscle.

(4) The **superior thyroid, facial,** and **occipital** branches of the external carotid artery. The occipital artery courses posteriorly, deep to the sterno-cleidomastoid and splenius capitis muscles, and it becomes superficial on the posterior aspect of the scalp.

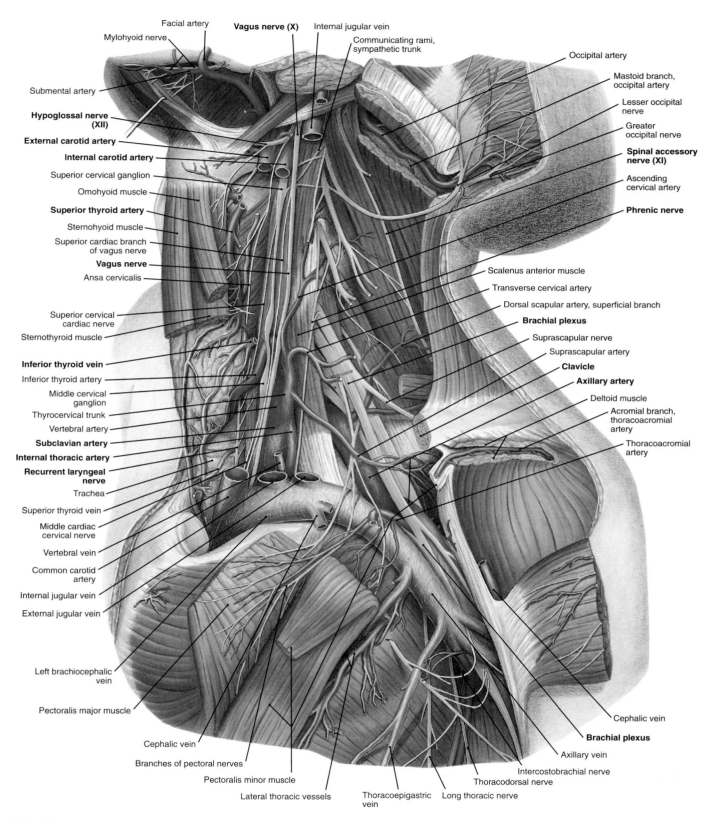

Facial artery
Mylohyoid nerve
Vagus nerve (X)
Internal jugular vein
Communicating rami, sympathetic trunk
Occipital artery
Mastoid branch, occipital artery
Submental artery
Lesser occipital nerve
Hypoglossal nerve (XII)
Greater occipital nerve
External carotid artery
Spinal accessory nerve (XI)
Internal carotid artery
Superior cervical ganglion
Ascending cervical artery
Omohyoid muscle
Phrenic nerve
Superior thyroid artery
Sternohyoid muscle
Superior cardiac branch of vagus nerve
Scalenus anterior muscle
Vagus nerve
Transverse cervical artery
Ansa cervicalis
Dorsal scapular artery, superficial branch
Brachial plexus
Superior cervical cardiac nerve
Suprascapular nerve
Sternothyroid muscle
Suprascapular artery
Inferior thyroid vein
Clavicle
Inferior thyroid artery
Axillary artery
Middle cervical ganglion
Deltoid muscle
Thyrocervical trunk
Acromial branch, thoracoacromial artery
Vertebral artery
Subclavian artery
Thoracoacromial artery
Internal thoracic artery
Recurrent laryngeal nerve
Trachea
Superior thyroid vein
Middle cardiac cervical nerve
Vertebral vein
Common carotid artery
Internal jugular vein
External jugular vein
Left brachiocephalic vein
Pectoralis major muscle
Cephalic vein
Cephalic vein
Brachial plexus
Branches of pectoral nerves
Axillary vein
Intercostobrachial nerve
Pectoralis minor muscle
Thoracodorsal nerve
Lateral thoracic vessels
Thoracoepigastric vein
Long thoracic nerve

FIGURE 534 **Nerves and Blood Vessels of the Neck, Stage 6: Brachial Plexus**

NOTE: (1) With the carotid arteries, jugular veins, and clavicle removed, the roots and trunks of the **brachial plexus** are exposed as they divide into cords that surround the axillary artery in the axilla.

(2) The **sympathetic trunk** lying deep to the carotid arteries and coursing with the vagus nerve and the superior cardiac branch of the vagus nerve.

(3) The **thyroid gland, superior** and **inferior thyroid arteries,** and the **thyroid veins.** Also note the proximity of the **recurrent laryngeal nerve** to the thyroid gland.

PLATE 535 Neck: Jugular System of Veins

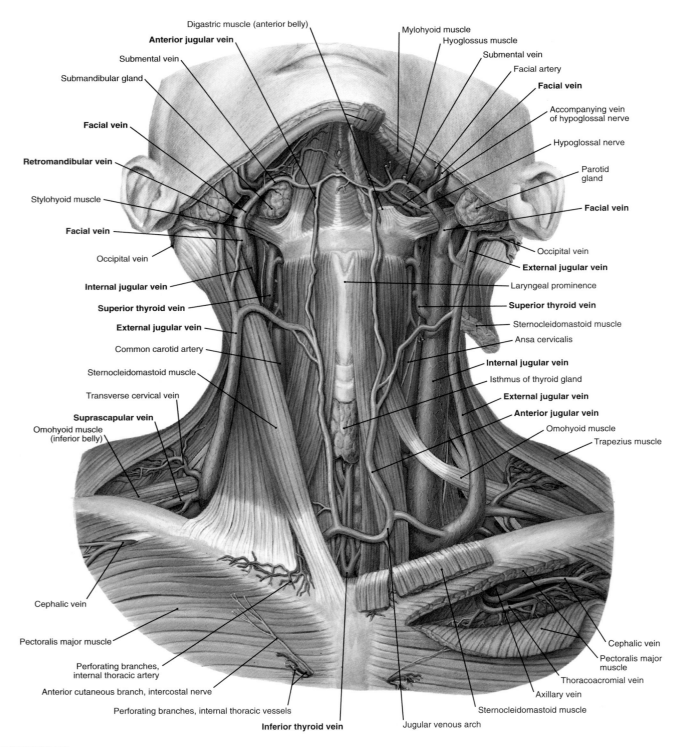

Digastric muscle (anterior belly)
Anterior jugular vein
Submental vein
Submandibular gland
Facial vein
Retromandibular vein
Stylohyoid muscle
Facial vein
Occipital vein
Internal jugular vein
Superior thyroid vein
External jugular vein
Common carotid artery
Sternocleidomastoid muscle
Transverse cervical vein
Suprascapular vein
Omohyoid muscle
(inferior belly)
Cephalic vein
Pectoralis major muscle
Perforating branches,
internal thoracic artery
Anterior cutaneous branch, intercostal nerve
Perforating branches, internal thoracic vessels
Inferior thyroid vein

Mylohyoid muscle
Hyoglossus muscle
Submental vein
Facial artery
Facial vein
Accompanying vein
of hypoglossal nerve
Hypoglossal nerve
Parotid
gland
Facial vein
Occipital vein
External jugular vein
Laryngeal prominence
Superior thyroid vein
Sternocleidomastoid muscle
Ansa cervicalis
Internal jugular vein
Isthmus of thyroid gland
External jugular vein
Anterior jugular vein
Omohyoid muscle
Trapezius muscle
Cephalic vein
Pectoralis major
muscle
Thoracoacromial vein
Axillary vein
Sternocleidomastoid muscle
Jugular venous arch

FIGURE 535 **Veins of the Neck and Infraclavicular Region**

NOTE: (1) The **jugular system of veins** consists of anterior, external, and internal jugular veins, all shown on the left side, where the sternocleido-mastoid muscle was removed.

(2) The **anterior jugular** descends close to the midline, is frequently small, and drains laterally into the external jugular. The **external jugular** courses along the surface of the sternocleidomastoid muscle. It forms within the parotid gland and enlarges because of its occipital, retroman-dibular, and posterior auricular tributaries. The external jugular flows into the subclavian vein after it receives tributaries from the scapular and clavicular regions.

(3) The **internal jugular** is large and collects blood from the brain, face, and neck. At its junction with the subclavian, the **brachiocephalic vein** is formed.

Chapter 7 The Neck and Head

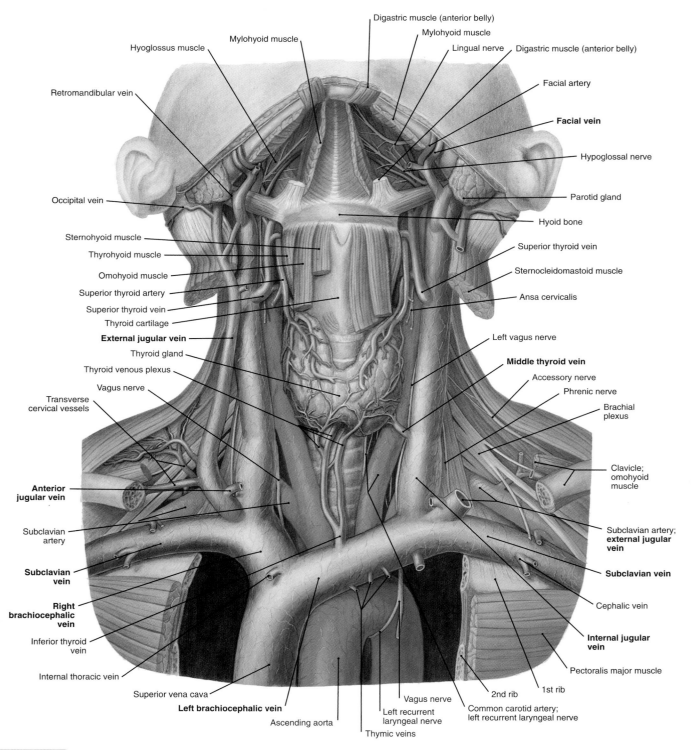

Digastric muscle (anterior belly)
Mylohyoid muscle
Mylohyoid muscle
Lingual nerve
Digastric muscle (anterior belly)
Hyoglossus muscle
Facial artery
Retromandibular vein
Facial vein
Hypoglossal nerve
Occipital vein
Parotid gland
Hyoid bone
Sternohyoid muscle
Superior thyroid vein
Thyrohyoid muscle
Sternocleidomastoid muscle
Omohyoid muscle
Superior thyroid artery
Ansa cervicalis
Superior thyroid vein
Thyroid cartilage
Left vagus nerve
External jugular vein
Thyroid gland
Middle thyroid vein
Thyroid venous plexus
Accessory nerve
Vagus nerve
Phrenic nerve
Transverse cervical vessels
Brachial plexus
Anterior jugular vein
Clavicle; omohyoid muscle
Subclavian artery
Subclavian artery; **external jugular vein**
Subclavian vein
Subclavian vein
Right brachiocephalic vein
Cephalic vein
Inferior thyroid vein
Internal jugular vein
Internal thoracic vein
Pectoralis major muscle
Superior vena cava
2nd rib
1st rib
Left brachiocephalic vein
Vagus nerve
Common carotid artery; left recurrent laryngeal nerve
Ascending aorta
Left recurrent laryngeal nerve
Thymic veins

FIGURE 536 **Deep Arteries and Veins of the Neck and Great Vessels of the Thorax**

NOTE: (1) The sternocleidomastoid and strap muscles have been removed from the neck, thereby exposing the carotid arteries, internal jugular veins, and thyroid gland.
(2) The middle portion of the anterior thoracic wall has been resected to show the aortic arch and its branches, the brachiocephalic veins and their tributaries, the superior vena cava and the vagus nerves.
(3) In the submandibular region, the mylohyoid and anterior digastric muscles have been cut, revealing the lingual and hypoglossal nerves.

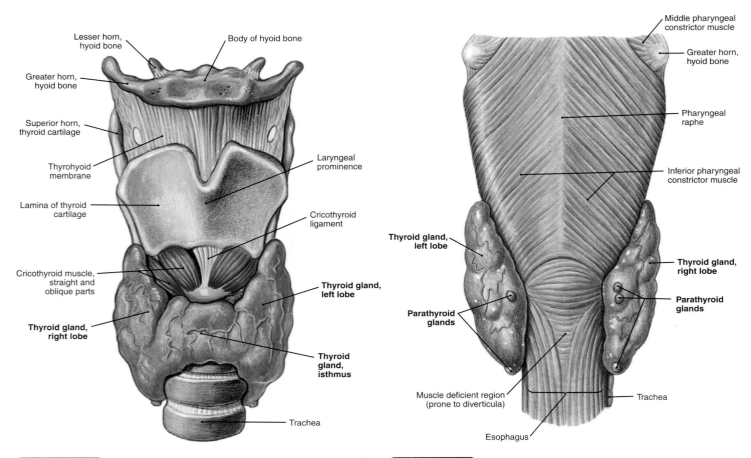

FIGURE 537.1 Ventral View of Thyroid Gland Showing Relation to Larynx and Trachea

FIGURE 537.2 Dorsal View of Thyroid Gland Showing Relation to Pharynx and Parathyroids

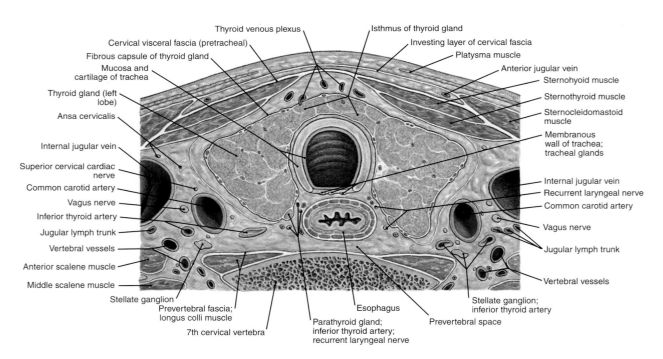

FIGURE 537.3 Cross Section of the Anterior Neck at the Level of the C7 Vertebra

NOTE: Observe the relationship of the isthmus and lobes of the thyroid gland to the trachea. Also observe the location of the parathyroid glands, the recurrent laryngeal nerves, and the inferior thyroid arteries along the posteromedial border of the thyroid gland.

FIGURE 538.1 Scintiscan of the Thyroid Gland ▶

NOTE: (1) A scintiscan (scintigram, scintigraph, or gamma image) is the visual representation of the distribution in an entire body (whole-body scan) or in an organ of a gamma-emitting radioactive substance as detected by a scintillation scanner or gamma camera.

(2) Radioactive iodine (^{123}I) and technetium-99m (^{99m}Tc) have excellent properties for imaging the thyroid gland, and the latter radionuclide was used to obtain this image 35 minutes after injection.

(3) This technique is used to detect thyroid nodules and tumors of thyroid glandular tissue in the bed of the thyroid and throughout the body as a follow-up technique after the removal of a thyroid cancer.

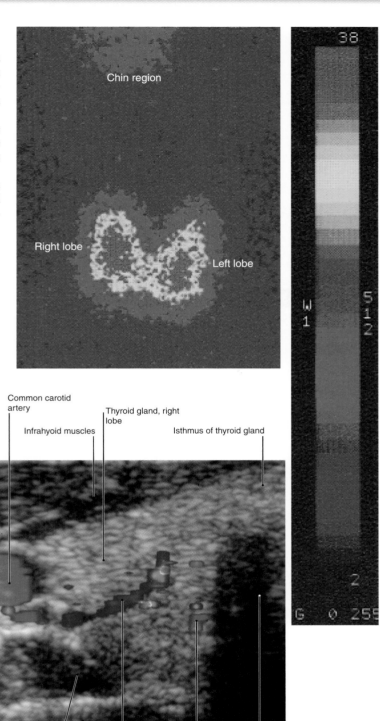

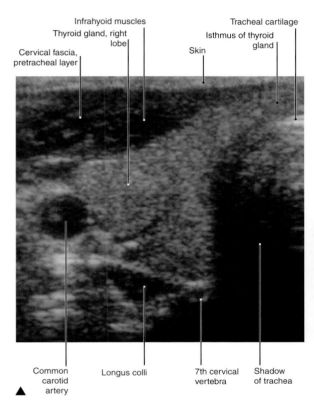

FIGURE 538.2 Ultrasound Scan of the Thyroid Gland

NOTE: This is a horizontal ultrasound scan with the sound being administered in a ventrodorsal direction.

FIGURE 538.3 Ultrasound Scan of the Thyroid Gland

NOTE: This scan shows the direction of blood flow (color flow Doppler sonogram).

Red = toward the transducer (arteries)
Blue = away from the transducer (veins)

◀

FIGURE 538.4 Enlarged Thyroid (often called Graves' disease)

NOTE that common symptoms of Graves' disease include goiter (seen here), fine tremor, increased nervousness and emotional instability, intolerance to heat, increased sweating, loss of weight, and diminished strength. (From Harrison, T.R., and Isselbacher, K.J. *Harrison's Principles of Internal Medicine*, 9th Edition. New York: McGraw-Hill, 1980.)

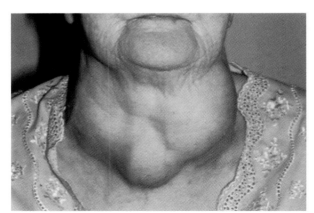

PLATE 539 Patterns of Lymph Drainage (Adult) and Chains of Nodes (Child)

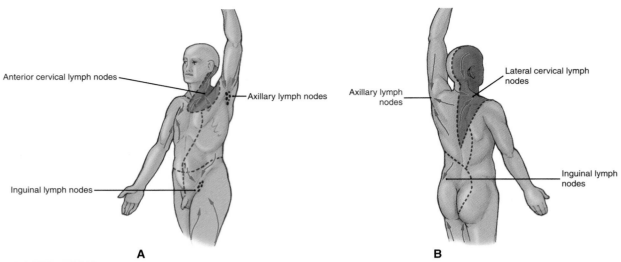

FIGURE 539.1A and B Drainage Patterns of Lymph Nodes on the Anterior (A) and Posterior (B) Aspects of the Body

Anterior cervical lymph nodes

Axillary lymph nodes

Inguinal lymph nodes

Lateral cervical lymph nodes

Axillary lymph nodes

Inguinal lymph nodes

A

B

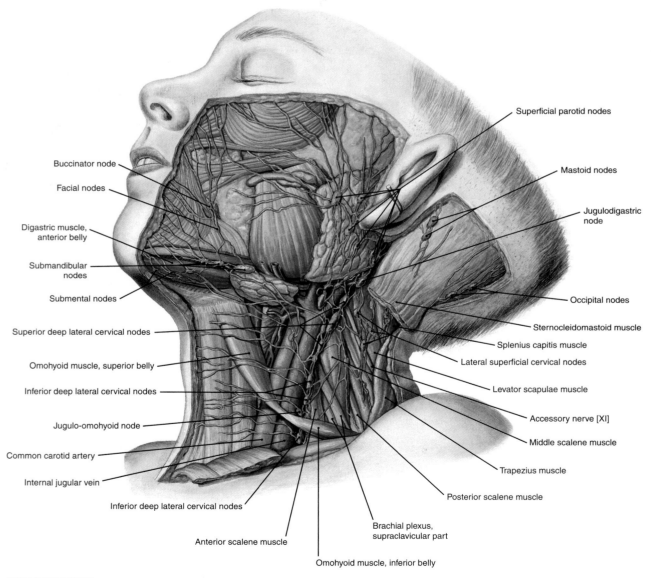

FIGURE 539.2 Superficial Nodes of the Face and Neck in an 8-Year-Old Boy

NOTE: The platysma muscle has been removed and the sternocleidomastoid muscle has been sectioned.

Buccinator node
Facial nodes
Digastric muscle, anterior belly
Submandibular nodes
Submental nodes
Superior deep lateral cervical nodes
Omohyoid muscle, superior belly
Inferior deep lateral cervical nodes
Jugulo-omohyoid node
Common carotid artery
Internal jugular vein
Inferior deep lateral cervical nodes
Anterior scalene muscle
Omohyoid muscle, inferior belly
Brachial plexus, supraclavicular part
Posterior scalene muscle
Trapezius muscle
Middle scalene muscle
Accessory nerve [XI]
Levator scapulae muscle
Lateral superficial cervical nodes
Splenius capitis muscle
Sternocleidomastoid muscle
Occipital nodes
Jugulodigastric node
Mastoid nodes
Superficial parotid nodes

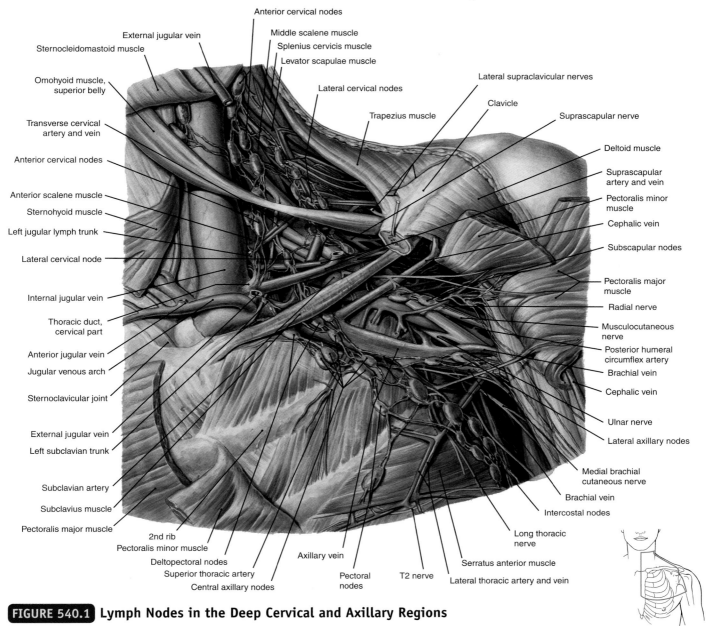

Anterior cervical nodes
External jugular vein
Sternocleidomastoid muscle
Middle scalene muscle
Splenius cervicis muscle
Levator scapulae muscle
Omohyoid muscle, superior belly
Lateral cervical nodes
Lateral supraclavicular nerves
Transverse cervical artery and vein
Trapezius muscle
Clavicle
Suprascapular nerve
Anterior cervical nodes
Deltoid muscle
Anterior scalene muscle
Suprascapular artery and vein
Sternohyoid muscle
Pectoralis minor muscle
Left jugular lymph trunk
Cephalic vein
Lateral cervical node
Subscapular nodes
Internal jugular vein
Pectoralis major muscle
Thoracic duct, cervical part
Radial nerve
Musculocutaneous nerve
Anterior jugular vein
Posterior humeral circumflex artery
Jugular venous arch
Brachial vein
Sternoclavicular joint
Cephalic vein
External jugular vein
Ulnar nerve
Left subclavian trunk
Lateral axillary nodes
Medial brachial cutaneous nerve
Subclavian artery
Brachial vein
Subclavius muscle
Intercostal nodes
Pectoralis major muscle
2nd rib
Long thoracic nerve
Pectoralis minor muscle
Serratus anterior muscle
Deltopectoral nodes
Axillary vein
Superior thoracic artery
Pectoral nodes
T2 nerve
Lateral thoracic artery and vein
Central axillary nodes

FIGURE 540.1 **Lymph Nodes in the Deep Cervical and Axillary Regions**

NOTE: Most of the clavicle and pectoralis muscles have been removed.

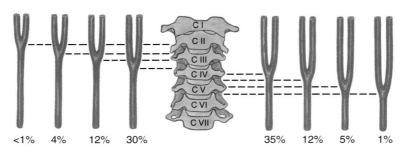

C I
C II
C III
C IV
C V
C VI
C VII

<1%   4%   12%   30%   35%   12%   5%   1%

FIGURE 540.2 **Variations in the Vertebral Level for the Bifurcation of the Common Carotid Artery**

PLATE 541 Neck: Anterior Vertebral Muscles

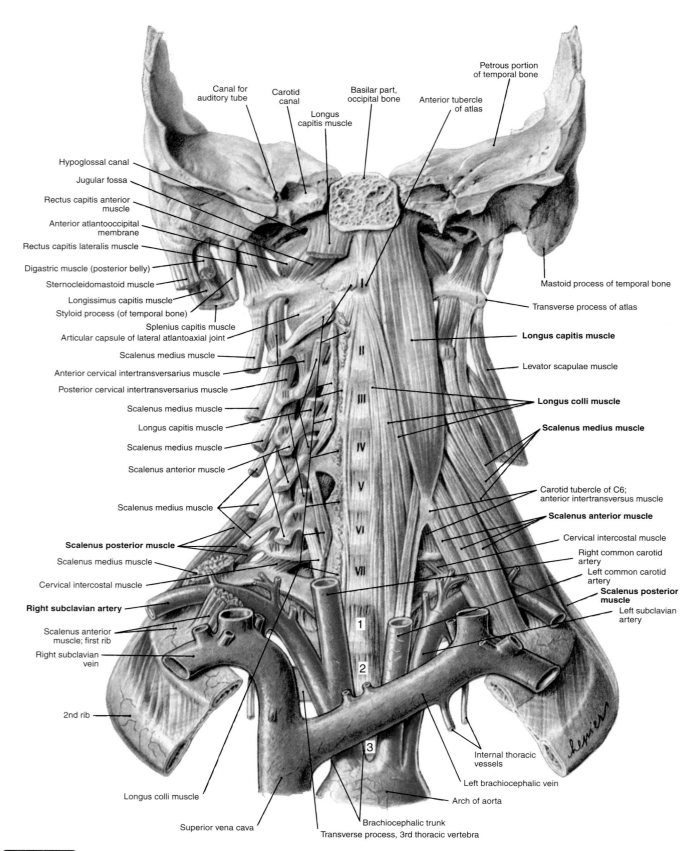

Canal for auditory tube

Carotid canal

Basilar part, occipital bone

Longus capitis muscle

Petrous portion of temporal bone

Anterior tubercle of atlas

Hypoglossal canal

Jugular fossa

Rectus capitis anterior muscle

Anterior atlantooccipital membrane

Rectus capitis lateralis muscle

Digastric muscle (posterior belly)

Sternocleidomastoid muscle

Longissimus capitis muscle

Styloid process (of temporal bone)

Splenius capitis muscle

Articular capsule of lateral atlantoaxial joint

Scalenus medius muscle

Anterior cervical intertransversarius muscle

Posterior cervical intertransversarius muscle

Scalenus medius muscle

Longus capitis muscle

Scalenus medius muscle

Scalenus anterior muscle

Scalenus medius muscle

Scalenus posterior muscle

Scalenus medius muscle

Cervical intercostal muscle

Right subclavian artery

Scalenus anterior muscle; first rib

Right subclavian vein

2nd rib

Longus colli muscle

Superior vena cava

Mastoid process of temporal bone

Transverse process of atlas

Longus capitis muscle

Levator scapulae muscle

Longus colli muscle

Scalenus medius muscle

Carotid tubercle of C6; anterior intertransversus muscle

Scalenus anterior muscle

Cervical intercostal muscle

Right common carotid artery

Left common carotid artery

Scalenus posterior muscle

Left subclavian artery

Internal thoracic vessels

Left brachiocephalic vein

Arch of aorta

Brachiocephalic trunk

Transverse process, 3rd thoracic vertebra

FIGURE 541 **Prevertebral Region and Root of the Neck (Anterior View)**

NOTE: (1) On the specimen's right, the longus colli, longus capitis, and scalene muscles have been removed, exposing the transverse processes of the cervical vertebrae onto which these muscles are seen to attach.

(2) There are two long (longus colli and longus capitis) and two short (rectus capitis anterior and lateralis) prevertebral muscles. These flex the head and neck forward and bend the head and neck laterally.

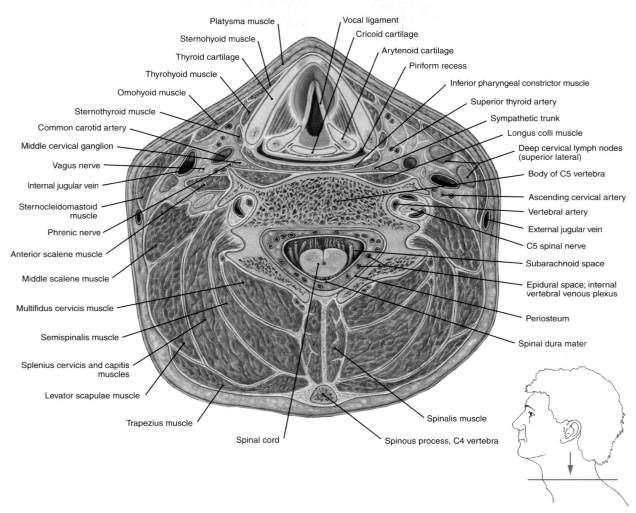

FIGURE 542 Cross Section of the Neck at the C5 Vertebral Level

ANTERIOR VERTEBRAL MUSCLES				
Muscle	Origin	Insertion	Innervation	Action
SUPERIOR OBLIQUE PART				
Longus colli	Anterior tubercles of transverse processes of third, fourth, and fifth cervical vertebrae	Tubercle of the anterior arch of the atlas	Ventral rami of the C2 to C6 spinal nerves	
INFERIOR OBLIQUE PART				
	Anterior surface of the bodies of the first two or three thoracic vertebrae	Anterior tubercles of the transverse processes of the fifth and sixth cervical vertebrae		Weak flexor of the neck; slightly rotates and bends neck laterally
VERTICAL PART				
	Anterolateral surfaces of the last three cervical and upper three thoracic vertebrae	Anterior surfaces of the bodies of second, third, and fourth cervical vertebrae		
Longus capitis	By tendinous slips from the transverse processes of the third, fourth, fifth, and sixth cervical vertebrae	Inferior surface of the basilar part of the occipital bone	Branches from the anterior rami of C1, C2, and C3 nerves	Flexes the head and the upper cervical spine
Rectus capitis anterior	Anterior surface of the lateral mass of the atlas and its transverse process	Inferior surface of the basilar part of the occipital bone	Fibers from the anterior rami of C1 and C2	Flexes the head and helps stabilize the atlantooccipital joint
Rectus capitis lateralis	Superior surface of the transverse process of the atlas	Inferior surface of the jugular process of the occipital bone	Anterior rami of the C1 and C2 nerves	Bends the head laterally to the same side

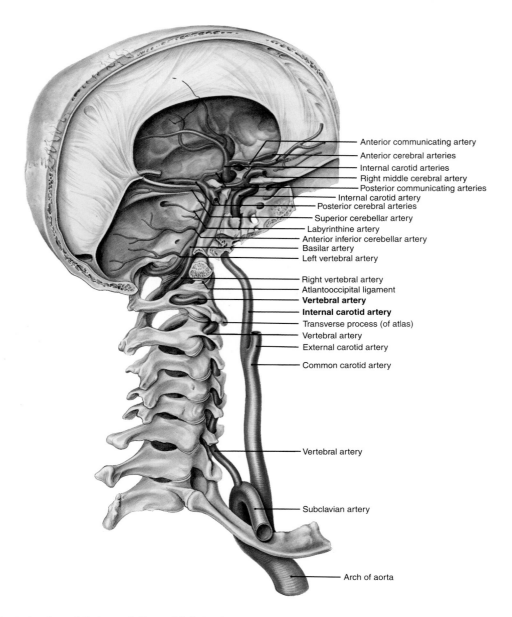

Anterior communicating artery
Anterior cerebral arteries
Internal carotid arteries
Right middle cerebral artery
Posterior communicating arteries
Internal carotid artery
Posterior cerebral arteries
Superior cerebellar artery
Labyrinthine artery
Anterior inferior cerebellar artery
Basilar artery
Left vertebral artery

Right vertebral artery
Atlantooccipital ligament
Vertebral artery
Internal carotid artery
Transverse process (of atlas)
Vertebral artery
External carotid artery

Common carotid artery

Vertebral artery

Subclavian artery

Arch of aorta

FIGURE 543.1 Vertebral and Internal Carotid Arteries

NOTE: (1) Both the internal carotid and the vertebral arteries ascend in the neck to enter the cranial cavity to supply blood to the brain. Although the vertebral arteries give off some spinal and muscular branches in the neck prior to entering the skull, the internal carotid arteries do not have branches in the neck.

(2) The origin of the **vertebral artery** from the subclavian ascends in the neck through the foramina in the transverse processes of the cervical vertebrae.

(3) The two vertebral arteries join to form the **basilar artery**. This vessel courses along the ventral aspect of the brainstem.

(4) The **internal carotid artery** begins at the bifurcation of the common carotid and ascends to its entrance in the carotid canal in the petrous part of the temporal bone. After a somewhat tortuous course, it enters the cranial cavity.

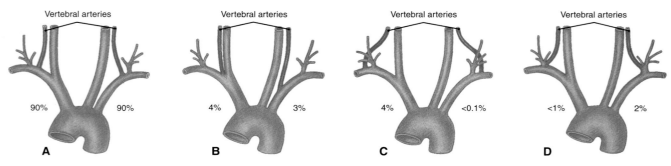

Vertebral arteries   Vertebral arteries   Vertebral arteries   Vertebral arteries

90%   90%   4%   3%   4%   <0.1%   <1%   2%

A   B   C   D

FIGURE 543.2 Variations (and Percentages) in the Origin of the Vertebral Arteries

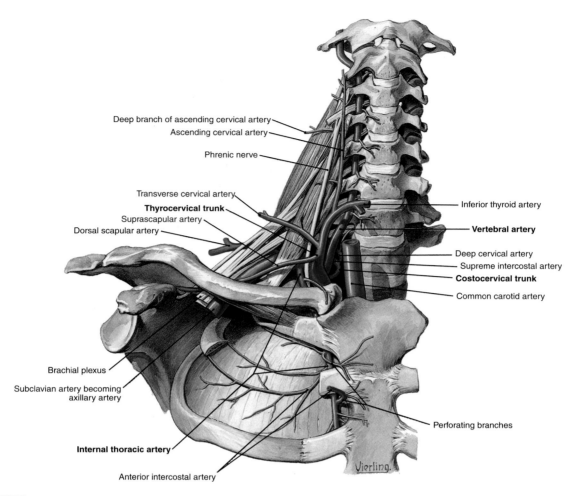

Deep branch of ascending cervical artery
Ascending cervical artery
Phrenic nerve
Transverse cervical artery
Thyrocervical trunk
Suprascapular artery
Dorsal scapular artery
Brachial plexus
Subclavian artery becoming axillary artery
Internal thoracic artery
Anterior intercostal artery
Inferior thyroid artery
Vertebral artery
Deep cervical artery
Supreme intercostal artery
Costocervical trunk
Common carotid artery
Perforating branches

FIGURE 544.1 **Right Subclavian Artery and Its Branches**

NOTE: (1) The right subclavian artery arises from the brachiocephalic trunk, although on the left it branches from the aorta. It ascends into the root of the neck, arches laterally, and then descends between the first rib and clavicle to become the axillary artery.

(2) The subclavian artery generally has four major branches and sometimes five. These are the **vertebral artery,** the **internal thoracic artery,** the **thyrocervical trunk,** and the **costocervical trunk**.

(3) In about 40% of bodies, there is also a **dorsal scapular artery** arising directly from the subclavian. Thus, in this region there is considerable variation in the origin of vessels such as the suprascapular artery, the transverse cervical artery, and this latter vessel's superficial and deep branches, the superficial cervical artery and the descending scapular artery. (For a complete description of these vessels see: Clemente CD, ed. *Gray's Anatomy of the Human Body,* 30th Edition, Lea & Febiger, Philadelphia, 1985:703–709.)

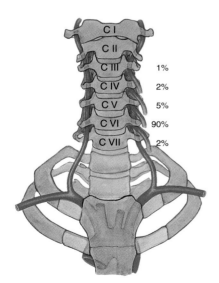

C I
C II
C III — 1%
C IV — 2%
C V — 5%
C VI — 90%
C VII — 2%

◀ **FIGURE 544.2** **Variations in the Level of Entry of the Vertebral Artery into the Transverse Foramina of Cervical Vertebrae**

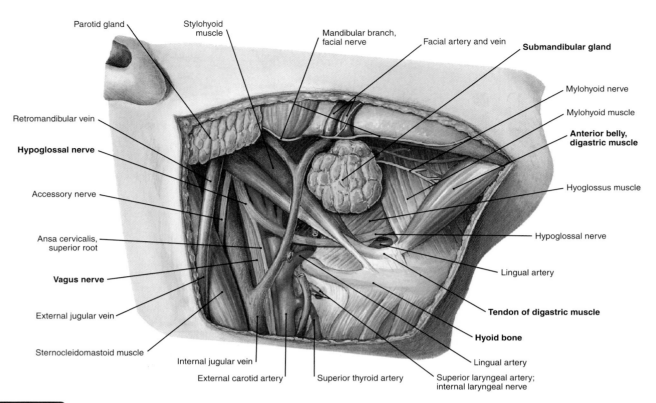

Parotid gland
Stylohyoid muscle
Mandibular branch, facial nerve
Facial artery and vein
Submandibular gland
Mylohyoid nerve
Mylohyoid muscle
Anterior belly, digastric muscle
Retromandibular vein
Hypoglossal nerve
Hyoglossus muscle
Accessory nerve
Hypoglossal nerve
Lingual artery
Ansa cervicalis, superior root
Vagus nerve
Tendon of digastric muscle
External jugular vein
Hyoid bone
Sternocleidomastoid muscle
Lingual artery
Internal jugular vein
External carotid artery
Superior thyroid artery
Superior laryngeal artery; internal laryngeal nerve

FIGURE 545.1 **Right Submandibular Triangle and Submandibular Gland**

NOTE: The **submandibular triangle** is bounded by the two bellies of the digastric muscle and by the lower border of the mandible. The floor of the triangle is formed by the mylohyoid and hyoglossus muscles, between which the **hypoglossal nerve** enters the oral cavity.

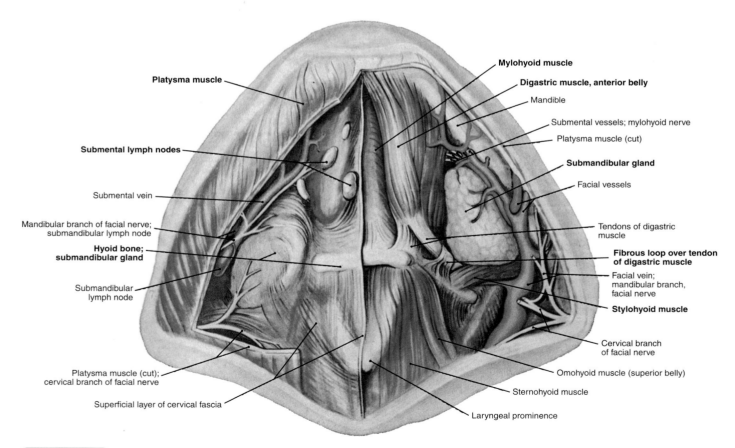

Platysma muscle
Mylohyoid muscle
Digastric muscle, anterior belly
Mandible
Submental vessels; mylohyoid nerve
Platysma muscle (cut)
Submental lymph nodes
Submandibular gland
Facial vessels
Submental vein
Mandibular branch of facial nerve; submandibular lymph node
Tendons of digastric muscle
Hyoid bone; submandibular gland
Fibrous loop over tendon of digastric muscle
Facial vein; mandibular branch, facial nerve
Submandibular lymph node
Stylohyoid muscle
Platysma muscle (cut); cervical branch of facial nerve
Cervical branch of facial nerve
Omohyoid muscle (superior belly)
Superficial layer of cervical fascia
Sternohyoid muscle
Laryngeal prominence

FIGURE 545.2 **Submandibular and Submental Regions (Dissection Stages 1 and 2)**

NOTE: In dissection **Stage 1** (reader's left), the superficial fascia with the platysma has been opened, showing the submandibular gland and lymph nodes. In dissection **Stage 2** (reader's right), the superficial layer of cervical fascia has been opened, showing the digastric, mylohyoid, and stylohyoid muscles.

Chapter 7 The Neck and Head

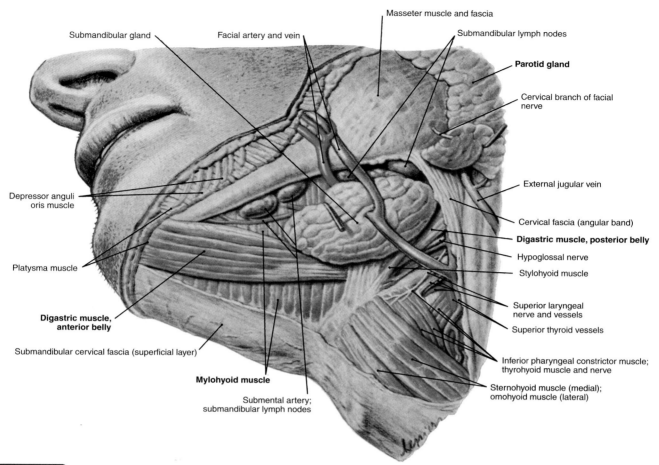

FIGURE 546.1 **Left Submandibular Triangle and Submandibular Gland (Viewed from Below)**

NOTE: Crossing the submandibular triangle are the **anterior facial vein** and the **facial artery**. Also observe the **submandibular** and **parotid glands** and the **submandibular lymph nodes**.

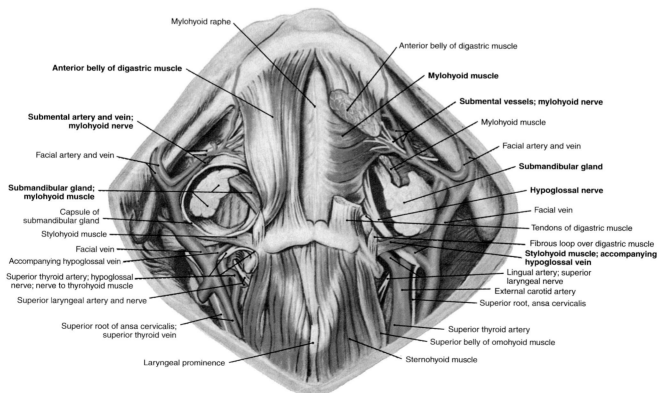

FIGURE 546.2 **Submandibular and Submental Regions (Dissection Stages 3 and 4)**

NOTE: In dissection **Stage 3** (reader's left), much of the submandibular gland has been removed, revealing the **submental nerve** and the **mylohyoid nerve**. In **Stage 4** (reader's right), the anterior digastric nerve and part of the mylohyoid nerve were removed, exposing the **hypoglossal nerve** and **accompanying vein**.

PLATE 547 Face: Superficial Muscles (Anterior View)

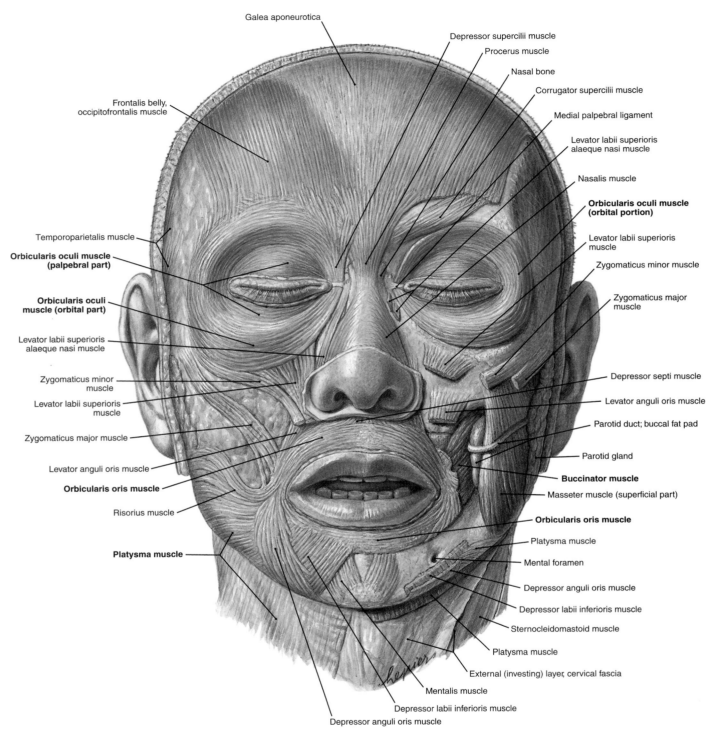

Galea aponeurotica

Depressor supercilii muscle

Procerus muscle

Nasal bone

Corrugator supercilii muscle

Medial palpebral ligament

Levator labii superioris alaeque nasi muscle

Nasalis muscle

Orbicularis oculi muscle (orbital portion)

Levator labii superioris muscle

Zygomaticus minor muscle

Zygomaticus major muscle

Depressor septi muscle

Levator anguli oris muscle

Parotid duct; buccal fat pad

Parotid gland

Buccinator muscle

Masseter muscle (superficial part)

Orbicularis oris muscle

Platysma muscle

Mental foramen

Depressor anguli oris muscle

Depressor labii inferioris muscle

Sternocleidomastoid muscle

Platysma muscle

External (investing) layer, cervical fascia

Frontalis belly, occipitofrontalis muscle

Temporoparietalis muscle

Orbicularis oculi muscle (palpebral part)

Orbicularis oculi muscle (orbital part)

Levator labii superioris alaeque nasi muscle

Zygomaticus minor muscle

Levator labii superioris muscle

Zygomaticus major muscle

Levator anguli oris muscle

Orbicularis oris muscle

Risorius muscle

Platysma muscle

Mentalis muscle

Depressor labii inferioris muscle

Depressor anguli oris muscle

FIGURE 547 Muscles of Facial Expression (Anterior View)

NOTE: (1) The muscles of facial expression are located within the layers of superficial fascia. Having developed from the mesoderm of the **second branchial arch**, they are innervated by the nerve of that arch, the seventh cranial or **facial nerve**.

(2) Facial muscles may be grouped into: (a) muscles of the **scalp**, (b) muscles of the **external ear**, (c) muscles of the **eyelid**, (d) the **nasal muscles**, and (e) the **oral muscles**. The borders of some facial muscles are not easily defined. The **platysma muscle** also belongs to the facial group, although it extends over the neck.

(3) The circular muscles surrounding the eyes (**orbicularis oculi**) and the mouth (**orbicularis oris**) assist in closure of the orbital and oral apertures and thus contribute to functions such as closing the eyes and the ingestion of liquids and food.

(4) Since facial muscles respond to thoughts and emotions, they aid in communication.

(5) The **buccinator muscles** are flat and are situated on the lateral aspects of the oral cavity. They assist in mastication by pressing the cheeks against the teeth, preventing food from accumulating in the oral vestibule.

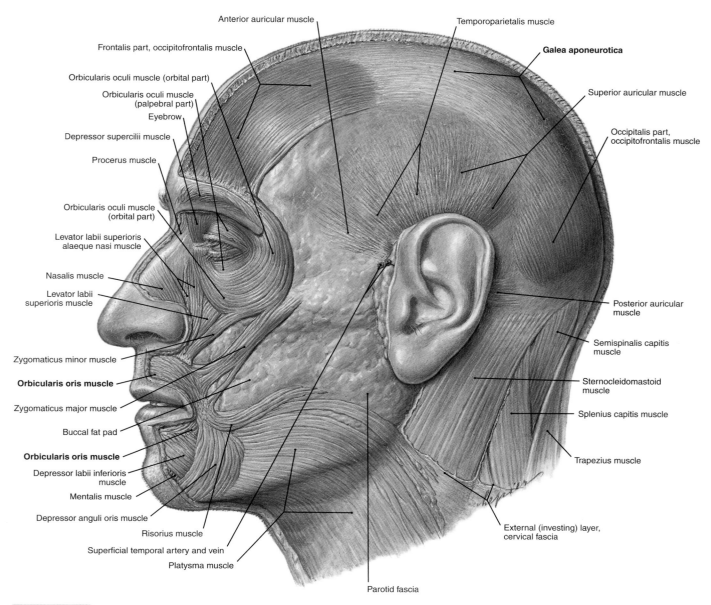

Anterior auricular muscle

Frontalis part, occipitofrontalis muscle

Orbicularis oculi muscle (orbital part)

Orbicularis oculi muscle (palpebral part)

Eyebrow

Depressor supercilii muscle

Procerus muscle

Orbicularis oculi muscle (orbital part)

Levator labii superioris alaeque nasi muscle

Nasalis muscle

Levator labii superioris muscle

Zygomaticus minor muscle

Orbicularis oris muscle

Zygomaticus major muscle

Buccal fat pad

Orbicularis oris muscle

Depressor labii inferioris muscle

Mentalis muscle

Depressor anguli oris muscle

Risorius muscle

Superficial temporal artery and vein

Platysma muscle

Parotid fascia

Temporoparietalis muscle

Galea aponeurotica

Superior auricular muscle

Occipitalis part, occipitofrontalis muscle

Posterior auricular muscle

Semispinalis capitis muscle

Sternocleidomastoid muscle

Splenius capitis muscle

Trapezius muscle

External (investing) layer, cervical fascia

FIGURE 548.1 Muscles of Facial Expression and the Superficial Posterior Cervical Muscles

NOTE: (1) The **frontalis** and **occipitalis** portions of the occipitofrontalis muscle are continuous with an epicranial aponeurosis called the **galea aponeurotica**.

(2) The **orbicularis oculi** consists of orbital, palpebral, and lacrimal (not shown) portions.

(3) Into the **orbicularis oris** merge a number of facial muscles in a somewhat radial manner.

Temporal branches

Zygomatic branches

Parotid plexus

Posterior auricular branch

Facial nerve

Buccal branches

Mandibular branch

Cervical branch

FIGURE 548.2 Branches of the Facial Nerve Supplying ▶ the Superficial Facial Muscles

NOTE: All the muscles of facial expression are innervated by branches of the seventh cranial nerve, the **facial nerve.** These branches are the **temporal, zygomatic, buccal, mandibular, cervical,** and **posterior auricular nerves.**

Chapter 7 The Neck and Head

SUPRAHYOID MUSCLES

Muscle	Origin	Insertion	Innervation	Action
Digastric	Anterior belly: Digastric fossa on inner aspect of lower border of mandible Posterior belly: Mastoid notch of the temporal bone	Ends by an intermediate tendon between the two bellies that attaches to the hyoid bone	Anterior belly: Mylohyoid branch of trigeminal nerve (V) Posterior belly: Digastric branch of the facial nerve (VII)	Opens the mouth by depressing the mandible; elevates the hyoid bone
Stylohyoid	Posterior and lateral surface of styloid process of temporal bone	Body of the hyoid bone near the greater horn	Stylohyoid branch of the facial nerve (VII)	Elevates, fixes, and retracts the hyoid bone
Mylohyoid The two mylohyoid muscles form the floor of the oral cavity	Entire length of the mylohyoid line of the mandible	Posterior fibers: Into body of the hyoid bone Middle and anterior fibers: The median raphe between the muscles of both sides	Mylohyoid branch of the trigeminal nerve (V)	During swallowing, both muscles raise floor of mouth, elevate the hyoid bone, and depress the mandible in opening the mouth
Geniohyoid	Inferior mental spine on the inner surface of the symphysis menti	Anterior surface of the body of hyoid bone	First cervical nerve carried along the hypoglossal nerve	Elevates and draws hyoid bone forward; when hyoid is fixed, it retracts and depresses mandible

SUPERFICIAL MUSCLES OF THE FACE AND HEAD

MUSCLES OF THE SCALP

Muscle	Origin	Insertion	Innervation	Action
Occipitofrontalis	Occipital belly: Lateral two-thirds of superior nuchal line on occipital bone and mastoid part of temporal bone	Into the galea aponeurotica	Posterior auricular branch of the facial nerve (VII)	Draws scalp back; raises eye brow and wrinkles forehead in expression of surprise
	Frontal belly: Fibers continuous with those of procerus medially and orbicularis oculi laterally	Into the galea aponeurotica	Temporal branch of the facial nerve (VII)	
Temporoparietalis	From temporal fascia above and in front of auricle of ear	Onto the temporal fascia and skin on the side of the head	Temporal branch of the facial nerve (VII)	Tightens the scalp and draws back the skin of the temples

EXTRINSIC MUSCLES OF THE EAR

Muscle	Origin	Insertion	Innervation	Action
Anterior auricular	Anterior part of the temporal fascia	Onto the spine of the helix	Temporal branch of the facial nerve (VII)	Draws auricle of ear forward and upward (minimal action)
Superior auricular	Epicranial aponeurosis on the side of the head	Upper part of the cranial surface of auricle of ear	Temporal branch of the facial nerve (VII)	Draws the auricle of the ear upward (minimal action)
Posterior auricular	Mastoid process of the temporal bone	Medial surface of auricle at convexity of concha	Posterior auricular branch of the facial nerve (VII)	Draws the auricle backward (minimal action)

MUSCLES OF EYELIDS

Muscle	Origin	Insertion	Innervation	Action
Orbicularis oculi: Palpebral part	Medial palpebral ligament	Cross the eyelids and interlace to form the lateral palpebral raphe	Temporal and zygomatic branches of the facial nerve (VII)	Closes the eyelids gently as in sleeping and blinking
Orbital part	Nasal part of frontal bone; frontal process of the maxilla; medial palpebral ligament	Forms ellipse around orbit without being interrupted on the lateral side	Temporal and zygomatic branches of the facial nerve (VII)	Closes the eyelids when a more forceful contraction is necessary, as in winking one eye
Corrugator supercilii	Medial end of the superciliary arch	Deep surface of the skin above the middle of the supraorbital margin	Temporal branch of the facial nerve (VII)	Draws the eyebrow medially and down

SUPERFICIAL MUSCLES OF THE FACE AND HEAD (Continued)

MUSCLES OF THE NOSE

Muscle	Origin	Insertion	Innervation	Action
Procerus	From fascia over the lower part of the nasal bone	Into the skin of the lower part of the forehead between eyebrows	Buccal branch of the facial nerve (VII)	Draws down the medial angle of eyebrow such as in frowning or concentration
Nasalis	Transverse part: From the maxilla lateral to the nasal notch	Ascends to bridge of nose; meshes with opposite insertion	Buccal branch of the facial nerve (VII)	Compresses the nasal aperture
	Alar part: From the maxilla above the lateral incisor tooth	Attaches to the cartilaginous ala of the nose	Buccal branch of the facial nerve (VII)	Assists in opening the nasal aperture in deep inspiration
Depressor septi	From the maxilla above the medial incisor	Into the mobile part of the nasal septum	Buccal branch of the facial nerve (VII)	Assists alar part of nasalis muscle in widening nares

MUSCLES OF THE MOUTH

Muscle	Origin	Insertion	Innervation	Action
Levator labii superioris	Along lower part of orbit from maxilla and zygomatic bones	Upper lip between levators anguli oris and labii superioris alaeque nasi	Buccal branch of the facial nerve (VII)	Raises the upper lip and carries it forward
Levator labii superioris alaeque nasi	Upper part of the frontal process of the maxilla	Inserts by two slips: into alar cartilage and into upper lip with levator labii superioris	Buccal branch of the facial nerve (VII)	Raises the upper lip and dilates the nostril
Levator anguli oris	Canine fossa of the maxilla just below the infraorbital foramen	Into angle of mouth merging with orbicularis oris, depressor anguli oris, and zygomaticus major	Buccal branch of the facial nerve (VII)	Raises the angle of the mouth and forms the nasolabial furrow
Zygomaticus minor	Lateral surface of the zygomatic bone	Upper lip between levator labii superioris and zygomaticus major	Buccal branch of the facial nerve (VII)	Elevates the upper lip and helps form the nasolabial furrow
Zygomaticus major	From the zygomatic bone in front of the zygomatico-temporal suture	Into angle of mouth with levator and depressor anguli oris and orbicularis oris muscles	Buccal branch of the facial nerve (VII)	Draws the angle of the mouth upward and backward as in laughing
Risorius	From parotid fascia over masseter muscle	Into the skin at the angle of the mouth	Buccal branch of the facial nerve (VII)	Retracts the angle of the mouth
Depressor labii inferioris	Oblique line of mandible between symphysis menti and the mental foramen	Into lower lip and at midline blending with muscle from other side	Mandibular branch of the facial nerve (VII)	Draws the lower lip downward and a bit laterally
Depressor anguli oris	From oblique line of mandible, lateral and below depressor labii inferioris	Into the angle of the mouth blending with orbicularis oris and risorius	Mandibular branch of the facial nerve (VII)	Draws angle of mouth down and laterally as in expression of sadness
Mentalis	From the incisive fossa of the mandible	Into the skin of the chin	Mandibular branch of the facial nerve (VII)	Raises and protrudes lower lip; wrinkles chin in expression of doubt or disdain
Orbicularis oris	Fibers derived from other facial muscles (buccinator, levators, and depressors of lips and angles, zygomatic muscles) pass into lips; also some intrinsic muscle fibers make up orbicularis oris	Several strata of muscle fibers form a sphincter-like muscle with fibers that decussate at the angles of the mouth	Buccal branch of the facial nerve (VII)	Closes the lips, and its deep fibers can press the lips against the teeth; also it protrudes the lips and is important in speech
Buccinator	Alveolar processes of mandible and maxilla opposite upper and lower molar teeth; posteriorly, it arises from the pterygomandibular raphe opposite superior constrictor	Fibers course forward to blend into the formation of the orbicularis oris, decussating at the angles of the mouth	Buccal branch of the facial nerve (VII)	Compresses the cheeks during chewing; also compresses the distended cheeks as in blowing a horn

PLATE 551 **Face: Muscles of Mastication; Parotid Gland**

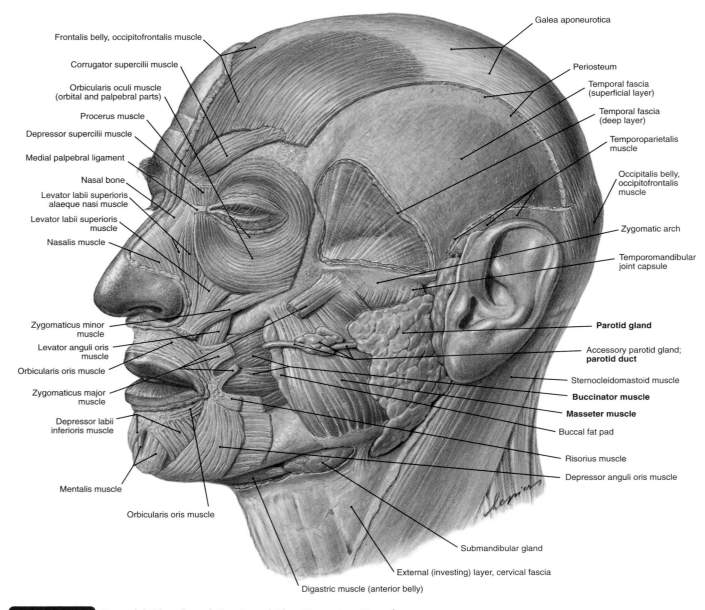

Galea aponeurotica

Frontalis belly, occipitofrontalis muscle

Corrugator supercilii muscle

Orbicularis oculi muscle
(orbital and palpebral parts)

Procerus muscle

Depressor supercilii muscle

Medial palpebral ligament

Nasal bone

Levator labii superioris
alaeque nasi muscle

Levator labii superioris
muscle

Nasalis muscle

Zygomaticus minor
muscle

Levator anguli oris
muscle

Orbicularis oris muscle

Zygomaticus major
muscle

Depressor labii
inferioris muscle

Mentalis muscle

Orbicularis oris muscle

Periosteum

Temporal fascia
(superficial layer)

Temporal fascia
(deep layer)

Temporoparietalis
muscle

Occipitalis belly,
occipitofrontalis
muscle

Zygomatic arch

Temporomandibular
joint capsule

Parotid gland

Accessory parotid gland;
parotid duct

Sternocleidomastoid muscle

Buccinator muscle

Masseter muscle

Buccal fat pad

Risorius muscle

Depressor anguli oris muscle

Submandibular gland

External (investing) layer, cervical fascia

Digastric muscle (anterior belly)

FIGURE 551.1 **Parotid Gland and Duct and the Masseter Muscle**

NOTE: (1) The **parotid gland** extends from the zygomatic arch to below the angle of the mandible. It lies anterior to the ear and superficial to the **masseter muscle**. It is enclosed in a tight fascial sheath, and its duct courses medially across the face to enter the oral cavity through the fibers of the **buccinator muscle**.

(2) The masseter muscle extends from the zygomatic bone to the ramus, angle, and body of the mandible. It elevates the mandible (closes the mouth) and is supplied by the trigeminal nerve.

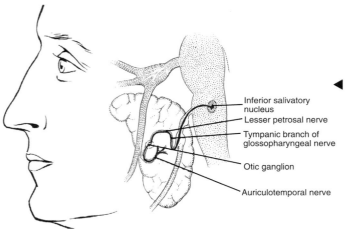

Inferior salivatory
nucleus

Lesser petrosal nerve

Tympanic branch of
glossopharyngeal nerve

Otic ganglion

Auriculotemporal nerve

◄ **FIGURE 551.2** **Parasympathetic Innervation of the Parotid Gland**

NOTE: (1) Preganglionic parasympathetic fibers that innervate the parotid gland emerge from the brainstem in the ninth (glossopharyngeal) nerve.

(2) These fibers then travel along the **tympanic nerve** to the middle ear and then form the **lesser petrosal nerve** that joins the **otic ganglion**.

(3) Postganglionic fibers then travel within the **auriculotemporal nerve** to reach the parotid gland.

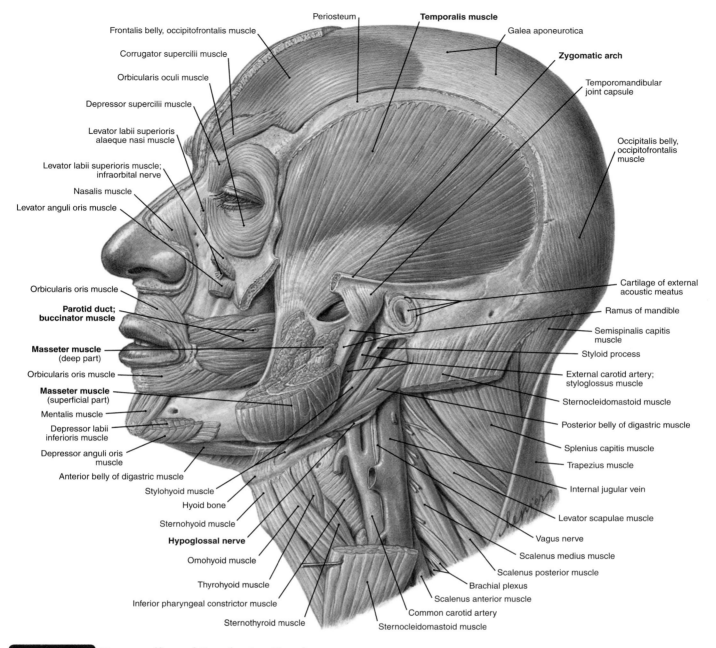

Frontalis belly, occipitofrontalis muscle

Corrugator supercilii muscle

Orbicularis oculi muscle

Depressor supercilii muscle

Levator labii superioris alaeque nasi muscle

Levator labii superioris muscle; infraorbital nerve

Nasalis muscle

Levator anguli oris muscle

Orbicularis oris muscle

Parotid duct; buccinator muscle

Masseter muscle (deep part)

Orbicularis oris muscle

Masseter muscle (superficial part)

Mentalis muscle

Depressor labii inferioris muscle

Depressor anguli oris muscle

Anterior belly of digastric muscle

Stylohyoid muscle

Hyoid bone

Sternohyoid muscle

Hypoglossal nerve

Omohyoid muscle

Thyrohyoid muscle

Inferior pharyngeal constrictor muscle

Sternothyroid muscle

Periosteum

Temporalis muscle

Galea aponeurotica

Zygomatic arch

Temporomandibular joint capsule

Occipitalis belly, occipitofrontalis muscle

Cartilage of external acoustic meatus

Ramus of mandible

Semispinalis capitis muscle

Styloid process

External carotid artery; styloglossus muscle

Sternocleidomastoid muscle

Posterior belly of digastric muscle

Splenius capitis muscle

Trapezius muscle

Internal jugular vein

Levator scapulae muscle

Vagus nerve

Scalenus medius muscle

Scalenus posterior muscle

Brachial plexus

Scalenus anterior muscle

Common carotid artery

Sternocleidomastoid muscle

FIGURE 552.1 Temporalis and Buccinator Muscles

NOTE: (1) The external ear and zygomatic arch have been removed, along with most of the masseter muscle to demonstrate the origin of the temporalis muscle from the temporal fossa and its insertion on the coronoid process of the mandible. Similar to the masseter, the temporalis is innervated by the mandibular branch of the trigeminal nerve.

(2) The various fiber bundles of the buccinator muscle as they extend directly into the orbicularis oris at both the upper and lower lips. Similar to the other facial muscles, the buccinator is supplied by the facial nerve (VII, buccal branch).

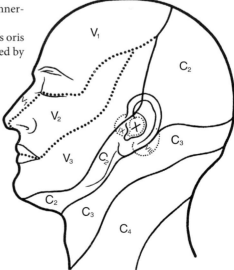

FIGURE 552.2 Cutaneous Nerve Patterns (Dermatomes) of the ▶ Head and Neck

NOTE: (1) The anterior and lateral surfaces of the head and face are supplied by the divisions of the trigeminal nerve.

(2) The posterior and lateral surfaces of the head and neck are supplied by the cervical nerves. Small areas of skin around the ear are innervated by the facial (VII), glossopharyngeal (IX), and vagus (X) nerves.

PLATE 553 Face: Superficial Vessels and Nerves (Dissection 1)

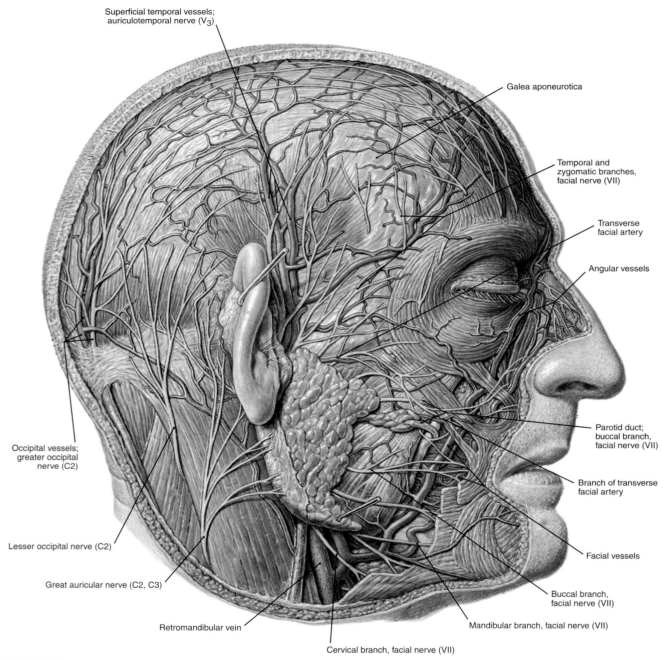

Superficial temporal vessels;
auriculotemporal nerve (V₃)

Galea aponeurotica

Temporal and
zygomatic branches,
facial nerve (VII)

Transverse
facial artery

Angular vessels

Parotid duct;
buccal branch,
facial nerve (VII)

Branch of transverse
facial artery

Occipital vessels;
greater occipital
nerve (C2)

Facial vessels

Lesser occipital nerve (C2)

Great auricular nerve (C2, C3)

Buccal branch,
facial nerve (VII)

Retromandibular vein

Mandibular branch, facial nerve (VII)

Cervical branch, facial nerve (VII)

FIGURE 553 Superficial Dissection of the Face: Vessels and Nerves (Dissection 1)

NOTE: (1) In this dissection the capsule of the parotid gland has been opened to reveal the substance of the gland and the branches of the **facial nerve** that emerge from under its borders. These cross the face to supply the muscles of facial expression (see Fig. 554) for a more complete view of the facial branches.

(2) The cervical nerves. The **greater occipital nerve** is a sensory nerve from the *posterior* primary ramus of C2, and it courses upward with the occipital vessels to supply the posterior scalp. The **lesser occipital (C2)** and **great auricular (C2, C3) nerves** are from the anterior primary rami and are also sensory nerves. They supply the posterolateral neck region and the lateral scalp behind the ear.

(3) The course of the **facial artery and vein** is partially covered by the muscles of facial expression. These vessels have been exposed to demonstrate their ascent lateral to the nose to reach the medial side of the orbit where they are called the **angular artery and vein**.

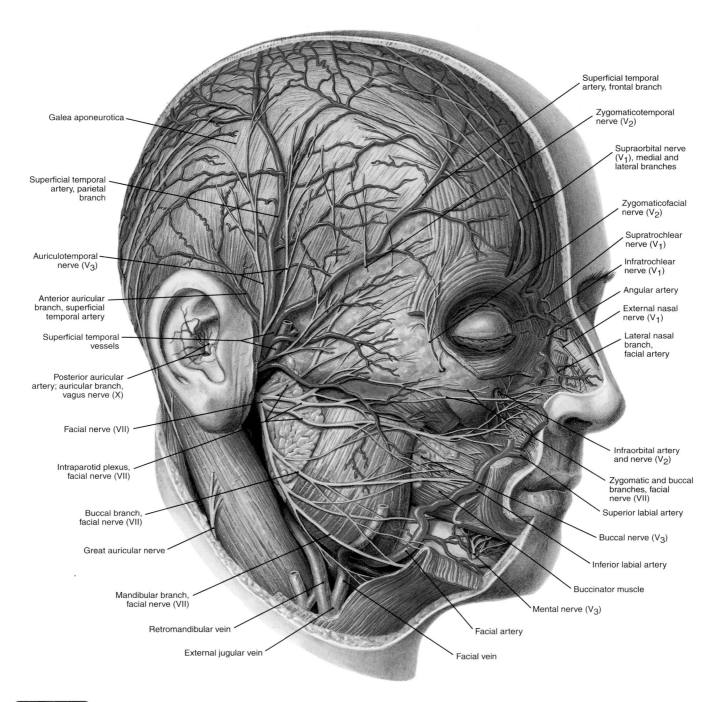

Galea aponeurotica

Superficial temporal artery, parietal branch

Auriculotemporal nerve (V₃)

Anterior auricular branch, superficial temporal artery

Superficial temporal vessels

Posterior auricular artery; auricular branch, vagus nerve (X)

Facial nerve (VII)

Intraparotid plexus, facial nerve (VII)

Buccal branch, facial nerve (VII)

Great auricular nerve

Mandibular branch, facial nerve (VII)

Retromandibular vein

External jugular vein

Superficial temporal artery, frontal branch

Zygomaticotemporal nerve (V₂)

Supraorbital nerve (V₁), medial and lateral branches

Zygomaticofacial nerve (V₂)

Supratrochlear nerve (V₁)

Infratrochlear nerve (V₁)

Angular artery

External nasal nerve (V₁)

Lateral nasal branch, facial artery

Infraorbital artery and nerve (V₂)

Zygomatic and buccal branches, facial nerve (VII)

Superior labial artery

Buccal nerve (V₃)

Inferior labial artery

Buccinator muscle

Mental nerve (V₃)

Facial artery

Facial vein

FIGURE 554 **Superficial Dissection of the Face: Vessels and Nerves (Dissection 2)**

NOTE: (1) The superficial part of the parotid gland has been removed to show the branches of the **facial nerve**, which emerge from the substance of the gland. Identify the **temporal, zygomatic, buccal, mandibular,** and **cervical** branches. The **posterior auricular** branch is not shown.

(2) The superficial sensory branches of the **trigeminal nerve**:

    (a) From the **ophthalmic division**: the supraorbital, supratrochlear, the ascending and descending branches of the infratrochlear, and the external nasal.

    (b) From the **maxillary division**: the zygomaticotemporal, the zygomaticofacial, and the infraorbital.

    (c) From the **mandibular division**: the buccal, mental, and auriculotemporal.

(3) The general distribution of **superficial temporal artery**. Also observe the course of the **facial artery** as it ascends on the face to become the **angular artery**. Among other structures, the facial artery supplies the chin and the upper and lower lips and it anastomoses with vessels emerging from the orbit.

PLATE 555 Muscles of Mastication

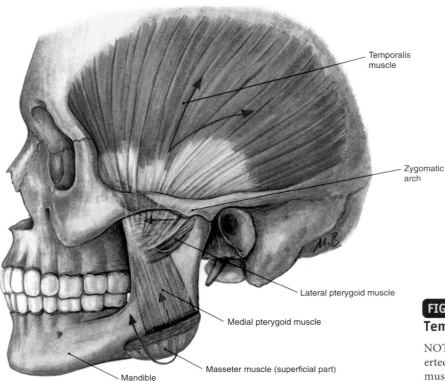

Temporalis
muscle

Zygomatic
arch

Lateral pterygoid muscle

Medial pterygoid muscle

Masseter muscle (superficial part)

Mandible

FIGURE 555.1 **Actions of the Masseter and Temporalis Muscles**

NOTE that the arrows indicate the directions of force exerted by the temporalis, masseter, and medial pterygoid muscles in closing the jaw.

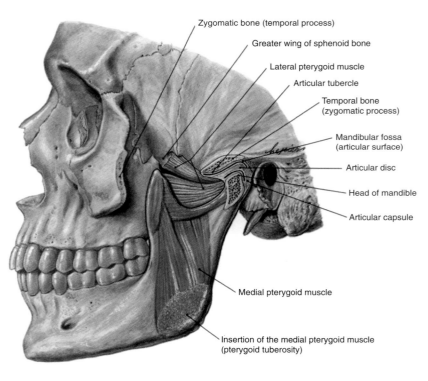

Zygomatic bone (temporal process)

Greater wing of sphenoid bone

Lateral pterygoid muscle

Articular tubercle

Temporal bone
(zygomatic process)

Mandibular fossa
(articular surface)

Articular disc

Head of mandible

Articular capsule

Medial pterygoid muscle

Insertion of the medial pterygoid muscle
(pterygoid tuberosity)

FIGURE 555.2 **Medial and Lateral Pterygoid Muscles (Lateral View)**

NOTE: (1) The left zygomatic arch has been removed. Posteriorly, the bone has been cut to show the **temporomandibular joint** and the articular disk. The medial pterygoid muscle and part of the lateral pterygoid muscle on the inner aspect of the mandible are represented as though the bone was transparent.

(2) The **medial pterygoid muscle** arises from the medial surface of the lateral pterygoid plate of the sphenoid as well as from the palatine bone and inserts on the medial surface of the ramus and angle of the mandible. It assists the masseter and temporalis in closing the jaw.

(3) The lateral pterygoid arises by two heads, one from the sphenoid bone and one from the palatine bone. It inserts on the medial ramus and angle of the mandible. It assists the masseter and temporalis to close the jaw.

MUSCLES OF MASTICATION				
Muscle	**Origin**	**Insertion**	**Innervation**	**Action**
Masseter	Zygomatic surface of maxilla and the zygomatic arch	Lateral surface of ramus of mandible and the coronoid process of mandible	Masseteric branch of mandibular nerve	Closes the jaw by elevating the mandible
Temporalis	Temporal fossa and deep surface of the temporal fascia	Medial surface of anterior border of coronoid process; anterior border of ramus of mandible	Deep temporal branches of the mandibular nerve	Elevates mandible and closes the jaw; posterior fibers retract mandible

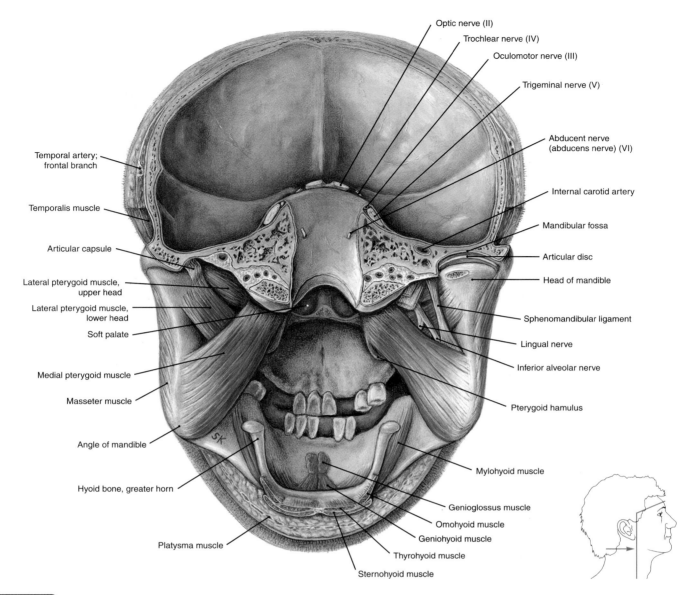

FIGURE 556 **Pterygoid, Mylohyoid, and Geniohyoid Muscles as Seen from Below and Behind**

NOTE: (1) A muscular sling is formed around the ramus of mandible to its angle by the insertions of the **medial pterygoid** and **masseter muscles** (seen on the left). The medial pterygoid muscle descends to attach along the medial aspect of the mandible, while the masseter courses down to insert on the outer aspect of the jaw.

(2) The fibers of the lateral pterygoid course principally in the horizontal plane. The **mylohyoid** and **geniohyoid muscles** attach the mandible to the hyoid bone. Other muscles shown are the **tensor** and **levator veli palatini muscles**.

MUSCLES OF MASTICATION (Continued)				
Muscle	**Origin**	**Insertion**	**Innervation**	**Action**
Lateral pterygoid	**Superior head:** Infratemporal crest and lateral surface of greater wing of sphenoid bone **Inferior head:** Lateral surface of lateral pterygoid plate of sphenoid	Neck of condyle of mandible; articular disk and capsule of temporomandibular joint	Lateral pterygoid branch of mandibular nerve	Opens mouth by drawing condyle and disk forward Acting together: protrudes mandible Acting alternately: grinding action
Medial pterygoid	**Deep head:** Medial surface of lateral pterygoid plate of sphenoid; pyramidal process of palatine bone **Superficial head:** Pyramidal process of palatine bone; tuberosity of maxilla	Lower and posterior part of medial surface of ramus and angle of mandible	Medial pterygoid branch of mandibular nerve	Elevates mandible closing jaw Acting together: protrudes mandible Acting alone: protrudes one side Acting alternately: grinding action

PLATE 557 Temporomandibular Joint and Mandibular Ligaments

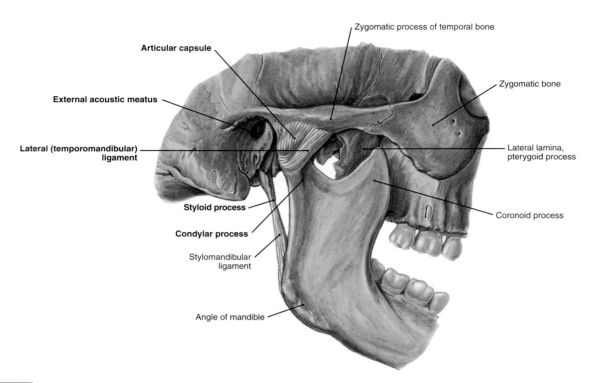

FIGURE 557.1 Right Temporomandibular Joint (Lateral View)

NOTE: (1) The articular capsule and the **lateral** (temporomandibular) **ligament** extend between the zygomatic process of the temporal bone above and the neck of the condylar process of the mandibular ramus below.

(2) The articular capsule is a loose sac that is fused anteriorly and laterally with the **lateral ligament.** Also note the **stylomandibular ligament** extending from the tip of the styloid process to the angle and posterior border of the mandible.

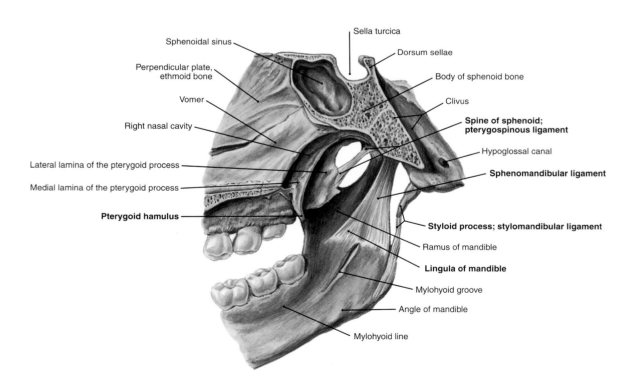

FIGURE 557.2 Right Temporomandibular Region (Medial View)

NOTE: Medial to the temporomandibular joint, the **pterygospinous ligament** extends from the sphenoidal spine to the posterior margin of the lateral pterygoid plate. The **sphenomandibular ligament** descends from the sphenoidal spine to the lingula of the mandible.

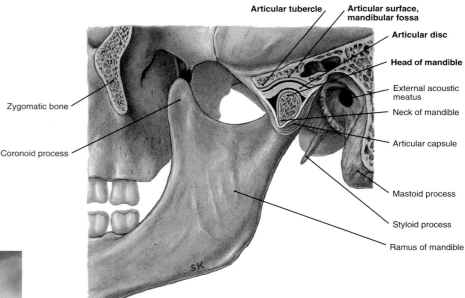

▲

FIGURE 558.1 Sagittal Section of the Temporomandibular Joint with the Jaw Closed

NOTE: (1) An **articular disk** is interposed between the mandibular fossa of the temporal bone and the mandibular condyle, creating two joint cavities.

(2) With the jaw closed, the head of the condyle of the mandible and the articular disk lie totally within the mandibular fossa.

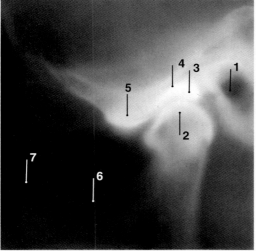

◀ ## FIGURE 558.2 Arthrograph of the Temporomandibular Joint with the Jaw Closed

Key for Figures 558.2 and 558.4
1. External acoustic meatus
2. Condylar process
3. Articular disk
4. Mandibular fossa, temporal bone
5. Articular tubercle, temporal bone
6. Mandibular notch
7. Coronoid process
▼

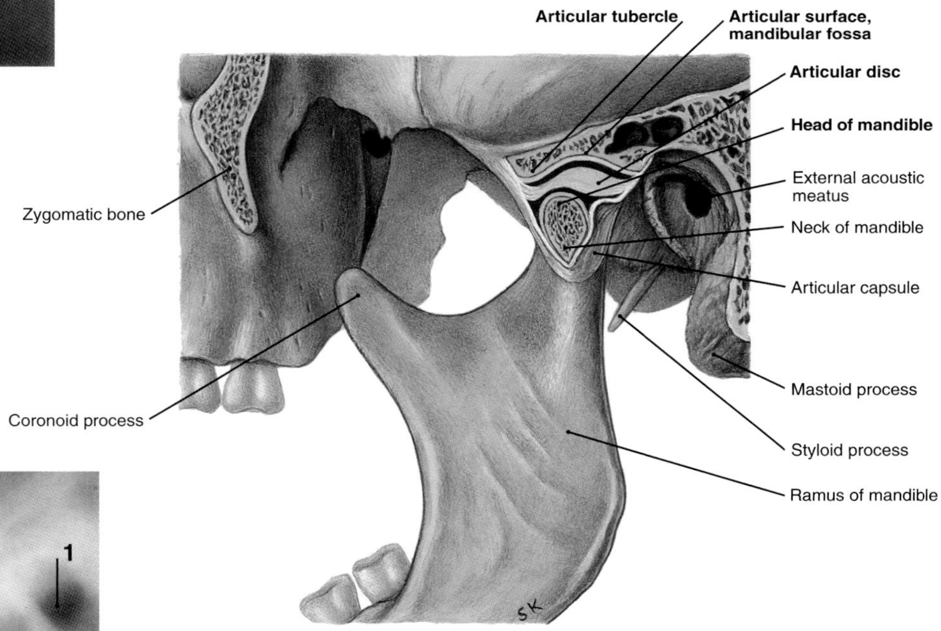

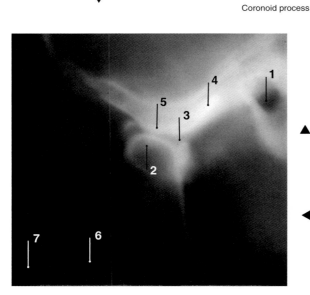

▲ ## FIGURE 558.3 Sagittal Section of the Temporomandibular Joint with the Jaw Opened

NOTE: When the jaw is opened, the condyle **glides forward** within the joint capsule to lie opposite the **articular tubercle** of the temporal bone.

◀ ## FIGURE 558.4 Arthrograph of the Temporomandibular Joint with the Jaw Opened

NOTE: The mandibular condyle moves forward significantly when the jaw is opened. In Figures 558.2 and 558.4, compare the distance between the condyle (2) and the external acoustic meatus (1).

PLATE 559 Face: Superficial and Deep Arteries

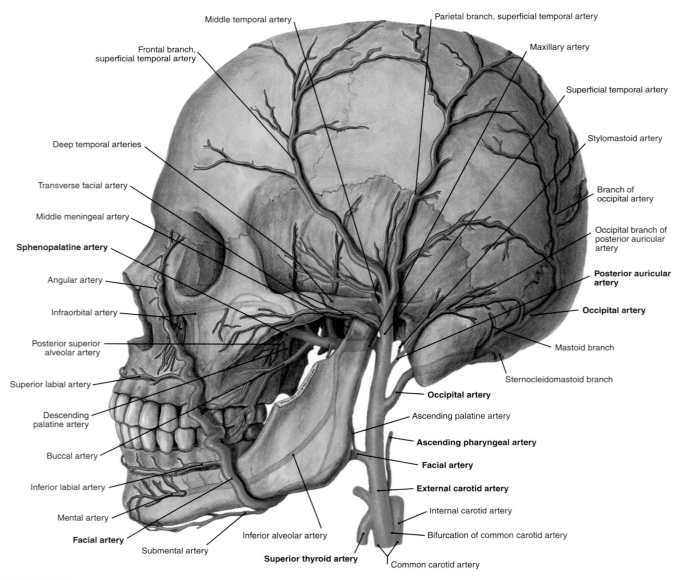

Middle temporal artery

Parietal branch, superficial temporal artery

Frontal branch, superficial temporal artery

Maxillary artery

Superficial temporal artery

Deep temporal arteries

Stylomastoid artery

Transverse facial artery

Branch of occipital artery

Middle meningeal artery

Occipital branch of posterior auricular artery

Sphenopalatine artery

Posterior auricular artery

Angular artery

Infraorbital artery

Occipital artery

Posterior superior alveolar artery

Mastoid branch

Superior labial artery

Sternocleidomastoid branch

Occipital artery

Descending palatine artery

Ascending palatine artery

Ascending pharyngeal artery

Buccal artery

Facial artery

Inferior labial artery

External carotid artery

Internal carotid artery

Mental artery

Bifurcation of common carotid artery

Facial artery

Inferior alveolar artery

Submental artery

Superior thyroid artery

Common carotid artery

FIGURE 559 External Carotid Artery and Its Branches

NOTE: (1) The **external carotid artery** branches from the common carotid and is the principal artery that supplies the anterior neck, the face, the scalp, the walls of the **oral** and **nasal cavities**, the bones of the skull, and the dura mater, but not the orbit or brain.

(2) Its main branches from inferior to superior are:

(a) The **superior thyroid**, which courses downward to supply the thyroid gland. It also supplies the sternocleidomastoid and infrahyoid muscles and the inner aspect of the larynx by way of the **superior laryngeal artery**.

(b) The **ascending pharyngeal**, which ascends to supply the pharyngeal constrictor muscles and other small branches to the prevertebral muscles, middle ear, and dura mater.

(c) The **lingual**, which is the principal artery of the tongue. It also gives branches to suprahyoid muscles and the sublingual gland.

(d) The **facial**, which ascends to supply the anteromedial aspect of the face. It also gives branches to the palatine tonsil, the submandibular gland, and on the face, to both lips and the nose. It ends as the **angular artery**, which anastomoses with the infraorbital.

(e) The **occipital**, which courses to the back of the head to supply the scalp. On its way it sends branches to the sternocleidomastoid and other muscles and to the dura mater.

(f) The **posterior auricular**, which courses behind the external ear. It helps supply the scalp, the middle ear, and the external auricle.

(g) The **superficial temporal**, which supplies the side of the head and gives off the **transverse facial artery**, which courses across the face.

(h) The **maxillary**, which is the principal artery of the deep face. It has three parts and many branches. It supplies the tympanic membrane, gives rise to the **middle meningeal artery**, and supplies the muscles of mastication, all lower and some upper teeth, the infraorbital region, the hard and soft palate, and the walls of the nasal cavity.

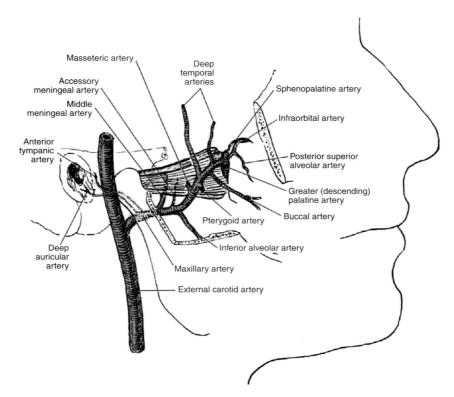

FIGURE 560.1 Branches of the Maxillary Artery (after Grant, J.C.B., Atlas of Anatomy, 6th Edition. Baltimore: Williams and Wilkins, 1972)

NOTE: Branches from the maxillary artery are given off from all three parts of the vessel: from the first part: **anterior tympanic, deep auricular, middle and accessory meningeal,** and **inferior alveolar;** from the second part: **masseteric, deep temporal, pterygoid,** and **buccal;** and from the third part: **sphenopalatine, infraorbital, greater (descending) palatine, posterior superior alveolar,** and **the artery of the pterygoid canal.**

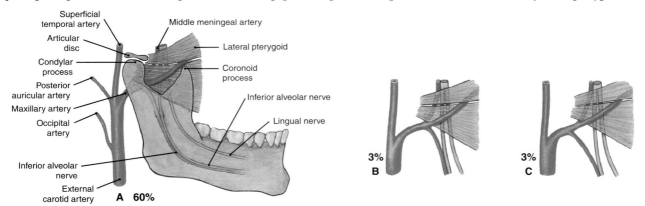

FIGURE 560.2 Variations in the Maxillary Artery Passing Lateral to the Lateral Pterygoid Muscle

NOTE: The maxillary artery courses lateral (superficial) to the lateral pterygoid muscle in about two-thirds of the cases. In 60% of these cadavers (**A**), the middle meningeal artery arises proximal to the inferior alveolar artery. In 3% of these cadavers (**B**), the middle meningeal artery arises opposite the inferior alveolar artery. In 3% of these cadavers (**C**), the middle meningeal artery arises distal to the inferior alveolar artery.

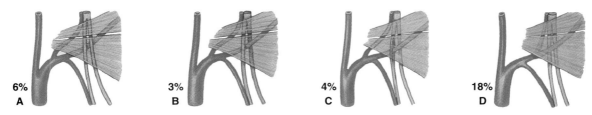

FIGURE 560.3 Variations in the Maxillary Artery Passing Medial to the Lateral Pterygoid Muscle

NOTE: The maxillary artery courses medial to the lateral pterygoid muscle in about 31% to 33% of cadavers. In **A**, the maxillary artery courses medial to the lingual and inferior alveolar nerves in 6%; in **B**, the maxillary artery courses between the lingual and inferior alveolar nerves in 3%; in **C**, the maxillary artery courses through a loop in the inferior alveolar nerve in 4%; and in **D**, the maxillary artery gives origin to the middle meningeal artery distal to the inferior alveolar artery.

PLATE 561 Superficial Veins of the Face and Skull

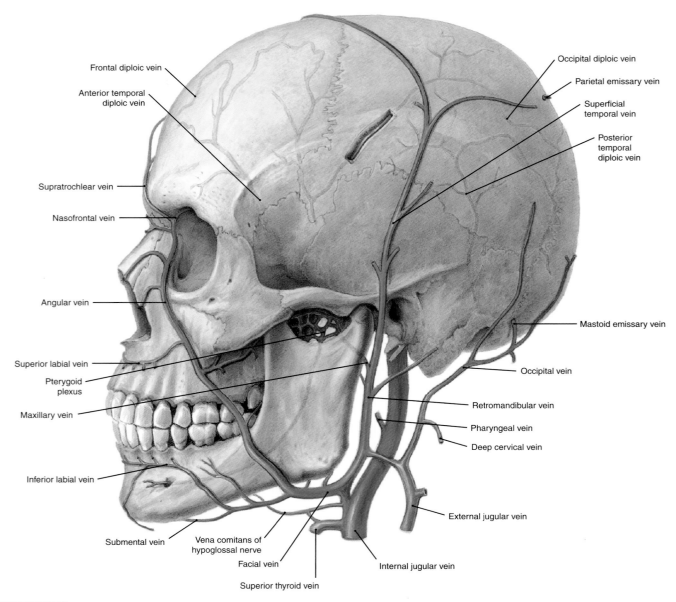

Frontal diploic vein

Anterior temporal diploic vein

Supratrochlear vein

Nasofrontal vein

Angular vein

Superior labial vein

Pterygoid plexus

Maxillary vein

Inferior labial vein

Submental vein

Vena comitans of hypoglossal nerve

Facial vein

Superior thyroid vein

Occipital diploic vein

Parietal emissary vein

Superficial temporal vein

Posterior temporal diploic vein

Mastoid emissary vein

Occipital vein

Retromandibular vein

Pharyngeal vein

Deep cervical vein

External jugular vein

Internal jugular vein

FIGURE 561 **Principal Superficial Veins of the Face and Head, Showing Connections to Deeper Veins**

NOTE: (1) The **angular vein** is formed at the root of the nose and courses inferolaterally to become the **facial vein**. The angular-facial trunk communicates by way of deeper vessels with the **cavernous sinus** within the cranial cavity and with **pterygoid plexus** of veins in the infratemporal fossa.

(2) The **superficial temporal vein**, which drains the lateral aspect of the superficial head and the **maxillary vein**, which drains the deep face. They join to form the **retromandibular vein**.

(3) The **occipital vein**, which forms on the posterolateral aspect of the scalp and which courses downward into the **external jugular vein**. The diploic veins and the various emissary veins (condylar, mastoid, and parietal veins) interconnect the superficial veins with the **dural sinuses**.

(4) Within the cranial cavity, the **sigmoid sinus**, draining most of the other dural sinuses, terminates at the jugular foramen. Just below this foramen, the sigmoid sinus becomes the **internal jugular vein**, which descends in the neck to the thorax.

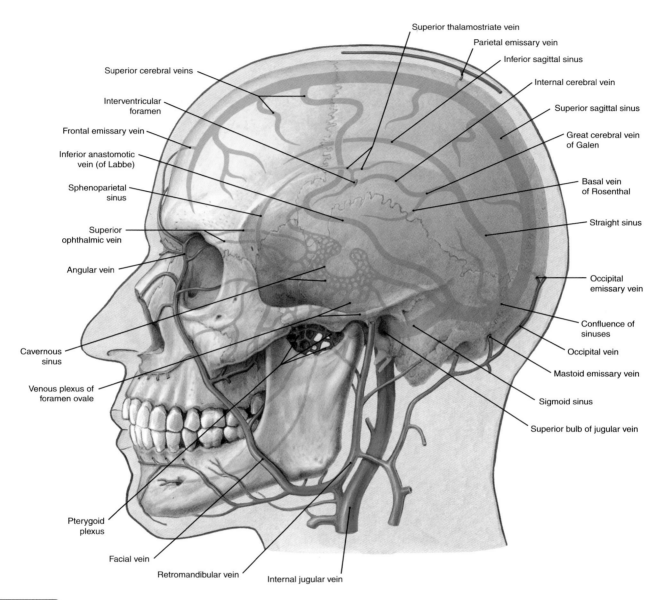

Superior thalamostriate vein
Parietal emissary vein
Inferior sagittal sinus
Internal cerebral vein
Superior sagittal sinus
Great cerebral vein of Galen
Basal vein of Rosenthal
Straight sinus
Occipital emissary vein
Confluence of sinuses
Occipital vein
Mastoid emissary vein
Sigmoid sinus
Superior bulb of jugular vein

Superior cerebral veins
Interventricular foramen
Frontal emissary vein
Inferior anastomotic vein (of Labbe)
Sphenoparietal sinus
Superior ophthalmic vein
Angular vein
Cavernous sinus
Venous plexus of foramen ovale
Pterygoid plexus
Facial vein
Retromandibular vein
Internal jugular vein

FIGURE 562 **Internal Jugular Vein and Its Extracranial Tributaries**

NOTE: (1) The superficial face is drained by the **angular vein** and the **superior** and **inferior labial** veins. These flow into the large facial vein that descends obliquely adjacent to the facial (not shown) artery (see Fig. 563).

(2) The internal jugular vein forms at the base of the skull. Within the skull, blood in the **sigmoid sinus** drains through the jugular foramen, and as the sigmoid sinus emerges from the jugular foramen in the neck it becomes the **internal jugular vein**.

(3) Within the skull, observe the confluence of sinuses. This large venous channel receives blood from the **superior sagittal sinus**, the **straight sinus,** and **the inferior anastomotic vein** (of Labbé).

(4) The **cavernous sinus** and its communications with the ophthalmic veins of the orbit and the pterygoid plexus of veins in the deep face.

(5) The many emissary veins passing through the skull and forming many connections between the dural sinuses and the veins on the exterior of the skull.

PLATE 563 Face: Deep Vessels and Nerves (Dissection 1)

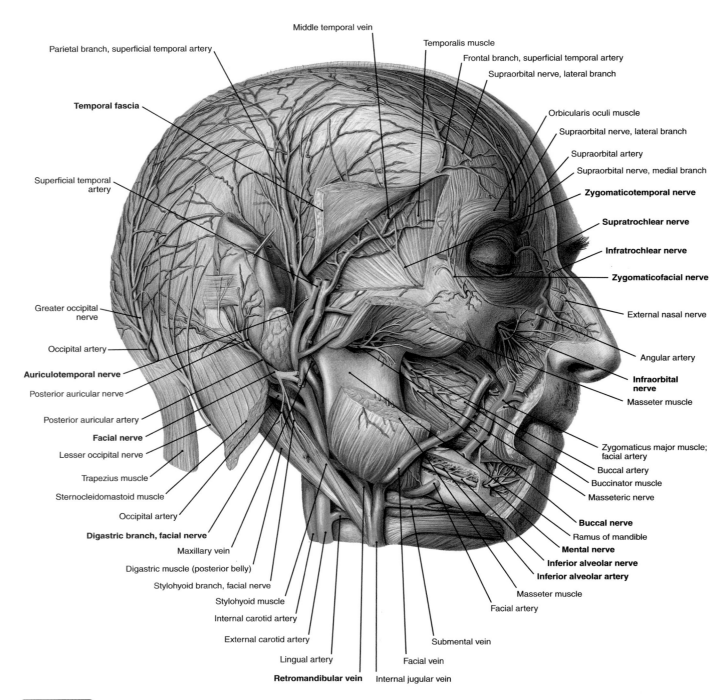

Middle temporal vein
Parietal branch, superficial temporal artery
Temporalis muscle
Frontal branch, superficial temporal artery
Supraorbital nerve, lateral branch
Temporal fascia
Orbicularis oculi muscle
Supraorbital nerve, lateral branch
Supraorbital artery
Supraorbital nerve, medial branch
Superficial temporal artery
Zygomaticotemporal nerve
Supratrochlear nerve
Infratrochlear nerve
Zygomaticofacial nerve
Greater occipital nerve
External nasal nerve
Occipital artery
Angular artery
Auriculotemporal nerve
Infraorbital nerve
Posterior auricular nerve
Masseter muscle
Posterior auricular artery
Facial nerve
Zygomaticus major muscle; facial artery
Lesser occipital nerve
Buccal artery
Buccinator muscle
Trapezius muscle
Masseteric nerve
Sternocleidomastoid muscle
Occipital artery
Buccal nerve
Ramus of mandible
Digastric branch, facial nerve
Mental nerve
Maxillary vein
Inferior alveolar nerve
Digastric muscle (posterior belly)
Inferior alveolar artery
Stylohyoid branch, facial nerve
Masseter muscle
Stylohyoid muscle
Facial artery
Internal carotid artery
External carotid artery
Submental vein
Lingual artery
Facial vein
Retromandibular vein
Internal jugular vein

FIGURE 563 Vessels and Nerves of the Deep Face (Dissection 1)

NOTE: (1) The temporal fascia has been cut and partially reflected. The superficial muscles on the side of the face and the parotid gland have been removed. The main trunk of the facial nerve has been cut and its branches across the face removed. The masseter muscle was severed and reflected upward to show the masseteric artery and nerve.

(2) The following are branches of the **trigeminal nerve**:
  (a) **Ophthalmic division**: supraorbital, supratrochlear, infratrochlear, and external nasal branches.
  (b) **Maxillary division**: zygomaticotemporal, zygomaticofacial, and infraorbital branches.
  (c) **Mandibular division**: auriculotemporal, masseteric, buccal, inferior alveolar, and mental branches.

(3) The posterior auricular, digastric, and stylohyoid branches of the facial nerve arise from the facial nerve trunk prior to its division within the parotid gland.

(4) The anastomosis of arteries above and at the medial aspect of the orbit. The vessels involved include the frontal branch of the superficial temporal, the supraorbital, supratrochlear, and angular arteries and their branches.

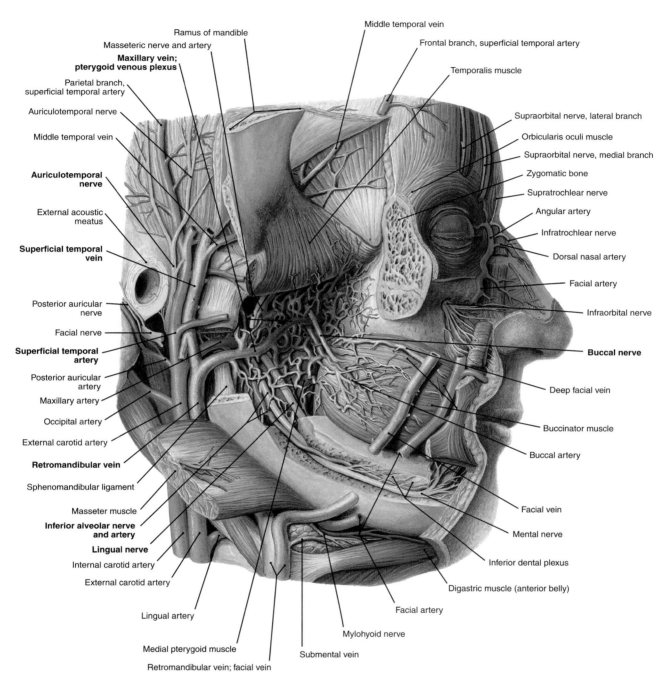

Ramus of mandible
Masseteric nerve and artery
**Maxillary vein;
pterygoid venous plexus**
Parietal branch,
superficial temporal artery
Auriculotemporal nerve
Middle temporal vein
**Auriculotemporal
nerve**
External acoustic
meatus
**Superficial temporal
vein**
Posterior auricular
nerve
Facial nerve
**Superficial temporal
artery**
Posterior auricular
artery
Maxillary artery
Occipital artery
External carotid artery
Retromandibular vein
Sphenomandibular ligament
Masseter muscle
**Inferior alveolar nerve
and artery**
Lingual nerve
Internal carotid artery
External carotid artery
Lingual artery
Medial pterygoid muscle
Retromandibular vein; facial vein

Middle temporal vein
Frontal branch, superficial temporal artery
Temporalis muscle
Supraorbital nerve, lateral branch
Orbicularis oculi muscle
Supraorbital nerve, medial branch
Zygomatic bone
Supratrochlear nerve
Angular artery
Infratrochlear nerve
Dorsal nasal artery
Facial artery
Infraorbital nerve
Buccal nerve
Deep facial vein
Buccinator muscle
Buccal artery
Facial vein
Mental nerve
Inferior dental plexus
Digastric muscle (anterior belly)
Facial artery
Mylohyoid nerve
Submental vein

FIGURE 564 **Infratemporal Region of the Deep Face (Dissection 2)**

NOTE: (1) The zygomatic arch has been cut and reflected upward along with the insertion of the temporalis muscle. A portion of the mandible has also been removed to show the course of the **maxillary vein** and **artery** deep to the mandible. The branches of the artery in the infratemporal region can better be seen in Figure 565.

(2) The maxillary vein forms from the **pterygoid plexus** of veins, which lies adjacent to the pterygoid muscles and which anastomoses with the facial vein by way of the **deep facial vein**. This plexus also anastomoses with the cavernous sinus through communicating veins in the foramen lacerum and foramen ovale and by way of the inferior ophthalmic vein.

(3) The body of the mandible has been opened to expose the inferior alveolar artery and nerve.

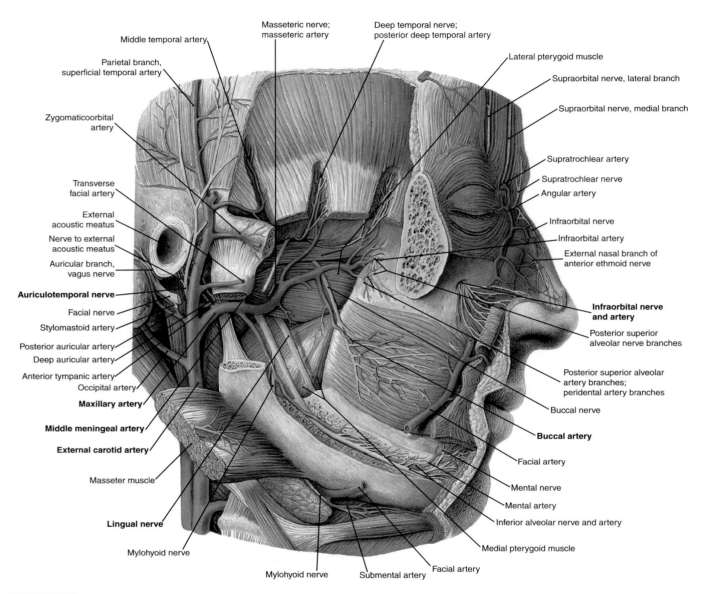

Masseteric nerve; masseteric artery

Deep temporal nerve; posterior deep temporal artery

Middle temporal artery

Lateral pterygoid muscle

Parietal branch, superficial temporal artery

Supraorbital nerve, lateral branch

Supraorbital nerve, medial branch

Zygomaticoorbital artery

Supratrochlear artery

Supratrochlear nerve

Transverse facial artery

Angular artery

External acoustic meatus

Infraorbital nerve

Nerve to external acoustic meatus

Infraorbital artery

Auricular branch, vagus nerve

External nasal branch of anterior ethmoid nerve

Auriculotemporal nerve

Infraorbital nerve and artery

Facial nerve

Posterior superior alveolar nerve branches

Stylomastoid artery

Posterior auricular artery

Deep auricular artery

Posterior superior alveolar artery branches; peridental artery branches

Anterior tympanic artery

Occipital artery

Maxillary artery

Buccal nerve

Middle meningeal artery

Buccal artery

External carotid artery

Facial artery

Masseter muscle

Mental nerve

Mental artery

Lingual nerve

Inferior alveolar nerve and artery

Mylohyoid nerve

Medial pterygoid muscle

Mylohyoid nerve   Submental artery   Facial artery

FIGURE 565 Infratemporal Region of the Deep Face: Maxillary Artery (Dissection 3)

NOTE: (1) The **infratemporal fossa** has been opened laterally to show the pterygoid muscles, the maxillary artery and its branches, and some of the branches of the mandibular division of the trigeminal nerve.

(2) In this dissection, the following branches of the **maxillary artery** are shown: (a) deep auricular, (b) anterior tympanic, (c) inferior alveolar, (d) middle meningeal, (e) masseteric (cut), (f) deep temporal, (g) pterygoid (not labeled), (h) buccal, (i) posterior superior alveolar, and (j) infraorbital. **NOT** shown in this view are the descending palatine branch, the artery of the pterygoid canal, and the pharyngeal and sphenopalatine branches.

(3) The following are branches of the **mandibular division** of the **trigeminal nerve:** (a) auriculotemporal, (b) lingual, (c) inferior alveolar, (d) mylohyoid, (e) masseteric, (f) deep temporal, and (g) buccal. Observe the course of the inferior alveolar nerve, accompanied by the inferior alveolar artery within the mandible.

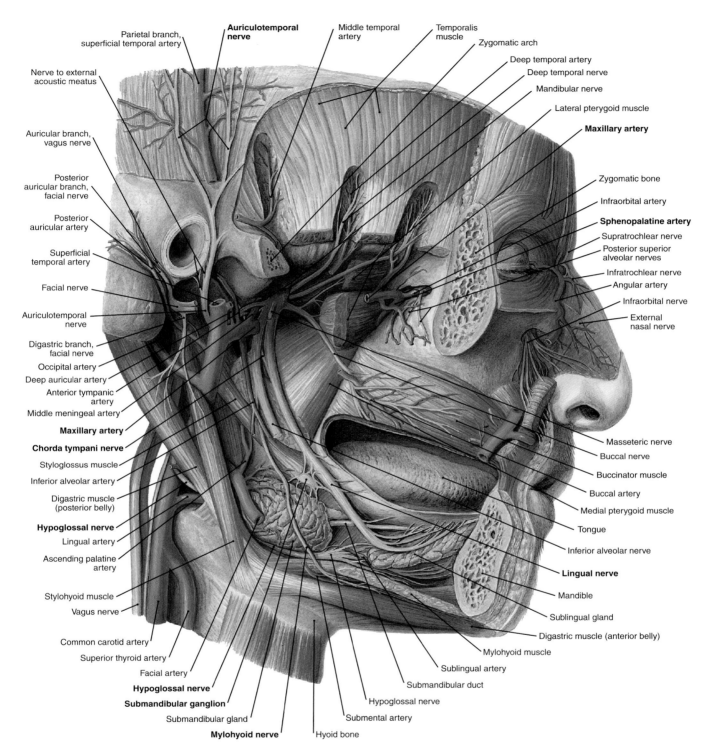

Parietal branch, superficial temporal artery
Auriculotemporal nerve
Middle temporal artery
Temporalis muscle
Zygomatic arch
Nerve to external acoustic meatus
Deep temporal artery
Deep temporal nerve
Mandibular nerve
Lateral pterygoid muscle
Maxillary artery
Auricular branch, vagus nerve
Posterior auricular branch, facial nerve
Zygomatic bone
Infraorbital artery
Posterior auricular artery
Sphenopalatine artery
Supratrochlear nerve
Posterior superior alveolar nerves
Superficial temporal artery
Infratrochlear nerve
Facial nerve
Angular artery
Auriculotemporal nerve
Infraorbital nerve
External nasal nerve
Digastric branch, facial nerve
Occipital artery
Deep auricular artery
Anterior tympanic artery
Middle meningeal artery
Maxillary artery
Chorda tympani nerve
Masseteric nerve
Buccal nerve
Styloglossus muscle
Buccinator muscle
Inferior alveolar artery
Buccal artery
Digastric muscle (posterior belly)
Medial pterygoid muscle
Hypoglossal nerve
Tongue
Lingual artery
Inferior alveolar nerve
Ascending palatine artery
Lingual nerve
Mandible
Stylohyoid muscle
Vagus nerve
Sublingual gland
Digastric muscle (anterior belly)
Common carotid artery
Mylohyoid muscle
Superior thyroid artery
Sublingual artery
Facial artery
Submandibular duct
Hypoglossal nerve
Hypoglossal nerve
Submandibular ganglion
Submental artery
Submandibular gland
Mylohyoid nerve
Hyoid bone

FIGURE 566 **Infratemporal Region of the Deep Face: Mandibular Nerve Branches (Dissection 4)**

NOTE: (1) The zygomatic arch, much of the right mandible, and the lateral pterygoid muscle have been removed in this dissection. Also, a portion of the maxillary artery has been cut away, along with the distal part of the inferior alveolar nerve beyond the point where the mylohyoid nerve branches.

(2) The **lingual nerve** coursing to the tongue. High in the infratemporal fossa, the **chorda tympani nerve** (a branch of the facial) joins the lingual. The chorda tympani carries both special sensory **taste** fibers from the anterior two-thirds of the tongue and **preganglionic parasympathetic** fibers from the facial to the **submandibular ganglion**.

(3) The distal part of the maxillary artery as it courses toward the sphenopalatine foramen. After giving off the infraorbital artery, the sphenopalatine branch enters the nasal cavity through the foramen and serves as the principal vessel to the nasal mucosa.

PLATE 567 **Skull and Orbital Cavity (Anterior View)**

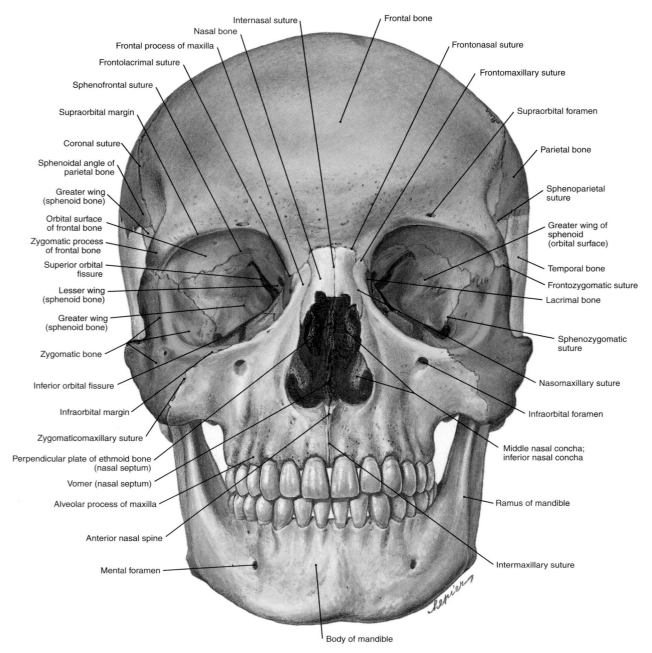

Internasal suture
Nasal bone
Frontal process of maxilla
Frontolacrimal suture
Sphenofrontal suture
Supraorbital margin
Coronal suture
Sphenoidal angle of parietal bone
Greater wing (sphenoid bone)
Orbital surface of frontal bone
Zygomatic process of frontal bone
Superior orbital fissure
Lesser wing (sphenoid bone)
Greater wing (sphenoid bone)
Zygomatic bone
Inferior orbital fissure
Infraorbital margin
Zygomaticomaxillary suture
Perpendicular plate of ethmoid bone (nasal septum)
Vomer (nasal septum)
Alveolar process of maxilla
Anterior nasal spine
Mental foramen

Frontal bone
Frontonasal suture
Frontomaxillary suture
Supraorbital foramen
Parietal bone
Sphenoparietal suture
Greater wing of sphenoid (orbital surface)
Temporal bone
Frontozygomatic suture
Lacrimal bone
Sphenozygomatic suture
Nasomaxillary suture
Infraorbital foramen
Middle nasal concha; inferior nasal concha
Ramus of mandible
Intermaxillary suture
Body of mandible

FIGURE 567.1 **Anterior Aspect of the Skull**

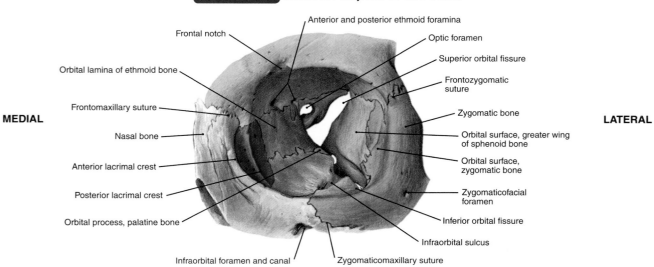

Frontal notch
Anterior and posterior ethmoid foramina
Optic foramen
Superior orbital fissure
Frontozygomatic suture
Orbital lamina of ethmoid bone
Frontomaxillary suture
Nasal bone
Anterior lacrimal crest
Posterior lacrimal crest
Orbital process, palatine bone
Infraorbital foramen and canal
Zygomaticomaxillary suture
Zygomatic bone
Orbital surface, greater wing of sphenoid bone
Orbital surface, zygomatic bone
Zygomaticofacial foramen
Inferior orbital fissure
Infraorbital sulcus

MEDIAL

LATERAL

FIGURE 567.2 **Left Bony Orbital Cavity (Anterior View)**

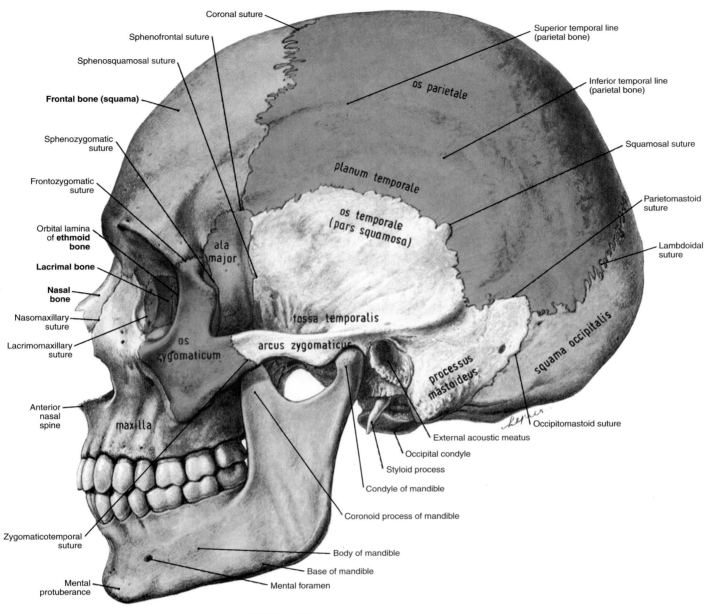

Coronal suture

Sphenofrontal suture

Sphenosquamosal suture

Frontal bone (squama)

Sphenozygomatic suture

Frontozygomatic suture

Orbital lamina of **ethmoid bone**

Lacrimal bone

Nasal bone

Nasomaxillary suture

Lacrimomaxillary suture

Anterior nasal spine

Zygomaticotemporal suture

Mental protuberance

Superior temporal line (parietal bone)

os parietale

Inferior temporal line (parietal bone)

planum temporale

Squamosal suture

os temporale (pars squamosa)

Parietomastoid suture

ala major

Lambdoidal suture

fossa temporalis

arcus zygomaticus

os zygomaticum

maxilla

processus mastoideus

squama occipitalis

Occipitomastoid suture

External acoustic meatus

Occipital condyle

Styloid process

Condyle of mandible

Coronoid process of mandible

Body of mandible

Base of mandible

Mental foramen

FIGURE 568.1 Lateral Aspect of the Skull

ANTERIOR

Zygomatic arch

POSTERIOR

Zygomaticofacial foramen

Infratemporal fossa

Foramen ovale

Foramen spinosum

Spine of greater wing, sphenoid bone

Pterygoid process

Zygomaticoalveolar crest

Perpendicular plate of palatine bone; **pterygopalatine fossa**

Pyramidal process of palatine bone

Hamulus of pterygoid process, sphenoid bone

Alveolar foramina

FIGURE 568.2 Inferolateral Aspect of the Skull with the Zygomatic Arch Removed

NOTE: The pterygopalatine fossa and the pterygoid process of the sphenoid bone.

PLATE 569 Calvaria from Above; Occipital Bone (Posterior View)

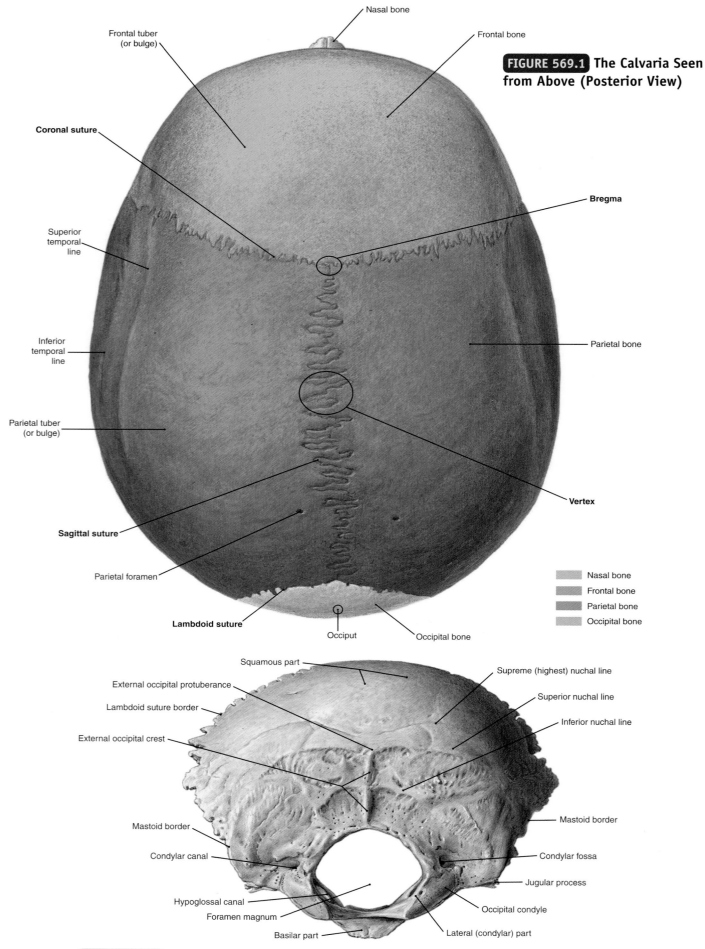

Nasal bone

Frontal tuber
(or bulge)

Frontal bone

FIGURE 569.1 The Calvaria Seen
from Above (Posterior View)

Coronal suture

Bregma

Superior
temporal
line

Inferior
temporal
line

Parietal bone

Parietal tuber
(or bulge)

Vertex

Sagittal suture

Parietal foramen

Nasal bone
Frontal bone
Parietal bone
Occipital bone

Lambdoid suture

Occiput

Occipital bone

Squamous part

Supreme (highest) nuchal line

External occipital protuberance

Superior nuchal line

Lambdoid suture border

Inferior nuchal line

External occipital crest

Mastoid border

Mastoid border

Condylar canal

Condylar fossa

Jugular process

Hypoglossal canal

Foramen magnum

Occipital condyle

Basilar part

Lateral (condylar) part

FIGURE 569.2 Occipital Bone from Behind Showing Some Posterior Features of the Skull

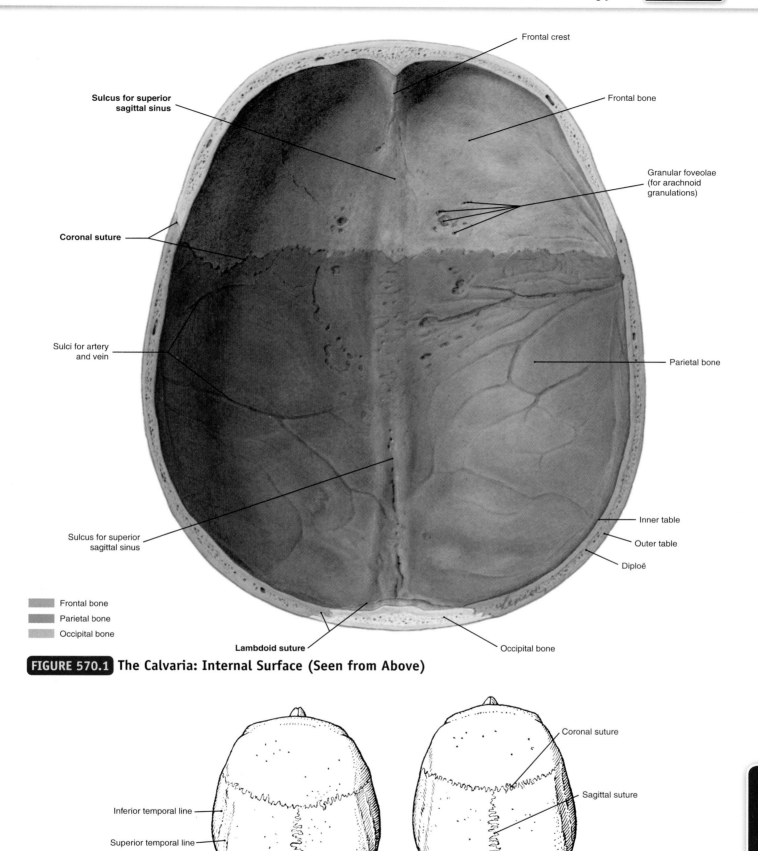

FIGURE 570.1 The Calvaria: Internal Surface (Seen from Above)

FIGURE 570.2 Brachycephalic Skull (A) and Dolichocephalic Skull (B)

NOTE: Skulls are classified by comparing their width to their length. When the greatest width exceeds 80% of the length, the skull is more round and called **brachycephalic (A)**. When the width is less than 75% of length, the more oblong skull is called **dolichocephalic (B)**. When the comparison is between 75% and 80%, the skull is classified as **mesaticephalic**.

PLATE 571 Newborn Skull (Anterior and Lateral Views)

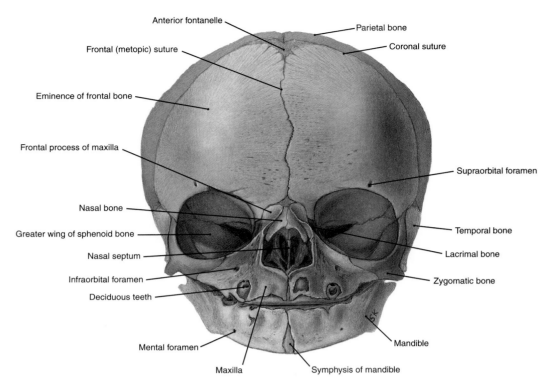

FIGURE 571.1 Skull at Birth (Frontal View)

NOTE: (1) The bones that enclose the cranial cavity (neurocranium) include the **frontal, parietal, occipital, temporal** and **sphenoid bones,** and the **cribriform plate** of the **ethmoid bone**.

(2) The bones that form the face and hard palate and enclose the nasal cavity are the **mandible, maxilla, zygomatic, lacrimal, nasal** and **palatine bones, inferior concha,** most of the **ethmoid bone,** and the **vomer.**

(3) The skull at birth is large in comparison to the size of the rest of the body because of the precocious growth of the brain; the facial bones, however, are still not well developed.

(4) The maxilla and mandible are rudimentary at birth and the teeth have yet to erupt. In addition, the maxillary sinuses and nasal cavity are small, as are the frontal, ethmoid and sphenoid sinuses.

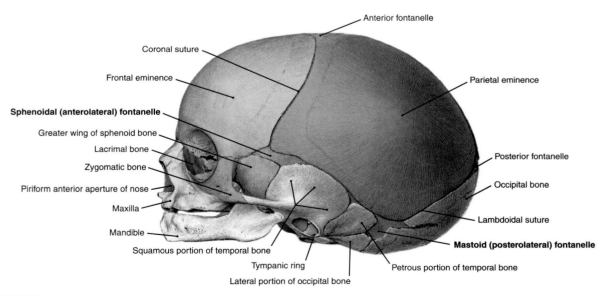

FIGURE 571.2 Skull at Birth (Lateral View)

NOTE: (1) Ossification of the maturing **flat bones of the skull** is accomplished by the intramembranous process of bone formation. At birth this process is incomplete, thereby leaving soft membranous sites between the growing bones. Bones forming the base of the cranial cavity develop by ossification in cartilage.

(2) The incompletely ossified nature of the skull just prior to birth is of some benefit, however, since the mobility of the bones permits changes in skull shape, as may be required during the birth process.

(3) The **sphenoidal** (or anterolateral) fontanelle located at the pterion and the **mastoid** (or posterolateral) found at the asterion.

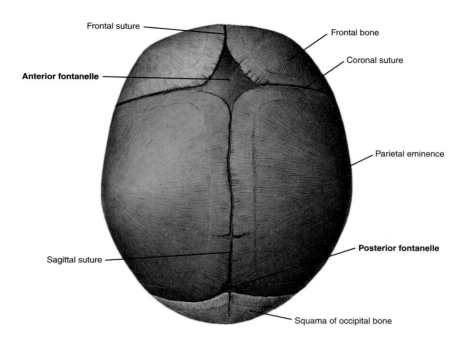

Frontal suture — Frontal bone

Coronal suture

Anterior fontanelle —

Parietal eminence

Posterior fontanelle

Sagittal suture —

Squama of occipital bone

FIGURE 572.1 Skull at Birth (Seen from Above)

NOTE: (1) The soft sites on the skull of the newborn infant are called **fontanelles**. From this superior view can be seen the **anterior** and **posterior fontanelles**.
(2) The largest of the fontanelles at birth is the **anterior fontanelle** located at the bregma and interconnecting the frontal and parietal bones. It is approximately diamond-shaped and is situated at the junction of the coronal and sagittal sutures.
(3) Following the sagittal suture to its junction with the occipital bone will locate the **posterior fontanelle** (at the lambda). This is generally triangular in shape and is small at birth.

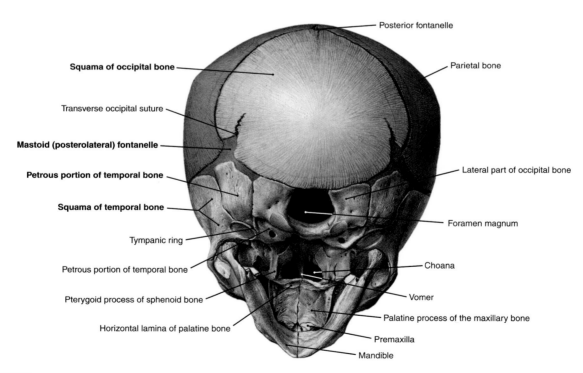

Posterior fontanelle

Squama of occipital bone —
Parietal bone

Transverse occipital suture —

Mastoid (posterolateral) fontanelle —

Petrous portion of temporal bone —
Lateral part of occipital bone

Squama of temporal bone —

Foramen magnum

Tympanic ring —

Petrous portion of temporal bone —
Choana

Pterygoid process of sphenoid bone —
Vomer

Horizontal lamina of palatine bone —
Palatine process of the maxillary bone

Premaxilla

Mandible

FIGURE 572.2 Skull at Birth (Posteroinferior View)

NOTE: (1) The separate ossification of the petrous and squamous portions of the temporal bone as well as the basilar and squamous parts of the occipital bone.
(2) The **mastoid (posterolateral) fontanelles** are found at the articulation of the occipital, temporal, and parietal bones.
(3) Growth and ossification of the bones that encase the brain are more precocious than the bones that form the facial skeleton. Facial bones continue growth through puberty. This differential accounts for the marked differences in facial features seen in a 4- or 5-year-old child with that same person at 15 or 16 years of age.

PLATE 573 Scalp and Frontal Section of Scalp, Skull, and Meninges

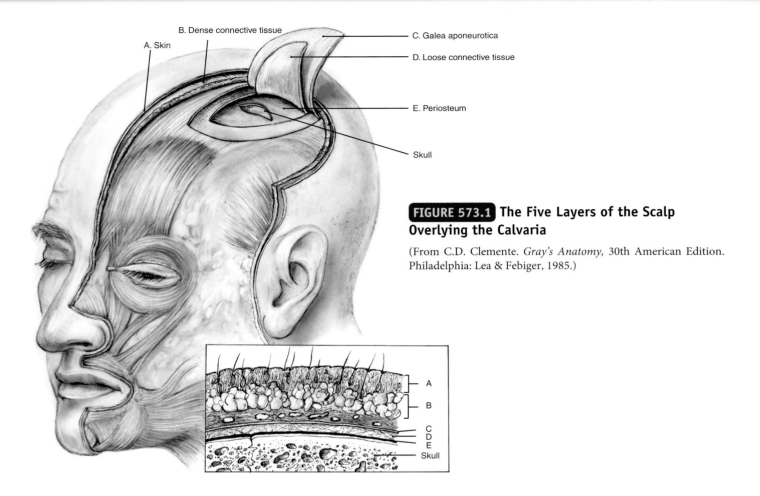

FIGURE 573.1 **The Five Layers of the Scalp Overlying the Calvaria**

(From C.D. Clemente. *Gray's Anatomy*, 30th American Edition. Philadelphia: Lea & Febiger, 1985.)

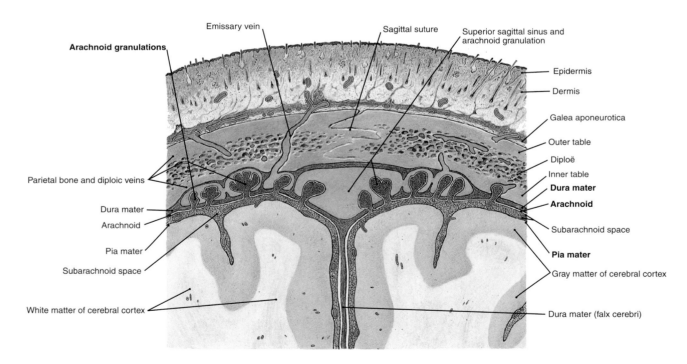

FIGURE 573.2 **Scalp, Skull, Meninges, and Brain**

NOTE: (1) This is a frontal section through the cranium and upper cerebrum and shows the bony and soft coverings of the brain. The veins and dural sinuses are colored in blue while the bone is light brown.

(2) Superficial to the dura mater, arachnoid, and pia mater that encase the neural tissue of the brain are found the bony skull and the layers of the scalp.

(3) The **arachnoid granulations**. Tufts of arachnoid (sometime called arachnoid villi) lie next to the endothelium of the sinuses and allow passage of the cerebrospinal fluid from the subarachnoid space into the venous system.

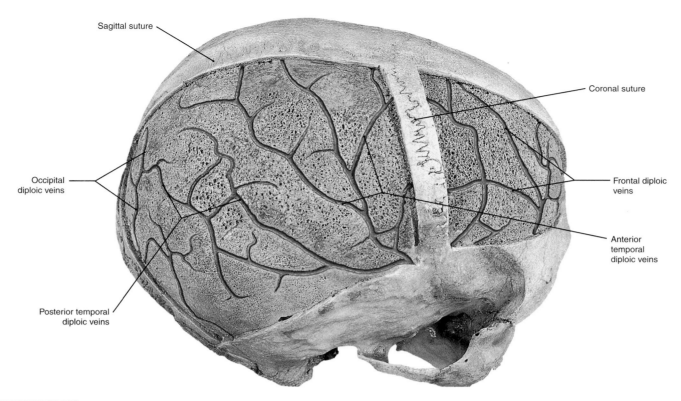

FIGURE 574.1 **Diploic Veins**

NOTE: (1) Removing the outermost table of compact bone reveals a more spongy layer of bone. Within this latter layer course venous channels called the **diploic veins**. These veins communicate with the scalp on the exterior and the dural sinuses within the skull.

(2) The diploic veins are named according to their location: **frontal, temporal,** and **occipital.**

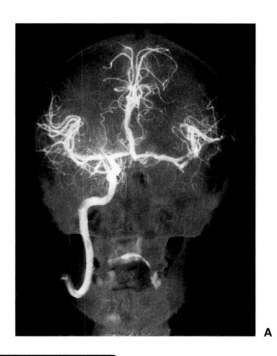

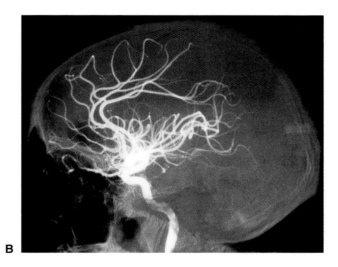

FIGURE 574.2A and B **Radiograph Showing the Distribution of the Internal Carotid Artery**

NOTE: (1) Contrast medium injected into one internal carotid artery (in this case, the left artery) becomes distributed to both sides of the brain. This points to the fact that the contralateral side of the brain can receive blood when the medium is injected ipsilaterally.

(2) This occurs because of the vascular arrangement at the circle of Willis so that each carotid artery has some bilateral distribution.

(These radiographs were achieved with digital subtraction angiography, which diminishes all other tissues and concentrates on demonstrating [in this case] only the arterial tree.)

A. Anterior–posterior radiograph. **B.** Lateral radiograph.

PLATE 575 Dura Mater and Meningeal Vessels from Above

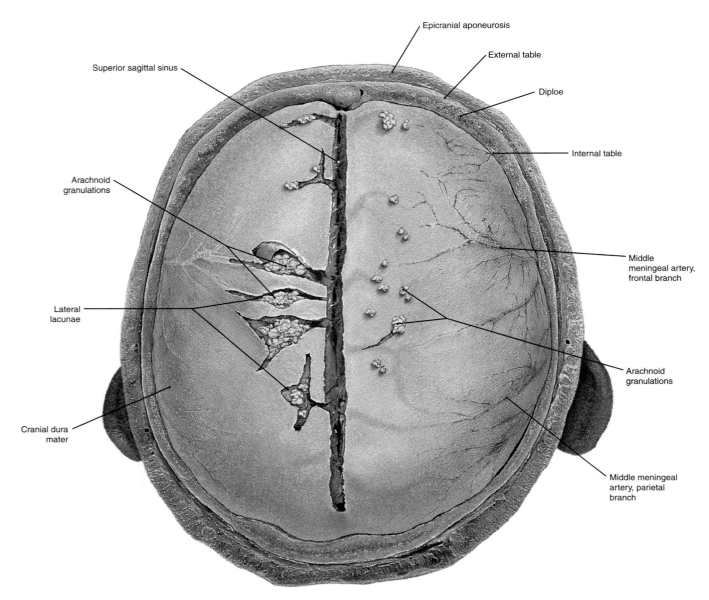

Epicranial aponeurosis

External table

Superior sagittal sinus

Diploe

Internal table

Arachnoid granulations

Middle meningeal artery, frontal branch

Lateral lacunae

Arachnoid granulations

Cranial dura mater

Middle meningeal artery, parietal branch

FIGURE 575 Surface of the Dura Mater with the Superior Sagittal Sinus Opened (Viewed from Above)

NOTE: (1) The skull cap (also called the **calvaria**) has been removed, leaving the **dura mater** intact. The dura is a two-layered structure (an inner **meningeal layer** and an outer **periosteal layer**), but these layers are inseparably fused throughout much of their expanse. In this dissection the "two layers" were stripped from the skull as a single membrane.

(2) In some regions, the meningeal and periosteal layers are separated to form the cavities for the **venous sinuses** in the dura mater. In this dissection the longitudinally oriented **superior sagittal sinus** has been opened, as have a number of lateral venous lacunae that communicate with this sinus.

(3) The **arachnoid granulations**. These are elevated bulbous protrusions of the arachnoid into the dura mater and, since they grow from infancy through childhood, they eventually form pits on the inner surface of the skull (see Fig. 570.1).

(4) The projections from the arachnoid are called **arachnoid villi** and appear as diverticula of the subarachnoid space into the venous sinuses. Cerebrospinal fluid passes from the subarachnoid space through the arachnoid villi into the venous blood of the dural sinus (see also Fig. 573.2).

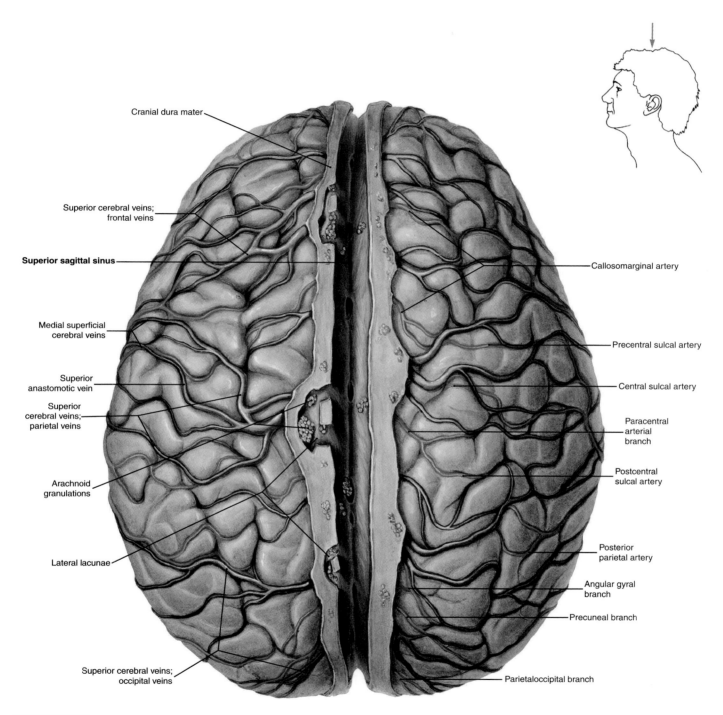

Cranial dura mater

Superior cerebral veins; frontal veins

Superior sagittal sinus

Medial superficial cerebral veins

Superior anastomotic vein

Superior cerebral veins; parietal veins

Arachnoid granulations

Lateral lacunae

Superior cerebral veins; occipital veins

Callosomarginal artery

Precentral sulcal artery

Central sulcal artery

Paracentral arterial branch

Postcentral sulcal artery

Posterior parietal artery

Angular gyral branch

Precuneal branch

Parietaloccipital branch

FIGURE 576 Arteries and Veins on the External Surface of the Cerebral Cortex

NOTE: (1) The **superior sagittal sinus** into which drain the superficial veins on the surface of the cerebral cortex.
(2) The **precentral, central, and postcentral sulcal arteries** that supply much of the parietal lobe of the cortex.
(3) The **arachnoid granulations** through which filters the cerebrospinal fluid that is returned to the venous system.

PLATE 577 **Dura Mater and Dural Venous Sinuses (Lateral View)**

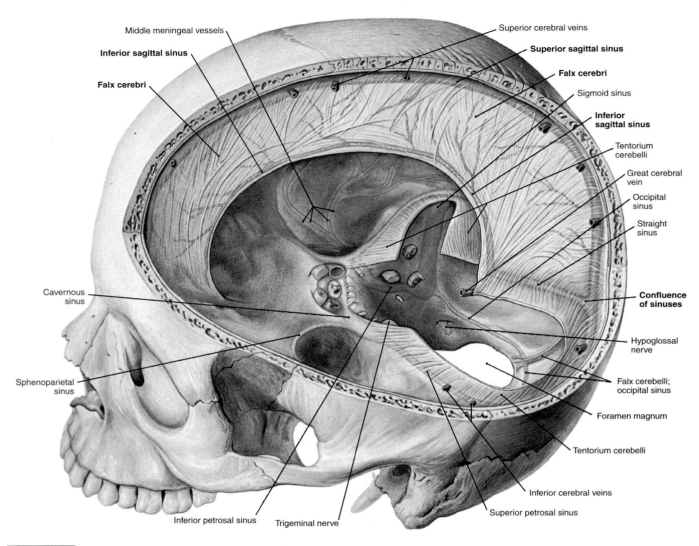

Middle meningeal vessels

Inferior sagittal sinus

Falx cerebri

Cavernous sinus

Sphenoparietal sinus

Inferior petrosal sinus

Trigeminal nerve

Superior cerebral veins

Superior sagittal sinus

Falx cerebri

Sigmoid sinus

Inferior sagittal sinus

Tentorium cerebelli

Great cerebral vein

Occipital sinus

Straight sinus

Confluence of sinuses

Hypoglossal nerve

Falx cerebelli; occipital sinus

Foramen magnum

Tentorium cerebelli

Inferior cerebral veins

Superior petrosal sinus

FIGURE 577 **Intracranial Dura Mater and the Dural Sinuses**

NOTE: (1) With the skull opened and the brain removed, the reflections of the dura mater are exposed. The sinuses are colored blue, the arteries red. Most of the left **tentorium cerebelli** and part of the right were cut away to open the posterior cranial fossa.

(2) The six **unpaired sinuses**: the **superior** and **inferior sagittal sinuses**, the **occipital sinus**, and the **straight sinuses**. Two other unpaired sinuses (not labeled) at the base of the skull are the **intercavernous** and **basilar sinuses**. These can be seen in Figure 578.

(3) The six **paired sinuses**: **transverse, sigmoid, superior** and **inferior petrosal, cavernous**, and **sphenoparietal**. The dural sinuses consist of spaces between the two layers of dura, which drain the cerebral blood, returning it to the **internal jugular vein**.

(4) The **sphenoparietal sinuses** course near the posterior margin of the lesser wings of the sphenoid bone and help form the boundary between the anterior and middle cranial fossae. Similarly, the **superior petrosal sinuses** course along the superior margins of the petrous parts of the temporal bone at the boundary between the middle and posterior cranial fossae.

(5) The sickle-shaped **falx cerebri**. This double-layered, midline reflection of dura mater extends from the crista galli anteriorly to the tentorium cerebelli posteriorly. It also extends vertically between the two cerebral hemispheres. Within the layers of the falx, observe the **superior** and **inferior sagittal sinuses** and the **straight sinus**, all of which flow into the **transverse sinus** or the **confluence of sinuses**.

(6) The **tentorium cerebelli** is a tentlike reflection of dura mater that forms a partition between the occipital lobes of the cerebral cortex and the cerebellum. The **falx cerebelli** extends vertically between the two cerebellar hemispheres.

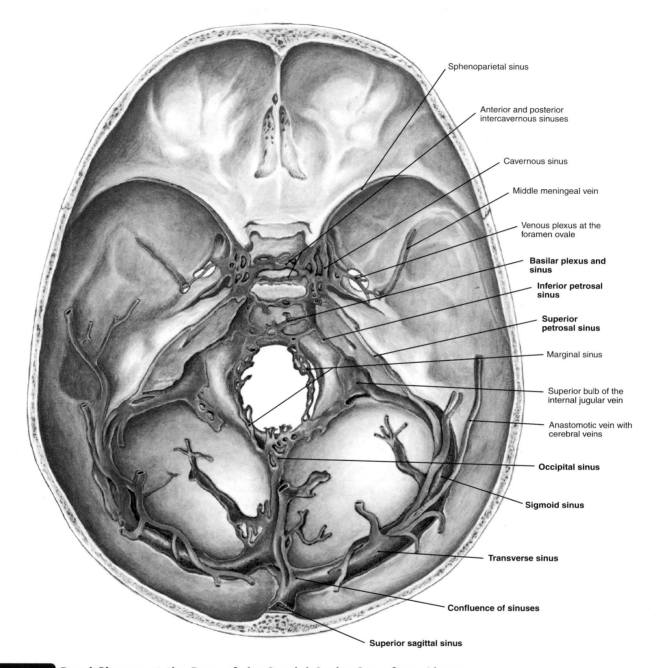

Sphenoparietal sinus

Anterior and posterior intercavernous sinuses

Cavernous sinus

Middle meningeal vein

Venous plexus at the foramen ovale

Basilar plexus and sinus

Inferior petrosal sinus

Superior petrosal sinus

Marginal sinus

Superior bulb of the internal jugular vein

Anastomotic vein with cerebral veins

Occipital sinus

Sigmoid sinus

Transverse sinus

Confluence of sinuses

Superior sagittal sinus

FIGURE 578 **Dural Sinuses at the Base of the Cranial Cavity Seen from Above**

NOTE: (1) The falx cerebri and the tentorium cerebelli and other dural reflections at the base of the cranial cavity have been removed to expose the venous sinuses from above.

(2) On both sides, the **transverse sinus** courses laterally from the **confluence of sinuses** and then continues as the **sigmoid sinus**. Just above the jugular foramen, the sigmoid sinus enlarges as the **superior bulb of the internal jugular vein**. Below the jugular foramen it becomes the **internal jugular vein** (see Fig. 562).

(3) Venous blood also flows to the transverse-sigmoid sinus from the **occipital sinus** and the **superior** and **inferior petrosal sinuses**. In addition, the **cavernous, intercavernous,** and **basilar sinuses** adjacent to the body of the sphenoid bone and the basilar part of the occipital bone also drain posteriorly and laterally into the sigmoid sinus at the jugular foramen.

(4) Anastomoses between these internal sinuses and the external veins occur through the various foramina, such as the superior orbital fissure (with the ophthalmic veins) and through the foramen lacerum and the foramen ovale (with the pterygoid plexus of veins). Other anastomoses occur with the cerebral, meningeal, and emissary veins.

PLATE 579 **Internal Carotid and Vertebral Arteries**

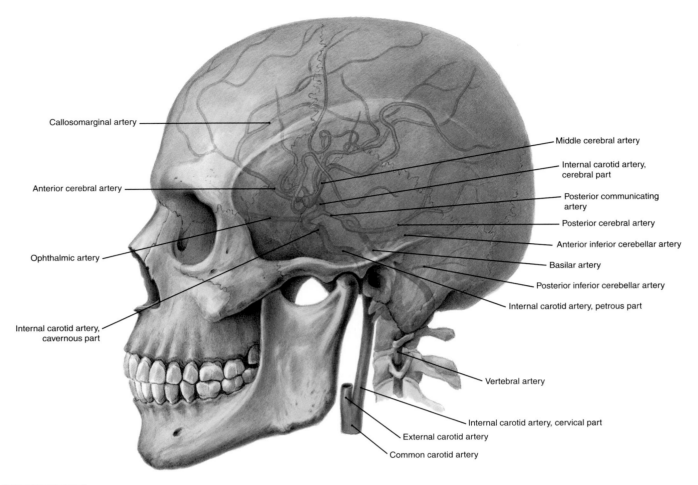

Callosomarginal artery

Anterior cerebral artery

Ophthalmic artery

Internal carotid artery, cavernous part

Middle cerebral artery

Internal carotid artery, cerebral part

Posterior communicating artery

Posterior cerebral artery

Anterior inferior cerebellar artery

Basilar artery

Posterior inferior cerebellar artery

Internal carotid artery, petrous part

Vertebral artery

Internal carotid artery, cervical part

External carotid artery

Common carotid artery

FIGURE 579.1 **Internal Carotid and Vertebral Arteries: Intracerebral Branches**

NOTE: The direct branches off of the internal carotid artery in the skull are the ophthalmic arteries; the anterior and middle cerebral arteries; and the posterior communicating branch to the circle of Willis.

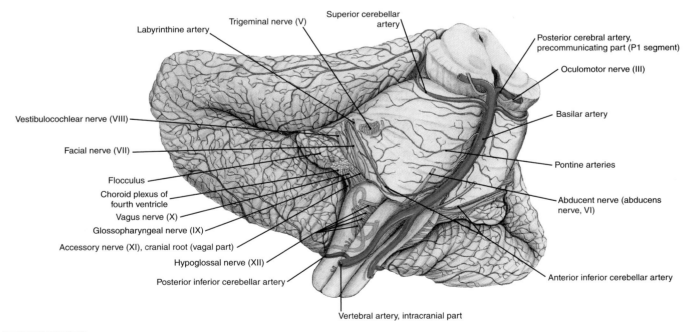

Labyrinthine artery

Trigeminal nerve (V)

Superior cerebellar artery

Posterior cerebral artery, precommunicating part (P1 segment)

Oculomotor nerve (III)

Vestibulocochlear nerve (VIII)

Basilar artery

Facial nerve (VII)

Pontine arteries

Flocculus

Choroid plexus of fourth ventricle

Vagus nerve (X)

Glossopharyngeal nerve (IX)

Accessory nerve (XI), cranial root (vagal part)

Hypoglossal nerve (XII)

Posterior inferior cerebellar artery

Abducent nerve (abducens nerve, VI)

Anterior inferior cerebellar artery

Vertebral artery, intracranial part

FIGURE 579.2 **Basilar Artery and Its Branches**

NOTE: The two vertebral arteries join to form the **basilar artery**, which ascends on the ventral surface of the brainstem. These vessels supply the cerebellum, medulla oblongata, pons, and posterior aspect of the cerebral cortex. The vertebral arteries also send descending branches to supply the spinal cord.

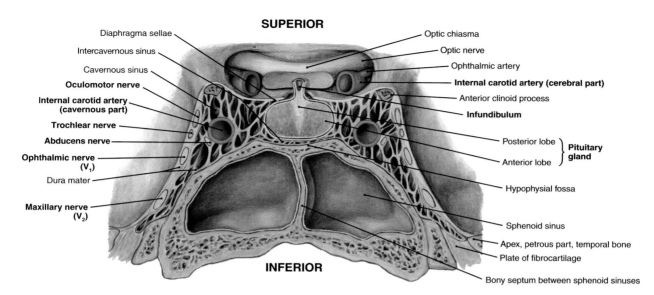

SUPERIOR

Diaphragma sellae
Intercavernous sinus
Cavernous sinus
Oculomotor nerve
Internal carotid artery (cavernous part)
Trochlear nerve
Abducens nerve
Ophthalmic nerve (V₁)
Dura mater
Maxillary nerve (V₂)

Optic chiasma
Optic nerve
Ophthalmic artery
Internal carotid artery (cerebral part)
Anterior clinoid process
Infundibulum
Posterior lobe } **Pituitary gland**
Anterior lobe }
Hypophysial fossa
Sphenoid sinus
Apex, petrous part, temporal bone
Plate of fibrocartilage
Bony septum between sphenoid sinuses

INFERIOR

FIGURE 580.1 **Frontal Section through the Cavernous Sinus and Base of the Skull Showing the Internal Carotid Artery**

NOTE: (1) This is an anterior view of the cavernous sinus and shows the internal carotid artery (which is seen to have turned back on itself) and the oculomotor, trochlear, V₂, V₃, and abducens nerves all within the cavernous sinus.
(2) Upon traversing the carotid canal, the internal carotid artery courses anteriorly, medially, and superiorly to enter the cavernous sinus.
(3) **Within the sinus,** the artery initially courses forward (medial to the abducens nerve and the sphenoid bone, as shown in this figure). The vessel then curves superiorly and then posteriorly in a U-shaped manner and pierces the dura mater medial to the anterior clinoid process. At this site the **ophthalmic artery** branches from the main stem.
(4) The internal carotid artery then gives off the **anterior** and **middle cerebral arteries,** as shown in Figure 580.2.

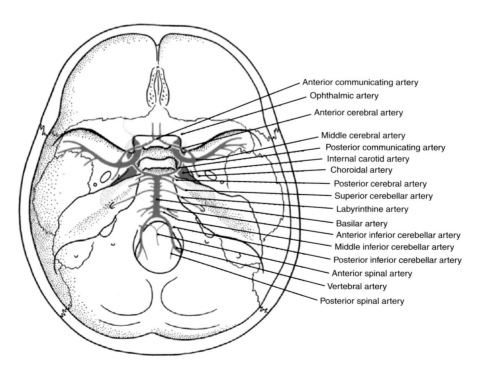

Anterior communicating artery
Ophthalmic artery
Anterior cerebral artery
Middle cerebral artery
Posterior communicating artery
Internal carotid artery
Choroidal artery
Posterior cerebral artery
Superior cerebellar artery
Labyrinthine artery
Basilar artery
Anterior inferior cerebellar artery
Middle inferior cerebellar artery
Posterior inferior cerebellar artery
Anterior spinal artery
Vertebral artery
Posterior spinal artery

FIGURE 580.2 **Cerebral Part of the Internal Carotid Artery and Other Vessels at the Base of the Brain**

NOTE: The two internal carotid arteries (cerebral parts) and the basilar artery (formed by the two vertebral arteries) give rise to all the named vessels in this figure (see also Fig. 581.2).

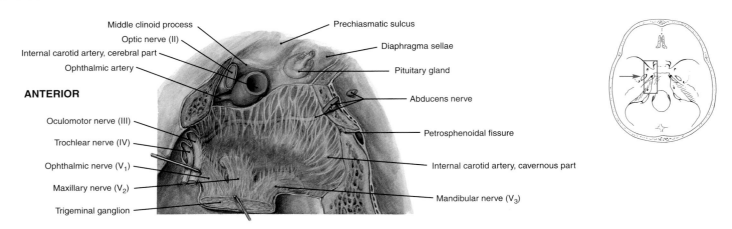

Middle clinoid process
Optic nerve (II)
Internal carotid artery, cerebral part
Ophthalmic artery

ANTERIOR

Oculomotor nerve (III)
Trochlear nerve (IV)
Ophthalmic nerve (V$_1$)
Maxillary nerve (V$_2$)
Trigeminal ganglion

Prechiasmatic sulcus
Diaphragma sellae
Pituitary gland
Abducens nerve
Petrosphenoidal fissure
Internal carotid artery, cavernous part
Mandibular nerve (V$_3$)

FIGURE 581.1 Internal Carotid Artery within the Cavernous Sinus

NOTE: The lateral dural wall of the cavernous sinus has been removed and the trigeminal ganglion has been pulled laterally. Observe the loop formed by the internal carotid artery before entering the base of the skull and the ophthalmic artery branching anteriorly to enter the orbit in the optic canal with the optic nerve.

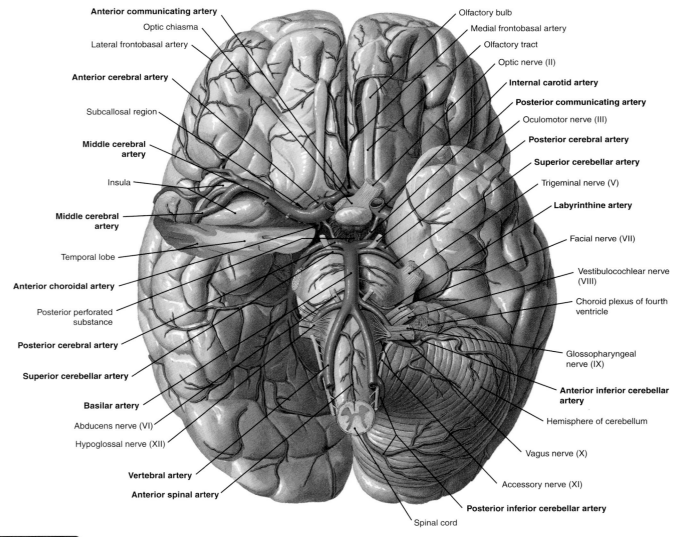

Anterior communicating artery
Optic chiasma
Lateral frontobasal artery
Anterior cerebral artery
Subcallosal region
Middle cerebral artery
Insula
Middle cerebral artery
Temporal lobe
Anterior choroidal artery
Posterior perforated substance
Posterior cerebral artery
Superior cerebellar artery
Basilar artery
Abducens nerve (VI)
Hypoglossal nerve (XII)
Vertebral artery
Anterior spinal artery

Olfactory bulb
Medial frontobasal artery
Olfactory tract
Optic nerve (II)
Internal carotid artery
Posterior communicating artery
Oculomotor nerve (III)
Posterior cerebral artery
Superior cerebellar artery
Trigeminal nerve (V)
Labyrinthine artery
Facial nerve (VII)
Vestibulocochlear nerve (VIII)
Choroid plexus of fourth ventricle
Glossopharyngeal nerve (IX)
Anterior inferior cerebellar artery
Hemisphere of cerebellum
Vagus nerve (X)
Accessory nerve (XI)
Posterior inferior cerebellar artery
Spinal cord

FIGURE 581.2 Arteries at the Base of the Brain

NOTE: (1) Branches of the **vertebral arteries** form the anterior spinal artery medially and the posterior inferior cerebellar arteries *laterally*.
(2) The **basilar artery** is formed near the pontomedullary junction and gives off the anterior inferior cerebellar, labyrinthine, pontine (not labeled), superior cerebellar, and posterior cerebral arteries successively as it ascends.
(3) The **internal carotid arteries** connect with the posterior cerebral by way of the posterior communicating arteries and then give off the middle and anterior cerebral arteries. The anterior cerebral arteries are joined by the anterior communicating artery.

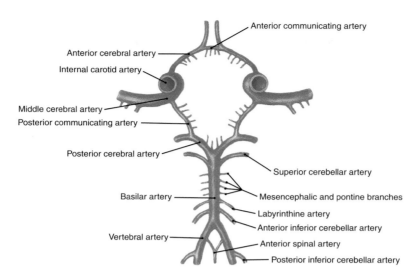

FIGURE 582.1 Circle of Willis

NOTE: The circle of Willis is formed by the **posterior cerebral, posterior communicating, internal carotid, anterior cerebral,** and **anterior communicating arteries.**

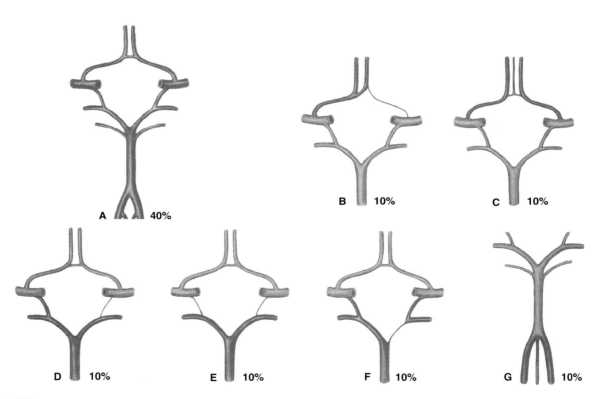

FIGURE 582.2 Variations in the Formation of the Circle of Willis

NOTE: Only about 40% of cadavers show the "normal" pattern of formation seen in **A.**

 A shows the "normal" textbook pattern.
 B shows a narrow anterior cerebral artery on one side.
 C shows a small branch coursing forward from the anterior communicating artery.
 D shows a narrow posterior communicating artery on one side.
 E shows narrow posterior communicating arteries on both sides.
 F shows a narrow posterior cerebral artery on one side. The posterior cerebral artery on the side with the anomaly is substituted for by a continuation of the posterior communicating artery of that same side.
 G shows a low junction of the two vertebral arteries in the formation of the basilar artery.

PLATE 583 Carotid Arteriogram (Lateral View)

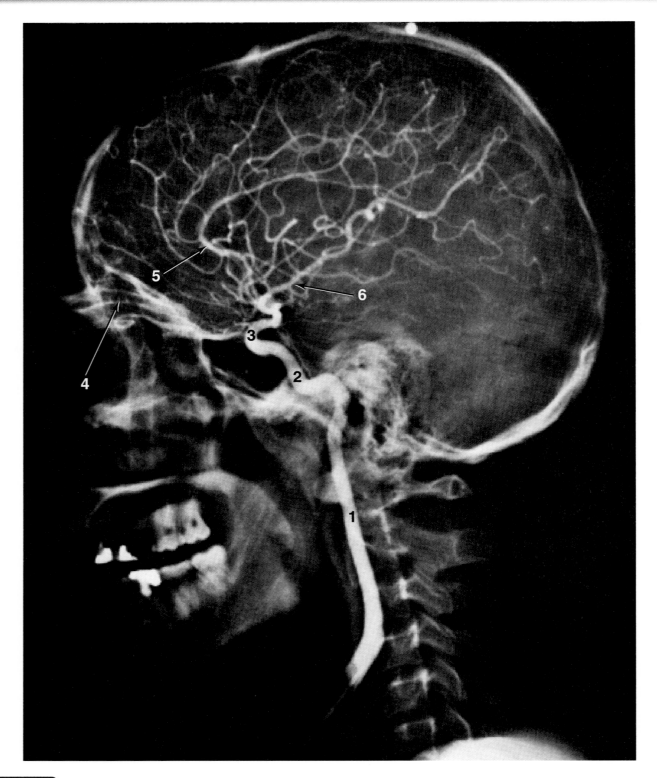

FIGURE 583 Carotid Arteriogram (Lateral View)

NOTE: (1) This is a lateral view of a left carotid arteriogram showing the internal carotid artery and its **cervical, petrous,** and **cavernous** parts before entering the cranial cavity as the **cerebral** part.
(2) The cervical part courses in the carotid canal, whereas the cavernous part courses through the cavernous sinus.
(3) The ophthalmic artery is a branch of the internal carotid artery that enters the orbital cone posteriorly. Also note the anterior and middle cerebral arteries that branch from the anterior end of the circle of Willis.

1. Internal carotid artery (cervical part)
2. Internal carotid artery (petrous part)
3. Internal carotid artery (cavernous part)
4. Ophthalmic artery
5. Anterior cerebral artery
6. Middle cerebral artery

(From Wicke, 6th ed.)

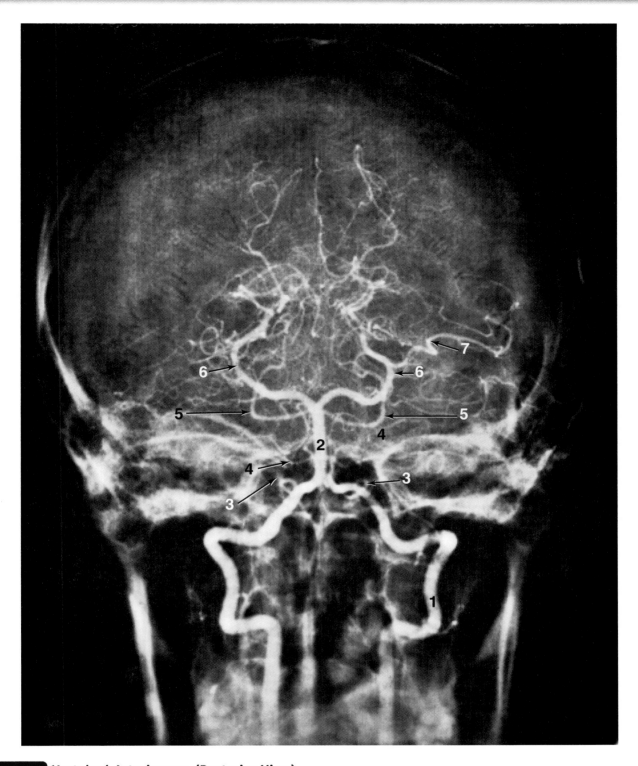

FIGURE 584 **Vertebral Arteriogram (Posterior View)**

NOTE: (1) The two vertebral arteries ascend in the neck through foramina in the transverse processes of the first six cervical vertebrae. Above the atlas the arteries bend medially and lie in a groove on the superior surface of the atlas.

(2) The two vessels perforate the atlantooccipito membrane and join on the ventral surface of the medulla oblongata to form the **basilar artery.** This vessel ascends along the pons and finally terminates as it divides into the two **posterior cerebral arteries.**

(3) On their ascent, the vertebral and basilar arteries supply the cerebellum, the medulla, and pons and also give off the branches that form the **anterior spinal artery.**

1. Vertebral artery
2. Basilar artery
3. Posterior inferior cerebellar artery
4. Anterior inferior cerebellar artery
5. Superior cerebellar artery
6. Posterior cerebral artery (sometimes referred to as the artery of sight)
7. Occipital branch of the posterior cerebral artery

(From Wicke, 6th ed.)

PLATE 585 Paramedian Section of the Skull

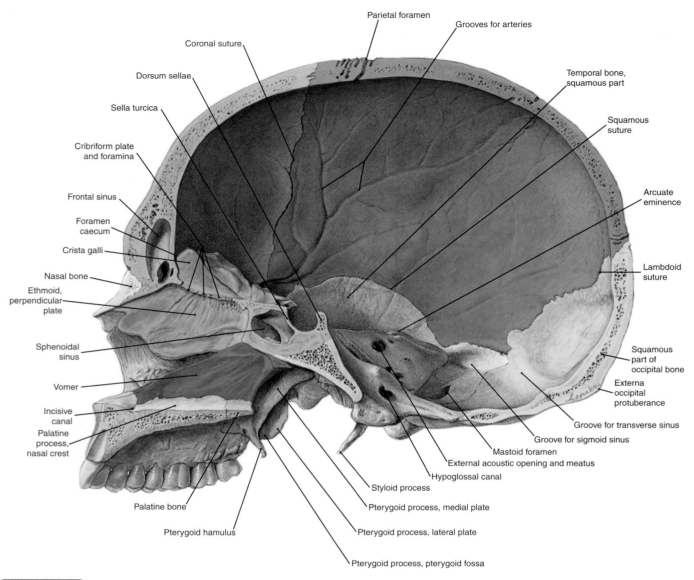

Parietal foramen

Grooves for arteries

Coronal suture

Dorsum sellae

Temporal bone,
squamous part

Sella turcica

Squamous
suture

Cribriform plate
and foramina

Frontal sinus

Arcuate
eminence

Foramen
caecum

Crista galli

Nasal bone

Lambdoid
suture

Ethmoid,
perpendicular
plate

Sphenoidal
sinus

Squamous
part of
occipital bone

Vomer

Externa
occipital
protuberance

Incisive
canal

Groove for transverse sinus

Palatine
process,
nasal crest

Groove for sigmoid sinus

Mastoid foramen

External acoustic opening and meatus

Hypoglossal canal

Styloid process

Palatine bone

Pterygoid process, medial plate

Pterygoid hamulus

Pterygoid process, lateral plate

Pterygoid process, pterygoid fossa

FIGURE 585.1 Paramedian Section of the Skull

NOTE: This section was made slightly to the left of the midline so that a medial view of the right half of the skull is presented. Observe that the vomer (a midline bone) is shown in its entirety and the palatine and maxilla are cut slightly to the left of the midline.

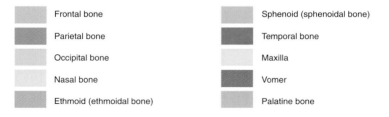

Frontal bone	Sphenoid (sphenoidal bone)
Parietal bone	Temporal bone
Occipital bone	Maxilla
Nasal bone	Vomer
Ethmoid (ethmoidal bone)	Palatine bone

FIGURE 585.2 Base of the Skull: Internal Aspect (Superior View)

NOTE: There are important structures that traverse the foramina at the base of the skull.
(1) **Anterior cranial fossa**:
  (a) **Foramen cecum**: a small vein
  (b) **Cribriform plate**: filaments of olfactory receptor neurons to the olfactory bulb
  (c) **Anterior ethmoid foramen**: anterior ethmoidal vessels and nerve
  (d) **Posterior ethmoid foramen**: posterior ethmoidal vessels and nerve
(2) **Middle cranial fossa**:
  (a) **Optic foramen**: optic nerve; ophthalmic artery
  (b) **Superior orbital fissure**: oculomotor nerve; trochlear nerve; ophthalmic nerve; abducens nerve; sympathetic nerve fibers; superior ophthalmic vein; orbital branch of middle meningeal artery; dural recurrent branch of the lacrimal artery
  (c) **Foramen rotundum**: maxillary nerve

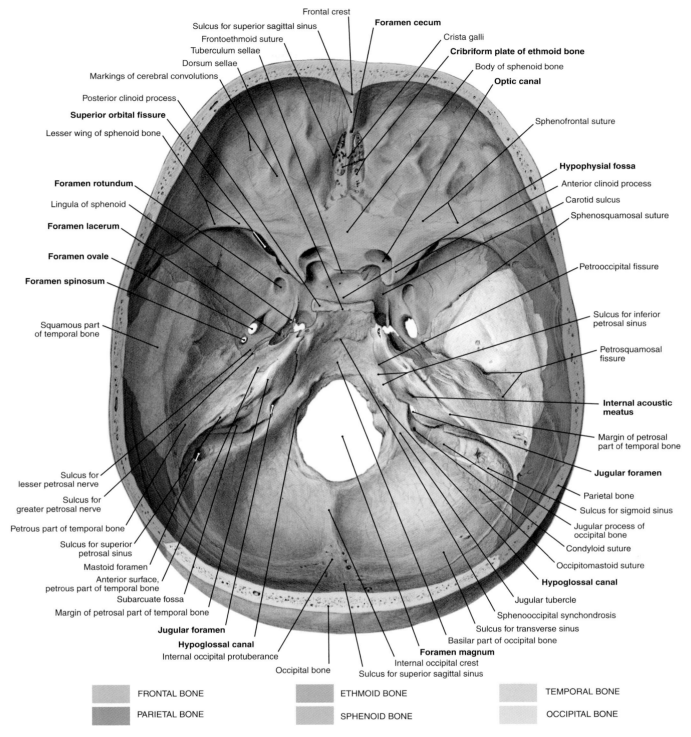

Frontal crest
Sulcus for superior sagittal sinus
Frontoethmoid suture
Tuberculum sellae
Dorsum sellae
Markings of cerebral convolutions
Posterior clinoid process
Superior orbital fissure
Lesser wing of sphenoid bone
Foramen rotundum
Lingula of sphenoid
Foramen lacerum
Foramen ovale
Foramen spinosum
Squamous part of temporal bone
Sulcus for lesser petrosal nerve
Sulcus for greater petrosal nerve
Petrous part of temporal bone
Sulcus for superior petrosal sinus
Mastoid foramen
Anterior surface, petrous part of temporal bone
Subarcuate fossa
Margin of petrosal part of temporal bone
Jugular foramen
Hypoglossal canal
Internal occipital protuberance
Occipital bone

Foramen cecum
Crista galli
Cribriform plate of ethmoid bone
Body of sphenoid bone
Optic canal
Sphenofrontal suture
Hypophysial fossa
Anterior clinoid process
Carotid sulcus
Sphenosquamosal suture
Petrooccipital fissure
Sulcus for inferior petrosal sinus
Petrosquamosal fissure
Internal acoustic meatus
Margin of petrosal part of temporal bone
Jugular foramen
Parietal bone
Sulcus for sigmoid sinus
Jugular process of occipital bone
Condyloid suture
Occipitomastoid suture
Hypoglossal canal
Jugular tubercle
Sphenooccipital synchondrosis
Sulcus for transverse sinus
Basilar part of occipital bone
Foramen magnum
Internal occipital crest
Sulcus for superior sagittal sinus

FRONTAL BONE
PARIETAL BONE
ETHMOID BONE
SPHENOID BONE
TEMPORAL BONE
OCCIPITAL BONE

FIGURE 586 **Base of the Skull: Internal Aspect (Continued from Previous Page)**

  (d) **Foramen ovale**: mandibular nerve; accessory meningeal artery
  (e) **Foramen spinosum**: middle meningeal artery; a recurrent dural branch of mandibular nerve
  (f) **Foramen lacerum**: The internal carotid artery passes across the foramen above the fibrocartilaginous plate but does *not* traverse it. The nerve of the pterygoid canal emerges from the foramen to enter the pterygoid canal. The meningeal branch of the ascending pharyngeal artery actually traverses the foramen
(3) **Posterior cranial fossa**:
  (a) **Internal acoustic meatus**: facial nerve; vestibulocochlear nerve; labyrinthine artery
  (b) **Jugular foramen**: sigmoid sinus, which becomes internal jugular vein; meningeal branches of occipital and ascending pharyngeal arteries; glossopharyngeal nerve; vagus nerve; accessory nerve
  (c) **Hypoglossal canal**: hypoglossal nerve
  (d) **Foramen magnum**: spinal cord; spinal part of accessory nerve; anterior and posterior spinal arteries; vertebral arteries; tectorial membrane

PLATE 587 Bony Floor of the Cranial Cavity; The Pituitary Gland

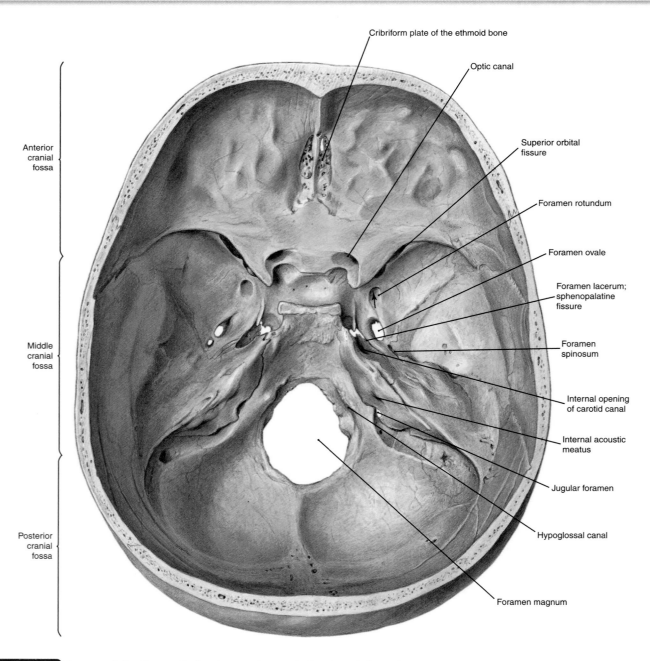

Cribriform plate of the ethmoid bone

Optic canal

Superior orbital fissure

Foramen rotundum

Foramen ovale

Foramen lacerum; sphenopalatine fissure

Foramen spinosum

Internal opening of carotid canal

Internal acoustic meatus

Jugular foramen

Hypoglossal canal

Foramen magnum

Anterior cranial fossa

Middle cranial fossa

Posterior cranial fossa

FIGURE 587.1 **Internal Surface of the Bony Floor of the Cranial Cavity**

NOTE the anterior, middle, and posterior cranial fossae. The **anterior fossa** sustains the frontal lobes, while the **middle fossa** holds the temporal lobes. The **posterior fossa** is continuous with the vertebral column, and it houses the cerebellum, pons, and medulla oblongata. The latter is continuous with the spinal cord.

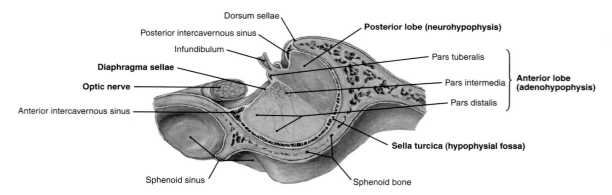

Dorsum sellae

Posterior intercavernous sinus

Infundibulum

Diaphragma sellae

Optic nerve

Anterior intercavernous sinus

Sphenoid sinus

Sphenoid bone

Posterior lobe (neurohypophysis)

Pars tuberalis

Pars intermedia

Pars distalis

Anterior lobe (adenohypophysis)

Sella turcica (hypophysial fossa)

FIGURE 587.2 **Median Sagittal Section through the Pituitary Gland and the Sella Turcica of the Sphenoid Bone**

NOTE: The **sella turcica** (hypophysial fossa) in the sphenoid bone is lined and covered (**diaphragma sellae**) by dura mater. The anterior and posterior lobes form a single organ that lies below and slightly behind the optic chiasma.

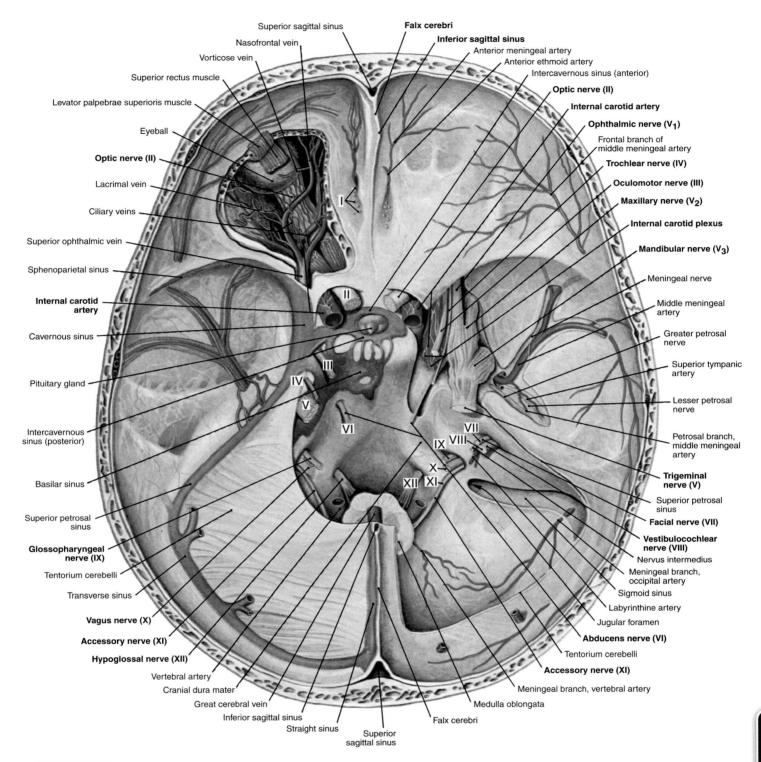

FIGURE 588 Base of the Cranial Cavity: Vessels, Nerves, and Dura Mater

NOTE: (1) The anterior, middle, and posterior **cranial fossae** in the floor of the cranial cavity. In the anterior fossae rest the **frontal lobes** of the brain, whereas the **temporal lobes** lie in the middle fossae and the **brainstem** and **cerebellum** rest in the posterior fossa.

(2) The dura mater and the orbital plate of the frontal bone have been removed to expose the left orbit from above. The **superior ophthalmic vein** drains posteriorly into the cavernous sinus and the **optic nerve** is seen to course from the orbit through the optic canal.

(3) The medial aspect of the middle fossa shows the cavernous sinus, the internal carotid artery, the third, fourth, fifth, and sixth cranial nerves coursing toward the orbit or the face, and the middle meningeal artery traversing the foramen spinosum.

(4) The foramina for the last six pairs of cranial nerves in the posterior fossa. The 7th and 8th nerves pass through the internal acoustic meatus, whereas the 9th, 10th, and 11th nerves traverse the jugular foramen and the 12th nerve traverses at the hypoglossal canal.

PLATE 589 Inferior Surface of the Brain: Cranial Nerves

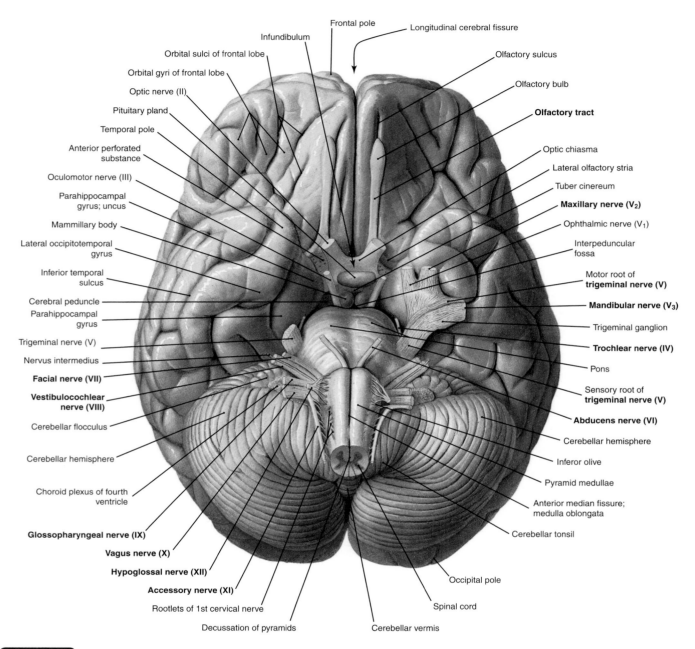

Frontal pole

Infundibulum

Longitudinal cerebral fissure

Orbital sulci of frontal lobe

Olfactory sulcus

Orbital gyri of frontal lobe

Olfactory bulb

Optic nerve (II)

Olfactory tract

Pituitary pland

Temporal pole

Optic chiasma

Anterior perforated
substance

Lateral olfactory stria

Oculomotor nerve (III)

Tuber cinereum

Parahippocampal
gyrus; uncus

Maxillary nerve (V₂)

Mammillary body

Ophthalmic nerve (V₁)

Lateral occipitotemporal
gyrus

Interpeduncular
fossa

Inferior temporal
sulcus

Motor root of
trigeminal nerve (V)

Cerebral peduncle

Mandibular nerve (V₃)

Parahippocampal
gyrus

Trigeminal ganglion

Trigeminal nerve (V)

Trochlear nerve (IV)

Nervus intermedius

Pons

Facial nerve (VII)

Sensory root of
trigeminal nerve (V)

**Vestibulocochlear
nerve (VIII)**

Abducens nerve (VI)

Cerebellar flocculus

Cerebellar hemisphere

Cerebellar hemisphere

Inferor olive

Choroid plexus of fourth
ventricle

Pyramid medullae

Anterior median fissure;
medulla oblongata

Glossopharyngeal nerve (IX)

Cerebellar tonsil

Vagus nerve (X)

Hypoglossal nerve (XII)

Accessory nerve (XI)

Occipital pole

Rootlets of 1st cervical nerve

Spinal cord

Decussation of pyramids

Cerebellar vermis

FIGURE 589 Ventral View of the Brain Showing the Origins of the Cranial Nerves

NOTE: (1) The cranial nerves attach to the base of the brain. The **olfactory tracts** and **optic nerves** (**I** and **II**) subserve receptors of special sense in the nose and eye, and as cranial nerve trunks attach to the base of the forebrain in contrast to all other cranial nerves that attach to the midbrain, pons, or medulla of the brainstem.

(2) The **oculomotor (III), trochlear (IV)**, and **abducens (VI) nerves** are motor nerves to the extraocular muscles. The **trigeminal nerve (V)** is the largest of the cranial nerves, and the **trochlear** is the smallest. The abducens nerve attaches to the brainstem at the junction of the pons and medulla (pontomedullary junction) medial to the attachments of the **facial (VII)** and **vestibulocochlear (VIII) nerves**.

(3) The **glossopharyngeal (IX)** and **vagus (X) nerves** emerge from the medulla laterally in a line comparable to the spinal and medullary parts of the **accessory nerve (XI)**. In contrast, the **hypoglossal nerve (XII)** rootlets emerge from the ventral medulla in a line consistent with the ventral rootlets of the cervical nerves of the spinal cord.

(4) The cranial nerves are of the utmost importance as signposts in localizing disorders both inside and outside the cranial cavity. The functions of most cranial nerves are tested in each complete physical examination performed by competent physicians.

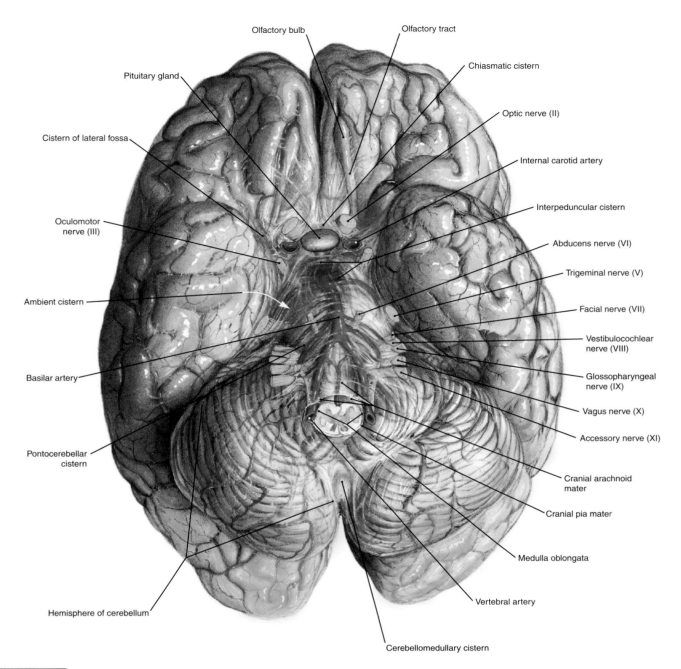

Olfactory bulb

Olfactory tract

Chiasmatic cistern

Pituitary gland

Optic nerve (II)

Cistern of lateral fossa

Internal carotid artery

Interpeduncular cistern

Oculomotor nerve (III)

Abducens nerve (VI)

Trigeminal nerve (V)

Ambient cistern

Facial nerve (VII)

Vestibulocochlear nerve (VIII)

Basilar artery

Glossopharyngeal nerve (IX)

Vagus nerve (X)

Accessory nerve (XI)

Cranial arachnoid mater

Pontocerebellar cistern

Cranial pia mater

Medulla oblongata

Hemisphere of cerebellum

Vertebral artery

Cerebellomedullary cistern

FIGURE 590 **Base of the Brain: Arteries and Cranial Nerves with the Arachnoid Mater Intact**

NOTE: (1) The dura mater has been completely removed from the brain, leaving intact the arachnoid mater and pia mater. Observe the vertebral arteries joining to form the basilar artery and, anteriorly, the internal carotid arteries severed upon entering the cranial cavity at the base of the brain.

(2) Between the arachnoid mater and the pia mater and the cerebral vessels is the **subarachnoid space**, within which is found the cerebrospinal fluid that is formed in the choroid plexuses. At certain sites the arachnoid mater separates from the pia mater to form pools of cerebrospinal fluid called **cisterns**.

(3) In this figure are seen the cisterns on the ventral aspect of the brainstem; however, they also are located on the dorsal aspect of the brainstem, especially between the cerebellum and the pons and medulla oblongata.

(4) Identify the following cisterns:

(a) The **cistern of the lateral fossa** extends between the orbital surface of the frontal lobe and the anteromedial surface of the temporal lobe. It contains the internal carotid artery.

(b) The **ambient cistern** (also called the **cistern of the great cerebral vein**) is located between the splenium of the corpus callosum and the rostral surface of the cerebellum. It contains the great cerebral vein and the pineal gland.

(c) The **pontocerebellar cistern** on the anterior surface of the pons containing the basilar artery. It communicates superiorly with the interpeduncular cistern and inferiorly with the subarachnoid space of the spinal cord.

(d) The large **cerebellomedullary cistern** (also called the **cisterna magna**) between the medulla oblongata and the inferior surface of the cerebellum.

(e) The **interpeduncular cistern** contains the circle of Willis; it also continues anteriorly as the **chiasmatic cistern** anterior to the pituitary gland and adjacent to the optic chiasma.

PLATE 591 Base of Skull: Inferior Surface, Foramina, and Markings

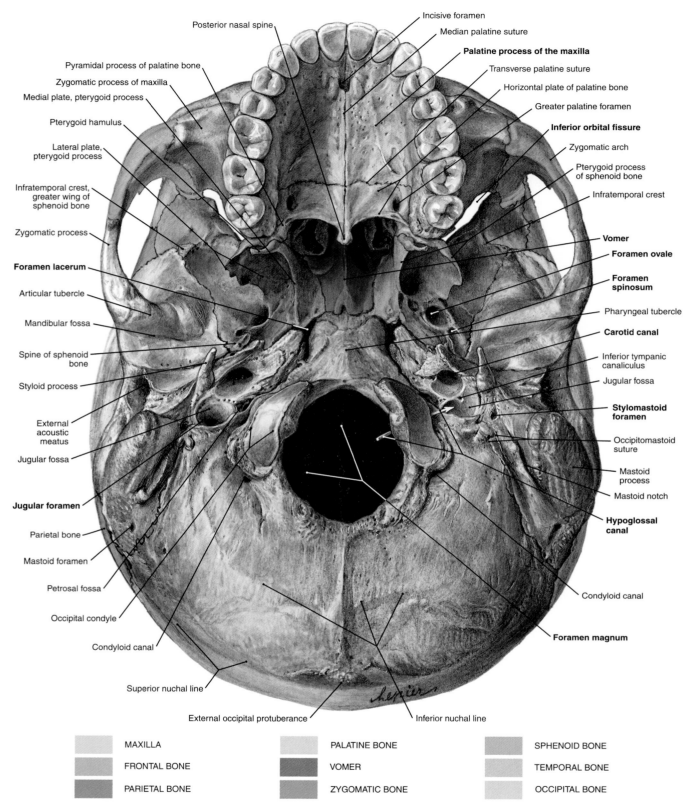

Posterior nasal spine
Pyramidal process of palatine bone
Zygomatic process of maxilla
Medial plate, pterygoid process
Pterygoid hamulus
Lateral plate, pterygoid process
Infratemporal crest, greater wing of sphenoid bone
Zygomatic process
Foramen lacerum
Articular tubercle
Mandibular fossa
Spine of sphenoid bone
Styloid process
External acoustic meatus
Jugular fossa
Jugular foramen
Parietal bone
Mastoid foramen
Petrosal fossa
Occipital condyle
Condyloid canal
Superior nuchal line
External occipital protuberance

Incisive foramen
Median palatine suture
Palatine process of the maxilla
Transverse palatine suture
Horizontal plate of palatine bone
Greater palatine foramen
Inferior orbital fissure
Zygomatic arch
Pterygoid process of sphenoid bone
Infratemporal crest
Vomer
Foramen ovale
Foramen spinosum
Pharyngeal tubercle
Carotid canal
Inferior tympanic canaliculus
Jugular fossa
Stylomastoid foramen
Occipitomastoid suture
Mastoid process
Mastoid notch
Hypoglossal canal
Condyloid canal
Foramen magnum
Inferior nuchal line

MAXILLA   PALATINE BONE   SPHENOID BONE
FRONTAL BONE   VOMER   TEMPORAL BONE
PARIETAL BONE ZYGOMATIC BONE   OCCIPITAL BONE

FIGURE 591 Base of the Skull: External Aspect (Inferior View)

NOTE: (1) The posterior part of the base of the skull consists of the **occipital** and **temporal bones**. Anteriorly are the facial bones: the **maxilla, palatine, zygomatic,** and **vomer**. Interposed between these two groups of bones is the **sphenoid bone.**

(2) The bony palate is formed by the transverse processes of the two maxillae and the horizontal plates of the palatine bones.

(3) The medial and lateral plates of the pterygoid process of the sphenoid bone, behind which are the foramen ovale and foramen spinosum in the greater wings of the sphenoid.

(4) The **foramen lacerum, carotid canal, jugular foramen, styloid process** (of temporal bone), **hypoglossal canal** (arrow), and the **foramen magnum**.

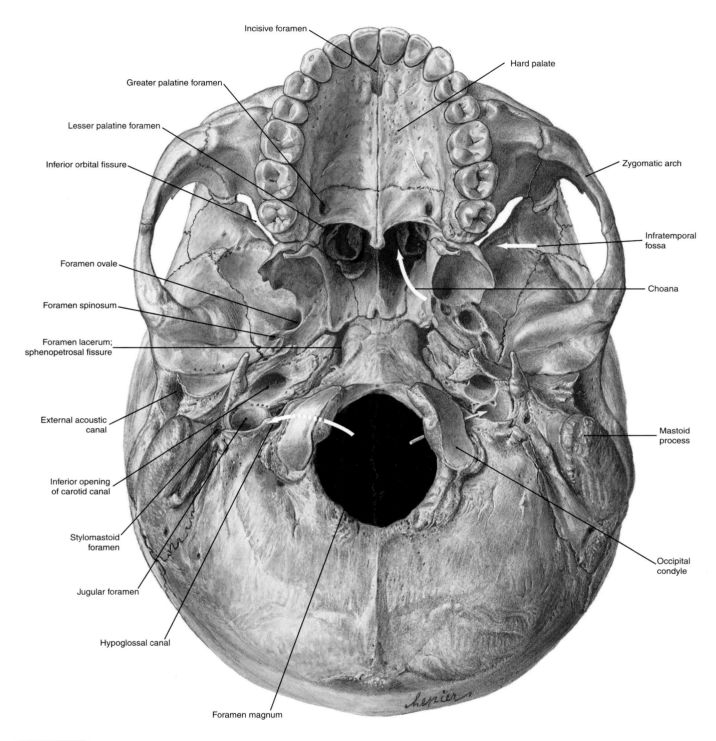

Incisive foramen

Hard palate

Greater palatine foramen

Lesser palatine foramen

Inferior orbital fissure

Zygomatic arch

Foramen ovale

Infratemporal fossa

Foramen spinosum

Choana

Foramen lacerum; sphenopetrosal fissure

External acoustic canal

Mastoid process

Inferior opening of carotid canal

Stylomastoid foramen

Jugular foramen

Occipital condyle

Hypoglossal canal

Foramen magnum

FIGURE 592 Inferior Surface of the Bony Skull

NOTE: (1) The white arrows indicate the **infratemporal fossa**, one **choana**, and the **two hypoglossal canals**. Also observe the **greater and lesser palatine foramina** through which course the greater and lesser palatine arteries and nerves that serve the palate in the oral cavity.

(2) The **foramen lacerum** that is covered inferiorly by a small plate of cartilage across which the internal carotid artery passes prior to its ascending course lateral to the body of the sphenoid bone. The vessel then opens into the floor of the cranial cavity adjacent to the optic nerves.

PLATE 593 Eye: Surface Anatomy (Anterior View)

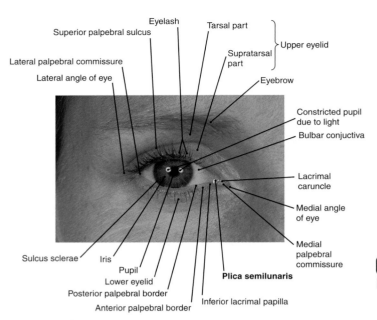

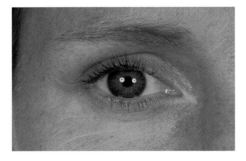

FIGURE 593.2 Photograph of Living Eye Identical to Figure 593.1

FIGURE 593.1 Right Eye and Eyelids

NOTE: (1) The eyeball, protected in front by two movable and thin **eyelids** or **palpebrae**, is covered by a transparent mucous membrane, the **conjunctiva**, which reflects along the inner surface of both eyelids as the **palpebral conjunctiva**.

(2) At the medial angle of the eye is located a small, reddish island of tissue called the **lacrimal caruncle**.

(3) The **pupil** is the opening in the **iris**. Constriction and dilation of the pupil is controlled autonomically. Parasympathetic fibers in the oculomotor nerve innervate the constrictor muscle of the pupil, whereas sympathetic fibers from the superior cervical ganglion supply the pupillary dilator muscle.

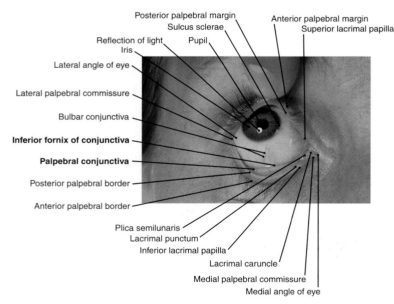

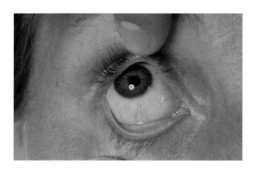

FIGURE 593.4 Photograph of Living Eye Identical to Figure 538.3

FIGURE 593.3 Right Lower Eyelid and Medial Angle

NOTE: (1) The right lower eyelid has been pulled downward to show the inner surface of the lower lid (i.e., the palpebral conjunctiva) and to enlarge the exposure of the medial angle (also called the **medial canthus**).

(2) The conjunctiva is highly vascular, and its bulbar part (over the eyeball) and inferior palpebral part (on the inner surface of the lower eyelid) are continuous along a line of reflection called the **inferior conjunctival fornix**. A similar reflection line, the **superior conjunctival fornix**, lies between the eyeball and the upper eyelid.

(3) When the medial angle is more completely exposed, a pair of small openings, the **lacrimal puncta**, can be found located above and below the lacrimal caruncle. These openings lead into small **lacrimal canals** through which tears enter the **lacrimal sac**.

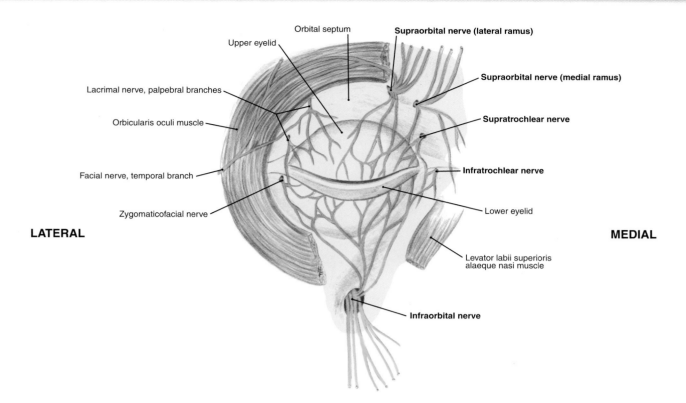

FIGURE 594.1 Innervation of the Eyelids (Anterior View, Right Eye)

NOTE: (1) The rich cutaneous innervation found around the anterior orbit is derived from the ophthalmic and maxillary divisions of the trigeminal nerve, which achieve the anterior orbital region through foramina in the frontal, zygomatic, and maxillary bones.

(2) Superomedially are found the large rami of the **supraorbital** branch of the frontal nerve (V_1), which emerges through the supraorbital foramen or notch. Also note the **supratrochlear** branch of the frontal nerve, which appears through a small foramen above the trochlea of the superior oblique muscle.

(3) The **infratrochlear nerve** is a terminal branch of the nasociliary nerve (V_1) that becomes superficial below the trochlea of the superior oblique. Along with palpebral branches of the **infraorbital nerve** (V_2), it sends fibers to the lower eyelid.

(4) The **lacrimal nerve** (V_1) superolaterally, supplying the upper eyelid; the **zygomaticofacial nerve** (V_2) to the lower eyelid and skin over the cheek bone; the **temporal branch of the facial nerve,** which is a motor nerve to the orbicularis oculi muscle.

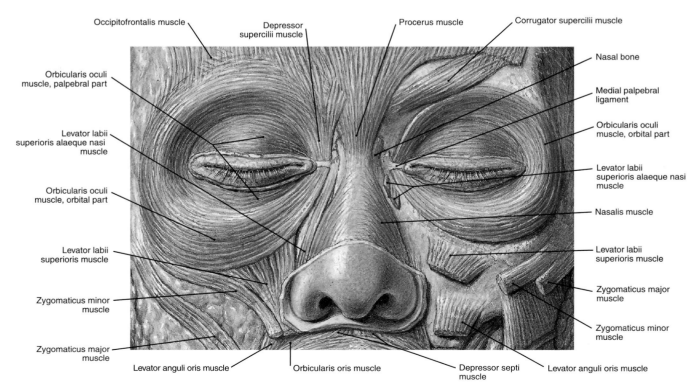

FIGURE 594.2 Superficial Facial Muscles around the Orbit (Anterior View)

PLATE 595 **Bony Orbit (Anterior View and Frontal Section)**

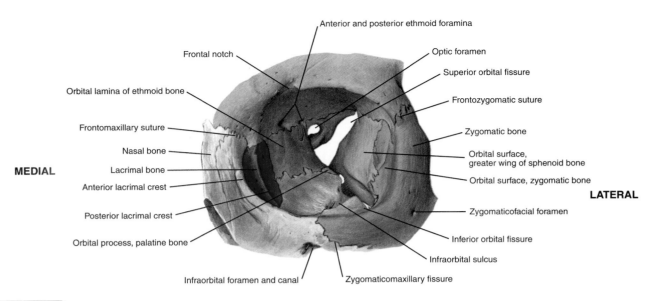

FIGURE 595.1 **Bones That Form the Orbital Cavity (Left Side, Anterior View)**

NOTE: (1) The bony structure of the orbit is composed of parts of seven bones: the **maxilla, zygomatic, frontal, lacrimal, palatine, ethmoid,** and **sphenoid.**

(2) The **roof** of the orbit is formed by the orbital plate of the **frontal bone**; the **floor** consists of the orbital plate of the **maxilla,** the **palatine,** and the **zygomatic bones**; the **medial wall** is thin and delicate and is formed by the frontal process of the **maxilla,** the orbital lamina of the **ethmoid,** and the **lacrimal bone**; and the strong **lateral wall** consists of the orbital processes of the **sphenoid** and **zygomatic bones.**

(3) The **optic foramen,** the **superior** and **inferior orbital fissures,** and the **anterior** and **posterior ethmoid foramina.**

Key for Figures 595.1 and 595.2:

NASAL BONE	VOMER	TEMPORAL BONE
FRONTAL BONE	ZYGOMATIC BONE	INFERIOR NASAL CONCHA
PALATINE BONE	MAXILLA	SPHENOID BONE
ETHMOID BONE		LACRIMAL BONE

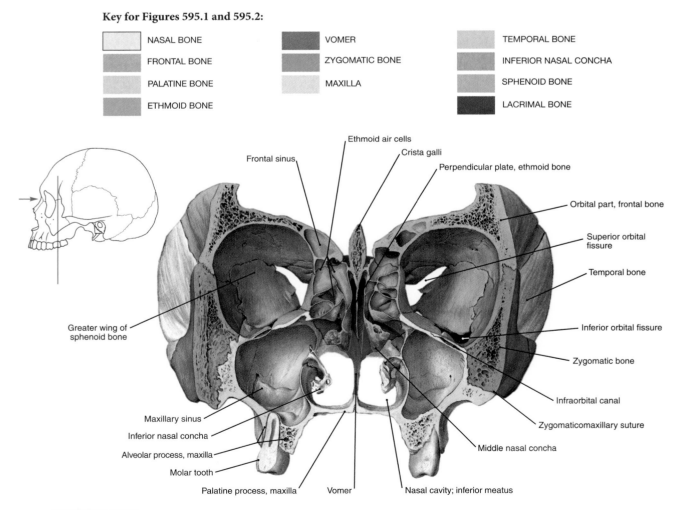

FIGURE 595.2 **Frontal Section through the Orbital and Nasal Cavities and the Maxillary Sinus**

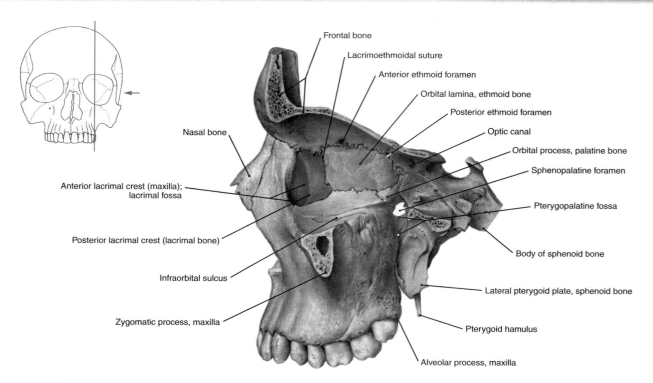

Frontal bone
Lacrimoethmoidal suture
Anterior ethmoid foramen
Orbital lamina, ethmoid bone
Posterior ethmoid foramen
Optic canal
Orbital process, palatine bone
Sphenopalatine foramen
Pterygopalatine fossa
Body of sphenoid bone
Lateral pterygoid plate, sphenoid bone
Pterygoid hamulus
Alveolar process, maxilla

Nasal bone
Anterior lacrimal crest (maxilla); lacrimal fossa
Posterior lacrimal crest (lacrimal bone)
Infraorbital sulcus
Zygomatic process, maxilla

FIGURE 596.1 Medial Wall of the Left Orbital Cavity and a Lateral View of the Pterygopalatine Fossa

NOTE: (1) Anteriorly on the thin medial wall of the orbital cavity is found the **lacrimal fossa** for the **lacrimal sac**. The fossa is limited in front by the anterior lacrimal crest of the maxilla and behind by the posterior lacrimal crest of the lacrimal bone.

(2) The medial wall is formed by the orbital lamina of the **ethmoid bone** and the **lacrimal bone**. The **maxilla** inferiorly and the **sphenoid** and **palatine bones** posteriorly also contribute to this wall. Also observe the **anterior** and **posterior ethmoidal foramina**.

Key for Figures 596.1 and 596.2:

FRONTAL BONE	NASAL BONE	MAXILLA
LACRIMAL BONE	PALATINE BONE	TEMPORAL BONE
SPHENOID BONE	ETHMOID BONE	ZYGOMATIC BONE

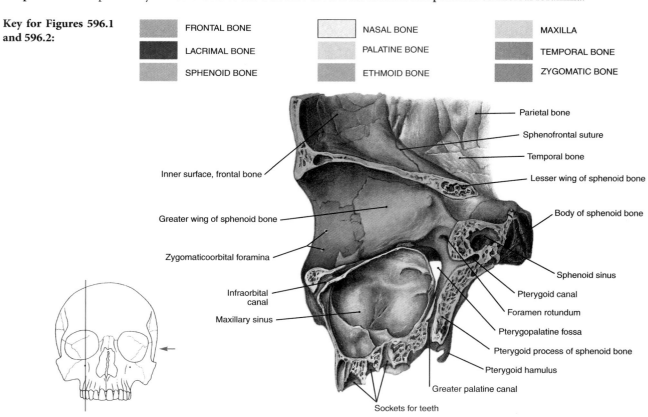

Parietal bone
Sphenofrontal suture
Temporal bone
Lesser wing of sphenoid bone
Body of sphenoid bone
Sphenoid sinus
Pterygoid canal
Foramen rotundum
Pterygopalatine fossa
Pterygoid process of sphenoid bone
Pterygoid hamulus
Greater palatine canal

Inner surface, frontal bone
Greater wing of sphenoid bone
Zygomaticoorbital foramina
Infraorbital canal
Maxillary sinus
Sockets for teeth

FIGURE 596.2 Lateral Wall of the Right Orbital Cavity Bond a Medial View of the Pterygopalatine Fossa

NOTE: (1) The lateral wall of the orbit is formed by the orbital surface of the greater wing of the **sphenoid bone** and the frontal process of the **zygomatic bone**. Note the small zygomaticoorbital foramina through which course the **zygomaticofacial** and **zygomaticotemporal** branches of the maxillary nerve (sensory nerves).

(2) The **foramen rotundum** and the **infraorbital canal** for the **maxillary nerve**. Also note the **maxillary sinus** below the orbit and the **pterygo-palatine fossa** and **greater palatine canal** behind the maxillary sinus and below the apex of the orbit.

PLATE 597 Orbital Septum, Eyelids, and Tarsal Plates

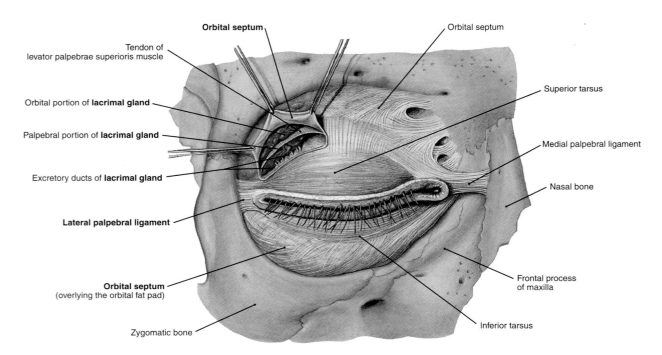

FIGURE 597.1 Orbital Septum, Lacrimal Gland, and Tarsi of the Right Eye

NOTE: (1) With the skin, superficial fascia, and orbicularis oculi muscle removed, the orbital septum has been exposed anteriorly. The septum attaches to the periosteum of the bone peripherally around the orbit and to the tarsi of the eyelids centrally.

(2) The lacrimal gland and its excretory ducts in the upper lateral aspect of the anterior orbit lying just beneath the orbital septum.

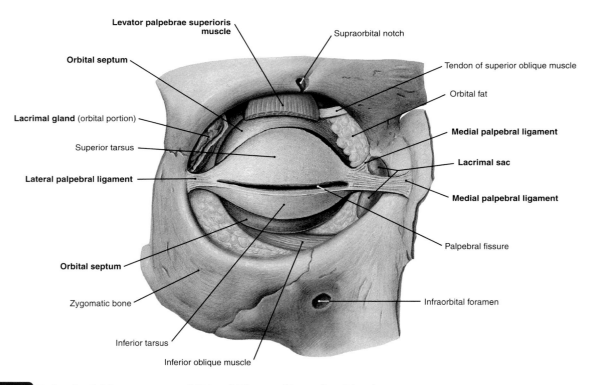

FIGURE 597.2 Palpebral Ligaments and Tarsal Plates (Anterior View)

NOTE: (1) The superficial structures of the orbit have been removed along with the orbital septum and the tendon of the levator palpebrae superioris muscle.

(2) The lateral and medial margins of the tarsal plates are attached to the lateral and medial palpebral ligaments, which in turn are attached to bone. The medial ligament is located just anterior to the lacrimal sac.

(3) From this anterior view, both the tendon of the superior oblique muscle and the inferior oblique muscle can be visualized. Also note the location of the orbital portion of the lacrimal gland in the upper lateral part of the orbit.

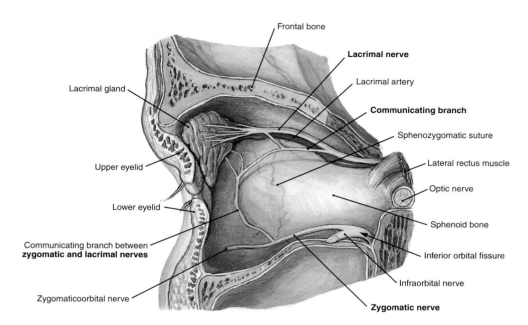

FIGURE 598.1 **Innervation of the Lacrimal Gland**

NOTE: (1) The lacrimal gland is supplied by the lacrimal artery, which is a thin, tortuous branch of the ophthalmic artery that courses anteriorly in the orbital cavity.

(2) The lacrimal gland receives postganglionic parasympathetic fibers that are secretomotor in type. Preganglionic fibers are said to emerge from the brain in the nervus intermedius part of the facial nerve (VII). These fibers then synapse with the cell bodies of the postganglionic neurons in the pterygopalatine ganglion.

(3) The preganglionic parasympathetic fibers reach the pterygopalatine ganglion by way of the greater petrosal nerve, which then becomes part of the nerve of the pterygoid canal. The postganglionic fibers leave the ganglion and travel for a short distance with the zygomatic nerve, a branch of the infraorbital nerve. From this nerve, in the inferior part of the orbit, the parasympathetic fibers, by way of a communicating branch to the lacrimal nerve, travel to the lacrimal gland.

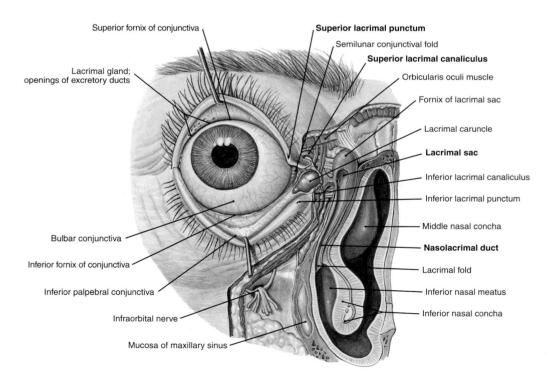

FIGURE 598.2 **Lacrimal Canaliculi, Lacrimal Sac, and Nasolacrimal Duct**

NOTE: From the ducts of the lacrimal gland, tears moisten the surface of the eyeball and drain medially through the lacrimal canaliculi to the lacrimal sac and then descend to the nasal cavity by way of the nasolacrimal duct.

Chapter 7 The Neck and Head

PLATE 599 **Lacrimal Apparatus**

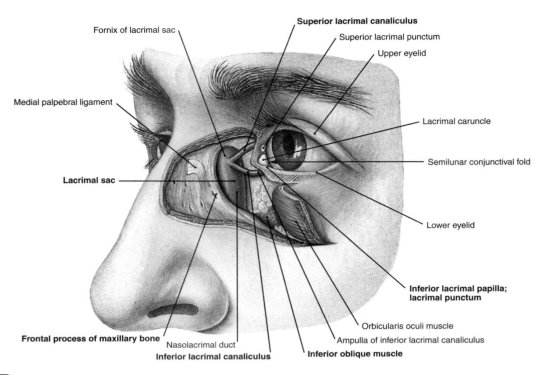

Superior lacrimal canaliculus
Fornix of lacrimal sac
Superior lacrimal punctum
Upper eyelid
Medial palpebral ligament
Lacrimal caruncle
Semilunar conjunctival fold
Lacrimal sac
Lower eyelid
Inferior lacrimal papilla;
lacrimal punctum
Orbicularis oculi muscle
Frontal process of maxillary bone
Nasolacrimal duct
Ampulla of inferior lacrimal canaliculus
Inferior lacrimal canaliculus
Inferior oblique muscle

FIGURE 599.1 **Lacrimal Canaliculi and Lacrimal Sac (Left Side, Superficial Dissection)**

NOTE: (1) The skin and superficial fascia have been removed over the medial angle of the orbit. Observe the cut orbicularis oculi muscle and medial palpebral ligament. The latter structure is still attached to the frontal process of the maxilla.

(2) Severance of the medial palpebral ligament exposes the underlying lacrimal sac, which is located in a small fossa formed by the maxilla and lacrimal bone. This sac receives a lacrimal canaliculus from each eyelid, and each of these two ducts is about 1 cm long.

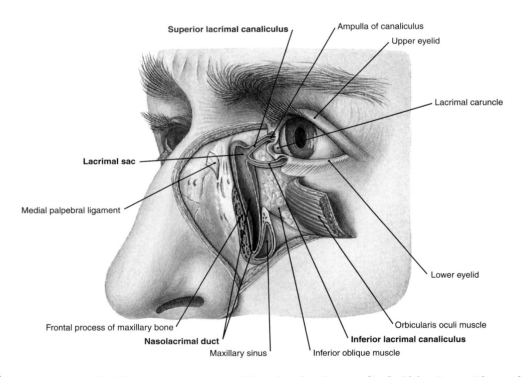

Superior lacrimal canaliculus
Ampulla of canaliculus
Upper eyelid
Lacrimal caruncle
Lacrimal sac
Medial palpebral ligament
Lower eyelid
Orbicularis oculi muscle
Frontal process of maxillary bone
Inferior lacrimal canaliculus
Nasolacrimal duct
Maxillary sinus
Inferior oblique muscle

FIGURE 599.2 **Lacrimal Canaliculi, Lacrimal Sac, and Nasolacrimal Duct (Left Side, Deep Dissection)**

NOTE: (1) At the medial edge of both eyelids are found single minute orifices (lacrimal puncta) of the lacrimal canaliculi, which lead from the eyelids to the lacrimal sac.

(2) The lacrimal sac forms the upper end of the nasolacrimal duct, which then extends about 2 cm into the inferior meatus of the nasal cavity.

(3) Lacrimal secretions pass across the surface of the eyeball toward the canaliculi and then are transported to the nasal cavity by the nasolacrimal duct. Excessive secretions, as in crying, roll over the edge of the lower eyelid as tears.

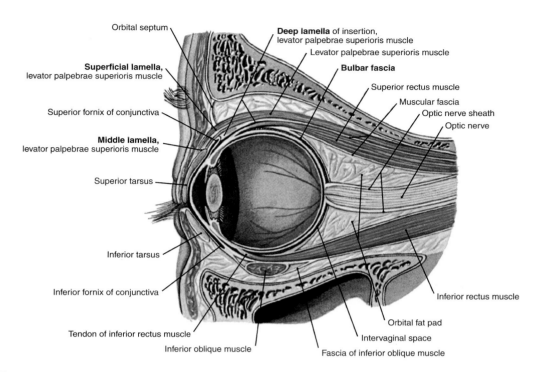

FIGURE 600.1 Sagittal View of the Orbital Cavity and Eyeball

NOTE: (1) The **bulbar fascia** is a thin membrane that encloses the posterior three-fourths of the eyeball and separates the eyeball from the orbital fat and other contents of the orbital cavity.

(2) The bulbar fascia is prolonged over the bellies of the ocular muscles but then is pierced by the tendons of these muscles as they insert on the outer coat of the eyeball.

(3) The insertion of the **levator palpebrae superioris** is trilaminar. The superficial layer inserts into the upper eyelid, the middle layer into the superior tarsus, and the deep layer into the superior fornix of the conjunctiva.

(4) The palpebral **conjunctiva** is a thin transparent mucous membrane on the innermost aspect of the eyelid. At the conjunctival angle (fornix), it reflects over the eyeball as far as the sclerocorneal junction.

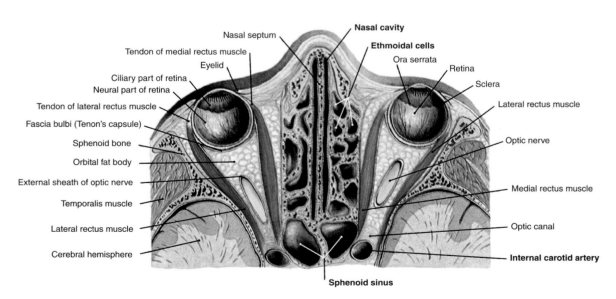

FIGURE 600.2 Horizontal Section through Both Orbits at the Level of the Sphenoid Sinus

NOTE: (1) Between the orbital cavities is situated the **ethmoid bone**, containing the ethmoidal air sinuses (air cells). The vertically oriented perpendicular plate of the ethmoid serves as part of the nasal septum, and it subdivides the nasal cavity into two chambers.

(2) The posterior portion of the orbits is separated by the **sphenoid sinuses**, located within the body of the sphenoid bone. These sinuses frequently are not symmetrical.

PLATE 601 Orbit from Above: Ophthalmic Nerve and Artery (Dissection 1)

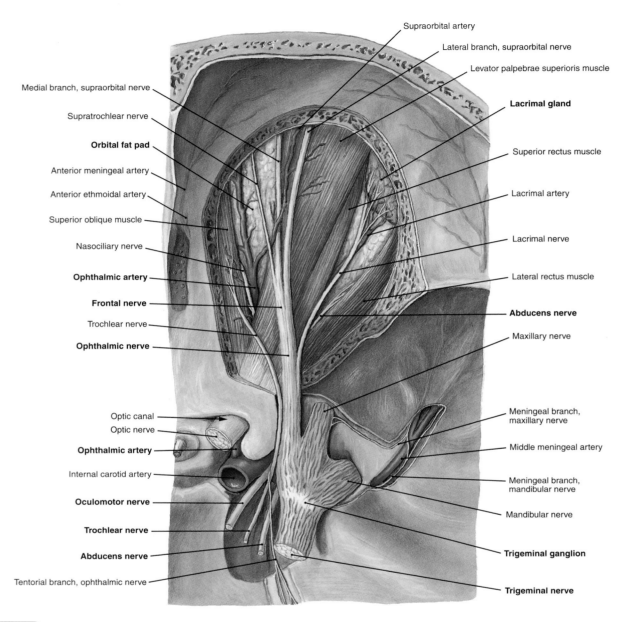

Supraorbital artery

Lateral branch, supraorbital nerve

Levator palpebrae superioris muscle

Lacrimal gland

Medial branch, supraorbital nerve

Supratrochlear nerve

Orbital fat pad

Superior rectus muscle

Anterior meningeal artery

Anterior ethmoidal artery

Lacrimal artery

Superior oblique muscle

Nasociliary nerve

Lacrimal nerve

Ophthalmic artery

Lateral rectus muscle

Frontal nerve

Trochlear nerve

Abducens nerve

Ophthalmic nerve

Maxillary nerve

Optic canal

Optic nerve

Meningeal branch, maxillary nerve

Ophthalmic artery

Middle meningeal artery

Internal carotid artery

Meningeal branch, mandibular nerve

Oculomotor nerve

Mandibular nerve

Trochlear nerve

Abducens nerve

Trigeminal ganglion

Tentorial branch, ophthalmic nerve

Trigeminal nerve

FIGURE 601 Nerves and Arteries of the Orbit (Stage 1), Superior View: Ophthalmic Nerve and Artery

NOTE: (1) The orbital plate of the frontal bone has been removed and the superior orbital fissure opened to expose the structures of the right orbit from above. The ophthalmic division of the trigeminal nerve divides into **lacrimal, frontal,** and **nasociliary branches**.

(2) The **lacrimal nerve** courses anteriorly and laterally in the orbit and accompanies the lacrimal branch of the ophthalmic artery to supply the lacrimal gland.

(3) The **frontal nerve** overlies the levator palpebrae superioris muscle and soon divides into a delicate **supratrochlear branch** and larger medial and lateral **supraorbital branches**. These course to the front of the orbit, where they emerge on the forehead.

(4) The **nasociliary nerve** crosses the orbit from lateral to medial, deep to the superior rectus muscle, and accompanies the ophthalmic artery for a short distance.

(5) The **trochlear nerve** enters the orbit medial to the ophthalmic nerve to supply the superior oblique muscle.

(6) The **optic nerve** leaves the orbit and enters the cranial cavity just medial to the internal carotid artery and the ophthalmic artery enters the orbit through the optic canal.

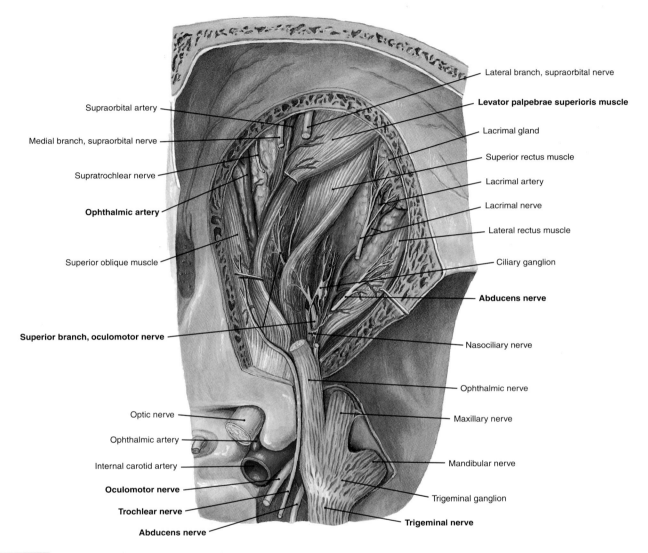

Lateral branch, supraorbital nerve

Supraorbital artery

Levator palpebrae superioris muscle

Medial branch, supraorbital nerve

Lacrimal gland

Supratrochlear nerve

Superior rectus muscle

Ophthalmic artery

Lacrimal artery

Lacrimal nerve

Lateral rectus muscle

Superior oblique muscle

Ciliary ganglion

Abducens nerve

Superior branch, oculomotor nerve

Nasociliary nerve

Ophthalmic nerve

Optic nerve

Maxillary nerve

Ophthalmic artery

Internal carotid artery

Mandibular nerve

Oculomotor nerve

Trigeminal ganglion

Trochlear nerve

Trigeminal nerve

Abducens nerve

FIGURE 602 **Nerves and Arteries of the Orbit (Stage 2), Superior View: Trochlear and Abducens Nerves**

NOTE: (1) With the right orbit opened from above, the ophthalmic division of the trigeminal nerve and its lacrimal, supratrochlear, and frontal branches have been cut. The levator palpebrae superioris and superior rectus muscles have been pulled medially to reveal their inferior surfaces, where filaments from the **superior branch of the oculomotor nerve** innervate the two muscles.

(2) The **nasociliary branch** of the ophthalmic nerve is still intact as it is seen turning medially deep to the superior rectus muscle. Also note that a fine communicating filament containing sensory fibers interconnects the ciliary ganglion and nasociliary nerve.

(3) The **trochlear nerve** supplies the superior oblique muscle along its upper surface. If this nerve is injured, a patient has difficulty turning the eyeball laterally and down; when asked to look inferolaterally, the affected eye rotates medially, resulting in double vision, or diplopia.

(4) The **abducens nerve** supplies the lateral rectus muscle along its medial surface. After emerging from the brainstem at the pontomedullary junction, this nerve follows a long course in the floor of the cranial cavity and enters the orbit through the superior orbital fissure.

(5) Injury to the abducens nerve produces a diminished ability to move the eyeball laterally. From the resulting medial or convergent gaze of the affected eyeball, the patient experiences diplopia (double vision).

PLATE 603 **Orbit from Above: Optic Nerve; Ciliary Ganglion (Dissection 3)**

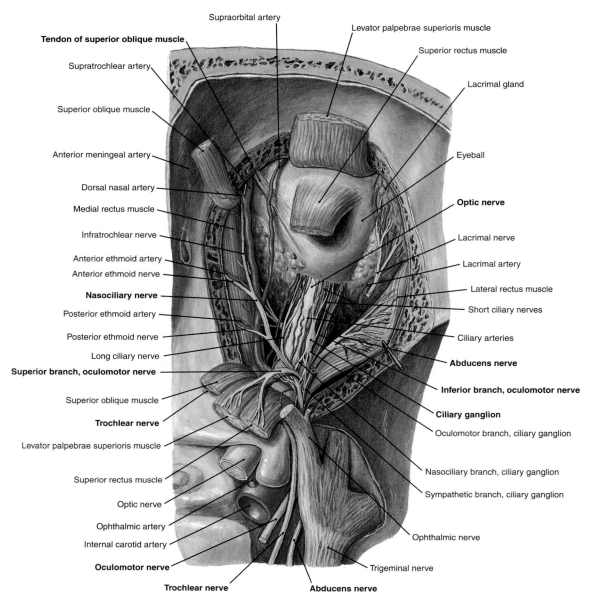

Supraorbital artery

Levator palpebrae superioris muscle

Superior rectus muscle

Tendon of superior oblique muscle

Lacrimal gland

Supratrochlear artery

Superior oblique muscle

Anterior meningeal artery

Eyeball

Dorsal nasal artery

Optic nerve

Medial rectus muscle

Infratrochlear nerve

Lacrimal nerve

Anterior ethmoid artery

Lacrimal artery

Anterior ethmoid nerve

Lateral rectus muscle

Nasociliary nerve

Short ciliary nerves

Posterior ethmoid artery

Ciliary arteries

Posterior ethmoid nerve

Abducens nerve

Long ciliary nerve

Inferior branch, oculomotor nerve

Superior branch, oculomotor nerve

Ciliary ganglion

Superior oblique muscle

Oculomotor branch, ciliary ganglion

Trochlear nerve

Levator palpebrae superioris muscle

Nasociliary branch, ciliary ganglion

Superior rectus muscle

Sympathetic branch, ciliary ganglion

Optic nerve

Ophthalmic artery

Internal carotid artery

Ophthalmic nerve

Oculomotor nerve

Trigeminal nerve

Trochlear nerve

Abducens nerve

FIGURE 603 **Nerves and Arteries of the Orbit (Stage 3), Superior View: Optic Nerve and Ciliary Ganglion**

NOTE: (1) With the levator palpebrae superioris, superior rectus, and superior oblique muscles cut and reflected, the **nasociliary nerve** and **ophthalmic artery** are seen crossing over the **optic nerve** from lateral to medial.

(2) The relationship to the optic nerve of the longitudinally oriented **long posterior ciliary arteries** (from the ophthalmic) and the **long ciliary nerves** (two or three branches from the nasociliary nerve).

(3) The **ciliary ganglion** lies lateral to the optic nerve. Its **parasympathetic root** comes from the oculomotor nerve and its **sensory root** from the nasociliary nerve. Postganglionic parasympathetic fibers reach the eyeball by the **short ciliary nerves**.

(4) Postganglionic parasympathetic nerve fibers supply the **sphincter of the pupil** and the muscle responsible for accommodation of the lens, the **ciliary muscle**.

(5) Some **sympathetic fibers** that arrive in the orbit along the ophthalmic artery also course through the ciliary ganglion. These are principally vasoconstrictor fibers to arteries that supply the eyeball. Sympathetic fibers that supply the **dilator of the pupil** course to the posterior pole of the eyeball by way of the **long ciliary nerves**.

(6) Although the supratrochlear nerve is derived from the frontal branch of the ophthalmic nerve, the **infratrochlear nerve** (as well as the **anterior** and **posterior ethmoid nerves**) is derived from the nasociliary branch of the ophthalmic nerve.

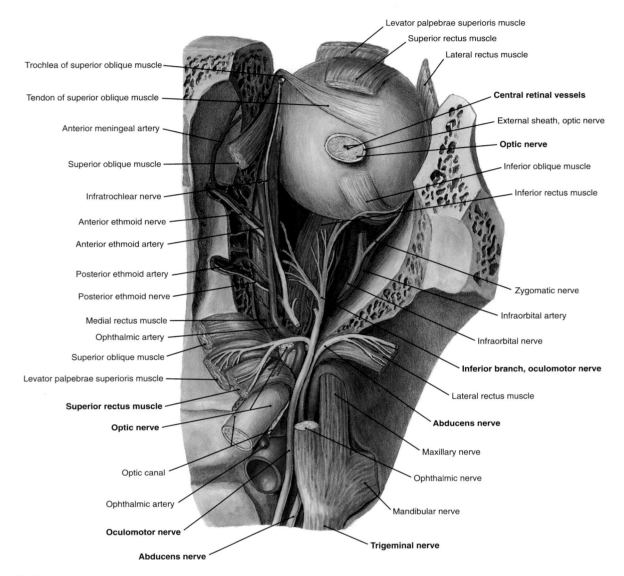

Levator palpebrae superioris muscle

Superior rectus muscle

Lateral rectus muscle

Trochlea of superior oblique muscle

Tendon of superior oblique muscle

Anterior meningeal artery

Central retinal vessels

External sheath, optic nerve

Optic nerve

Superior oblique muscle

Infratrochlear nerve

Inferior oblique muscle

Anterior ethmoid nerve

Inferior rectus muscle

Anterior ethmoid artery

Posterior ethmoid artery

Posterior ethmoid nerve

Zygomatic nerve

Medial rectus muscle

Infraorbital artery

Ophthalmic artery

Infraorbital nerve

Superior oblique muscle

Levator palpebrae superioris muscle

Inferior branch, oculomotor nerve

Superior rectus muscle

Lateral rectus muscle

Optic nerve

Abducens nerve

Maxillary nerve

Optic canal

Ophthalmic nerve

Ophthalmic artery

Mandibular nerve

Oculomotor nerve

Trigeminal nerve

Abducens nerve

FIGURE 604 Nerves and Arteries of the Orbit (Stage 4), Superior View: Oculomotor Nerve (Inferior Branch)

NOTE: (1) The levator palpebrae superioris, superior rectus, superior oblique, and lateral rectus muscles have been cut and reflected; the optic nerve has also been severed. The anterior half of the eyeball has been depressed and its posterior pole directed upward. Observe the **central retinal vessels** as well as the insertions of the superior oblique and inferior oblique muscles.

(2) The **oculomotor nerve** courses through the superior orbital fissure and the common tendinous ring. It quickly gives off its **superior branch**, which courses upward in the orbit to supply the levator palpebrae superioris and superior rectus muscles. The **inferior branch** of the oculomotor nerve courses anteriorly in the deep part of the orbit to supply the inferior rectus, medial rectus, and inferior oblique muscles.

(3) The anterior and posterior ethmoid arteries and nerves and the infratrochlear nerve all located medially in the orbit. Also note the **infraorbital nerve** and **artery** in the infraorbital groove more laterally.

(4) The **ophthalmic artery** is the first branch of the internal carotid artery within the cranial cavity; it immediately enters the orbit through the optic canal with the optic nerve. Probably, the most important of the branches of the ophthalmic artery is the **central retinal artery**, which courses with its **vein** within the optic nerve.

(5) The central artery is the **only** source of blood to the neural retina and an increase in pressure on the posterior part of the orbital cavity or edema of the optic nerve caused by an inflammatory process can seriously compromise vision either by blockage of the artery or by diminishing the flow in the **central retinal vein.**

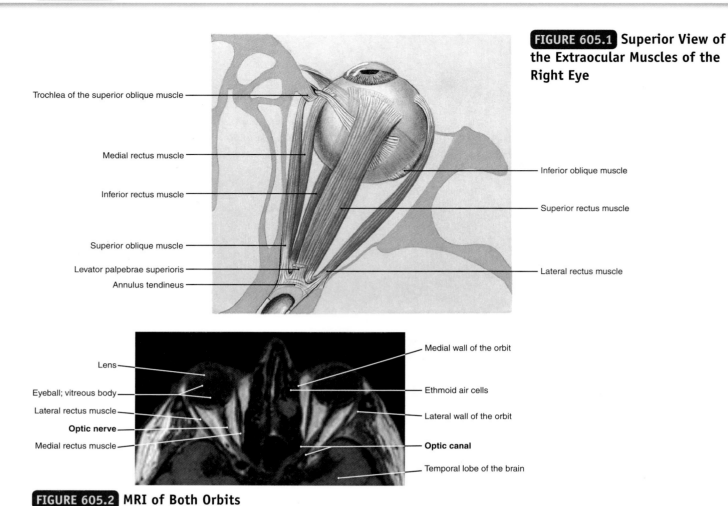

FIGURE 605.1 Superior View of the Extraocular Muscles of the Right Eye

Trochlea of the superior oblique muscle

Medial rectus muscle

Inferior rectus muscle

Superior oblique muscle

Levator palpebrae superioris

Annulus tendineus

Inferior oblique muscle

Superior rectus muscle

Lateral rectus muscle

Lens

Eyeball; vitreous body

Lateral rectus muscle

Optic nerve

Medial rectus muscle

Medial wall of the orbit

Ethmoid air cells

Lateral wall of the orbit

Optic canal

Temporal lobe of the brain

FIGURE 605.2 **MRI of Both Orbits**

NOTE the optic nerve seen in the left orbit and the optic canal seen in the right orbit.

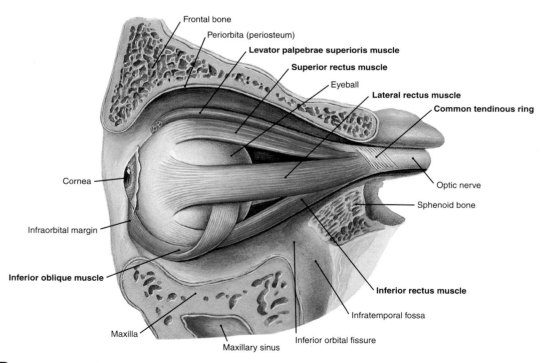

Frontal bone

Periorbita (periosteum)

Levator palpebrae superioris muscle

Superior rectus muscle

Eyeball

Lateral rectus muscle

Common tendinous ring

Cornea

Infraorbital margin

Inferior oblique muscle

Maxilla

Maxillary sinus

Inferior orbital fissure

Inferior rectus muscle

Infratemporal fossa

Sphenoid bone

Optic nerve

FIGURE 605.3 **Eye Muscles (Left Lateral View)**

NOTE: (1) With the lateral wall of the left orbit removed along with the bulbar fascia and eyelids, five of the seven extraocular muscles become exposed. Those evident from this view are the superior, lateral, and inferior rectus muscles, along with the levator palpebrae superioris and inferior oblique. Not seen are the medial rectus and superior oblique.

(2) Of the seven muscles, all except the levator palpebrae superioris and the inferior oblique take origin from the common tendinous ring that surrounds the optic nerve.

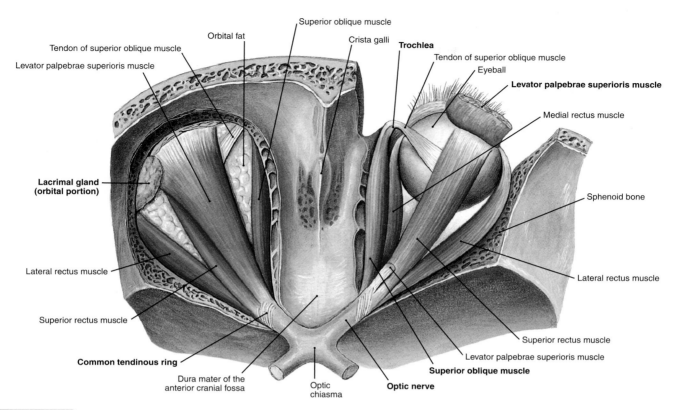

FIGURE 606.1 Muscles of the Orbital Cavity (Seen from Above)

NOTE: (1) The orbital plates of the frontal bones have been removed from within the cranial cavity. On the left side, only the bony roof of the orbit has been opened and the muscles, orbital fat, and lacrimal gland have been left intact.

(2) On the right side, the levator palpebrae superioris muscle has been resected and the orbital fat removed to expose the ocular muscles.

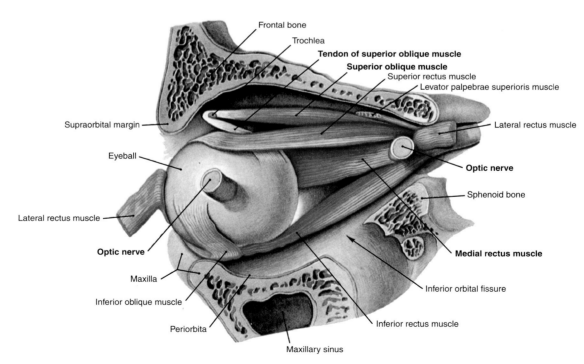

FIGURE 606.2 Eye Muscles, Left Lateral View (Lateral Rectus Muscle and Optic Nerve Cut)

NOTE: The eyeball has been rotated 90 degrees so that its posterior pole is directed laterally. This reveals to advantage the insertion of the inferior oblique muscle and the superior oblique muscle and tendon as it bends around the trochlea to insert on the eyeball.

Chapter 7 The Neck and Head

PLATE 607 **Orbit: Extraocular Muscles, Insertions and Actions**

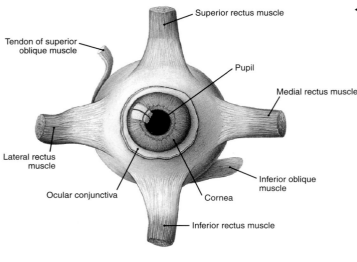

Superior rectus muscle

Tendon of superior oblique muscle

Pupil

Medial rectus muscle

Lateral rectus muscle

Inferior oblique muscle

Ocular conjunctiva

Cornea

Inferior rectus muscle

◀ **FIGURE 607.1** Right Eyeball and Muscle Insertions (Front)

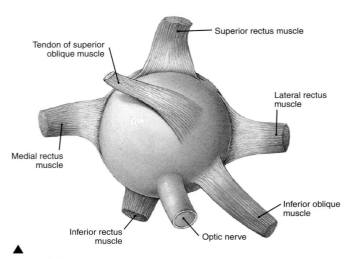

Tendon of superior oblique muscle

Superior rectus muscle

Lateral rectus muscle

Medial rectus muscle

Inferior oblique muscle

Inferior rectus muscle

Optic nerve

▲

FIGURE 607.2 Right Eyeball and Muscle Insertions (Behind and Above)

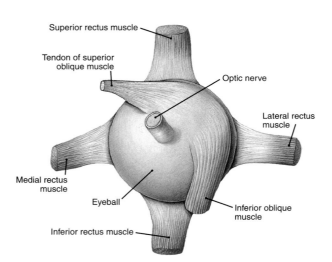

Superior rectus muscle

Tendon of superior oblique muscle

Optic nerve

Lateral rectus muscle

Medial rectus muscle

Eyeball

Inferior oblique muscle

Inferior rectus muscle

◀ **FIGURE 607.3** Right Eyeball and Muscle Insertions (Behind and Below)

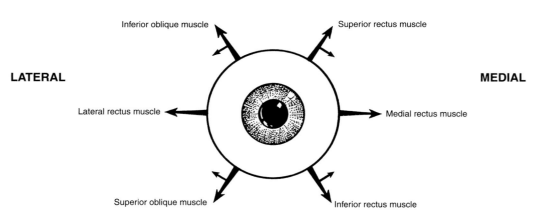

Inferior oblique muscle

Superior rectus muscle

LATERAL

MEDIAL

Lateral rectus muscle

Medial rectus muscle

Superior oblique muscle

Inferior rectus muscle

FIGURE 607.4 Schema of Extraocular Muscle Actions

NOTE:
(1) The **lateral rectus** *abducts* the eyeball only.
(2) The **superior oblique** *abducts*, *depresses*, and *medially rotates* the eyeball.
(3) The **inferior oblique** *abducts*, *elevates*, and *laterally rotates* the eyeball.
(4) The **medial rectus** *adducts* the eyeball only.
(5) The **inferior rectus** *adducts*, *depresses*, and *laterally rotates* the eyeball.
(6) The **superior rectus** *adducts*, *elevates*, and *medially rotates* the eyeball.

NOTE the following muscle innervations:
(1) The **oculomotor nerve (III)**: levator palpebrae superioris, superior rectus, medial rectus, inferior rectus, inferior oblique muscles.
(2) The **trochlear nerve (IV)**: superior oblique muscle.
(3) The **abducens nerve (VI)**: lateral rectus muscle.

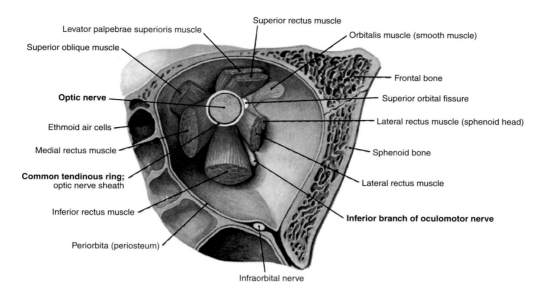

FIGURE 608.1 Origins of the Ocular Muscles, Apex of Left Orbit

NOTE: (1) This anterior view of the apex of the left orbit shows the stumps of the ocular muscles, which have been cut close to their origins.
(2) The four rectus muscles arise from a tendinous ring surrounding the optic canal. The levator palpebrae superioris and superior oblique arise from the sphenoid bone close to the tendinous ring, whereas the inferior oblique (not shown here, see Fig. 597.2) arises from the orbital surface of the maxilla.

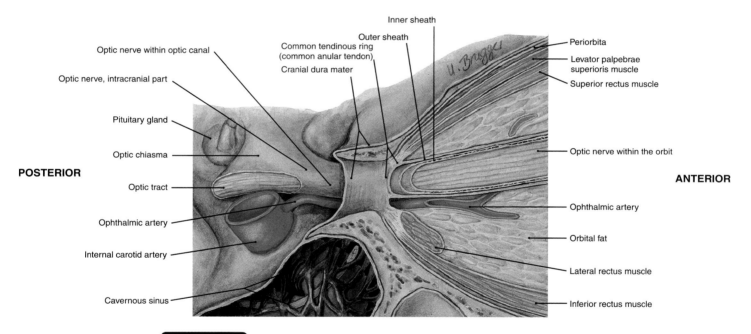

FIGURE 608.2 Ophthalmic Artery and Optic Nerve in the Optic Canal

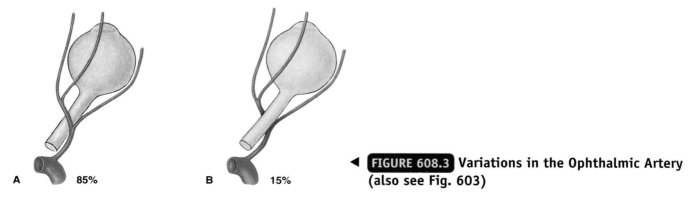

◀ **FIGURE 608.3** Variations in the Ophthalmic Artery (also see Fig. 603)

PLATE 609 Eyeball: Horizontal Section; Iris

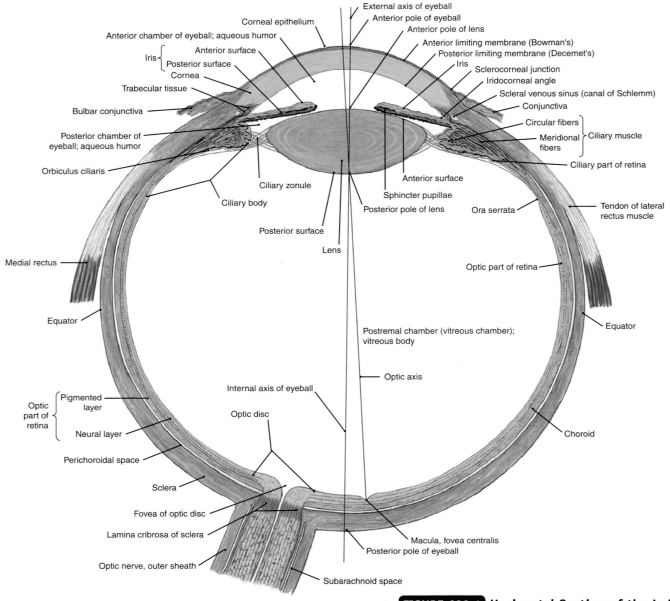

External axis of eyeball
Anterior pole of eyeball
Anterior pole of lens
Corneal epithelium
Anterior chamber of eyeball; aqueous humor
Anterior limiting membrane (Bowman's)
Posterior limiting membrane (Decemet's)
Anterior surface
Iris
Iris {
Posterior surface
Sclerocorneal junction
Cornea
Iridocorneal angle
Trabecular tissue
Scleral venous sinus (canal of Schlemm)
Conjunctiva
Bulbar conjunctiva
Circular fibers
Meridional fibers } Ciliary muscle
Posterior chamber of eyeball; aqueous humor
Ciliary part of retina
Orbiculus ciliaris
Anterior surface
Ciliary zonule
Sphincter pupillae
Tendon of lateral rectus muscle
Ciliary body
Posterior pole of lens
Ora serrata
Posterior surface
Lens
Medial rectus
Optic part of retina
Equator
Equator
Postremal chamber (vitreous chamber); vitreous body
Optic axis
Internal axis of eyeball
Optic part of retina { Pigmented layer
Optic disc
Neural layer }
Choroid
Perichoroidal space
Sclera
Fovea of optic disc
Lamina cribrosa of sclera
Macula, fovea centralis
Posterior pole of eyeball
Optic nerve, outer sheath
Subarachnoid space

▲ **FIGURE 609.1** Horizontal Section of the Left Eyeball through the Optic Disk and Nerve

NOTE: The eyeball is composed of three concentric layer or tunics:
(1) An **outer fibrous tunic,** which consists of the tough **sclera** posteriorly and the translucent **cornea** anteriorly **(brown).**
(2) The **middle vascular tunic** including the **choroid** posteriorly and the **ciliary body** and **iris** anteriorly **(blue).**
(3) The **inner neural tunic,** which is **retina.** It consists of a **neural part** posteriorly, and a **nonneural part** that underlies the ciliary body and iris. The junction between these two parts is the **ora serrata (yellow).**

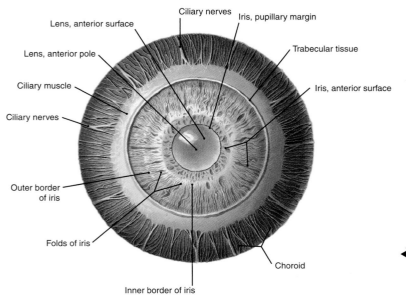

Ciliary nerves
Iris, pupillary margin
Lens, anterior surface
Lens, anterior pole
Trabecular tissue
Ciliary muscle
Iris, anterior surface
Ciliary nerves
Outer border of iris
Folds of iris
Choroid
Inner border of iris

◀ **FIGURE 609.2** Iris and Pupil (Anterior View)

NOTE: The anterior pole of the lens is located behind the iris.

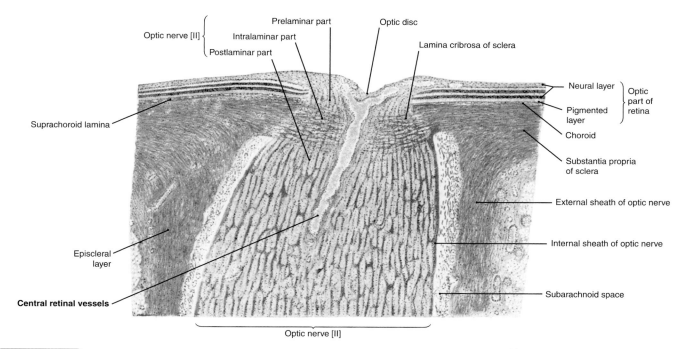

FIGURE 610.1 Horizontal Section of the Optic Disk Region of the Eyeball

NOTE: The axons of the optic nerve leave the eyeball at the **optic disk,** or blind spot, where there are no visual receptors.

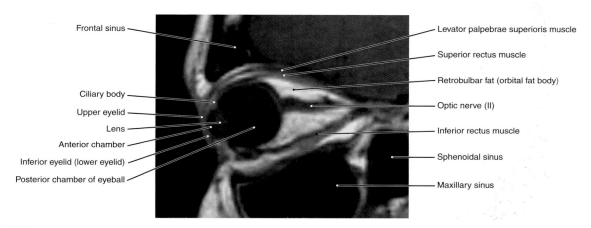

FIGURE 610.2 Magnetic Resonance Image through the Right Orbit: Lateral View

NOTE: This is a sagittal section through the optic nerve.

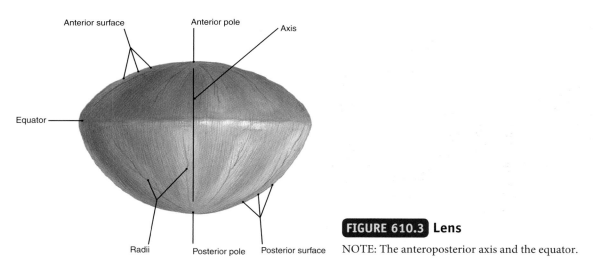

FIGURE 610.3 Lens

NOTE: The anteroposterior axis and the equator.

PLATE 611 **Arteries and Veins within the Orbital Cavity**

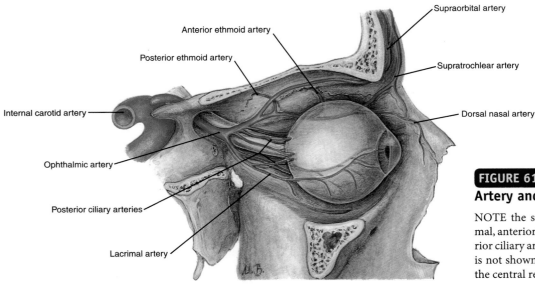

Supraorbital artery

Anterior ethmoid artery

Posterior ethmoid artery

Supratrochlear artery

Internal carotid artery

Dorsal nasal artery

Ophthalmic artery

Posterior ciliary arteries

Lacrimal artery

FIGURE 611.1 **The Ophthalmic Artery and Its Branches**

NOTE the supraorbital, supratrochlear, lacrimal, anterior and posterior ethmoid, and posterior ciliary arteries, but the central retinal artery is not shown or labeled. See some branches of the central retinal artery in **Figure 611.2.**

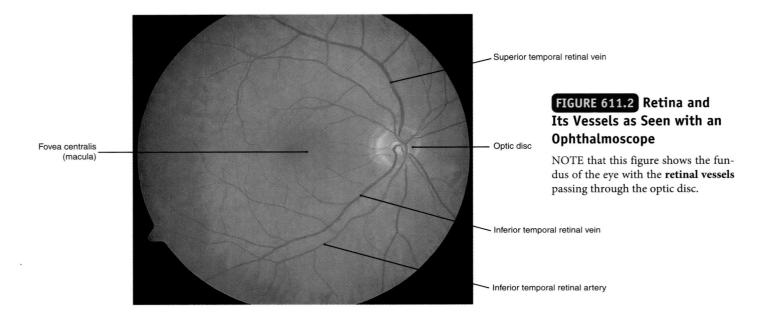

Superior temporal retinal vein

Fovea centralis (macula)

Optic disc

Inferior temporal retinal vein

Inferior temporal retinal artery

FIGURE 611.2 **Retina and Its Vessels as Seen with an Ophthalmoscope**

NOTE that this figure shows the fundus of the eye with the **retinal vessels** passing through the optic disc.

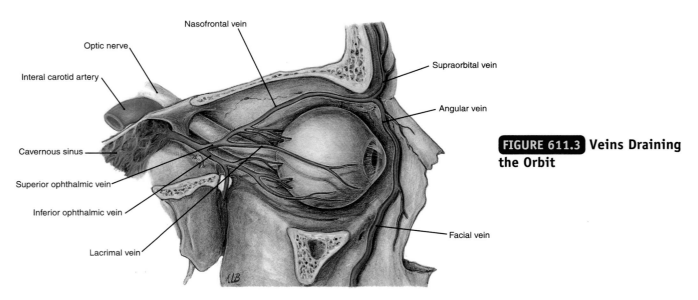

Nasofrontal vein

Optic nerve

Supraorbital vein

Interal carotid artery

Angular vein

Cavernous sinus

Superior ophthalmic vein

Inferior ophthalmic vein

Facial vein

Lacrimal vein

FIGURE 611.3 **Veins Draining the Orbit**

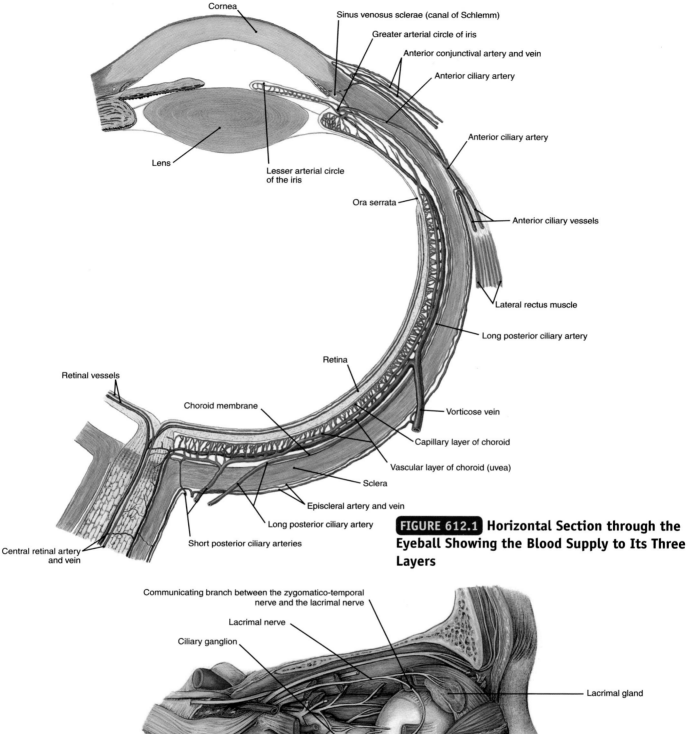

Cornea

Sinus venosus sclerae (canal of Schlemm)

Greater arterial circle of iris

Anterior conjunctival artery and vein

Anterior ciliary artery

Anterior ciliary artery

Lens

Lesser arterial circle of the iris

Ora serrata

Anterior ciliary vessels

Lateral rectus muscle

Long posterior ciliary artery

Retina

Retinal vessels

Choroid membrane

Vorticose vein

Capillary layer of choroid

Vascular layer of choroid (uvea)

Sclera

Episcleral artery and vein

Long posterior ciliary artery

Short posterior ciliary arteries

Central retinal artery and vein

FIGURE 612.1 Horizontal Section through the Eyeball Showing the Blood Supply to Its Three Layers

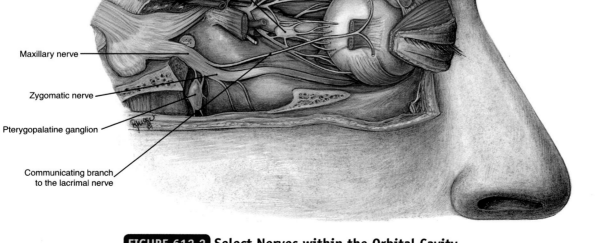

Communicating branch between the zygomatico-temporal nerve and the lacrimal nerve

Lacrimal nerve

Ciliary ganglion

Lacrimal gland

Maxillary nerve

Zygomatic nerve

Pterygopalatine ganglion

Communicating branch to the lacrimal nerve

FIGURE 612.2 Select Nerves within the Orbital Cavity

PLATE 613 External Nose; Lateral Wall of the Nasal Cavity

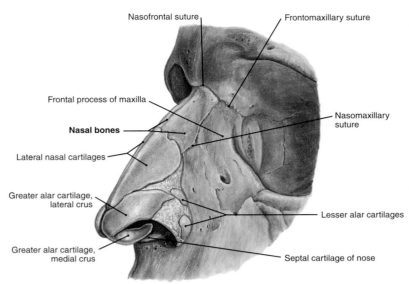

Nasofrontal suture

Frontomaxillary suture

Frontal process of maxilla

Nasomaxillary suture

Nasal bones

Lateral nasal cartilages

Greater alar cartilage, lateral crus

Lesser alar cartilages

Greater alar cartilage, medial crus

Septal cartilage of nose

FIGURE 613.1 Cartilages and Bones of the External Nose

NOTE: (1) The distal and lateral parts of the external nose consist mostly of nasal cartilages. The bony framework that forms the base of the nose consists of the nasal bones and the nasal processes of the maxillary and frontal bones.

(2) The oval-shaped external openings are called the external nares (or nostrils). These lead into the nasal vestibules, which are continuous with the nasal cavities.

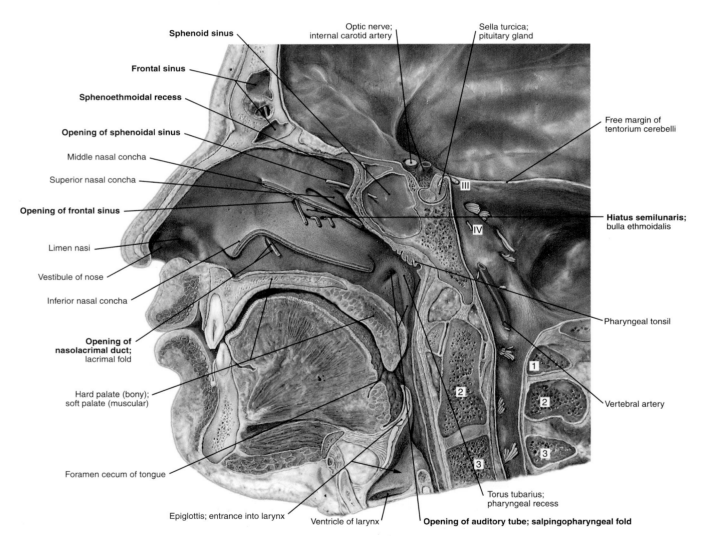

Sphenoid sinus

Optic nerve; internal carotid artery

Sella turcica; pituitary gland

Frontal sinus

Sphenoethmoidal recess

Free margin of tentorium cerebelli

Opening of sphenoidal sinus

Middle nasal concha

Superior nasal concha

III

Opening of frontal sinus

Hiatus semilunaris; bulla ethmoidalis

IV

Limen nasi

Vestibule of nose

Inferior nasal concha

Pharyngeal tonsil

1

Opening of nasolacrimal duct; lacrimal fold

2

2

Vertebral artery

Hard palate (bony); soft palate (muscular)

3

Foramen cecum of tongue

3

Torus tubarius; pharyngeal recess

Epiglottis; entrance into larynx

Ventricle of larynx

Opening of auditory tube; salpingopharyngeal fold

FIGURE 613.2 Lateral Wall of the Right Nasal Cavity Showing Openings of the Paranasal Air Sinuses and the Nasopharynx

NOTE: (1) This paramedian sagittal section of the head shows the right nasal cavity after the middle and inferior nasal conchae were removed. The nasal cavity communicates anteriorly with the exterior through the nostril and posteriorly with the nasopharynx.

(2) The openings of the paranasal sinuses and other structures:

    (a) The **sphenoid sinus**, which drains into the **sphenoethmoid recess** above the superior concha.

    (b) The **frontal** and **maxillary sinuses**, both of which open in a groove called the **hiatus semilunaris** in the middle meatus below the middle concha.

    (c) The **nasolacrimal duct**, which opens into the inferior meatus below the inferior concha.

    (d) The **auditory tube**, which opens into the nasopharynx just behind the inferior concha.

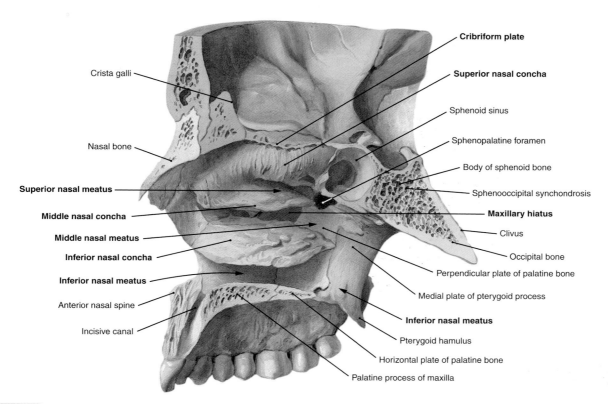

FIGURE 614.1 Bony Lateral Wall of the Right Nasal Cavity

NOTE: (1) The nasal septum has been removed and the mucosa stripped from the irregular lateral wall of the nasal cavity and the hard palate. Also note that in front of the nasal conchae are the **nasal bone** (gray) and the **maxilla,** and behind is the **perpendicular plate** of the **palatine bone** (blue).

(2) The **crista galli, cribriform plate,** and the **superior** and **middle nasal conchae** are all parts of the **ethmoid bone** (light orange). Below these is the **inferior nasal concha,** which is a separate bone (gray). The bony floor of the nasal cavity is the hard palate, formed by the **palatine process** of the **maxilla** and the **horizontal plate** of the **palatine bone.**

(3) The arrows that follow the courses of the **superior, middle,** and **inferior meatuses,** each under its respective nasal concha. Also note the **sphenoid sinus,** the **sphenopalatine foramen,** and the opening of the maxillary sinus **(maxillary hiatus).**

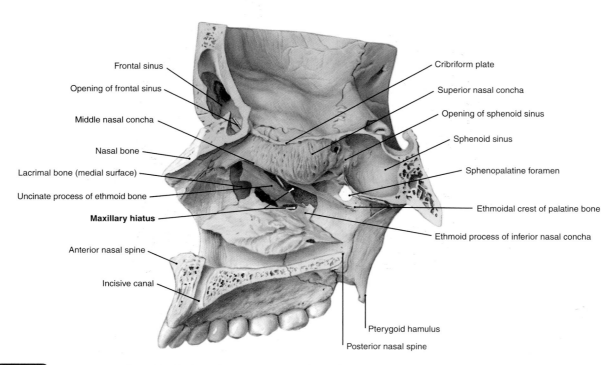

FIGURE 614.2 Bony Lateral Wall of the Right Nasal Cavity with the Middle Nasal Concha Removed

NOTE: More complete exposure of the **maxillary hiatus** and the bony structures deep to (lateral to) the middle nasal concha. Compare with Figure 614.1.

PLATE 615 Nasal Septum: Skeletal Parts; Lateral Nasal Wall

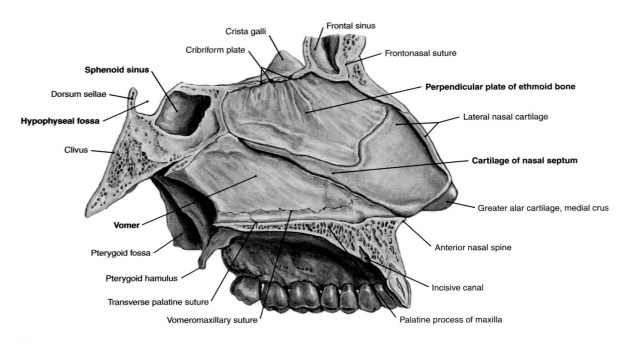

FIGURE 615.1 Nasal Septum: Structure and Blood Supply (Notes)

NOTE: (1) The skeletal structure of the nasal septum includes the **perpendicular plate of the ethmoid bone,** the **vomer bone,** and the **cartilage of the nasal septum**.

(2) The arteries of the septum include: superior and posterior—the **anterior and posterior ethmoid arteries** and the **posterior septal branches** of the **sphenopalatine artery**; inferior and anterior—the **septal branch** of the **superior labial artery**, which enters through the nostrils, and the **septal branch** of the **greater palatine artery**, which enters the nasal cavity by way of the incisive foramen.

(3) The **septal nerves** include: branches of the **anterior ethmoid nerve** (from the ophthalmic nerve), the **nasopalatine nerve** (from the maxillary nerve), and the **internal nasal branches** of the infraorbital nerves that enter the nasal cavities through the nostrils.

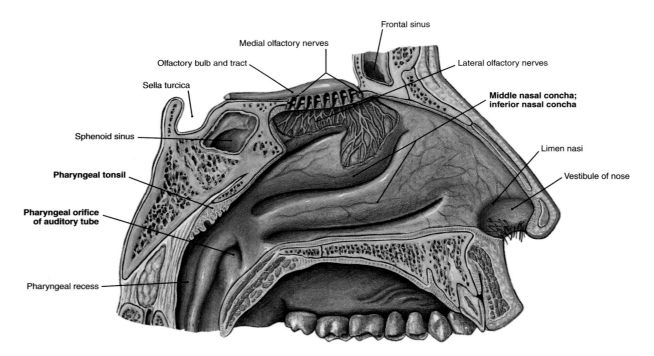

FIGURE 615.2 Lateral Wall of the Left Nasal Cavity Showing the Olfactory Nerves

NOTE: The mucous membrane overlying the **lateral olfactory nerves** has been removed. The lateral wall of the nasal cavity is marked by the **superior, middle,** and **inferior nasal conchae**. Beneath each concha courses the corresponding nasal passage, or **meatus**.

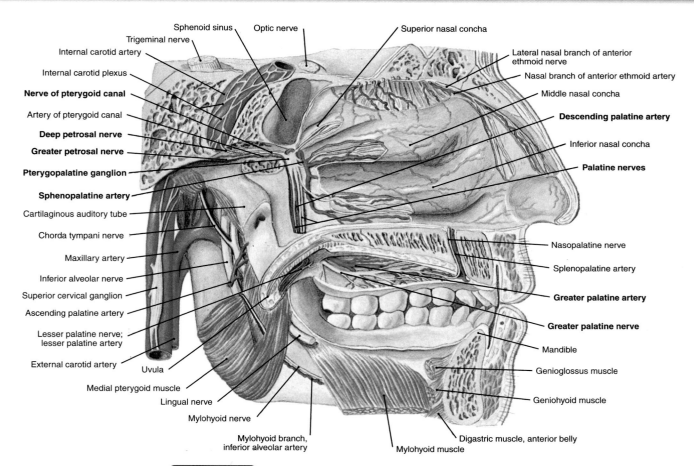

FIGURE 616.1 Pterygopalatine Ganglion and Its Branches

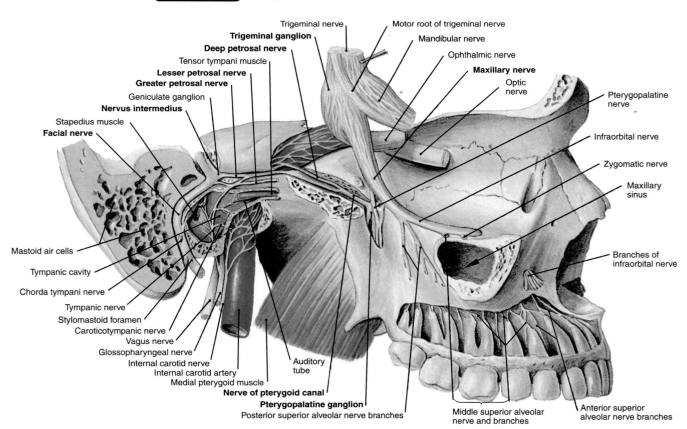

FIGURE 616.2 Maxillary Nerve, Petrosal Nerves, and Facial Nerve

NOTE: The **nerve of the pterygoid canal** is formed by the union of the **deep petrosal nerve** (postganglionic sympathetic) and the **greater petrosal nerve** (sensory and preganglionic, **VII**, parasympathetic fibers). The **lesser petrosal nerve** carries preganglionic, **IX**, parasympathetic fibers to the **otic ganglion**.

PLATE 617 Paranasal Sinuses

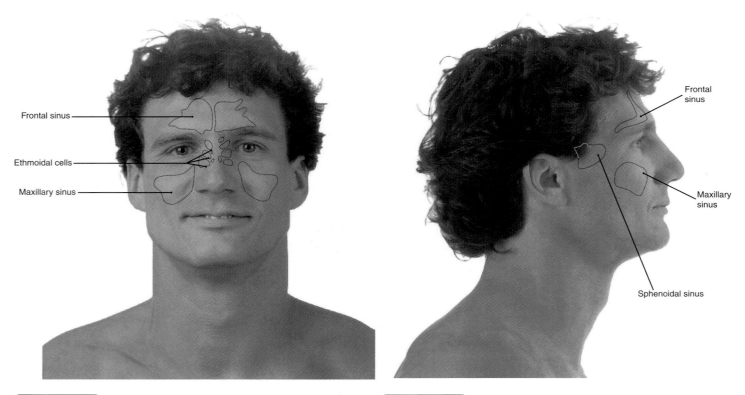

Frontal sinus

Ethmoidal cells

Maxillary sinus

Frontal sinus

Maxillary sinus

Sphenoidal sinus

FIGURE 617.1 Surface Projection of the Paranasal Sinuses onto the Anterior Aspect of the Face

NOTE: The sphenoid sinus is not shown in this figure.

FIGURE 617.2 Surface Projection of the Paranasal Sinuses onto the Lateral Aspect of the Face

NOTE: The ethmoid sinuses are not shown in this figure.

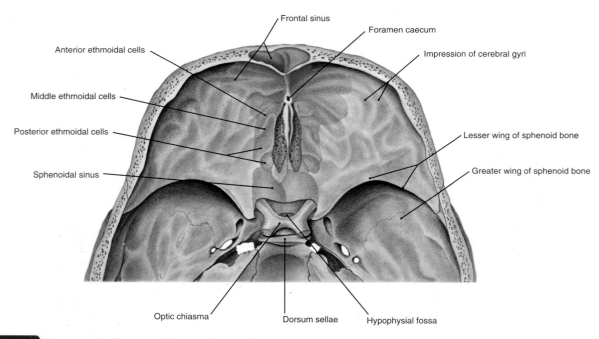

Frontal sinus

Foramen caecum

Anterior ethmoidal cells

Impression of cerebral gyri

Middle ethmoidal cells

Posterior ethmoidal cells

Lesser wing of sphenoid bone

Sphenoidal sinus

Greater wing of sphenoid bone

Optic chiasma

Dorsum sellae

Hypophysial fossa

FIGURE 617.3 Paranasal Sinuses Viewed from Above

NOTE: (1) The frontal anterior ethmoid, middle ethmoid, posterior ethmoid, and sphenoid sinuses are projected onto the base of the anterior cranial fossa; the maxillary sinus is not shown.

(2) The sinuses are named for the bones that contain them.

(3) The **frontal sinus** drains into the middle meatus of the nasal cavity through the ethmoidal infundibulum or the frontonasal duct; the **anterior ethmoid air cells** open into the ethmoidal infundibulum or the frontonasal duct, **the middle ethmoid cells** open onto the ethmoid bulla in the middle meatus, and the **posterior ethmoid air cells** open into the superior meatus; the **sphenoid sinus** opens into the sphenoethmoidal recess posterior to the superior concha.

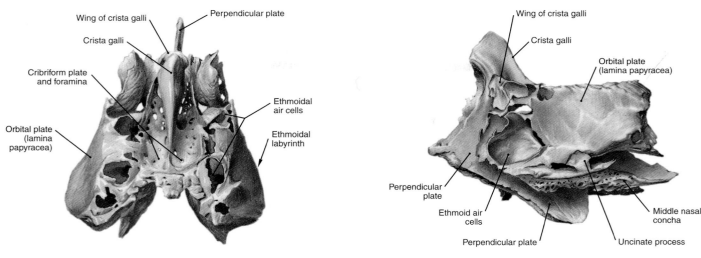

FIGURE 618.1 Superior Surface of the Ethmoid Bone

FIGURE 618.2 Ethmoid Bone (Left Lateral View)

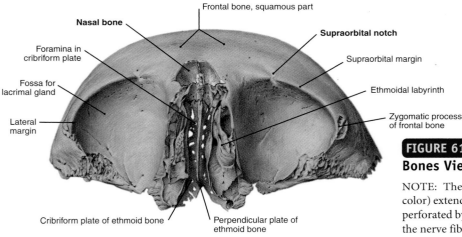

FIGURE 618.3 Frontal, Ethmoid, and Nasal Bones Viewed from Above

NOTE: The cribriform plate of the ethmoid bone (orange color) extends laterally from the midline on both sides and it is perforated by many foramina. Through these foramina course the nerve fibers of the primary olfactory receptor cells.

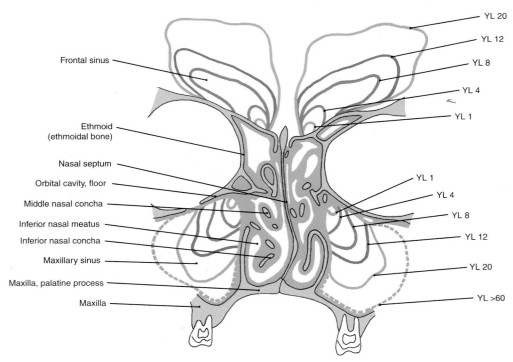

FIGURE 618.4 Enlargement of the Frontal and Maxillary Sinuses

NOTE: The growth of the frontal sinus is indicated from the 1st year of life (YL) to the 20th year, whereas the maxillary sinus is shown from the 1st year of life to the 20th year, and then at the 60th year.

Chapter 7 The Neck and Head

PLATE 619 Oral Cavity: Palate and Tongue (Anterior View); Oral Muscles

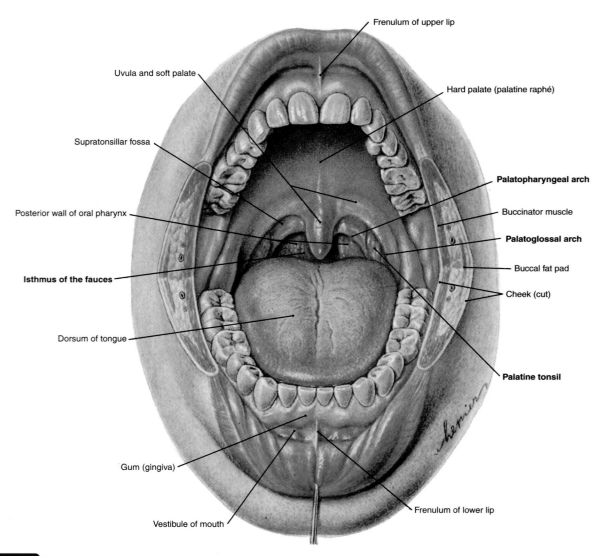

Frenulum of upper lip

Uvula and soft palate

Hard palate (palatine raphé)

Supratonsillar fossa

Palatopharyngeal arch

Buccinator muscle

Posterior wall of oral pharynx

Palatoglossal arch

Buccal fat pad

Isthmus of the fauces

Cheek (cut)

Dorsum of tongue

Palatine tonsil

Gum (gingiva)

Frenulum of lower lip

Vestibule of mouth

FIGURE 619.1 Oral Cavity

NOTE: (1) The position of the **palatine tonsils** located on each side of the oral cavity within fossae between the **palatoglossal** and **palatopharyngeal folds** (or **arches**).

(2) The passage between the oral cavity and the oral pharynx is called the **fauces**. This aperture or isthmus commences anteriorly at the palatoglossal arches on each side and is also bounded by the soft palate superiorly and the dorsum of the tongue inferiorly.

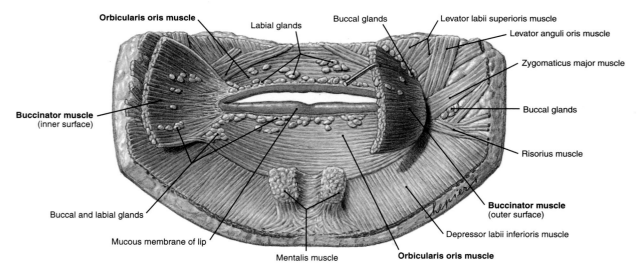

Orbicularis oris muscle

Labial glands

Buccal glands

Levator labii superioris muscle

Levator anguli oris muscle

Zygomaticus major muscle

Buccinator muscle
(inner surface)

Buccal glands

Risorius muscle

Buccal and labial glands

Buccinator muscle
(outer surface)

Mucous membrane of lip

Depressor labii inferioris muscle

Mentalis muscle

Orbicularis oris muscle

FIGURE 619.2 Lips Viewed from within the Oral Cavity

NOTE: The contour of the lips depends on the arrangement of the muscular bundles, which interlace at the labial margins. These include the elevators and depressors of the lips and their angles along with the **orbicularis oris** and **buccinator muscles**.

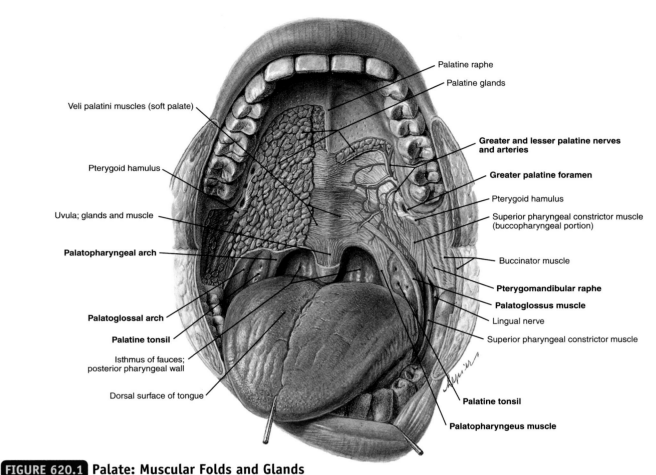

Palatine raphe
Palatine glands

Veli palatini muscles (soft palate)

**Greater and lesser palatine nerves
and arteries**

Greater palatine foramen

Pterygoid hamulus

Pterygoid hamulus

Superior pharyngeal constrictor muscle
(buccopharyngeal portion)

Uvula; glands and muscle

Buccinator muscle

Palatopharyngeal arch

Pterygomandibular raphe

Palatoglossus muscle

Lingual nerve

Palatoglossal arch

Superior pharyngeal constrictor muscle

Palatine tonsil

Isthmus of fauces;
posterior pharyngeal wall

Dorsal surface of tongue

Palatine tonsil

Palatopharyngeus muscle

FIGURE 620.1 **Palate: Muscular Folds and Glands**

NOTE: The oral mucosa has been removed from both the hard and soft palate, revealing the palatal musculature, vessels, and glands. Observe the **palatoglossus** and **palatopharyngeus muscles**, along with the **greater** and **lesser palatine nerves** and **vessels**.

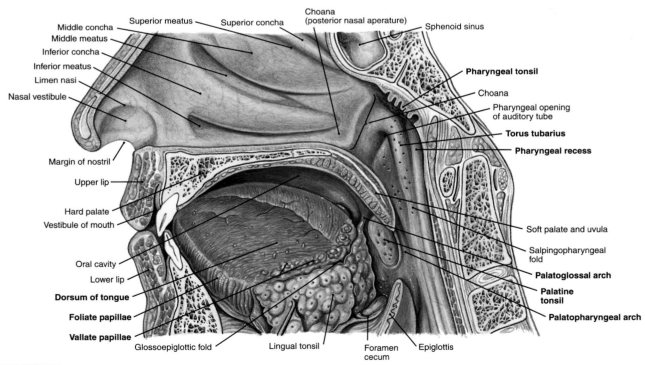

Choana
(posterior nasal aperature)

Superior meatus — Superior concha

Sphenoid sinus

Middle concha
Middle meatus
Inferior concha
Inferior meatus
Limen nasi
Nasal vestibule

Pharyngeal tonsil

Choana

Pharyngeal opening
of auditory tube

Torus tubarius

Pharyngeal recess

Margin of nostril

Upper lip

Hard palate
Vestibule of mouth

Soft palate and uvula

Salpingopharyngeal
fold

Oral cavity

Palatoglossal arch

Lower lip

**Palatine
tonsil**

Dorsum of tongue

Foliate papillae

Palatopharyngeal arch

Vallate papillae

Glossoepiglottic fold   Lingual tonsil   Foramen   Epiglottis
cecum

FIGURE 620.2 **Tongue, Palatine Tonsil, and the Oropharynx**

NOTE: (1) In this sagittal view, the tongue has been deviated to demonstrate the right palatoglossal arch and right palatine tonsil. Observe the
large **vallate papillae**.
(2) The opening of the **auditory tube** in the nasopharynx, behind which is a cartilaginous elevation of the tube called the **torus tubarius**. Also note
the **pharyngeal tonsil** (**adenoid**).

PLATE 621 Oral Cavity: Sublingual Region and Parotid Duct Orifice

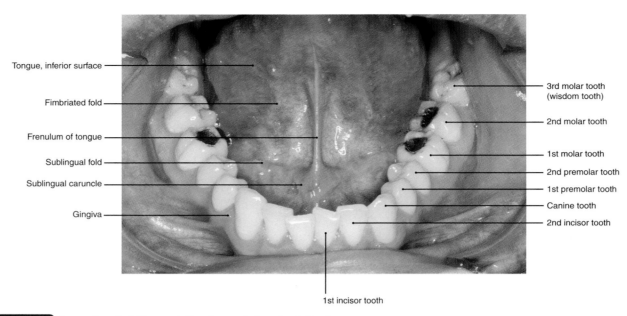

Tongue, inferior surface

Fimbriated fold

Frenulum of tongue

Sublingual fold

Sublingual caruncle

Gingiva

3rd molar tooth (wisdom tooth)

2nd molar tooth

1st molar tooth

2nd premolar tooth

1st premolar tooth

Canine tooth

2nd incisor tooth

1st incisor tooth

FIGURE 621.1 **Anterior Sublingual Region of the Oral Cavity**

NOTE: (1) The mucous membrane covering the floor of the oral cavity continues over the inferior surface of the tongue and meets at the midline as an elevated fold called the **frenulum of the tongue.**

(2) The **sublingual folds**. Along these open the **ducts of the sublingual glands**, and at their anterior end on each side is an orifice for the **submandibular duct** called the **sublingual caruncle.**

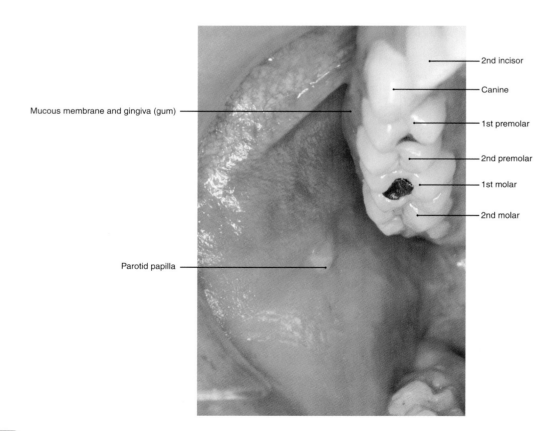

Mucous membrane and gingiva (gum)

Parotid papilla

2nd incisor

Canine

1st premolar

2nd premolar

1st molar

2nd molar

FIGURE 621.2 **Orifice of the Parotid Duct**

NOTE: The opening of the parotid duct (sometimes called Stensen's duct) in the oral cavity is marked by a small elevation called the parotid papilla, which is located opposite the upper (maxillary) second molar tooth.

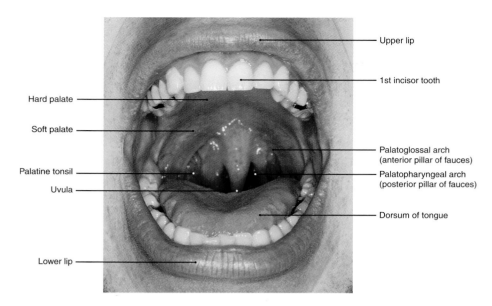

Upper lip

1st incisor tooth

Hard palate

Soft palate

Palatoglossal arch (anterior pillar of fauces)

Palatine tonsil

Palatopharyngeal arch (posterior pillar of fauces)

Uvula

Dorsum of tongue

Lower lip

FIGURE 622.1 Oral Cavity; Anterior View of the Palate and Dorsum of the Tongue

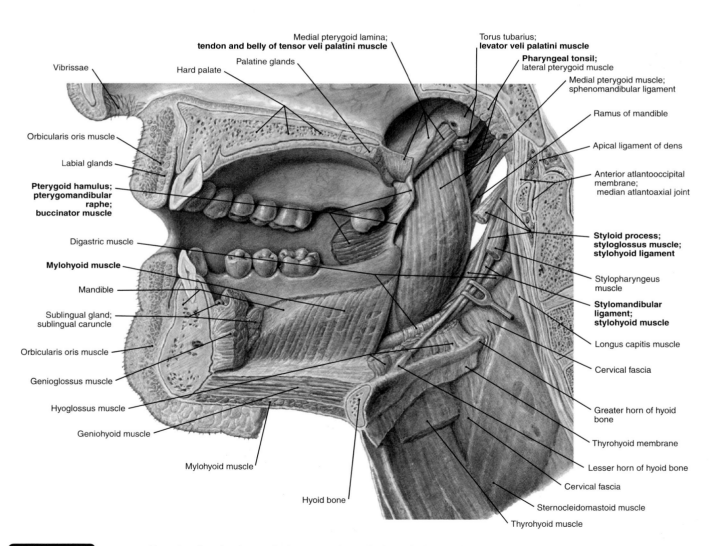

Vibrissae

Medial pterygoid lamina; **tendon and belly of tensor veli palatini muscle**

Palatine glands

Hard palate

Torus tubarius; **levator veli palatini muscle**

Pharyngeal tonsil; lateral pterygoid muscle

Medial pterygoid muscle; sphenomandibular ligament

Orbicularis oris muscle

Labial glands

Ramus of mandible

Apical ligament of dens

Pterygoid hamulus; pterygomandibular raphe; buccinator muscle

Anterior atlantooccipital membrane; median atlantoaxial joint

Digastric muscle

Styloid process; styloglossus muscle; stylohyoid ligament

Mylohyoid muscle

Mandible

Stylopharyngeus muscle

Sublingual gland; sublingual caruncle

Stylomandibular ligament; stylohyoid muscle

Orbicularis oris muscle

Longus capitis muscle

Genioglossus muscle

Cervical fascia

Hyoglossus muscle

Greater horn of hyoid bone

Geniohyoid muscle

Thyrohyoid membrane

Mylohyoid muscle

Lesser horn of hyoid bone

Cervical fascia

Hyoid bone

Sternocleidomastoid muscle

Thyrohyoid muscle

FIGURE 622.2 Paramedian Sagittal View of the Interior of the Right Oral Cavity and the Upper Neck (Muscles and Ligaments)

NOTE: In this dissection, the right half of the oral cavity was exposed and the mucous membrane removed from the floor of the mouth to reveal the **mylohyoid muscle**. Also observe the **pterygomandibular raphe** and **buccinator muscle**.

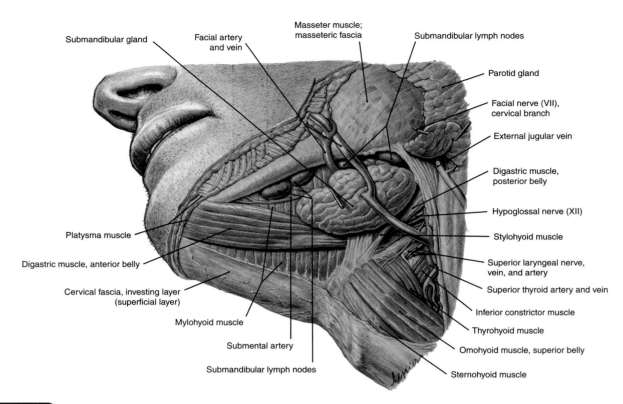

Submandibular gland — Facial artery and vein — Masseter muscle; masseteric fascia — Submandibular lymph nodes — Parotid gland — Facial nerve (VII), cervical branch — External jugular vein — Digastric muscle, posterior belly — Hypoglossal nerve (XII) — Stylohyoid muscle — Superior laryngeal nerve, vein, and artery — Superior thyroid artery and vein — Inferior constrictor muscle — Thyrohyoid muscle — Omohyoid muscle, superior belly — Sternohyoid muscle

Platysma muscle — Digastric muscle, anterior belly — Cervical fascia, investing layer (superficial layer) — Mylohyoid muscle — Submental artery — Submandibular lymph nodes

FIGURE 623.1 Floor of the Oral Cavity: Intact and Viewed from the Submandibular Region in the Upper Neck

NOTE: (1) The **submandibular** and **parotid glands** that produce saliva that is transported by secretory ducts to the oral cavity.
(2) The **submandibular triangle** bounded by the anterior and posterior bellies of the digastric muscle and the mandible.
(3) The **mylohyoid muscle** forming the largest part of the floor of the oral cavity. Compare this figure with Figures 626.1 and 626.2.

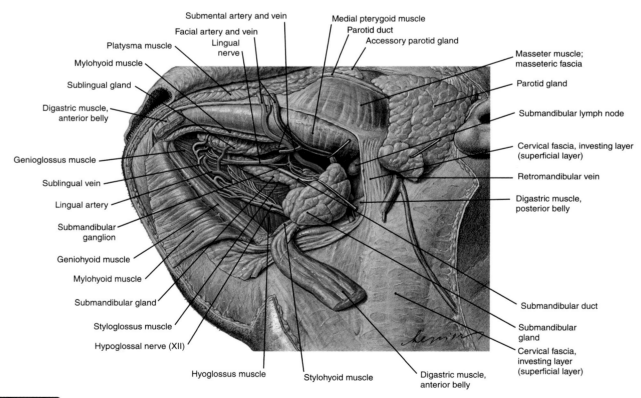

Platysma muscle — Mylohyoid muscle — Sublingual gland — Digastric muscle, anterior belly — Genioglossus muscle — Sublingual vein — Lingual artery — Submandibular ganglion — Geniohyoid muscle — Mylohyoid muscle — Submandibular gland — Styloglossus muscle — Hypoglossal nerve (XII)

Submental artery and vein — Facial artery and vein — Lingual nerve — Medial pterygoid muscle — Parotid duct — Accessory parotid gland — Masseter muscle; masseteric fascia — Parotid gland — Submandibular lymph node — Cervical fascia, investing layer (superficial layer) — Retromandibular vein — Digastric muscle, posterior belly — Submandibular duct — Submandibular gland — Cervical fascia, investing layer (superficial layer)

Hyoglossus muscle — Stylohyoid muscle — Digastric muscle, anterior belly

FIGURE 623.2 Floor of the Oral Cavity: Opened Inferiorly from the Submandibular Region

NOTE: (1) The anterior belly of the digastric and mylohyoid muscles has been reflected to reveal: the **sublingual gland, lingual nerve, submandibular ganglion** and **duct, hypoglossal nerve** and **vein,** and **lingual artery**.
(2) The hypoglossal nerve is the motor nerve to all tongue muscles *except* the palatoglossus. The lingual nerve supplies the anterior two-thirds of the tongue with general sensation.
(3) The three salivary glands are all shown in this figure: the **parotid gland** on the side of the face, the **submandibular gland** in the suprahyoid region, and the **sublingual gland**, which lies in its entirety within the oral cavity. Compare this figure with Figures 623.1, 624.1, and 624.2.

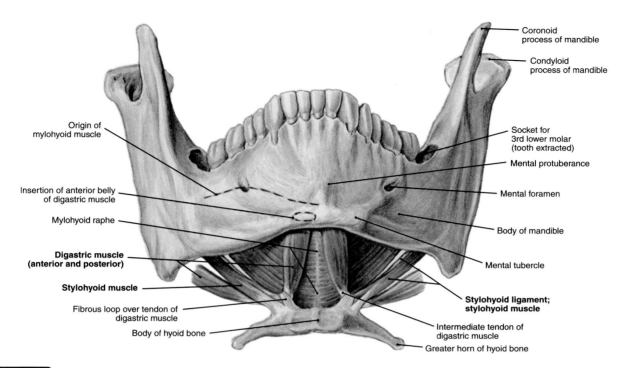

FIGURE 624.1 Suprahyoid Muscles and Floor of the Mouth (Viewed from Below)

NOTE: (1) On the mandible are the inner attachments of the **mylohyoid muscle** (broken line) and the **anterior belly of the digastric muscle** (circle). Observe the attachments of the **mylohyoid, digastric,** and **stylohyoid muscles** and the **stylohyoid ligament** on the hyoid bone.

(2) The tendon between the anterior and posterior bellies of the digastric muscle is anchored by a fibrous loop to the hyoid bone.

(3) The stylohyoid muscle is supplied by the facial (or seventh) cranial nerve, as is the posterior belly of the digastric muscle. The action of the stylohyoid muscle is to retract and elevate the hyoid bone, thus, elongating the floor of the mouth.

(4) The two bellies of the digastric muscle also elevate the hyoid bone, while the mylohyoid muscle raises the floor of the mouth when swallowing and is capable of pushing the tongue upward in the mouth and protruding the tongue forward.

(5) In addition, the mylohyoid muscles depress the mandible in chewing, swallowing, sucking, and blowing air out of the mouth.

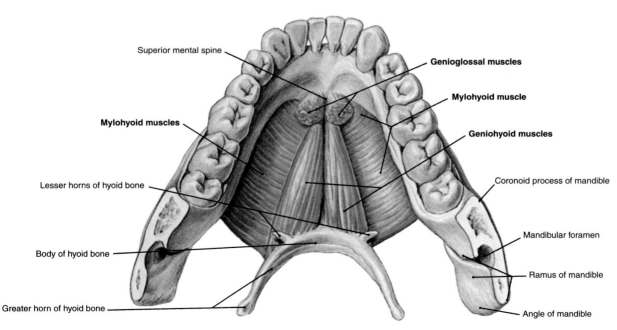

FIGURE 624.2 Mylohyoid and Geniohyoid Muscles (Viewed from Above)

NOTE: The **mylohyoid** and **geniohyoid muscles** form the floor of the oral cavity. The mylohyoids arise along the mylohyoid lines of the mandible and insert into the median raphe, which extends from the hyoid bone to the symphysis menti. The genioglossal muscles have been severed near their origin.

PLATE 625 Oral Cavity: Salivary Glands

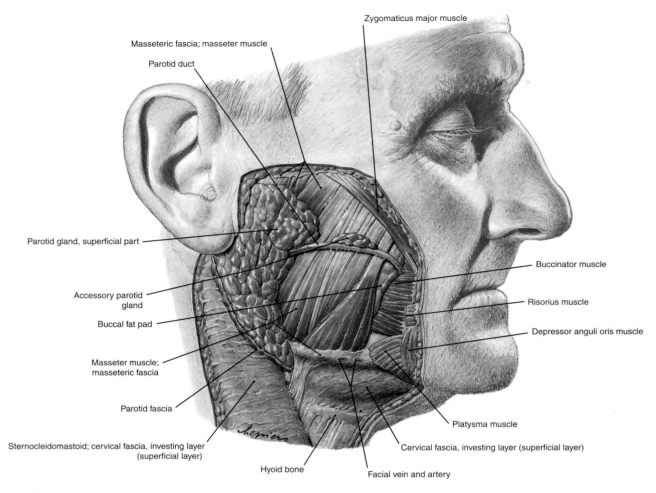

Zygomaticus major muscle

Masseteric fascia; masseter muscle

Parotid duct

Parotid gland, superficial part

Accessory parotid gland

Buccal fat pad

Masseter muscle; masseteric fascia

Parotid fascia

Sternocleidomastoid; cervical fascia, investing layer (superficial layer)

Hyoid bone

Facial vein and artery

Buccinator muscle

Risorius muscle

Depressor anguli oris muscle

Platysma muscle

Cervical fascia, investing layer (superficial layer)

FIGURE 625 Lateral View of the Parotid Gland and an Accessory Parotid Gland Attached to the Parotid Duct

PAROTID GLAND

DEVELOPMENT: Arises during the sixth week of gestation as an epithelial outgrowth from the mouth and forms a tube that grows backward toward the ear. The posterior part of the tube branches into lobes that become the gland, and it enmeshes the facial nerve. The tube remains as the **parotid duct**, which opens into the mouth opposite the second upper molar tooth.

ADULT GLAND: A serous gland, weighing about 25 g, on either side of the face in front of the ear. Located between the mandible and the sternocleidomastoid muscle.

ARTERIES: Branches of the external carotid artery as it passes behind the gland.

VEINS: Empty into the external jugular vein.

INNERVATION: *Sympathetic*: Postganglionic vasomotor fibers come from the superior cervical ganglion by way of the external carotid plexus. *Parasympathetic*: Preganglionic secretomotor fibers course in the **glossopharyngeal nerve** and then the **lesser petrosal nerve** to the **otic ganglion**, where they synapse. Postganglionic fibers course to the parotid gland by way of the **auriculotemporal nerve (V)**.

LYMPH DRAINAGE: Superficial and deep parotid nodes drain into cervical lymph nodes.

SUBMANDIBULAR GLAND

DEVELOPMENT: Arises during the sixth week of gestation from an epithelial ridge in a groove between the tongue and the lower jaw. The caudal end of the ridge forms numerous branches that extend backward and ventrally beneath the mandible as glandular lobules. The main stalk, connected to the deep part of the gland persists as the **submandibular duct**.

ADULT GLAND: A seromucous gland of about 8 g on each side. The **superficial part** is the size of a walnut and is located in the digastric triangle of the upper neck. The **deep part** extends above the mylohyoid muscle into the oral cavity. The **submandibular duct** extends forward from the deep part and opens at the **sublingual caruncle** at the side of the frenulum below the tongue.

ARTERIES: Submental branches of the **facial artery** in neck and of **lingual artery** in oral cavity.

VEINS: Drain into the facial and lingual veins and then into the **internal jugular vein**.

INNERVATION: *Sympathetic*: Postganglionic vasomotor fibers come from the superior cervical ganglion by way of the external carotid plexus. *Parasympathetic*: Preganglionic fibers course in the **nervus intermedius** part of the **facial nerve**. They travel to the **submandibular ganglion** by way of the **chorda tympani nerve** and then the **lingual nerve**. Postganglionic fibers from the ganglion **course directly** to the gland.

LYMPH DRAINAGE: Into submandibular nodes and then into upper and lower deep cervical nodes.

FIGURE 626.1 Submandibular and Sublingual Glands

NOTE: (1) With the tongue removed and the genioglossus and geniohyoid muscles cut, the submandibular and sublingual glands are exposed and their relationship to the inner aspect of the mandible is demonstrated.

(2) The submandibular duct measures about 5 cm and courses anteriorly between the sublingual gland and the genioglossus muscle (cut). It opens in the floor of the mouth at the sublingual caruncle.

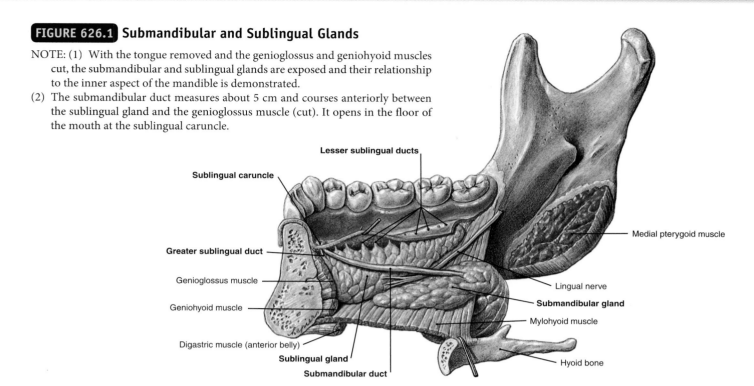

SUBLINGUAL GLAND

DEVELOPMENT: Appears as a series of epithelial buds along the groove between the lower jaw and the tongue during the eighth week of gestation, just lateral to the submandibular primordium. The buds enlarge and some of the more anterior ones join to form a duct that opens near the submandibular duct. The remaining buds open by separate ducts (8–10) in the floor of the mouth above the sublingual fold.

ADULT GLAND: A seromucous gland on each side (30% serous, 70% mucous) weighing about 4 g. It is narrow and flattened and located deep to the mucous membrane in the floor of the mouth. Its ducts (10–20) open in a line along the surface of the sublingual fold. Several anterior ducts join to form the main sublingual duct. This opens near the caruncle of the submandibular duct.

ARTERIES: **Sublingual branch** of the **lingual artery**, which anastomoses with the **submental branch** of the **facial artery**.

VEINS: Drain into lingual vein and then into internal jugular vein.

INNERVATION: Same as for the submandibular gland.

LYMPH DRAINAGE: Superficial and deep submandibular nodes and then into deep cervical nodes.

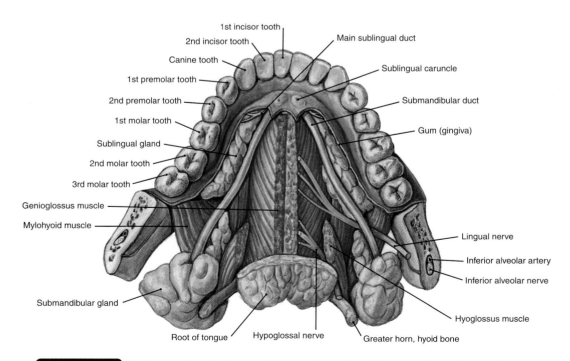

FIGURE 626.2 Salivary Glands in the Floor of the Oral Cavity (Seen from Above)

PLATE 627 Oral Cavity: Midsagittal Section, the Tongue

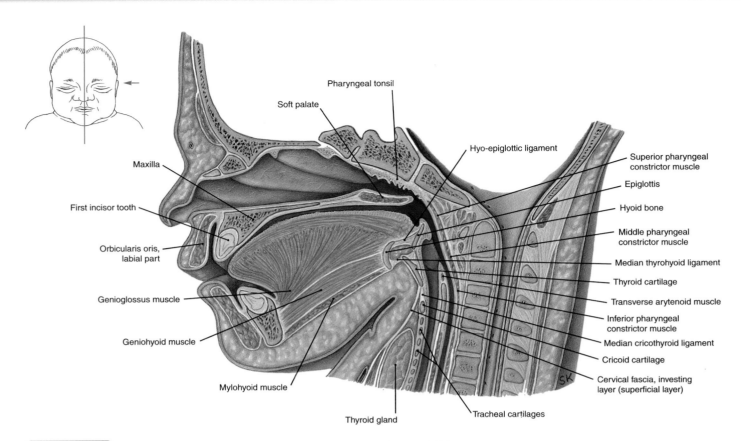

FIGURE 627.1 Median Section through the Head of a Newborn Child

NOTE: (1) The midline section of the tongue and its underlying muscles, the geniohyoid and the mylohyoid.
(2) In the newborn, the larynx is considerably higher than in the adult.
(3) The genioglossus muscle is shown in this figure and in Figure 627.2.

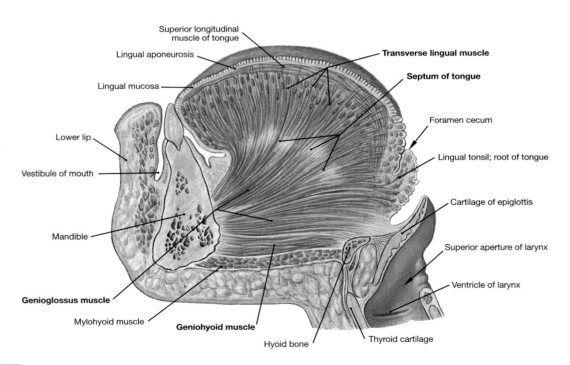

FIGURE 627.2 Genioglossus and Intrinsic Muscles of the Tongue

NOTE: (1) In this midsagittal section can be seen the median fibrous septum of the tongue and the **intrinsic** tongue musculature, which includes the longitudinal, transverse, and vertical muscles of the tongue.
(2) The **genioglossus** constitutes most of the tongue musculature, and its fibers radiate backward and upward in a fanlike manner from the uppermost of the mental spines (genial tubercles) on the inner surface of the mandible, just above the origin of the geniohyoid muscle.

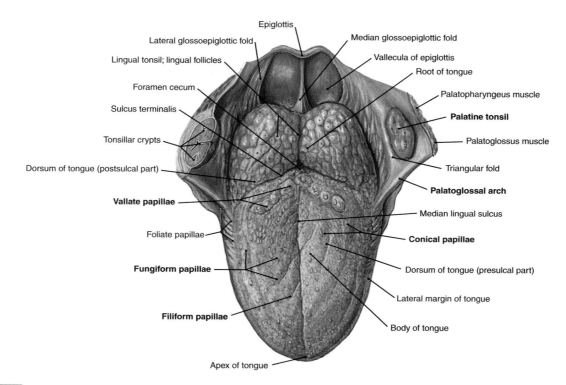

Epiglottis
Lateral glossoepiglottic fold
Lingual tonsil; lingual follicles
Foramen cecum
Sulcus terminalis
Tonsillar crypts
Dorsum of tongue (postsulcal part)
Vallate papillae
Foliate papillae
Fungiform papillae
Filiform papillae
Apex of tongue

Median glossoepiglottic fold
Vallecula of epiglottis
Root of tongue
Palatopharyngeus muscle
Palatine tonsil
Palatoglossus muscle
Triangular fold
Palatoglossal arch
Median lingual sulcus
Conical papillae
Dorsum of tongue (presulcal part)
Lateral margin of tongue
Body of tongue

FIGURE 628.1 **Dorsal Surface of the Tongue**

NOTE: (1) The dorsum of the tongue is marked by numerous elevations called papillae. These serve as location sites of receptors for the special sense of **taste**. Observe the inverted V-shaped group of large **vallate papillae**.
(2) The **fungiform papillae** are found principally at the sides and apex of the tongue. These are large, round, and deep red.
(3) The **filiform** (conical) **papillae**. These are small and arranged in rows that course parallel to the vallate papillae.
(4) The parallel vertical folds (about five in number) called the **foliate papillae** on the lateral border of the tongue just anterior to the palatoglossal arch. These are studded with taste receptors.

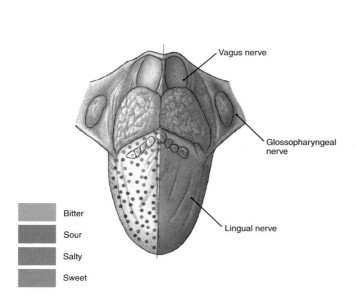

Vagus nerve
Glossopharyngeal nerve
Lingual nerve

Bitter
Sour
Salty
Sweet

FIGURE 628.2 **Innervation and Location of Taste Qualities on the Dorsum of the Tongue**

NOTE: On the right: fields of innervation by the **lingual, glossopharyngeal** and **vagus nerves**. On the left: Receptors for the basic tastes of **salt** and **sweet** are clustered anterior to those for **bitter** and **sour**.

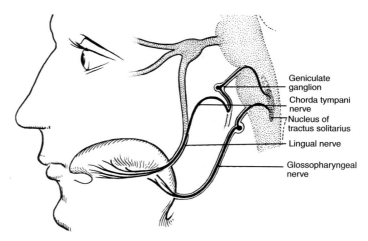

Geniculate ganglion
Chorda tympani nerve
Nucleus of tractus solitarius
Lingual nerve
Glossopharyngeal nerve

FIGURE 628.3 **Principal Pathways for Taste**

NOTE: (1) The two principal pathways for taste are along the **lingual nerve** to the **chorda tympani nerve** for the anterior two-thirds of the tongue and the **glossopharyngeal nerve** for the posterior third of the tongue.
(2) Two lesser pathways (not shown) are:
  (a) From the epiglottis along the **internal laryngeal branch** of the **vagus**.
  (b) From the palate along the **palatine nerves** and the **nerve of the pterygoid canal** to the **greater petrosal nerve** and then the **nervus intermedius part** of the **facial nerve**.

Chapter 7 The Neck and Head

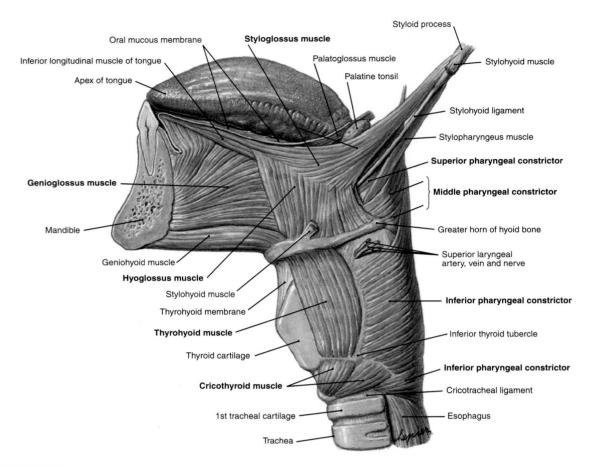

FIGURE 629.1 Extrinsic Tongue Muscles; External Larynx and Pharynx (Lateral View 1)

NOTE: The tongue is attached to the hyoid bone, the mandible, the styloid process, the soft palate, and the pharyngeal wall.

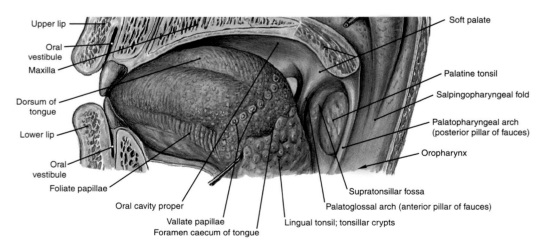

FIGURE 629.2 Paramedian Section of the Oral Cavity, Oral Pharynx, and Tongue

NOTE: (1) The lingual tonsil covering the posterior third of the tongue. Also observe the vallate papillae located in a line between the anterior two-thirds of the tongue and the posterior third.

(2) The palatine tonsil in the tonsillar bed located between the palatoglossal and palatopharyngeal folds.

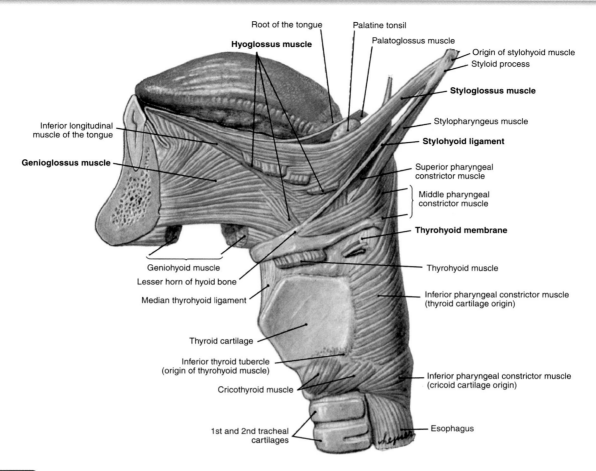

FIGURE 630.1 Extrinsic Tongue Muscles; External Larynx and Pharynx (Lateral View 2)

NOTE: (1) In this dissection, the hyoglossus muscle has been removed, revealing the attachments of the **stylohyoid ligament** and the **middle pharyngeal constrictor muscle** along the hyoid bone. The geniohyoid muscle has been cut and the thyrohyoid **muscle removed.**

(2) The blending of the fibers of the styloglossus, hyoglossus, and genioglossus at the base of the **tongue.**

(3) The penetration through the **thyrohyoid membrane** by the **superior laryngeal vessels** and **nerve.**

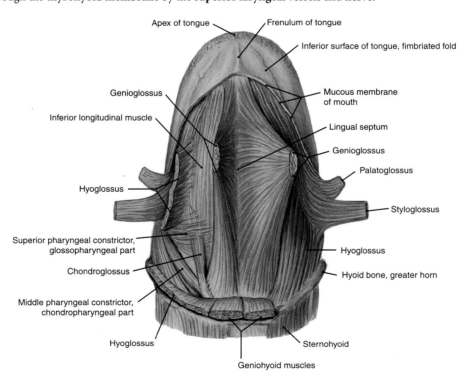

FIGURE 630.2 Ventral View of the Muscles of the Tongue

NOTE: The large genioglossus muscle detached from the mandible and the hyoglossus muscle inserting into the side of the tongue from its origin on the hyoid bone. Also observe the insertions of the palatoglossus and styloglossus muscles.

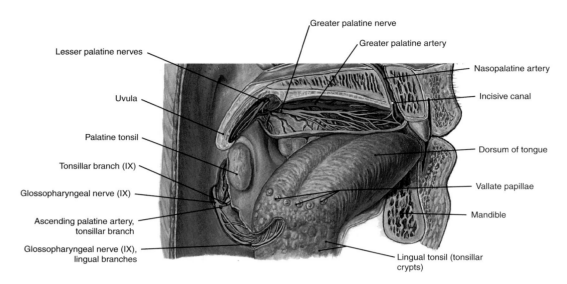

FIGURE 631.1 Nerves and Arteries of the Posterior Tongue and Palate

NOTE: (1) The **glossopharyngeal nerve** supplies both general sensation and the special sense of taste to the posterior third of the tongue.
(2) The **greater palatine artery** and **nerve** supply the palate in the roof of the oral cavity and the **ascending** pharyngeal artery, one of several vessels that supply the palatine tonsil located in the oropharynx.

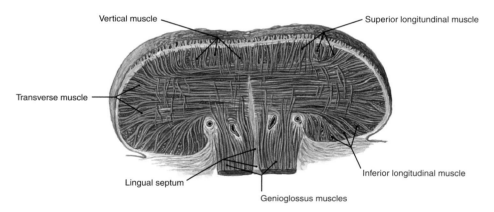

FIGURE 631.2 Transverse Section through the Middle of the Tongue (Anterior View)

NOTE: The transverse and vertical fibers of the intrinsic tongue muscles can best be seen in a transverse section. Observe, however, the cut longitudinal fibers both superiorly and inferiorly.

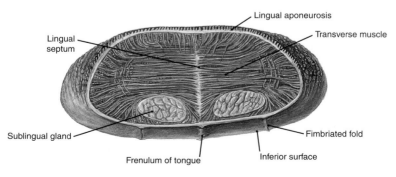

FIGURE 631.3 Transverse Section through the Tip of the Tongue

NOTE: The sublingual glands deep to the anterior part of the tongue.

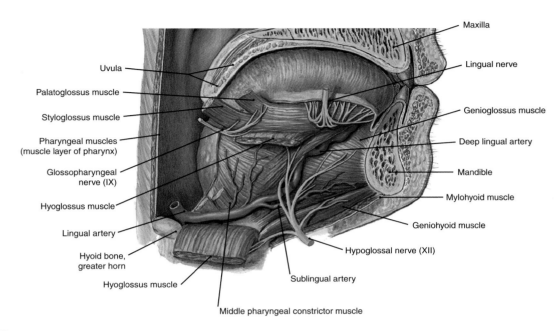

FIGURE 632 **Opened Oral Cavity Showing the Tongue and Its Nerves and Arterial Supply**

NOTE: (1) The longitudinal and medial course of the **lingual artery**. Also observe the **lingual, glossopharyngeal,** and **hypoglossal nerves**.

(2) The **hypoglossal nerve** supplies the genioglossus, hyoglossus, and styloglossus muscles as well as all of the intrinsic muscles of the tongue.

(3) The **lingual nerve** is sensory to the anterior two-thirds of the tongue (both general sensation and taste, the latter by way of the **chorda tympani** nerve fibers), while the **glossopharyngeal nerve** supplies the posterior third of the tongue (both general sensation and taste).

(4) The **geniohyoid muscle** extending from the mental spine of the mandible (posterior to the symphysis menti) to the anterior surface of the hyoid bone.

(5) The **hyoglossus muscle** has been severed in order to show the forward course of the lingual artery.

EXTRINSIC MUSCLES OF THE TONGUE				
Muscle	**Origin**	**Insertion**	**Innervation**	**Action**
Genioglossus	Upper part of the mental spine of mandible	In a fanlike manner along the ventral surface of tongue; anterior surface of body of hyoid bone	Hypoglossal nerve	Draws the tongue forward and protrudes the apex of the tongue
Hyoglossus	Entire length of the greater horn of hyoid bone and lateral part of body of hyoid bone	Into the side of tongue	Hypoglossal nerve	Depresses the tongue
Styloglossus	Styloid process of temporal bone and the stylohyoid ligament	Side and inferior aspect of the tongue	Hypoglossal nerve	Draws the tongue upward and backward
Palatoglossus	Oral surface of the palatine aponeurosis	Side and dorsum of the tongue	Pharyngeal branch of the vagus nerve (fibers emerge from brain in cranial part of accessory nerve [i.e., XI via X])	Elevates the posterior part of the tongue

In addition, the tongue contains longitudinal, transverse, and vertical muscles whose fibers commence and terminate within the tongue itself and, hence, are considered **intrinsic tongue muscles**. These are all supplied by the **hypoglossal nerve**.

PLATE 633 Teeth: Innervation of Upper and Lower Teeth; Mandible

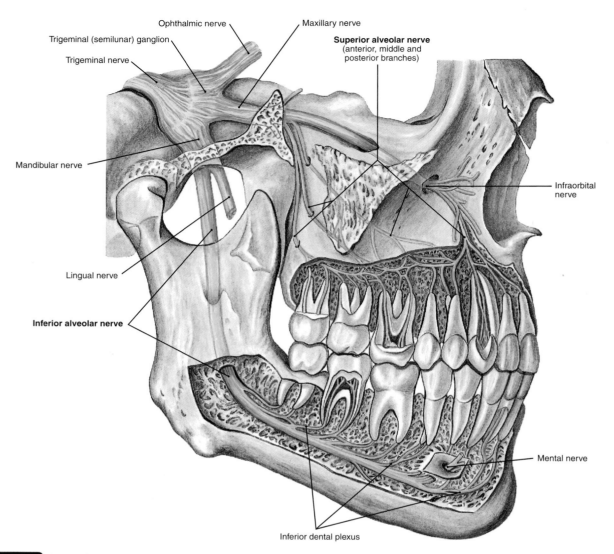

Ophthalmic nerve

Maxillary nerve

Trigeminal (semilunar) ganglion

Superior alveolar nerve
(anterior, middle and
posterior branches)

Trigeminal nerve

Mandibular nerve

Infraorbital
nerve

Lingual nerve

Inferior alveolar nerve

Mental nerve

Inferior dental plexus

FIGURE 633.1 Superior Alveolar Nerves (Maxillary) and Inferior Alveolar Nerve (Mandibular) and Their Branches to the Upper and Lower Teeth

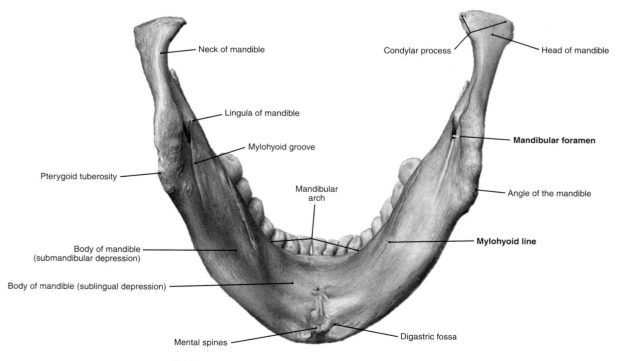

Neck of mandible

Condylar process

Head of mandible

Lingula of mandible

Mandibular foramen

Mylohyoid groove

Pterygoid tuberosity

Mandibular
arch

Angle of the mandible

Body of mandible
(submandibular depression)

Mylohyoid line

Body of mandible (sublingual depression)

Mental spines

Digastric fossa

FIGURE 633.2 Mandible as Seen from Below

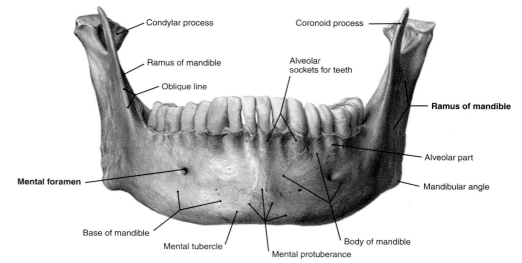

Condylar process

Coronoid process

Ramus of mandible

Alveolar sockets for teeth

Oblique line

Ramus of mandible

Alveolar part

Mental foramen

Mandibular angle

Base of mandible

Mental tubercle

Body of mandible

Mental protuberance

FIGURE 634.1 Mandible (Seen from Front)

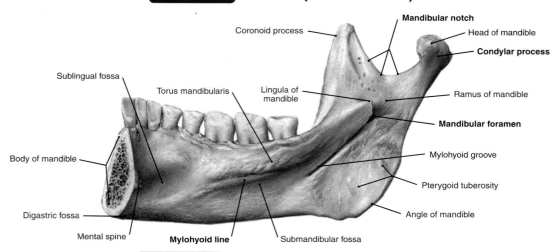

Coronoid process

Mandibular notch

Head of mandible

Condylar process

Sublingual fossa

Torus mandibularis

Lingula of mandible

Ramus of mandible

Mandibular foramen

Body of mandible

Mylohyoid groove

Pterygoid tuberosity

Digastric fossa

Angle of mandible

Mental spine

Mylohyoid line

Submandibular fossa

FIGURE 634.2 Right Mandible (Inner Surface)

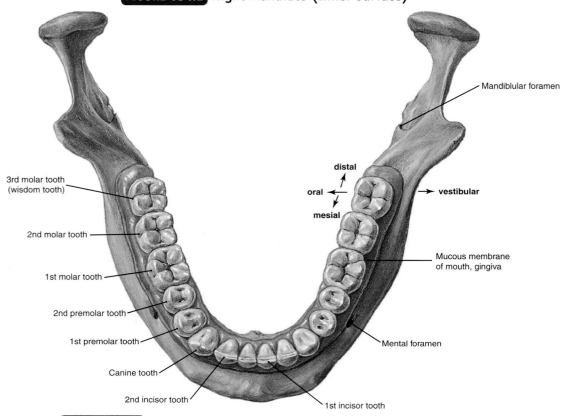

Mandiblular foramen

3rd molar tooth (wisdom tooth)

distal

oral

vestibular

mesial

2nd molar tooth

1st molar tooth

Mucous membrane of mouth, gingiva

2nd premolar tooth

1st premolar tooth

Mental foramen

Canine tooth

2nd incisor tooth

1st incisor tooth

FIGURE 634.3 Mandibular Arch and the Lower Teeth (Seen from Above)

PLATE 635 Upper Teeth and Palate from Below

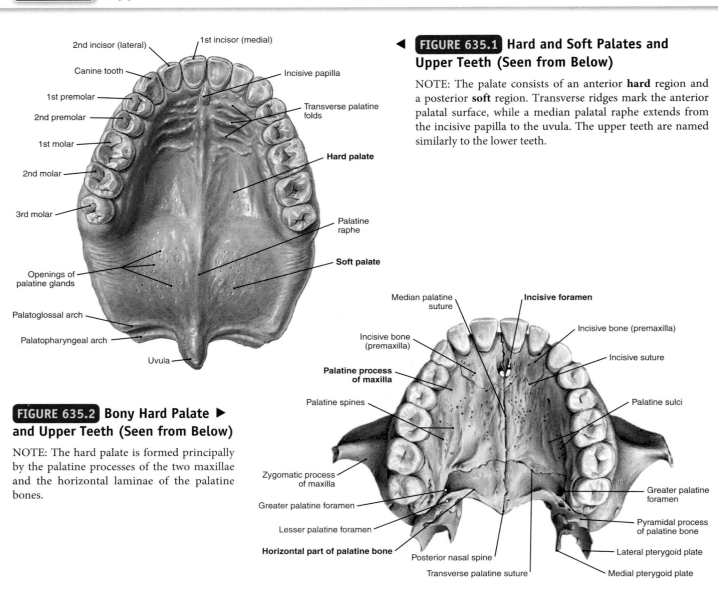

2nd incisor (lateral)
1st incisor (medial)
Canine tooth
1st premolar
2nd premolar
1st molar
2nd molar
3rd molar
Openings of palatine glands
Palatoglossal arch
Palatopharyngeal arch
Uvula
Incisive papilla
Transverse palatine folds
Hard palate
Palatine raphe
Soft palate

◄ **FIGURE 635.1** Hard and Soft Palates and Upper Teeth (Seen from Below)

NOTE: The palate consists of an anterior **hard** region and a posterior **soft** region. Transverse ridges mark the anterior palatal surface, while a median palatal raphe extends from the incisive papilla to the uvula. The upper teeth are named similarly to the lower teeth.

FIGURE 635.2 Bony Hard Palate ► and Upper Teeth (Seen from Below)

NOTE: The hard palate is formed principally by the palatine processes of the two maxillae and the horizontal laminae of the palatine bones.

Median palatine suture
Incisive foramen
Incisive bone (premaxilla)
Incisive bone (premaxilla)
Incisive suture
Palatine process of maxilla
Palatine spines
Palatine sulci
Zygomatic process of maxilla
Greater palatine foramen
Lesser palatine foramen
Horizontal part of palatine bone
Posterior nasal spine
Transverse palatine suture
Greater palatine foramen
Pyramidal process of palatine bone
Lateral pterygoid plate
Medial pterygoid plate

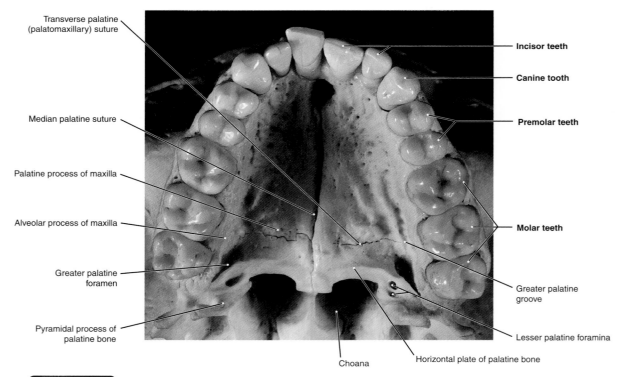

Transverse palatine (palatomaxillary) suture
Median palatine suture
Palatine process of maxilla
Alveolar process of maxilla
Greater palatine foramen
Pyramidal process of palatine bone
Choana
Horizontal plate of palatine bone
Incisor teeth
Canine tooth
Premolar teeth
Molar teeth
Greater palatine groove
Lesser palatine foramina

FIGURE 635.3 Photograph of the Bony Palate Showing the Maxillary Arch and Upper Teeth

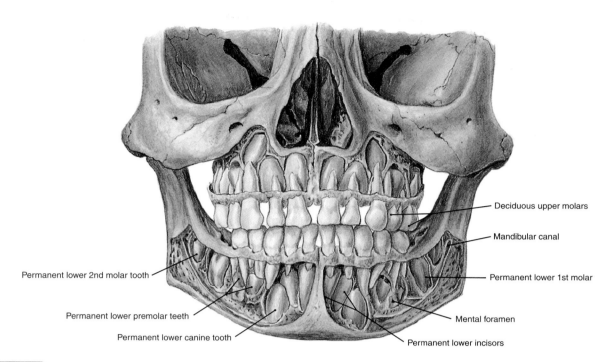

Deciduous upper molars

Mandibular canal

Permanent lower 2nd molar tooth

Permanent lower 1st molar

Permanent lower premolar teeth

Mental foramen

Permanent lower canine tooth

Permanent lower incisors

FIGURE 636.1 Facial Skeleton of a 5-Year-Old Child Showing Full Deciduous Dentition (20 Teeth)

NOTE: (1) The **deciduous teeth** are shown as white, whereas the rudiments of the **permanent teeth**, shown in blue, have been exposed by removing the outer walls of the alveolar processes of both maxillae and the mandible.

(2) All 20 deciduous teeth have erupted: eight incisors, four canines, and eight molars. Normally all deciduous teeth are replaced by the 12th year.

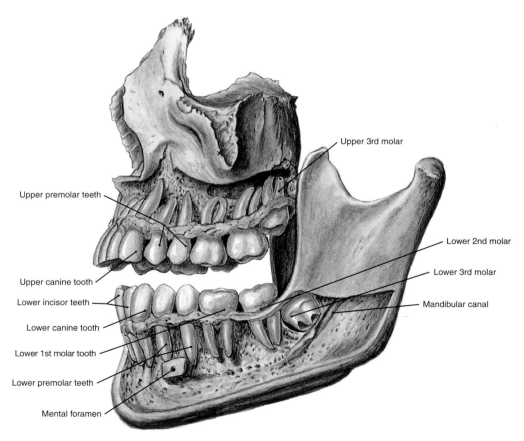

Upper 3rd molar

Upper premolar teeth

Lower 2nd molar

Lower 3rd molar

Upper canine tooth

Lower incisor teeth

Mandibular canal

Lower canine tooth

Lower 1st molar tooth

Lower premolar teeth

Mental foramen

FIGURE 636.2 Dentition of a 20-Year-Old Person (Seen from Left Side)

NOTE: (1) The roots of the permanent teeth have been exposed by removing the alveolar walls. All of the permanent teeth have erupted through the gums, with the exception of the lower third molar.

(2) The canines and incisors have but one root, as generally do the premolars, although the latter may have two roots. The first and second molars usually have three roots, whereas the smaller third molar may have less than three and may even be single-rooted.

PLATE 637 **Left Adult Permanent Teeth (Vestibular and Medial Aspects)**

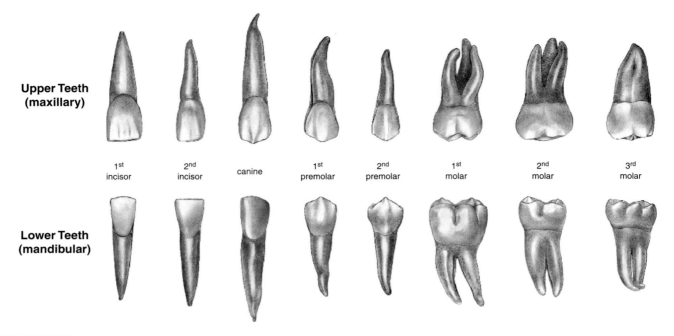

Upper Teeth (maxillary)

1st incisor | 2nd incisor | canine | 1st premolar | 2nd premolar | 1st molar | 2nd molar | 3rd molar

Lower Teeth (mandibular)

FIGURE 637.1 **Left Adult Permanent Teeth: Vestibular View**

NOTE: (1) The orientations of **"vestibular,"** **"medial** or **mesial,"** **"oral,"** and **"distal"** are shown in Figure 634.3.

(2) The **incisor teeth** have a sharp edge and a single root. Observe that the first maxillary incisor is larger than the first mandibular incisor, and the roots of the maxillary incisors are rounded, whereas the roots of the mandibular incisors are flattened.

(3) The **canine tooth** is somewhat larger than the incisors, and it has a single cusp. It is also the longest of all the teeth.

(4) The **premolar teeth** have a buccal and a palatal cusp (hence they are often called bicuspids). The upper first premolar usually has two roots and the upper second premolar usually has one root, but it may have two. Both lower premolars have a single root, but the root of the first lower premolar may be bifid.

(5) Vestibular refers to the vestibule of the mouth, and depending on the tooth is either from the anterior direction or from the lateral direction.

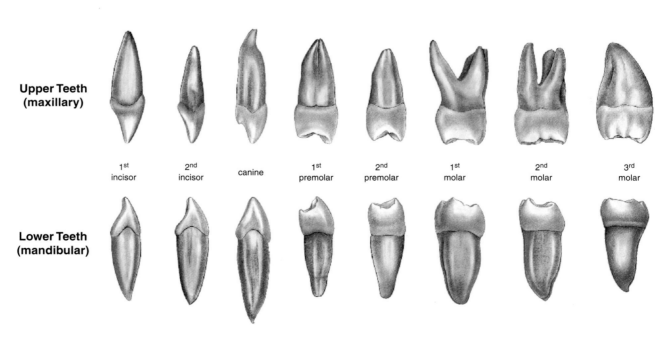

Upper Teeth (maxillary)

1st incisor | 2nd incisor | canine | 1st premolar | 2nd premolar | 1st molar | 2nd molar | 3rd molar

Lower Teeth (mandibular)

FIGURE 637.2 **Left Adult Permanent Teeth: Medial or Mesial View**

NOTE: The **molar teeth** decrease in size posteriorly. They have four or five cusps. The first and second molars generally have three roots, whereas the third molar (wisdom tooth) often may have only a single root.

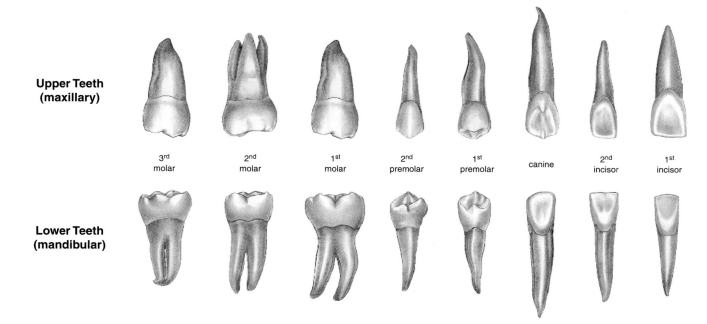

Upper Teeth (maxillary)

| 3rd molar | 2nd molar | 1st molar | 2nd premolar | 1st premolar | canine | 2nd incisor | 1st incisor |

Lower Teeth (mandibular)

FIGURE 638.1 Left Adult Permanent Teeth: Oral View

NOTE that "oral" in the mandibular region means **"lingual,"** whereas in the maxillary region, oral refers to **"palatal."**

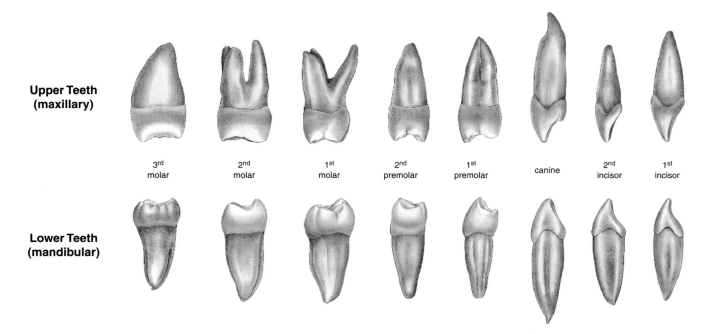

Upper Teeth (maxillary)

| 3rd molar | 2nd molar | 1st molar | 2nd premolar | 1st premolar | canine | 2nd incisor | 1st incisor |

Lower Teeth (mandibular)

FIGURE 638.2 Left Adult Permanent Teeth: Distal View

See Fig. 634.3.

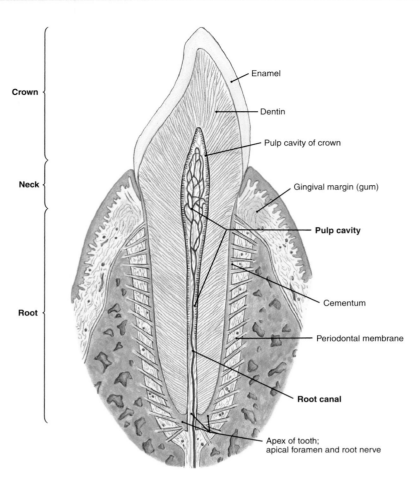

FIGURE 639.1 **Longitudinal Section of the Tooth**

NOTE: (1) The crown of the tooth is covered with **enamel** and projects from the **gingiva,** or gum. The root is embedded within the alveolar bony **socket** and covered by a thin layer of **cementum.**

(2) The main portion of the tooth consists of **dentin,** which surrounds the **root canal** and **pulp cavity** containing the **dental artery** and **nerve.**

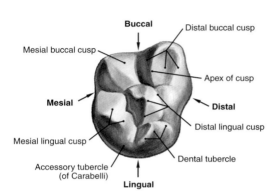

FIGURE 639.2 **Occlusal Surface of the Right Upper First Molar**

NOTE: The upper first molar may have a fifth cusp, the tubercle of Carabelli, on the mesiolingual surface of the crown.

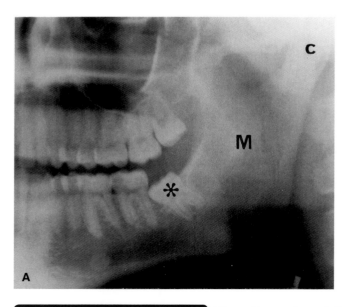

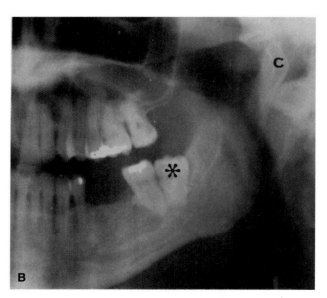

FIGURE 639.3, 639.4, and 640.3 **Three Examples of Commonly Encountered Patterns of Impacted Lower Third Molar Teeth: A. Mesioangular Impaction (Fig. 639.3); B. Distoangular Impaction (Fig. 639.4); C. Horizontal Impaction (See Fig. 640.3, next plate)**

Asterisk (*) = impacted molar tooth; M = mandible; c = condyloid process
(Contributed by Edward J.H. Nathanial, MD, PhD, Department of Anatomy, University of Manitoba, Winnipeg, Canada.)

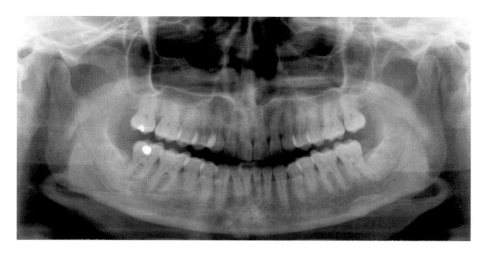

FIGURE 640.1 Radiograph of the Maxilla and Mandible. Plain Film with No Labels. For Labels, See Below (Fig. 640.2)

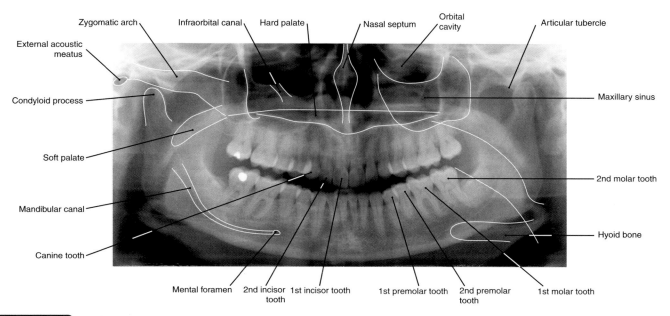

FIGURE 640.2 Radiograph of the Maxilla and Mandible

NOTE: the locations of adjacent structures to the oral cavity such as the nasal septum, maxillary sinus, hyoid bone, mandibular canal, infraorbital canal, and hard palate.

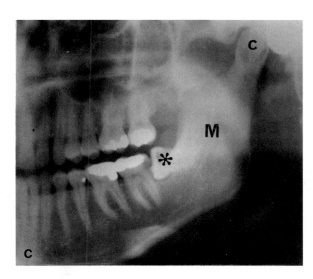

FIGURE 640.3 Horizontal Impaction

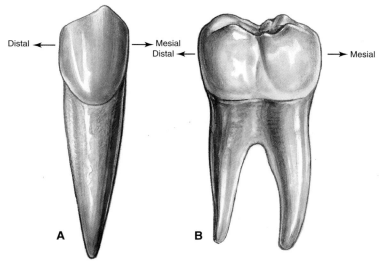

FIGURE 640.4 A. Lower Canine (Vestibular Surface); B. Lower Second Molar (Vestibular Surface)

PLATE 641 Pharynx: External Muscles (Lateral View)

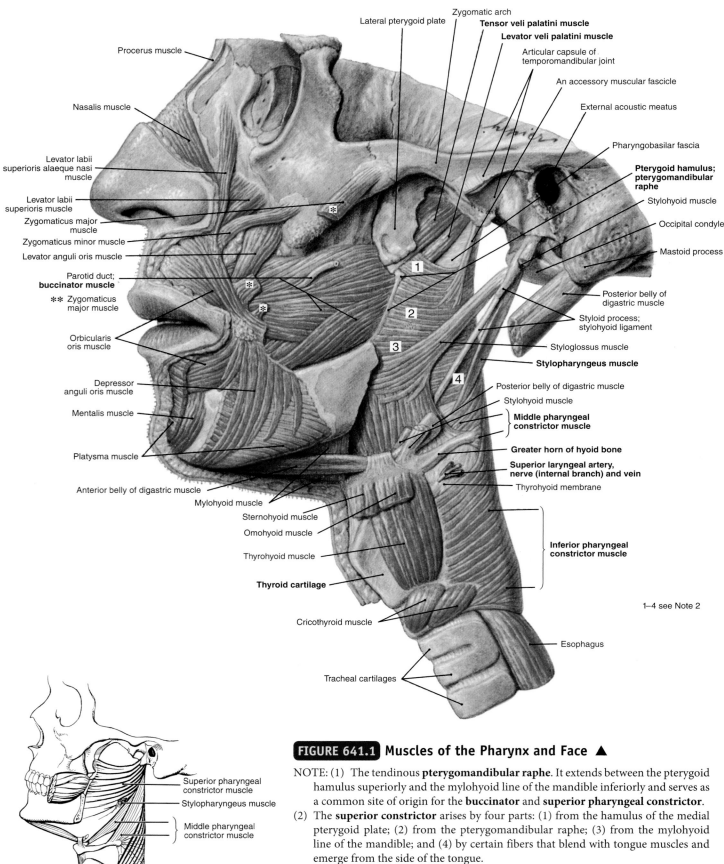

Zygomatic arch

Lateral pterygoid plate

Tensor veli palatini muscle

Levator veli palatini muscle

Articular capsule of temporomandibular joint

An accessory muscular fascicle

External acoustic meatus

Pharyngobasilar fascia

Pterygoid hamulus; pterygomandibular raphe

Stylohyoid muscle

Occipital condyle

Mastoid process

Posterior belly of digastric muscle

Styloid process; stylohyoid ligament

Styloglossus muscle

Stylopharyngeus muscle

Posterior belly of digastric muscle

Stylohyoid muscle

Middle pharyngeal constrictor muscle

Greater horn of hyoid bone

Superior laryngeal artery, nerve (internal branch) and vein

Thyrohyoid membrane

Inferior pharyngeal constrictor muscle

Procerus muscle

Nasalis muscle

Levator labii superioris alaeque nasi muscle

Levator labii superioris muscle

Zygomaticus major muscle

Zygomaticus minor muscle

Levator anguli oris muscle

Parotid duct; **buccinator muscle**

✳✳ Zygomaticus major muscle

Orbicularis oris muscle

Depressor anguli oris muscle

Mentalis muscle

Platysma muscle

Anterior belly of digastric muscle

Mylohyoid muscle

Sternohyoid muscle

Omohyoid muscle

Thyrohyoid muscle

Thyroid cartilage

Cricothyroid muscle

Tracheal cartilages

Esophagus

1–4 see Note 2

FIGURE 641.1 Muscles of the Pharynx and Face ▲

NOTE: (1) The tendinous **pterygomandibular raphe**. It extends between the pterygoid hamulus superiorly and the mylohyoid line of the mandible inferiorly and serves as a common site of origin for the **buccinator** and **superior pharyngeal constrictor**.

(2) The **superior constrictor** arises by four parts: (1) from the hamulus of the medial pterygoid plate; (2) from the pterygomandibular raphe; (3) from the mylohyoid line of the mandible; and (4) by certain fibers that blend with tongue muscles and emerge from the side of the tongue.

(3) The **middle constrictor** arises from the greater and lesser horns of the hyoid bone, whereas the larger and thicker **inferior constrictor** arises from the thyroid and cricoid cartilages.

Superior pharyngeal constrictor muscle

Stylopharyngeus muscle

Middle pharyngeal constrictor muscle

Inferior pharyngeal constrictor muscle

Cricothyroid muscle

◄ **FIGURE 641.2** Diagram of the Origins of the Pharyngeal Constrictor Muscles

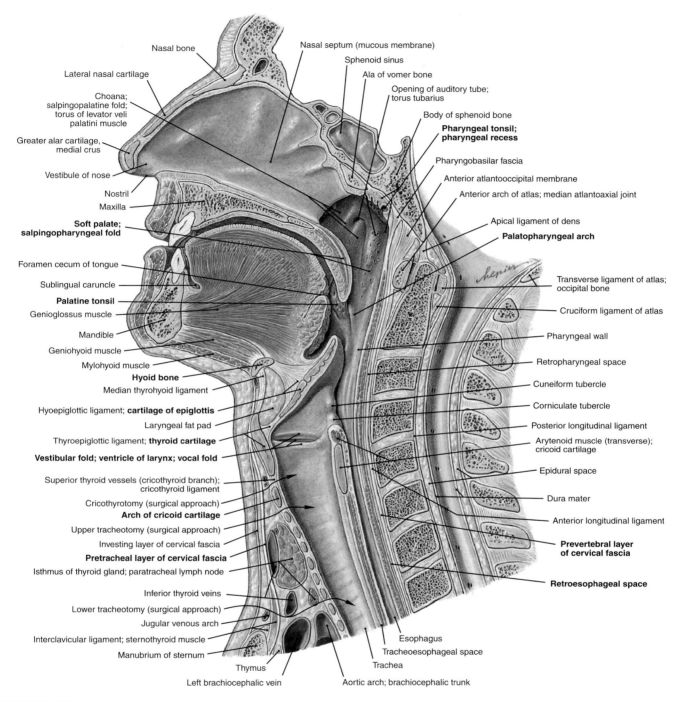

Nasal bone

Nasal septum (mucous membrane)

Sphenoid sinus

Lateral nasal cartilage

Ala of vomer bone

Choana; salpingopalatine fold; torus of levator veli palatini muscle

Opening of auditory tube; torus tubarius

Body of sphenoid bone

Pharyngeal tonsil; pharyngeal recess

Greater alar cartilage, medial crus

Pharyngobasilar fascia

Anterior atlantooccipital membrane

Vestibule of nose

Anterior arch of atlas; median atlantoaxial joint

Nostril

Maxilla

Apical ligament of dens

Soft palate; **salpingopharyngeal fold**

Palatopharyngeal arch

Foramen cecum of tongue

Transverse ligament of atlas; occipital bone

Sublingual caruncle

Palatine tonsil

Cruciform ligament of atlas

Genioglossus muscle

Mandible

Pharyngeal wall

Geniohyoid muscle

Retropharyngeal space

Mylohyoid muscle

Cuneiform tubercle

Hyoid bone

Median thyrohyoid ligament

Corniculate tubercle

Hyoepiglottic ligament; **cartilage of epiglottis**

Posterior longitudinal ligament

Laryngeal fat pad

Arytenoid muscle (transverse); cricoid cartilage

Thyroepiglottic ligament; **thyroid cartilage**

Vestibular fold; ventricle of larynx; vocal fold

Epidural space

Superior thyroid vessels (cricothyroid branch); cricothyroid ligament

Dura mater

Cricothyrotomy (surgical approach)

Arch of cricoid cartilage

Anterior longitudinal ligament

Upper tracheotomy (surgical approach)

Investing layer of cervical fascia

Pretracheal layer of cervical fascia

Prevertebral layer of cervical fascia

Isthmus of thyroid gland; paratracheal lymph node

Inferior thyroid veins

Retroesophageal space

Lower tracheotomy (surgical approach)

Jugular venous arch

Interclavicular ligament; sternothyroid muscle

Esophagus

Manubrium of sternum

Tracheoesophageal space

Trachea

Thymus

Left brachiocephalic vein

Aortic arch; brachiocephalic trunk

FIGURE 642 **Midsagittal Section of the Mouth, Pharynx, Larynx, and Other Head and Neck Viscera**

NOTE: (1) The closed oral cavity is occupied principally by the tongue. The posterior end of the oral cavity opens into the **oropharynx**. Superiorly, the posterior nasal cavities are continuous with the **nasopharynx**, whereas inferiorly the **laryngeal part of the pharynx** (between the levels of the epiglottis and cricoid cartilages) communicates with the larynx.

(2) The pharynx continues inferiorly as the **esophagus**, whereas the larynx becomes the **trachea** below the level of the cricoid cartilage.

(3) During **deglutition** (swallowing) food gets directed toward the posterior part of the oral cavity. The soft palate is then elevated and tensed (levator and tensor veli palatini muscles) thereby closing off the nasopharynx so that food enters the oropharynx. At the same time the larynx is drawn upward toward the epiglottis and the pharynx ascends as well. This action closes off the laryngeal orifice (aditus) and prevents food from entering the larynx.

(4) The arrows indicate surgical approaches to the airway (larynx and trachea).

PLATE 643 Pharynx from Behind: Muscles

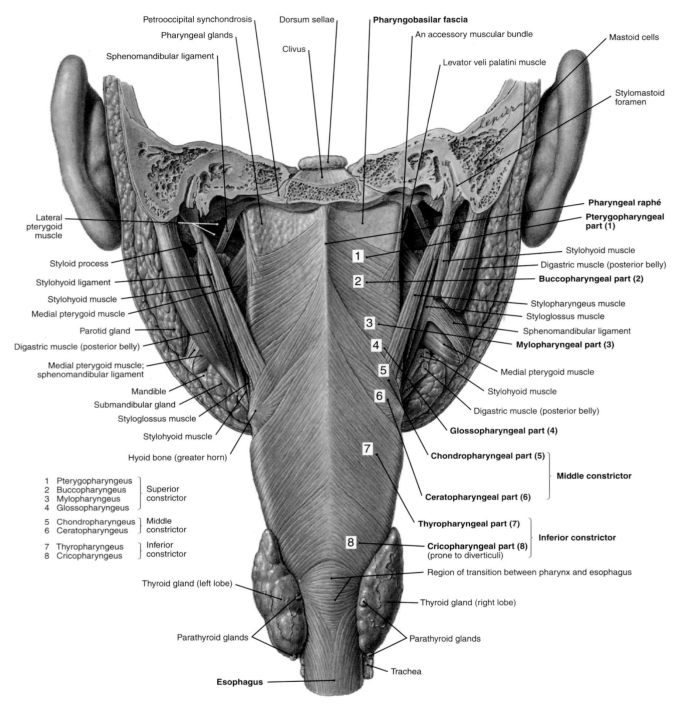

Petrooccipital synchondrosis
Pharyngeal glands
Sphenomandibular ligament
Dorsum sellae
Clivus
Pharyngobasilar fascia
An accessory muscular bundle
Levator veli palatini muscle
Mastoid cells
Stylomastoid foramen
Pharyngeal raphé
Pterygopharyngeal part (1)
Stylohyoid muscle
Digastric muscle (posterior belly)
Buccopharyngeal part (2)
Stylopharyngeus muscle
Styloglossus muscle
Sphenomandibular ligament
Mylopharyngeal part (3)
Medial pterygoid muscle
Stylohyoid muscle
Digastric muscle (posterior belly)
Glossopharyngeal part (4)
Chondropharyngeal part (5)
Middle constrictor
Ceratopharyngeal part (6)
Thyropharyngeal part (7)
Inferior constrictor
Cricopharyngeal part (8)
(prone to diverticuli)
Region of transition between pharynx and esophagus
Thyroid gland (right lobe)
Parathyroid glands
Trachea

Lateral pterygoid muscle
Styloid process
Stylohyoid ligament
Stylohyoid muscle
Medial pterygoid muscle
Parotid gland
Digastric muscle (posterior belly)
Medial pterygoid muscle; sphenomandibular ligament
Mandible
Submandibular gland
Styloglossus muscle
Stylohyoid muscle
Hyoid bone (greater horn)
Thyroid gland (left lobe)
Parathyroid glands
Esophagus

1	Pterygopharyngeus	
2	Buccopharyngeus	Superior
3	Mylopharyngeus	constrictor
4	Glossopharyngeus	
5	Chondropharyngeus	Middle
6	Ceratopharyngeus	constrictor
7	Thyropharyngeus	Inferior
8	Cricopharyngeus	constrictor

FIGURE 643 Dorsal View of the Pharyngeal Muscles

NOTE: (1) This posterior view of the pharynx was achieved by making a frontal transection through the petrous and mastoid parts of the temporal bone and through the body of the occipital bone. The styloid processes and their muscular attachments are left intact.

(2) The divisions of the **pharyngeal constrictors**. Their muscle fibers arise laterally to insert in a posterior raphe in the midline. The **superior constrictor** is divisible into four parts, whereas the **middle and inferior constrictors** are each divisible into two.

(3) Above the superior constrictor is found the fibrous **pharyngobasilar fascia**, which attaches to the basal portion of the occipital bone and to the temporal bones. Below the inferior constrictor, the pharynx is continuous with the muscular esophagus.

(4) The superior and middle constrictor muscles and the thyropharyngeal part of the inferior constrictor are innervated by the **pharyngeal branch of the vagus nerve**. These fibers have their cell bodies in the nucleus ambiguus in the medulla oblongata; they emerge from the brain in the rootlets of the bulbar part of the accessory nerve and then, by a communicating branch, join the vagus nerve.

(5) The cricopharyngeal part of the inferior constrictor is supplied by the recurrent laryngeal branch of the vagus nerve.

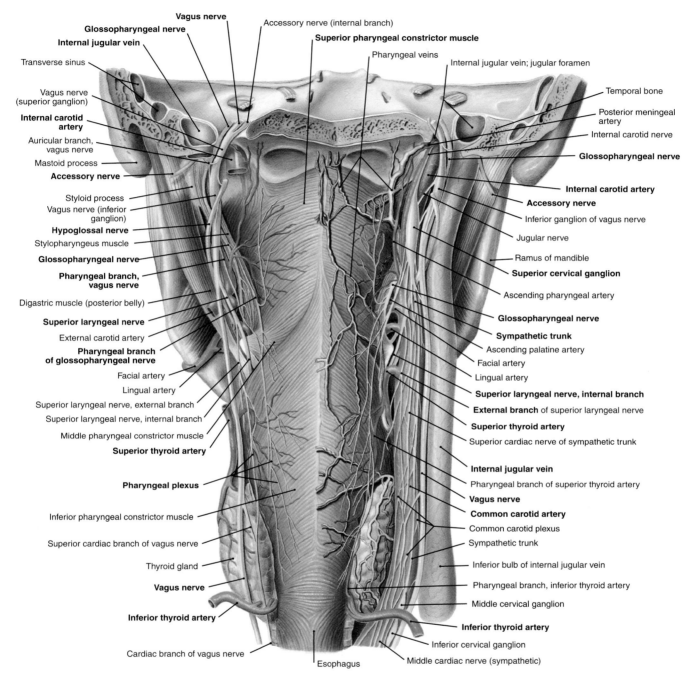

Vagus nerve
Glossopharyngeal nerve
Internal jugular vein
Transverse sinus
Vagus nerve (superior ganglion)
Internal carotid artery
Auricular branch, vagus nerve
Mastoid process
Accessory nerve
Styloid process
Vagus nerve (inferior ganglion)
Hypoglossal nerve
Stylopharyngeus muscle
Glossopharyngeal nerve
Pharyngeal branch, vagus nerve
Digastric muscle (posterior belly)
Superior laryngeal nerve
External carotid artery
Pharyngeal branch of glossopharyngeal nerve
Facial artery
Lingual artery
Superior laryngeal nerve, external branch
Superior laryngeal nerve, internal branch
Middle pharyngeal constrictor muscle
Superior thyroid artery
Pharyngeal plexus
Inferior pharyngeal constrictor muscle
Superior cardiac branch of vagus nerve
Thyroid gland
Vagus nerve
Inferior thyroid artery
Cardiac branch of vagus nerve

Accessory nerve (internal branch)
Superior pharyngeal constrictor muscle
Pharyngeal veins
Internal jugular vein; jugular foramen
Temporal bone
Posterior meningeal artery
Internal carotid nerve
Glossopharyngeal nerve
Internal carotid artery
Accessory nerve
Inferior ganglion of vagus nerve
Jugular nerve
Ramus of mandible
Superior cervical ganglion
Ascending pharyngeal artery
Glossopharyngeal nerve
Sympathetic trunk
Ascending palatine artery
Facial artery
Lingual artery
Superior laryngeal nerve, internal branch
External branch of superior laryngeal nerve
Superior thyroid artery
Superior cardiac nerve of sympathetic trunk
Internal jugular vein
Pharyngeal branch of superior thyroid artery
Vagus nerve
Common carotid artery
Common carotid plexus
Sympathetic trunk
Inferior bulb of internal jugular vein
Pharyngeal branch, inferior thyroid artery
Middle cervical ganglion
Inferior thyroid artery
Inferior cervical ganglion
Middle cardiac nerve (sympathetic)
Esophagus

FIGURE 644 **Nerves and Vessels on the Dorsal and Lateral Walls of the Pharynx**

NOTE: (1) The head has been split longitudinally. The pharynx, larynx, and facial structures were separated from the vertebral column and its associated muscles. This posterior view of the pharynx also shows the large nerves and blood vessels that course through the neck. On the right side, observe the **carotid artery, internal jugular vein, vagus nerve,** and the **sympathetic trunk**.

(2) On the left side are the **glossopharyngeal** and **hypoglossal nerves,** which were exposed by removing the carotid arteries and internal jugular vein. In addition to the jugular vein, the **jugular foramen** transmits the 9th, 10th, and 11th cranial nerves.

(3) The **thyroid gland** and its **superior and inferior thyroid arteries**. The superior and middle thyroid veins drain into the internal jugular vein, whereas the inferior thyroid veins (not shown) usually drain into the left brachiocephalic vein.

PLATE 645 Pharynx, Opened from Behind; Lymphatic Ring

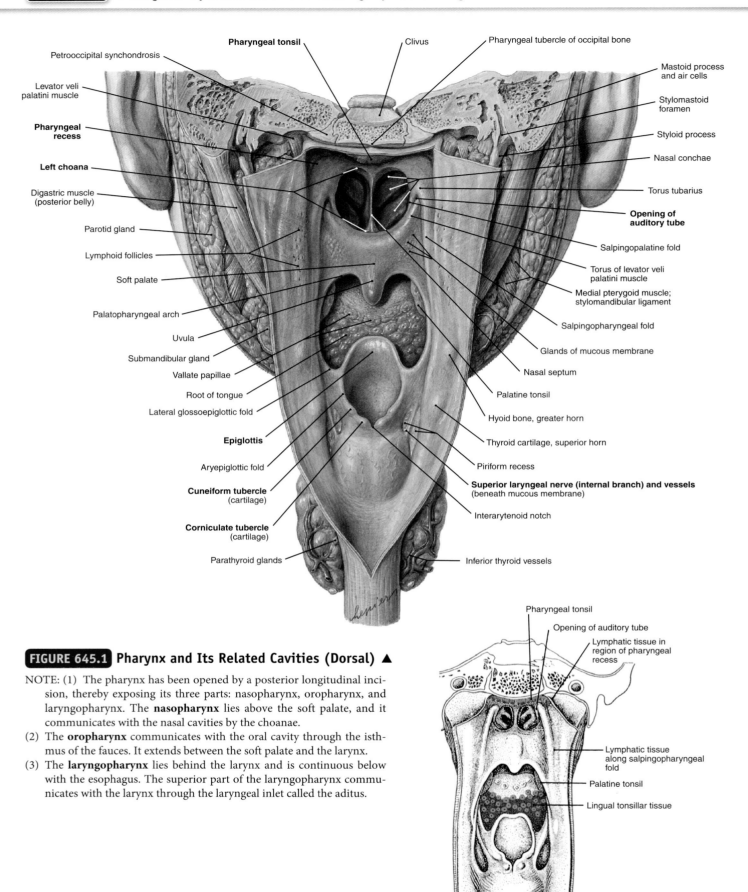

Petrooccipital synchondrosis

Pharyngeal tonsil

Clivus

Pharyngeal tubercle of occipital bone

Mastoid process and air cells

Levator veli palatini muscle

Stylomastoid foramen

Pharyngeal recess

Styloid process

Left choana

Nasal conchae

Digastric muscle (posterior belly)

Torus tubarius

Opening of auditory tube

Parotid gland

Salpingopalatine fold

Lymphoid follicles

Torus of levator veli palatini muscle

Soft palate

Medial pterygoid muscle; stylomandibular ligament

Palatopharyngeal arch

Salpingopharyngeal fold

Uvula

Glands of mucous membrane

Submandibular gland

Nasal septum

Vallate papillae

Palatine tonsil

Root of tongue

Hyoid bone, greater horn

Lateral glossoepiglottic fold

Thyroid cartilage, superior horn

Epiglottis

Piriform recess

Aryepiglottic fold

Superior laryngeal nerve (internal branch) and vessels
(beneath mucous membrane)

Cuneiform tubercle
(cartilage)

Interarytenoid notch

Corniculate tubercle
(cartilage)

Parathyroid glands

Inferior thyroid vessels

FIGURE 645.1 Pharynx and Its Related Cavities (Dorsal) ▲

NOTE: (1) The pharynx has been opened by a posterior longitudinal incision, thereby exposing its three parts: nasopharynx, oropharynx, and
laryngopharynx. The **nasopharynx** lies above the soft palate, and it
communicates with the nasal cavities by the choanae.

(2) The **oropharynx** communicates with the oral cavity through the isthmus of the fauces. It extends between the soft palate and the larynx.

(3) The **laryngopharynx** lies behind the larynx and is continuous below
with the esophagus. The superior part of the laryngopharynx communicates with the larynx through the laryngeal inlet called the aditus.

Pharyngeal tonsil

Opening of auditory tube

Lymphatic tissue in region of pharyngeal recess

Lymphatic tissue along salpingopharyngeal fold

Palatine tonsil

Lingual tonsillar tissue

FIGURE 645.2 Oronasopharyngeal Lymphatic Ring ▶

NOTE: The lymphatic ring is shown in red. This circular accumulation of lymphatic tissue includes the lingual tonsil (which consists of lymphoid follicles on the
posterior third of the tongue), the palatine tonsils, the pharyngeal tonsil, and more
diffuse lymphoid tissue in the wall of the nasopharynx along the salpingopharyngeal fold.

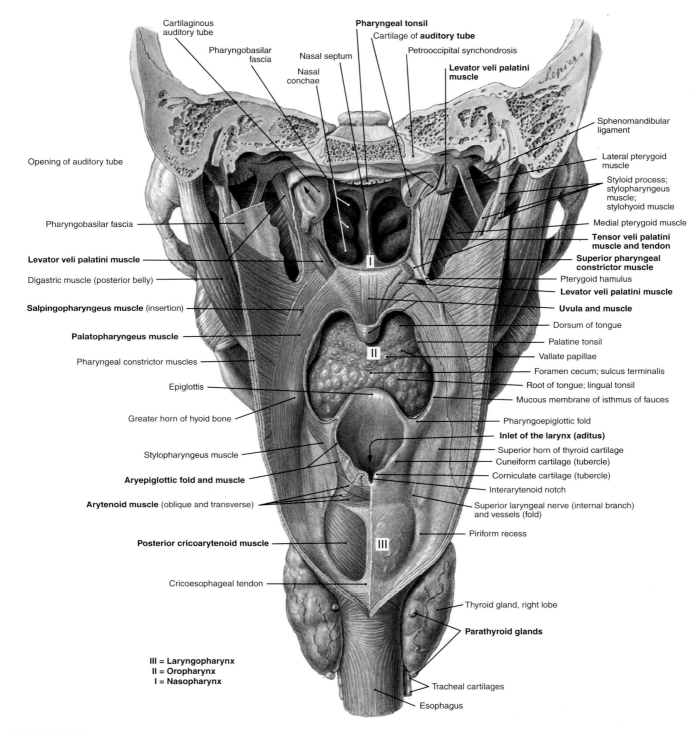

Cartilaginous auditory tube
Pharyngobasilar fascia
Nasal septum
Nasal conchae
Pharyngeal tonsil
Cartilage of **auditory tube**
Petrooccipital synchondrosis
Levator veli palatini muscle

Opening of auditory tube

Sphenomandibular ligament
Lateral pterygoid muscle
Styloid process; stylopharyngeus muscle; stylohyoid muscle
Medial pterygoid muscle

Pharyngobasilar fascia
Tensor veli palatini muscle and tendon
Superior pharyngeal constrictor muscle
Levator veli palatini muscle
Digastric muscle (posterior belly)
Pterygoid hamulus
Levator veli palatini muscle
Salpingopharyngeus muscle (insertion)
Uvula and muscle
Dorsum of tongue
Palatopharyngeus muscle
Palatine tonsil
Pharyngeal constrictor muscles
Vallate papillae
Foramen cecum; sulcus terminalis
Epiglottis
Root of tongue; lingual tonsil
Mucous membrane of isthmus of fauces
Greater horn of hyoid bone
Pharyngoepiglottic fold
Inlet of the larynx (aditus)
Stylopharyngeus muscle
Superior horn of thyroid cartilage
Cuneiform cartilage (tubercle)
Aryepiglottic fold and muscle
Corniculate cartilage (tubercle)
Interarytenoid notch
Arytenoid muscle (oblique and transverse)
Superior laryngeal nerve (internal branch) and vessels (fold)
Posterior cricoarytenoid muscle
Piriform recess
Cricoesophageal tendon
Thyroid gland, right lobe
Parathyroid glands

III = **Laryngopharynx**
II = **Oropharynx**
I = **Nasopharynx**

Tracheal cartilages
Esophagus

FIGURE 646 **Muscles of the Soft Palate, Pharynx, and Posterior Larynx**

NOTE: (1) This dissection is similar to that in Figure 645. The pharynx has been opened dorsally by a midline incision and the mucous membrane has been removed from the soft palate, pharynx, and left posterior larynx. On the right, a part of the levator veli **palatini muscle** has been removed to expose the adjacent **tensor veli palatini muscle**.

(2) The **muscles of the soft palate**. Both the muscle of the uvula and the levator veli palatini muscle are innervated by the pharyngeal branch of the vagus nerve, whereas the tensor veli palatini is supplied by the mandibular division of the trigeminal nerve.

(3) The **palatopharyngeus muscle** arises by two fascicles from the soft palate. The muscle fibers of these fascicles arise posterior and anterior to the insertion of the levator veli palatini muscle. The fascicles descend and merge and then insert into the posterior border of the thyroid cartilage and onto the adjacent pharyngeal wall.

PLATE 647 Pharynx and Soft Palate from Behind: Vessels and Nerves

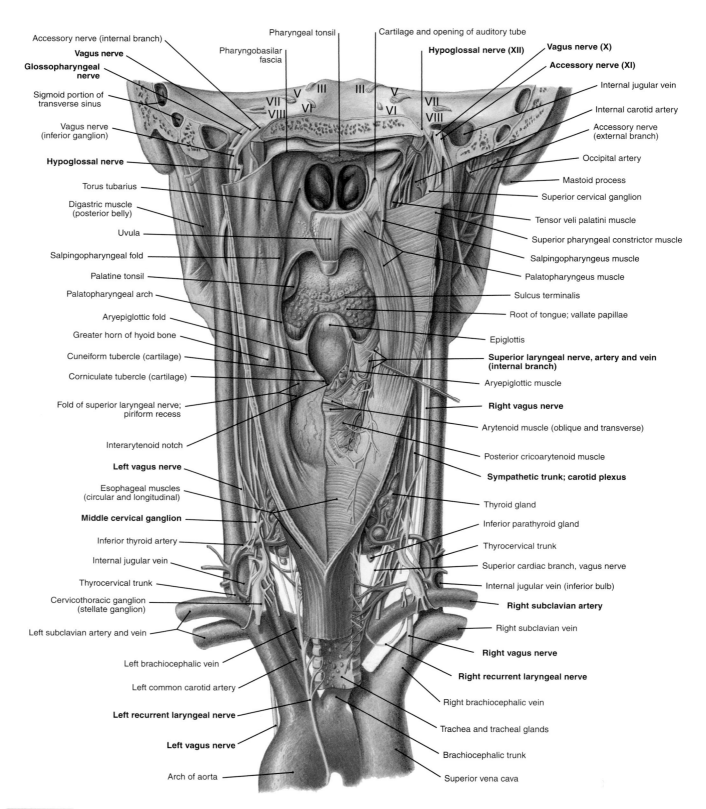

Accessory nerve (internal branch)
Vagus nerve
Glossopharyngeal nerve
Sigmoid portion of transverse sinus
Vagus nerve (inferior ganglion)
Hypoglossal nerve
Torus tubarius
Digastric muscle (posterior belly)
Uvula
Salpingopharyngeal fold
Palatine tonsil
Palatopharyngeal arch
Aryepiglottic fold
Greater horn of hyoid bone
Cuneiform tubercle (cartilage)
Corniculate tubercle (cartilage)
Fold of superior laryngeal nerve; piriform recess
Interarytenoid notch
Left vagus nerve
Esophageal muscles (circular and longitudinal)
Middle cervical ganglion
Inferior thyroid artery
Internal jugular vein
Thyrocervical trunk
Cervicothoracic ganglion (stellate ganglion)
Left subclavian artery and vein
Left brachiocephalic vein
Left common carotid artery
Left recurrent laryngeal nerve
Left vagus nerve
Arch of aorta

Pharyngeal tonsil
Pharyngobasilar fascia
Cartilage and opening of auditory tube
Hypoglossal nerve (XII)
Vagus nerve (X)
Accessory nerve (XI)
Internal jugular vein
Internal carotid artery
Accessory nerve (external branch)
Occipital artery
Mastoid process
Superior cervical ganglion
Tensor veli palatini muscle
Superior pharyngeal constrictor muscle
Salpingopharyngeus muscle
Palatopharyngeus muscle
Sulcus terminalis
Root of tongue; vallate papillae
Epiglottis
Superior laryngeal nerve, artery and vein (internal branch)
Aryepiglottic muscle
Right vagus nerve
Arytenoid muscle (oblique and transverse)
Posterior cricoarytenoid muscle
Sympathetic trunk; carotid plexus
Thyroid gland
Inferior parathyroid gland
Thyrocervical trunk
Superior cardiac branch, vagus nerve
Internal jugular vein (inferior bulb)
Right subclavian artery
Right subclavian vein
Right vagus nerve
Right recurrent laryngeal nerve
Right brachiocephalic vein
Trachea and tracheal glands
Brachiocephalic trunk
Superior vena cava

VII V III III V VII
VIII VI VI VIII

FIGURE 647 Pharynx Opened from Behind: Cervical Viscera, Muscles, Vessels, and Nerves

NOTE: (1) The nasal, oral, and laryngeal orifices communicate with the pharynx. Observe the **superior laryngeal artery, vein,** and **nerve (internal branch)** entering the larynx from above.

(2) The **recurrent laryngeal nerves** ascend to the larynx from the thorax. The left nerve courses around the arch of the aorta, while on the right side the recurrent laryngeal nerve curves around the subclavian artery.

(3) The **inferior cervical ganglion** at the level of the seventh cervical vertebra is fused with the first thoracic ganglion (in about 80% of cases). When fused, the joint ganglion is called the **stellate ganglion.**

MUSCLES OF THE PALATE

Muscle	Origin	Insertion	Innervation	Action
Musculus uvulae	Posterior nasal spine (palatine bone); palatine aponeurosis	Descends into the mucous membrane of the uvula	Pharyngeal branch of the vagus nerve	Pulls the uvula up and contracts the uvula on its own side
Tensor veli palatini	Scaphoid fossa of pterygoid process; cartilaginous part of auditory tube; spine of sphenoid	Tendon courses around the pterygoid hamulus and then inserts into the palatine aponeurosis	Branch of the mandibular division of the trigeminal nerve	Tenses the soft palate; acting singly, it pulls the soft palate to one side
Levator veli palatini	Inferior surface of temporal bone; cartilaginous part of auditory tube	Upper surface of the palatine aponeurosis	Pharyngeal branch of the vagus nerve	Elevates the soft palate
Palatoglossus	Oral surface of the palatine aponeurosis	Into the side of the tongue	Pharyngeal branch of the vagus nerve	Elevates root of tongue; two muscles together close off oral cavity from oropharynx
Palatopharyngeus	Posterior border of the hard palate; palatine aponeurosis	Posterior border of thyroid cartilage; lateral wall of pharynx	Pharyngeal branch of the vagus nerve	Pulls the pharynx upward during swallowing

MUSCLES OF THE PHARYNX

Superior pharyngeal constrictor	**Pterygopharyngeal Part**		Motor fibers: Pharyngeal branch of vagus nerve (fibers originating in the medullary part of accessory nerve)	The constrictor muscles act as sphincters of the pharynx and induce peristaltic waves during swallowing
	Pterygoid hamulus of sphenoid bone	Pharyngobasilar fascia and the midline raphe		
	Buccopharyngeal Part			
	Pterygomandibular raphe	Posterior midline pharyngeal raphe		
	Mylopharyngeal Part			
	Mylohyoid line of mandible	Posterior midline pharyngeal raphe		
	Glossopharyngeal Part		Sensory fibers of mucosa: Glossopharyngeal nerve and some trigeminal nerve fibers	
	A few fibers arise from the side of tongue	Posterior midline pharyngeal raphe		
Middle pharyngeal constrictor	**Chondropharyngeal Part**			
	Lesser horn of hyoid bone	Posterior midline pharyngeal raphe		
	Ceratopharyngeal Part			
	Greater horn of hyoid bone	Posterior midline pharyngeal raphe		
Inferior pharyngeal constrictor	**Thyropharyngeal Part**			
	Oblique line on the lamina of thyroid cartilage	Posterior midline pharyngeal raphe		
	Cricopharyngeal Part			
	Side of the cricoid cartilage	Posterior midline pharyngeal raphe	Cricopharyngeus: Recurrent laryngeal branch of vagus	
Stylopharyngeus	Medial side of base of styloid process	Lateral wall of pharynx between the superior and middle constrictors	Glossopharyngeal nerve	Elevates the lateral wall of the pharynx during swallowing and speech
Salpingopharyngeus	Inferior part of the cartilage of the auditory tube	Blends with the palatopharyngeus on the lateral wall of the pharynx	Pharyngeal branch of vagus nerve	Raises upper lateral wall of the pharynx
Palatopharyngeus	Described with the palatal muscles above			

PLATE 649 Larynx: Anterior Relationships, Vessels and Nerves

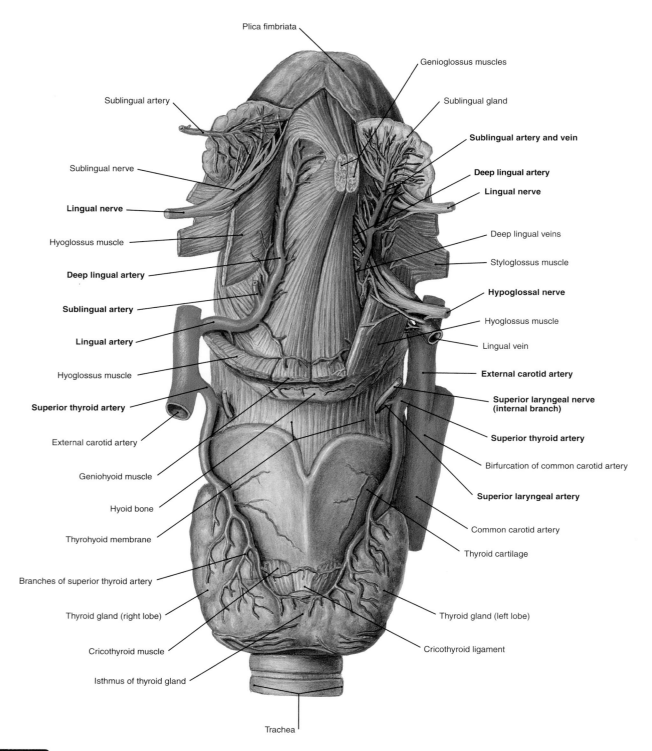

Plica fimbriata
Genioglossus muscles
Sublingual artery
Sublingual gland
Sublingual artery and vein
Sublingual nerve
Deep lingual artery
Lingual nerve
Lingual nerve
Deep lingual veins
Hyoglossus muscle
Styloglossus muscle
Deep lingual artery
Hypoglossal nerve
Sublingual artery
Hyoglossus muscle
Lingual artery
Lingual vein
Hyoglossus muscle
External carotid artery
Superior thyroid artery
Superior laryngeal nerve (internal branch)
External carotid artery
Superior thyroid artery
Geniohyoid muscle
Birfurcation of common carotid artery
Hyoid bone
Superior laryngeal artery
Thyrohyoid membrane
Common carotid artery
Thyroid cartilage
Branches of superior thyroid artery
Thyroid gland (left lobe)
Thyroid gland (right lobe)
Cricothyroid muscle
Cricothyroid ligament
Isthmus of thyroid gland
Trachea

FIGURE 649 Anterior View of Larynx, Tongue and Thyroid Gland, Vessels, and Nerves

NOTE: (1) The **superior thyroid arteries** descend to the thyroid gland. In their course, they give off the **superior laryngeal arteries**, which penetrate the thyrohyoid membrane to enter the interior of the larynx. They are accompanied by the **internal laryngeal branch** of the **superior laryngeal nerve**.

(2) The cranial and medial course of the **lingual artery** deep to the hyoglossus muscle and its suprahyoid (not labeled), sublingual, and deep lingual branches.

(3) The **lingual nerves** as they enter the tongue to supply its anterior two-thirds with general sensation. The motor nerve to the tongue is the **hypoglossal**, seen coursing along with its accompanying veins. It enters the base of the tongue just above the hyoid bone, passing anteriorly across the external carotid and lingual arteries.

(4) The **common carotid artery** bifurcates at about the level of the upper border of the thyroid cartilage. The lingual artery branches from the external carotid above the hyoid bone, while the superior laryngeal arises at the level of the thyrohyoid membrane.

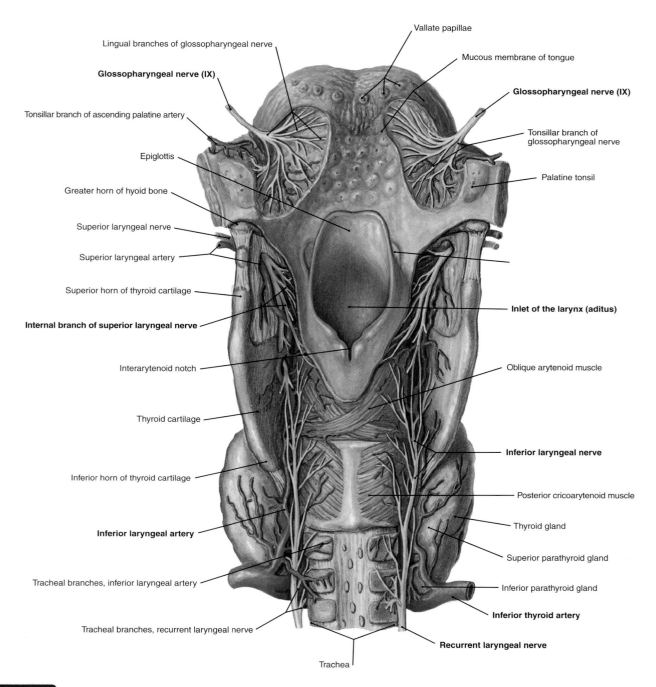

Vallate papillae

Lingual branches of glossopharyngeal nerve

Mucous membrane of tongue

Glossopharyngeal nerve (IX)

Glossopharyngeal nerve (IX)

Tonsillar branch of ascending palatine artery

Tonsillar branch of glossopharyngeal nerve

Epiglottis

Palatine tonsil

Greater horn of hyoid bone

Superior laryngeal nerve

Superior laryngeal artery

Superior horn of thyroid cartilage

Inlet of the larynx (aditus)

Internal branch of superior laryngeal nerve

Interarytenoid notch

Oblique arytenoid muscle

Thyroid cartilage

Inferior laryngeal nerve

Inferior horn of thyroid cartilage

Posterior cricoarytenoid muscle

Thyroid gland

Inferior laryngeal artery

Superior parathyroid gland

Tracheal branches, inferior laryngeal artery

Inferior parathyroid gland

Inferior thyroid artery

Tracheal branches, recurrent laryngeal nerve

Recurrent laryngeal nerve

Trachea

FIGURE 650 **Posterior View of the Larynx, Tongue and Thyroid Gland, Vessels, and Nerves**

NOTE: (1) The **glossopharyngeal nerves (IX)** enter the root or pharyngeal part of the tongue to supply the posterior third of the surface of the tongue with both general sensation and the special sense of taste. Also note the **tonsillar branch** of the **ascending palatine artery** (from facial artery) supplying the palatine tonsil.

(2) The course of the **internal branch** of the **superior laryngeal nerve**. It is sensory to the laryngeal mucous membrane on the interior of the larynx as far down as the vocal folds.

(3) The **recurrent laryngeal nerve** is the principal motor nerve to the larynx, and it supplies all of the laryngeal muscles *except* the cricothyroid muscle (which is supplied by the external branch of the superior laryngeal nerve). In addition, the recurrent laryngeal nerve supplies sensory innervation to the interior of the larynx below the vocal folds.

(4) The **important relationship** of the recurrent laryngeal nerves to the inferior thyroid artery and its inferior laryngeal branches. Also observe the proximity of the recurrent laryngeal nerves to the posterior aspect of the thyroid glands.

PLATE 651 Larynx: Cartilages and Membranes

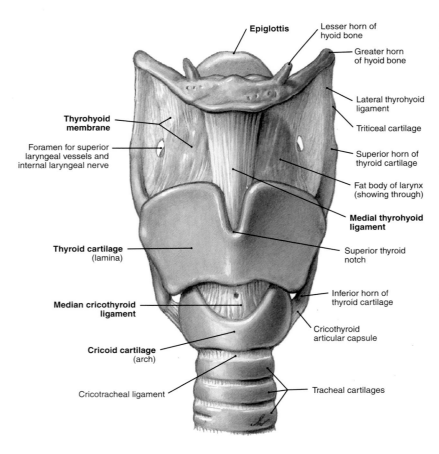

Epiglottis

Lesser horn of hyoid bone

Greater horn of hyoid bone

Lateral thyrohyoid ligament

Thyrohyoid membrane

Triticeal cartilage

Foramen for superior laryngeal vessels and internal laryngeal nerve

Superior horn of thyroid cartilage

Fat body of larynx (showing through)

Medial thyrohyoid ligament

Thyroid cartilage (lamina)

Superior thyroid notch

Median cricothyroid ligament

Inferior horn of thyroid cartilage

Cricothyroid articular capsule

Cricoid cartilage (arch)

Cricotracheal ligament

Tracheal cartilages

FIGURE 651.1 **Cartilages and Ligaments of the Larynx (Ventral View)**

NOTE: (1) The laryngeal cartilages form the skeleton of the larynx, and they are interconnected by ligaments and membranes. There are three larger **unpaired** cartilages (**cricoid, thyroid,** and **epiglottis**) and three sets of **paired** cartilages (**arytenoid, corniculate,** and **cuneiform**). In this anterior view, the unpaired cricoid, thyroid, and epiglottis are all visible.

(2) The **thyrohyoid membrane** and the centrally located thyrohyoid ligament. Attached to the upper border of the thyroid cartilage, this membrane stretches across the posterior surfaces of the greater horns of the hyoid bone. The medial thyrohyoid ligament extends from the thyroid notch to the body of the hyoid bone. The membrane is pierced by the **superior laryngeal vessels** and the **internal laryngeal branch of the superior laryngeal nerve**.

(3) The **cricothyroid ligament** attaches the apposing margins of the cricoid and thyroid cartilages. This ligament underlies the cricothyroid muscles.

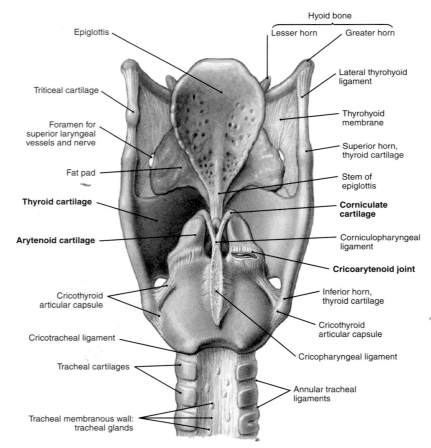

Hyoid bone

Lesser horn

Greater horn

Epiglottis

Lateral thyrohyoid ligament

Triticeal cartilage

Thyrohyoid membrane

Foramen for superior laryngeal vessels and nerve

Superior horn, thyroid cartilage

Fat pad

Stem of epiglottis

Thyroid cartilage

Corniculate cartilage

Arytenoid cartilage

Corniculopharyngeal ligament

Cricoarytenoid joint

Cricothyroid articular capsule

Inferior horn, thyroid cartilage

Cricotracheal ligament

Cricothyroid articular capsule

Tracheal cartilages

Cricopharyngeal ligament

Annular tracheal ligaments

Tracheal membranous wall: tracheal glands

FIGURE 651.2 **Cartilages and Ligaments of the Larynx (Dorsal View)**

NOTE: (1) The articulation of the paired arytenoid cartilages with the cricoid cartilage below. These synovial cricoarytenoid joints are surrounded by articular capsules and strengthened by the posterior cricoarytenoid ligaments.

(2) The cricoarytenoid joints allow for: (a) **rotation of the arytenoid cartilage** on an axis that is nearly vertical and (b) the **horizontal gliding movement** of the arytenoid cartilages.

(3) Rotation of the arytenoid cartilages results in medial or lateral displacement of the vocal folds, thereby increasing or decreasing the size of the opening between the folds, the **rima glottis**.

(4) Horizontal gliding of the arytenoid cartilages permits the bases of these cartilages to be approximated or moved apart. Medial rotation and medial gliding of the arytenoid cartilages occur simultaneously, as do the two lateral movements.

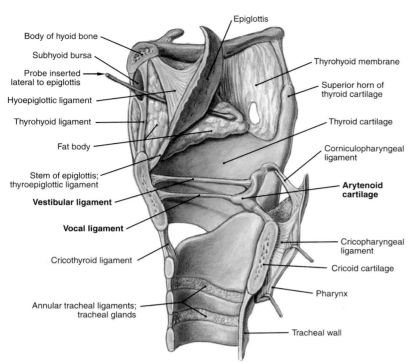

Body of hyoid bone
Subhyoid bursa
Probe inserted lateral to epiglottis
Hyoepiglottic ligament
Thyrohyoid ligament
Fat body
Stem of epiglottis; thyroepiglottic ligament
Vestibular ligament
Vocal ligament
Cricothyroid ligament
Annular tracheal ligaments; tracheal glands

Epiglottis
Thyrohyoid membrane
Superior horn of thyroid cartilage
Thyroid cartilage
Corniculopharyngeal ligament
Arytenoid cartilage
Cricopharyngeal ligament
Cricoid cartilage
Pharynx
Tracheal wall

◀ **FIGURE 652.1** Right Half of the Larynx Showing the Cartilages and Vestibular and Vocal Ligaments

NOTE: (1) The **vestibular ligament** is a compact band of fibrous tissue attached anteriorly to the thyroid cartilage and posteriorly to the anterior and lateral surface of the arytenoid cartilage. It is enclosed by mucous membrane to form the vestibular fold (or false vocal fold).

(2) The **vocal ligament** consists of elastic tissue and is attached anteriorly to the thyroid cartilage and posteriorly to the vocal process of the arytenoid cartilage. It, too, is covered by mucous membrane, which, along with the vocalis muscle forms the vocal fold. Laryngeal sounds are produced by oscillations of the vocal folds initiated by puffs of air.

FIGURE 652.2 Vocal Ligaments and Conus ▶ Elasticus (Seen from Above)

NOTE: (1) The **conus elasticus** is a membrane consisting principally of yellow elastic fibers; it interconnects the thyroid, cricoid, and arytenoid cartilages. It underlies the mucous membrane below the vocal folds and is overlaid to some extent by the thyroarytenoid and cricothyroid muscles on the exterior of the larynx.

(2) The symmetry of the arytenoid cartilages and their related vocal ligaments.

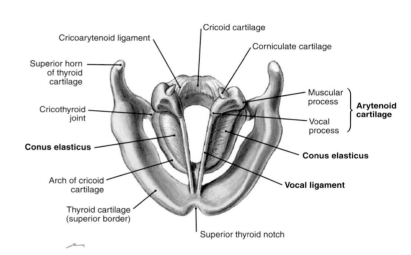

Cricoarytenoid ligament
Superior horn of thyroid cartilage
Cricothyroid joint
Conus elasticus
Arch of cricoid cartilage
Thyroid cartilage (superior border)
Superior thyroid notch

Cricoid cartilage
Corniculate cartilage
Muscular process
Vocal process   **Arytenoid cartilage**
Conus elasticus
Vocal ligament

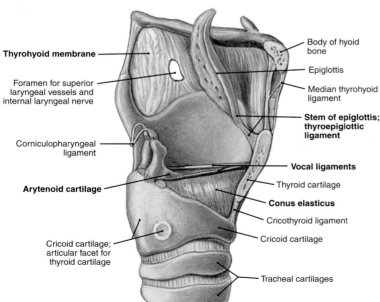

Thyrohyoid membrane
Foramen for superior laryngeal vessels and internal laryngeal nerve
Corniculopharyngeal ligament
Arytenoid cartilage
Cricoid cartilage; articular facet for thyroid cartilage

Body of hyoid bone
Epiglottis
Median thyrohyoid ligament
Stem of epiglottis; thyroepiglottic ligament
Vocal ligaments
Thyroid cartilage
Conus elasticus
Cricothyroid ligament
Cricoid cartilage
Tracheal cartilages

◀ **FIGURE 652.3** Upper Left Part of the Larynx

NOTE: (1) The right halves of the hyoid bone, epiglottis, and thyroid cartilage have been removed to open the upper left portion of the larynx. The two vocal ligaments, the arytenoid cartilages, and the conus elasticus are also displayed.

(2) The attachment of the stem of the epiglottis to the thyroid cartilage by means of the thyroepiglottic ligament.

(3) The conus elasticus as it forms the vocal ligament and attaches to the arytenoid, thyroid, and cricoid cartilages.

(4) Although sounds are initiated at the vocal folds, the pitch, range, quality, volume, tone, and overtones of the human voice also incorporate structures in the mouth (tongue, teeth, and palate), nasal sinuses, pharynx, rest of the larynx, lungs, diaphragm, and abdominal muscles.

Chapter 7 The Neck and Head

PLATE 653 Larynx: Muscles

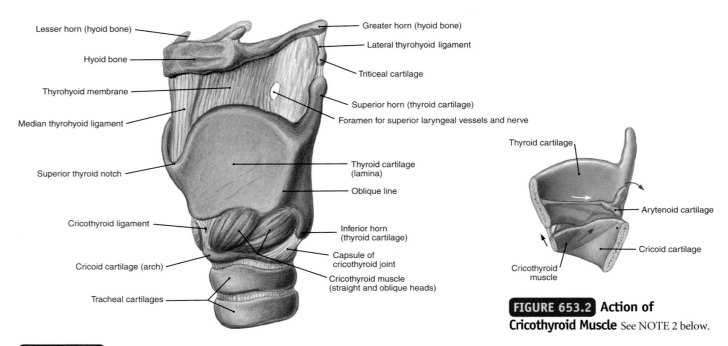

FIGURE 653.2 Action of Cricothyroid Muscle See NOTE 2 below.

FIGURE 653.1 Ventrolateral View of the Exterior Larynx and the Cricothyroid Muscle

NOTE: (1) The **cricothyroid muscle** consists of **straight** and **oblique** heads. The straight head is more vertical and inserts onto the lower border of the lamina of the thyroid cartilage, whereas the oblique head is more horizontal and inserts onto the inferior horn of the thyroid cartilage.

(2) The cricothyroid muscle tilts the anterior part of the cricoid cartilage upward. In so doing, the arytenoid cartilages (which are attached to the cricoid) are pulled dorsally. In addition, the thyroid cartilage is pulled forward and downward. These actions increase the distance between the arytenoid and thyroid cartilages, thereby increasing the tension of and elongating the vocal folds (see insert diagram above).

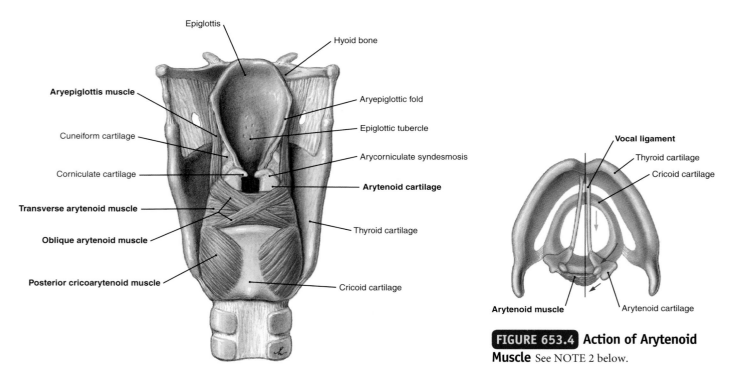

FIGURE 653.4 Action of Arytenoid Muscle See NOTE 2 below.

FIGURE 653.3 Posterior View of the Larynx: Muscles

NOTE: (1) The **arytenoid muscle** consists of a **transverse portion** that spans the zone between the arytenoid cartilages and an **oblique portion** that consists of muscular fascicles that cross posterior to the transverse fibers. Each of the fascicles of the oblique part extends from the base of the one arytenoid cartilage to the apex of the other cartilage. Some oblique fibers continue to the epiglottis as the **aryepiglottic muscle**.

(2) The transverse arytenoid approximates the arytenoid cartilages closing the posterior part of the rima glottis. The oblique arytenoid and the aryepiglottic muscles tend to close the inlet into the larynx by pulling the aryepiglottic folds together and approximating the arytenoid cartilages and epiglottis.

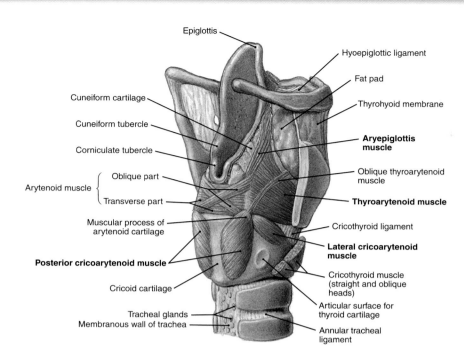

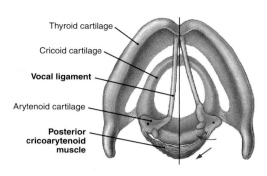

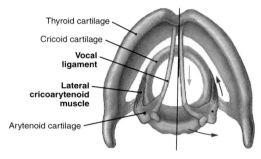

FIGURE 654.1 Posterolateral View of the Laryngeal Muscles

FIGURE 654.2 **Action of Posterior Cricoarytenoid** See NOTE 3 below.

FIGURE 654.3 **Action of Lateral Cricoarytenoid** See NOTE 3 below.

NOTE: (1) The right lamina of the thyroid cartilage and the thyrohyoid membrane have been partially cut away to expose the lateral cricoarytenoid and thyroarytenoid muscles.

(2) The **posterior cricoarytenoid muscle** extends from the lamina of the cricoid cartilage to the muscular process of the arytenoid cartilage, whereas the **lateral cricoarytenoid muscle** arises laterally from the arch of the cricoid cartilage and inserts with the posterior cricoarytenoid muscle onto the arytenoid cartilage.

(3) The posterior cricoarytenoids are the only **abductors** of the vocal folds, whereas the lateral cricoarytenoids act as antagonists and **adduct** the vocal folds. The posterior muscle abducts by pulling the base of the arytenoid cartilages medially and posteriorly, whereas the lateral muscle adducts by pulling these same cartilages anteriorly and laterally.

(4) The **thyroarytenoid muscle** is a thin sheet of muscle radiating from the thyroid cartilage backward toward the arytenoid cartilage. Its upper fibers continue to the epiglottis and, joining the aryepiglottic fibers, become the **thyroepiglottic muscle.** Its deepest and most medial fibers form the **vocalis muscle** which is attached to the lateral aspect of the vocal fold. The thyroarytenoid muscles draw the arytenoid cartilages toward the thyroid cartilage and, thus shorten (relax) the vocal folds.

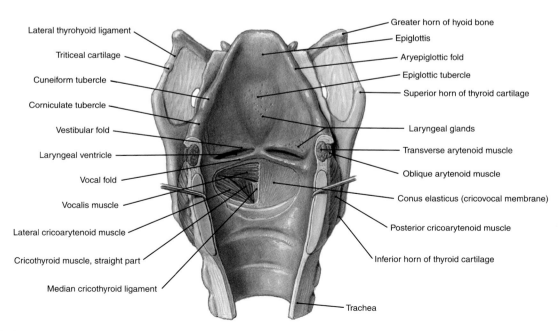

FIGURE 654.4 Larynx Opened from Behind (Posterior View)

NOTE: The lateral walls of the larynx have been opened widely, and the left part of the conus elasticus has been removed.

PLATE 655 Larynx (Frontal and Midsagittal Sections)

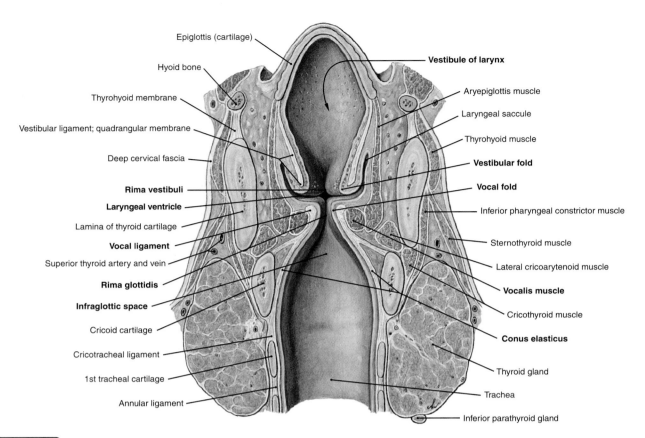

Epiglottis (cartilage)

Hyoid bone

Thyrohyoid membrane

Vestibular ligament; quadrangular membrane

Deep cervical fascia

Rima vestibuli

Laryngeal ventricle

Lamina of thyroid cartilage

Vocal ligament

Superior thyroid artery and vein

Rima glottidis

Infraglottic space

Cricoid cartilage

Cricotracheal ligament

1st tracheal cartilage

Annular ligament

Vestibule of larynx

Aryepiglottis muscle

Laryngeal saccule

Thyrohyoid muscle

Vestibular fold

Vocal fold

Inferior pharyngeal constrictor muscle

Sternothyroid muscle

Lateral cricoarytenoid muscle

Vocalis muscle

Cricothyroid muscle

Conus elasticus

Thyroid gland

Trachea

Inferior parathyroid gland

FIGURE 655.1 Frontal Section through the Larynx Showing the Laryngeal Folds and Cavities in Its Anterior Half

NOTE: (1) The paired **vocal folds** consist of mucous membrane overlying the **vocal ligaments** and **vocalis muscles**. Just superior to the vocal folds observe the **vestibular folds**, which are separated from the vocal folds by a recess called the **laryngeal ventricle** (or sinus).

(2) Above the vestibular folds is the **vestibule** of the larynx, which lies just below the laryngeal inlet. Below the vocal folds is the **infraglottic space**, which communicates with the trachea below and is limited above by the **rima glottis** between the two vocal folds.

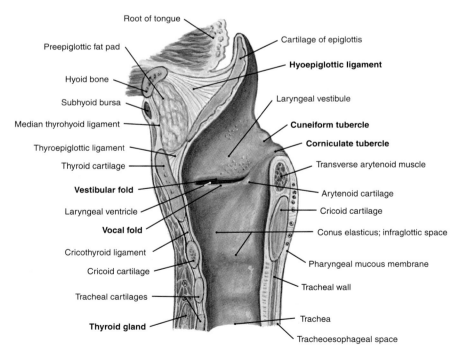

Root of tongue

Preepiglottic fat pad

Hyoid bone

Subhyoid bursa

Median thyrohyoid ligament

Thyroepiglottic ligament

Thyroid cartilage

Vestibular fold

Laryngeal ventricle

Vocal fold

Cricothyroid ligament

Cricoid cartilage

Tracheal cartilages

Thyroid gland

Cartilage of epiglottis

Hyoepiglottic ligament

Laryngeal vestibule

Cuneiform tubercle

Corniculate tubercle

Transverse arytenoid muscle

Arytenoid cartilage

Cricoid cartilage

Conus elasticus; infraglottic space

Pharyngeal mucous membrane

Tracheal wall

Trachea

Tracheoesophageal space

FIGURE 655.2 Midsagittal Section of Larynx

NOTE: (1) The laryngeal inlet leads to the laryngeal vestibule, the anterior border of which is the epiglottis. The **aryepiglottic folds**, marked by oval elevations (cuneiform and corniculate cartilages), define the borders of the laryngeal inlet.

(2) The epiglottis attaches **superiorly** to the hyoid bone (by the hyoepiglottic ligament); **inferiorly** to the thyroid cartilage (by the thyroepiglottic ligament); and **laterally** to the arytenoid cartilages (by the aryepiglottic folds).

FIGURE 656.1 Cross Section of Larynx ▶
at the Vocal Folds

NOTE: (1) The orientation of the arytenoid cartilages
and their articulations with the cricoid cartilage.

(2) The vocal folds consist of mucous membrane
over the vocal ligaments, lateral to which extend
the deeper part of the thyroarytenoid muscle.

(3) By drawing the arytenoid cartilages forward,
the thyroarytenoids shorten and relax the vocal
folds. At the same time, they medially rotate
the arytenoid cartilages and, thus, approximate
the vocal folds.

(4) The intercartilaginous part of the rima glottidis
is bounded by the arytenoid and cricoid cartilages, whereas the intermembranous part is
bounded by the vocal fold mucous membrane.

I = intermembranous part of the rima glottidis
II = intercartilaginous part of the rima glottidis

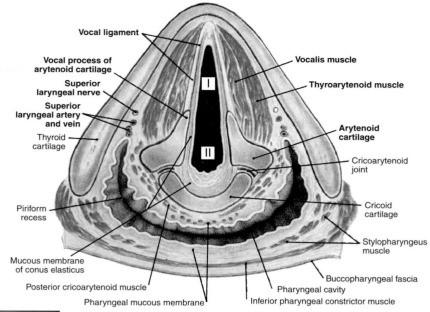

Vocal ligament
Vocal process of arytenoid cartilage
Superior laryngeal nerve
Superior laryngeal artery and vein
Thyroid cartilage
Piriform recess
Mucous membrane of conus elasticus
Posterior cricoarytenoid muscle
Pharyngeal mucous membrane

Vocalis muscle
Thyroarytenoid muscle
Arytenoid cartilage
Cricoarytenoid joint
Cricoid cartilage
Stylopharyngeus muscle
Buccopharyngeal fascia
Pharyngeal cavity
Inferior pharyngeal constrictor muscle

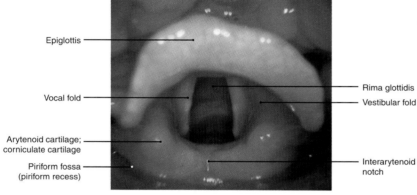

Epiglottis
Vocal fold
Arytenoid cartilage; corniculate cartilage
Piriform fossa (piriform recess)

Rima glottidis
Vestibular fold
Interarytenoid notch

◀ **FIGURE 656.2** Rima Glottidis in Forced or
Deep Inspiration (Direct Laryngoscopy)

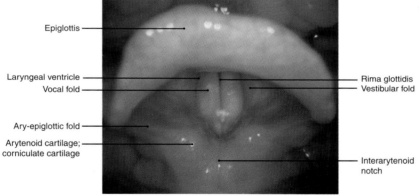

Epiglottis
Laryngeal ventricle
Vocal fold
Ary-epiglottic fold
Arytenoid cartilage; corniculate cartilage

Rima glottidis
Vestibular fold
Interarytenoid notch

◀ **FIGURE 656.3** Rima Glottidis during Shrill
Tone Phonation (Direct Laryngoscopy)

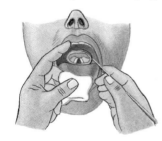

FIGURE 656.5 Indirect Laryngoscopy ▲

NOTE: Protraction of the tongue creates space for a
laryngoscopic mirror so that the vocal folds can be
visualized indirectly by their reflection in the mirror.

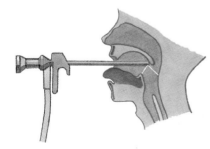

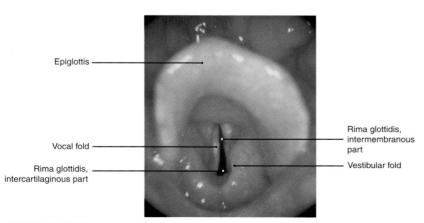

Epiglottis
Vocal fold
Rima glottidis, intercartilaginous part

Rima glottidis, intermembranous part
Vestibular fold

FIGURE 656.4 Rima Glottidis during Whispering: Intercartilaginous
Part Open (Direct Laryngoscopy)

FIGURE 656.6 Direct Laryngoscopy ▲

NOTE: The use of an endoscope allows visualization of the vocal folds directly.

PLATE 657 External Ear: Surface Anatomy, Cartilage, and Muscles

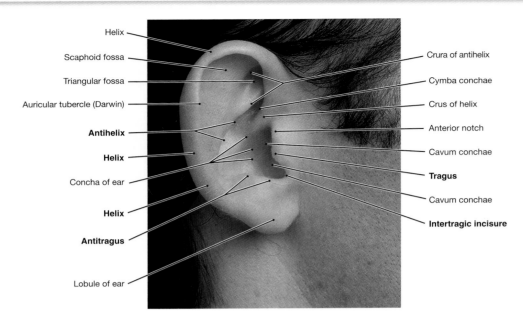

Helix
Scaphoid fossa
Triangular fossa
Auricular tubercle (Darwin)
Antihelix
Helix
Concha of ear
Helix
Antitragus
Lobule of ear

Crura of antihelix
Cymba conchae
Crus of helix
Anterior notch
Cavum conchae
Tragus
Cavum conchae
Intertragic incisure

FIGURE 657.1 **Right External Ear (Lateral View)**

NOTE: (1) The external ear (or auricle) consists of skin overlying an irregularly shaped elastic fibrocartilage. The ear lobe, or lobule, does not contain cartilage but is soft and contains connective tissue and fat.

(2) The **external acoustic meatus** courses through the auricle to the tympanic membrane. It is an oval canal that extends for about 2.5 cm in an S-shaped curve to the tympanic membrane. It consists of an outer cartilaginous part (1 cm) and a narrower more medial part that is osseous (1.5 cm).

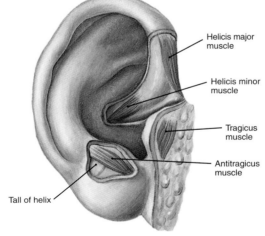

Helicis major muscle
Helicis minor muscle
Tragicus muscle
Antitragicus muscle
Tall of helix

FIGURE 657.3 **Intrinsic Muscles of External Ear (Lateral Surface)**

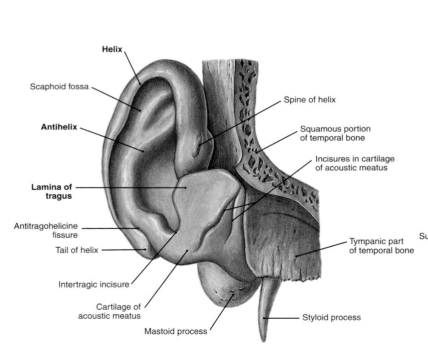

Helix
Scaphoid fossa
Antihelix
Lamina of tragus
Antitragohelicine fissure
Tail of helix
Intertragic incisure
Cartilage of acoustic meatus
Mastoid process

Spine of helix
Squamous portion of temporal bone
Incisures in cartilage of acoustic meatus
Tympanic part of temporal bone
Styloid process

FIGURE 657.2 **Cartilage of the Right External Ear ▲ (Seen from Front)**

NOTE: (1) With the skin of the external ear removed, the contours of the single cartilage conform generally with those of the intact auricle. The cartilage is seen to be absent inferiorly at the site of the ear lobe.

(2) The external rim of the auricle is called the **helix.** Another curved prominence anterior to the helix is the **antihelix.** A notch inferiorly (intertragic incisure) separates the **tragus** anteriorly from the **antitragus** posteriorly.

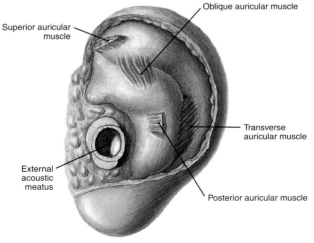

Oblique auricular muscle
Superior auricular muscle
Transverse auricular muscle
External acoustic meatus
Posterior auricular muscle

FIGURE 657.4 **Muscles Attaching to the Medial Surface of External Ear**

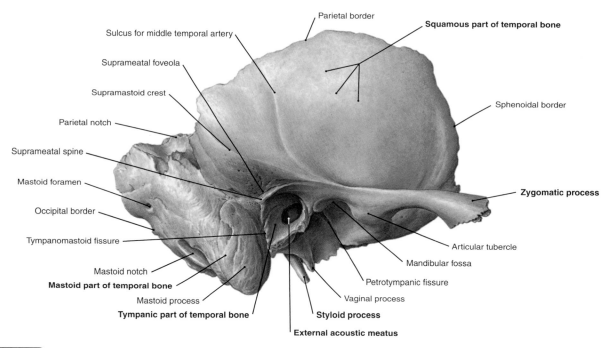

FIGURE 658.1 Right Temporal Bone (Lateral View)

NOTE: (1) The temporal bone forms the osseous encasement for the middle and internal ear and consists of three parts: **squamous, tympanic, and petrous.**

(2) The **squamous part** is broad in shape, and it is thin and flat. From it extends the zygomatic process. The **tympanic part** is interposed below the squamous and anterior to the petrous parts. The external acoustic meatus, which leads to the tympanic membrane, is surrounded by the tympanic part of the temporal bone.

(3) The hard **petrous part** contains the organ of hearing and the vestibular canals. Its mastoid process is not solid but contains many air cells, and its external surface affords attachment to several muscles.

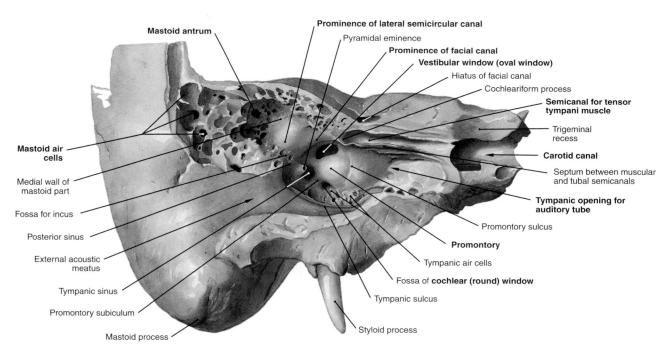

FIGURE 658.2 Lateral Dissection of the Right Temporal Bone Showing the Tympanic Cavity

NOTE: (1) The tympanic cavity (middle ear) communicates posteriorly with the mastoid antrum and, in turn, with the mastoid air cells. It also is in communication with the nasopharynx by way of the auditory tube.

(2) The **lateral wall** of the tympanic cavity is formed by the tympanic membrane (not shown), while the **medial wall** (or labyrinthine wall) presents the following important structures: the **promontory** (projection of the first turn of the cochlea); the **vestibular window** (oval window); the **cochlear window** (round window); the bony prominence of the **facial canal;** and posteriorly, the prominence of the **lateral semicircular canal** and the **pyramidal eminence.**

PLATE 659 Ear: External and Middle Ear (Frontal Sections)

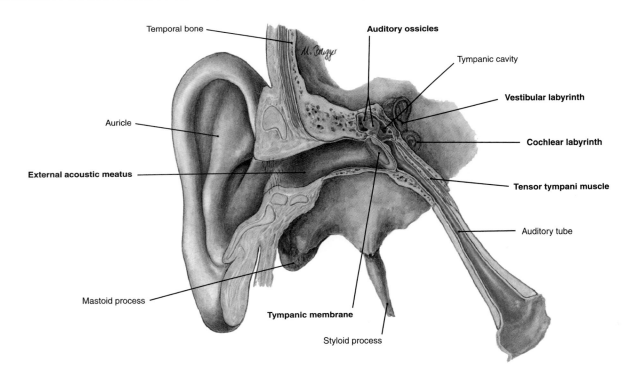

Temporal bone

Auditory ossicles

Tympanic cavity

Vestibular labyrinth

Auricle

Cochlear labyrinth

External acoustic meatus

Tensor tympani muscle

Auditory tube

Mastoid process

Tympanic membrane

Styloid process

FIGURE 659.1 Frontal Section through the Right External, Middle, and Internal Ear

NOTE: (1) The external acoustic meatus commences at the auricle and leads to the external surface of the tympanic membrane. Through the meatus course the sound waves that cause vibration of the tympanum.

(2) The **middle ear** (or tympanic cavity) contains three ossicles (malleus, incus, and stapes) and two muscles (tensor tympani and stapedius; the latter is not shown).

(3) The cavity of the middle ear communicates with the **mastoid antrum** and **mastoid air cells** posteriorly, and the nasopharynx by way of the **auditory tube**. This tube courses downward, forward, and medially from the middle ear.

(4) The ossicles interconnect the tympanic membrane with the inner ear. The inner ear contains the coiled **cochlea** (or organ of hearing) and the three **semicircular canals** (the vestibular organ) and their associated vessels and nerves.

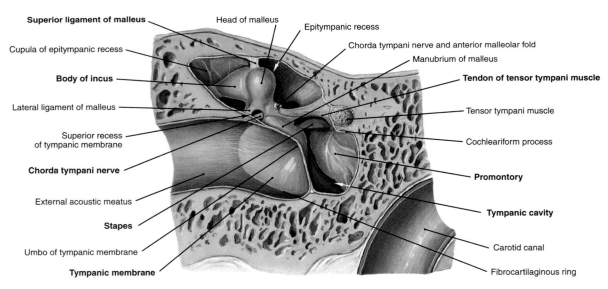

Superior ligament of malleus

Head of malleus

Epitympanic recess

Cupula of epitympanic recess

Chorda tympani nerve and anterior malleolar fold

Manubrium of malleus

Body of incus

Tendon of tensor tympani muscle

Lateral ligament of malleus

Tensor tympani muscle

Superior recess of tympanic membrane

Cochleariform process

Chorda tympani nerve

Promontory

External acoustic meatus

Tympanic cavity

Stapes

Carotid canal

Umbo of tympanic membrane

Tympanic membrane

Fibrocartilaginous ring

FIGURE 659.2 Frontal Section through the Right External and Middle Ear

NOTE: (1) The slender tendon of the *tensor tympani muscle* turns sharply upon reaching the tympanic cavity to terminate on the manubrium of the malleus.

(2) The tympanic cavity is extended superiorly by the epitympanic recess located above the level of the tympanic membrane. On the medial wall of the middle ear observe the promontory that protrudes into the tympanic cavity. This bony prominence is formed by the spiral cochlea of the internal ear.

(3) The lateral and superior ligaments attaching to the head of the malleus. The anterior ligament of the malleus, which interconnects the neck of the malleus to the anterior wall of the tympanic cavity, is not shown.

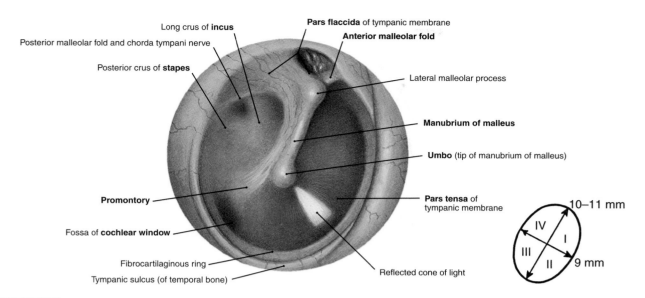

Long crus of **incus**

Posterior malleolar fold and chorda tympani nerve

Posterior crus of **stapes**

Pars flaccida of tympanic membrane

Anterior malleolar fold

Lateral malleolar process

Manubrium of malleus

Umbo (tip of manubrium of malleus)

Promontory

Pars tensa of tympanic membrane

Fossa of **cochlear window**

10–11 mm

IV

I

III

II

9 mm

Fibrocartilaginous ring

Tympanic sulcus (of temporal bone)

Reflected cone of light

FIGURE 660.1 Right Tympanic Membrane as Seen with an Otoscope in a Living Person

NOTE: (1) The tympanic membrane is oval and measures about 9 mm across and from 10 to 11 mm vertically; it often is described as consisting of four quadrants (see lower inset diagram).

(2) The **anterior** and **posterior malleolar folds**. The more lax part (pars flaccida) of the tympanic membrane lies above and between these folds, whereas the rest is more tightly stretched (pars tensa).

(3) The blood supply of the membrane is derived from the **deep auricular** and **anterior tympanic branches** of the maxillary artery and the **stylomastoid branch** of the posterior auricular artery.

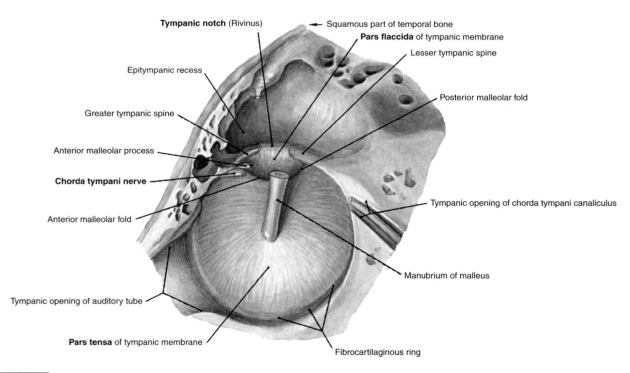

Tympanic notch (Rivinus)

Squamous part of temporal bone

Pars flaccida of tympanic membrane

Lesser tympanic spine

Epitympanic recess

Posterior malleolar fold

Greater tympanic spine

Anterior malleolar process

Chorda tympani nerve

Tympanic opening of chorda tympani canaliculus

Anterior malleolar fold

Tympanic opening of auditory tube

Manubrium of malleus

Pars tensa of tympanic membrane

Fibrocartilaginous ring

FIGURE 660.2 Lateral Wall of the Right Middle Ear (Tympanic Membrane Viewed from within the Tympanic Cavity)

NOTE: (1) The **manubrium** of the **malleus** has been severed from the remainder of the ossicle and left attached to the tympanic membrane. The fibrocartilaginous tympanic ring is deficient superiorly, forming the **tympanic notch** (of Rivinus). The looser portion of the tympanic membrane (**pars flaccida**) covers this zone.

(2) The tympanic membrane below the malleolar folds is the **pars tensa**. This portion is made taut by the **tensor tympani muscle**, which attaches to the manubrium of the malleus.

(3) The external surface of the tympanic membrane is innervated by the **auriculotemporal branch** of the mandibular nerve (V) and the **auricular branch** of the vagus nerve (X). The internal surface of the membrane is supplied by the **tympanic branch** of the glossopharyngeal nerve (ix).

PLATE 661 Ear: Lateral Wall of Tympanic Cavity; Middle Ear Ossicles

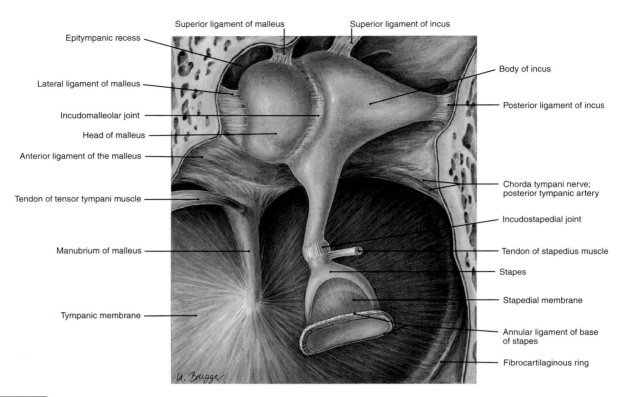

FIGURE 661.1 Middle Ear Ossicles and Attachment of Muscle Tendons (Right Side)

NOTE: (1) The tendon of the **tensor tympani muscle** inserts on the manubrium of the malleus and the short tendon of the **stapedius muscle** inserts onto the neck of the stapes close to its articulation with the incus.

(2) The tensor tympani draws the manubrium medially, thereby making the tympanic membrane taut. At the same time its action pushes the base of the stapes more securely into the vestibular window. The tensor is innervated by the mandibular division of the **trigeminal nerve.**

(3) The stapedius opposes the action of the tensor at the vestibular window, tilting the head of the stapes away from the window. Its denervation results in hyperacusis, a condition in which sounds are perceived as unduly loud. The stapedius is supplied by the **facial nerve.**

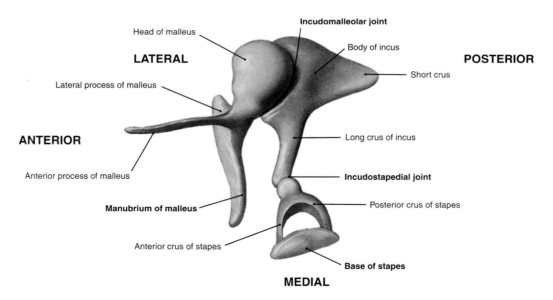

FIGURE 661.2 Right Auditory Ossicles

NOTE: (1) When sound waves are received at the tympanic membrane, they cause a **medial** displacement of the manubrium of the malleus. The head of the malleus is then tilted **laterally**, pulling with it the body of the incus. At the same time the long process of the incus is displaced **medially**, as is the articulation between the incus and the stapes.

(2) The base of the stapes rocks as if it were on a fulcrum at the vestibular window, thereby establishing waves in the perilymph. These waves stimulate the auditory receptors and become dissipated at the secondary tympanic membrane covering the cochlear window.

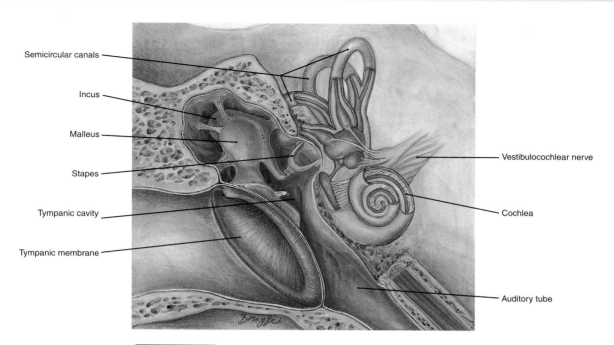

Semicircular canals

Incus

Malleus

Stapes

Tympanic cavity

Tympanic membrane

Vestibulocochlear nerve

Cochlea

Auditory tube

FIGURE 662.1 Structures in the Middle and Internal Ear

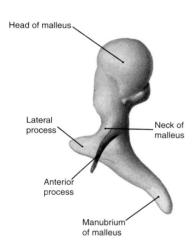

Head of malleus

Lateral process

Neck of malleus

Anterior process

Manubrium of malleus

FIGURE 662.2 Malleus: Anterior View

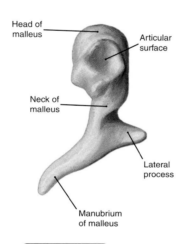

Head of malleus

Articular surface

Neck of malleus

Lateral process

Manubrium of malleus

FIGURE 662.3 Malleus: Posterior View

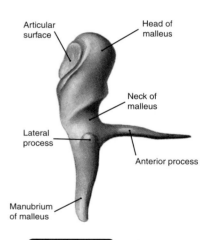

Articular surface

Head of malleus

Neck of malleus

Lateral process

Anterior process

Manubrium of malleus

FIGURE 662.4 Malleus: Lateral View

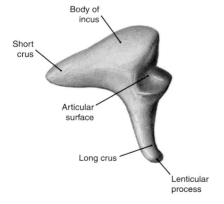

Body of incus

Short crus

Articular surface

Long crus

Lenticular process

FIGURE 662.5 Incus: Lateral View

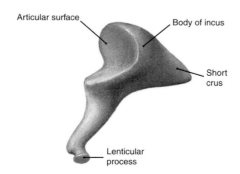

Articular surface

Body of incus

Short crus

Lenticular process

FIGURE 662.6 Incus: Medial View

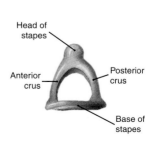

Head of stapes

Anterior crus

Posterior crus

Base of stapes

FIGURE 662.7 Stapes: Superior View

PLATE 663 **Ear: Lateral Wall of Tympanic Cavity; Chorda Tympani Nerve**

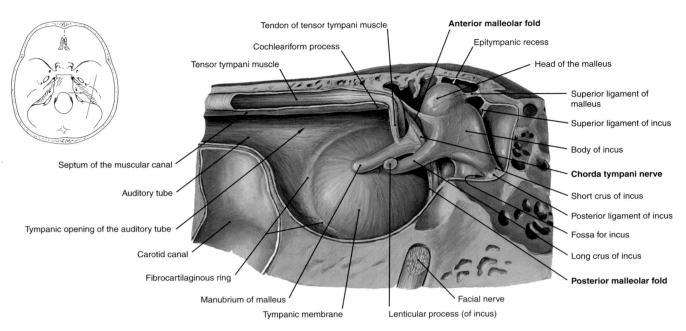

Tendon of tensor tympani muscle
Anterior malleolar fold
Cochleariform process
Epitympanic recess
Tensor tympani muscle
Head of the malleus
Superior ligament of malleus
Superior ligament of incus
Body of incus
Septum of the muscular canal
Chorda tympani nerve
Auditory tube
Short crus of incus
Posterior ligament of incus
Tympanic opening of the auditory tube
Fossa for incus
Carotid canal
Long crus of incus
Fibrocartilaginous ring
Posterior malleolar fold
Manubrium of malleus
Facial nerve
Tympanic membrane
Lenticular process (of incus)

FIGURE 663.1 **Lateral Wall of the Right Tympanic Cavity (Viewed from the Medial Aspect)**

NOTE: (1) The tympanic cavity is completely lined with a mucous membrane that attaches onto the surface of all the structures of the middle ear. This tympanic mucosa is continuous with that lining the mastoid air cells posteriorly and the auditory tube anteriorly.

(2) Reflections of the tympanic mucous membrane form the **anterior** and **posterior malleolar folds.** These are also reflected around the **chorda tympani nerve** as it curves along the medial side of the manubrium of the malleus.

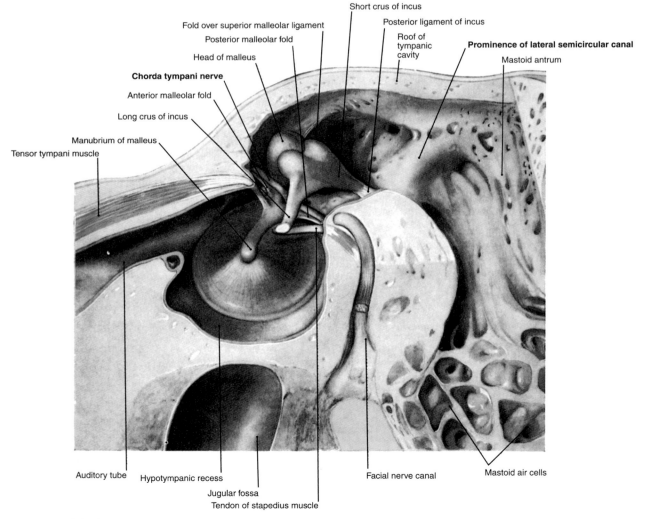

Short crus of incus
Fold over superior malleolar ligament
Posterior ligament of incus
Posterior malleolar fold
Roof of tympanic cavity
Prominence of lateral semicircular canal
Head of malleus
Mastoid antrum
Chorda tympani nerve
Anterior malleolar fold
Long crus of incus
Manubrium of malleus
Tensor tympani muscle
Auditory tube   Hypotympanic recess
Facial nerve canal
Mastoid air cells
Jugular fossa
Tendon of stapedius muscle

FIGURE 663.2 **Tensor Tympani and Stapedius Muscles and Chorda Tympani Nerve (Right Side)**

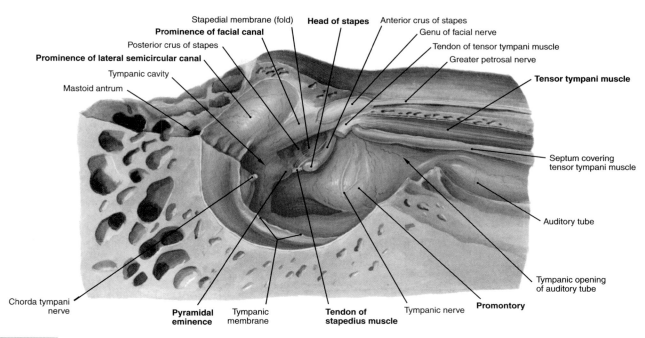

Stapedial membrane (fold) **Head of stapes** Anterior crus of stapes
Prominence of facial canal Genu of facial nerve
Posterior crus of stapes Tendon of tensor tympani muscle
Prominence of lateral semicircular canal Greater petrosal nerve
Tympanic cavity **Tensor tympani muscle**
Mastoid antrum

Septum covering
tensor tympani muscle

Auditory tube

Tympanic opening
of auditory tube

Chorda tympani
nerve **Pyramidal** Tympanic **Tendon of** Tympanic nerve **Promontory**
eminence membrane **stapedius muscle**

FIGURE 664.1 **Medial Wall of the Right Tympanic Cavity (Viewed from Lateral Aspect)**

NOTE: (1) The tympanic membrane has been removed, along with the bony roof of the tympanic cavity. The malleus and incus have also been removed and the tendon of the tensor tympani severed. Observe the **stapes** with its base directed toward the vestibular window and the **stapedius muscle** still attached to its neck.

(2) Several bony markings: (a) the prominence containing the **lateral semicircular canal,** (b) the curved prominence of the **facial canal** with its facial nerve, (c) the **promontory,** which is a rounded thin bony covering over the **cochlea,** and (d) the hollow **pyramidal eminence,** from which arises the **stapedius muscle.**

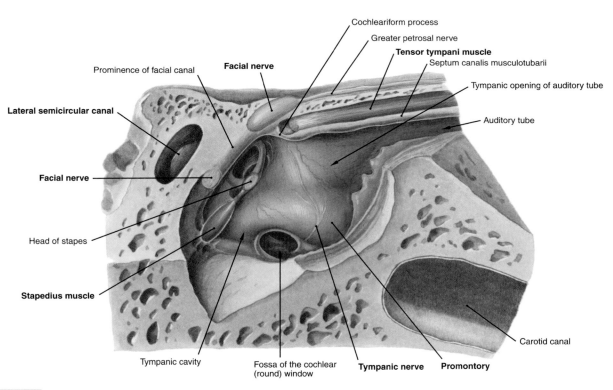

Cochleariform process
Greater petrosal nerve
Tensor tympani muscle
Prominence of facial canal **Facial nerve** Septum canalis musculotubarii

Tympanic opening of auditory tube

Lateral semicircular canal
Auditory tube

Facial nerve

Head of stapes

Stapedius muscle

Carotid canal

Tympanic cavity Fossa of the cochlear **Tympanic nerve** **Promontory**
(round) window

FIGURE 664.2 **Medial Wall of the Right Tympanic Cavity Showing the Stapedius Muscle**

NOTE: (1) The stapedius muscle emerges through the apex of the pyramidal eminence and it is about 4 mm in length. It pulls the base of the stapes laterally and protects the inner ear from damage caused by loud sounds.

(2) The **tympanic** branch of the **glossopharyngeal nerve** (IX) coursing along the promontory. This nerve is sensory to the mucous membrane of the middle ear and is also known as the nerve of Jacobson. Its fibers are joined by sympathetic fibers to form the **tympanic plexus.**

PLATE 665 Ear: Facial Canal; Nerves of External and Middle Ear

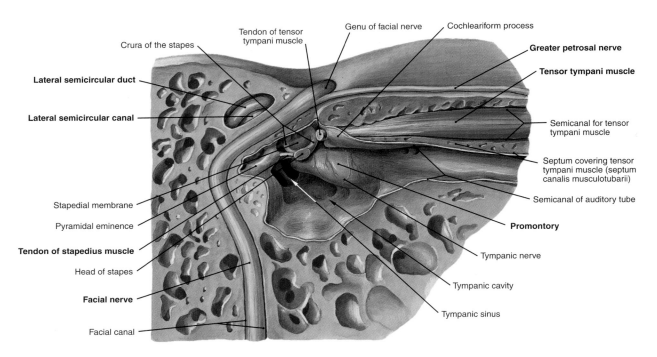

FIGURE 665.1 Medial Wall of Right Tympanic Cavity (Lateral View)

NOTE: (1) The bone forming the prominences of the **lateral semicircular canal** and the **facial canal** has been removed to reveal their internal structures.
(2) The **greater petrosal nerve** carries preganglionic parasympathetic fibers from the facial nerve to the pterygopalatine ganglion as well as many taste fibers from the soft palate.
(3) Coursing along the surface of the promontory can be seen the **tympanic branch** of the **glossopharyngeal nerve** and the tympanic vessels along with sympathetic fibers from the carotid plexus (caroticotympanic nerves).

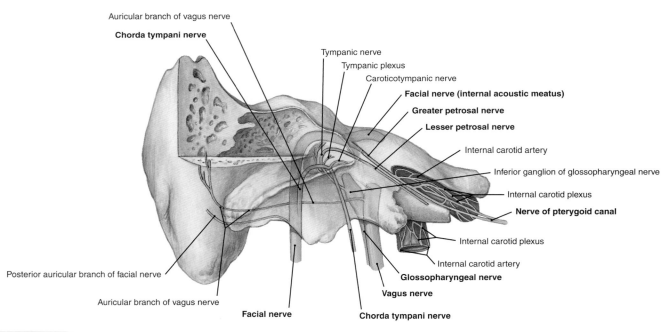

FIGURE 665.2 Facial, Glossopharyngeal, and Vagus Nerves Projected on Temporal Bone

NOTE: (1) From the tympanic plexus (see NOTE 3, Fig. 665.1) emerges the **lesser petrosal nerve**, which courses to the **otic ganglion**.
(2) The **greater petrosal nerve** joins with sympathetic branches of the internal carotid plexus (actually the **deep petrosal nerve**) to form the nerve of the **pterygoid canal**.
(3) The **auricular branch** of the **vagus nerve** is distributed to the upper surface of the external auricle, to the posterior wall and floor of the external acoustic meatus, and to part of the lateral (outer) surface of the tympanic membrane.

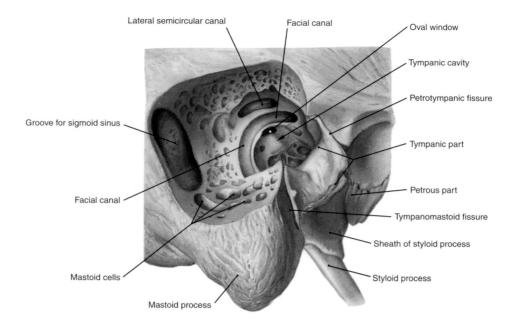

FIGURE 666.1 Dissected Right Temporal Bone

NOTE: (1) Through the facial canal courses the **facial nerve**. The canal commences at the internal auditory meatus and continues through the petrous part of the temporal bone to its exit at the stylomastoid foramen (see Fig. 665.1).

(2) In its descent, the facial canal courses posterior to the cavity of the middle ear (tympanic cavity), where the facial nerve gives off the nerve to the stapedius muscle and the chorda tympani branch.

(3) The location of the lateral semicircular canal superiorly and the groove for the sigmoid sinus posteriorly.

(4) Within the tympanic cavity is located the oval window adjacent to which would be found the base of the stapes.

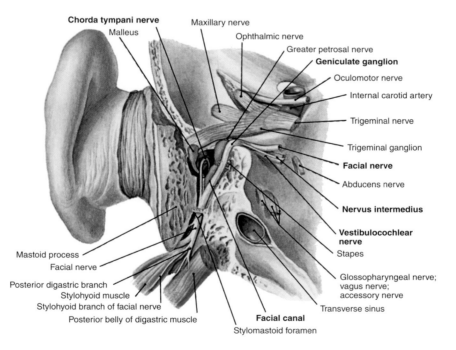

FIGURE 666.2 Intracranial Course of the Facial Nerve Viewed Posteriorly

NOTE: (1) This is a frontal section of the temporal bone that opens the facial canal from behind. Observe the **chorda tympani nerve** coursing from the **facial nerve** across (from posterior to tanterior) the tympanic cavity along the inner surface of the tympanic membrane.

(2) The internal acoustic meatus in the floor of the skull transmits the facial nerve (and **nervous intermedius**) and the **vestibulocochlear nerve**.

(3) Distal to the **geniculate ganglion** (the sensory ganglion of the facial nerve) the facial nerve enters the facial canal where it first courses laterally and then turns sharply backward and inferiorly (see Fig. 665.1).

(4) Beyond the chorda tympani branch, the trunk of the facial nerve descends in the temporal bone to emerge on the side of the face through the stylomastoid foramen posterior to the ear lobe.

PLATE 667 **Internal Ear Projected onto the Bony Base of the Skull**

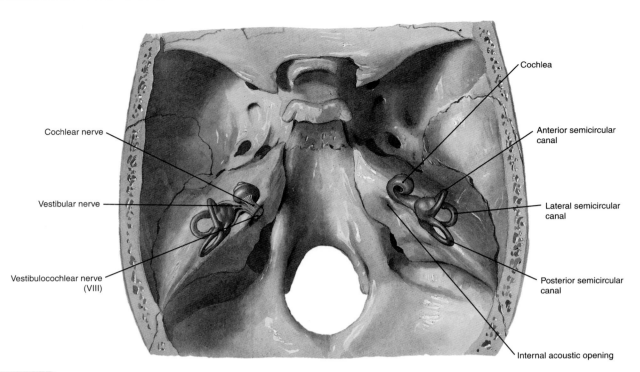

Cochlea

Cochlear nerve

Anterior semicircular canal

Vestibular nerve

Lateral semicircular canal

Vestibulocochlear nerve (VIII)

Posterior semicircular canal

Internal acoustic opening

FIGURE 667.1 **Cochlea and Semicircular Canals Projected onto the Petrous Part of the Temporal Bone**

NOTE: (1) The internal ear lies in the petrous part of the temporal bone just deep to the crest of that bone (called the arcuate eminence [not labeled]) that separates the middle cranial fossa from the posterior cranial fossa. Also observe the internal acoustic (auditory) meatus on the posterior aspect of the arcuate eminence through which pass the facial and vestibulocochlear nerves.

(2) The orientation of the anterior, lateral, and posterior semicircular canals, and the cochlea is positioned slightly medial and anterior to the canals. Also note (on the reader's left) the vestibular and cochlear divisions of the vestibulocochlear nerve that carries impulses from the vestibular receptors in the semicircular canals that inform the brain of the position of the head in space and the receptors in the cochlea that transmit the special sense of hearing.

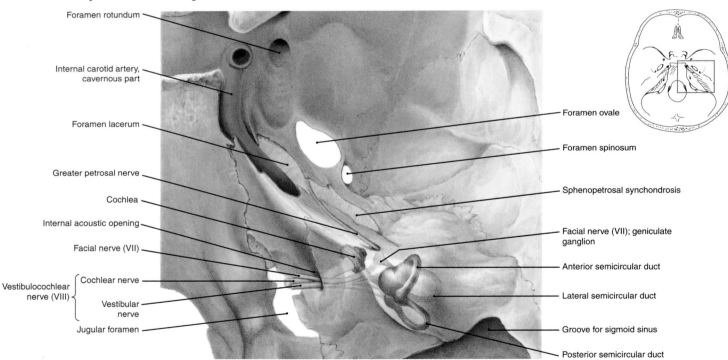

Foramen rotundum

Internal carotid artery, cavernous part

Foramen lacerum

Greater petrosal nerve

Cochlea

Internal acoustic opening

Facial nerve (VII)

Vestibulocochlear nerve (VIII) { Cochlear nerve / Vestibular nerve }

Jugular foramen

Foramen ovale

Foramen spinosum

Sphenopetrosal synchondrosis

Facial nerve (VII); geniculate ganglion

Anterior semicircular duct

Lateral semicircular duct

Groove for sigmoid sinus

Posterior semicircular duct

FIGURE 667.2 **Structures of the Right Inner Ear and the Vestibulocochlear and Facial Nerves Visualized from Above**

NOTE: (1) The semicircular canals and the cochlea of the inner ear are projected onto the superior surface of the petrous portion of the temporal bone. Also observe the **facial nerve** and **the vestibular and cochlear divisions** of the **vestibulocochlear nerve** traversing the internal acoustic (auditory) meatus.

(2) The orientation of the cochlea is similar to that in Figure 667.1. Also note the **geniculate ganglion** through which course the fibers that form the greater petrosal nerve. This ganglion contains the cell bodies for the taste fibers in the chorda tympani nerve for the anterior two-thirds of the tongue.

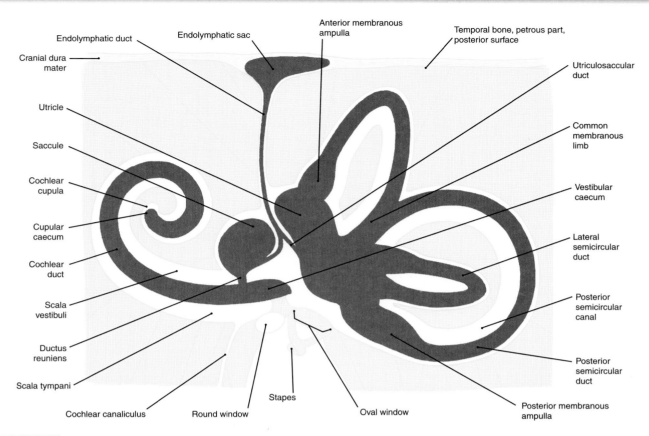

Cranial dura mater
Endolymphatic duct
Endolymphatic sac
Anterior membranous ampulla
Temporal bone, petrous part, posterior surface
Utriculosaccular duct
Utricle
Saccule
Common membranous limb
Cochlear cupula
Vestibular caecum
Cupular caecum
Lateral semicircular duct
Cochlear duct
Posterior semicircular canal
Scala vestibuli
Ductus reuniens
Posterior semicircular duct
Scala tympani
Cochlear canaliculus
Round window
Stapes
Oval window
Posterior membranous ampulla

FIGURE 668.1 **Membranous Labyrinth of the Inner Ear**

NOTE: The membranous labyrinth is a closed system of ducts and sacs surrounded by the bony labyrinth of the inner ear. It contains endolymph surrounded by perilymph and consists of the ducts of the semicircular canals, the utricle, the saccule, the endolymphatic duct, and the duct of the cochlea.

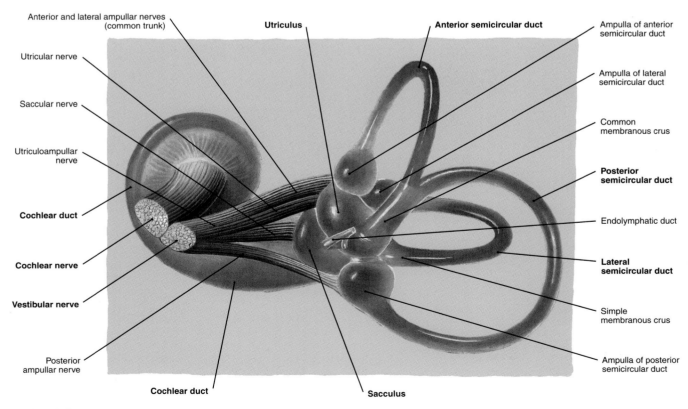

Anterior and lateral ampullar nerves (common trunk)
Utriculus
Anterior semicircular duct
Ampulla of anterior semicircular duct
Utricular nerve
Ampulla of lateral semicircular duct
Saccular nerve
Common membranous crus
Utriculoampullar nerve
Posterior semicircular duct
Cochlear duct
Cochlear nerve
Endolymphatic duct
Vestibular nerve
Lateral semicircular duct
Simple membranous crus
Posterior ampullar nerve
Cochlear duct
Sacculus
Ampulla of posterior semicircular duct

FIGURE 668.2 **Right Membranous Labyrinth (Medial View)**

NOTE: The ampullae of the three semicircular ducts, the sacculus, the utriculus, and the cochlear duct, and the connections of the endolymphatic duct to the utriculus and sacculus.

CHAPTER 8 Cranial Nerves

Plates

669 Cranial Nerve Attachments to the Base of the Brain

670 Apertures in the Base of the Skull Transmitting the Cranial Nerves

671 Olfactory Nerve (CN I); Olfactory Bulb and Tract

672 Olfactory Nerve; Olfactory Bulb and Tract (Continued)

673 Optic Nerve (CN II)

674 Optic Nerve and Tract (Continued)

675 Oculomotor (CN III), Trochlear (CN IV), and Abducens (CN VI) Nerves

676 Oculomotor, Trochlear, and Abducens Nerves (Continued)

677 Trigeminal Nerve (CN V)

678 Ophthalmic Division of the Trigeminal Nerve

679 Maxillary Division of the Trigeminal Nerve

680 Mandibular Division of the Trigeminal Nerve

681 Facial Nerve (CN VII)

682 Facial Nerve (Continued): Branches to Muscles of Facial Expression

683 Facial Nerve (Continued): Greater Petrosal Nerve

684 Facial Nerve (Continued): Chorda Tympani Branch

685 Vestibulocochlear Nerve (CN VIII)

686 Vestibulocochlear Nerve (Continued)

687 Glossopharyngeal Nerve (CN IX)

688 Glossopharyngeal Nerve (Continued)

689 Vagus Nerve (CN X)

690 Vagus Nerve (Continued)

691 Accessory Nerve (CN XI)

692 Accessory Nerve (Continued)

693 Hypoglossal Nerve (CN XII)

694 Hypoglossal Nerve (Continued)

PLATE 669 **Cranial Nerve Attachments to the Base of the Brain**

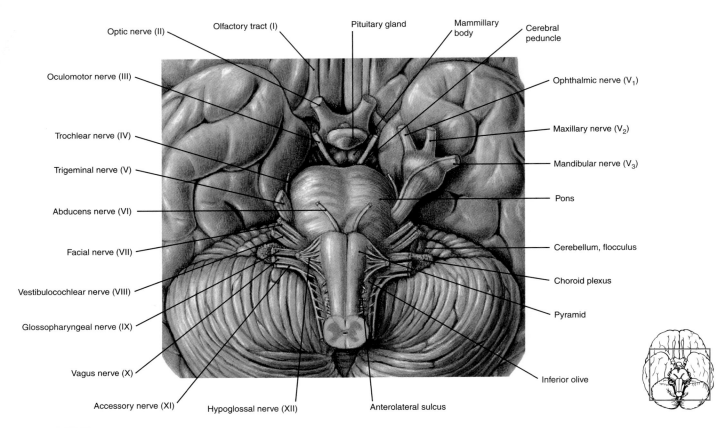

Optic nerve (II)

Olfactory tract (I)

Pituitary gland

Mammillary body

Cerebral peduncle

Oculomotor nerve (III)

Ophthalmic nerve (V₁)

Trochlear nerve (IV)

Maxillary nerve (V₂)

Trigeminal nerve (V)

Mandibular nerve (V₃)

Abducens nerve (VI)

Pons

Facial nerve (VII)

Cerebellum, flocculus

Vestibulocochlear nerve (VIII)

Choroid plexus

Glossopharyngeal nerve (IX)

Pyramid

Vagus nerve (X)

Inferior olive

Accessory nerve (XI)

Hypoglossal nerve (XII)

Anterolateral sulcus

FIGURE 669 **Ventral View of the Brain and the Sites of Attachment of the Cranial Nerves**

NOTE: (1) The cranial nerves (CN) supply motor and sensory innervation to the head and, in some instances, to other region of the body. There are 12 pairs of cranial nerves, and these are attached to the brain from the basal forebrain to the medulla oblongata.

(2) The cranial nerves pass through openings in the skull to (or from) extracranial structures, and they are subject to damage along their paths due to vascular or traumatic incidents or from infections or neoplasms.

SITES OF ATTACHMENT OF THE CRANIAL NERVES TO THE BRAIN

  I **Olfactory Nerves:** These are neurons from receptors for the special sense of smell in the nasal cavity that pierce through foramina in the cribriform plate of the ethmoid bone and terminate on neurons of the olfactory bulb (about 20 bundles). The axons from neurons in the olfactory bulbs (which are second-order neurons in the olfactory pathway) form the **olfactory tracts** that attach to the basal forebrain.

 II **Optic Nerves:** These join at the optic chiasma. The **anterior cerebral artery** lies anterior to the optic chiasma and the **internal carotid artery** is located lateral to the chiasma. The optic tracts then course posteriorly and laterally to enter the diencephalon.

III **Oculomotor Nerve:** Emerges on the medial side of the ventral midbrain and passes between the posterior cerebral artery (superior to the nerve) and the superior cerebellar artery (inferior to the nerve).

 IV **Trochlear Nerve:** Most slender of cranial nerves. It is the only cranial nerve that emerges from the posterior aspect of the brainstem. It attaches to the brain immediately below the inferior colliculus in the upper pons.

  V **Trigeminal Nerve:** It is attached to the anterior surface of the pons near its upper border. The smaller motor root is covered by the large sensory root.

 VI **Abducens Nerve:** Emerges at the lower border of the pons, in a furrow between the pons and the pyramid of the medulla oblongata (the pontomedullary junction).

VII **Facial Nerve:** Also attaches at the lower border of the pons (at the cerebellopontine angle) medial and slightly anterior to the vestibulocochlear nerve.

VIII **Vestibulocochlear Nerve:** Attaches in the same groove as the facial nerve but lateral to the facial nerve.

 IX **Glossopharyngeal Nerve:** Attached to the upper aspect of the medulla oblongata in front of the vagus nerve in a groove between the medulla and the cerebellar peduncle.

  X **Vagus Nerve:** Attached by 8 to 10 filaments in the same groove as the glossopharyngeal nerve but just posterior to it.

 XI **Accessory Nerve:** The **cranial root** is formed by filaments that emerge just caudal to the rootlets that form the vagus nerve. The **spinal root** arises from fibers from the upper five segments of the spinal cord.

The fibers from the cranial root join the **vagus nerve** and become distributed in the pharyngeal and laryngeal branches of the vagus. The fibers of the spinal root leave the cranial fibers and descend from base of the jugular foramen to supply the sternocleidomastoid and trapezius muscles.

XII **Hypoglossal Nerve:** Fibers emerge from the ventrolateral aspect of the caudal medulla in line with the ventral roots spinal cord. They represent the four fused precervical nerves.

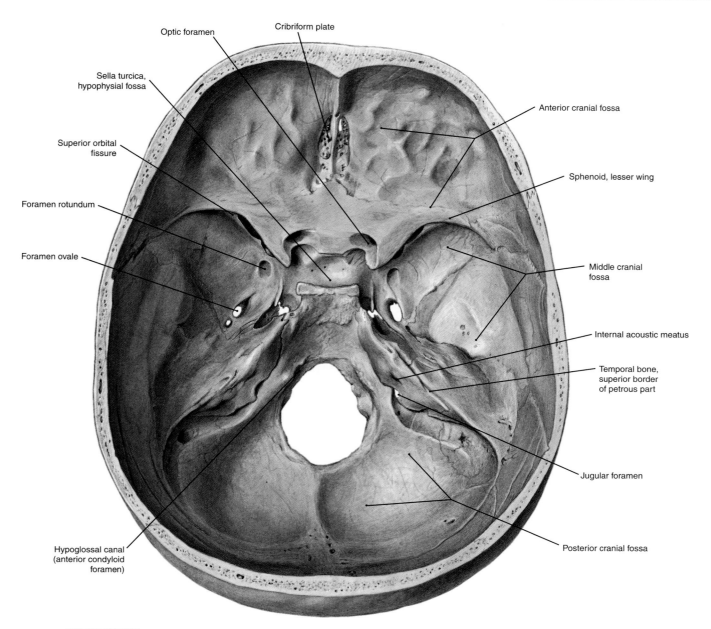

Optic foramen

Cribriform plate

Sella turcica, hypophysial fossa

Anterior cranial fossa

Superior orbital fissure

Sphenoid, lesser wing

Foramen rotundum

Foramen ovale

Middle cranial fossa

Internal acoustic meatus

Temporal bone, superior border of petrous part

Jugular foramen

Hypoglossal canal (anterior condyloid foramen)

Posterior cranial fossa

FIGURE 670 **Base of the Skull Showing Foramina through Which the Cranial Nerves Traverse**

	Nerve	Location
I	**Olfactory**	**Cribriform plate** of the ethmoid bone
II	**Optic**	**Optic foramen** of sphenoid bone (with the ophthalmic artery)
III	**Oculomotor**	
IV	**Trochlear**	**Superior orbital fissure** of sphenoid bone
V_1	**Ophthalmic division, trigeminal**	
V_2	**Maxillary division, trigeminal**	**Foramen rotundum** of sphenoid bone
V_3	**Mandibular division, trigeminal**	**Foramen ovale** of sphenoid bone
VI	**Abducens**	**Superior orbital fissure** of sphenoid bone
VII	**Facial**	
VIII	**Vestibulocochlear**	**Internal acoustic meatus** of temporal bone (petrous part)
IX	**Glossopharyngeal**	
X	**Vagus**	**Jugular foramen,** between the occipital bone and the petrous portion of temporal bone
XI	**Accessory**	
XII	**Hypoglossal**	**Hypoglossal Canal** (anterior condylar foramen)

PLATE 671 Olfactory Nerve (CN I); Olfactory Bulb and Tract

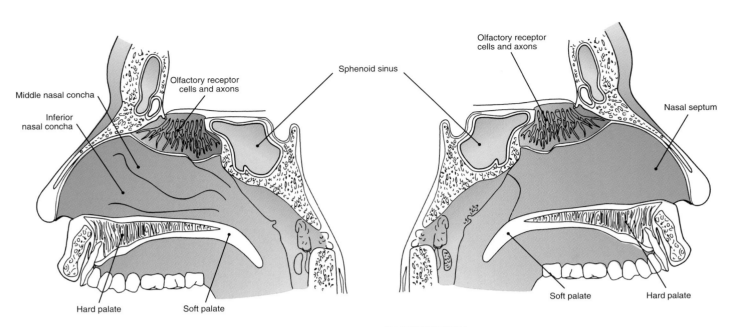

FIGURE 671.1 Lateral Wall of the Nasal Cavity and Olfactory Receptors (Olfactory Nerve/Cranial Nerve I)

FIGURE 671.2 Nasal Septum and Olfactory Receptors (Olfactory Nerve/Cranial Nerve I)

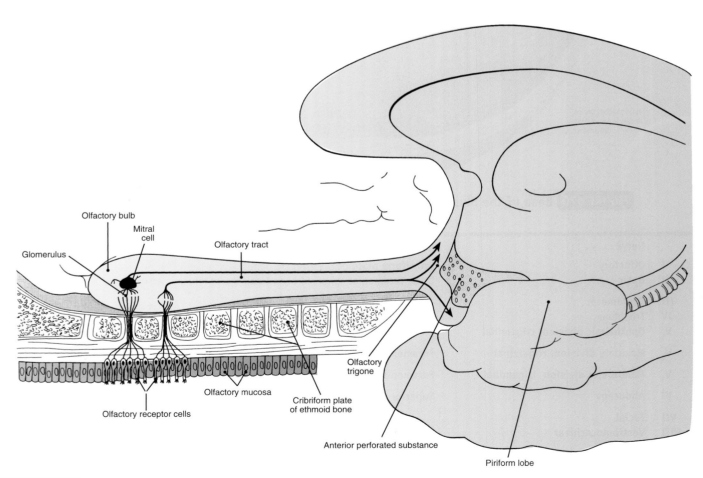

FIGURE 671.3 Olfactory Mucosa, Receptors, and Nerves (CN I) and Olfactory Bulb and Tract of the Central Nervous System (CNS)

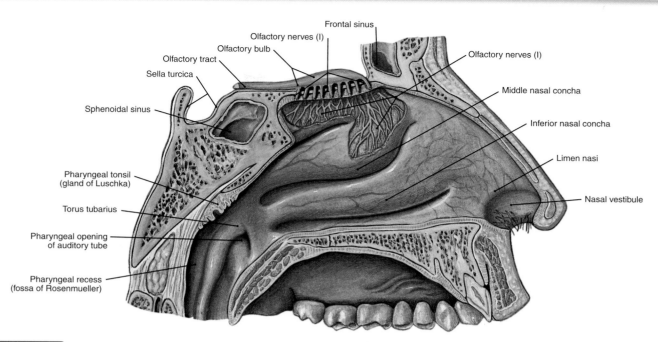

FIGURE 672.1 Lateral Wall of the Nasal Cavity: Olfactory Nerves (CN I) and Olfactory Bulb and Tract

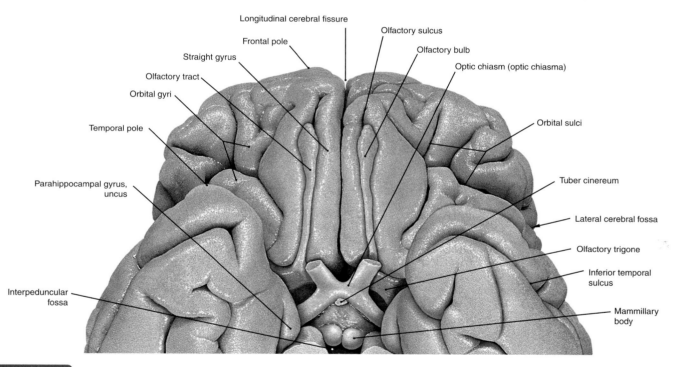

FIGURE 672.2 Basal Forebrain Showing the Olfactory Bulb, Olfactory Tract, and Olfactory Trigone (Central Nervous System)

FIGURES 672.1 and 672.2

NOTE: (1) The olfactory receptor cells and their axons that enter the olfactory bulb constitute the first cranial nerve. These are peripheral nerves, while the olfactory bulb and olfactory tract are brain (central nervous system [CNS]) structures.

(2) The olfactory receptors are located in the **olfactory epithelium** that overlies the superior concha in the lateral wall of the nasal cavity and the adjoining mucosa that covers the superior aspect of the nasal septum (see Figs. 671.1 and 671.2).

(3) About 20 small bundles of nerve fibers from the receptor cells enter the olfactory bulbs on each side by passing through the foramina of the cribriform plate of the ethmoid bone (see Fig. 671.3).

(4) The receptor neuron fibers synapse with tufted and mitral cells in the olfactory bulb and project their axons centrally to form the olfactory tracts (see Figs. 671.3 and 672.2). These tracts are often mistakenly considered the first pair of cranial nerves. The receptor cells and their axons form the first cranial nerve. Second-order neurons (such as the tufted cells and mitral cells in the olfactory bulb) send their axons posteriorly to form the olfactory tract, which is completely a CNS tract.

(5) Damage to the olfactory filaments or the olfactory tracts may occur following fractures of the skull in the anterior cranial fossa or by tumors or inflammation in this fossa. This can result in anosmia (loss of the sense of smell).

Chapter 8 Cranial Nerves

PLATE 673 | Optic Nerve (CN II)

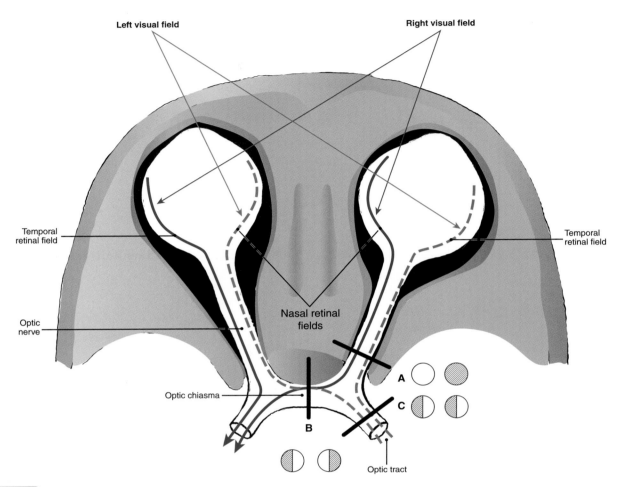

FIGURE 673 **Visual Fields; Retinal Fields; Retina; Optic Nerve; Optic Chiasma (Diagram)**

NOTE: (1) The **optic nerves** transmit visual impulses from the retina posteriorly to the brainstem. The fibers that form the optic nerves are axons from the ganglion cells in the retina. These cells form the innermost layer of the retina and emerge from the bulb of the eye at the optic disk (see Plates 609–612).

(2) A **visual field** is the area in space that is visible to an eye at a given position. A visual field is also called a field of vision. The **nasal retina** is the nasal half of the retina medial to the optic disk (sometimes called the **nasal retinal field**); the **temporal retina** is the outer half of the retina lateral to the optic disk (sometimes called the **temporal retinal field**).

(3) As the optic nerves course posteriorly from the eyeball, half of its fibers cross to the opposite side of the brain at the **optic chiasma.** Fibers from the temporal retina of both eyes DO NOT cross at the optic chiasma, whereas fibers from the nasal retinas of the two eyes CROSS at the optic chiasma.

(4) Posterior to the optic chiasma the optic fibers form the **optic tracts** that carry the fibers to the midbrain, where they synapse with neurons in the lateral geniculate body. These latter neurons send their fibers to the cerebral cortex.

(5) Because of the crossed and uncrossed fibers in the optic chiasma, different lesions in the visual pathway will result in varying losses of vision:

   (a) An **optic nerve** lesion results in a loss of vision in that eye; thus, there is a loss of both nasal and temporal field vision in that one eye **(A).**

   (b) An **optic chiasma [B]** lesion that cuts though the middle of the optic chiasma results in a loss of vision from the nasal half of the retina of the right eye (right temporal visual field) and the nasal half of the retina of the left eye (left temporal visual field). This condition is called **bitemporal hemianopia** because both temporal visual fields are lost and indicates that the crossed fibers at the optic chiasma are cut, whereas the uncrossed fibers are intact.

   (c) A lesion in the **optic tract [C]** on one side (e.g., in the right optic tract) will eliminate vision from the temporal half of the retina of the right eye and the nasal half of the retina of the left eye. This means that there is a loss of input from the contralateral visual fields to both eyes, resulting in a loss of input to the left nasal retinal field and to the right temporal retinal field. This is called **homonymous hemianopia.**

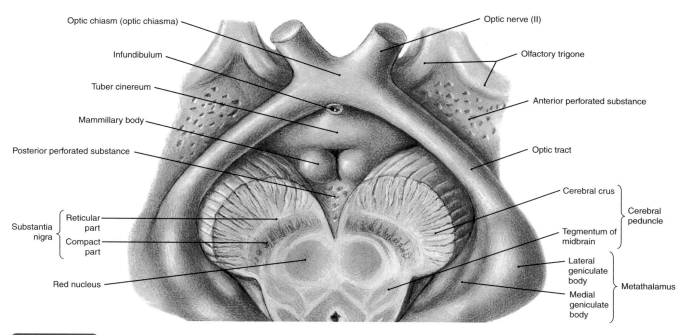

FIGURE 674.1 Optic Chiasma, Optic Tract, and Lateral Geniculate Body; Severed Midbrain (Caudal View)

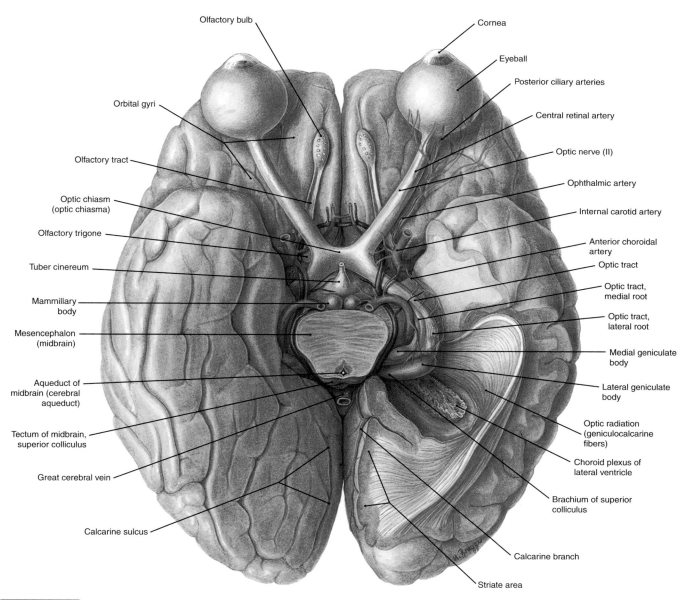

FIGURE 674.2 Visual Pathway from the Optic Nerve to the Cerebral Cortex; Ophthalmic Artery

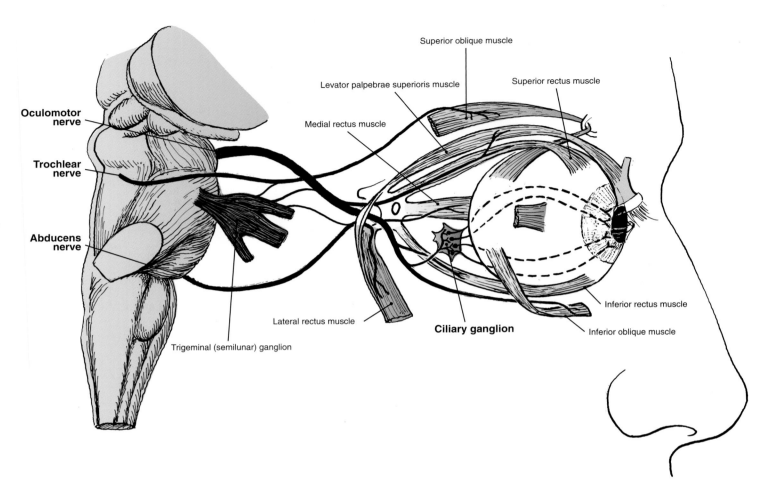

Superior oblique muscle

Levator palpebrae superioris muscle

Superior rectus muscle

Medial rectus muscle

Oculomotor nerve

Trochlear nerve

Abducens nerve

Lateral rectus muscle

Ciliary ganglion

Inferior rectus muscle

Inferior oblique muscle

Trigeminal (semilunar) ganglion

FIGURE 675 Oculomotor (CN III), Trochlear (CN IV), and Abducens (CN VI) Nerves: Lateral View (Diagram)

OCULOMOTOR NERVE (III)

NOTE: (1) The **oculomotor nerve** principally carries **somatomotor fibers** to five extraocular muscles and **preganglionic parasympathetic fibers** to the **ciliary ganglion**. These fibers have their cell bodies in the midbrain: those to the extraocular muscles in the **main oculomotor nucleus**, while the preganglionic parasympathetic fibers have their cell bodies in the **accessory** or **autonomic nucleus** (of Edinger–Westphal).

(2) The oculomotor nerve emerges from the midbrain between the posterior cerebral artery (superior to the nerve) and the superior cerebellar artery (just caudal to the nerve). Hardening of these pulsating arteries and plaques within them can injure the nerve.

(3) The oculomotor nerve courses through the cavernous sinus and enters the orbit by way of the superior orbital fissure and within the annulus tendinous; the nerve then divides into **superior and inferior divisions** and within the orbit supplies five extraocular muscles.

(4) The **superior division** is the smaller of the two and ascends lateral to the optic nerve to supply the **levator palpebrae superioris** and the **superior rectus muscles**; the **inferior division** divides into three branches to supply the **medial rectus**, the **inferior rectus**, and the **inferior oblique muscles**.

(5) The **preganglionic parasympathetic fibers** emerge from the midbrain with the somatomotor fibers and course in the inferior division of the oculomotor nerve in the branch to the inferior oblique muscle. The parasympathetic fibers then leave the nerve to the inferior oblique and pass directly to the **ciliary ganglion,** where they synapse with postganglionic parasympathetic cell bodies.

(6) The postganglionic parasympathetic fibers emerge from the ganglion and course along the **short ciliary nerves** to supply the **ciliary muscle** and the **constrictor of the pupil**. The ciliary muscle controls the shape of the lens, whereas the constrictor of the pupil controls the size of the pupil by reducing its diameter.

(7) Lesions of the oculomotor nerve result in a condition called **ophthalmoplegia.** Its symptoms include (a) **strabismus,** which is the inability to direct both eyes to the same object; this effect results in a downward and abducted eyeball, (b) **a dilated pupil,** (c) **a droopy eyelid** because the levator muscle is denervated, and (d) **a loss of accommodation.**

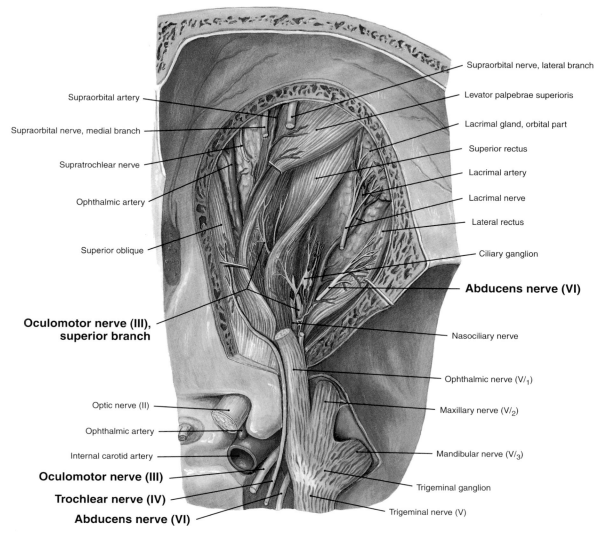

Supraorbital nerve, lateral branch

Supraorbital artery

Levator palpebrae superioris

Supraorbital nerve, medial branch

Lacrimal gland, orbital part

Supratrochlear nerve

Superior rectus

Lacrimal artery

Ophthalmic artery

Lacrimal nerve

Superior oblique

Lateral rectus

Ciliary ganglion

Oculomotor nerve (III), superior branch

Abducens nerve (VI)

Nasociliary nerve

Ophthalmic nerve (V/₁)

Optic nerve (II)

Maxillary nerve (V/₂)

Ophthalmic artery

Internal carotid artery

Mandibular nerve (V/₃)

Oculomotor nerve (III)

Trochlear nerve (IV)

Trigeminal ganglion

Abducens nerve (VI)

Trigeminal nerve (V)

FIGURE 676 **Oculomotor, Trochlear, and Abducens Nerves as They Enter the Orbital Cavity (Superior View)**

TROCHLEAR NERVE (IV)

NOTE: (1) The **trochlear nerve** is the smallest of all the cranial nerves and it supplies only the **superior oblique muscle** in the orbit. It is the only cranial nerve to emerge from the central nervous system on the dorsal aspect of the brain.

(2) The fibers of the trochlear nerve cross to the contralateral side before leaving the dorsal midbrain; after emerging, the nerve is directed laterally around the brainstem immediately above the pons between the posterior cerebral and superior cerebellar arteries.

(3) The nerve then passes rostrally in the lateral wall of the **cavernous sinus** below the oculomotor nerve and superior to the ophthalmic division of the trigeminal nerve (see Fig. 580.1). Anteriorly, it crosses the oculomotor nerve from lateral to medial and it enters the orbit through the **superior orbital fissure** outside the annulus tendineus. In the orbit, the nerve lies superior to the extraocular muscles and it pierces the superior surface of the superior oblique muscle.

(4) **If the oculomotor nerve is injured**, the superior oblique muscle is denervated and it causes an impairment in turning the eye downward and outward. The eye is extorted (outward rotation) because the inferior oblique muscle is acting unopposed.

ABDUCENS NERVE (VI)

NOTE: (1) The **abducens nerve** supplies only the **lateral rectus muscle** within the orbit. Its fibers descend from the abducens nucleus located in the caudal pons, just deep to the fourth ventricle.

(2) The abducens fibers emerge from the ventral surface of the brainstem in the sulcus between the anterior medulla and the posterior border of the pons.

(3) The nerve then courses superiorly, anteriorly, and laterally through the pontine cistern. It then bends acutely forward to traverse the cavernous sinus and it enters the orbital cavity through the **superior orbital fissure** and within the annulus tendineus. It pierces the lateral rectus along the medial surface of the muscle.

(4) The nerve travels a long course from the lower pons to the orbit and is subject to damage due to skull fractures or in cases involving increased intracranial pressure.

(5) If the lateral rectus muscle is denervated, the medial rectus acts unopposed **(internal strabismus).**

PLATE 677 Trigeminal Nerve (CN V)

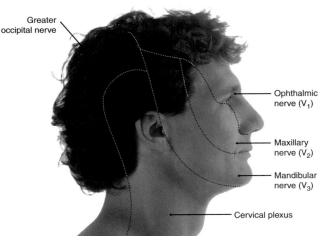

Greater occipital nerve

Ophthalmic nerve (V₁)

Maxillary nerve (V₂)

Mandibular nerve (V₃)

Cervical plexus

FIGURE 677.1 **Lateral View of the Face: Surface Areas Supplied by the Three Divisions of the Trigeminal Nerve**

NOTE: (1) The **ophthalmic nerve** supplies the skin of nose, the upper eyelid, and the scalp from the eyebrow posteriorly to the vertex or top of the skull cap.
(2) The **maxillary nerve** supplies the region between the eyelid and the upper lip, including the skin over the cheek bone.
(3) The **mandibular nerve** supplies the skin of the lower jaw, the lateral part of the face anterior to the ear, and the skin of the temple region on the lateral side of the head.

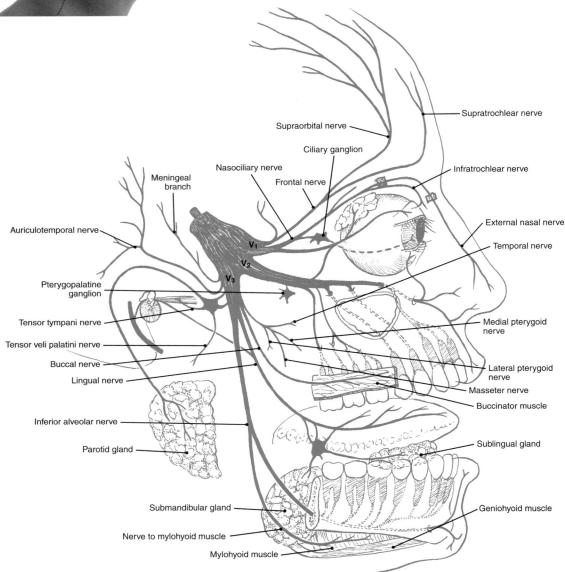

Supratrochlear nerve

Supraorbital nerve

Ciliary ganglion

Nasociliary nerve

Meningeal branch

Frontal nerve

Infratrochlear nerve

External nasal nerve

Auriculotemporal nerve

Temporal nerve

V₁

V₂

V₃

Pterygopalatine ganglion

Medial pterygoid nerve

Tensor tympani nerve

Tensor veli palatini nerve

Lateral pterygoid nerve

Buccal nerve

Masseter nerve

Lingual nerve

Buccinator muscle

Inferior alveolar nerve

Parotid gland

Sublingual gland

Submandibular gland

Geniohyoid muscle

Nerve to mylohyoid muscle

Mylohyoid muscle

FIGURE 677.2 **Diagrammatic Representation of the Trigeminal Nerve and Its Branches**

NOTE: (1) The trigeminal nerve is the largest of the cranial nerves, and it is the great sensory nerve of the face and of the orbital, oral and nasal cavities; it also supplies much of the anterior scalp and all of the teeth.
(2) In addition to its sensory functions the trigeminal nerve, through its mandibular division, supplies the **four muscles of mastication**, as well as the **mylohyoid muscle**, the **anterior belly of the digastric muscle,** and two tensors: the **tensor veli palatini** and the **tensor tympani** muscles.
(3) The cell bodies of the sensory fibers in the o**phthalmic, maxillary,** and **mandibular divisions** of the **trigeminal** nerve are located within the trigeminal (or semilunar) **ganglion.** The ganglion is located in a cleft or recess covered by dura mater, called the **trigeminal cave,** on the anterior aspect of the petrous portion of the temporal bone in the middle cranial fossa of the bony base of the skull.

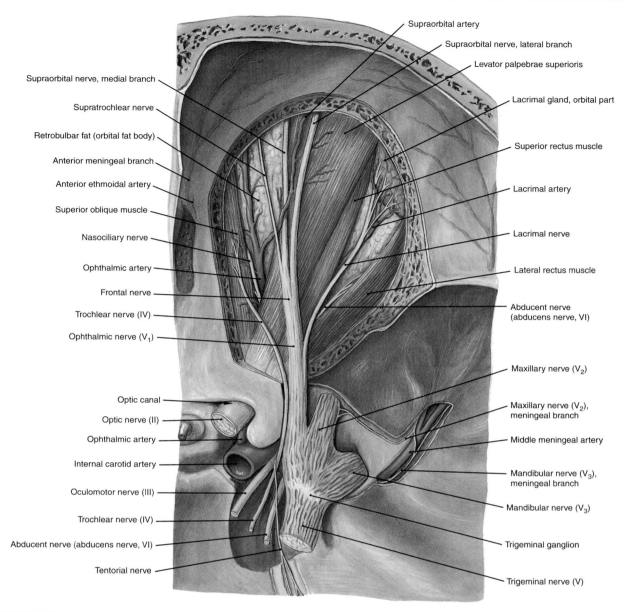

FIGURE 678.1 Branches of the Ophthalmic Division of the Trigeminal Nerve upon Its Entrance into the Orbit

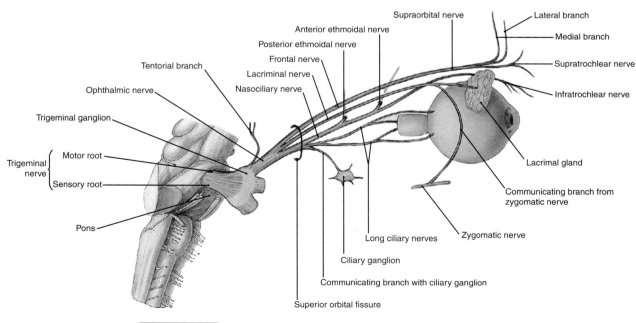

FIGURE 678.2 Ophthalmic Division of the Trigeminal Nerve

PLATE 679 Maxillary Division of the Trigeminal Nerve

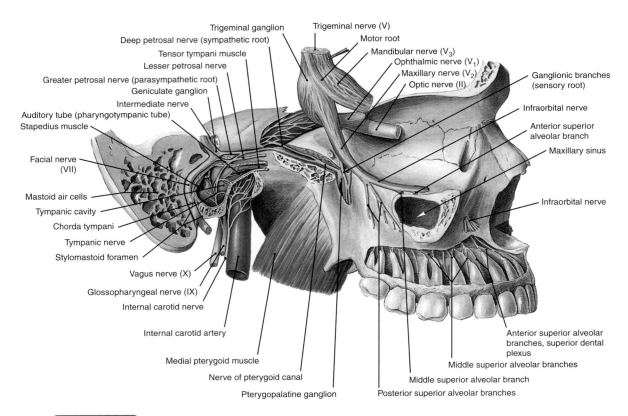

FIGURE 679.1 Maxillary Nerve and Its Infraorbital and Superior Alveolar Branches

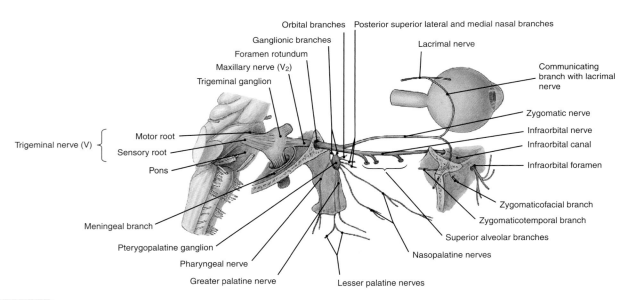

FIGURE 679.2 Maxillary Division of the Trigeminal Nerve

NOTE: (1) The **zygomatic, infraorbital, nasopalatine, greater** and **lesser palatine, lateral** and **medial nasal,** and **pharyngeal** branches derive from the trunk of the maxillary nerve. These are all sensory nerves.

(2) This nerve supplies all of the upper teeth through the superior alveolar branches that come off of the infraorbital nerve. After emerging on the face, the infraorbital nerve supplies the skin from the upper lip to the lower eyelid.

(3) The nasopalatine and greater and lesser palatine branches supply the nasal septum and the hard and soft palates, whereas the pharyngeal nerve supplies the mucosa of the nasopharynx.

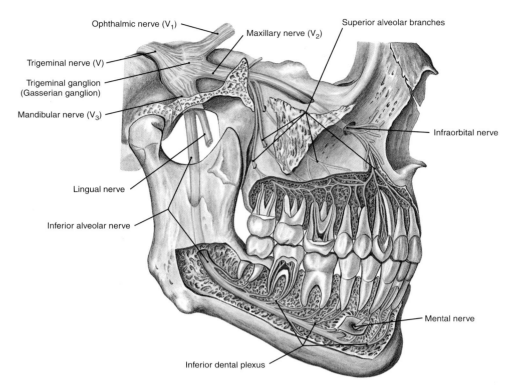

FIGURE 680.1 **Maxillary and Mandibular Nerves**

NOTE: (1) In this figure, only the **inferior alveolar nerve** and the proximal stump of the cut **lingual nerve** from the mandibular nerve are shown.

(2) The infraorbital and superior alveolar branches of the maxillary nerve are seen supplying structures in the maxillary region.

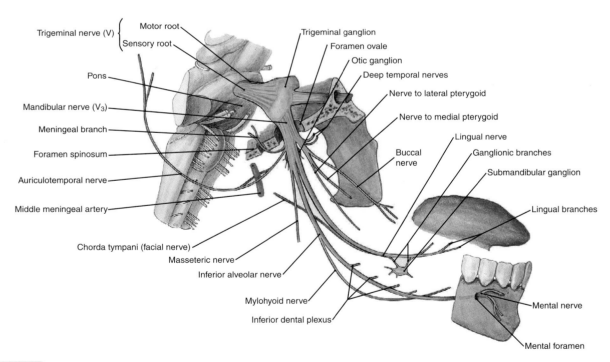

FIGURE 680.2 **Mandibular Division of the Trigeminal Nerve**

NOTE: (1) The **auriculotemporal, inferior alveolar,** and **lingual nerves** and the branches that supply the muscles of mastication: the **masseteric** and **deep temporal nerves** and the **nerves to the lateral and medial pterygoid muscles**.

(2) The mylohyoid branch of the inferior alveolar nerve that supplies the mylohyoid muscle and the anterior belly of the digastric muscle.

(3) Not shown in this figure but shown in Figure 677.2, are the small, delicate branches that supply two tensor muscles: the **tensor veli palatini** that tenses the soft palate and the **tensor tympani muscle** that tenses the tympanic membrane in the middle ear.

(4) The mandibular nerve supplies sensory innervation to all of the lower teeth, the skin of the chin, lower lip, and the side of the face and head anterior to the external ear.

PLATE 681 Facial Nerve (CN VII)

FIGURE 681.1 **Facial Nerve Descending in the Facial Canal**

NOTE: (1) The facial nerve emerges from the brainstem by motor and sensory roots. The cells bodies of the fibers in the sensory root are located in the **geniculate ganglion**.

(2) The sensory fibers of the facial nerve are of two types: **general sensation** and **special sense** of **taste** from the anterior two-thirds of the tongue that course centrally in chorda tympani nerve.

(3) The motor fibers of the facial nerve also are of two types: **somato-motor** to the muscles of facial expression, the stapedius muscle, and to the posterior belly of the digastric muscle and stylohyoid muscle and **visceromotor** (preganglionic parasympathetic) that go to the pterygopalatine and submandibular ganglia.

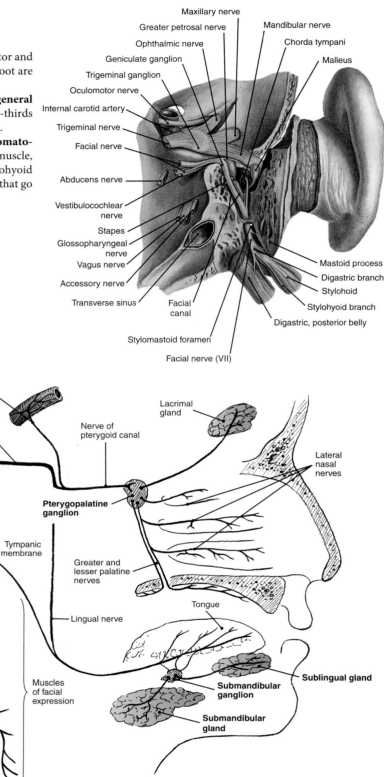

FIGURE 681.2 **Diagrammatic View of the Facial Nerve**

NOTE: (1) The **greater petrosal nerve** branches from the main stem of the facial nerve at the genu of the facial nerve (i.e., where the nerve turns about 90 degrees inferiorly from its horizontal course through the internal acoustic meatus).

(2) The **chorda tympani nerve** branches along the facial canal posterior to the middle ear. It then enters the middle ear cavity courses across the tympanic membrane and emerges in the deep face. It joins the **lingual nerve** (a branch of the trigeminal nerve) and descends to the submandibular ganglion.

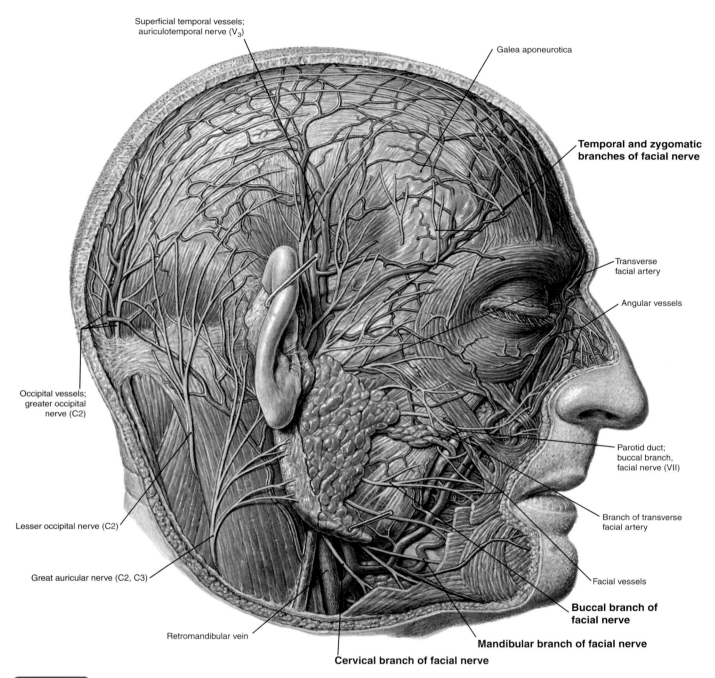

Superficial temporal vessels;
auriculotemporal nerve (V₃)

Galea aponeurotica

Temporal and zygomatic branches of facial nerve

Transverse facial artery

Angular vessels

Occipital vessels;
greater occipital
nerve (C2)

Parotid duct;
buccal branch,
facial nerve (VII)

Lesser occipital nerve (C2)

Branch of transverse facial artery

Great auricular nerve (C2, C3)

Facial vessels

Buccal branch of facial nerve

Retromandibular vein

Mandibular branch of facial nerve

Cervical branch of facial nerve

FIGURE 682 **Facial Nerve on the Side of the Face**

NOTE: (1) The facial nerve emerges from the facial canal at the stylomastoid foramen behind the ear lobe, courses through the parotid gland, and divides into muscular branches for the muscles of facial expression.

(2) The following branches of the facial nerve supply the muscles of facial expression: **temporal, zygomatic, buccal, mandibular,** and **cervical** branches. These nerves contain somatomotor fibers that are under voluntary control.

(3) Injury to the facial nerve or dysfunction of the facial nerve on one side because of paralysis (Bell's palsy) leaves that side of the face expressionless and results in a loss of tone of the superficial facial muscles. This is usually recognizable because of a loss of firmness and a sagging of the face on the afflicted side compared with the normal side.

(4) Because the branches of the facial nerve cross the face horizontally, any incision that might be necessary should be a horizontal one and *not vertical.*

(5) The parotid gland overlies the facial nerve anterior and inferior to the external ear.

(6) The posterior aspect of the scalp is supplied by sensory fibers from the greater occipital nerve (posterior primary ramus of C2), and the skin posterior to the ear and on the lateral side of the upper neck is supplied with sensory fibers from lesser occipital nerve and the great auricular nerve from the cervical plexus and not from either the facial or trigeminal nerves.

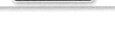 **PLATE 683** Facial Nerve (Continued): Greater Petrosal Nerve

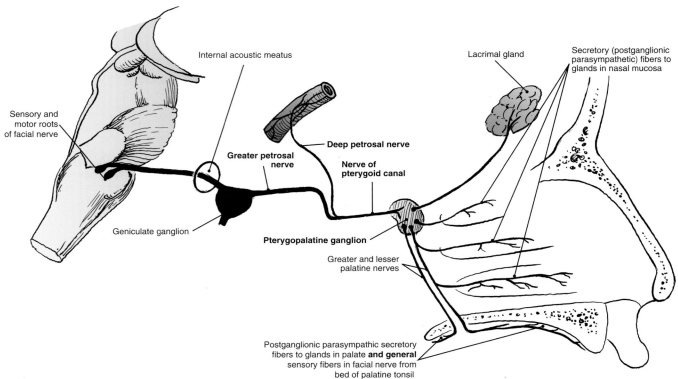

FIGURE 683.1 **Diagrammatic Representation of the Facial Nerve and Its Connections**

NOTE: (1) The **greater petrosal nerve** commences at the **geniculate ganglion** and is joined by the **deep petrosal nerve** to form the nerve of the pterygoid canal. The greater petrosal nerve is carrying preganglionic parasympathetic fibers to the pterygopalatine ganglion and taste fibers from the palate. It receives postganglionic sympathetic fibers from the **deep petrosal nerve**, and together these various fibers form the **nerve of the pterygoid canal.**

(2) From the pterygopalatine ganglion postganglionic parasympathetic fibers course (a) to the lacrimal gland by way of the zygomatic branch of the maxillary nerve and then the lacrimal branch of the ophthalmic nerve, (b) to mucous glands in the lining of the lateral wall of the nasal cavity and septum, and (c) to mucous glands in the lining of the soft and hard palate by way of the greater and lesser palatine nerves. It is also thought that these nerves carry taste fiber from the palate as well.

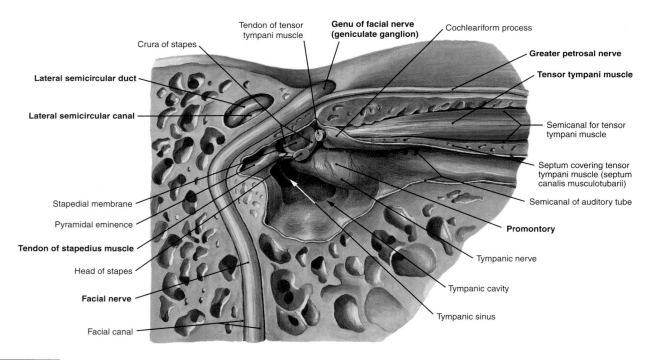

FIGURE 683.2 **Facial Nerve in the Facial Canal and Its Greater Petrosal Branch**

NOTE: The greater petrosal nerve branches from the facial nerve at the genu (90-degree turn). It carries preganglionic parasympathetic fibers and taste fibers from the palate.

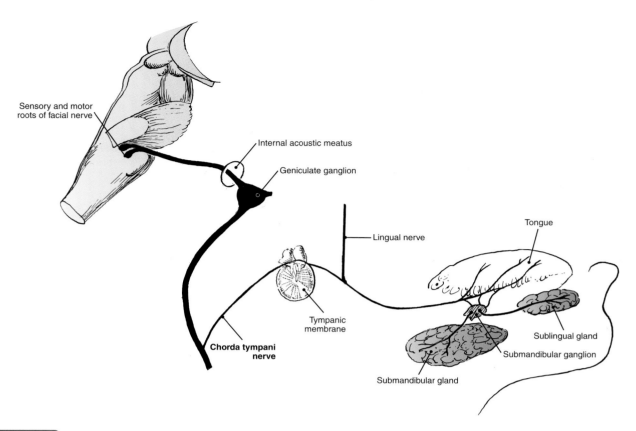

FIGURE 684.1 **Diagrammatic Representation of the Facial Nerve and Its Chorda Tympani Branch**

NOTE: (1) The facial nerve descends in the facial canal and at the level of the tympanic cavity it gives off the chorda tympani nerve that pierces the bone to enter the tympanic cavity.

(2) This nerve carries visceromotor (preganglionic parasympathetic) nerve fibers that synapse in the submandibular ganglion to supply the submandibular and sublingual glands. It also carries special sensory taste fibers from the anterior two-thirds of the tongue.

(3) Within the tympanic cavity the nerve courses over the medial surface of the tympanic membrane adjacent to the superior border of the membrane.

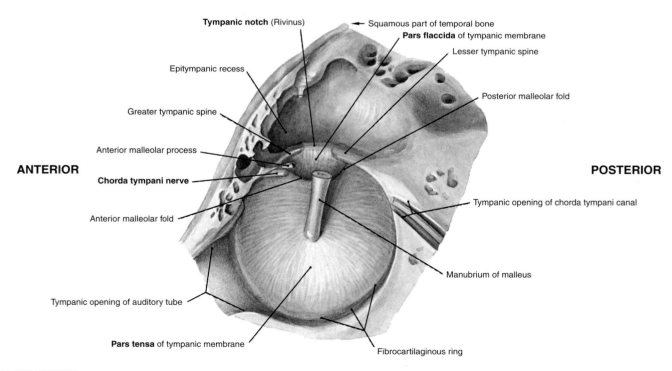

FIGURE 684.2 **Medial View of the Tympanic Membrane in the Middle Ear Cavity**

NOTE: The chorda tympani nerve enters the posterior aspect of the tympanic cavity and after crossing the tympanic membrane, it leaves the cavity anteriorly to enter the superior aspect of the deep face (see Fig. 566).

PLATE 685 Vestibulocochlear Nerve (CN VIII)

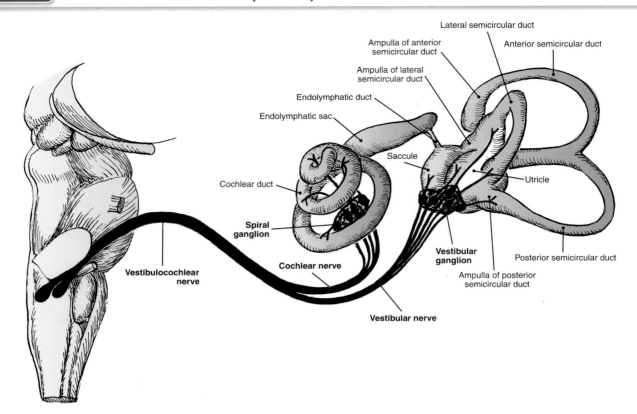

FIGURE 685.1 **Vestibulocochlear Nerve (CN VIII)**

NOTE: (1) The **spiral organ of Corti** within the internal ear contains the receptor cells for the special sense of hearing. These receptors, called **hair cells**, are in the **cochlear duct**, and they are innervated by the peripheral processes of sensory neurons whose cell bodies are in the **spiral ganglion**. The central processes of these neurons form the **cochlear nerve**.

(2) The **vestibular apparatus** of the eighth cranial nerve consists of three semicircular canals, the utricle, the saccule, receptors within these structures, and the neurons in the **vestibular ganglion**. These neurons send peripheral processes to these receptor cells and their central processes to the brain by way of the **vestibular nerve**.

(3) The cochlear and vestibular nerves join to form the **vestibulocochlear** or **eighth cranial nerve**.

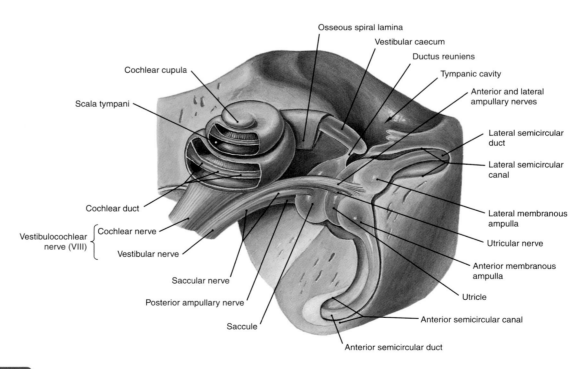

FIGURE 685.2 **Right Vestibulocochlear Nerve, the Cochlea, and the Membranous Labyrinth of the Internal Ear**

NOTE: (1) The anterior, lateral, and posterior **ampullary nerves** of the semicircular canals and the delicate **saccular** and **utricular nerves** all join to form the **vestibular nerve**.

(2) The fibers of the cochlear nerve receive input from the cochlear receptor cells in the **spiral organ of Corti**.

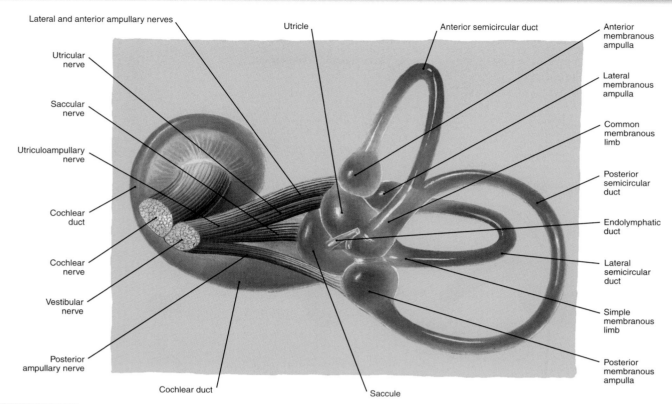

Lateral and anterior ampullary nerves

Utricular nerve

Saccular nerve

Utriculoampullary nerve

Cochlear duct

Cochlear nerve

Vestibular nerve

Posterior ampullary nerve

Cochlear duct

Utricle

Saccule

Anterior semicircular duct

Anterior membranous ampulla

Lateral membranous ampulla

Common membranous limb

Posterior semicircular duct

Endolymphatic duct

Lateral semicircular duct

Simple membranous limb

Posterior membranous ampulla

FIGURE 686.1 **Membranous Labyrinth, the Organ of Corti, and the Vestibular and Cochlear Nerves**

NOTE: (1) The vestibular nerve is the nerve of equilibrium, and because of its connections in the brain, sensory input from this nerve is able to alter eye movements and movements of the head and body that might counteract a loss of balance in an attempt to prevent a fall and thereby maintain equilibrium.

(2) The membranous labyrinth lies within the walls of the bony or osseous labyrinth.

(3) The receptors within the saccule and utricle are able to sense the position of the head with respect to gravity and are sometimes called the **static labyrinthine receptors.** These receptors (**maculae**) contain ciliated hair cells with a gelatinous substance over them and small crystals (**otoliths**) within the gel; since they react to head position in relationship to gravity, they are considered the organ of **static balance.**

(4) The receptors on the ampullae of the semicircular canals are related to kinetic balance and are stimulated by angular acceleration of the head. These are referred to as organs of **kinetic balance.**

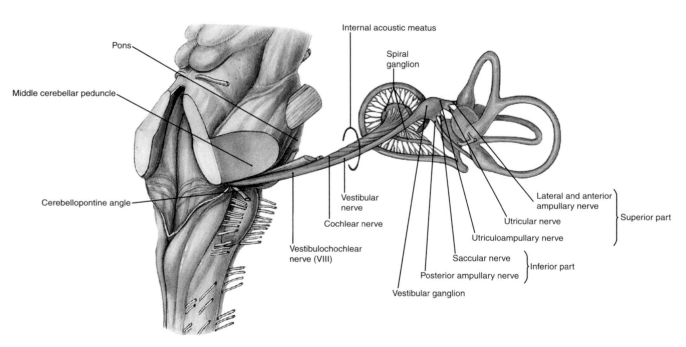

Pons

Middle cerebellar peduncle

Cerebellopontine angle

Internal acoustic meatus

Spiral ganglion

Vestibular nerve

Cochlear nerve

Vestibulochochlear nerve (VIII)

Saccular nerve

Posterior ampullary nerve

Vestibular ganglion

Lateral and anterior ampullary nerve

Utricular nerve

Utriculoampullary nerve

Superior part

Inferior part

FIGURE 686.2 **Diagrammatic Schema of the Vestibulocochlear Nerve**

NOTE: The vestibulocochlear and facial nerves attach to the brain at the cerebellopontine angle just posterior to the middle cerebellar peduncle.

PLATE 687 Glossopharyngeal Nerve (CN IX)

FIGURE 687.1 Sensory Innervation of the Pharynx ▶

NOTE: The glossopharyngeal nerve supplies the oral pharynx with sensory innervation and is the afferent limb of the gag reflex.

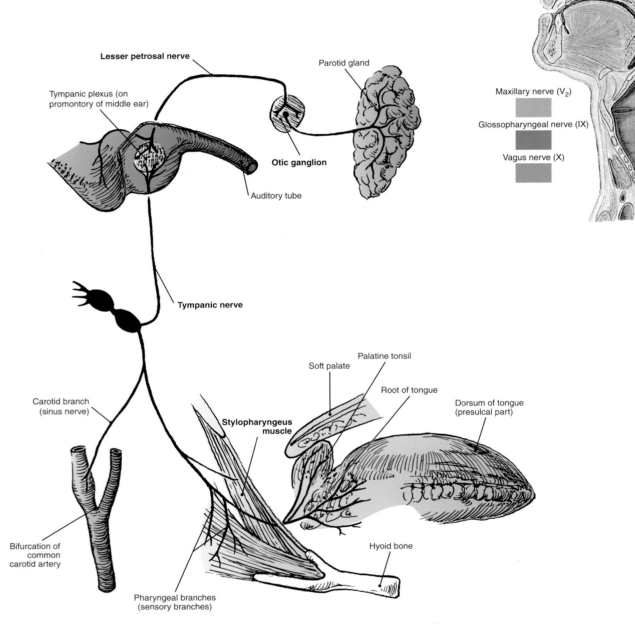

Lesser petrosal nerve

Parotid gland

Tympanic plexus (on promontory of middle ear)

Maxillary nerve (V₂)

Otic ganglion

Glossopharyngeal nerve (IX)

Auditory tube

Vagus nerve (X)

Tympanic nerve

Palatine tonsil

Soft palate

Root of tongue

Dorsum of tongue (presulcal part)

Carotid branch (sinus nerve)

Stylopharyngeus muscle

Bifurcation of common carotid artery

Hyoid bone

Pharyngeal branches (sensory branches)

FIGURE 687.2 Diagrammatic Representation of the Glossopharyngeal Nerve

NOTE: (1) The glossopharyngeal nerve supplies one voluntary muscle, the **stylopharyngeus.** This muscle (on both sides) elevates the pharynx during the act of swallowing. After supplying this muscle, the nerve supplies the posterior third of the tongue with both general sensory fibers and fibers of the special sense of **taste.**

(2) The glossopharyngeal nerve also has preganglionic parasympathetic nerve fibers that ascend in the **tympanic branch** to the middle ear and divide to form the **tympanic plexus** over the surface of the promontory.

(3) From this plexus, the fibers reassemble to form the **lesser petrosal nerve**, which enters the base of the skull on the superior surface of the temporal bone. It leaves the skull base through a small foramen adjacent the greater petrosal nerve and passes through the foramen ovale to join the **otic ganglion.**

(4) From the otic ganglion, postganglionic parasympathetic fibers join the **auriculotemporal nerve** and innervate the parotid gland.

(5) The **pharyngeal branches** of the glossopharyngeal nerve supply sensory innervation to the mucosa of the oropharynx and participate in the **gag reflex** (see Fig. 687.1).

(6) The **carotid branch** contains visceral afferent fibers and with the vagus nerve supplies the carotid body.

(After Grant, J.C.B., Atlas of Anatomy, 6th Edition. Baltimore: Williams & Wilkins, 1972).

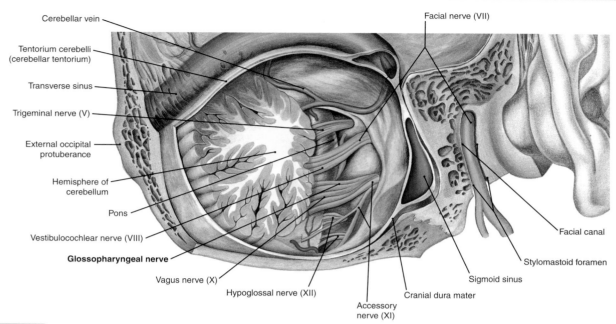

FIGURE 688.1 Glossopharyngeal Nerve Coursing from the Skull Base through the Jugular Foramen

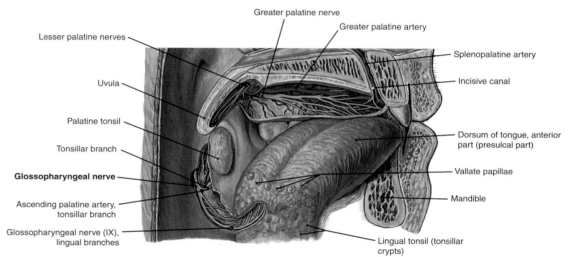

FIGURE 688.2 Glossopharyngeal Nerve in the Oropharynx and Penetrating the Posterior Third of the Tongue

NOTE: At this site the glossopharyngeal nerve is sensory and carries general sensory and special sensory fibers (taste) to the posterior third of the tongue.

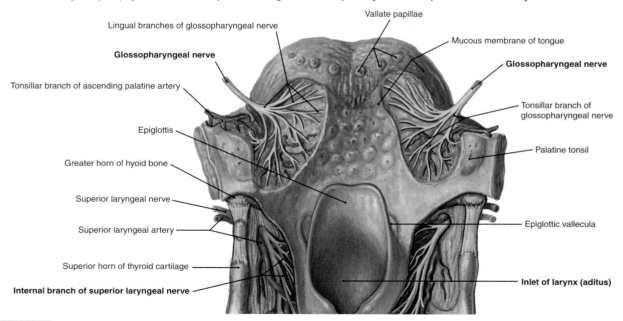

FIGURE 688.3 Glossopharyngeal Nerve and Its Lingual Branches to the Posterior Tongue and to the Vallate Papillae

PLATE 689 Vagus Nerve (CN X)

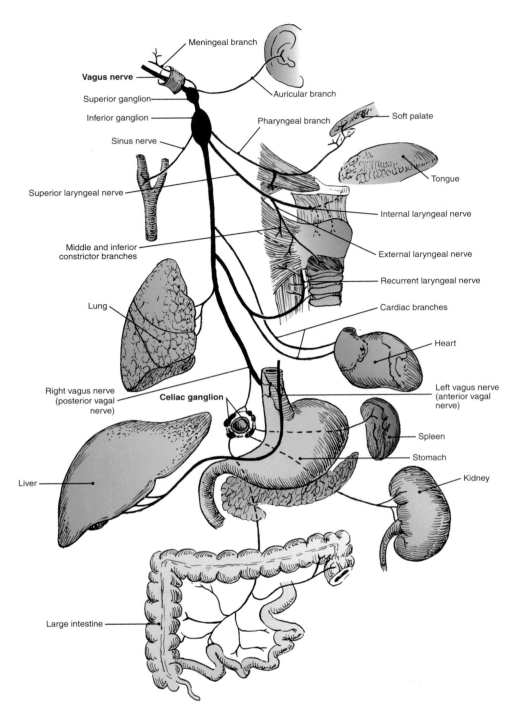

Meningeal branch

Vagus nerve

Auricular branch

Superior ganglion

Inferior ganglion

Pharyngeal branch

Soft palate

Sinus nerve

Tongue

Superior laryngeal nerve

Internal laryngeal nerve

Middle and inferior
constrictor branches

External laryngeal nerve

Recurrent laryngeal nerve

Lung

Cardiac branches

Heart

Right vagus nerve
(posterior vagal
nerve)

Celiac ganglion

Left vagus nerve
(anterior vagal
nerve)

Spleen

Stomach

Liver

Kidney

Large intestine

FIGURE 689 **Diagrammatic Representation of the Vagus Nerve**

NOTE: (1) The vagus nerve contains both visceromotor and viscerosensory fibers as well as somatomotor fibers. The latter come from the medullary part of the accessory nerve, and they supply voluntary muscles in the larynx, pharynx, and soft palate.

(2) The visceromotor fibers are preganglionic parasympathetic fibers that innervate the organs in the neck, the thorax, and the abdomen as far as the splenic flexure of the transverse colon.

(3) The vagus also contains a few somatosensory fibers in its **auricular branch** that supply some skin of the external ear; other sensory fibers are in the **superior laryngeal** and **recurrent laryngeal** branches that supply the internal mucosa of the larynx. In addition, the vagus contains visceral afferent fibers from organs in the neck, thorax, and abdomen. All of these sensory fibers have their cell bodies in the **superior and inferior ganglia** of the vagus.

(4) Visceral afferent fibers in the **carotid sinus** nerve are from pressoreceptor cells that respond to blood pressure changes.

(5) The **pharyngeal branch** of the vagus supplies motor fibers to the pharyngeal constrictor muscles as well as to the muscles of the soft palate (except the tensor veli palatini muscle). These motor fibers in the vagus are from the accessory nerve and are often described as 11 via 10 (i.e., accessory via the vagus).

(6) The **superior laryngeal branch** has an **external branch** supplying the cricothyroid muscle and an **internal branch** to the mucosa of the upper larynx. All other muscles of the larynx are supplied by the recurrent laryngeal branch.

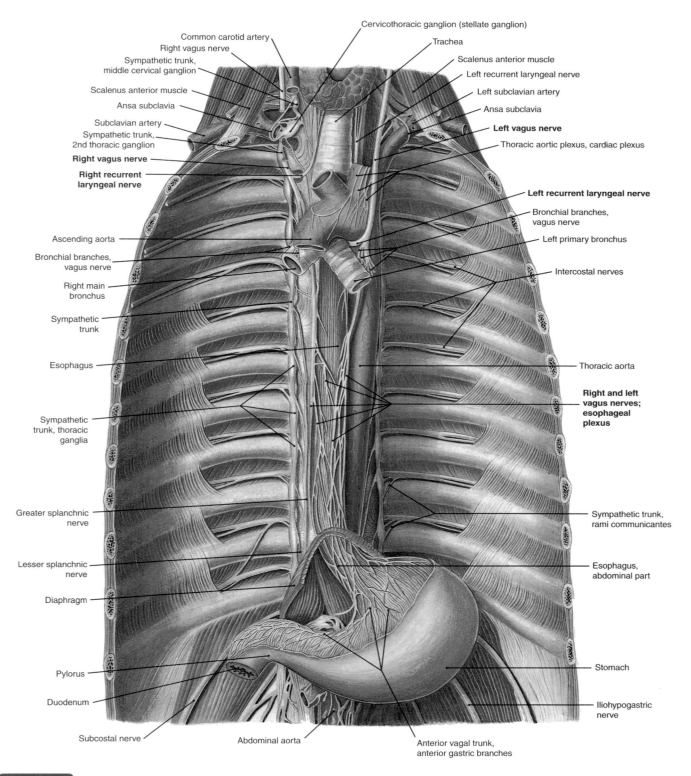

FIGURE 690 Vagus Nerve in the Thorax

NOTE: (1) The vagus nerves enter the superior mediastinum, give off the recurrent laryngeal nerves, and then course medially toward the bronchi, where they form bronchial plexuses, and then toward the esophagus.

(2) The **left vagus nerve** splits into branches and forms the **anterior** esophageal plexus, while the **right vagus nerve** forms the **posterior** esophageal plexus.

(3) The fibers of these plexuses enter the abdomen through the esophageal hiatus. The left vagal fibers become the **anterior gastric branches** and the right vagal fibers become the **posterior gastric branches.** The anterior branches supply the anterosuperior aspect of the stomach, whereas the posterior branches supply the posteroinferior aspect of the stomach.

PLATE 691 Accessory Nerve (CN XI)

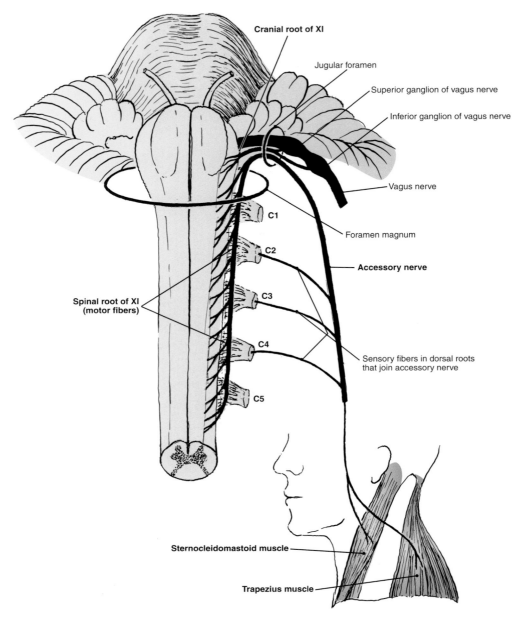

Cranial root of XI

Jugular foramen

Superior ganglion of vagus nerve

Inferior ganglion of vagus nerve

Vagus nerve

C1

Foramen magnum

C2

Accessory nerve

C3

Spinal root of XI
(motor fibers)

C4

Sensory fibers in dorsal roots
that join accessory nerve

C5

Sternocleidomastoid muscle

Trapezius muscle

FIGURE 691 **Diagrammatic Representation of the Accessory Nerve (XI Cranial Nerve)**

NOTE: (1) The **accessory nerve** (sometimes called the spinal accessory nerve) is formed by the brief union of fibers that originate in the spinal cord and others that emerge from the medulla oblongata.

(2) Motor nerve fibers leave the spinal cord from cervical segmental levels down as far as C5. The fibers from these upper cervical segments join to form a single trunk that ascends in the spinal canal and enters the cranial cavity through the foramen magnum. This constitutes the **spinal root**.

(3) Within the cranial cavity the spinal root is joined by the smaller **cranial root**, which consists of five or six delicate rootlets that leave the medulla oblongata just inferior to the rootlets of the vagus nerve.

(4) The cranial root briefly joins the spinal root and then **separates from it and merges with the rootlets of the vagus nerve**, with which it descends through the jugular foramen.

(5) The spinal root (now consisting of the original spinal motor fibers) turns inferiorly and also leaves the cranial cavity through the jugular foramen to enter the neck, where it supplies the **sternocleidomastoid muscle,** and crosses the posterior triangle to innervate the **trapezius muscle**.

(6) The medullary fibers that join the vagus nerve become distributed in its pharyngeal and recurrent laryngeal branches to supply striated fibers of the pharyngeal and laryngeal muscles and the muscles of the soft palate (except for the tensor veli palatini muscle).

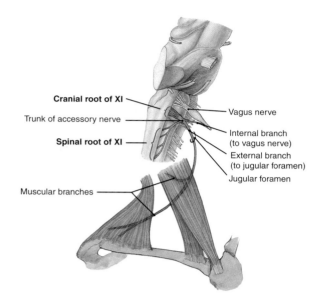

FIGURE 692.1 Schema of the Accessory Nerve

NOTE: (1) The spinal and cranial roots of the accessory nerve join for a short distance within the cranial cavity.

(2) The "internal branch" (cranial root) joins the vagus nerve, and the "external branch" (spinal root) descends in the neck as the **accessory nerve** to supply motor innervation to the **sternocleidomastoid** and the **trapezius** muscles.

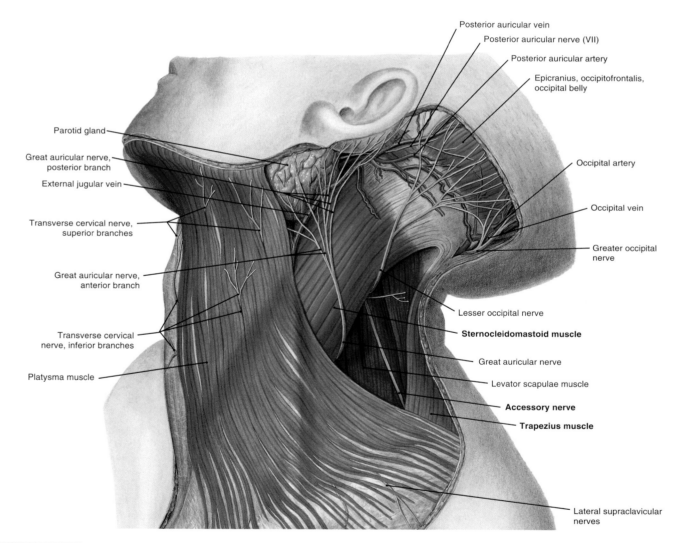

FIGURE 692.2 **Accessory Nerve Traversing the Posterior Triangle of the Neck**

NOTE: (1) Distal to the jugular foramen, the accessory nerve descends in the neck deep to the **sternocleidomastoid muscle** as it innervates it. Then it crosses the posterior triangle of the neck to the deep surface of the **trapezius muscle**, which it also supplies.

(2) Sensory fibers from the **C3, C4,** and **C5** segments also join the nerve. Some of these supply proprioceptors that allow the individual to know the positions of the head and shoulder as the muscles act.

PLATE 693 Hypoglossal Nerve (CN XII)

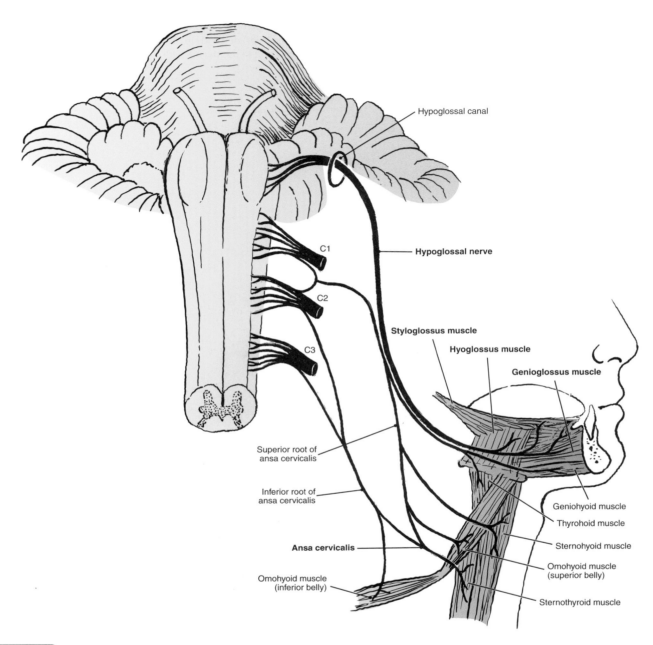

Hypoglossal canal

C1

C2

Hypoglossal nerve

C3

Styloglossus muscle

Hyoglossus muscle

Genioglossus muscle

Superior root of
ansa cervicalis

Inferior root of
ansa cervicalis

Geniohyoid muscle

Thyrohoid muscle

Sternohyoid muscle

Ansa cervicalis

Omohyoid muscle
(superior belly)

Omohyoid muscle
(inferior belly)

Sternothyroid muscle

FIGURE 693 **Hypoglossal Nerve (Diagrammatic Representation)**

NOTE: (1) The hypoglossal nerve is the motor nerve of the tongue. Its fibers emerge from the medulla oblongata in a line with the oculomotor, trochlear, and abducens nerves and the anterior roots (motor) of the spinal cord.

(2) This nerve supplies all the **intrinsic muscles** (longitudinal, transverse, and vertical) of the tongue and all of the **extrinsic muscles** (except the palatoglossus) that move the tongue (i.e., the **styloglossus, hyoglossus,** and **genioglossus).**

(3) The palatoglossus muscle is innervated by the pharyngeal branch of the vagus and forms the anterior pillar of the fauces in the oral cavity. It is the only muscle with the term "glossus" in its name not supplied by the hypoglossal nerve.

(4) In the upper neck, the hypoglossal nerve takes a 270-degree turn deep to the posterior belly of the digastric muscle and enters the oral cavity between the hypoglossus and mylohyoid muscles (see Fig. 694.2).

(5) The C1, C2, and C3 nerves emerge from the spinal cord and form two descending nerve trunks: the **superior** and **inferior roots** of the **ansa cervicalis.** The superior root (C1 and C2 fibers) courses with the hypoglossal nerve for a short distance, *but they are NOT hypoglossal fibers.*

(6) The superior root (C1 and C2) joins the inferior root (C2 and C3) and together they join as a loop called the **ansa cervicalis.** From this cervical nerve formation the strap muscles of the neck are innervated.

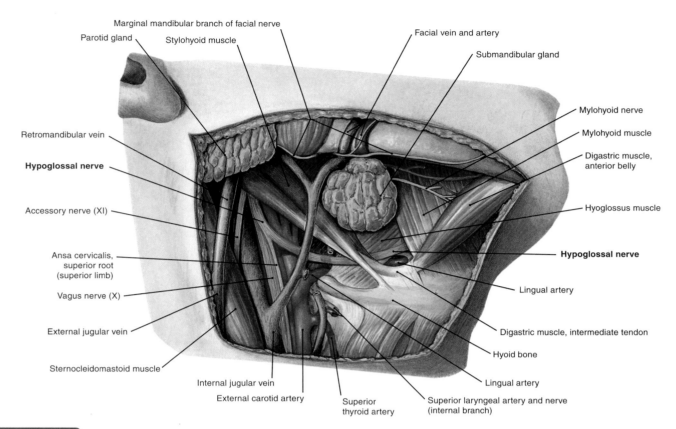

FIGURE 694.1 Hypoglossal Nerve in the Superior Neck Region

NOTE that in the submandibular triangle, the hypoglossal nerve courses superficial to the hyoglossus muscle and deep to the mylohyoid muscle to enter the oral cavity

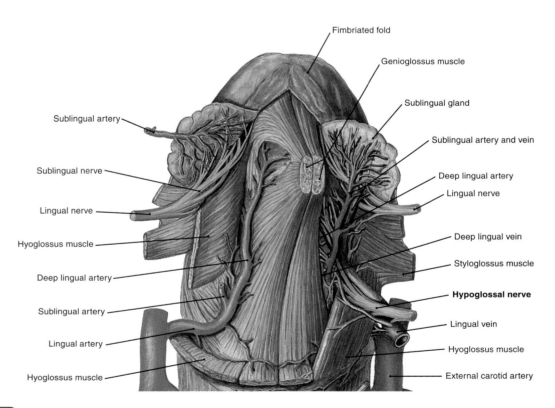

FIGURE 694.2 Hypoglossal Nerve as It Enters the Tongue (Inferior View)

NOTE that when the hypoglossal nerve is injured, the muscles on that side of the tongue are denervated. When the patient is asked to protrude the tongue, it is directed to the paralyzed side because the innervated muscles on the normal side act unopposed.

Index

Numbers refer to Plates.
Numbers in **boldface** type indicate main references.
*Muscle chart describes action, innervation, insertion, and origin.

A

Abdomen, 3, **219–322**
  anterior wall of, 238
    deep dissection of, 242
    epigastric anastomosis, **231**
    external oblique muscle, **221**
    inguinal region of, 232
    inner surface of, **222**
    internal oblique muscle of, **224, 225**
    male, inguinal region, 236
    rectus abdominis muscles of, **225, 227**
    rectus sheath of, **226, 230**
    second muscle layer of, **226**
    superficial musculature of, 221
    superficial vessels and nerves of, **220**
    transverse sections of, 230
    transversus abdominis muscles of, **227**
  caudal aspect, 318, 319
  cavity of, 250, 251, **288**
    celiac trunk and its branches, **252, 256**
    duodenojejunal junction and large intestine, 290
    female, posterior abdominal peritoneum, 306
    gastroduodenal vessels, **253**
    greater omentum, 243, 246, 247, 248, 250, **250,** 251, 252, 253 254, **264,** 288
    inferior mesenteric vessels and their branches, **294**
    jejunum, ileum, and ascending, 288
    large intestine, **251, 290,** 300
    lumbar, sacral, and coccygeal plexuses
    male, retroperitoneal organs, 307
    mesenteries, 300
    mesocolons and mesentery of small intestine, **300**
    omentum reflected, **251**
    roots of mesocolons/mesentery, **306**
    sigmoid colons, 290
    small intestine, **251**
    splenic vessels, **253**
    superior mesenteric vessels and their branches, **292**
    transverse colons, 288
  computerized tomography scans of, **273,** 320, **322**
    pancreatitis, spleen, diaphragmatic surface, **286**
    spleen, visceral surface, **287**
    splenic hemorrhage, **287**
    transverse section and, **318–321**
  cross section of, 322
  dorsal wall, 315
  female urogenital organs, **245**
  frontal section of, 229
  greater splanchnic nerves, 317
  iliac crest, frontal section of, 229
  inferior part of, 223
  intercostal nerves of, 220
  large intestine of, **304**
  lumbar and sacral plexuses of, **316**

  lumbar vertebra of, 284
  male
    bladder, 354
    median sagittal section, **246**
    paramedian section, **247**
    and pelvis, **246**
    urogenital organs, **244**
  median sagittal section of, **246, 342**
  muscles of, 229
    deep layer of, 227
    frontal section, **229**
    lumbar vertebra, 229
    middle layer of, 226
    rectus, 228
    right internal oblique, 223
    transverse sections, **228**
    transversus, 222
    umbilicus, 229
  in newborn, 243
  omental bursa, 249
  pancreas, 276
  pancreatitis, CT of, **286**
  parasagittal ultrasound of, 280, 281
  and pelvis, 240
  posterior wall of, 290
    diaphragm, **314, 315**
    lymph nodes and channels, **352**
    muscles of, **314**
    retroperitoneal organs, **307**
    vessels and nerves, **317**
  sacroiliac joint, 322
  second lumbar vertebra, 284
  small intestine, 288, **300**
  splenic hemorrhage, CT, **287**
  superficial inguinal ring, 223
  surface projections
  symphysis pubis, frontal section of, 229
  testis, 369
  transverse colon, 305
  transverse diameter of, 243
  transverse section of, 228, **228, 230,** 318, 319, **320, 321**
    CT of, 319
    lumbar level, 322
  transverse ultrasound of, 277
  upper
    CT of, **275, 287**
    radiograph of, 256
    transverse section of, 320
    transverse ultrasound of, 277
  wall of
    blood vessels, **147**
    epigastric anastomosis, **231**
    inner surface, **147,** 222
    muscles, **11, 15,** 147, 314
    newborn child, **242**
    projection of the skeleton, **144**
    superficial vessels and nerves, **220**
    transversus and rectus abdominis muscles, **227**
    vessels and nerves, **317**

    of young female, **5, 139**
    in young male, **139**
Abdominal aorta, 293, 320
Abdominal organs, 244
  muscle, 317
  surface projection of
    anterior view, 244
    left lateral view, 245
    posterior view, 244
    right lateral view, 245
  venous drainage of, 298
Abdominal sympathetic chain, 317
Abdominal viscera, 249, 296
Abdominopelvic cavity, **316**
Accessory breast, 4
Acetabular labrum, 481
Acetabulum, 481
  bones, 323
  bony, 481
  border of, 324
  limbus of, 364
  lunate surface of, 324, 345
  pelvis, 478
  rim of, 323
Acromion, 18, 22, 30, 32, 42, 44, 45, 55, 60, 61, 112, 114–116, 118, 119, 371, 373, 529
Adductor magnus
  ischiocondylar part of, 437
  tendinous opening on, 424
Adult female pelvis
  median sagittal section, 342
  viscera of, 330
Adult right hip bone
  lateral view of, 323
  medial view of, 324
Alar ligaments of dens, 390
Ampullae, 357
Ampulla of uterine tube, 333
Anal
  canal, 219
    inner surface of, 359
    median section, 360
  column, 359, 360
  muscles, chart of, **346**
  region, 347
  sinuses, 359
  sphincter muscle, external, 359
Anastomosis
  acromial, 22
  cubital, 66
  at elbow joint, 88
  epigastric arterial, 25, **231**
  in hand, 445
  in hip and knee regions, 413
  internal thoracic–epigastric, **25**
  palmar carpal, 110
  between portal vein and superior vena cava, 204
  at rectum, 12
  superior and inferior epigastric vessels, 231
  vascular, 66
Angiogram of aortic arch, 205

Angle
cerebellopontine, 669, 686
costal, 142
costodiaphragmatic, 149
of eye, 593
of eyebrow, 550
between femoral neck and shaft, 482
inferior, 32, 33, 112, 371
infrasternal, 5, 139, 144
lateral, 379, 593
of mandible, 555, 633
of mouth, 550
and posterior border of mandible, 557
of 3rd and 5th ribs, 143
sternal, 3, 5, 18, 19, 139
subcostal, 5
superior, 55, 117
of scapula, 30
of 4th rib, 143, 168
Ankle
articular surface of, **499**
bones of, 504
joint of (*See* Ankle joints)
ligaments of, **503, 504**
movements at, **453**
posterior tibial artery at, 467
radiographs of, 508
retinaculum of
extensor, 456, 457
flexor, 456, 463, 465, 466, 498
tendons at, 456, 461
viewed from behind
Ankle joints
bony structures in, 498
dorsiflexion and plantar flexion of foot at, 453
on dorsum of foot, 456
lateral ligaments of, 502
synovial fold of, 499
X-ray of, **498**
Ankle region
muscles and tendons of, 462
synovial sheaths of, 456, 457
tendons of, 456, 457
Annulus fibrosus, 398
Anocutaneous line, 360
Ansa
cervicalis
inferior root of, 532
superior root of, 532, 534, 545
subclavia, 206, 208
Antebrachial fascia, 62
Antecubital fossa, 41
Anterior intercostal vessels, 147
Antrum
cardiac, 197
mastoid, 658, 659, 663, 664
pyloric, 255, 261, 267, 268
Anus, 219, 344, 347, 349, 359, 360, 361, 365
Aorta, 282
abdominal, 194, 248, 264, 293, 294, 307, 308, 315,
320, 352
arch of, 151, 164, 175, 197, 215, 543, 647
ascending, 189, 192, 205, 206, 208, 213, 218, 318,
536, 690
bifurcation of, 340, 351, 422
computed tomography of, 218
descending, 198, 216, 404
posterior view, 199
thoracic, 198, 199, 201, 206
trigones, 186
ultrasound of, 273
variations in branches from arch of, 205
Aortic hiatus, 210
Aortic valve, 185

Apical ligaments of dens, 390
Aponeurosis
bicipital, 41, 43, 54, 56, 58, 70, 76, 84, 134
external oblique, 11, 15, 148, 223, 229, 232
palmar, 94
Appendicitis, 302
Appendix(ces)
epididymis, 238
epiploicae, 251, 304, 307, 353
fibrosa hepatis, 271
inflammation of, 302
location, variations in, 302, 303
surfaces of
vermiform, **302, 303,** 321
blood supply, **303**
vermiform, blood supply, 303
vesicular, 332, 334, 335
Arch
aortic, 47, 149, 170, 175, 193
of atlas, 381, 390, 391, 400, 642
of axis, 388, 389
carpal, 110
costal, 44, 144
of cricoid cartilage, 642
deep plantar, 474
dental, 391
iliopectineal, 314, 315
lumbocostal, 314, 315
mandibular, 634
maxillary, 635
palatoglossal, 619, 620
palatopharyngeal, 619, 620, 622
palmar, 28, 106, 107, **108,** 110
deep, 28
deep, variations in, **109**
superficial, 28
plantar, 413, 474, 476
pubic, 325–327
tendinous, 464, 479
venous
dorsal, 195, 454
jugular, 530, 535, 540, 642
vertebral, 380, 388, 389, 393, 397, 401, 408
zygomatic, 551, 555, 568, 592, 641
Arcuate
arteries, 310
line, 230
Arm, 2
anterior, **59**
artery of, 59, 66
brachial, **58**
muscles of, **54, 56–57, 63**
posterior dissection of, **60**
nerves in, 59, 66
cutaneous, 36, 37
median, **58**
ulnar, **58**
posterior
heads of triceps muscle of, **63**
vessels and nerves of, **66**
superficial dissection
anterior view, **36**
posterior view, **37**
superficial veins in, 36, 37
transverse section through lower third of,
133
Arteries
abdominal, **296**
anterior labial, 232
anterior perforating, 220
appendicular, 303
axillary, 23, **24,** 27, 58
at base of brain, 581
basilar, 543, 579

brachial, 28, 67, 76, 78, 124
deep, 58
profunda, 28
branches, 264
carotid
bifurcation, 540
common, 25
external, and branches, 559
internal, 579
within the cavernous sinus, 581
cerebral part, 580
radiograph, 574
vertebral and internal, 543
central retinal, 604
colic, 294, 297
common hepatic, 257
coronary, **178–180**
cremasteric, 239
cystic, 280
deep, of posterior compartment of leg, 467
deferential, 234
descending genicular, 445
digital
common palmar, 28, 94
dorsal, 92, 93
plantar, 470
dorsal, 367
dorsalis pedis, 450, 459, 476
epigastric
superficial, 13
superior, 13, 25, 231
external iliac, 25, 147, 231
femoral, 220
adductor hiatus and, 423
deep, 425
superficial branches of, 416
variations in position of deep, 422
fibular
branching of, 467
from posterior tibial, 444
variations in branching pattern of, 444
gastroduodenal, 253, 256, 264, 269
gastroepiploic, 254, 256, 257
gastric branches of, 264
gastroomental, 257
hepatic, 247, 256, 257, 259
humeral circumflex
anterior, 58
posterior, 33, 67
ileal, 292
ileocolic, 293
inferior epigastric, 13, 25, 147, 231, 339
inferior mesenteric, 295, 296
branches of, 295
radiograph of, **295**
inferior mesenteric, radiograph of, **295**
inferior suprarenal, 309
intercostal, **14**
anterior, 25, 231
interlobar, 310
internal iliac, 341, 351
divisions of, 339
internal thoracic, 231
interosseous
anterior, 28, 78
common, 78
posterior, 78, 89
recurrent, 89
jejunal, 292
left pulmonary, 160
of male, 194
mammary, medial and lateral, **8**
maxillary, 560, 565
median, 78

mesenteric, **297**
metatarsal, 470
  plantar, 474
middle colic, 292
musculophrenic, 25, 147, 231
obturator
  aberrant, 339
  aberrant origin of, 339
ophthalmic, 601, 604, 674
  its branches, 611
  in optic canal, 608
  variations in, 608
ovarian, 341
  diagram of, 335
palmar digital
  proper, 28
pancreaticoduodenal, 253
perforating branches of deep femoral, 413
pericardiacophrenic, 147
phrenic, inferior, 317
plantar
  deep, 459, 474
  lateral, 473, 476
  medial, 473, 476
popliteal, 413, 423
  branches of, 444
  superior genicular, middle genicular and single
    inferior genicular, 445
princeps pollicis, 93
pyloric-duodenal region, **269**
  anterior view, 269
  posterior view, 269
radial, 28, 76, 78, 93, 95, 98, 105, 107, 108, 110,
    124
radial collateral, 67, 76, 78, 89
radial indicis, 94
radial recurrent, 78
renal
  inferior phrenic, 309
of right hip region, 422
right renal
  arteriogram of, 310
right subclavian and branches, 544
scapular
  circumflex, 26, 67
  dorsal, 27, 28, 544
of scapular and posterior brachial regions, **67**
spinal
  anterior, 404, 406
  posterior, 406
  and their sulcal branches, 406
splenic, 252, 256, 260
subclavian, 24, 25, 27, 533
superficial epigastric
  branches of, 220
superficial external pudendal, 13
superficial iliac circumflex, 13
superior and inferior gluteal, 439
superior epigastric, 231
superior mesenteric, 296
  branching of, 297
  radiograph of, **293**
superior pancreaticoduodenal, 280
superior rectal, 294, 295, 341
suprascapular, 33, 67
supreme intercostal, 231
supreme thoracic, 24
systemic, in adult, **194**
testicular, 239, 367
of thigh, 422
thoracic
  internal, 13, 25, 147
  lateral, 4, 16, 27, 28
thoracoacromial, 16, 22, 24, 28

thoracodorsal, 26, 27
tibial
  anterior, 413, 444, 449, 450, 459
  anterior, variations in branching pattern of, 444
  posterior, 413, 444, 476
transverse cervical, 28
ulnar, 28, 76, 78, 94, 105, 106, 107, 108, 124
ulnar collateral
  inferior, 67, 76, 89
  superior, 76, 78
ulnar recurrent, 67
umbilical, 242
to upper extremity, **28**
urethral, 370
uterine, 335
vaginal, 335
variations in origins of femoral circumflex, 422
variations of, 310
vertebral, 27, 383, 543, 579
  nerves of
    occipital, 384
  of suboccipital region
    ventral surface of medulla oblongata, 384
  of suboccipital triangle, 384
Arteriograms, 180–181
  brachial, 79
  carotid, 583
  celiac trunk, 256
  femoral-popliteal-tibial, 445
  iliac, 339, 340
  left coronary, 180
  of left femoral—popliteal—tibial arterial tree, 445
  limb, upper, 38
  mesenteric, 293, 295
  right coronary, 181
  vertebral, 583, 584
Arthrograph, 558
Arthroscopy of knee joint, 491
Articular capsule, 119
  of hip joint, 481
  posterior aspect of, 487
Articular cartilage, 138
Articular cavity, 124
Articular disc, 131, 140
Articular surface, 324
  of ankle, **499**
  of right talocalcaneonavicular joint, 505
  of talocrural (ankle) joint, 499
  of tibia, 499
Articulations. See Joints
Atlantoaxial joints
  cruciform ligament of, 390
  median, 390, 391
  posterior view of, 389
  radiographs of, 391
Atlantooccipital joints
  cruciform ligament of, 390
  median sagittal section of, 391
  posterior view of, 389
Atlas
  anterior arch of, 391, 400
  caudal view, 388
  cruciform ligament of, 642
  dens of, 390
  lateral mass, 389
  posterior arches, 390
  posterior arch of, 385
  posterior tubercle of, 378
  transverse process, 384
  transverse process o, 378
  and vertebral artery, 148
  viewed from above, 388
  X-ray of, **391**
Auditory ossicles, right, 661

Auricle
  of ear, 549, 657, 659
  external rim of, 657
  of heart
    light, 176
    right, 176
Autonomic nervous system, **208, 209**
  parasympathetic division, 208
  sympathetic division of, 208
Autonomic nucleus, 675
Axilla
  artery, 46
  cords of brachial plexus, **46**
  dissection of, **26, 27**
  lateral thoracic wall and superficial, **20**
  musculature, 224
  nerves, 26
  vessels and nerves of
    deep, **27**
    superficial, **26**
Axillary fascia, 15
Axillary fat pad, 4
Axillary fossa, 1
Axillary sweat glands, 4
Axis
  bone, 31
  eyeball, 609
  heart, 149
  posterior view of, 388
  spinous process of, 381, 390
  stomach, 249
  transverse process, 384
  vagina, 332
  vertebral arch, 389

B

Back, **371–386**. See also Vertebra(e)
  dermatomes and cutaneous nerve of, **372**
  muscles of
    deep, **376**, 379–380, 386
    erector spinae, **375, 377**
    intermediate, **374, 376**, 379
    latissimus dorsi, **374**
    multifidus, 380
    rotatores, 380
    semispinalis, 380
    semispinalis muscles, **375**
    superficial, **373**
    thoracolumbar fascia, 386
    transversospinal groups, **378**
  primary rami of spinal nerves, **386**
  skeletal structures in, 371
  superficial muscles of, **373**
  surface anatomy of, **371**
  vessels and nerves of
    deep, **383**
    superficial, **382**
Biceps femoris
  short head of, 438
  tendon of, 438
Bifurcation
  aorta, 340
  of brachial artery, 77
  bronchoscopy, **165**
  common carotid artery, 559
  diaphragm, 197
  pulmonary trunk, 216
Bile ducts, 280
  branching of, 272
Biliary ducts
  radiograph of, 279
Biliary tract, 281
Birth process, 336

Bitemporal hemianopia, 673
Bladder, urinary, 193, 235, 243–247, 288, 300, 303,
    304, 306, 307, 315, 325, 330, 334, 341,
    351, 353, 356
  apex of, 354, 355
  base of, 355
  on computed tomography
  fundus of, 368
  internal iliac artery, branches of, **351**
  membranous urethra, 368
  midsagittal section of, 355
  mucosal folds of, 356
  mucous membrane of, 354
  muscular layer of, 354
  position during pregnancy, 330
  posterior surface of, 354
  radiograph of, 356
  trigone of, 354, 355
  uvula of, 356
Bones
  acetabulum, 323
  capitate, 130, 131
  carpal, 128, 129
  hamate, 130, 131
  lunate, 130, 131
  metacarpal, 128, 138
  occipital, 569
  pisiform, 130
  projections onto anterior body wall, **144**
  scaphoid, 130, 131
  sesamoid, 130, 138
  trapezium, 131
  triquetral, 130, 131
  of upper limb: radius and ulna, **122**
  of wrist and hand
    dorsal aspect, **129**
    palmar aspect, **128**
Bony acetabulum, 481
Bony palate
  and maxillary arch, 635
  and upper teeth, 635
Brachial fascia, 4, 15, 16, 30, 132
Brachial plexus, 26, 30
  complete diagram, **48**
  formation, 48
  in posterior lateral neck region, 47
  roots of origin and general schema, **47**
  and three cords, **46**
Brachiocephalic trunk, 25
Brain
  attachment of cranial nerves, 669
  base of, 590
  external surface of, 576
  inferior surface of, 589
  of newborn child, 402
  precocious growth, 571
  soft coverings of, 573
  ventral view, 589, 669
Breast
  areola, **6**
  cancer of, 6
  fat body, 6
  female, 4
    cancer, 6
    nipple and areola, **6**
  lobular nature, 4
  lymph drainage, 7
  milk line and accessory nipples, 4
  nipple, **6,** 9
  pectoral fascia, 6
  radiograph of, 6
Bronchi, **157, 162**
  anterior aspect of, 162
  left primary bronchus, 162
  in living person, 163

  opened, 163
  right primary bronchus, 162
  Surface Projection, 163
Bronchial tree, **157**
  bronchogram, 165
Bronchogram, 165
Bronchoscopy, 165
Bulb
  ampulla, 268
  artery of, 345
  duodenal, 265, 267
  internal jugular vein, 578
  penile urethra, 356
  penis, 235, 356
  superior duodenum, 261
Bulbourethral glands, 235, 356
Bursa
  acromial, 17
  anserine, 424
  bicipitoradial, 71, 125
  coracobrachial, 55
  iliopectineal, 421, 424
  infrapatellar, 414, 447, 484
  intermuscular, 432, 438
  ischial, 479
  omental, 248, 249, 258, 259, **259, 260,** 319
    porta hepatis, **259, 260**
    stomach, lymphatics of, **260**
  between pectoralis major muscle, 54
  popliteus, 494
  prepatellar, 414, 447, 541
  radial, 96, 134
  subacromial, 55, 116, 119
  subcoracoid, 30, 54
  subcutaneous, 124, 134
  subdeltoid, 30, 32, 54, 55, 60, 63
  subgastrocnemius, 463
  subhyoid, 652
  subsartorial, 424
  subtendinous, 114, 479, 510
  suprapatellar, 485, 488, 490, 492, 512
  synovial, 114, 432
  trochanteric, 431, 432, 437, 438, 479, 480
  ulnar, 96

C

Calcaneal region, 1
Calcaneal tuberosity, 409
Canal
  adductor (of Hunter), 420, 423, 443
  anal, 219, 342, 346, 359, 362
    inner surface of, 359
    median section, 360
  carotid, 543, 580, 583, 587, 591, 658, 663
  cochlea, 667
  cochlear, 668
  condylar, 569
  condyloid, 591
  facial, 658, 664, **665–666,** 681, 682, 684
  femoral, 425
  gastric, 255
  gastrointestinal, 248
  hypoglossal, 541, 557, 569, 585, 586, 588, 670,
    693
  incisive, 614, 615, 631
  infraorbital, 595, 640, 679
  inguinal, 226, 234, 237, 240, **241,** 357, 369
    direct inguinal hernias, **241**
    indirect inguinal hernias, **241**
  lacrimal, 593, 599
  mandibular, 636, 640
  obturator, 326, 343, 360, 424, 480, 481
  optic, 581, 586, 587, 588, 596, 601, 608, 678
  osseous–aponeurotic, 471

  palatine, 596
  pterygoid, 560, 565, 586, 596, 598, 616, 665, 679,
    681, 683
    nerve of, 616
  pudendal (of Alcock), 345, 348, 361, 365, 366,
    433
  pyloric, 263, 265, 267, 268
  root, 639
  sacral, 328, 351, 398, 399, 481
  of schlemm, 609, 612
  semicanal, 658
    of auditory tube, 683, 686
  spinal, 402, 691
  vertebral, 386, 387, 397, 398, 402, 405, 406, 407
Canine, lower, 640
Capitulum, 113, 122
Capsule, 33, 64, 114, 119, 124, 130, 145, 424, 462,
    480, 494, 553, 556
  articular, 124
  of cricothyroid, 653
  cricothyroid articular, 651
  of elbow joint, 134
  fibrous renal, 309
  of intervertebral joints, 378
  of lateral atlantoaxial, 389
  of left shoulder joint, 114
  metacarpophalangeal joint, 92
  musculotendinous, 61
  renal
  rotator cuff tendinous, 61
  of submandibular gland, 546
Cardiac incisure, 262
Cardiac notch, 158, 254
Carotid arteriogram, **583**
Carpal tunnel, 84
  distal cross section of middle finger, **105**
  superficial palmar arterial arch, **106**
  syndrome, 105
  transverse section, through right wrist showing,
    106
Cartilage
  articular, 138, 482, 490
  arytenoid, 163, 542, 651, 652, 655
  of auditory tube, 645
  bronchial, 162, 165
  corniculate, 163, 646, 652, 656
  costal, 140, 143, 144, 146, 147, 169, 199, 217, 226,
    227, 230, 519
  cricoid, 149, 162, 163, 400, 542, 627, 630, 641,
    642, 651, 652
  cuneiform, 646, 654
  of epiglottis, 654
  of external acoustic meatus, 658
  of external ear, **657**
  hyaline, 115, 398
  of larynx, 651–652
  nasal, 613, 615, 642
  thyroid, 149, 162, 163, 519, 537, 542, 627, 630,
    641, 642, 645, 646, 649, 650, 651, 653, 688
  tracheal, 162, 163, 199, 538, 627, 629, 641, 646,
    651
  triticeal, 651, 654
Cauda equina, 246, 405
  lumbar injection into, 408
  sacral puncture into, 408
  within vertebral canal, 407
Cavernous sinus, 676
Cavity
  abdominal, 250, 251, 252, 253, 288, **288,** 290,
    292, 300, 306, 307
    celiac trunk and its branches, **252, 256**
    duodenojejunal junction and large intestine,
      290
    female, posterior abdominal peritoneum, 306
    gastroduodenal vessels, **253**

greater omentum, 243, 246, 247, 248, 250, **250,** 251, 252, 253 254, **264,** 288
  inferior mesenteric vessels and their branches, **294**
  jejunum, ileum, and ascending, 288
  large intestine, **251, 290,** 300
  lumbar, sacral, and coccygeal plexuses
  male, retroperitoneal organs, 307
  mesenteries, 300
  mesocolons and mesentery of small intestine, **300**
  omentum reflected, **251**
  roots of mesocolons/mesentery, **306**
  sigmoid colons, 290
  small intestine, **251**
  splenic vessels, **253**
  superior mesenteric vessels and their branches, **292**
  transverse colons, 288
amniotic, 192, 492
cranial, 604, 606, 691, 692
glenoid, 112, 114, 115, 118, 140
joint, 492
middle ear, 684
nasal, 600, **613, 614**
oral, 549, 551, **619–628,** 626, 648, 693
orbital, 596, 598, 604, 606, 611, 612
pericardial, 170, 196, 216
peritoneal, 319, 320, 321, 353
pharyngeal, 656
pleural, 152, 153, 154
of tunica vaginalis testis,
tympanic, 658, 659, 661, 662, 664, 666, 679, 683, 685
Cecum, **301**
  large intestine, 304
  radiograph of, 291
  surface projection of, 302
Celiac trunk, 252, 296
  arteriogram, 256
  branches, **256,** 264
Central axillary nodes, 7
Central nervous system, 402, 671
Cephalic vein, 4, 13, 15, 16, 17, 23, 29, 36, 41, 86, 90
Cerebral cortex, 674
  arteries and veins on, 576
Cerebrospinal fluid, 405
Cervical enlargements, causes of, 403
Cervical intervertebral disks, frontal section through, 398
Cervical intervertebral joints, median sagittal section of, 397
Cervical spinal column
  dorsal view of, 389
  lateral view of, 400
Cervical spinal cord, 403
Cervical vertebrae, **388–389**
  and atlantooccipital membranes, **389**
  fifth, 388
  intervertebral disks and ligaments, 397
  seventh, 388
  spinous processes of, 397
  ventral view of, 389
Cervical viscera, 647
Childbearing, function of, 326
Ciliary ganglion, 675
  parasympathetic root, 603
Circle of Willis
  variations in formation of, 582
  vascular arrangement at, 574
Circumflex scapular vein, 23, 26
Cirrhosis, 12
Cisterna chyli, 203, 211, 352
  intestinal trunk, 211
  lumbar vertebra, 210
  lymph channels, 352

Cisterna magna, 590
Clavicle
  acromial end, 121
  anterolateral view, 118
  axillary artery, 11, 24, 42, 44, 117, 224, 544
  bones, 42
  inferior view, 145
  jugular veins, 534
  muscle, 54
  subclavius muscle, 54
Clavicular notch, 19, 141
Clavipectoral fascia, 17
Cleft
  anal, 350
  clavicular and sternocostal heads, 17
  pudendal, 344, 350
  uncovertebral, 398
Clitoris, 344
  cavernous nerves of, 233
  crus, 349
  glans, 344
  superficial dorsal vein of, 232
Coccyx, segments of, 399
Cochlea, 685
Colic flexure, 293, 305
Colic impression, 287
Collateral circulation, 361
Colles' fascia, 347
Colon
  ascending, 251, 291, 295, 298
    radiograph of, 291
  descending, 209, 219, 243, 248, 251, 290, 294, 295, 297, 304, 305, 319, 321, 322
  haustra of, 250, 251, 288, 301
  sigmoid, 219, 246, 248, 249, 251, 290, 292, 297, 298, 307, 330, 353, 361
  splenic flexure of, 283
  taenia of, 251
  transverse, 219, 246, 251, 258, 288, 308, 689
Column(s)
  iliocostalis, 375
  longissimus, 375
  spinalis, 375
Common bile duct, 283, 284, 286
  union of, 285
Compartments
  anterior, 513
    tendons, 514
  deep perineal, 347, 358
  lateral, 514
  posterior, superficial and deep parts of, 513
Computerized tomographs
  of thorax, 218
  of wrist, **136**
Concha(e)
  nasal, 567
    inferior, 595, 598
    middle, 595, 598, 614
    superior, 613
Condyles
  femoral lateral, 485
  medial and lateral, 479, 497
Conus
  arteriosus, 183
  medullaris, membranous continuation of, 405
Cord
  brachial plexus, **46**
  of brachial plexus axilla, **46**
  cervical spinal, 403
  spermatic, 15, 223, **223,** 236, 369, **369**
    cremaster muscle, **237**
    in inguinal region, **234**
    male inguinal region, **236**
    vessels and nerves of, 367

spinal, 14, 321, **402–408**
  anterior dissection, 207
  anterior median fissure of, 403
  arterial supply of, **403**
  and brain of newborn child, 402
  cauda equina of, **405**
  with dura mater, 404
  horns, 209
  lumbar puncture into, 408
  meninges, at cervical level, 406
  sacral puncture into, 408
  and segments in adult, 402
  spinal arteries of, **406**
  spinal roots of, **403**
  termination of neural part of, 405
  ventral view, 403
  within vertebral canal, 403
  umbilical, 192
Coronary arterial system, 178–179
Coronary arteriogram, 180–181
Coronary sinus, 177, 179
Coronary vessels, 176
Coronoid process, 122, 125
Corpus, 235, 237, 246
Corpus spongiosum penis, 370
Costal margin, 5, 139
Costocervical trunk, 544
Costotransverse joints, 394
Costovertebral joints
  and ligaments, **394–395**
  lower, 394
  sagittal section through spinal column showing, 395
  transverse section of, 393
Cranial cavity, 587, 588
Cranial nerve
  abducens (VI), 675, 676
  accessory (XI)
    diagrammatic representation of, 691
    schema of, 692
  apertures in base of skull transmitting, 670
  attachments to base of brain, **669**
  facial (VII)
    chorda tympani branch of, **684**
    diagrammatic view of, 681
    in facial canal, 681
    greater petrosal branch of, **683**
    on side of face, 682
  glossopharyngeal (IX)
    coursing from skull base through jugular foramen, 688
    in oropharynx, 688
    sensory innervation of, 687
  hypoglossal (XII)
    diagrammatic representation of, 693
    in superior neck region, 694
  location of, 670
  olfactory (I)
    olfactory bulb and tract, **671–672**
    somatomotor fibers of, 675
  optic (II)
    tract and, 674
    visual fields and, 673, 674
  trigeminal (V)
    and its branches, 677
    mandibular division of, 680
    maxillary division of, **679**
    ophthalmic division of, **678**
  trochlear (IV), 675, 676
  vagus (X)
    diagrammatic representation of, 689
    in thorax, 690
  vestibulocochlear (VIII)
    connections in brain, 686
    diagrammatic schema of, 686
    vestibular apparatus of, 685

Cremasteric fascia, 236
Cremasteric reflex, 237
Crest
    ethmoidal of palatine bone, 614
    frontal, 586
    iliac, 401, 408, 415, 427, 429, 434, 435
    infratemporal, 591
    intertrochanteric, 325
    lacrimal, 595, 596
    obturator, 324
    occipital, 569, 586
    pubic, 324
    sacral, 399
    supinator, 87
    supraepicondylar, 133
    zygomaticoalveolar, 568
Cross-sections
    of anterior neck at level of C7 vertebra, 537
    of deep back, 386
    of foot through metatarsal bones, 515
    of lower right leg and proximal right foot, 514
    of lower third of arm, 133
    of middle finger through middle phalanx, 105
    of neck at C5 vertebral level, 542
    of right hand through metacarpal bones, 137
    of right upper extremity through middle of
        humerus, 132
    of thorax, 214
    through distal end of right femur, 512
    through middle of right leg, 513
    through middle of right thigh, 511
    through middle third of right forearm, 135
    through proximal third of right forearm, 134
    through right upper extremity at level of elbow
        joint, 134
    through superior aspect of right thigh, 510
    of upper limb, 132
        arm, 132
        elbow and upper forearm, 134
        wrist and hand, 137
Crus
    atrioventricular bundle, 182
    clitoris, 331, 350
    cranial margin and medial, 237
    diaphragm, 309, 315
    helix, 657
    incus, 660, 663
    penis, 353
    right medial, 314
    of superficial inguinal ring, 15
Cubital fossa, 34, 42
Cusps
    aortic valve, 185, 190, 190
    mitral valve, 187
    right commissure, 191
    tricuspid valve, 182
Cystic duct, 278
Cystic vessel, 280

D

DB. See Duodenal bulb
Dentition, 636
Dermatomes, 9
    and cutaneous nerves of back, 372
    of upper limb, 35
Descending colon, 308
Diaphragm, 147, 149, 151, 152, 160, 166, 168–170,
    196, 197, 204, 213, 218, 218, 314, 315, 318
    abdominal surface of, 270
    central tendon of, 146, 229
    costal part of, 318, 319, 320
    crura of, 204
    dome of, 149, 261
    lumbar part of, 213, 247, 273, 318, 319

pelvic, 362
    posterior abdominal wall structures, 314
    urogenital, 345, 358
Diaphragmatic attachment, 271
Diaphysis, 123
Diploic veins, 574
Disc
    articular, 126, 140, 328, 555
    interpubic, 336, 345
    intervertebral, 326, 389, 395
    optic, 610, 611
Disk problem, causes of, 398
Distal phalanx, 138
Dorsal carpal network, 93
Dorsal foot, 1
Dorsal interossei, 476
Dorsal mesogastrium, 248, 249
Dorsiflexion, 453
Duct(us)
    aberrant inferior, 239
    bile, 247, 255, 257, 258, 259, 268, 271, 272, 283,
        284
    biliary, 278
        radiographs of, 279
    cochlear, 668, 685, 686
    cystic, 254, 257, 271, 278, 280, 319
        variations, 278
    efferent, 238
    ejaculatory, 355, 357
    endolymphatic, 668, 685, 686
    of epididymis, 357
    of epoöphoron, 332, 334
    excretory, 349, 358
    frontonasal, 617
    gallbladder, 278
        radiographs of, 279
    hepatic, 254, 257, 272, 278, 279, 280
        variations, 278
    hepatopancreatic, 285
    lactiferous, 6, 9
    lymphatic, 210, 211
    mesonephric, 331, 357
    nasolacrimal, 598, 599, 615
    pancreatic, 246, 247, 255, 268, 283, 284, 284
        common bile, 284, 285
    pancreatic system, 283
    paramesonephric (Müllerian), 331, 357
    paraurethral, 344
    parotid, 522, 553, 621, 625
    semicircular, 667, 668, 685
    of seminal vesicle, 368
    sublingual, 626
    submandibular, 566, 625, 626
    system, 9
    thoracic, 167, 203, 207, 210, 211, 217, 319, 352,
        540
    vitelline, 248
    wolffian, 357
Ductus arteriosus, 192, 193
Ductus deferens, 234, 235, 237, 317, 354
    ampulla of, 355
    artery of, 239
    beginning of, 239
Ductus venosus, 192
Duodenal ampulla, 291
Duodenal bulb, 265
Duodenal ulcers, 267
Duodenojejunal junction, 300
Duodenum, 206, 244, 247, 248, 249, 251, 254, 255,
    258, 259, 262, 266, 266, 278, 279, 282,
    284, 285, 288, 291, 292, 306, 307, 690
    anterior view, 268
    bulb of superior, 261
    cross-sections through,
    descending, 261, 262, 282, 283, 303, 308

head of, 283
    horizontal, 254, 304
        3rd part of, 255, 307
    inferior part, 282
    internal structure, 255
    longitudinal section of, 268
    pancreas, 283
    pylorus opening into, 268
    superior (1st) part of, 283, 306
    surface projection of, 282
    upper, 255
Dural sinuses, 561, 562, 574, 577–578
Dura mater, 403, 408, 573
    cranial, 668, 688
    dorsal and ventral roots to, 404
    dorsal root ganglion with, 207
    and dural venous sinuses, 577
    intracranial, 577
    meningeal (See Meningeal dura mater)
    periosteal layer of, 406
    relationship of dorsal and ventral roots to, 404
    removal of, 590
    spinal cord with, 404

E

Ear, 657–668
    external, 547, 552, 559, 657, 681, 689 (See also
        External ear)
    extrinsic muscles, 549
    internal, 662, 667 (See also Internal ear)
    lateral wall, 663
    middle, 659, 661, 662, 687 (See also Middle ear)
    right tympanic cavity of
        lateral wall of, 663
        medial wall of, 664
    structures, 662
    surface anatomy, 657
    tympanic membrane, 660
Ejaculatory ducts, 355, 356, 356
Elbow
    arteries, 79
    bones of, 125
    brachial arteriogram, 79
    nerves, 79
    radiograph, 123
Embryo, 338
Embryonic liver, 248
Eminence
    hypothenar, 34, 95, 136
    iliopubic, 324
    intercondylar, 486, 493
    lateral plantar, 470
    thenar, 42, 136
Epicondyle
    humerus, 37, 134
    lateral, 43
    medial, 34, 54
    ulnar nerve, 79
Epididymis, 235, 238, 244, 247, 357
    anterior view, 238
    appendix, 238
    and beginning of ductus deferens, 239
    blood supply, schematic representation of, 239
    body of, 240
    head, 237, 238, 355, 357
    inferior ligament of, 238
    lateral view, 238
    longitudinal section of, 238
    sinus of, 238, 240
    tail of, 238, 239, 355, 357
    testis and, 238, 239, 353
Epigastric anastomosis, schematic diagram of, 231
Epigastric region, 219
Epiphysis, 123, 397, 398

Eponychium, 138
Esophagus, 196, **197**, 202, 203, 212, 215–217, 219,
        244, 246, 537, 629, 630, 641, 642
    abdominal part, 197, 206, 213
    anterior aspect of, 167
    aorta and lower, 197
    arterial blood supply, 198
    beneath pericardium, 175
    cervical part, 197, 198
    common sites of diverticula, **201**
    CT of, 275
    dome of, 166
    esophageal hiatus, 218
    esophagoscope, superior view, 200
    locations of diverticula, 201
    muscular layer, **262**
    posterior view, 198, 199
    posterior view of, 198
    radiograph, 200, **200,** 261
    relationship, to aorta and trachea, 197
    seen through esophagoscope, 200
    sites of constrictions, **201**
    thoracic part, 167, 197, 198
    traversing esophageal hiatus, 315
    veins of, **204**
    venous plexus, 204
Ethmoid bone
    left lateral view of, 618
    superior surface of, 618
Extensor retinaculum, 89, 92
External ear
    cartilage of right, 657
    frontal section through, 659
    muscles of
        attaching to medial surface, 657
        intrinsic, 657
    nerves of, **665**
External genitalia, 351
External nares. *See* Nostrils
External nose
    cartilages and bones of, 613
    nasal cavities (*See* Nasal cavities)
Eye, 593–612
    muscles of, 605–606
    right
        eyelids and, 593
        tarsi of, 597
    superficial nerves and muscles of, **594**
    surface anatomy of, **593**
Eyeball
    blood supply to layers of, 612
    horizontal section of, 609, 612
    and muscle insertions, 607
    sagittal view of, 600
Eyelids
    innervation of, 594
    and medial angle, 593

F

Face
    branches of the facial nerve, 548
    infratemporal region of the deep, 564, 566
    mandibular nerve branches, 566
    masseter and temporalis muscles, 555
    of mastication, **555**
    maxillary artery, 565
    medial and lateral pterygoid muscles, 555
    muscles of, 641
        facial expression, 548
        mastication, 551, 556
        superficial, 547
    nerves of, 524
    pterygoid muscles, 556
    superficial and deep arteries, **559**

    superficial nodes of, 539
    superficial posterior cervical muscles, 548
    superficial veins of, 561
    vessels and nerves of
        deep, 563
        superficial, **553–554**
Facial canal, 665
Facial muscles, superficial, 594
Fascia
    bulbar, 600
    cremasteric muscle, 236
    crural, 461
    deep, 447
    deltoid, 4, 16
    lata, 429
Fat body of breast, 6
Fauces, 619
Female breast, 4, 5
    anterior view, 5
    lateral view, 5
    lateral view of, **9**
    lymph channels from, 7
    normal, radiograph of, 6
    in reclined thorax, lateral view, **9**
Female external genitalia, **344**
Female genital organs, innervation of, **233**
Female genitourinary organs, 331
Female inguinal region, **232**
Female lesser pelvis, 326
Female pelvic floor, **343**
Female pelvic organs
    anterosuperior view, 333
    arterial supply, 335
Female pelvis, **326**
    blood supply, ovary, uterus,and vagina, **335**
    blood vessels of, 341
    bones and ligaments, **329**
    cross section of, 363
    CT of, **334,** 363
    hemisected pelvis, **328**
    iliac arteriogram, **339**
    internal iliac artery
        branches of, **340**
    joints and ligaments, 329
    midsagittal view, **342**
    muscular floor of, 343
    musculature of, 345
    pelvic ligaments, 328
    pelvis organs, arteries, and veins, **341**
    peritoneal ligaments, **333**
    peritoneal reflections, **333**
    posteroinferior view, 328
    reproductive organs, **334**
    sacroiliac joint, **329**
    uterosalpingogram, **330**
Female perineum
    inferior view of, 345
    muscles of, 347
    nerves and blood vessels of, 348
    vessels and nerves, **348**
Female sacral
    posteroinferior view, 350
    surface anatomy of, 350
Female urogenital triangle anal region, surface
        anatomy of, **350**
Femoral nerves, 316
Femoral–popliteal–tibial arteriogram, 445
Femoral sheath, 417
Femoral triangle, 1, 219
Femoral vein, 220
Femoral vessels
    superficial inguinal lymphatic nodes into,
        417
Femur
    adductor brevis muscles, 427

    anterior view, **478**
    blood supply, **483**
    body of, 484
    cross section through distal end of, **512**
    epicondyle of, 468
    head of, 325, 363, 364
    hip joint and head of, **482**
    lateral condyle of, 486, 491, 493
    lateral rotators of, 435
    lesser trochanter of, 314
    ligament of head of, 481, 482, 483
    medial condyle of, 418, 421
    MRI showing, 489
    muscle attachments, 478, 479
    neck of, 325, 363
    patella on, 421
    posterior view, **479**
    right, 479
    superior end of, 482
    synovial membrane, 494
    thigh bone, 443, 511
    tuberosity of, 431
    upper, blood supply to, 483
Fetal roentgenogram, 337
Fibers
    abdominal, 17
    afferent, 687
    autonomic, 362
    clavicular, 18
    from dorsal and ventral roots, 386
    of iliofemoral and pubofemoral ligaments,
        480
    intercrura, 15
    of interspinous ligaments, 397
    of ischiofemoral ligament, 480
    of long plantar ligament, 506
    motor, 232
    muscle, 146, 163, 169
    optic, 673
    parasympathetic, 233, 593, 675, 683, 687
    postganglionic, 209, 598
    preganglionic, 209, 233, 598
    preganglionic parasympathetic, 598
    Purkinje, 189
    sensory, 52, 681, 682, 687, 689, 691
    of soleus, 463
    somatomotor, 675, 682, 689
    sternocostal, 17
    sympathetic, 233, 235, 603
    transverse, 329
    visceromotor, 689
    viscerosensor, 689
Fibula, 337, 456
    anterior ligament of head, 452
    body of, 484
    calcaneofibular ligament of, 502
    distal, 498
    head of, 451, 493
    proximal ends of, 496
    right, 497
    shaft (body), 493
    at talocrural (ankle) joint, 499
    and tibia, 496
Fibular retinacula, superior and inferior, 456
Filum terminale, 246
Finger
    anatomy of, **92**
    cross section, 104, 105
    injection site, **90**
    joints and ligaments, 131
    longitudinal section through flexed, 138
    sagittal section through, 110
    site for local anesthesia, 90
    tendon insertions, 104
    tendons and cross section of middle, **104**

Fingernail
  bed exposed, 138
  normal position, 138
  removed from nail bed, 138
Fingernails, **138**
Fishhook stomach, 261
Fissure
  anterior median, 403
  horizontal, 154, 158
  inferior orbital, 567
  longitudinal cerebral, 589
  oblique, 149, 212, 217
  oral, 219
  palpebral, 597
  petrooccipita, 586
  right portal, 274
  sphenopetrosal, 592
  tympanomastoid, 658
  zygomaticomaxillary, 595
Flexure
  duodenojejunal, 268, 282, 294
  hepatic, 258
  left colic, 149
  perineal, 359
  rectum, perineal, 353
  right colic, 149
  sigmoid colon, 291
  splenic, 212, 213
Fold
  axillary, 2
  glossoepiglottic, 645
  laryngeal, 655
  lateral umbilical, 222
  longitudinal, 283
  median umbilical, 222
  mucosal, 356
  myocardial, 186
  palatoglossal and palatopharyngeal, 619
  salpingopalatine, 642
  sublingual, 626
  superior ileocecal, 303
  synovial, 499
  umbilical, 222, 228, 241, 250, 368
  vestibular, 655
  vocal, 652
Foot, 2, **454–459**
  attachments of muscles, 501
  bones of, muscles attachments
    dorsal aspect of, 500
    plantar aspect of, 501
  deep fascia investing, 447
  dorsal, 1
  dorsal right
    cutaneous innervation of, 454
    deep vessels and nerves of, **459**
    intrinsic muscles of, 458
    lateral ligaments of, 502
    muscles and tendons on, **457–458**
    superficial muscles and tendon sheaths of, **455**
    superficial veins and cutaneous nerves of, 460
    superficial vessels and nerves of, **454**
    tendons and synovial sheaths of, 456
  dorsiflexion and plantar flexion of, 453
  dorsum of, **455**
  inversion and eversion of, 453
  longitudinal arches of, **509**
  longitudinal axis, 458
  medial ligaments of, 504
  muscles of, 474
  plantar aspect of, 458, **471, 473,** 477
  sagittal section of, 504, 507
  skeleton of, 500
  sole of, 471
    muscles of, 477
    right, 475

Foot, plantar
  aponeurosis of, **470**
  arteries of, **473**
    deep, **474**
    variations in, 476
  nerves of, **470, 473**
  plantar muscles of
    *chart of, 477
    first layer of, 471
    second layer of, 472
    third layer of, 475
  vessels of, **470**
    deep, **474**
Foot, right
  bones of, 500–501, 503
  compartments of, 516
  frontal section through metatarsal bones of, 515
  ligaments on plantar surface of, 506
  oblique section through calcaneus and talus of, 514
  skeleton of, 502
  sole of, 470
    plantar arch and deep vessels and nerves of, 474
    plantar nerves and arteries of, 473
    second layer of plantar muscles of, 472
Foramen
  costotransverse, 394
  epiploic, 258
  intervertebral, 405
  jugular, 591, 592
  magnum, 586
  mandibular, 633
  mastoid, 586
  mental, 547
  nutrient, 145, 497
  omental, 258
  sciatic, 348, 433
  sphenopalatine, 596, 614
  supraorbital, 567
  transverse, 388
  vertebral, 218, 388
Foramen ovale, 193
Forearm, 2
  anterior
    deep muscles, 72
    muscles, **73**
    pronator teres and flexor digitorum superficialis, **71**
    superficial muscles, **70**
    vessels and nerves
      deep dissection, **78**
      intermediate dissection, **77**
      superficial dissection, **76**
  arteries, 88, **89**
  bones, 126
  cutaneous nerves, 69
  extensor muscles of, **85**
  interosseous membrane of, 110
  left anterior, muscles, 72
  middle (cross section and MRI), **135**
  muscles of, 83
    deep, **72**
    deep extensor, **82, 83,** 87
    dorsal, 85
    flexor, 73, 74
    posterior, 80
    radial extensor, 85
    superficial, 70
    supinator, 85
  nerves, 76, 77, 78, **88, 89**
  pronated, **84**
  superficial dissection, 69
    of anterior, **68**
    of posterior, **69**

  superficial extensor muscles, **80, 81**
  superficial veins, 69
  supination and pronation, **84**
  vessels, 76, 77, 78
Fossa
  acetabular, 325
  antecubital, 41
  axillary, 1
  coronoid, 113
  cranial, 577, 585
  cubital, 42, 68, 78
  digastric, 519
  glenoid, 19
  iliac, 426
  infraclaviculcar, 42
  infratemporal, 605
  intercondylar, 484
  intersigmoid, 290
  ischioanal, 363
  ischiorectal, 365
  mandibular, 558, 591
  olecranon, 123
  popliteal, 409, 442, 512
  radial, 113
  scaphoid, 657
  subscapular, 30
  supraclavicular, 527
Fovea
  centralis, 609, 611
  for dens, 388, 390
  head of femur, 325, 478, 479, 480
  optic disc, 609
Frenulum, 301
Frontal section
  MRI of thorax, **212, 213**
  of thorax and abdomen from behind, 196
  through cavernous sinus and base of skull, 580
  through lower left thorax, **213**
    and upper left abdomen, **213**
  through thoracic cavity, 212
  through thorax, **212**

G

Gag reflex, 687
Gallbladder, 250, 258, 270, 272, 274, 280, 284, 303, 306, 320
  biliary ducts and, 279
  disease, **281**
  fundus of, 149
  inflammation of, 281
  radiograph of, 279, **284**
    biliary duct system, 278
    blood supply, **280**
    cholycystitis, **281**
    fossa of, 259
    multiple gallstones, **281**
    posterior surface of, 271
  serous coat, neck of, 278
  ultrasound of, **280**
Gallstones, **281**
Ganglion
  cervical, 644
  cervicothoracic, 47, 209
  ciliary, **603**
  2nd thoracic, 166
  pterygopalatine, 209, 683
  root, 207
  spinal, 384, 403
  submandibular, 566
  sympathetic, 206
  trigeminal, 666, 678, 680
Gastric, **267**
  arteries, 254, 256, 257, 264
  impression, 287

Gastrointestinal system
    development of, 248
    organs of, **219**
Gastrointestinal tube, 248
Gastropancreatic fold, 259
Genitalia, superficial tissues of, 417
Genital system, 341
Gland
    adrenal, 276, 319
    areolar, 5
    axillary sweat, 4
    bulbourethral, 235, 356, 358
    greater vestibular, 350
    lacrimal, 606, 676
    mammary, 6, 217
    parotid, 219, 645
    pituitary, 669
        chiasmatic cistern anterior to, 590
        median sagittal section through, 587
    prostate, 235, 357
    salivary, 626
    seminal, 246
    seromucous, 625
    sublingual, 219, 559, 626
    submandibular, 531, 535, 546, 623, 625, 626
    suprarenal, **309**
    thyroid, 149, 152, 197, 528, 537, 650
    tracheal, 647
    vestibular, 331
Glans
    clitoris, 331, 336, 344, 350
    penis, 235, 247, 356, 367–370
        section midway, 370
Glenoid cavity, 118
Glenoid fossa, 118
Glenoid labrum, **118,** 119
Gluteal fascia, 11
Gluteal region
    deep muscles of, 431, 437
    gluteus maximus of, 431–432
    and lateral rotators, 432
    muscles of, **434**
    safe quadrant for injections into, 435
    vessels and nerves of, 439
        deep, **433**
Gluteus maximus and iliotibial tract, 435
Gluteus minimus and lateral rotators of
        femur,435
Greater duodenal papilla, 255, 283
Great saphenous vein, 12, 13
Groove
    bicipital, 26
    costal, 142
    intertubercular, 114
    interventricular, 186
    malleolar, 497
    mylohyoid, 634
    radial, 63, 113
    supra-acetabular, 324
Gubernaculum testis, 357

H

Hand, 2
    adductor pollicis muscle, 101
    arteries of left dorsal, 93
    bones, showing attachment of muscles, 128
    deep flexor tendons, 100
    deep muscles, 99
    dermatomes, **91**
    digital arteries of, 106
    dorsum of
        and arteries, **93**
        dermatomes, 91
        extensor tendons on, 91

    and interosseous muscles, **91**
    nerves of, 90
    superficial veins, 90
    tendons and interosseous muscles, **91**
    tendons, arteries, and digital nerves, 93
    veins and nerves, **90**
    finger of, 90
    hypothenar muscles, 97, 98
    index finger of
        nerves and arteries, 92
        tendon insertions, 92
    joints and ligaments of, 130, **131**
    muscles of, 98, 100
    palm of, 94
    radial side, arteries and superficial nerves, **111**
    radiograph of, 127, 131
    skeleton of, 128, 129
    superficial nerves, arteries, and tendons, 111
    superficial palmar arch, 106
    supination and pronation, **84**
    synovial tendon sheathes, variations, 99
    thenar muscles, 97
Haustrae, 251
Head, 3
    midsagittal section of, 642
    Superficial Lymph Nodes, 526
    temporal and facial regions of, 522
    Vessels of, 526
Heart
    arteriogram, **180–181**
    atrioventricular bundle dissected, 189
    atrioventricular bundle system, **190**
    blood supply, **176**
        to interventricular septum, 178
    blood vessels, **177**
    chordae tendineae, **187**
    conduction system, **188, 189**
    coronary arteries, **178**
    coronary sinus, 177
    coronary vessels, 177
    diaphragmatic surface, 177
    frontal section, 188, **188**
    and great vessels, **172, 173, 174**
    interior of pericardium, 175
    left and right coronary arteries, 179
    left atrium and ventricle, **184**
    left ventricle and ascending aorta, **185**
    left ventricular and aortic junction, 190
    mitral valve, 187
    muscular anatomy, **186**
    papillary muscles, **187**
    positions, during full inspiration, 169
    projection, onto anterior thoracic wall, 169
    pulmonary trunk, 183
    right atrium, 182
    right ventricle, 182, 183
    shadow outline of, 149
    sinoatrial and atrioventricular nodes, 190
    surface projection, **171**
    tricuspid valve, 187
    valves, **167,** 176, **191**
    variations in coronary artery distribution, **179**
    veins, drain into, 171
    venous drainage of ventricles, 177
    ventral view of, 172
Hemorrhoidal zone, 360
Hepatopancreatic duct, 285
Hernia, 241
    indirect/congenital, 240
Herpes zoster (shingles), mapping of skin areas
        affected by, 372
Hiatus
    adductor, 421, 443
    anal, 343
    aortic, 197, 210, 314, 315

    esophageal, 199, 314
    maxillary, 614
    sacral, 408
    urogenital, 343
Hilton's line, 359
Hilum, of left lung, **164**
Hip bone
    adult
        anterior view of, 324
        medial view of, 324
    5-year-old child, 323
        medial view, 324
Hip joints
    arterial supply to, 483
    articular capsule of, 480
    frontal section of, 482
        pelvis showing, 481
    radiograph of, 325, 483
    right
        anterior exposure of, 481
        frontal section and opened socket of, 481
        frontal section through, 480
        posterior view of, 480
        socket of, 481
Horizontal section
    through thorax
        at bifurcation of pulmonary trunk, 216
        at level of arch of aorta, 215
        at level of eighth thoracic vertebra, 217
        at level of left atrium, 216
        at level of seventh thoracic vertebra, 217
Horns
    coccygeal, 399
    hyoid bone, 537, 630, 641
    of hyoid bone, 622
    lateral meniscus, 488, 489
    spinal cord, 209
    thyroid cartilage, 537, 650
Horse's tail. *See* Cauda equina
Humerus, 42, 54, 60, 64, 71, 84, **113,** 115, 116, 117,
        133, 337, 387
    head of, 18
    rotation, 31
    shaft of, 121
    surgical neck of, 120
    trochlea of, 125
Hyaline cartilage, 398
Hyoid bone, 519, 520, 523, 537, 545, 549, 556, 622,
        624, 630, 632, 649, 651–653, 655
    ansa cervicalis, 519
    body of, 537, 549, 632
    fibrous loop, 624
    horn, 537
    hyoglossus muscle, 148
    lesser horns, 624
    stylohyoid ligament, 624
    stylohyoid muscle, 624
    thyrohyoid membrane, 528
Hypogastric plexus, 235
Hypothenar eminence, 95

I

Ileocecal junction, 288, 292, 300, 301, **301**
Ileum
    with contrast medium, 289
    radiograph of, 291
Iliac crest, 324
Iliac vessels, 290
Iliococcygeus, 345
Ilioinguinal branches, 316
Iliotibial tract, 429
Immune-lymphoid system, 150
Incus, 662
Index finger, **138**

Inferior vena cava, 175, 239, 247, 273, 275, 276, 282, 285, **299,** 321
Infraspinatus fascia, 44
Infraspinatus fossa, 117
Infrasternal angle, 139
Inguinal canal, 237
  diagram of, 241
  walls of, 234
Inguinal hernias, 241
Inguinal region, 220
Intercostal vein, 14
Intercrural fibers, 15, 223
Internal ear, 685
  frontal section through, 659
  projected onto bony base of skull, 667
  right membranous labyrinth of, 668
  structures in, 662, 667
Internal iliac
  nodes, 211
  visceral branches of, 351
Internal intercostal membrane, 146
Internal pudendal vessels, 366
Internal spermatic fascia, 237
Internal strabismus, 676
Internal thoracic anastomosis, 25
Internal thoracic vein, 13, 147
Interosseous membrane, 89, 93, 99, 126
Intersigmoid fossa, 290
Interspinales, 378
Intertransversarii, 378
Intervertebral disks, 395
  cervical and lumbar, 398
  and ligaments of cervical vertebrae, 397
  median sagittal section of, 397
Intervertebral foramina, 395
Intestine. See Small intestine
Intramuscular gluteal injection, safe zone for, 434
Intraoperative cholangiogram, radiograph of, 279
Iris and pupil, 609
Ischial spines, 323, 325, 328
Ischial tuberosity, 323, 324, 328
Ischiorectal fossae, 347
IVC. See Inferior vena cava

J

Jaundice, 281
Jejunum, 320, 321
  with contrast medium, 289
  radiograph of, 291
Joints
  acromioclavicular, 42, 61, **116**
  ankle (talocrural), 497
    articular surface of, 499
    bony structures in, 498
    dorsiflexion and plantar flexion of foot at, 453
    on dorsum of foot, 456
    fibula at, 499
    lateral ligaments of, 502
    ligaments on medial aspect of, 504
    medial aspect of, 503
    sagittal section of, **507**
    synovial fold of, 499
    X-ray of, **498**
  atlantoaxial
    cruciform ligament of, 390
    median, 390, 391
    posterior view of, 389
    radiographs of, 391
  atlantooccipital
    cruciform ligament of, 390
    median sagittal section of, 391
    posterior view of, 389
  between atlas and odontoid process, 391

calcaneocuboid, 507
capsule, 33
carpometacarpal, 42
costovertebral
  and ligaments, **394–395**
  lower, 394
  sagittal section through spinal column showing, 395
  transverse section of, 393
craniovertebral, **390–391**
distal radioulnar, 42
elbow, 42, **124**
  bones, ligaments (medial view), **125**
  flexed and supinated, 125
  left, 124
  radiographs, adult and child, **123**
frontal section of joint, **119**
glenohumeral, 42
hip
  arterial supply to, 483
  articular capsule of, 480
  frontal section of, 482
    pelvis showing, 481
  radiograph of, 325, 483
  right
    anterior exposure of, 481
    frontal section and opened socket of, 481
    frontal section through, 480
    posterior view of, 480
    socket of, 481
interphalangeal, 131
intertarsal, **505**
knee, **485** (See also Knee joints)
metacarpophalangeal, 42
midcarpal, 42
radiocarpal, 131
radioulnar, 125, **126**
  bones of, 125
  CT of, 136
scapuloclavicular, 118
shoulder (glenohumeral), **116, 119**
sternoclavicular, 5, 139, 140
sternocostal, 140
sternomanubrial, 140
subtalar, 498, 502, 507
talocalcaneonavicular
  anteriorly, 507
  right, 505
tarsometatarsal, **505**
  intertarsal and, 507
temporomandibular, **557**
transverse tarsal (midtarsal), 507
wrist, 42, **131**
  joints and ligaments of, **131**
  transverse section through, 137
J-shaped stomach. See Fishhook stomach
Jugular notch, 5, 19, 139, 141
Junction
  aortic valve, 190
  cartilages, 145
  cecum, **301**
  dorsal and ventral spinal roots, 14
  duodenojejunal, 290
  duodenum, 262
  esophageal-diaphragmatic, 201
  ileocecal, 288
  manubrium, 144
  pharynx, 200
  spinal nerve, 14
  splenic and superior mesenteric veins, 253
  splenic vein, 283
  stomach, 255
  superior vena cava, 166
  xiphisternal, 3, 141
  xiphoid process, 19, 141

K

Kidneys, 196, 209, 248, 276, 282, 306, 307, 308, 313, 331, 357, 689
  anterior surface contact relationships, 308
  cortex of, 312
  dorsal view, 311
  fetal lobulation, 313
  hilar structures, **311**
  hilum of, 307
  horseshoe, anterior view of, 313
  internal structure, **312**
  lateral margins of, 313
  left, 276
    frontal section, 312
    suprarenal, 309
  malformations, **313**
  perinephric fat (perineal fat capsule), 319
  posterior abdominal wall, 319
  projection of, 311
  relationship of, 386
  retrograde pyelogram, **313**
  ribs, 276
  segmentation, **308**
  suprarenal glands, **309**
  surface projection, **311**
  ventral and dorsal relationship, **308**
Knee joints
  anteriorly opened, 485
  arthroscopy of, 491
  articular capsule of, 487
  fibrous capsule of, 492
  flexed right, 485
  "locked," 485
  magnetic resonance images of, 489
  movement, **494**
  posterior superficial view of, 487
  radiographs of, **493**
  right
    anterior view of, 484
    arthrogram of, 490
    frontal section through, 486
    synovial membrane within capsule of, **494**
    tibial collateral ligament and, 486
  sagittal section through, 488
  synovial cavity and bursae of, **492**
  transverse section through, 488
Knee region
  medial surface of, 443
  muscles and tendons of, 462

L

Labium majus, 344
Lacrimal apparatus, **598–599**
Lacrimal canaliculi, 598, 599
Lacrimal gland
  innervation of, 598
  and its excretory ducts, 597
  and lacrimal apparatus, **598**
Lacrimal sac, 598, 599
Lactiferous ducts, 6, 9
Lactiferous sinus, 6, 9
Lamina
  cricoid cartilage, 163, 400, 654
  dorsal vertebral arches, 395
  ethmoid bone, 567
  lumbar vertebra, 405
  pterygoid process, 557
  separation of, 396
  thyroid cartilage, 163, 537, 653
  tragus, 527
  vertebral arch, 388, 393, 394, 395, 396, 397, 401
Lanzmann's point, 302
Laryngopharynx, 219

Laryngoscopy, 656
Larynx, **649–656**
    cartilages and ligaments of, 651–652
    cross section, at vocal folds, 656
    external, 629–630
    frontal section through, 655
    midsagittal section of, 642, 655
    muscles of, 646
        posterior view of, 653
        posterolateral view of, 654
        ventrolateral view of, 653
    opened from behind, 654
    upper left part of, 652
    vessels and nerves of, **649–650**
Lateral axillary nodes, 7
Lateral cubital sulcus, 42
Lateral epicondyle, 62
Lateral intermuscular septum, 81
Lateral malleolus, 1
Lateral sternal line, 2
Lateral thoracic vein, 4, 12, 27
Lateral umbilical folds, 222, 250
Latissimus dorsi
    intermediate back muscles and, **374**
    removal of, 374
    superficial muscles, 373
    and trapezius, 373
Latissimus dorsi fascia, 16
Left internal jugular vein, 210
Left kidney, dorsal view of, 311
Left subclavian vein, 210
Leg, 2
    anterior compartment of, **449**
    crural fascia of, 414
    deep fascia of, 461
    fibularis muscles of, 410
    medial view of, 462
    muscles of lateral compartment of, 448
    right, 513
    tendons of, right, 452
Leg, anterior
    deep fascia investing, 447
    muscles of, 447
        *chart of, 448
        deep, 451
    superficial vessels and nerves of, **446**
    vessels, lymphatics, and muscles of, **449**
Leg, lateral
    muscles of
        deep, 451
        fibular, 452
        fibularis brevis, 448
        fibularis longus, 448
    trauma to, 452
Leg, posterior
    arteries and nerves of, **465**
    muscles of
        deep, 466
        soleus and plantaris, **463**
        superficial calf, 461
        tibialis posterior and flexor hallucis longus,
        469
    nerves and vessels of, 464
    soleus muscle level of, 464
    superficial veins and cutaneous nerves of, 460
    tibial nerve in, 465
Leg, posterior compartment of
    deep muscle group of, **466**
    deep vessels and nerves of, **467**
    muscles of
        attachments of, **468**
        *chart of, **468**
    soleus muscle level of, 464
    tibial nerve in, 465
Lens, 610

Levator scapulae, 379
Ligamenta flava
    between adjacent lumbar vertebrae, 396
    of dorsal vertebral arches, 395
Ligament(s)
    acromioclavicular, 116, 117
    annular, 126
    anococcygeal raphe, 345, 350
    anterior (inferior) tibiofibular, 502
    anterior longitudinal, 146, 389
        fibers of, 395
    anterior sacroiliac, 327, 329
    anterior sternoclavicular, 140
    anteroinferior view, 326
    associated, 327
    bifurcation, 502
    bones
        female pelvis, **326**
        male pelvis, **327**
    calcaneocuboid, 506
    of calcaneofibular, 502
    calcaneonavicular, 502
        long, 509
        plantar, 509
    cardinal, 332
    clavicular and scapular, **118**
    collateral, 130, 131, 138
    connecting gliding joints, 394
    coracoacromial, 116
    coracoclavicular, 54, 116
    coracohumeral, 61, 116
    coronary, 270
    costoclavicular, 140
    costotransverse, 395
    costoxiphoid, 15
    cricothyroid, 162
    cruciate
        anterior, 485, 486
        attachments on tibia of, 495
        distal part of right anterior, 491
        posterior, 486
    deltoid, 503
    denticulate, 404
    dorsal carpometacarpal, 130
    dorsal intercarpal, 130
    dorsal metacarpal, 130
    falciform, 222, 250, 271
    female pelvis, **326**
    fudiform ligament of penis, 15
    gastrolienal, 248
    glenohumeral, 116
    of head of femur, 481
    of head of fibula, 496
    hepatoduodenal, 258
    hip joints, 326
    iliofemoral, 480
    inferior transverse scapular, 33, 67
    inguinal, 221, 223, 340, 409
    inguinal region, 234
    in inguinal region, **234**
    interclavicular, 140
    interosseous metacarpal, 131
    interosseous sacroiliac, 329
    interosseous talocalcaneal, 502
    interspinous
        fibers of, 397
        spinous processes of, 397
    intra-articular, 395
    ischiofemoral, 480
    lacunar, 223, 339
    of larynx, 651–652
    longitudinal
        anterior, 397
        posterior, 397
    long plantar, 506

    Mackenrodt's, 343
    mandibular, **557**
    medial, foot, 504
    medial talocalcaneal, 502
    medial umbilical, 13, 193
    oblique and arcuate popliteal, 487
    of ovaries, 332
    palmar carpal, 94
    palmar radiocarpal, 130
    palmar ulnocarpal, 130
    palpebral, 597
    patellar, 484
    pectineal, 234
    pisometacarpal, 130
    plantar calcaneocuboid, 503
    plantar calcaneonavicular, 506
    on plantar surface of right foot, 506
    posterior tibiofibular, 502
    pubofemoral, 480
    pulmonary, 160
    radial annular, 121, 124
    radial collateral, 121, 124
    radiate carpal, 130
    radiate sternocostal, 140
    reflected inguinal, 15
    right knee joint and tibial collateral, 486
    of right shoulder, 114
    sacroiliac, 329
    sacrospinous, 328
    sacrotuberous, 328
    splenorenal, 260
    superficial transverse metacarpal, 94
    superior transverse scapular, 116, 117
    suspensory, 9, 15
    transverse acetabular, 481
    trapezoid, 116
    ulnar collateral, 124
    uterine, 343
    viewed from above, 327
    viewed from front, 326
    vocal, 652
Ligamentum arteriosum, 172, 175
Ligamentum flavum, 397
Ligamentum venosum, 193
Ligamentum venosus, 271
Limb, lower, **409–516**
    anterior and medial nerves of, **440**
    anterior aspect of
        dermatomes and, 410
        muscles and fasciae on, **414**
        photograph of, 409
    arteries of, **413**
    bones of, **412, 413,** 479
        fibula, 497
        tibia, 496–497
    bony landmarks of, 409
    femoral vessels and nerves of, **423**
    foot (*See* Foot)
    hip region of
        anterior muscles of, 426
        arteries of, **422**
        deep muscles of, 431
    joints of, **412**
        hip, 480–482
        knee, 484 (*See also* Knee joints)
        ligaments, 506
        menisci, 495
        patella, 495
        talocrural (ankle), 498
        tibiofibular, 496
    leg (*See also* Leg)
        crural fascia of, 414, 415
        muscles of posterior, 414
    nerves of
        anterior aspect of, 440

Limb, lower (*continued*)
  cutaneous, **410**
    posterior, **441**
  posterior aspect of
    muscles and fasciae on, **415**
    photograph of, 409
  surface anatomy and peripheral nerve fields
      of, **410**
  thigh, anterior
    deep fasciae of, 414
    deep layer of, **424**
    deep vessels and nerves of, **425**
    movements of, **426**
    muscles of, 414, 415, 418, **418–421, 426**
    superficial vessels and nerves of, **416**
  thigh, lateral
    muscles of, 427
  thigh, medial
    deep fasciae of, 414
    deep layer of, **424**
    deep vessels and nerves of, **425**
    muscles of, 414, **421,** 427
  thigh, posterior
    fascia lata of, 415
    hamstring muscles of, 430, 437
    muscles of, 427, **437**
    sciatic nerve and popliteal vessels of, 436
    superficial vessels and nerves of, 428
  thigh, superficial
    gluteal muscles and, 429
Limb, upper, 2, **33**
  abduction, 37
  arteries, **28,** 38
  arteriogram, 38
  attachments of muscles, **65**
  blood vessels, 38
  bones, **42,** 64, 65, **122**
  cross sections of, **137**
  cutaneous innervation, 35
  cutaneous nerves, **40**
  dermatomes, **35, 86**
  muscles, **44, 45**
  muscular contours, **43**
  nerves, **39,** 66
  posterior muscles, **86**
  posterior, muscles and dermatomes (review), **86**
  radial nerve distribution, 53
  superficial venous patterns in, **41**
  surface anatomy, **34, 42**
  surface and skeletal anatomy, **42**
Linea alba, 15
Liver, 149, 196, 258
  anterior body wall, 248
  anterior surfaces of, 271
  arterial supply, 257
  bare area, 249, 270, 271
  blood supply, **257**
  caudate lobe of, 259, 260
  cirrhosis of, 12
  diaphragmatic furrows, 275
  diaphragmatic surface, 274
  diaphragmatic surface of, 271
  division of, 274
  dorsocranial view of, 270
  embryonic, 248
  and falciform, 248
  gallbladder, 306
  and gallbladder, 306
  hepatic divisions, 274
  inferior margin, 288
  left lobe of, 243, 250, 257, 270, 320
  left triangular ligament, 270
  metastatic tumor in, **277**
  in the neonate, 243
  position of, 270

    posterior surface of, 271
    right lobe of, 252, 264, 270
    round ligament of, 274
    segments of, 272, **274**
    shape of, 275
    spleen, 318
    superior mesenteric artery of, 257
    surface projection of, **270**
    surgery, 272
    tumor mass, 277
    visceral surface, 274, 278
Long thoracic vein, 23
Lower limb. *See* Limb, lower
Lumbar enlargements, 403
Lumbar intervertebral disk
    median sagittal section through, 398
    mucoid material of, 398
    photograph of, 398
Lumbar lymph nodes, 352
Lumbar puncture, 408
Lumbar triangle, 11
Lumbar vertebrae
    anterior view of, 396
    cranial view of, 396
    CT of, **284**
    intervertebral disks and ligaments, 397
    lateral view of, 396
    ligamenta flava between adjacent, 396
    magnetic resonance image of, 398
    median sagittal section of, 397
    zygapophyseal joints ligamenta flava between
        adjacent, 396
Lumbosacral plexus
    anterior thigh, 316
    posterior abdominal wall, 316
Lumbosacral trunk, 316
Lunar months, 336
Lung(s), **157**
    bronchopulmonary segments
        lateral view, **159**
        medial view, **161**
    costodiaphragmatic recess, 164
    development into pleural membranes, 153
    diaphragmatic surfaces, 160
    dissected hilum of, 164
    lateral (sternocostal) view, **158**
    lateral view, 157
    medial (mediastinal) view, **160**
    mediastinal surfaces, 160
    sternocostal view, 158
Lunula, 138
Lymphangiogram
    of axilla, **7**
    of pectoral and axillary lymph nodes, 7
Lymphatic channel flow, 210
Lymphatic drainage
    adult female breast from, **8**
    on lateral scalp and face, **525**
    patterns of, **525, 539**
    thoracic duct, **210**
Lymphatic vessels, **266**
Lymph channels, 7
Lymph drainage, 7
Lymph nodes
    axillary, 20, 211
        apical, **8**
        fascia, 4
    bronchopulmonary, 174
    central axillary, **8**
    deep cervical, 8
    in deep cervical and axillary regions, 540
    drainage patterns of, 525, 539
    iliac, 211
    inframammary, 8
    inguinal, 211

        deep, 417
        superficial, 417
    paraesophageal and tracheobronchial, 198
    parasternal, 8
    regional, **211**
    sacral, 211
    superficial axillary, 16
    supraclavicular, 8
    that drain breast, **7**
Lymph vessels, **211,** 260

M

Magnetic resonance images
    of ankle, subtalar, and talonavicular joints,
        508
    cross section at lower third of arm, 133
    of foot through metatarsal bones, 515
    of knee joint, 489
    of lumbar vertebrae, 398
    of orbit, 605, 610
    of right femur, 512
    of right upper limb through middle of humerus,
        132
    of thorax
        at level of aortic valve, 213
        at level of superior vena cava, 212
        through distal part of right thigh, 512
        through metatarsal bones of right foot, 515
        through middle of right thigh, 511
Male external genitalia, surface anatomy of, 367
Male genital organs
    autonomic innervation of, 235
    innervation of, **235**
Male genitourinary system, diagram of, 357
Male inguinal region, **236**
Male nipple, 2
Male pelvic organs, 353, **353**
Male pelvis, **326, 351**
    anteroinferior aspect, 327
    blood vessels of, 351
    cross section, **364**
    cross section of, 364
    CT image of, 364
    inferior outlet, 327
    median sagittal section of, 355
    midsagittal section, **355**
    pelvic diaphragm, 362
    rectum, internal iliac artery of, **351**
    visceral innervation, **362**
Male perineum
    muscles, **365**
    nerves, **358**
    nerves and blood vessels, 366
    penis, surface anatomy; dorsal vessels and
        nerves, **367**
    superficial muscles of, 365
    surface anatomy of, 365
    vessels and nerves, **366**
Male thorax, surface contours on, 2
Male urethra, 356
Male urogenital diaphragm, **358**
Male urogenital organs, 252
Malleoli, 455
Malleus, 662
Mammary lobes, 4, 6
Mandible, 571, 629, 633, 643, 688
    angle of, 557, 634
    body of, 205
    in chewing, swallowing, 624
    condyle of, 568
    inner surface, 634
    mylohyoid line of, 641, 648
    neck of, 633
    protrudes, 556

radiograph of, 640, **640**
ramus of, 564, 644
Mandibular arch and lower teeth, 634
Mandibular nodes, 211
Manubrium, 19, 140
Maxilla, radiograph of, 640
Maxillary arch
  and bony palate, 635
Maxillary sinus, 595
McBurney's point, 302
Medial bicipital furrow, 34
Medial crus of superficial inguinal ring, 15
Medial epicondyle, 70, 125
Medial intermuscular septum, 58, 70
Medial rectus, 675
Medial umbilical fold, 222
Median antebrachial vein, 36, 41
Median cubital vein, 29, 36
Median umbilical fold, 222, 250
Mediastinum, **166, 167**
  great vessels, **170**
  with the mediastinal pleura, 166, 167
  subdivisions, **170,** 176
Medulla, 312
Membranes, 119, 126, 356, 651, 652, 660, 684
  acoustic
    external, 557, 564, 565, 568, 657, 658, 659,
      665
    internal, 586, 588, 666, 670, 681
  antebrachial interosseous, 87
  anterior atlantooccipital, 389
  atlantooccipital, 384, 584
  cricovocal, 654
  interosseous, 496
  nasal
    inferior, 598, 614, 618
    middle, 614
    superior, 614
  perineal, 345, 347, 348, 350
  pleural, 153
  posterior atlantooccipital, 384, 389, 391
  quadrangular, 655
  tectorial, 390, 391, 586
Membranous labyrinth, 668, 685, 686
Meningeal dura mater, 406
Menisci
  arterial supply of, 495
  C-shaped, 495
  lateral, 495
  medial, 495
Mesenteric vein joins, 299
Mesoappendix, 288
Mesocolon, 251
Mesogastria, 248, 249
Mesonephric duct, 331, 357
Metacarpal bones, 73, 83, 85, 87, 91, 92, 96, 103,
  109, 110, 128, 129, 130, 131, 137, 138
Metatarsophalangeal joint, 454
Midclavicular line, 2
Middle ear
  frontal section through, 659
  lateral wall of right, 660
  nerves of, **665**
  ossicles, 661
  structures in, 662
Midrespiratory phase, 270
Milk line, 4
Mitral valve, 187
Molar tooth, 595, 621, 626, 634, 635, 636, 637,
  640
  impacted lower third, 639
  lower, 550
  lower second, 640
  upper, 625
Mons pubis, 344

Mouth
  floor of, 624
  midsagittal section of, 642
Mucous membrane, 213, 255, 278, 349, 354, 359, 360,
    621, 622, 626, 642, 645, 646, 648, 652, 655
  of conus elasticus, 656
  of isthmus of fauces, 646
  laryngeal, 650
  of lip, 619
  of mouth, 630, 634
  pharyngeal, 655, 656
  thin transparent, 600
  of tongue, 650, 688
  transparent, 593
  vocal fold, 656
Muscle fibers, 18, 169, 237, 421, 431, 643, 646
  cardiac, 189
  intercostal
    external, 146
    internal, 146
  intrinsic, 550
  nonstriated, 163
Muscles, 24, 45, 60, 100, 101, 262, 314, 346, 349,
    362, 374, 378, 453, 477, 550, 646, 648
  of abdominal walls, 15
  abduct, 137, 458
  abductor digiti minimi, 97, 128, 471, 477, 516
  abductor hallucis, 471, 473, 477
  abductor pollicis brevis, 96, 97, 110, 128
  abductor pollicis longus, 44, 71, 83, 87, 89, 128
  accessory, 18
  acromial, 33
  acromion, 42, 44
  adductor, 247, 419, 425
  adductor hallucis, 472, 474, 475, 507
  adductor hallucis transverse head, 477
  adductor longus, 410, 421
  adductor pollicis, 44, 93, 96, 105, 107, 128
  adjacent tensor veli palatini, 646
  anconeus, 44, 45, 81, 83, 86, 87, 89
  anterior abdominal wall, 169, 224
  of anterior arm, **56, 57**
  anterior auricular, 523
  anterior cervical intertransversarius, 541
  anterior compartment, 449
  of anterior compartment of leg, 447
  anterior digastric, 536
  anterior forearm, 70, 72
  anterior intertransversus, 541
  anterior scalene, 21
  anterior vertebral, 542
  aryepiglottic, 647, 653
  attachments
    bones of right foot, 500–501
    on fibula and tibia, 468
    right pelvis and femur, 479
  back
    erector spinae and semispinalis, **375**
    superficial, **373**
  biceps, 20, 30, 32, 54, 56, 58, 61, 62, 70, 76, 81,
    86, 116
  biceps brachii, 2, 11, 17, 21, 23, 34, 49, 56, 58, 84
  biceps femoris, 429
  brachialis, 11, 32, 45, 49, 56, 57, 59, 62, 76, 78, 81,
    124, 134
  brachioradialis, 34, 45, 56, 62, 70, 71, 76, **80,** 81,
    83, 84, 85, 86, 89
  buccinator, 552, 619
  bulbocavernosus, 368
  bulbospongiosus, 347, 350
  carpi ulnaris, 74
  cervical, 148
    intercostal, 541
    interspinous, 385
  ciliary, 603, 609, 675

circular, 255, 547
coccygeus, 343, 362
coracobrachialis, 17, 20, 23, 30, 49, 56, 57, 58, 86
cremaster, 15, 230, 236, 237, 369
  testis, 237
cricothyroid, posterior view of, 653
cruropedal, 466
deep lateral thoracic, **22**
deep, of posterior leg, 466
of deep palmar hand region, **100, 101**
deep posterior compartment, 466
deep transverse perineal, 358, 365
deltoid, 2, 15, 17, **17,** 21, 23, 27, 30, 32, 33, 42, 44,
  45, 58, 62, 86, 119, 148, 221
deltopectoral triangle, 1, 2, 15, **22**
digitorum superficialis, 45
dorsal forearm, 73
dorsal interosseous, 102, **102,** 458, 500
  of ear, 549
epicranius, 522, 523
erector spinae, 318, 320
  iliocostalis, longissimus, and spinalis parts
    of, 377
  and its overlying fascia, 374
    quadratus lumborum and psoas major muscles
      of, 386
  and semispinalis capitis muscles, 375
  and semispinalis muscles, **375**
extensor carpi radialis, 66, 134
extensor carpi radialis brevis, 56, 62, 81, 86, 89
extensor carpi radialis longus, 45, 56, 62, 71, 81,
  89
extensor carpi ulnaris, 81, 86
extensor digiti minimi, 86
extensor digitorum, 44, 81, 86, 89
extensor digitorum brevis, 457, 458, 500
extensor digitorum longus, 448
extensor forearm, 87, 88
extensor hallucis, 414
extensor hallucis brevis, 457, 458
extensor hallucis longus, 451
  *chart, 448
extensor pollicis brevis, 44, 83, 89, 93
extensor pollicis longus, 81, 83, 89
extensors carpi radialis longus, 86
external anal sphincter, 348, 358, 366
external intercostal, 21, 146, 148
external oblique, 4, 11, 13, 15, 21, 27, 44, 139,
  224, 225
  fibers of, 221, 224
extraocular, 589, **605,** 605–607, 606–607, 675,
  676
of eyelids, 549
facial, 547, 548, 550, 552, 594, 682
of facial expression, 681
fascia over
  latissimus dorsi, 4
  triceps, 4
femoral, 316
femorotibial, 466
fibular, 452
fibularis brevis, 451
  *chart, 448
fibularis longus, 448
fibularis tertius, 448
flexor capri radialis, 45, 70, 71, 73, 76, 128
flexor carpi ulnaris, 45, 70, 71, 73, 76, 78, 81, 83,
  87, 128
flexor digiti minimi, 97, 101, 105, 106, 477
flexor digiti minimi brevis, 128
flexor digitorum, 105
flexor digitorum brevis, 471, 477
flexor digitorum longus, 465, 469
flexor digitorum profundus, 74, 128
flexor digitorum superficialis, 45, 70, 71, 73, 76, 128

Muscles (*continued*)
flexor hallucis brevis, 477
flexor hallucis longus, 465, 466, 469
flexor pollicis brevis, 96, 97, 98, 128, 138
flexor pollicis longus, 44, 70, 71, 74, 128
flexor retinaculum, 45, 96, 462
of forearm, 83
  deep, **72**
  deep extensor, **82, 83,** 87
  dorsal, 85
  flexor, 73, 74
  posterior, 80
  radial extensor, 85
  superficial, 70
  supinator, 85
of forearm, flexor muscle chart, **73**
four-sided, 315
gastrocnemius, 461, 468
gemellus, 431
  inferior, 431, 479
genioglossal, 624
geniohyoid, 556
gluteal, 429
  *chart of, 434
  deep, 438
  middle and deep, 432
  safe gluteal quadrant of, **435**
  superficial thigh and, 429
gluteus maximus, 11, 429, 430
  abductors and medial rotators, 431
  right, 431
gluteus medius, 432, 433
gluteus minimus, 433
gracilis, 419, 424
hamstring, 415, 427, 430, 436, 437, 510, 512
of hip, 426
hyoglossus, 224, 545
hypothenar, 45, **97**
iliacus, 315, 426
iliococcygeus, 247, 343, 362
iliocostalis, 379
iliocostalis lumborum, 375, 377
iliocostalis thoracis, 319, 375, 376, 377
iliopsoas, 419, 421
  flexor of thigh, 420
inferior gemellus, 432, 435, 437, 438
inferior oblique, 675
inferior rectus, 675
infrahyoid, 519, 538, 559
infraspinatus, 11, 32, 33, 116
innervated, 694
innervations of, 607
intercostal, 228, 318
of intermediate compartment, 516
internal abdominal oblique, 234
internal anal sphincter, 359
internal intercostal, 21, 146
internal oblique, 148, 223, 224, 226
internal oblique muscle abdominis, 230
interossei
  dorsal, 476, 477
  plantar, 476, 477
involuntary, 209
ischiocavernosus, 350, 365, 368
laryngeal, 650, 654, 691
lateral, 414, 447
on lateral and posterior aspect of arm, **62**
of lateral compartment, 516
lateral rectus, 606, 676
lateral thoracic, 11
latissimus dorsi, 3, 10, 11, 15, 20, 21, 22, 23, 26,
    27, 30, 44, 54, 58, 321
left anterior forearm, 70
left psoas, 317
levator anguli oris, 523, 547, 551, 552, 594, 619, 641

levator ani, 343, 361, 363
  fibers of, 359
levator costae, 377
levator palpebrae superioris, 675
levator scapulae, 21, 32, 54
levator scapuli, 526
longissimus capitis, 375, 377, 378, 381–384, 541
longissimus thoracis, 319, 375, 376, 377
longus capitis, 148, 541, 542, 622
longus colli, 146, 542
lower limb, 2
lumbrical, 98, 104, **104,** 108, 472
  first, second, third, and fourth, 477
magnus, 421
major, 11, 15, 17, 18, 20–22, 26, 32, 44, 54, 64, 65,
    148, 215, 216
masseter, 556
of medial compartment, 516
medial head of gastrocnemius, 462
medial lumbar intertransverse, 380
median nerve supplies, 50
middle scalene, 21, 47, 384, 526, 528, 537, 539,
    540, 542
minimus, 364, 432
minor, **18**
of mouth, 549
multifidus, 380, 383, 384
muscle deltoid, 20
mylohyoid, 556, 624, 677
nasal, 547
of nose, 549
oblique auricular, 657
oblique head, 477
obturator externus, 424
obturator internus, 363, 364
obturator nerve supplies, 440
occipitofrontal, 383
ocular, origin of, 608
omohyoid, 21, 30, 54
opponens digiti minimi, 97, 98
opponens pollicis, 96, 97, 98, 128
oral, 547, 619
palatal, 648
palatopharyngeus, 620
palmar interossei, 128
palmar interosseous, 103
palmaris brevis, 94, 95
palmaris longus, 45, 70, 71, 73, 76
pectinate, 182
pectineus, 410, 419
  quadrangular and flat, 420
pectoralis major, 2, 3, 4, 9, 10, 11, 15, **18,** 21, 26,
    27, 30, 44, 56, 58, 62, 139, 148
  cut margin, 224
pectoralis major and minor, 224
pectoralis minor, **18,** 20–23, 27, 54, 56, 58, 148,
    224
pectoral, pectoralis major and deltoid muscles, **17**
perineal, 346
peroneus logus, 414
pharyngeal, 199, 201, 632, 643
pharyngeal constrictor, 641
piriformis, 432
plantar
  *chart of, 477
  first layer of, 471, 477
  second layer of, 472, 477
  third layer of, 475, 477
plantaris, 463
  *chart, 468
platysma, 15, **17,** 521
popliteal, 487, 488, 492
popliteus, 466
  *chart, 468
posterior auricular, 523, 548, 657

posterior cervical intertransversarius, 541
posterior cervical intertransverse, 384
posterior compartment, 462, 466, 468
posterior forearm, 70, 79, 89
posterior scalene, 21
posterior scapular, **32**
postural, 468
prevertebral, 541, 559
procerus, 547, 548, 551, 641
pronator quadratus, 70, 71, 74, 78, 84, 99, 105,
    128
pronator teres, 71, 73, 75, **75,** 78, 124
psoas, 196, 316
psoas major, 315, 426
psoas minor, 426
pterygoid, 556
pubococcygeus, 246, 247, 343, 362
puborectalis, 343, 345
pupillary dilator, 593
pyloric sphincter, 255, 268, 283
pyramidalis, 13, 230
quadratus femoris, 432
quadratus lumborum, 315
quadratus plantae, 472–475, 477, 498, 507, 516
quadriceps, 418, 511
quadriceps femoris, 419
  constituents of, 420
  innervation of, 418
radial antebrachial, 57
radial extensor, 85
radialis brevis, 45
of radius and ulna, muscle chart, **74**
rami communicantes, 206
rectus abdominis, 2, 3, 13, 139, 147, 230, 231
rectus abdominus, 7, 16
rectus capitis anterior, 542
rectus capitis lateralis, 542
rectus femoris, 421, 426
rhomboid, 374, 375, 382
  removal of, 374
rhomboideus major, 32, 54
rhomboideus minor, 32, 54
risorius, 521, 547, 548, 551, 619, 625
rotator cuff, 32, 61, 113
rotatores, 378, 380
sacrospinalis, 376
sartorius, 11, 418, 419, 424, 426
scalene, 519, 528, 541
scalenus anterior, 25
scalenus medius, 146
of scalp, 549
scapulae, 383
semimembranosus, 438
semispinalis, **375**
semispinalis capitis, 380
  and erector spinae muscle, 375
  medial and lateral fascicles of, 377
  and suboccipital triangle, 381
semispinalis thoracis, 377, 378, 381
semitendinosus, 424
semitendinosus-semimembranosus, 510
serratus anterior, 3, 4, 9, 10, 15, 19, 20, 21, 22, 27,
    30, 54, 139, 148, 221, 224
serratus anterior fascia, 16
serratus posterior, 376
sheath of rectus abdominis, 25
of shoulder, **55**
shoulder and arm, **54**
smooth, 301, 359, 608
soleus, 463, 467
  tibial nerve and, 465
spinalis, 379
spinous processes, 375
splenius capitis, 224
stapedius, 663, 664

sternocleidomastoid, 15, 19, 21, 44, 148, 224
sternothyroid, 146
strap, 519, 527, 532, 536, 693
styloglossus, 630, 632
stylohyoid, 148, 545, 624
subcapularis, 55
subclavius, 19, 21, 54, 56, 58, 148, 224
suboccipital, 385
subscapularis, 19, 21, 23, 30, 31, 46, 54, 56–58,
        61, 64, 112, 116, 117, 119, 215
superficial dorsal, 85
superficial extensor muscles of forearm,
        80, 81
superficial thigh, 429
of superficial thoracic, 15
superficial thoracic and abdominal wall, **11, 15**
superior, 374–378, 381, 383–385, 431
superioris alaeque nasi, 594
superior rectus, 675
supinator, 71, 76, 83, 85, 87, 89
supinator muscle extensor digiti minimi, 134
suprahyoid, 549, 624
supraspinatus, 30, 33, 54, 61, 62, 67, 116, 117
temporalis, 552
tensor fasciae latae, 11, 363, 364, 409, 410, 418,
        420, 429, 437, 479, 480
tensor fascia lata, 414, 415, 419
tensor tympani, 663
tensor veli palatini, 622, 641, 642, 646, 647, 689,
        691
teres major, 3, 11, 26, 30, 32, 33, 44, 54, 62
teres minor, 11, 32, 33, 44, 116, 117
tertius, 447
thenar, 45, 50, 96, **97,** 105, 107, 137
thumb, 83
thyroarytenoid, 654, 656
thyroepiglottic, 654
tibialis anterior, 449
    in anterior compartment, 449
    *chart, 448
tibialis posterior, 466, 469
    *chart, 468
trachealis, 163
tragicus, 527, 657
transverse auricular, 657
transverse lingual, 627
transverse perineal, 343, 345, 347, 350, 358,
        365
transversospinal, 386
transversus, 230
transversus abdominis, 148, 227, 230, 241
transversus thoracis, 146, 147, 217
transverus abdominis, 25
trapezius, 11, 19, 30, 44, 527, 669, 691, 692
triceps, 30, 32, 33, 42, 44, 45, 54, 58, 62, 70, 81, 86
triceps brachii, 11, 53, 116, 124
upper fibers of popliteus, 495
of upper limb
    anterior and posterior views, **45**
    anterior view, **64**
    lateral view, **44**
    posterior view, **65**
urethral sphincter, 347, 353, 358
urogenital, 358
vaginal sphincter, 345
vastus, 420
vastus lateralis, 429
vocalis, 655
voluntary, 687, 689
zygomatic, 550
Muscular floor, sagittal section of, 622
Muscular folds, 620
Musculocutaneous nerve, 23
Musculophrenic, 231
Musculophrenic vessels, 147

N

Nail matrix, 138
Nasal cavities, 671
    frontal section through, 595
    lateral wall of, **613,** 672
    right
        bony lateral wall of, 614
Nasal septum, 671
    structure and blood supply, 615
Nasolacrimal duct, 598, 599, 613
    drainage routes of, 615
Neck, 3
    anterior triangle of, **523,** 531
    anterior view of musculature, **519**
    brachial plexus, 534
    chains of lymph nodes in, 526
    deep arteries and veins of, 536
    external investing and pretracheal fascial layers,
        527
    fascial planes, 527
    infraclavicular region, 535
    infrahyoid muscles of, 519
    large vessels, 532
    muscles of
        deeper layers, 224
        posterior triangle, 528
        semispinalis capitis and suboccipital
            triangle, 381
        splenius cervicis, splenius capitis, and
            semispinalis capitis, 376
        transversospinal groups, 378
    muscular floor of posterior triangle of, 528
    nerves of, 522, 524
    platysma layer, 529
    posterior, 382
    posterior triangle of, **523**
    scalene muscles, 528
    sternocleidomastoid layer, 530
    subclavian artery, 533
    superficial lateral vessels, 522
    superficial lymph nodes, 526
    superficial nodes of, 539
    suprahyoid submandibular region, 545, **546**
    triangles of, 520
    veins of, 535
    vessels of, 526
Neck viscera, midsagittal section of, 642
Nerve(s)
    abducens, 602, 669
    abducens (VI), 675, 676
    accessory, 669, **691**
        Schema of, 692
        traversing posterior triangle of neck, 692
    accessory (XI)
        diagrammatic representation of, 691
        schema of, 692
    alveolar
        inferior, 633
        superior, 633
    anterior and posterior ethmoid, 603
    anterior cutaneous, 10, 13, 27, 220
    anterior cutaneous intercostal, 220
    anterior femoral cutaneous, 13
    anterior gastric, 206
    anterior scrotal, 236
    anterior thoracic segmental, **10**
    anus, 349
    apertures in base of skull transmitting, 670
    and arteries of the posterior forearm (deep
        dissection), **89**
    arteries of the posterior forearm (superficial
        dissection), **88**
    attachments to base of brain, **669**
    auriculotemporal, 551, 687

axillary, 26, 33, 39, 40, **52,** 67
    distribution, 52
    spinal segments forming, 52
cervical
    eighth, 403
    first, 403
        dorsal root ganglion of, 402
cervical spinal, 382
chorda tympani, 663
cluneal, 411
    medial, posterior primary rami (boldface) of,
        372
    superior, posterior primary rami (boldface)
        of, 372
cochlear, 686
common fibular, 411, 441, 450
common plantar digital, 470
cutaneous, 39, 220
    of anterior thigh, 416
    branches of, 409, 411
    branches of medial brachial, 36
    distribution, 372
    lateral dorsal, 454
    lateral sural, 442
    medial sural, 442
    patterns, 552
cutaneous, distribution, 372
deep
    of posterior compartment of leg, 467
    of suboccipital region, 383
    of upper back, 383
deep fibular, 459
deep radial, 78, 89
dorsal digital, 90, 92, 93
facial (VII)
    chorda tympani branch of, **684**
    diagrammatic view of, 681
    in facial canal, 681
    greater petrosal branch of, **683**
    on side of face, 682
femoral, 440
fibular, 441, 453
    common, 411
    deep, 454
    superficial, 454
    superficial and deep, 411, 453
fibular (superficial and deep), 441
frontal, 601
    supraorbital branch of, 594
    supratrochlear branch of, 594
fused precervical, 669
genitofemoral, 234, 316
glossopharyngeal, 669, 687
    and its lingual branches, 688
glossopharyngeal (IX)
    coursing from skull base through jugular fora-
        men, 688
    in oropharynx, 688
    sensory innervation of, 687
hypoglossal (XII)
    diagrammatic representation of, 693
    in superior neck region, 694
ilioinguinal, 13
iliohypogastric, 220, 236, 411
iliohypogastric lumbar, 316
ilioinguinal, 220, 234, 367
iliopubic, 229, 411, 440
inferior cervical cardiac, 208
inferior gluteal, 363, 432–434, 439, 441, 510
inferior laryngeal, 650
infraorbital, 594
infratrochlear, 594, 603
intercostal, 220
intercostobrachial, 13, 16, 20, 26, 27, 29, 36, 40
intermediate supraclavicular, 16

Nerve(s) (*continued*)
  internal laryngeal, 545, 651, 652, 689
  lacrimal, 594, 601
  lateral ampullary, 685
  lateral antebrachial cutaneous, 29, 36, 39, 49, 59, 67
  lateral brachial cutaneous, 33
  lateral cutaneous, 10, 26, 220
  lateral femoral cutaneous, 440
  lateral plantar, 470, 473
  lateral supraclavicular, 16, 29
  lateral sural, 411
  lesser petrosal, 551, 586, 588, 616, 625, 665, 679, 687
  of limbs, 372
  lingual, 649, 680
  location of, 670
  of lower limb, 440
  lower surface, 148
  male perineum, **358**
  mandibular, 677, 680
  masseter, 677
  masseteric, 563–566, 680
  maxillary, 677, 680
  medial and lateral plantar, 470
  medial antebrachial cutaneous, 29, 34, 36
  medial brachial cutaneous, 29, 36, 58
  medial calcaneal, 470
  medial cluneal, 372, 428, 430
  medial pterygoid, 677
  medial supraclavicular, 16
  median, 23, 34, 40, **50**, 76, 78, 86, 97, 106, 107, 124
    distribution, 50
    distribution, spinal segments, and palsy, **50**
    palsy, 50
    spinal segments forming, 50
  meningeal, 588
  middle cardiac, 644
  middle cervical cardiac, 208
  middle cluneal, 411, 436
  musculocutaneous, 39, 49, 58, 86
    distribution, 49
  nasociliary, 594, 601–603, 603, 676–678
  obturator, 316, 425
    diagrammatic representation of, 440
    of medial thigh, 440
  occipital
    greater, 383, 385
    lesser, 383
    third, 385
  oculomotor
    inferior branch of, 604
  olfactory (I)
    olfactory bulb and tract, **671–672**
    somatomotor fibers of, 675
  ophthalmic, 601
  optic, 601, 603
  optic (II)
    tract and, 674
    visual fields and, 673, 674
  ovarian autonomic, 330
  palmar digital, 39, 92
  of penis, 366
  perineal, 348, 358, 366
  perineal vessels, 366
  peripheral, 386, 672
  petrosal
    deep, 616
    greater, 616
    lesser, 616
  pharyngeal, 679
  phrenic, 27, 150
  plantar, 473

plantar digital
    common, 473
    proper, 473
  of popliteal fossa, 442
  posterior abdominal vessels, 317
  posterior ampullar, 668
  posterior antebrachial, 37, 66
  posterior antebrachial cutaneous, 36, 39, 67
  posterior brachial cutaneous, 39, 67
  posterior ethmoidal, 678
  posterior femoral cutaneous, 441
  posterior gastric, 206
  posterior interosseous, 89, 135
  of posterior lower trunk, 372
  posterior scrotal, 366
  posterior vagal, 689
  presacral, 208, 233, 235
  proper plantar digital, 470
  pterygopalatine, 616
  radial, 29, 39, 40, **53,** 58, 67, 76, 86, 88
    distribution, 53
    distribution, spinal segments, and palsy, **53**
    palsy, 53
    spinal segments forming, 53
  root, 639
  sacral, 209, 233, 247, 316, 321, 399, 403
  saphenous, 411, 423, 440, 441, 446, 460
    cutaneous branch of, 454
  scapular, 48
  sciatic, 432, 441
    diagrammatic representation of, 441
    of popliteal fossa, 442
    in posterior thigh, 510
    of posterior thigh, 436, 439
    tibial division of, 437
  segmental, 372
  sensory, 36, 68, 89, 232, 366, 382, 383, 446, 553, 596, 677, 679
  septal, 615
  sinus, 687, 689
    carotid, 689
  spinal, 10, 14, 206, 207, 321, 362, 372, 379, 384, 386, 402, 404, 405, 406, 407, 542
    branching of, 386
    C3, 372
    cervical, 380, 528
    consecutive, 372
    cutaneous branches of, 10
    destruction of, 372
    formation of, 403
    lumbar, 379, 380, 405
    middle cervical, 380, 528
    mixed, 14, 404
    posterior primary rami of, 372
    and segments in adult, 402
    single, 35, 372
    upper cervical, 379
    upper thoracic, 379, 380
  sublingual, 649, 694
  submental, 546
  suboccipital
    suboccipital region, 385
    through suboccipital triangle, 383
  subscapular, 31, 48, 58
  superficial fibular, 450, 459
  superficial radial, 78
  superior alveolar, 566, 616, 633
  superior cluneal, 372, 411, 428, 436
  supraclavicular, 13, 16, 17, 40
  suprascapular, 33, 58, 61
  symphysis, 230
  of taste, **628**
  temporal branch of facial, 594
  tensor tympani, 677
  tensor veli palatini, 677

thoracic, 40
    lateral cutaneous branches, 10
    spinal, 382
    splanchnic, 166
  thoracodorsal, 26, 27, 58
  tibial, 464, 473
    in posterior leg, 465
  trigeminal (V)
    and its branches, 677
    mandibular division of, 680
    maxillary division of, **679**
    ophthalmic division of, **678**
  trochlear (IV), 601, 602, 675, 676
  ulnar, 20, 23, 29, 34, 40, 58, 67, 76, 78, 86, 89, 94
    distribution, 51
    palsy, 51, 52
    spinal segments forming, 51
  of upper limb, **39**
  vaginal, 233
  vagus (X), 150, 206, 669, **689**
    diagrammatic representation of, 689
    in thorax, 690
  to vastus medialis, 423
  vestibular, 667, 668, 685, 686
  vestibulocochlear (VIII)
    connections in brain, 686
    diagrammatic schema of, 686
    vestibular apparatus of, 685
  zygomaticofacial, 594
  zygomaticotemporal, 554, 563
  zygomatico-temporal, 612
Nerve supplies, 460, 631, 679, 687, 693
  abducens, 602, 676
  hypoglossal, 632
  lateral plantar, 473
  medial plantar, 473
  saphenous, 411, 460
  sciatic, 441
Neurovascular structures, 464, 467
Newborn child
  abdominal and thoracic viscera, 243
  anterior abdominal wall, **242**
  functional anatomy of, 243
  scrotum, **242**
  thoracic and abdominal viscera, **243**
  umbilical region in, 242
Nipple, 4, 6
Node(s), 6, 174, 178, 188, 198, 211, 212, 236, 260, 266, 417, 526, 539. *See also* Lymph nodes
  anterior axillary, 7
  anterior diaphragmatic, 174
  anterior mediastinal, 174
  apical, 215
  axillary, 7, 211
  celiac, 266
  deltopectoral, 7
  ileocolic, 247
  intercostal, 540
  mastoid, 539
  medial (apical) axillary, 7
  mesenteric, 211
  pancreaticoduodenal, 266
  parasternal mammary, 7
  paratracheal, 212, 215
  pectoral, 7, 540
  popliteal lymphatic, 442
  posterior mediastinal, 198
  pyloric, 266
  sinoatrial, 179, 189, 190
  splenic, 319
  submandibular, 211, 525, 539, 625, 626
  tracheobronchial, 164
  upper abdominal, 8
Nostrils, 613

Notch, 594, 657
  acetabular, 323, 324, 481
  angular, 254, 258, 261
  of apex of heart, 177
  of cardiac apex, 164
  greater sciatic, 325
  inferior vertebral, 393
  lesser sciatic, 324
  nasal, 550
  suprascapular, 519
  suprasternal, 19, 144, 162, 519
Nuchal line, 569
  superior, 373, 520, 528, 549, 569, 591
Nucleus pulposus, 398

O

Oblique fissure, 158
Oblique pericardial sinus, 173
Obliquus capitis inferior, 383, 385
Obliquus capitis superior, 383, 385
Obturator canal, 326
Obturator foramen, 325
Occipital bone, 379, 380, 385, 389, 390, 391, 402,
        404, 541, 542, 569, 571, 572, 585, 586, 643
  articulations of, 389
  inferior nuchal line of, 385
Occlusal surfaces, 639
Odontoid process
  anterior surface of, 388
  of axis, 390
  of axis and posterior articular facet, 388
  radiographs of, 391
Olecranon, 62, 83, 125
  fossa, 124
  processes, 122
Olfactory bulb, 671
  basal forebrain showing, 672
Olfactory epithelium, 672
Olfactory mucosa, 671
Olfactory tract, 672, 674
Olfactory trigone, 672
Omental bursa, 248, 249, 258, 259
Omental foramen, 258, 259
Ophthalmoplegia, 675
Opponens digiti minimi, 128
Optic canal, 608
Optic chiasma, 673, 674
Optic disk, 609
Oral cavity, 619–628
  anterior sublingual region of, 621
  floor
    inferior and superior views, 624
    viewed from neck, 623
  lips viewed from within, 619
  midsagittal section of, 627
  mouth, 622
  nerves and arterial supply of opened, 632
  palate
    muscular folds and glands, 620
    and tongue, 619
  paramedian sagittal view of interior of, 622
  paramedian section of, 629
  parotid duct orifice, 621
  passage between, 619
  salivary glands, 625–626
Oral mucosa, 620
Ora serrata (yellow), 609
Orbicularis oris, 619
Orbital cavity
  arteries and veins within, 611, 612
  bony structure of, 595
  frontal section through, 595
  horizontal section through, 600
  left, medial wall of, 596

muscles of, 606
right
  lateral wall of, 596
  MRI of, 610
  sagittal view of, 600
Orbital septum, 597
Orbit, bony
  anterior view and frontal section of, 595
  extraocular muscles of, 606–607
  medial and lateral walls of, 596
  nerve and artery of
    left lateral views of, 605
    superior view of, 601–604
    trochlear nerve, 602
  superficial facial muscles around, 594
Organ of Corti, 686
Oronasopharyngeal lymphatic ring, 645
Oropharynx, 620
Osseous–aponeurotic canals, 471
Otic ganglion, 687
Ovarian vessels, 306, 330
Ovary, 233, 245, 303, 306, 330–335, 342, 417
  arterial supply, 335
  frontal section of, 332
  medial surface, 333
  mesovarian border, 333
  suspensory ligament, 342

P

Palate, 592, 619, 620, 628, 631, 648, 652, 683
  anterior view of, 622
  bony
    and maxillary arch, 635
    and upper teeth, 635
  hard, 571, 592, 613, 614, 619, 620, 622, 635, 640,
        648, 671, 683
  muscles of
    *chart of, 648
    soft, 646
  posterior, nerves and arteries of, 631
  and upper teeth, 635
Palatine tonsils, 619, 620
Palm, 1, 34, 42, 84, 95–99, 107, 108, 109, 434
  deep dissection of muscles and fingers, 99
  deep palmar arch, 109
  muscles and flexor tendon insertions, 98
  muscles and tendon sheaths, 96
  muscles, synovial sheaths, and tendons, 96
  nerves and arteries, 107, 108
  palmar arterial arches, 108
  superficial dissection, 95
  superficial nerves and arteries of, 94
  superficial palmar arch, 107
  superficial vessels and nerves, 94
  surface projection of arteries, and nerves to, 109
Palmar cutaneous branches, 29, 94
Palpebral conjunctiva, 600
Pancreas, 247, 248, 249, 253, 259, 260, 266, 266,
        276, 282, 282, 282–286, 294, 306, 307
  body of, 259
  diffuse inflammation, CT, 286
  head of, 283
  retroperitoneal, 249
  surface projection of, 282
  tumor
    transaxial image, 285
  tumor, CT of, 285
  uncinate process of, 284
Pancreatic ampulla and papilla, 268
Pancreatic duct, 283, 284
  head of, 283
  union of, 285
Pancreatic necrosis, 286
Pancreaticoduodenal nodes, 266

Pancreatitis, 286
Papilla(e), 268, 285, 628
  filiform, 628
  fungiform, 628
  incisive, 635
  inferior lacrimal, 593, 599
  parotid, 621
  renal, 312, 313
Parasternal lines, 2
Parasternal mammary nodes, 7
Parasternal nodes, 7
Parasympathetic fibers, 235
Paraumbilical veins, 12, 299
Parietal branches, 351
Parietal layer, of pleura, 154
Parietal peritoneum, 248
Parietal pleurae, 153
Parotid duct
  accessory parotid gland attached to, 625
  orifice, 621
Parotid gland, 551
  lateral view of, 625
  parasympathetic innervation, 551
Parotid nodes, 211
Patella, 409, 410, 412, 414, 420, 421, 426, 445, 484,
        485, 488, 489, 490, 493, 495, 512
  right, anterior and posterior aspect of, 495
Patellar retinacula
  medial and lateral, 484
Patellar structures, 484
PC. See Pyloric canal
Pecten of pubis, 315, 420, 421
Pectoral fascia, 6, 9, 16, 17, 521
Pectoral nodes, 7
Peduncle
  cerebellar, 669
  cerebral, 589, 674
Pelvic brim, 306
Pelvic diaphragm, 362
  muscles, 346
Pelvic inlet, size of, 327
Pelvic organs, autonomic and visceral afferent in-
    nervation of, 362
Pelvic viscera external genitalia, 355
Pelvis, 3, 211, 246, 247, 313, 323–370, 325–328,
        330, 332, 336, 343, 348, 352, 362, 363
  bones
    lateral view of adult and child, 323
    medial and anterior views, 324
  female
    anteroinferior view, 326
    articulations of, 326
    hip joints, 326
  frontal section, diagram of, 361
  left side of, 336
  lymph nodes and channels, 352
  male, diagram of, 325
  median sagittal section of, 246
  muscular floor of, 362
  position of, 332
  radiograph of, 325, 325
  right half of, 336
  right, posterior view of, 479
  uterus, 332
Penile urethra, 355
Penis, 1, 15, 221, 223, 235, 236, 237, 349, 351, 355,
        356, 358, 366–370
  bulb of, 235, 368
  corpora cavernosa, 368
  corpus spongiosum, 368
  cross sections through, 370
  deep dorsal vein of, 369, 370
  distal end of, 370
  dorsal artery of, 369
  dorsal nerve of, 367

Penis (*continued*)
erectile bodies of, 368
fundiform ligament of, 220, 223
glans, 355, 370
longitudinal section, 369
section through middle of, 370
shaft of, **370**
skin of, 369, 370
superficial dorsal vein, 236
vascular circulation of, **369**
ventral aspect, **368**
vessels and nerves of, 367
Pericardiacophrenic vessels, 165
Pericardium, 164, 166, 170–173, 175, **175**, 176, 183, 196, 199, 207, 243
posterior view, 199
serous, 170, 177, 212
Perineal raphe, 344
Perineal structures, 344
Perineal vessels, 348
nerve, 366
Perineum, **323–370,** 340, 341, 343, 345, 347–353, 355, 358, 361, 365, 366
anterior, 347
blood vessels of, 351
central point of, 345
female
inferior view of, 345
muscles of, 347
nerves and blood vessels of, 348
vessels and nerves, **348**
frontal section, diagram of, 361
levator, 346
midsagittal section, **355**
pudendal nerve of, 358
Peritoneal cavity, 353
Peritoneal reflections, 333
Peritoneum, 230, 238, 240, 242, 248, 249, 250, 255, 259, 270, 283, 289, 290, 319, 333, 353
fold of, 250, 288
glistening, 288
urogenital, 359
Periumbilical veins, 13
Pes anserinus (goose's foot), 462
Pevator scapulae, 374
Phalanges, 128
Phalanx, 74, 96, 104, 127, 138, 472, 475, 500
coronoid, 73
Pharyngeal tonsil, 620
Pharynx, **641–647**
external, 629–630
and its related cavities, 645
midsagittal section of, 642
muscles of, 629, **641**, 643, 646
*chart of, 648
nerves and vessels of, 644, 647
paramedian section of, 629
and soft palate from behind, 647
Plane, 433, 513
anteroposterior, 196
horizontal, 556
transpyloric, 3
Plantar aponeurosis, 470
Plantar flexion, 453
Plantar interossei, 476
Plate, 338, 398, 592, 639
cribriform, 571, 585, 587, 614, 615, 618, 669, 670, 672
of fibrocartilage, 580
fibrocartilaginous, 586
horizontal, 591
lateral, 585, 591
Pleura, 149, 153–156, 160
diaphragmatic, 152, 153, 155, 166, 170, 175, 196, 207, 243, 314

layers of, 153, 154
partiel, 166
projection of pleural borders, 156
pulmonary, 164, 212, 213, 215
reflections of, **156**
Pleural cavity, 153, 154
Plexus, 152, 362, 407, 564, 687, 690
anastomoses, 364
anterior gastric, 206
basilar, 578
coccygeal, 316
coeliac, 208
esophageal, 166, 167, 204, 206, 690
external vertebral, 407
grouping of, 407
hypogastric, 235
inferior dental, 564, 633, 680
internal vertebral, 207, 407
intraparotid, 524, 554
lumbosacral, 386
pampiniform, 237, 239, 367, 369
prostatic, 235, 362, 364
rectal, 362
renal, 208, 233
subareolar, 7, 8
superior dental, 679
Pons, 208, 403, 404, 579, 584, 587, 589, 590, 669, 676, 678, 679, 680, 686, 688
caudal, 676
Popliteal fossa, 409
cross section of inferior thigh at level of, 512
deep muscles bounding, 443
femoral–popliteal–tibial arteriogram, 445
inferior thigh at level of, 512
nerves and vessels of, 442
popliteal artery of, 444
relationship of muscles, vessels, and nerves in, 488
subcutaneous dissection of, 442
sural branches of popliteal artery from, 464
tibial nerve and, 467
transverse section through, 488
Popliteal vein, 442
Popliteal vessels
within popliteal fossa, 442
of posterior thigh, 436
Porta hepatis, **259,** 260
structures, 258
Portal-caval shunt dissection, 204
Portal veins, 286
branches, ultrasound of, 273
branching, 272
branching patterns, **272**
formation of, 253
ultrasound scans, **273**
Portal venous systems (male), 195
Posterior brachial (arm) region, 1
Posterior cervical triangle, 1
Posterior humeral circumflex vein, 23
Posterior primary rami
of L1, L2, L3, S1, S2, and S3, 372
peripheral nerves derived from, 386
of spinal nerves, 386
Posterior superior iliac spine, 11, 311
Preaortic nodes, 260, 321
Preauricular nodes, 211
Preganglionic parasympathetic fibers, 675
Pregnancy
uterine growth, diagrammatic representation of, 336
uterus, sonogram, 338
Pregnant uterus
before birth, 336
fetal sonograms, **338**
fetal X-ray, **337**
midsagittal view, **336**

Prepuce, 246, 247, 344, 347, 355, 356, 367, 369, 370
of clitoris, 344, 349, 350
Principal lymph vessels, **211**
Process(es), 56, 73, 275, 314, 500, 571, 624, 685
accessory, 393, 396
acromial, 119
alveolar, 636
anterior clinoid, 580, 586
anterior malleolar, 660, 684
articular, 379, 380, 396
arytenoid cartilage, 652
condyloid, 639, 640
coronoid, 122
disease, 211
inflammatory, 105, 604
intramembranous, 571
jugular, 542, 569
mamillary, 380
middle clinoid, 581
nasal, 613
odontoid, 388, 390, 391
papillary, 319
peripheral, 685
pinous, 215
posterior clinoid, 586
styloid, 130, 643
uncinate, 247, 283, 284, 307, 398, 618
vaginal, 658
vocal, 652
Prominence
of facial canal, 658, 664
of lateral semicircular canal, 658, 663, 664
Promontory, 246, 325, 351, 387, 392, 401, 418, 420, 658, 659, 660, 664, 665, 683, 687
of sacrum, 315, 328, 399
subiculum, 658
Pronator teres, 71
Prostate gland, 235, 354, 357
Prostatic urethra incised anteriorly, 354
Proximal interphalangeal joints, 42
Proximal phalanx, 131, 138
Pterygopalatine fossa
lateral view of, 596
medial view of, 596
Pterygopalatine ganglion
and its branches, 616
Pubic arch, 326
Pubis, 227, 230, 246, 247, 315, 323–325, 336, 343, 346, 353, 363, 364, 368, 427
continuation, 230
fusion of, 323
ischial tuberosity, 324
mons, 344
pubovaginalis, 346
Pudendal canal, 348
Pudendal vessels
left internal, 351
Pulmonary trunk, 183
Pulmonary valve, 169
Pupil
constriction and dilation of, 593
dilator of, 603
sphincter of, 603
Pyloric antrum, 267
Pyloric canal, 265, 267
Pyloric sphincter, 255, 267
duodenal bulb, 265
Pyloroduodenal junction, 267

Q

Quadrangular space, 32
Quadrate lobes, 275
Quadriceps femoris, 421

R

Radial groove, 113
Radial notch, 122
Radial tuberosity, 122
Radiographs, 120, 121, 136, 161, 256, 261, 284, 291, 293, 490, 574
  anteroposterior, 498
  of atlantoaxial joints, 391
  of biliary duct system, 279
  of cervical spine, 400
  of duodenum, 261
  of hip joints, 325, 483
  of jejunum and ileum, **289**
  of knee joint, 493
  of large intestine, 305
  of lower esophagus, 261
  of lumbar spine, **401**
  of mandible and maxilla, 640
  and MRI of Ankle, 508
  of odontoid process, 391
  of pelvis, 325
  of proximal jejunum, 261
  of right knee, 484
  of right shoulder joint i, 120
  of right shoulder joint II, 121
  sacroiliac, 325
  of stomach, 261
  of subtalar and talocalcaneonavicular joints, 508
  of talocrural (ankle) joints, 498
  of thoracic spine, 400
  of veins, 23
  of the wrist and hand, 127
Radiopaque substance, 313
Radius, 42, 72, 74, 75, 83, 84, 87, 122–126, 129–131, 135, 136
  distal, 126
  distal aspect of, 126
  extensor muscles, 87
  fracture of, **75**
  fracture site, 75
  interosseous branch, 74
  muscle on anterior surface, 74
  pollicis, 87
Raphe, 345, 358
  compressing, 349
  lateral palpebral, 549
  median palatal, 635
  obturator anococcygeal, 346
  pterygomandibular, 550, 620, 622, 641
  short midline anococcygeal, 345
Recess, 290, 356, 491, 655, 677
  costodiaphragmatic, 164
  inferior duodenal, 290
  inferior ileocecal, 290
  pericardial, 172
  piriform, 200, 542, 645–647, 656
  sphenoethmoid, 613
  superior, 249, 319
Rectal ampulla, 304, 359
Rectouterine pouch, 333, 342
Rectovesical pouch, 355
Rectum, 219, 244, 245, 247, 297, 304, 306, 333, 342, 343, 353, 359–364
  arterial blood supply, 360
  arterial supply, **360**
  descending colon, 209
  external surface of, 359
  frontal section, 359
  inner surface of, 359
  internal and external surfaces, **359**
  internal iliac artery, branches of, **351**
  large intestine, 304
  median section, 360, **360**
  venous drainage of, 361

Rectus abdominis, 228
  sheath of, 230
Rectus capitis posterior major, 383, 385
Rectus capitis posterior minor, 385
Rectus sheath, 11, 16, 20, 147
  anterior layer, 4, 15, 221
  anterior layer of, 242
Reflections
  dorsal mesogastrium, 248
  peritoneal, 249, **353**
    adult female, 249
  of pleura, **154–156**
  primitive peritoneal, 248
Regions of body, 1, 22, 64, 90, 137, 164, 177, 186, 219, 220, 281, 286, 344, 358, 359, 517
  antebrachial, 42
  antecubital, 41
  anterior antebrachial, 1
  anterior brachial, 1
  anterior cervical, 219
  anterior cubital region, 1, 409
  anterior femoral, 1, 409
  anterior knee, 1, 409
  anterior neck, 1
  anterior shoulder, **31**
  anterior view, 219
  anterior wrist, 105
  axillary, 1, 23, 34, 42, 219
  of body, **1**
  buccal, 517
  cervical, anterior, 219
  clavicular, 535
  deltoid, 1
  elbow, vessels and nerves, **79**
  epigastric, 1
  frontal, 1
  gastrointestinal tract, **219**
  head and neck, **517**
  hypochondriac, 1
  hypogastric, 1
  infraclavicular, 1, 42
  inguinal, 1
  lateral abdominal, 1
  lateral pectoral, 1
  and longitudinal lines on male body, 2
  mental, 1
  nasal, 1
  oral, 1
  orbital, 1
  parietal, 1
  pectoral, 1, **17**
  pectoral, superficial vessels and cutaneous nerves, **16**
  posterior antebrachial, 1
  posterior brachial, 67
  posterior crural, 1
  posterior scapular, 33
  prevertebral, 541
  sternocleidomastoid, 1
  submandibular and submental, **545**
  temporomandibular, 557
  trochanteric, 1
  umbilical, 1
Renal arteriogram, **310**
Renal calyx, 312
Renal columns, 312
Renal impression, 287
Renal pelvis, 313, 331
Renal pyramids, 312
Renal segments, posterior surface of, 308
Renal sinus, 312
Renal vein, 309, 311
Renal vessels, 312

Retina, 600, 609, 610, 612, 673
  and its vessels, 611
  neural, 604
Retinacula, 456, 461, 462
  inferior extensor, 447
  inferior fibular, 456
  lateral patellar, 484
Retinaculum, 92, 96
  inferior fibular, 452, 455, 456, 498
Retrograde pyelogram, 313
Rhomboid major, 379
Rhomboid minor, 379
Ribs, 142, 143
  anterior surface, 19
  cage
    anterior surface, **19**
  and costal cartilages, **143**
  first, second, third, and eighth right, 142
  showing natural contour of thoracic cage, 143
  thoracic vertebrae articulation, 393
Right kidney, segments of, 308
Right lymphatic duct, 210
Right shoulder
  joint, anterior and posterior views of, **117**
  muscles, **54**
Right subclavian vein, 210
Right submandibular triangle, 545
Right testis
  anterior view, 238
  lateral view, 238
Rima glottidis, 656

S

Sacral hiatus, 399
Sacral plexus, 316
Sacroiliac joint, 322
  formation of, 387
  frontal section, 329
Sacrum, 30, 246, 247, 315, 322, 324, 325, 328, 329, 343, 373, 387, 392, 399, 409, 434
  anterior (pelvic) surface of, 399
  auricular (ear-shaped) surface of, 399
  and coccyx, **399**
  dorsal surface of, 399
Safe zone, 434
Sagittal section
  of temporomandibular joint, 558
  through pituitary gland and sella turcica, 587
  through the middle finger (ulnar view), **110**
Saphenous opening
  falciform margin of, 417
  in fascia lata, 417
Scalp, nerves of, 524
Scapula, 18, 20, 33, 42, 55, 112, 114, 115, 117, 120, 121, 141, 214, 371, 373, 379, 387
  dorsal surface, 112
  lateral view, 112
  skeleton of, **112**
  ventral surface, 112
Sciatic notches, 325
Scrotum, 236, 237, 238, 240–242, 241, 244, 246, 316, 353, 355, 357, 365, 367, 369
  cross section of, 240
  left, 237
  skin of, 237
  spermatic cord
    transverse section, 369
Semicircular canals, 667
Seminal vesicle, 235, 357
  ductus deferens, 364
Seminal vesicles, **354, 356,** 357
  radiograph of, 356
Semispinalis cervicis, 378, 380
  and thoracis, 377

Septa, 161, 238, 239, 240, 285, 355, 597, 615, 658, 663–665, 683
  canalis musculotubarii, 664, 665, 683
  connective-tissue, 161
  interatrial, 182, 184, 189
  intermuscular, 513
  interventricular, 178, 182–185, 188, 189, 193
  medial brachial intermuscluar, 133
  median fibrous, 627
  of penis, 370
  of scrotum, 246
  of tongue, 627
Serratus posterior inferior, 379
Serratus posterior superior, 379
Sheath, 16, 64, 221, 228, 230, 456, 477, 498, 608, 609
  carotid, 532
  digital, 92, 98
  digital fibrous, 471
  dural, 207
  fascial, 551
  femoral, 315, 316, 417
  of rectus abdominis muscle, 25, 44
  of styloid process, 666
  synovial, 455, 471
  tendinous, 110, 137
Shoulder, 30, 31, 33, 42, 52, 55, 64, 65, 115, 116, 119, 120, 520, 529, 692
  arteries, 67
  muscles of, **31**, 60, **63**
    anterior and posterior views, **55**
  nerves, **31**, 67
  posterior, 33
  region
    anterior aspect, muscles, **30**
    posterior aspect, muscles, **32**
    radiograph, 115
    rotator cuff capsule, **61**
    supraspinatus muscle, **61**
    supraspinatus muscle and rotator cuff capsule, **61**
  vessels, **30**, **31**
  and nerves, abduction of upper limb, **33**
Shoulder joint
  abduction, **31**
  and acromioclavicular joint, **116**
  adduction, **31**
  after removal of deltoid muscle, **119**
  bony structures, **114**
  extension, **31**
  flexion, **31**
  frontal section through, 119
  ligaments, 114, **114**
  radiograph, 120, 121
  rotation, **31**
  X-ray of right, **115**
Sigmoid colon, 290, 291, 297, 300, 305, 321
Sigmoid mesocolon, 290
Sinus, 175, 188, 355, 562, 573, 575, 577, 578, 580, 600, 617, 655
  anterior ethmoid, 615
  aortic, 185
  basilar, 577, 578, 588
  confluence of, 562, 577, 578
  dural, 561, 562, 573, 574, 575, 577, 578
  of epididymis, 238, 240
  ethmoidal air, 600
  frontal, 613
    growth of, 618
  inferior petrosal, 578, 586
  inferior sagittal, 562, 577, 588
  internal, 578
  lactiferous, 9
  maxillary, 613
    growth of, 618
  nasal, 652

oblique pericardial, 173, 175
paired, 577
paranasal
    openings of, 613, **615**
    surface projection of, 617
pericardial, 173
posterior intercavernous, 578
prostatic, 354, 356
of pulmonary trunk, 189
sphenoid, 600, 613
sphenoparietal, 562, 577, 578, 588
straight, 577
superior petrosal, 577
transverse pericardial, 173, 175, 176, 216
transverse-sigmoid, 578
unpaired, 577
venarum, 177, 182
venosus sclerae, 612
venous, 575, 578
Skeletal structures, 371
Skull
  anterior aspect of, 567
  base of, 585
    external aspect, 591
    internal aspect, 586
    superior view, 585
  at birth, 571–572
  brachycephalic, 570
  diploic veins, 574
  dolichocephalic, 570
  inferior surface of, 592
  inferolateral aspect of, 568
  internal jugular vein, 562
  lateral aspect of, 568
  layers of scalp overlying the calvaria, 573
  left bony orbital cavity, 567
  occipital bone, 569
  paramedian section of, 585
  superficial veins, 561
  surface of dura mater, 575
  zygomatic arch removed, 568
Small intestine
  image of, **291**
  mesentery of, 300
  mesocolons and mesentery, **300**
Soft tissues of right hip joints, 480
Spaces, 32, 60, 105, 143, 347, 358, 408, 516, 577, 656, 667, 673
  cavernous, 356
  diamond-shaped, 443
  infraglottic, 655
  intercostal, 10, 17, 27, 143, 149, 151, 169
  intervertebral disk, 401
  quadrangular, 32, 33, 55, 56, 60, 63, 67
  restricted, 105
  triangular, 30, 32, 33, 55, 56, 60
Spermatic cord, 15, 223, 236, **369**
  vessels and nerves of, 367
Spermatic cords, 369
Sphenoid, 555, 556, 557, 567, 585, 586, 591, 595, 596, 648, 670
Sphenoid bone, 555, 557, 567, 568, 571, 572, 577, 586, 587, 591, 595, 596, 600, 606, 617, 670
Sphenoid sinus, 571, 580, 587, 596, 600, 613, 614, 615, 616, 617, 620, 642, 671
Sphincter, 209, 336, 346, 356, 358, 603, 648
  of bladder, 235
  circular, 345
  complete sphincter, 346
  external anal, 345
  membranous, 343
  pupillae, 609
  pyloric, 255, 265, 267
  symphysis, 346

upper esophageal, 201
urethral, 346
Sphincter of pupil, 603
Spinal column
  lumbar region, 401
  thoracic region, 400
Spinal cord, 14, 321, **402–408**
  anterior dissection, 207
  anterior median fissure of, 403
  arterial supply of, **403**
  and brain of newborn child, 402
  cauda equina of, **405**
  lumbar puncture into, 408
  meninges, at cervical level, 406
  sacral puncture into, 408
  and segments in adult, 402
  spinal arteries of, **406**
  spinal roots of, **403**
  termination of neural part of, 405
  ventral view, 403
  within vertebral canal, 403
Spinal ganglia, spinal nerves of, 402
Spinal segments, **52**
Spine, 30, 33, 112, 117, 120, 302, 345, 373, 379, 380, 396, 407, 549, 648
  anterior inferior iliac, 323
  anterior superior iliac, 5, 15, 139, 323, 328
  of greater wing, 568
  of helix, 657
  iliac, 261, 314
  inferior posterior iliac, 329
  ischial, 323, 324, 328, 346, 348, 360, 361, 364, 387, 431, 434, 483
  of ischium, 324, 325
  mental, 549, 627, 632, 633, 634
  nasal, 567, 568, 591, 614, 615, 635, 648
  posterior inferior iliac, 435
  right, 302
  of scapula, 11, 32, 43, 44, 55, 60, 61, 112, 114, 115, 116, 119, 120, 121, 155, 214, 371, 379
  of sphenoid bone, 591
  upper cervical, 542
Spine of scapula, 11, 33, 44
Spinous process, 387
Spleen, 258, 286
  diaphragmatic surface, 286
  visceral surface, 287
Splenic vein, 276, 283, 287, 294, 298
Splenic vessels, 253
Splenius capitis, 374
Stellate ganglion, 647
Sternal angle, 5, 19, 139, 141
Sternal region, 1
Sternocleidomastoid region, 219
Sternum, 14, 18, 19, 140, 141, 143–146, 163, 169, 216, 217, 231, 246, 261, 387
  anterior surface, 19
  lower, 18
Stomach, 219, 258
  anterior surface layers, **262**
  anterior view of, 254, 262
  arteries and veins, **254**
  blood supply, **257**, **264**
  body of, 267
  cardiac portion of, 254
  duodenum, junction, 262
  external muscular layers of, 262
  fundus, 275
  greater omentum, 264, **264**
  lymphatic vessels, 266
  nodes of, 260, 266, **266**
  omental foramen, **258**
  posterior wall, 267
  radiograph of, **261**
  regional arterial supply, 254

in situ, **258**
  small ulcer, X-ray of, 265
  surface projection of, 261
  ulcers of, 265
  upper duodenum, internal structure, **255**
  X-ray of, 263
    ulcer, 265
Stomach bed, omental bursa and structures in, 260
Strabismus, 675
Styloid process, 34, 122
Subacromial bursa, 119
Subareolar plexus, 7
Subcoracoid bursa, 54
Subcostal plane, 3
Subcutaneous acromial bursa, 17
Subdeltoid bursa, 32, 54
Subinguinal nodes drain, 352
Submandibular gland, 545
Submandibular region, 623
Submandibulary gland, 219
Suboccipital region
  muscles of, **384,** 385
  nerves of, **384,** 385
    deep, 383
      greater occipital and third occipital, 385
      suboccipital, 385
    vertebral artery and occipital nerves, 384
    vessels of, **384**
      deep, 383
Suboccipital triangle, 383
  left, 381
  muscles of, 384
  and semispinalis capitis muscles, 381
  semispinalis muscle, 383
  vertebral artery of, 384
Subscapularis tendon, 119
Subscapular vein, 23, 26
Subtalar joint inversion, 453
Sulcus, 64, 501, 676
  anterior median, 406
  of aorta, 160
  inferior temporal, 589, 672
  intertubercular, 18, 64, 113, 373
  medial cubital, 42
  median lingual, 628
  posterior interventricular, 173, 177, 186, 187
  posterior palpebral margin, 593
  sclerae, 593
  of subclavian artery, 142, 160
  of subclavian vein crest, 142
  of superior vena cava, 160
  terminalis, 173, 177, 188, 628, 646, 647
Superficial branch, radial nerve, 89
Superficial cervical nodes, 211
Superficial circumflex iliac vein, 12
Superficial dissection of breast, milk line, **4**
Superficial epigastric vein, 12, 13, 232
Superficial external pudendal vein, 13
Superficial fascia, 15
Superficial iliac circumflex vein, 13, 232
Superficial inguinal nodes, 211, 352
Superficial inguinal ring
  female inguinal region, **232**
  spermatic cord, 223
  with spermatic cord, **223**
Superficial inguinal rings, 236
Superficial muscles of back
  intermediate and, 374
  trapezius and latissimus dorsi, 373, 376
Superficial veins
  of anterior trunk, **12**
  of the upper extremity, **29**
Superior epigastric vein, 13
Superior epigastric vessels, 147
Superior mesenteric arteriogram, 293

Superior mesenteric syndrome, 269
Superior mesenteric vein, 294, 298, 299
Superior orbital fissure, 676
Suprarenal gland, 309
  variations of, 310
Suprarenal glands, 308, 309
Suprarenal veins, variations of, 310
Suprarenal vessels, **310**
Supraspinatus fossa, 117
Suprasternal plane, 3
Surface anatomy, 140
  of back, **371**
  of the female and male anterior body
    walls, **139**
  of female body, **3**
  of female thoracic wall, **5**
  of male body, **2**
  thoracic and abdominal walls, 140
  of the upper limb, **34**
Surface projection, **261**
Sympathetic ganglion, 14
Sympathetic trunks, 206
Symphysis pubis, 305, 327
  level of, 363, 364
Symphysis pubis anteriorly, 347
Syndesmosis, 496
Synovial bursa, 114
Synovial cavity, 126
  of right knee joint, 492
Synovial fold, infrapatellar, 485
Synovial membrane, 492
  within capsule of right knee joint, 494
Synovial sheath, 64, 92, 96, 98, 99, 101, 104, 106,
    111, 119, 148, 452, 455, 456, 471
  of biceps muscle, 57
  of biceps tendon, 116
  of digital tendon, 104, 105
  of digital tendons, 96
  of flexor tendons, 96
  intertubercular, 61
  of little finger, 98
  of long biceps tendon, 54
  of tibialis anterior and extensor hallucis longus,
    456
Synovial tendon sheath, 92
Systemic venous systems in adult, **195**

T

Taenia, anterior, 250
Taenia coli, 251, 258, 260, 301
Taenia libera, 288, 290, 301, 302, 304
Taenia mesocolica, 301, 304
Talocrural joints. *See* Ankle joints
Talus, 497, 498, 499, 500, 501, 502, 503, 504, 505,
    507, 508, 509, 514
  articulation, 508
  bone, 499
  sustentaculum, 514
Tarsal plates, 597
Taste follicles, **628**
Taste, principal pathways for, 628
Tectorial membrane, 390, 391
Teeth, **633–639**
  canine, lower, 640
  crown of, 639
  deciduous, 636
  longitudinal section of, 639
  lower
    innervation of, 633
    mandibular arch and, 634
  mandible
    right, 634
    as seen from below, 633
    as seen from front, 634

permanent
  left adult, **637–638**
  rudiments of, 636
upper
  innervation of, 633
  palate and, 635
Temporal bone, 541, 549, 557, 558, 571, 572, 585,
    586, 591, 643, 657, 658, 660, 666, 667, 670
  auditory, 659
  dissection, **666**
  facial, glossopharyngeal, and vagus nerves
    projected on, 665
  forms, 658
  petrous part of, 667
  styloid process of, 384, 549
  tympanic cavity, 658
Temporal region, 1
Tendinous intersection, 139
Tendons
  of abductor pollicis longus, 44, 97, 137
  of adductor magnus, 424, 443, 487
  of ankle region, 456–457
  of biceps, 30, 56, 57, 134
  of biceps brachii, 46, 84, 119, 125
  of biceps femoris, 430, 438, 443, 461, 469
  of brachialis, 134
  of brachioradialis, 71
  calcaneal, 461, 463, 500, 514
  common anular, 608
  conjoined, 227
  of digastric muscles, 545
  of dorsal synovial sheaths, **92**
  of extensor, 91, 92, 122, 455
  of extensor carpi radialis brevis, 91
  of extensor carpi radialis longus, 91
  of extensor digiti minimi, 137
  of extensor digitorum, 44, 91, 136
  of extensor digitorum brevis, 458
  of extensor digitorum longus, 452, 455
  of extensor hallucis brevis, 452, 455, 458
  of extensor hallucis longus, 414, 447, 451, 452,
    455, 516
  of extensor pollicis brevis, 44, 71
  of extensor pollicis longus, 44, 86
  of external oblique, 378
  of fibularis, 447, 468
  of fibularis brevis, 455, 498, 506
  of fibularis longus, 475, 498, 505, 506, 507
  of fibularis tertius, 450, 452, 455, 514
  of flexor carpi radialis, 71, 72, 84, 97
  of flexor carpi ulnaris, 71, 84, 97
  of flexor digitorum, 105
  of flexor digitorum brevis, 472
  of flexor digitorum longus, 466, 467, 468, 469,
    472, 475
  of flexor hallucis longus, 466, 467, 468, 469,
    471–475, 506
  of flexor pollicis longus, 72, 105, 138
  of gastrocnemius, 462, 463
  of gluteus maximus, 480
  of gracilis, 424, 462, 488
  of iliopsoas, 438, 480
  of inferior rectus, 600
  of infraspinatus, 119
  insertions of, 506
  joint, 315
  of lateral head of gastrocnemius, 487
  of lateral rectus, 600, 609
  of latissimus dorsi, 30, 54
  of levator palpebrae superioris, 597
  of long head of biceps, 117, 118
  of medial head of gastrocnemius, 487
  of medial rectus, 600
  of obturator internus, 438, 479
  of palmaris longus, 71, 72, 95, 97

Tendons (*continued*)
of pectoralis major, 32
of plantaris, 461, 463, 464, 467, 514
of popliteus, 486, 487, 488, 492, 494, 495
of psoas minor, 315, 417
of quadriceps femoris, 414, 451, 486, 488, 494
of rectus femoris, 418, 452, 480, 481
of right dorsum of foot, 456–457
of sartorius, 421, 462, 488
of semimembranosus, 432, 437, 438, 443, 461, 462, 487, 488
of semitendinosus, 437, 438, 443, 461, 462, 488
of sheaths, 455
of sheaths of lateral malleolus, 456
of short and long flexors of toes, 471
of stapedius, 661, 663–665, 683
of sternocleidomastoid, 519
of stylohyoid, 527
of subscapularis, 54
of superior oblique, 597, 603, 604, 606, 607
of supraspinatus, 60, 114, 119
of tensor, 683
of tensor tympani, 659, 661, 663–665
of teres major, 54
of tibialis anterior and extensor hallucis longus, 455, 456
of trapezius muscle, 60
of triceps, 62
of vincula, 100
Testicular vessels, 237
Testis, 230, 235, 237–242, 244, 246, 353, 355, 357, 369
anterior views, **238**
blood supply, schematic representation of, 239
coverings of, 238
cross section of, 240
diagrammatic representation of, 240
efferent duct system, 238
epididymis, **239**
gubernaculum, 357
lateral views, **238**
longitudinal section of, 238
ovoid-shaped, 240
parietal layer, 240
right, 237, 365
in scrotum, **240**
Thigh, 1, 2, 219, 314, 316, 409, 418, 420, 426, 427, 429, 431, 434, 436, 439, 510
movements of, 426
muscles of, 429
Thigh, anterior
deep fasciae of, 414
deep layer of, **424**
deep vessels and nerves of, **425**
movements of, **426**
muscles of, 414, 415, **418–421, 426**
adductor, 419
*chart of, 426
deep layer of, 424
iliopsoas, 419, 420
intermediate layer of, 421
pectineus and gracilis, 419, 420
quadriceps femoris, 419, 420
superficial view of, 418
tensor fascia lata and sartorius, 419
sartorius, iliopsoas, pectineus, and femoral vessels and nerves in, 510
superficial vessels and nerves of, **416**
Thigh, lateral muscles of, 427
Thigh, medial
deep fasciae of, 414
deep layer of, **424**
deep vessels and nerves of, **425**
muscles of, 414, **421**, 427
*chart of, 427

deep layer of, 424
intermediate layer of, 421
Thigh, posterior
fascia lata of, 415
hamstring muscles of, 430, 437
muscles of, 427, 436, **437**
*chart of, 427
hamstring, 430, 437, 438
sciatic nerve and popliteal vessels of, **436**
sciatic nerve in, 510
vessels and nerves of, 439
superficial, 428
Thigh, right
cross section through middle of, 511
cross section through superior aspect of, 510
Thoracic, 244
cage, 140, 142
anterior view, **140**
internal surface of, 146, **146**
left clavicle, 145
posterior view, **141**
projection of thoracic and upper abdominal organs, **149**
radiograph of chest, **151**
ribs, **142**
sternocostal articulations, **145**
surface projection
anterior view, 244
left lateral view, 245
posterior view, 244
right lateral view, 245
Thoracic duct, 203, **210**, 211, 319, 352
Thoracic skeleton, 140, 141
Thoracic vertebra
costovertebral joints, 393
sixth, 393
tenth, 393
twelfth, 393
Thoracic viscera, 149
and root of neck, 152
Thoracic wall
anterior, **147, 148**
superficial dissection in male, 16
of young female, 5
blood vessels, 147, 202
muscles, 147
musculature, 148
nerves, 202
of pleural reflections, 154–155
projections of lungs, pleura, and heart onto, 153
pulmonary borders, 156
Thoracodorsal vein, 26, 27
Thoracoepigastric veins, 12, 16, 26, 27, 220
Thoracolumbar fascia, 11
cross section of, 386
removal of, 376
Thorax, 3
female, 3
great vessels of, 536
lymphatics of, 174
posteroanterior radiograph, 151, 168
skeleton of, **112**
surface projection of, 244
tomographic cross section, **218**
transverse sections through, **215–217**
truncated shape of, 243
young woman, surface contours on, 3
Thumb, **138**
Thymus, 147, 150, 152, 166, 167, 174, 243, 642
in adolescent, 150
2-year-old child, 150
Thyrocervical trunk, 25, 27, 544
Thyroid gland, 150
anterior view of, 649
dorsal view of, 537

enlarged, 538
posterior view of, 650
scintiscan of, 538
ultrasound scan, 538
ventral view of, 537
Tibia, 409, 427, 436, 447, 448, 451, 468, 484, 486, 489, 493, 495, 496, 497, 498, 499
distal end of, 498
inferior articular surface of, 499
lateral condyle of, 434, 436
right
condyles of, 495
posterior view of, 497
proximal ends of, 496
Tibial tuberosity, 490
Tibiofibular joint, inferior, 498
Tibiofibular syndesmosis, inferior, 498
Toes, 412, 447, 450, 453, 454, 458, 459, 466, 469, 470, 471, 472, 477, 500, 502, 509
fifth, 477, 501, 509
fourth, 457, 458, 476, 477, 500
lateral, 448, 455, 469, 471
Tongue, 566, 619–621, 626–632, 648, 649, 650, 687, 688
anterior view of, 620, 649
dorsum of, 622, **628**
midsagittal section of, 627
muscles of, **629**
*chart, 632
external larynx and pharynx, 629–630
extrinsic, 629
genioglossus and intrinsic, 627
ventral view of, 630
musculature, 627
paramedian section of, 629
posterior
nerves and arteries of, 631
posterior view of, 650
transverse section through, 631
Torus
of levator veli palatini muscle, 645
tubarius, 613, 620, 622, 642, 645, 647, 672
Trabeculae, 356
carneae, 184, 189
Trachea, 157, **157**, 162, **162**, 163, 165, 196–198, 201, 212, 215, 218, 520, 527, 537, 642, 655
bifurcation, 162, 163, 164, 165, 197, 198, 199, 218
bronchoscopy of, 165
carina, 165
cartilages, 162
Transpyloric plane, 3
Transversalis fascia, 147, 228, 230
Transverse colon, 219, 251
segment of, 304
Transverse pericardial sinus, 173, 175
Transverse section
MRI section through middle of forearm, 135
through lower third of arm, 133
through thorax, **215–216, 215–217**
through wrist joint, 137
Transversospinal groups, 379
Transversus abdominis, 228
Trapezius
and latissimus dorsi, 373
removal of, 374
superficial muscles, 373
Trauma to lateral side of leg, 452
Triangles, 383, 384, 520, 545
anterior cervical, 219
deltopectoral, 1, 2, 15, 22, 36, 219, 519, 521
posterior cervical, 1, 219
urogenital, 219, 345, 366
Triangular space, 30, 32
Tricuspid valve, 183, 187
Trigone of bladder, 354, 355

Trigones, 186, 191, 354, 356
Trochlear notch, 113, 122, 125, 126
Trunk, 3, 13, 47, 48, 148, 167, 210, 224, 225, 226, 314, 327, 338, 366, 371, 372, 426
  of accessory nerve, 692
  angular-facial, 561
  anterior (female)
    nerves of, **13**
    superficial vessels, **13**
    superficial vessels and nerves, **13**
  anterior vagal, 207, 208, 690
  arterial, 351
  celiac, 252, 296
    arteriogram, 256
    branches, **256,** 264
  costocervical, 198, 202, 544
  cranial nerve, 589
  descending nerve, 693
  ganglionated sympathetic, 206
  hepatic, 280
  hiocephalic, 215
  intestinal, 211, 352
  lateral, 372
  left bronchomediastinal, 211
  lower, 47, 48, 210, 240, 372
  lumbosacral, 316, 317
  musculature, deeper layers, 224
  posterior vagal, 207, 208
  right bronchomediastinal, 211
  right colic, 297
  right jugular, 211
  right subclavian, 211
  of spinal nerve, 386, 405
  upper, 47, 48, 529
Tuber
  cinereum, 589, 672, 674
  omentale, 259, 260
Tubercle, 56, 65, 96, 97, 115, 142, 143, 230, 379, 385, 393, 394, 478, 528, 542, 646
  abducts thumb brevis, 97
  accessory, 639
  adductor, 427, 437, 484
  anterior obturator, 323
  calcaneal, 503
  carotid, 146, 148, 541
  corniculate, 642, 645, 647, 654, 655
  costoxiphoid, 230
  cuneiform, 642, 645, 647, 654, 655
  genial, 627
  of ilium, 323
  inferior thyroid, 629, 630
  infraglenoid, 112, 118
  medial intercondylar, 484, 493, 496
  posterior obturator, 323, 324
  of rib, 142, 393, 395
  scalene, 528
  of scalenus anterior muscle, 142
  of superior lip, 518
  supraglenoid, 19, 112, 119
Tuberosity, 122, 125, 420, 461, 462, 471, 503, 556
  of calcaneus, 499, 504, 506
  of distal phalanx, 127
  of gluteus maximus muscle, 323
  of ilium, 324
  of navicular bone, 506
  of scalenus medial muscle, 142
  of scaphoid bone, 131
  of serratus anterior muscle, 142
  of tibia, 447, 449, 496
  transverse perineal, 349
  of ulna, 125
Tubes, 279, 312, 330, 334, 620, 625
  pharyngotympanic, 679
  preformed, 211
  primitive gastrointestinal, 248

Tunica albuginea, 238, 239
Tunica vaginalis testis, 237, 238, 240, 242, 357
Tympanic branch, 687
Tympanic cavity, 658
  lateral wall of, 663
  medial wall of, 664, 665
Tympanic membrane, **660,** 684
Tympanic plexus, 687

U

UG. *See* Urogenital
Ulcer, X-ray of, 265
Ulna, 42, 74, 83, 84, 87, 122–126, 128–131, 134–136
  distal aspect of, 126
  extensor muscles, 87
  muscle on anterior surface, 74
  posterior attachments of muscles, **87**
  shaft of, 85, 87
Umbilical ring, 139
Umbilical vein, 242, 271
Umbilicus, 2, 11, 15, 230
  above/at/below, 228
Upper abdomen
  CT, 287
  CT of, 275, 276, 287
  transverse section, 320
  transverse ultrasound of, 277
Upper abdominal viscera, 149
Upper back
  deep vessels and nerves of, 383
  nerves and vessels of superficial and intermediate muscle layers of, 382
Upper extremity
  cross section through middle of humerus, 132
  superficial veins, **29**
  venous pattern, **41**
Upper limb. *See* Limb, upper
Upper neck
  paramedian sagittal view of interior of, 622
  submandibular region in, 623
Ureter, 311, 312, 321
  course of, 306, 341
  ovarian vessels, 306
  retroperitoneal position of, 288
Urethra, 235, 237, 331, 336, 342–347, 344, 349, 355–357, **356,** 357, 362, 370
  bulbospongiosus, 235
  majus, 336
  membranous, 346, 355, 356, 358, 368
  penile, 355, 356, 368
  prostatic, 354, 355, 356
  voluntary constrictor, 346
Urethral orifice, 342, 344, 370
Urinary bladder, 353
  posterior aspect, 246
Urinary system, 357
Urogenital diaphragm, 343, 345, 355, 358
Urogenital region, 347
  muscle chart, **346**
  superficial muscles of, 349
Urogenital triangle, 219
Uterine, diagram of, 335
Uterine tube, 233, 331
  fimbriae of, 330
  frontal section of, 332
Uterine vessels, 341
Uterosalpingogram, 330
Uterus, 192, 223, 303, 306, 330–336, 331, 338, 341–343, 349
  angles and positions of, **332**
  arterial supply, 335
  frontal section of, 332
  interior of, **332**
  ligament of, 333, 334

  longitudinal axis of, 332
  pregnant, growth of, **336**
  round ligament of, 223, 232

V

Vagina, 192, 233, 245, 331–333, 335, 336, 342, 344–347, 349, 350, 363
  longitudinal axis of, 332
  perineal body, 349
  superficial urogenital muscle chart
    inner surface of, **349**
  upper, 343
Vaginalis process, 240
Vaginal muscular coat, 349
Vaginal opening, 347
Vaginal orifice, 331
Vaginal wall, 333
  internal anatomy of, 349
Valve(s), 169, 176, 183–185, 188, 196, 359
  of coronary sinus, 182, 189
  ileocecal, 289, 301
  of inferior vena cava, 182, 189
  left atrioventricular, 171, 184, 185, 188, 189, 191, 217
  left AV, 185
  of navicular fossa, 356
  right atrioventricular, 171, 188, 189, 191, 212, 217
  spiral, 279
  venous, 23
Vascular circulation, longitudinal section of, 369
Veins, 13, 26, 27, 174, 176, 204, 207, 232, 282, 307, 317, 321, 341, 417, 535, 546, 623
  accessory saphenous, 417, 442
  angular, 195, 561, 562, 611
  anterior cardiac, 176
  anterior interventricular, 177
  anterior tibial, 449
  axillary, 12, 20, **23,** 26, 27
  azygos, 203, 204
  basilic, 29, 34, 36, 41, 42, 68
  basivertebral, 246, 397, 407
    foramina for, 397
  brachial, 23, 26, 31, 36, 132–134, 195, 540
  central retinal, 604
  cerebral, 562, 576–578, 588, 590, 674
  circumflex scapular, 23
  digital, 454
  digital and metatarsal, 454
  diploic, 561, 573, 574
  dorsal scapular, 382
  external, 578
  femoral, 12, 423
  functions of, 407
  great saphenous, 416, 446
    superficial tributaries of, 417
  hepatic, 270, **298, 299**
    branching patterns, **272**
    distribution of, 275
    draining pattern of, 272
    ultrasound of, 273
  hepatic portal system of, **298,** 299
    inferior vena cava, relationship of, 299
    right branch of, 298
    tributaries, 298
  hypoglossal, 546
  ileal, 298
  ileocolic, 298
  iliac circumflex, 220
  illary, 23
  inferior basal, 217
  inferior epigastric, 13, 147

Veins (continued)
inferior gluteal, 361
inferior mesenteric, 195, 282, 294, 298, 299, 306, 307, 361
inferior mesentric, 298
inferior ophthalmic, 564, 611
inferior phrenic, 204, 299
internal iliac, 195, 299, 322, 341, 351, 353, 361, 364
intersegmental, 159
intervertebral, 407
jejunal, 292, 298
lacrimal, 588, 611
left gastroepiploic, 298
lingual, 625, 626, 649, 694
maxillary, 561, 563, 564
medial antebrachial, 41
medial femoral circumflex, 364
median antebrachial, 36, 41, 68, 135
middle cardiac, 164, 173, 176, 177
middle colic, 292, 298
middle meningeal, 578
middle thyroid, 536
obturator, 361
ophthalmic, 562, 578
pampiniform plexus of, 237, 239, 242, 367, 369
pancreatic, 298
phenous, 448
popliteal, 423
portal, 272
posterior humeral circumflex, 23
posterior interventricular, 164
posterior tibial, 449, 464
posterior ventricular, 173
pterygoid plexus of, 561, 562, 564, 578
pulmonary, 160, 166, 173, 175, 184, 188, 195, 217
radial, 195
rectal system of, 364
of right axilla, 23
right gastroepiploic, 298
saphenous, 460
great, 454
small, 454
scrotal, 236
sigmoid, 298, 299, 361
small saphenous, 460
sublingual, 623
superior mesenteric, 253
supraorbital, 611
suprascapular, 530, 535
supratrochlear, 561
systemic anterior abdominal wall, 12
testicular artery, 239, 321
thin-walled, 370
thoracoacromial, 535
thoracoepigastric, 220
transverse cervical, 524, 530, 535
tributaries, 23
ulnar, 195

of vertebral column, 407
vesical plexus of, 364
of vestibular bulb, 348
Vena caval foramen, 315
Venae comitantes, 449
Venous drainage, 177
Ventral mesogastrium, 248
Vermiform appendix
surface projection of, 302
Vertebra(e). See also Thoracic vertebra; Lumbar vertebrae
C5, 387
C7, 387
cervical, 388–389
and atlantooccipital membranes, 389
fifth, 388
intervertebral disks and ligaments, 397
seventh, 388
spinous processes of, 397
ventral view of, 389
Vertebral arches, 405
Vertebral arteriogram, **584**
Vertebral bodies, frontal section through, 398
Vertebral canal, 387
dorsal view of, 405
Vertebral column, 207
anterior dissection, 207
dorsally convex curvatures of, 392
functions of, 392
left lateral surface, in median plane, 387
left medial surface, in median plane, 387
lumbar vertebra of, 327
and pectoral and pelvic girdles, **387**
sacrum and coccyx, 392
veins of, 407
ventrally convex curvatures of, 392
Vertebral foramina, 395
Vertebral veins, third lumbar level, **407**
Vertebra prominens, 387, 388
Vesicouterine pouch, 333
Vessels
popliteal, 464
of popliteal fossa, 442
superficial, 416
trunks of plantar, 473
Vessels, deep
of suboccipital region, 383
of upper back, 383
Vestibular glands, 350
Vincula of tendons, 100
Visceral afferent fibers, 362
Viscera left intact, 250
Visceral layer, 153
Visceral peritoneum, 248
Visceral Pleurae, **153**
Vitelline duct, 248
Vocal folds
cross section of larynx at, 656

W
Wall
anterior abdominal, 238
deep dissection of, 242
epigastric anastomosis, **231**
external oblique muscle, **221**
inguinal region of, 232
inner surface of, **222**
internal oblique muscle of, **224, 225**
male, inguinal region, 236
rectus abdominis muscles of, **225, 227**
rectus sheath of, **226, 230**
second muscle layer of, **226**
superficial musculature of, 221
superficial vessels and nerves of, **220**
transverse sections of, 230
transversus abdominis muscles of, **227**
inguinal canal, 234
posterior abdominal, 290
diaphragm, **314, 315**
lymph nodes and channels, **352**
muscles of, **314**
retroperitoneal organs, **307**
vessels and nerves, **317**
thoracic
anterior, **147, 148**
superficial dissection in male, 16
of young female, 5
blood vessels, 147, 202
muscles, 147
musculature, 148
nerves, 202
of pleural reflections, 154–155
projections of lungs, pleura, and heart onto, 153
pulmonary borders, 156
superficial musculature of, 221
Wrist
arteries of left dorsal, 93
bones, showing attachment of muscles, 128
computerized tomographs of, **136**
coronal (frontal) section through, 131
extensor tendons and synovial sheaths, 92
and hand, ligaments and joints of, **130**
joints and ligaments of, 130
muscles, synovial sheaths, and tendons, 96
radiograph of, 127, 129
skeleton of, 128, 129

X
Xiphisternal junction, 141
Xiphisternal plane, 3
Xiphoid process, 19, 146, 318

Z
Zygapophyseal joints and ligamenta flava, 396